Discover Sherpath®

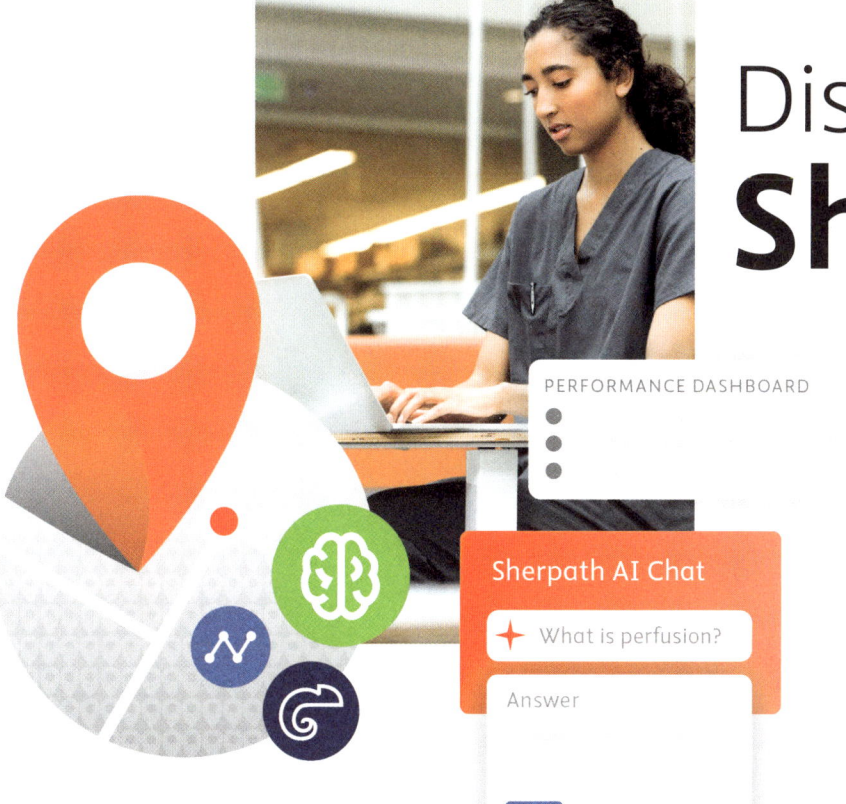

The digital teaching and learning technology built specifically for healthcare education.

Sherpath's all-in-one course delivery solution powers your textbook with innovative resources, including the following:

Digital lessons aligned with learning objectives create an interactive experience with multimedia, adaptive remediation, assignment assessments, and more. *Only available for select collections.*

Elsevier Adaptive Quizzing customizes quizzes based on performance and allows you to choose relevant quiz topics.

Sherpath AI conversational AI tool generates personalized answers to questions, sourced solely from Elsevier's vast library of trusted, evidence-based content.

eBook and resources are seamlessly accessible within Sherpath for quick access to relevant course materials, activities, and reading recommendations.

Performance dashboard offers a holistic view of course progress and areas of strength and weakness.

Enhanced test banks provide all-in-one access to your test bank from your Sherpath courses. *Only available for select collections.*

STUDENTS — Ask your instructor about enhancing your course experience with Sherpath!

INSTRUCTORS — Scan code or visit **myevolve.us/sphp** to learn more!

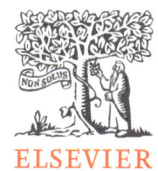

24-0461 TM/AF

ELSEVIER

MERRILL'S ATLAS OF
RADIOGRAPHIC POSITIONING & PROCEDURES

SIXTEENTH EDITION | VOLUME THREE

MERRILL'S ATLAS OF RADIOGRAPHIC POSITIONING & PROCEDURES

Jeannean Hall Rollins, MRC, BSRT(R)(CV)(M)
Associate Professor
Medical Imaging and Radiation Sciences Department
Arkansas State University
Jonesboro, Arkansas

Tammy Curtis, PhD, RT(R)(CT)(CHES)
Professor and Program Director
Radiologic Sciences and School of Allied Health
Northwestern State University
Shreveport, Louisiana

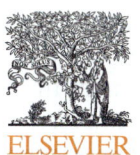

ELSEVIER

Elsevier
3251 Riverport Lane
St. Louis, Missouri 63043

MERRILL'S ATLAS OF RADIOGRAPHIC POSITIONING
AND PROCEDURES, SIXTEENTH EDITION

Set ISBN: 978-0-443-12041-1
Volume 1: 978-0-443-11717-6
Volume 2: 978-0-443-11689-6
Volume 3: 978-0-443-11690-2

Copyright © 2026 by Elsevier Inc. All rights are reserved, including those for text and data mining, AI training, and similar technologies.

Publisher's note: Elsevier takes a neutral position with respect to territorial disputes or jurisdictional claims in its published content, including in maps and institutional affiliations.

No part of this publication may be reproduced or transmitted in any form or by any means, electronic or mechanical, including photocopying, recording, or any information storage and retrieval system, without permission in writing from the publisher. Details on how to seek permission, further information about the Publisher's permissions policies and our arrangements with organizations such as the Copyright Clearance Center and the Copyright Licensing Agency, can be found at our website: www.elsevier.com/permissions.

This book and the individual contributions contained in it are protected under copyright by the Publisher (other than as may be noted herein).

Notice

Practitioners and researchers must always rely on their own experience and knowledge in evaluating and using any information, methods, compounds or experiments described herein. Because of rapid advances in the medical sciences, in particular, independent verification of diagnoses and drug dosages should be made. To the fullest extent of the law, no responsibility is assumed by Elsevier, authors, editors or contributors for any injury and/or damage to persons or property as a matter of products liability, negligence or otherwise, or from any use or operation of any methods, products, instructions, or ideas contained in the material herein.

Previous editions copyrighted 2023, 2019, 2016, 2012, 2007, 2003, 1999, 1995, 1991, 1986, 1982, 1975, 1967, 1959, and 1949.

Content Strategist: Margaret Benson, Luke Held
Senior Content Development Specialist: Rae Robertson
Publishing Services Manager: Julie Eddy
Senior Project Manager: Cindy Thoms
Design Direction: Brian Salisbury

Printed in Poland

Last digit is the print number: 9 8 7 6 5 4 3 2 1

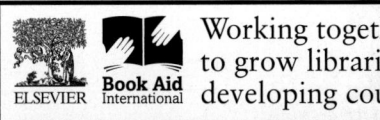

PREVIOUS AUTHORS

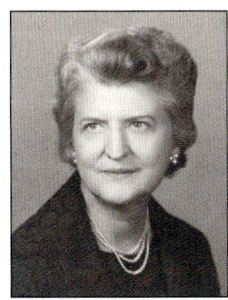

Vinita Merrill, 1905–1977. Vinita Merrill was born August 26, 1905, in the town of Asher, located in Pottawatomie County, Oklahoma. Ms. Merrill died on December 10, 1977, in New York City, New York. Her final resting place was in New Hampshire, where her ashes were spread along the scenic Mohawk River. Vinita began the compilation of *Merrill's* in 1936 while she worked as Technical Director and Chief Technologist in the Department of Radiology and Instructor in the School of Radiography at the New York Hospital. In 1949, while employed as Director of the Educational Department of Picker X-Ray Corporation, she wrote the first edition of the *Atlas of Roentgenographic Positions*. She completed three more editions from 1959 to 1975. Throughout her career, Vinita worked as a technologist, teacher, researcher, investigator, chief technologist, and radiology administrator. Seventy-six years later, Vinita's work lives on in the sixteenth edition of *Merrill's Atlas of Radiographic Positioning & Procedures*.

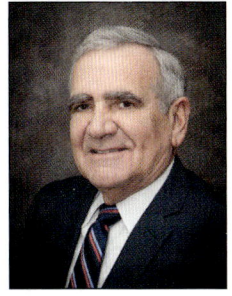

Philip W. Ballinger, PhD, RT(R), FASRT, FAEIRS, became the author of *Merrill's Atlas* in its fifth edition, which was published in 1982. He served as an author through the tenth edition, helping to launch successful careers for thousands of students who have learned radiographic positioning from *Merrill's*. Phil currently serves as Professor Emeritus in Radiologic Sciences and Therapy, Division of the School of Health and Rehabilitation Sciences, at The Ohio State University. In 1995, he retired after a 25-year career as Radiography Program Director and, after ably guiding *Merrill's Atlas* through six editions, he retired as *Merrill's* author. Phil continues to be involved in professional activities, such as speaking engagements at state, national, and international meetings.

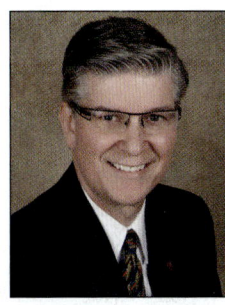

Eugene D. Frank, MA, RT(R), FASRT, FAEIRS, began working with Phil Ballinger on the eighth edition of *Merrill's Atlas* in 1995. He became the coauthor in its ninth, 50th-anniversary edition, published in 1999. He served as lead author for the eleventh and twelfth editions and mentored three coauthors. Gene retired from the Mayo Clinic/Foundation, Rochester, Minnesota, in 2001 after 31 years of employment. He was Associate Professor of Radiology in the College of Medicine and Director of the Radiography Program. He also served as Director of the Radiography Program at Riverland Community College, Austin, Minnesota, for 6 years before fully retiring in 2007. He is a Fellow of the American Society of Radiologic Technologists (ASRT) and the Association of Educators in Imaging and Radiologic Sciences (AEIRS). In addition to *Merrill's*, he is the coauthor of two radiography textbooks: *Quality Control in Diagnostic Imaging* and *Radiography Essentials for Limited Practice*. He continues to help radiography programs by teaching courses for sabbaticals and helps equip x-ray departments in West Africa with equipment.

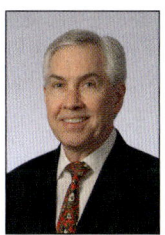

Bruce W. Long, MS, RT(R)(CV), FASRT, FAEIRS, began as a coauthor on the eleventh edition of *Merrill's Atlas*. He served as lead author for the thirteenth and fourteenth editions and coauthor on the fifteenth edition. Bruce retired in 2020 as Program Director and Associate Professor Emeritus from the Indiana University Radiologic and Imaging Sciences Program after 34 years of employment. He is a Fellow of the ASRT and AEIRS. In addition to *Merrill's*, he is the author of two radiography textbooks: *Orthopaedic Radiography* and *Radiography Essentials for Limited Practice*. His other publication activities include 28 articles in national professional journals.

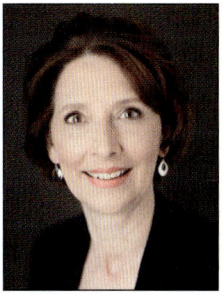

Barbara J. Smith, MS, RT(R)(QM), FASRT, FAEIRS, is an instructor in the Radiologic Technology program at Portland Community College, where she has taught for 34 years. The Oregon Society of Radiologic Technologists inducted her as a Life Member in 2003. She presents at state, regional, national, and international meetings; was a trustee with the American Registry of Radiologic Technologists (ARRT); and is involved in professional activities at these levels. Her publication activities include articles, book reviews, and chapter contributions. Currently, she serves as Chair of the Oregon Radiation Advisory Committee. As coauthor for four editions, Barb's role with the *Merrill's* team was to work with the contributing authors and to edit Volume 3.

THE MERRILL'S TEAM

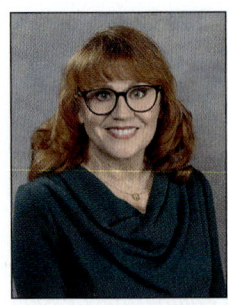

Jeannean Hall Rollins, MRC, BSRT(R)(CV)(M), is an Associate Professor in the Medical Imaging and Radiation Sciences department at Arkansas State University, where she has taught for 32 years. She presents regularly at national meetings. Her publication activities include articles, book reviews, and chapter contributions. The sixteenth edition is Jeannean's second as the lead author and sixth time on the *Merrill's* team. She is also sharing responsibility for revising the workbook with Dr. Tammy Curtis on this edition. Her first contribution to *Merrill's Atlas* was in the tenth edition as coauthor of the "Trauma Radiography" chapter. Prior to becoming a coauthor on the textbook, Jeannean was responsible for revising the workbook, *Mosby's Radiography Online,* and the *Evolve Instructor Electronic Resources* that accompany *Merrill's Atlas*.

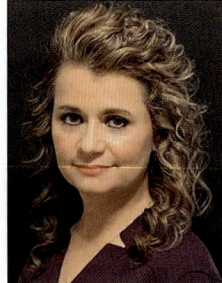

Tammy Curtis, PhD, RT(R)(CT) (CHES), is a Professor and Director of the Radiologic Sciences Program at Northwestern State University, where she has taught for 24 years. She presents at the state, regional, and national levels and is involved in professional activities at the state and national levels. Her publication activities include articles, book reviews, book contributions, and radiology education products. Previously, Tammy served on the advisory board and submitted several projects to the *Atlas*. In particular, for the twelfth edition, Tammy submitted an updated photo and biography of the original author, Vinita Merrill, which she discovered after a 3-year search of historical records. The fifteenth edition was Tammy's first as a coauthor of the textbook and third time as part of the *Merrill's* team. Her previous role on the *Merrill's* team was to update the workbook and work with the coauthors of the textbook to review content for all three volumes. In addition to serving as a coauthor on this edition of the textbook, Tammy also shares the workbook revision responsibilities with Jeannean Rollins.

ADVISORY BOARD

This edition of *Merrill's Atlas* benefits from the expertise of a special advisory board. The following board members have provided professional input and advice and have helped the authors make decisions about *Atlas* content throughout the preparation of the sixteenth edition.

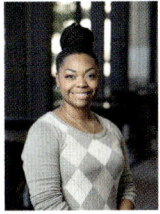

Darci K. Bray, MLS, BSRT, (R)(CT)(MR)
Epic Ambulatory Principal Trainer—OU Health University of Oklahoma Medical Center
Adjunct Faculty—University of Oklahoma Health Sciences Center
Oklahoma City, Oklahoma

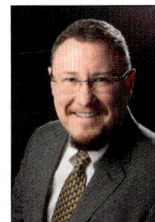

James G. Murrell, EdD, RT(R)(M)(QM)(CT), CRT(R)(F), FAEIRS
Dean of Imaging
Gurnick Academy of Medical Arts
Los Angeles, California

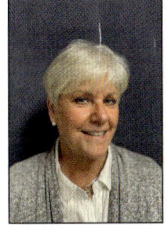

Kellie Cranfill, MSRS, RT(R)(BD)
Program Director of the IU Radiologic & Imaging Sciences Programs
Program Director for the IU Radiography Program
Assistant Professor of Clinical Radiologic and Imaging Sciences
Indiana University Purdue University at Indianapolis (IUPUI)
Indianapolis, Indiana

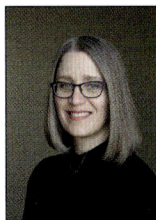

Christine Preachuk, RT(R), CAE
Manager
Diagnostic Imaging Program for X-Ray and Mammography
Health Sciences Centre, Shared Health Manitoba
Winnipeg, Manitoba, Canada

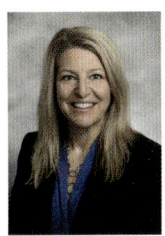

Kimberly Cross, PhD, RT(R)(CT)
Program Director
Emory University Medical Imaging Program
Emory Department of Radiology and Imaging Sciences
Atlanta, Georgia

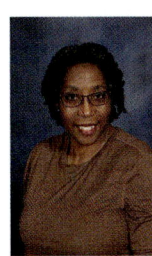

Marilyn J. Lewis Thompson, MBA, RT(R)(M)
Clinical Coordinator
Saint Luke's School of Radiologic Technology
Saint Luke's Hospital of Kansas City
Kansas City, Missouri

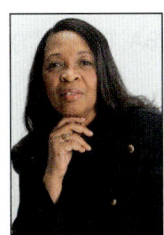

Parsha Y. Hobson, MPA, RT(R)
Professor, Program Director, and Chairperson
Radiography, Public Health, and Health Sciences
Passaic County Community College
Paterson, New Jersey

CHAPTER CONTENT EXPERTS

Richard E. Bass, BSRS (RT)(R)
Radiology, Louisiana
Shriners Children's Hospital
Shreveport

J. Tyler Carter, MS, RT(R)(CT)
Radiologic Technologist
Radiology
Piggott Community Hospital
Paragould, Arkansas

Derek P. Carver, MEd, RT(R)(MR)(ARRT)
Manager of Education and Training
Department of Radiology
Boston Children's Hospital
Boston, Massachusetts

Jennifer G. Chiu, EdD, MBA, RT(R)(CT)(ARRT)
Associate Professor and Program Director
Radiologic Science
St. John's University
Queens, New York

Rex Tom Christensen, MHA, RT(R)(MR)(CT)(ARRT), CIIP, MRSO
Associate Professor
Radiologic Sciences
Weber State University
Ogden, Utah

Jessica Cooper, MSRS, RT(R)(VI)(ARRT)
Assistant Professor, Special Programs Coordinator
Medical Imaging and Radiation Sciences
Arkansas State University
Jonesboro, Arkansas

Kristen Harper, MSRS, RT(R)(M)(CT)(BD)(ARRT)
Mammography/Bone Density Technologist
Radiology
NEA Baptist Memorial Hospital
Adjunct Professor and Clinical Instructor
Medical Imaging and Radiologic Sciences
Arkansas State University
Jonesboro, Arkansas

Garrett Johnson, BSRS RT(R)(ARRT)(RCIS)
Radiologic Technologist
Cath Lab
CHI St. Vincent Infirmary
Little Rock, Arkansas

Raymond James Johnson, BS, CNMT
Certified Nuclear Medicine Technologist
Radiology/Nuclear Medicine
John Peter Smith Health Network
Fort Worth, Texas

Becki Harris Keith, MS, RT(R)(CT)
Program Director
Radiologic Technology
Bon Secours Southside College of Health Sciences
Colonial Heights, Virginia

Machele D. Michels, RT(R)(T)(CT), CMD
Certified Medical Dosimetrist
Radiation Oncology
Mayo Clinic
Rochester, Minnesota

Zaidalynet Morales, MS, RT(R)(CT)(ARRT)
Associate Professor
Radiologic Science
St. John's University
Queens, New York

Cheryl Morgan-Duncan, MAS, RT(R)(M)
Assistant Professor and Clinical Coordinator
Radiography Program
Passaic County Community College
Staff Mammographer
Mammography
St. Joseph's Regional Medical Center
Paterson, New Jersey

Elizabeth Nelson, MSRS, RT(R)(MR), MRSO
Lead MRI Technologist
Radiology
Highland Clinic, APMC
Shreveport, Louisiana

Susanna Lynn Ovel, RT, RDMS, RVT
Senior Sonographer (Retired)
Medical Imaging
Sacramento, California

Richard R. Wall, PhD, RT(R)(CT)(CI), RCIS
Cardiac Interventional Technologist
Cardiology
Summerlin Hospital Medical Center
Las Vegas, Nevada
Adjunct Instructor
Radiologic Sciences
Northwestern State University of Louisiana
Shreveport, Louisiana
and
University of Missouri
Columbia, Missouri

Megan Wedgeworth, MBA, RT(R)(CT)
Assistant Professor
School of Allied Health
Northwestern State University
Shreveport, Louisiana

Haneen Zeidan, MSRS, RT(R)(M)
Mammography Technologist
Mammography
Newark University Hospital
Newark, New Jersey

PREFACE

Welcome to the sixteenth edition of *Merrill's Atlas of Radiographic Positioning & Procedures*. This edition continues the tradition of excellence begun in 1949, when Vinita Merrill wrote the first edition of what has become a classic text. For more than 76 years, *Merrill's Atlas* has provided a strong foundation in anatomy and positioning for thousands of students around the world who have gone on to successful careers as imaging technologists. *Merrill's Atlas* is also a mainstay for everyday reference in imaging departments all over the world. As the coauthors of the sixteenth edition, we are honored to follow in Vinita Merrill's footsteps.

Learning and Perfecting Positioning Skills

Merrill's Atlas has a tradition of helping students learn and perfect their positioning skills. After covering preliminary steps in radiography, radiation protection, and terminology in the introductory chapters, the first two volumes of the *Atlas* teach anatomy and positioning in separate chapters for each bone group or organ system. The student learns to position the patient properly so that the resulting radiograph provides the information the physician needs to correctly diagnose the patient's condition. The *Atlas* presents information for commonly requested projections, as well as for those less commonly requested, making it the only reference of its kind in the world.

The third volume provides basic information about a variety of special imaging modalities such as mobile and surgical imaging, pediatrics, geriatrics, computed tomography (CT), vascular radiology, magnetic resonance imaging (MRI), sonography, nuclear medicine technology, bone densitometry, and radiation therapy.

Merrill's Atlas is not only a comprehensive resource to help students learn but also an indispensable reference as they move into the clinical environment and ultimately into practice as imaging professionals.

New to This Edition

Since the first edition of *Merrill's Atlas* in 1949, many changes have occurred. This new edition incorporates many significant changes designed not only to reflect the technologic progress and advancements in the profession but also to meet the needs of today's radiography students. The major changes in this edition are highlighted as follows.

NEW PATIENT PHOTOGRAPHY

All patient positioning photographs have been replaced in Chapters 3, 4, 8, and 10. Additional new patient positioning photographs have been strategically added to replace or better illustrate diagrams. The new photographs show positioning detail to a greater extent and in some cases from a more realistic perspective. In addition, the updated equipment featured in the new photos provides students with a more realistic visual learning tool. The use of electronic central ray angle indicators enables a better understanding of where the central ray should enter the patient and the exact angle when required.

UPDATES IN THIS EDITION

"Essential" projections are now termed "Routine" projections. This terminology was chosen based on feedback from the Advisory Board, who polled educators and technologists from across the United States and Canada. Additionally, the routine projection icon ▲ is used to designate only those projections that are commonly performed in clinical practice. This represents a significant shift from the 15th edition, in which all projections listed in the ARRT Radiography Exam Content Specifications were designated with this icon.

In the positioning details, "Respiration" is a separate heading rather than a bullet point under the "Position of patient" heading. The author team and Advisory Board chose to emphasize proper breathing instructions based on feedback that these important instructions are often neglected in clinical practice. We hope this addition will improve the clinical practice of students and technologists by encouraging proper patient breathing instructions for every projection.

All units have been reformatted to follow the technical textbooks, as well as the ARRT. Units are presented as SI units with the traditional units in parentheses, e.g., 2.5 cm (1 inch). Additionally, SI units are most often rounded up to the nearest whole centimeter, as smaller measurements would be difficult to apply clinically. Therefore the equivalent traditional units may not be exact conversions. This is not an error, but a purposeful effort by the author team to provide realistic and applicable positioning guidelines. Fractions have been replaced by decimal equivalents (e.g., ½ inch [1.3 cm] is now presented as 1.3 cm [0.5 inch]).

Specific computed radiography (CR) image receptor sizes have been deleted in this edition. Again, feedback from our Advisory Board led the author team to simplify the image receptor sizes to comply with the most commonly used digital image receptors, which are large flat panel detectors. With this change, the author team focused on updating the collimated field size suggestions to emphasize radiation safety and optimum image quality. This is particularly important with the discontinuation of gonadal shielding in clinical practice.

Best practices that describe specific skills in each discipline were updated in all advanced modality chapters, allowing students more insight into the unique environment of each modality. All special imaging modality chapters have been updated to reflect current practices and technology, with nine chapters featuring new, updated figures. Chapter 25, Computed Tomography, features an updated examination protocol table. A safety section has been added to Chapter 26, Magnetic Resonance Imaging.

Learning Aids for the Student

POCKET GUIDE TO RADIOGRAPHY

The new edition of *Merrill's Pocket Guide to Radiography* complements this revision of *Merrill's Atlas*. Instructions for positioning the patient and the body part for all routine (formerly termed "essential") projections are presented in a complete yet concise manner. A new appendix with tips for positioning patients who are obese is new to this edition. Tabs are included to help the user locate the beginning of each section. Space is provided for the user to write in specifics of department techniques.

RADIOGRAPHIC POSITIONING AND PROCEDURES WORKBOOK

The new edition of this workbook features extensive review and self-assessment exercises that supplement the first 25 chapters in *Merrill's Atlas* in one convenient volume. Relevant material was updated to current practice and integrated into appropriate chapters. Terminology remains consistent to match the Content Specifications for the ARRT Radiography Examination, the ASRT Radiography Curriculum, and the evolution of digital imaging. New questions were developed to assess the newly added content in the textbook that reflects current ARRT content specifications. The features of the previous editions, including anatomy labeling exercises, positioning exercises, and self-tests, are still available. This edition features image evaluations to give students additional opportunities to evaluate radiographs for proper positioning and positioning questions to complement the workbook's strong anatomy review. The comprehensive multiple-choice tests at the end of each chapter help students assess their comprehension of the whole chapter. New exercises in this edition focus on improved understanding of essential projections and the need for appropriate collimated field sizes for digital imaging. Additionally, review and assessment exercises have been expanded for the chapters on pediatric imaging, the reproductive system, mobile radiography, surgical radiography, geriatric radiography, sectional anatomy, and vascular and interventional radiography. Exercises in these chapters help students learn the theory and concepts of these special techniques with greater ease. Answers to the workbook questions are found on the Evolve website.

Teaching Aids for the Instructor

EVOLVE INSTRUCTOR ELECTRONIC RESOURCES

This comprehensive resource provides valuable tools such as PowerPoint slides and an electronic test bank for teaching anatomy and positioning class. The test bank includes more than 2000 questions, including metadata enabling sorting by multiple categories.

Evolve may be used to publish the class syllabus, outlines, and lecture notes; set up "virtual office hours" and e-mail communication; share important dates and information through the online class calendar; and encourage student participation through chat rooms and discussion boards. Evolve allows instructors to post exams and manage their grade books online. For more information, visit www.evolve.elsevier.com or contact an Elsevier sales representative.

SHERPATH

Built specifically for health care education, this innovative teaching and learning technology offers interactive course content with a wealth of assignment types, assessment tools, and teaching resources to help engage students and achieve your learning objectives.

EVOLVE—ONLINE COURSE MANAGEMENT

Evolve is an interactive learning environment designed to work in coordination with *Merrill's Atlas*. Instructors may use Evolve to provide an Internet-based course component that reinforces and expands on the concepts delivered in class.

We hope you will find this edition of *Merrill's Atlas of Radiographic Positioning & Procedures* the best ever. Input from generations of readers has helped to keep the *Atlas* strong through 15 editions, and we welcome your comments and suggestions. We are constantly striving to build on Vinita Merrill's work, and we trust that she would be proud and pleased to know that the work she began over 70 years ago is still so appreciated and valued by the imaging sciences community.

Jeannean Hall Rollins
Tammy Curtis

ACKNOWLEDGMENTS

We must start by thanking our Elsevier team members Rae Robertson, Senior Content Development Specialist, and Meg Benson, Content Strategist. There is not sufficient space here to list the myriad ways in which they helped us during the revision process. Words are also insufficient to express our appreciation for their support, help, encouragement, and patience. Thank you both for making this sixteenth edition revision process as stress-free as possible!

In preparing for the sixteenth edition, our advisory board continually provided professional expertise and aid in the decision making on the revision of this edition. The advisory board members are listed on p. vii. We are most grateful for their input and contributions to this edition of the *Atlas*.

Contributors

The group of radiography professionals listed here contributed to this edition of the *Atlas* and made many insightful suggestions. These professionals are integral to maintaining the quality of *Merrill's Atlas* as a resource across all imaging sciences modalities. We are most appreciative of their willingness to share their expertise.

The author team extends special recognition to Jennifer G. Chiu, EdD, MBA, RT(R)(CT)(ARRT), Associate Professor and Program Director at St. John's University in Queens, New York; and Zaidalynet Morales, MS, RT(R)(CT)(ARRT), Associate Professor, also at St. John's University. We are honored to have their expertise on the revision of the *Evolve Instructor Electronic Resources* and other aspects for this sixteenth edition.

Our deepest appreciation to our faith, family, and colleagues, whose support and encouragement remain an indispensable part of this work. Finally, to all of our graduates and students, current and future, this edition is dedicated to you, our greatest teachers and inspiration. Thank you!

Jeannean Hall Rollins
Tammy Curtis

CONTENTS

VOLUME ONE

1. Preliminary Steps In Radiography, 1
2. General Anatomy and Radiographic Positioning Terminology, 45
3. Thoracic Viscera: Chest and Upper Airway, 81
4. Abdomen, 125
5. Upper Extremity, 141
6. Shoulder Girdle, 217
7. Lower Extremity, 267
8. Pelvis and Hip, 369
9. Vertebral Column, 409
10. Bony Thorax, 495

Addendum A: Summary of Abbreviations, 527

VOLUME TWO

11. Cranium, 1
12. Trauma Radiography, 103
13. Contrast Arthrography, 141
14. Myelography and Other Central Nervous System Imaging, 151
    Rebecca H. Keith
15. Digestive System: Salivary Glands, Alimentary Canal, and Biliary System, 169
16. Urinary System and Venipuncture, 273
17. Reproductive System, 327
18. Mammography, 347
    Haneen Zeidan
19. Bone Densitometry, 455
    Kristen E. Harper

Addendum B: Summary of Abbreviations, 495

VOLUME THREE

20. Mobile Radiography, 1
    Richard E. Bass
21. Surgical Radiography, 29
    J. Tyler Carter; Garrett Johnson
22. Pediatric Imaging, 71
    Derek Carver
23. Geriatric Radiography, 147
    Cheryl Morgan-Duncan
24. Sectional Anatomy for Radiographers, 171
    Rex T. Christensen
25. Computed Tomography, 227
    Megan Wedgeworth
26. Magnetic Resonance Imaging, 269
    Elizabeth Nelson
27. Vascular, Cardiac, and Interventional Radiography, 311
    Jessica Cooper; Richard Ryan Wall
28. Diagnostic Medical Sonography, 407
    Susanna L. Ovel
29. Nuclear Medicine and Molecular Imaging, 435
    Raymond J. Johnson
30. Radiation Oncology, 481
    Machele D. Michels

20
MOBILE RADIOGRAPHY
RICHARD E. BASS

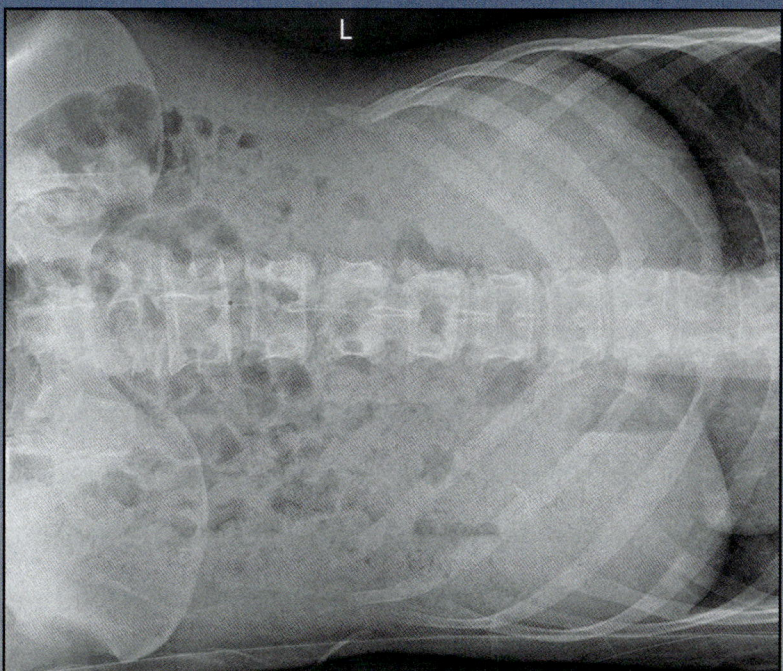

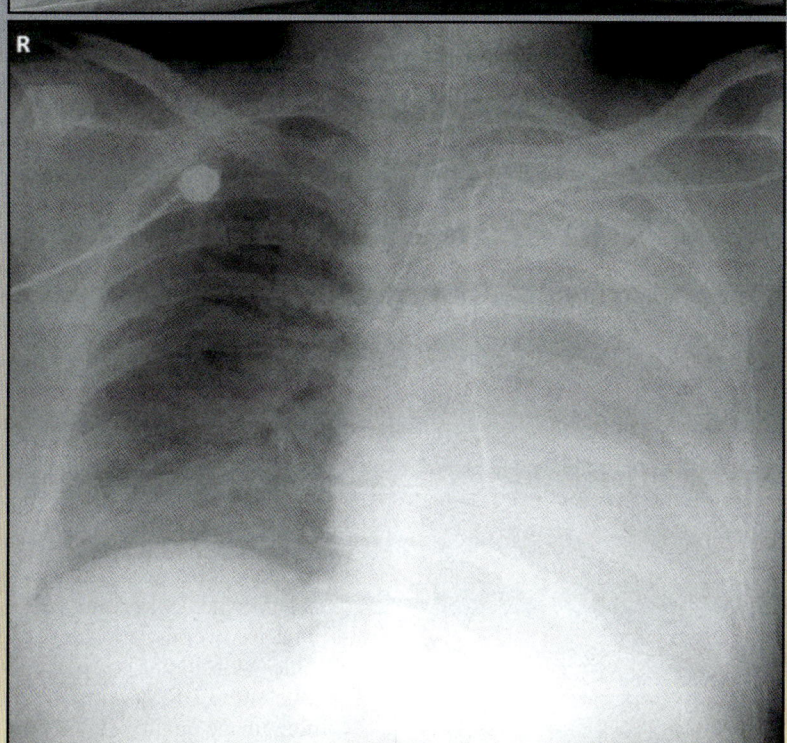

OUTLINE

Principles of Mobile Radiography, 2
Mobile X-Ray Machines, 2
Digital Radiography Mobile Units, 2
Technical Considerations, 3
Radiation Safety, 6
Isolation Considerations, 7
Performing Mobile Examinations, 7
RADIOGRAPHY, 10
Chest, 10
Abdomen, 14
Pelvis, 18
Femur, 20
Cervical Spine, 24
Best Practices in Mobile Imaging, 26

Principles of Mobile Radiography

This chapter focuses on mobile radiography and routine projections performed. The basic principles of mobile radiography are described, along with helpful hints for successfully performing portable examinations. The practice of mobile radiography was first introduced by Marie Curie during World War I. Curie was a chemist and physicist who conducted research on radioactivity. She is famous for discovering polonium and radium while working alongside her husband. In regard to the beginning of mobile radiography, Curie loaded automobiles with x-ray equipment and drove around on the battlefield to produce images of injured soldiers. Later, small portable units were designed for soldiers to carry and set up in field locations. Although mobile equipment is no longer "carried" to the patient, the term *portable* has persisted and is often used in reference to mobile procedures. Mobile radiography has progressed with technological advancements that range from film-based systems to computed radiography (CR) and the current practice of direct radiography (DR).

In general, mobile radiography allows imaging services to be brought to the patient. Compact mobile radiography units can produce diagnostic images in virtually any location (Fig. 20.1). Mobile radiography is commonly performed on patients with medical conditions that limit the patient from physically coming to the radiology department. Mobile exams can be performed in several areas throughout health care facilities: patients' rooms, emergency departments, trauma units, intensive care units, surgical suites, recovery rooms, the nursery, and neonatal units. Although there have been technological advances, exams performed in the radiology department using stationary equipment are still superior to exams performed with a mobile unit. Additional mobile imaging services include the performance of exams where patients reside, such as in their homes, assisted living residences, hospice accommodations, prisons, or nursing homes. Technologists operate mobile machines that are designed for transport by automobile or van. Technologists are also responsible for sending the images to radiologists and physicians for interpretation.

Mobile X-Ray Machines

Mobile x-ray machines are capable of producing images of most body parts. The design of the equipment varies in the exposure controls and power sources (generators). For example, some portable units need direct current plugged into an outlet, while others use a built-in battery system. Modern mobile x-ray machines have preset anatomic programs (APRs), similar to stationary units, in which the APR system adjusts the exposure techniques to predetermined values based on the selected examination. The radiographer can adjust these settings as needed to compensate for differences in the patient's body habitus or pathological condition.

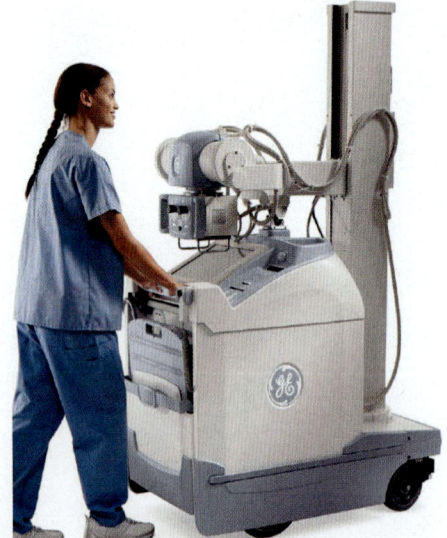

Fig. 20.1 Radiographer moving a battery-operated mobile radiography machine to a patient's room.

Older model x-ray machines have controls for setting kilovolt (peak) (kVp) and milliampere-seconds (mAs). The mAs control automatically adjusts milliamperage (mA) and time to preset values. Maximum settings differ among manufacturers. Both modern and older mobile x ray units typically have a range from 0.04 to 320 mAs, and from 40 to 130 kVp. The total power of the unit ranges from 15 to 25 kilowatts (kW), which is adequate for most mobile projections. By comparison, the power of a stationary radiography unit can reach 150 kW (150 kVp, 1000 mA) or more. Similar to stationary equipment, CR mobile units are being phased out and replaced with DR portables. As to radiation safety, the principle of ALARA (as low as reasonably achievable) still applies and is always a priority!

Digital Radiography Mobile Units

The advancement in digital imaging has evolved in both fixed x-ray rooms and bedside mobile units. Some mobile units have direct digital capability, wherein the image is acquired immediately on the unit. These machines have a flat-panel detector, similar to those found in a DR table bucky. The detector is connected to the portable unit by a tethered cord or communicates through wireless technology (Fig. 20.2). The bedside DR mobile unit converts digital data in real time, allowing images to be displayed on the mobile monitor within seconds after exposure. This practice enables the technologist to review the image before removing the wireless or tethered flat-panel IR from behind the patient or part. One of the benefits of using DR mobile units is improving workflow efficiency by displaying images after capture without having to process the IR in a separate reader housed in a different location. The images are sent wirelessly to the facility's picture archiving and communication system (PACS). Earlier DR mobile unit models used a physical cable to transfer images from the portable to PACS at designated wired ethernet network workstations. With current secure wireless systems, technologists can perform bedside imaging on multiple patients back-to-back and review the final images before leaving each patient's area. Another benefit when comparing CR to DR mobile units is lower radiation doses, as made possible with digital postprocessing software inherent to DR systems while maintaining high image quality.

Technical Considerations

Mobile radiography presents the radiographer with challenges different from those associated with performing examinations with stationary equipment in the radiology department. Although the positioning of the patient and placement of the central ray are essentially the same, several important technical matters must be clearly understood to perform optimal mobile examinations—for example, source-to-skin distance (SSD), grid application, *anode heel effect*, and source-to-image receptor distance (SID). In addition, exposure technique charts should be available (Fig. 20.3).

The SSD refers to the distance between the source of radiation (focal spot) in the x-ray tube and the nearest point on the patient's skin surface where the primary beam enters. In accordance with federal safety regulations, the SSD cannot be less than 30 cm (12 inches) to prevent unacceptable entrance skin exposure. Unlike stationary equipment, mobile units do not have automatic detents; therefore, the technologist manually adjusts tube height and distance to the patient.

STANDARD GRID

In older mobile units that still use CR plates, the image receptors are more sensitive to scatter radiation and background noise due to the lower K-edge values. Therefore, it is important to use a grid with CR plates, when needed, to help reduce scatter radiation to the image receptor.

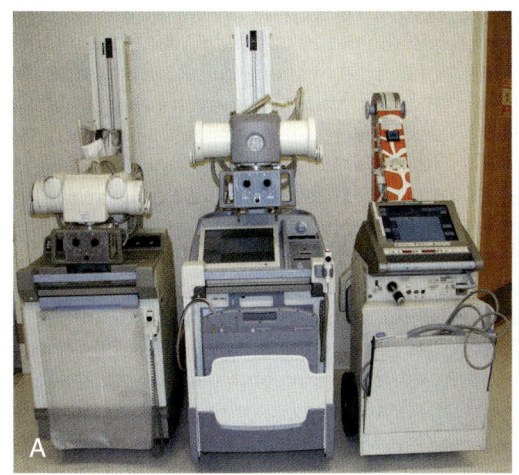 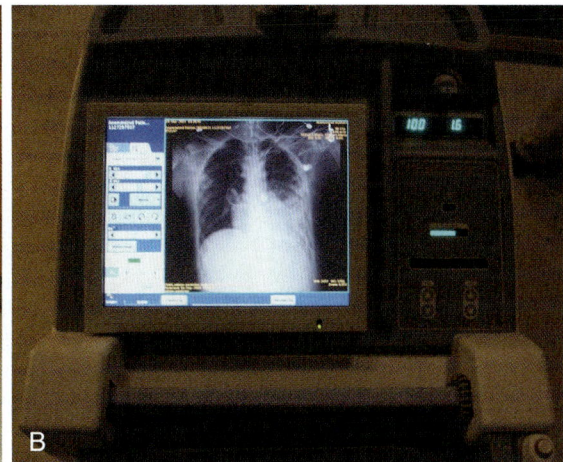 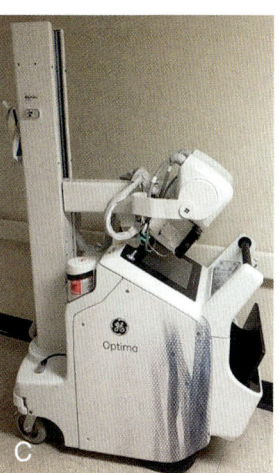

Fig. 20.2 (**A**) The machine on the left is an analog mobile unit, and the other two are digital units. Notice that the two digital mobile units have computer screens. (**B**) Mobile digital screen with a chest image. (**C**) DR mobile unit with wireless IR.

MOBILE RADIOGRAPHIC TECHNIQUE CHART

AMX—4   40-inch SID   CR IP   8:1 grid

Part	Projection	Position	cm—kVp	mAs	Grid
Chest	AP	Supine/upright	21—120	3.2	Yes
	AP	Lateral decubitus	21—85	6.25	Yes
Abdomen	AP	Supine	23—74	25	Yes
	AP	Lateral decubitus	23—74	32	Yes
Pelvis	AP	Supine	23—74	32	Yes
Femur (distal)	AP	Supine	15—70	10	Yes
	Lateral	Dorsal decubitus	15—70	10	Yes
C-spine	Lateral	Dorsal decubitus	10—62	20	Yes
NEONATAL					
Chest/abdomen	AP	Supine	7—64	0.8	No
	Lateral	Dorsal decubitus	10—72	1	No

Fig. 20.3 Sample radiographic technique chart showing manual technical factors used for the 10 common mobile projections described in this chapter. The kVp and mAs factors are for the specific centimeter measurements indicated. Factors vary depending on the actual centimeter measurement.

For optimal imaging, a grid must be level, centered to the central ray, and correctly used at the recommended focal distance (radius). When a grid is placed on a flexible surface such as the mattress of a bed, the weight of the patient can cause the grid to tilt "off level." If a longitudinal grid tilts transversely, the central ray forms an angle across the long axis. Image quality is then lost as a result of grid "cutoff" (Fig. 20.4). Off-level grid cutoff occurs most often when performing exams on patients who are lying on air mattresses, sandbag beds, bariatric beds, or saggy mattresses. The technologist must identify these obstacles before making an exposure. To help prevent grid cutoff, air mattresses and sandbag beds need to be fully inflated. If sandbag beds are not fully inflated, not only will unlevel grid cutoff occur, but an overlap of the sandbag onto the IR will cause an artifact. However, if the grid tilts longitudinally, the central ray angles through the long axis. In this case, grid cutoff is avoided; however, the image may be distorted or elongated.

Sometimes placing the grid under a patient can be difficult when centering the grid to the area of interest. If the central ray is directed to a point transversely off the midline of a grid more than 2.5 to 3.8 cm (1–1.5 inches), this causes a cutoff effect similar to that produced by off-level grid errors. The central ray can be directed longitudinally to any point along the midline of a grid without cutoff. Depending on the procedure, beam-restriction problems may occur; if this happens, a portion of the image is "collimated off," or patient exposure is excessive because of an oversized exposure field.

Grids used for mobile radiography are often of the focused type. However, some radiology departments continue to use older, parallel-type grids. All focused grids have a recommended focal range or radius that varies with the grid ratio. Projections taken at distances greater or less than the recommended focal range can produce a cutoff in which image quality is reduced on lateral margins. Grids with a lower ratio have a greater focal range but are less efficient for cleaning up scatter radiation. The radiographer must be aware of the *exact* focal range for the grid used. Most focused grids used for mobile radiography have a ratio of 6:1 or 8:1 and a focal range of about 91 to 112 cm (36 to 44 inches). The grid ratio can be found on the grid device itself. The technologist should verify which grid ratio they are using and adjust the appropriate technical factors. This focal range allows mobile examinations to be performed efficiently. Inverting a focused grid causes a pronounced cutoff effect similar to that produced by improper distance. Most grids are mounted on a protective frame, and the IR is easily inserted behind the grid (Fig. 20.5). The direction of the grid lines is usually marked to indicate whether it is transverse (short dimension) or longitudinal (long dimension).

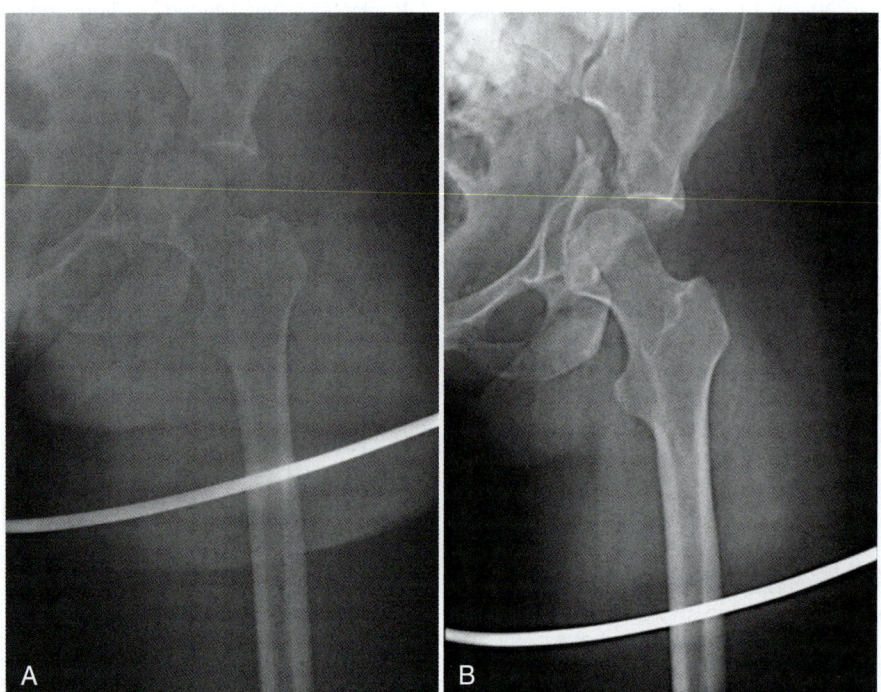

Fig. 20.4 Mobile radiograph of proximal femur and hip, showing comminuted fracture of left acetabulum. (**A**) Poor-quality radiograph resulted when grid was transversely tilted far enough to produce significant grid cutoff. (**B**) Excellent-quality repeat radiograph on the same patient, performed with grid accurately positioned perpendicular to central ray.

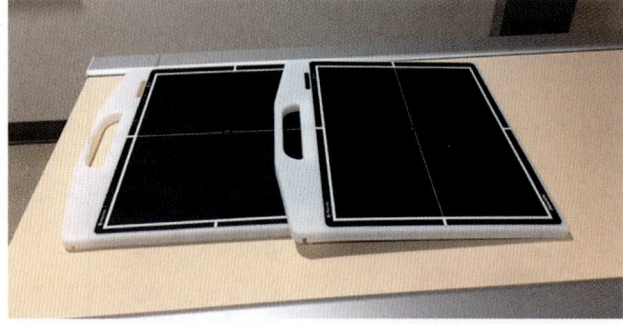

Fig. 20.5 The directions of the grid lines are marked on the front of the grid as either transverse *(short dimension)* or longitudinal *(long dimension)*. Focal ranges are clearly identified for proper use.

GRIDLESS IMAGING

With the evolution of DR mobile units, standard anti-scatter grids, and grid covers have been replaced with an alternate approach developed to compensate for image degradation through digital image processing. Vendors developed software that estimates the scattered radiation and provides scatter correction without the usage of standard grids. This technology enables the estimation of the scatter signal and calculation of the grid effect and improves image contrast reduction resulting from scatter by subtracting the estimated scatter from the raw image during postprocessing. The gridless imaging software, also referred to as virtual grid, eliminates artifacts caused by standard anti-scatter grids and the absorption of primary radiation, which negatively impacts image quality. Even though the virtual grid is built into the mobile unit systems, the technologist can activate or deactivate the use of this software. There are times when the virtual grid will not be sufficient and a standard grid is necessary, such as when imaging obese or bariatric patients. The examinations described in this chapter present methods of ensuring proper grid and IR placement for projections that require a grid.

ANODE HEEL EFFECT

Another consideration in mobile radiography is the *anode heel effect*. The heel effect causes a decrease in image intensity under the anode side of the x-ray tube, and is more pronounced with the following:
- Short SID
- Larger field sizes
- Small anode angles

Short SIDs and large field sizes are common in mobile radiography. The radiographer has control of the anode-cathode axis of the x-ray tube relative to the body part; correct placement of the anode-cathode axis with regard to the anatomy is essential. When performing a mobile examination, the radiographer may not always be able to orient the anode-cathode axis of the tube to the desired position due to limited space and maneuverability in the room. For optimal mobile radiography, the anode and cathode sides of the x-ray tube should be clearly marked to indicate where the high-tension cables enter the x-ray tube, and the radiographer should use the heel effect maximally (Table 20.1).

SOURCE-TO-IMAGE RECEPTOR DISTANCE

The SID should be maintained at 102 cm (40 inches) for most mobile examinations. A standardized distance for all patients and projections helps ensure imaging consistency. Longer SIDs— 102 to 122 cm (40–48 inches) —require increased mAs to compensate for the additional distance; the mA limitations of a mobile unit necessitate longer exposure times when the SID exceeds 102 cm (40 inches). Despite the longer exposure time, a radiograph with motion artifacts may result if the SID is greater than 102 cm (40 inches). In addition, motion artifacts may occur in the radiographs of critically ill adult patients and infants or small children who require chest and abdominal examinations but are unable to hold their breath.

RADIOGRAPHIC TECHNIQUE CHARTS

A radiographic technique chart should be available for use with every mobile machine. The chart should display, in an organized manner, the standardized technical factors for all the radiographic projections performed with the machine (see Fig. 20.3). Beginner radiographers may consider using a caliper ruler to measure the thickness of body parts to ensure that accurate and consistent exposure factors are used to penetrate the area of interest. Measuring the patient allows the radiographer to determine the optimal kVp level for all exposures (Fig. 20.6). However, with experience, radiographers can look at the part thickness and estimate the closest acceptable technique while practicing the ALARA principle.

TABLE 20.1
Cathode placement for mobile projections

Part	Projection	Cathode placement
Chest	AP	Diaphragm
	AP—decubitus	Down side of chest
Abdomen	AP	Diaphragm
	AP—decubitus	Down side of abdomen
Pelvis	AP	Upper pelvis
Femur	AP	Proximal femur
	Lateral	Proximal femur
Cervical spine	Lateral	Over lower vertebrae (102 cm [40 inches] SID only)
Chest and abdomen in neonate	All	No designation[a]

[a]Not necessary because of small field size of the collimator.
Note: The cathode side of the beam has the greatest intensity.
Just as in the department, the cathode side lines up with the thicker body parts.

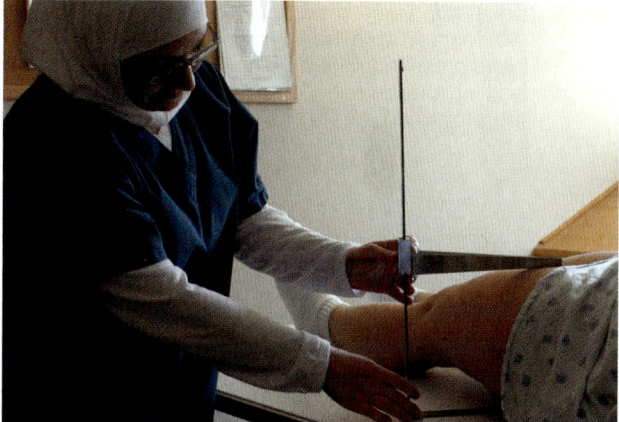

Fig. 20.6 Radiographer measuring the thickest portion of the femur to determine the exact technical factors needed for the examination.

Radiation Safety

Radiation protection for the radiographer, others in the immediate area, and the patient is paramount when performing mobile examinations. Mobile radiography produces some of the highest occupational radiation exposures for radiographers. For occupational safety, distance from the primary source of radiation should be considered before making an exposure. The National Council on Radiation Protection and Measurements (NCRP) recommends a minimum distance of 1.8 m (6 feet) from the radiation source.[1] While this is the minimal distance, the radiographer should stand as far away from the patient as possible while still observing the patient. In addition, the radiographer should inform all persons in the immediate area that an x-ray exposure is about to occur to allow bystanders to move away from the radiation source.

Radiographers should also position themselves to stand at a right angle (90 degrees) from the primary x-ray beam. The least amount of scatter radiation occurs at this position (Fig. 20.7). In situations in which the radiographer is unable to stand at a

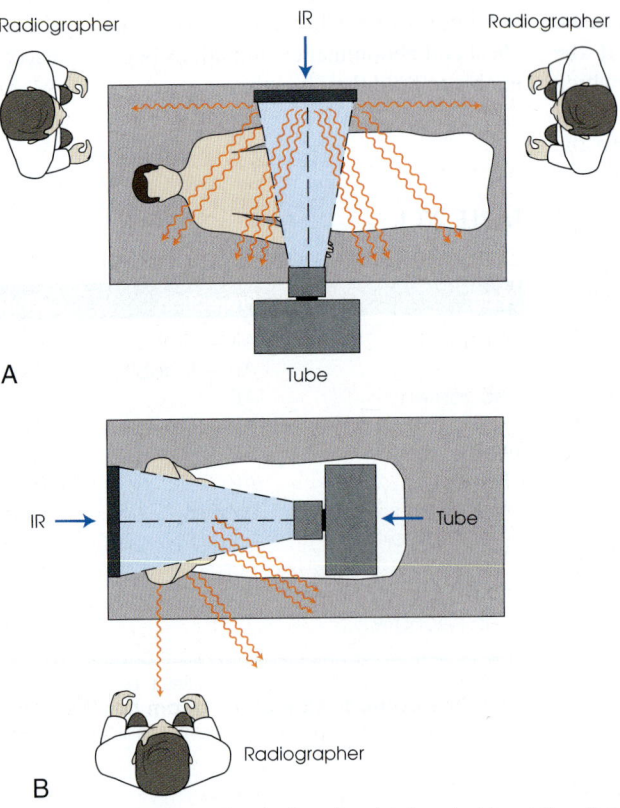

Fig. 20.7 Whenever possible, the radiographer should stand at least 2 m (6 feet) from the patient and useful beam. The lowest amount of scatter radiation occurs at a right angle (90 degrees) from the primary x-ray beam. **(A)** Note radiographer standing at either the head or the foot of the patient at a right angle to the x-ray beam for dorsal decubitus position lateral projection of the abdomen. **(B)** Radiographer standing at right angle to the x-ray beam for AP projection of the chest. *IR*, Image receptor.

90-degree angle, such as in confined spaces or small rooms, the radiographer should wear a lead apron and stand as far away as possible. When performing exams with a horizontal (cross-table) x-ray beam or during an upright AP chest, if the radiographer is unable to stand 2 m (6 feet) or at a right angle to the primary source, the radiographer should consider standing directly behind the x-ray tube. The x-ray tube is lead lined except for the window port. In addition, as previously mentioned, the SSD cannot be less than 30 cm (12 inches) in accordance with federal safety regulations.

Isolation Considerations

Two types of patients are often cared for in isolation units: (1) patients who have infectious microorganisms that could be spread to health care workers and visitors, and (2) patients who need protection from potentially lethal microorganisms that may be carried by health care workers and visitors. Optimally, a radiographer entering an isolation room should have full knowledge of the patient's disease, how the disease is transmitted, and the proper way to clean and disinfect equipment before and after use in the isolation unit. All patients must be treated with universal precautions.

If isolation is used to protect the patient from receiving microorganisms (reverse isolation), a different protocol may be required. Institutional policy regarding isolation procedures should be available and strictly followed.

In performing mobile procedures in an isolation unit, the radiographer should wear the required protective apparel for the specific situation: gown, cap, mask, shoe covers, face shield, and gloves. All persons entering a strict isolation unit must wear a mask, a gown, and gloves. Gloves are worn for drainage secretion precautions. Radiographers should always wash their hands with warm soapy water before putting on gloves. The x-ray machine is taken into the room and moved into position. The IR is placed into a clean protective cover. Pillowcase covers are insufficient in protecting the IR or the patient from body fluids soaking through the fabric. A clean, impermeable cover should be used in situations in which body fluids may come into contact with the IR. For examinations of patients in strict isolation, two radiographers may be required to maintain a safe barrier (see Chapter 1).

After finishing the examination, the radiographer should remove and dispose of the personal protective equipment (PPE) attire in accordance with institutional policies. All equipment that touched the patient or the patient's bed must be wiped with a disinfectant according to the appropriate aseptic technique. If necessary, the radiographer should wear new gloves while cleaning equipment. Handwashing is repeated before the radiographer leaves the room.

Performing Mobile Examinations

INITIAL PROCEDURES

Before leaving the radiology department, the radiographer should plan for the trip, ensuring that all of the necessary devices (e.g., IR, protective covers, grid, tape, markers, positioning blocks, masks, gowns, gloves, wipes) are transported with the mobile x-ray machine. This provides greater efficiency in performing examinations. Many mobile x-ray machines are equipped with storage areas for transporting IRs and supplies. If a battery-operated machine is used, the radiographer should check the machine to ensure that it is acceptably charged. An inadequately charged machine can interfere with performance and affect the quality of the radiograph.

When performing bedside mobile radiography, the radiographer should follow several important steps (Box 20.1). The radiographer begins by checking the patient's identification. The technologist should also validate that the examination ordered matches the patient's history and condition. The radiographer is responsible for verifying that everything is correct before starting the exam. After confirming the patient's identity, the radiographer enters the patient's room, makes an introduction as a radiographer, and informs the patient about the x-ray examinations to be performed. While in the room, the radiographer should observe any medical devices connected to the patient to avoid dislodging the devices when performing the imaging exam. For example, caution should be taken with patients who are being treated with the following medical devices: ventilators, chest tube drainage systems, extracorporeal membrane oxygenation (ECMO), feeding tubes, catheter bags, infusion pumps, traction mechanisms, and intravenous (IV) poles. Technologists should also avoid disrupting the patient's monitors, oxygen administration, blood pressure cuffs, cooling blankets, compression cuffs, pulse oximeters, continuous passive motion (CPM) apparatus, and other medical devices. Before positioning the portable unit or the patient, the radiographer should ask family members or visitors to step out of the room until the examination is finished. If necessary, the nursing staff should be alerted if assistance is required.

Communication and cooperation between the radiographer and nursing staff are essential for proper patient care during mobile radiography. For example, some patients cannot lie flat for an exam that is routinely performed in the supine position. The technologist should check with the patient's nurse to verify whether the patient can be moved into certain positions before performing the exam. In addition, communication with the patient is imperative, even if the patient appears to be unconscious or unresponsive.

EXAMINATION

When performing mobile exams, there will be obstacles the technologist must overcome. Chairs, stands, IV poles, wastebaskets, and other obstacles should be moved from the path of the mobile

---

BOX 20.1

Preliminary steps for the radiographer before mobile radiography is performed

- Announce your presence to the nursing staff and ask for assistance if needed.
- Determine that the correct patient is in the room.
- Introduce yourself to the patient and family as a radiographer and explain the examination.
- Observe the medical equipment in the room, other devices, and IV poles with fluids. Move the equipment if necessary.
- Ask family members and visitors to leave. (An exception would be that a family member may have to be present for the examination of a small child.)

machine. Lighting should be adjusted if necessary. The position of the portable machine should be taken into consideration for optimal maneuverability when performing various projections. If the patient is to be examined in the supine position, placing the base of the mobile machine near the middle of the longitudinal axis of the bed allows for a more direct AP projection of body parts. If the patient is to be seated upright, the base of the machine should be parked toward the foot of the bed to allow ease of tube angulation and sufficient SID. For lateral and decubitus projections, positioning the base of the mobile machine parallel or directly perpendicular to the longitudinal axis of the bed allows for ease of tube alignment to the part and IR. Room size can also influence the portable base position used.

For all projections, the primary x-ray beam must be collimated no larger than the size of the IR. When the central ray is correctly centered to the midline of the IR, the light field coincides with or fits within the outside borders of the IR. However, the collimation parameters should be coned down to just beyond the affected body part.

Unlike in the routine radiology department, during mobile radiography, technologists have limited resources in the immediate environment. Items such as tape, wedges, sheets, blankets, or pillows may be used as positioning aids while taking into consideration avoiding artifacts. Remember, the goal is to produce quality diagnostic images.

Standard marker placement of affected structures preexposure is still important. Most institutions require additional identification for mobile examinations. Typically, the time of the examination (especially for chest radiographs) and technical notes, such as the position of the patient or alternate projections, should be indicated.

For CR radiography, when multiple projections or exams are performed back to back, the technologist should establish a system for labeling and separating the exposed and unexposed IR plates. A common mistake is to "double expose" the CR plates, particularly if several examinations are performed at one time. In contrast, using DR imaging systems helps eliminate the chance of double exposure.

PATIENT CONSIDERATIONS

A brief but total patient assessment must be conducted before and during the examination. Some specific considerations to keep in mind are assessing the patient's condition, mobility, existing fractures, interfering devices, positioning, and asepsis.

Assessment of the patient's condition

A thorough assessment of the patient's condition and room allows the radiographer to make necessary adaptations to ensure the best possible patient care and imaging outcome. The radiographer assesses the patient's level of alertness and respiration and determines the extent to which the patient is able to cooperate, as well as the limitations that may affect the procedure. Some patients may be experiencing varying degrees of drowsiness because of their medications or medical condition. Many mobile examinations are performed in patients' rooms immediately after surgery. As a result, these patients may be under the influence of various anesthetics. It is always important to communicate with the patient even if they are not alert.

Patient mobility

The radiographer must never move a patient or part of the patient's body without assessing the patient's ability to move or tolerate movement. Gentleness and caution must prevail at all times. If unsure, the radiographer should always check with the nursing staff or physician. Many patients who undergo total joint replacement may be unable to move the affected joint for many days without assistance, but this may not be evident to the radiographer. Some patients may be able to indicate verbally their ability to move or their tolerance for movement. *The radiographer should never move a limb that had surgery or is fractured unless the nurse, the physician, or sometimes the patient grants permission.* Inappropriate movement of the patient by the radiographer during the examination may be harmful.

Fractures

Patients can have various types of fractures, ranging from one simple fracture to multiple fractures of many bones. A patient lying awake in a traction bed with a simple femoral fracture may be able to assist with a radiographic examination, while another patient may be unconscious and have multiple broken ribs, spinal fractures, or a severe closed head injury.

Few patients with multiple fractures are able to move or tolerate movement. The radiographer must be cautious, resourceful, and work in accordance with the patient's condition and pain tolerance level. If a patient's trunk or limb must be elevated into position for a projection, the radiographer should have ample assistance so that the part can be positioned safely without causing harm or intense pain.

Interfering devices

As previously mentioned, patients in intensive care units or orthopedic beds may be attached to various devices, wires, and tubing. These objects may be in the direct path of the x-ray beam and, consequently, produce artifacts on the image. Experienced radiographers know which objects can be moved out of the radiation field. When devices such as fracture frames cannot be moved, it may be necessary to angle the central ray or adjust the IR to obtain the best projection possible of the part. In many instances, the objects have to be radiographed along with the body part (Fig. 20.8). The radiographer must exercise caution in handling any of these devices and should never remove traction devices without the assistance of a physician.

Positioning and asepsis

During positioning, the IR placement can feel uncomfortable for the patient and is often cold and hard. Before the IR is placed, the radiographer should warn the patient of possible discomfort and assure them that the examination will be as brief as possible. The patient will appreciate the radiographer's concern and their efficiency in completing the examination.

When the surface of the IR inadvertently touches the patient's bare skin, it can stick. *The skin of older patients may be thin and dry and can be torn by manipulation of the IR if care is not taken.* An imaging plate cover over the IR protects the patient's skin, helps keep the IR clean, and assists with infection control. The IR must be enclosed in an appropriate, impermeable barrier where it may come in contact with blood, body fluids, or other potentially infectious material. IRs should be wiped off with a disinfectant for asepsis and infection control after each patient.

A contaminated IR can be difficult and sometimes impossible to clean. Approved procedures for disposing of used barriers must be followed.

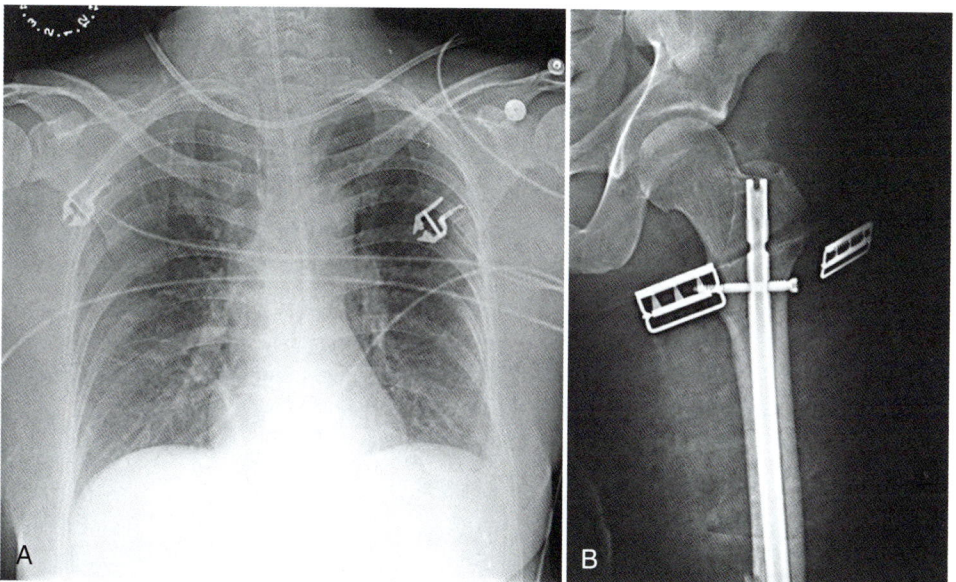

Fig. 20.8 (**A**) Mobile radiograph of chest. Note various objects in the image that could not be removed for the exposure. (**B**) Mobile radiograph of proximal femur and hip. Metal buckles could not be removed for the exposure.

RADIOGRAPHY
Chest

◆ AP PROJECTION[a]
Upright or supine

Image receptor: Positioned by manufacturer or department protocol for proper anatomy display orientation.

Position of patient

Depending on the condition of the patient, the projection should be performed with the patient in the upright position or to the greatest elevation that the patient can tolerate (if possible). Use the supine position for critically ill or injured patients.

---

[a]The nonmobile projection is described in Chapter 3.

Position of part
- Center the midsagittal plane to the IR.
- To include the entire chest, position the IR under the patient with the top about 5 cm (2 inches) above the relaxed shoulders. The exact distance depends on the size of the patient. When the patient is supine, the shoulders may move to a higher position relative to the lungs. Adjust accordingly.
- Make sure that the patient's shoulders are relaxed, then internally rotate the patient's arms forward. The dorsal surface of the hands should lie flat on the bed or stretcher to prevent scapular superimposition of the lung field if not contraindicated.
- Make sure that the patient's upper torso is not rotated or leaning toward one side (Fig. 20.9).

Respiration
- Inspiration unless otherwise requested. If the patient is receiving respiratory assistance, carefully watch the patient's chest to determine the inspiratory phase for the exposure.

Central ray
- Perpendicular to the long axis of the sternum and the center of the IR; the central ray should enter about 8 cm (3 inches) below the jugular notch at the level of T7.

Collimation
- Adjust to at least 35 × 43 cm (14 × 17 inches) on the collimator, less for smaller patients.

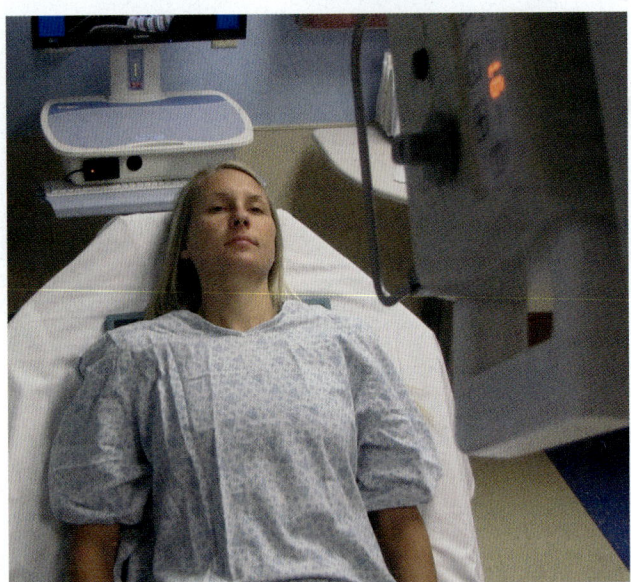

Fig. 20.9 Mobile AP chest: partially upright.

Chest

Structures shown

This projection shows the anatomy of the thorax, including the heart, trachea, diaphragmatic domes, and most importantly, the entire lung fields (including vascular markings) (Fig. 20.10).

EVALUATION CRITERIA

The optimum image obtained using correct positioning, CR-part-IR alignment, collimation, and exposure factors will demonstrate:

- The side marker placed clear of anatomy of interest
- Evidence of proper collimation
- No motion and well-defined (not blurred) diaphragmatic domes and lung fields
- Lung fields in their entirety from apices to costophrenic angles
- Approximately 2.5 cm (1 inch) of the pulmonary apices seen superior to the clavicles
- Pulmonary vascular markings from the hilar regions to the periphery of the lungs
- Ribs and thoracic intervertebral disk spaces faintly visible through heart shadow
- No rotation of the patient, with medial portion of clavicles and lateral border of ribs equidistant from vertebral column

NOTE: To ensure the proper angle from the x-ray tube to the IR, the radiographer can double-check the shadow of the shoulders from the field light projected onto the IR. If the shadow of the shoulders appears far above the upper edge of the IR, the angle of the tube must be corrected.

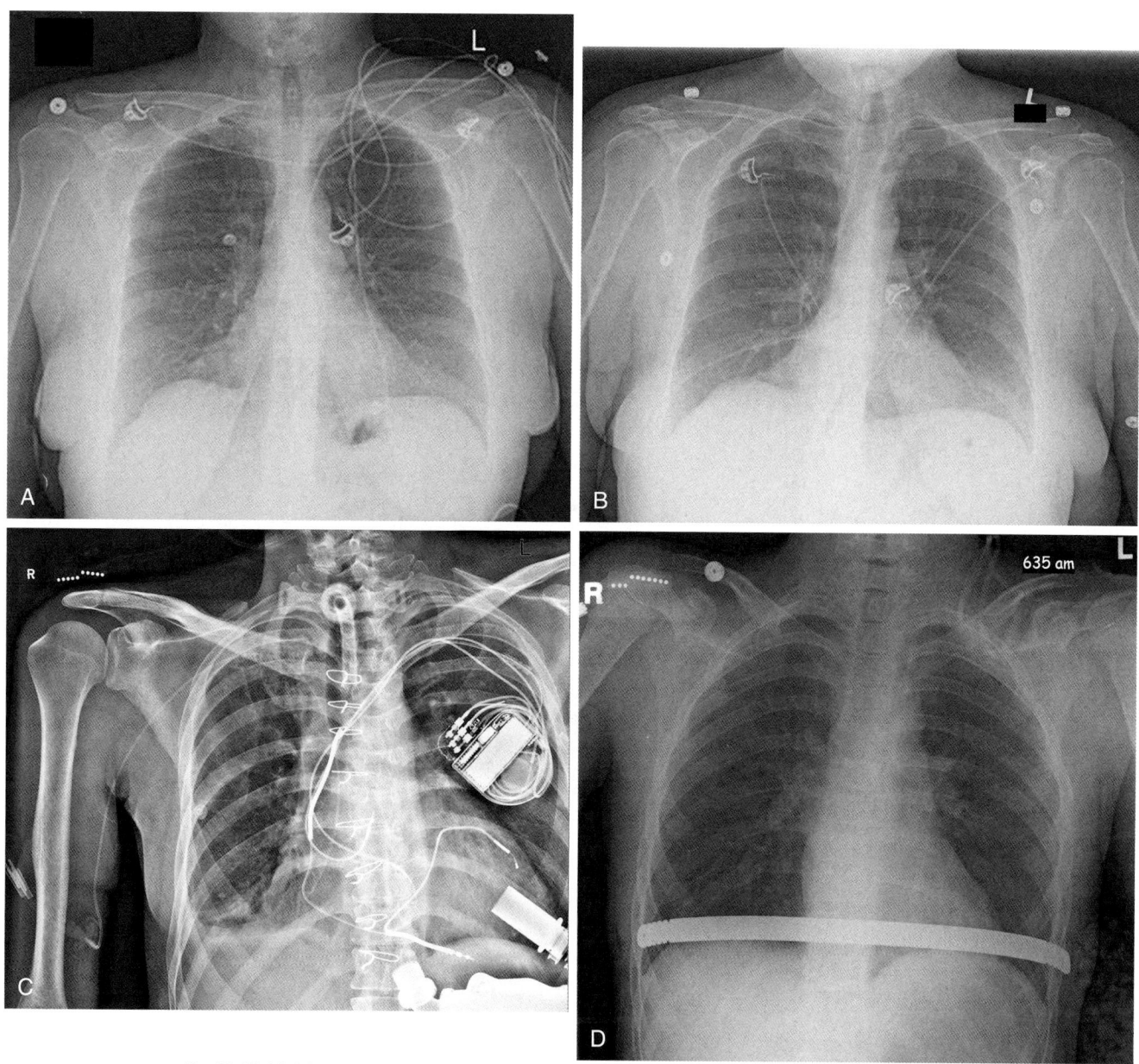

Fig. 20.10 Mobile AP chest radiographs. (**A**) AP chest image with incorrect cephalic tube angle resulting in an apical lordotic image in which the ribs appear boxy, the clavicles are projected too high, and the heart has a distorted silhouette. A tangle of lead wire is seen over the upper left chest. (**B**) Repeat image with the correct angle, central ray perpendicular to the long axis of the sternum. The radiographer has also positioned the lead wires appropriately. (**C**) Mobile peripherally inserted central catheter (PICC) placement image to visualize the PICC line from entrance to tip. Also seen are the tracheostomy, pacemaker, sternal wires, and ventricular assist device. (**D**) Adolescent postoperative patient with strut placed for pectus excavatum repair. Ice pack is seen in the lower right corner of the image.

Chest

AP OR PA PROJECTION[b]
Right or left lateral decubitus position

Image receptor + grid: Positioned by manufacturer or department protocol for proper anatomy display orientation.

Position of patient
- Place the patient in the lateral recumbent position.
- Flex the patient's knees to provide stabilization, if possible.
- Place a firm support under the patient to elevate the body 5 to 8 cm (2–3 inches) and prevent the patient from sinking into the mattress.
- Raise both of the patient's arms up and away from the chest region, preferably above the head. An arm lying on the patient's side can superimpose a region of free air.
- Make sure that the patient cannot roll off the bed.

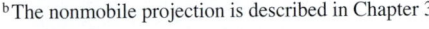
[b]The nonmobile projection is described in Chapter 3

Position of part
- Position the patient for the AP projection whenever possible. It is much easier to position an ill patient (particularly the arms) for an AP.
- Adjust the patient to ensure a lateral position. The coronal plane passing through the shoulders and hips should be vertical.
- Place the IR behind the patient and below the support so that the lower margin of the chest is visible.
- Adjust the grid so that it extends approximately 5 cm (2 inches) above the shoulders. In order to avoid distortion, the IR should be supported in position and not leaning against the patient (Fig. 20.11).

Respiration
- Inspiration unless otherwise requested.

Central ray
- Horizontal and perpendicular to the center of the IR, entering the patient at a level of 8 cm (3 inches) below the jugular notch for AP and T7 for PA.

Collimation
- Adjust to 35 × 43 cm (14 × 17 inches) on the collimator.

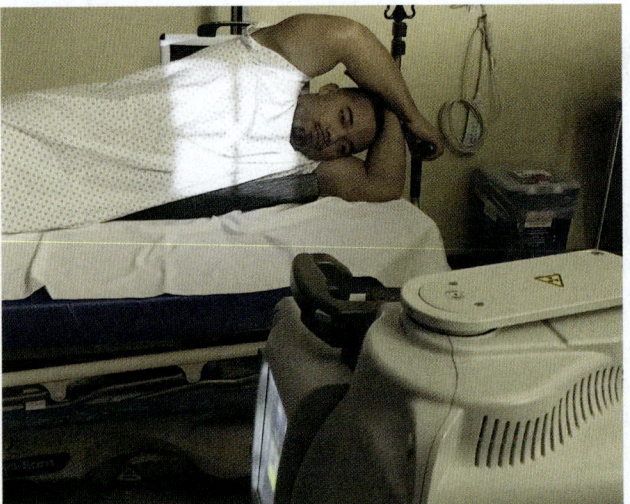

Fig. 20.11 Mobile AP chest: left lateral decubitus position. Note gray pad placed under the chest to elevate it. The block is necessary to ensure that the left side of chest is included on the image.

Chest

Structures shown

This projection shows the anatomy of the thorax, including the entire lung fields and any air or fluid levels that may be present (Fig. 20.12).

EVALUATION CRITERIA

The optimum image obtained using correct positioning, CR-part-IR alignment, collimation, and exposure factors will demonstrate:

- The side marker placed clear of anatomy of interest
- Evidence of proper collimation
- No motion
- No rotation of the patient, as demonstrated by the sternal ends of the clavicles equidistant from the spine
- Affected side in its entirety (upper lung for free air and lower lung for fluid)
- Patient's arms out of region of interest
- Faintly visible spine and pulmonary vascular markings from the hilar regions to the periphery of the lungs

NOTE: Fluid levels in the pleural cavity are best visualized with the affected side down, which also prevents mediastinal overlapping. Air levels are best visualized with the unaffected side down. The patient should be in position for at least 5 minutes before the exposure is made to allow air to rise and fluid levels to settle.

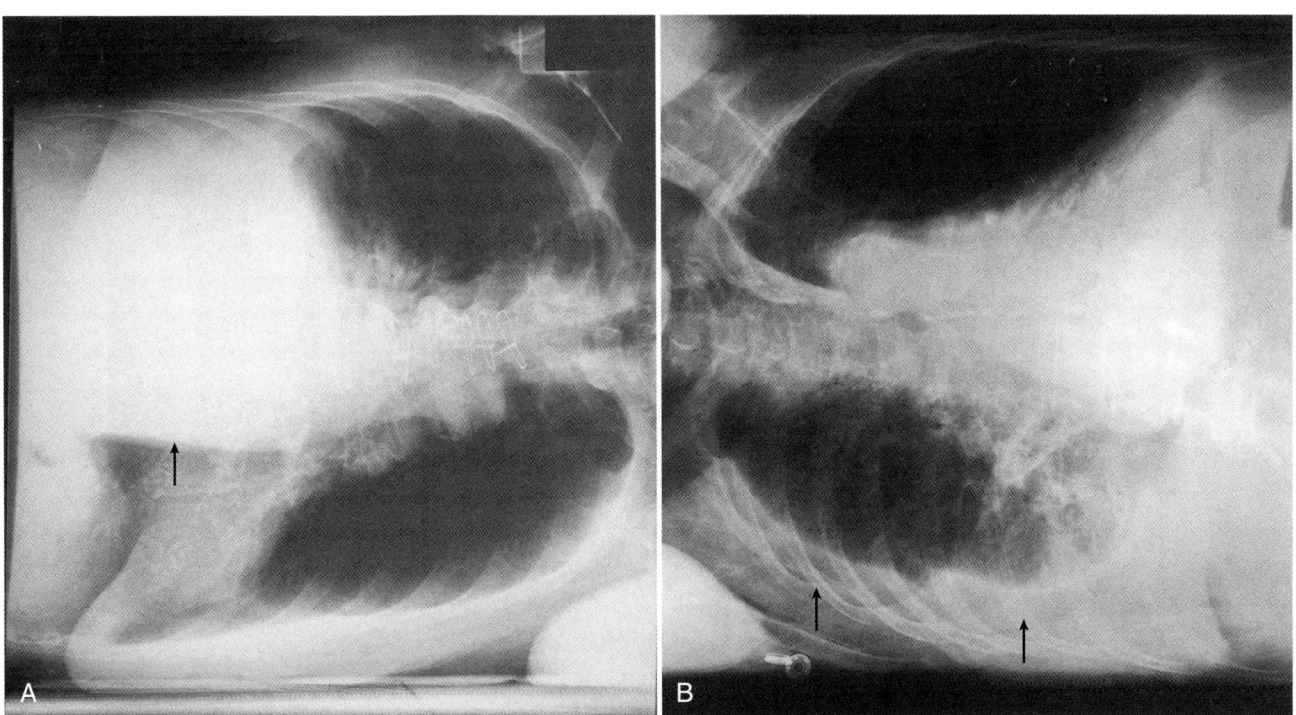

Fig. 20.12 Mobile AP chest radiographs performed in lateral decubitus positions in critically ill patients. **(A)** Left lateral decubitus position. The patient has a large right pleural effusion *(arrow)* and no left effusion. The complete left side of thorax is visualized because of elevation on a block. **(B)** Right lateral decubitus position. The patient has a right pleural effusion *(arrows)*, cardiomegaly, and mild pulmonary vascular congestion. The complete right side of thorax is visualized because of elevation on a block.

Abdomen

⚕ AP PROJECTION[c]

Image receptor + grid: Positioned by manufacturer or department protocol for proper anatomy display orientation.

Position of patient
- If necessary, adjust the patient's bed to achieve a horizontal bed position.
- Place the patient in a supine position.

Position of part
- Position the grid under the patient to show the abdominal anatomy from the pubic symphysis to the upper abdominal region.
- Keep the grid from tipping side to side by placing it in the center of the bed and, if necessary, stabilize it with blankets or towels.
- Use the patient's draw sheet to roll the patient; this makes it easier to shift the patient from side to side during positioning of the IR and provides a barrier between the patient's skin and the grid.
- Center the midsagittal plane of the patient to the midline of the grid.

[c]The nonmobile projection is described in Chapter 4.

- Center the grid to the level of the iliac crests. If the emphasis is on the upper abdomen, center the grid 5 cm (2 inches) above the iliac crests or high enough to include the diaphragm.
- Adjust the patient's shoulders and pelvis to lie in the same plane (Fig. 20.13).
- Move the patient's arms out of the region of the abdomen.

Respiration
- Expiration.

Central ray
- Perpendicular to the center of the grid along the midsagittal plane and at the level of the iliac crests or the 10th rib laterally.

Collimation
- Adjust to 35 × 43 cm (14 × 17 inches) on the collimator.

Structures shown
This projection shows the inferior margin of the liver, the spleen, kidneys, and psoas muscles, calcifications, and evidence of tumor masses. If the image includes the upper abdomen and diaphragm, the size and shape of the liver may be seen (Fig. 20.14).

EVALUATION CRITERIA
The optimum image obtained using correct positioning, CR-part-IR alignment, collimation, and exposure factors will demonstrate:
- The side marker placed clear of anatomy of interest
- Evidence of proper collimation
- No motion
- Outlines of the abdominal viscera
- Area from the pubic symphysis to the upper abdomen (two images may be necessary if the patient is tall or wide)
- Vertebral column in center of image
- Psoas muscles, lower margin of liver, and kidney margins
- No rotation
- Centered vertebral column
- Symmetric appearance of iliac wings

NOTE: Hypersthenic patients may require two separate projections using a crosswise grid. One grid is positioned for the upper abdomen and the other for the lower abdomen. Bariatric or morbid obesity patients may require up to four projections of each quad section: two crosswise uppers along with two crosswise lowers.

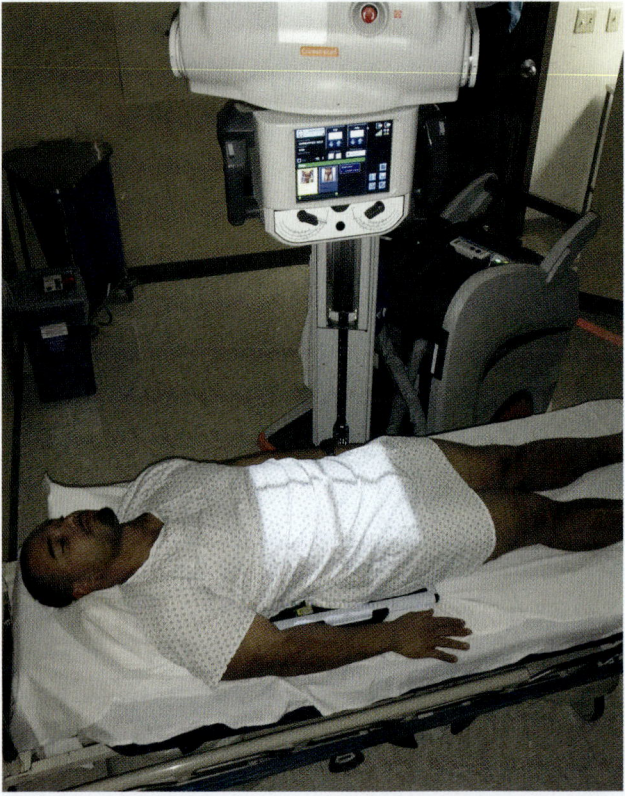

Fig. 20.13 Mobile AP of the abdomen.

Abdomen

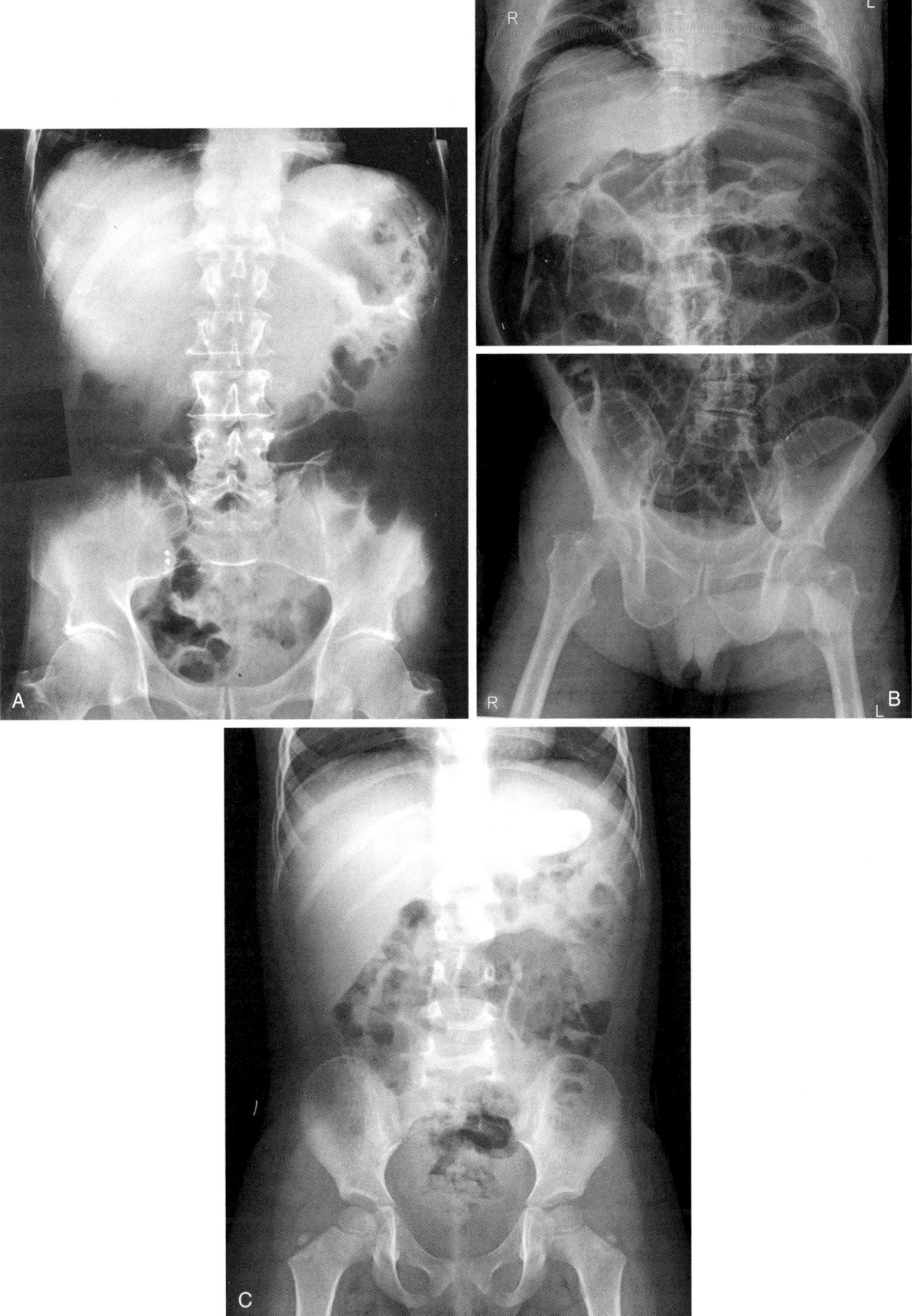

Fig. 20.14 Mobile AP abdominal radiographs. (**A**) Abdomen without pathology. The entire abdomen is seen in this patient. (**B**) Because of this patient's large body habitus, two crosswise (landscape) images of the abdomen were necessary to include all abdominal structures. Counting of vertebral bodies ensures adequate overlap. Note the large amount of free air, indicative of a perforated bowel. (**C**) Mobile AP abdominal image of a pediatric patient. Ingested jewelry bead is seen in the fundus of the stomach.

Abdomen

▲ AP OR PA PROJECTION[d]
Left lateral decubitus position

Image receptor + grid: Positioned by manufacturer or department protocol for proper anatomy display orientation.

Position of patient
- Place the patient in the left lateral recumbent position unless requested otherwise.
- Slightly flex the patient's knees to provide stabilization.
- If necessary, place a firm support under the patient to elevate the body and keep the patient from sinking into the mattress.
- If possible, raise both of the patient's arms away from the abdominal region. The right arm lying on the side of the abdomen may superimpose a region of free air.
- Make sure the patient cannot fall out of bed.

Position of part
- Use the PA or AP projection, depending on the room layout.
- Adjust the patient to ensure a true lateral position; the coronal plane passing through the shoulders and hips should be vertical.
- Place the grid vertically in front of the patient for a PA projection and behind the patient for an AP projection. The grid should be supported in position and not leaned against the patient to prevent grid cutoff.
- Position the grid so that its center is 5 cm (2 inches) above the iliac crests to ensure that the diaphragm is included. The pubic symphysis and lower abdomen do not have to be visualized (Fig. 20.15).
- Before making the exposure, ensure that the patient has been in the lateral recumbent position for at least 5 minutes to allow air to rise and fluid levels to settle.

Respiration
- Expiration.

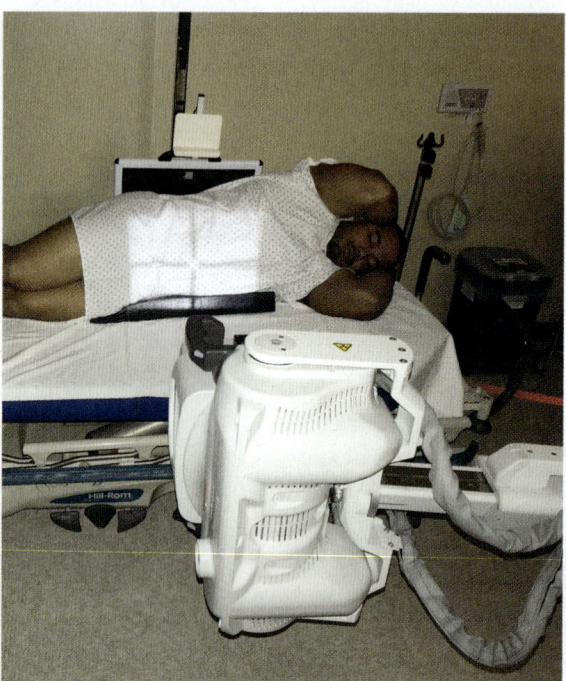

Fig. 20.15 Mobile AP abdomen: left lateral decubitus position. Note black blocks placed under the abdomen to level the abdomen and keep the patient from sinking into the mattress.

---

[d]The nonmobile projection is described in Chapter 4.

Abdomen

Central ray
- Horizontal and perpendicular to the center of the grid, entering the patient along the midsagittal plane.

Collimation
- Adjust to 35 × 43 cm (14 × 17 inches) on the collimator.

Structures shown
Air or fluid levels within the abdominal cavity are shown, and these projections are especially helpful in assessing free air in the abdomen. The right border of the abdominal region must be visualized (Fig. 20.16).

EVALUATION CRITERIA

The optimum image obtained using correct positioning, CR-part-IR alignment, collimation, and exposure factors will demonstrate:
- The side marker placed clear of anatomy of interest
- Evidence of proper collimation
- No motion
- Well-defined diaphragm and abdominal viscera
- Both sides of the abdomen. If abdomen is too wide:
  - Side down when fluid is suspected (ensure entire dependent side is included in the collimated field)
  - Side up when free air is suspected
- Right and left abdominal wall and flank structures
- No rotation
- Centered vertebral column
- Symmetric appearance of iliac wings

NOTE: Hypersthenic patients may require two projections using a 35 × 43 cm (14 × 17 inches) grid positioned crosswise to visualize the entire abdominal area. A patient with a long torso may require two projections with the grid lengthwise to visualize the entire abdominal region.

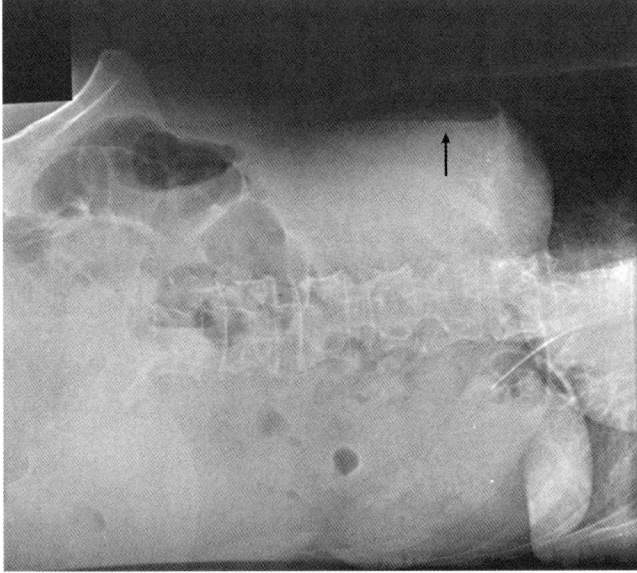

Fig. 20.16 Mobile AP of the abdomen: left lateral decubitus position. Free intraperitoneal air is seen on the upper or right side of the abdomen *(arrow)*. The radiograph is slightly underexposed to show free air more easily.

Pelvis

AP PROJECTION[e]

Image receptor + grid: Positioned by manufacturer or department protocol for proper anatomy display orientation.

Position of patient
- Adjust the patient's bed horizontally so that the patient is in a supine position.
- Move the patient's arms out of the region of the pelvis.

---

[e] The nonmobile projection is described in Chapter 8.

Position of part
- Position the grid under the pelvis so that the center is midway between the anterior superior iliac spine (ASIS) and the pubic symphysis. This is about 5 cm (2 inches) inferior to the ASIS and 5 cm (2 inches) superior to the pubic symphysis.
- Center the midsagittal plane of the patient to the midline of the grid. The pelvis should not be rotated.
- Rotate the patient's legs medially approximately 15 degrees when not contraindicated (Fig. 20.17).

Respiration
- Suspended.

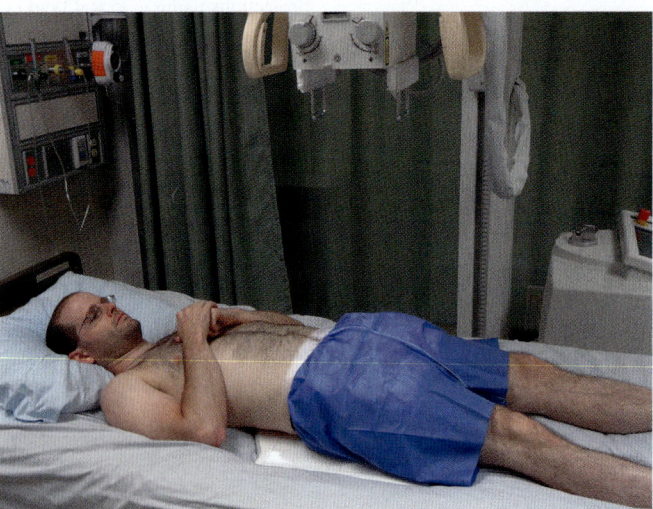

Fig. 20.17 Mobile of the AP pelvis. Grid is placed horizontally and perpendicular to the central ray.

Pelvis

Central ray
- Perpendicular to the midpoint of the grid, entering the midsagittal plane. The central ray should enter the patient 5 cm (2 inches) above the pubic symphysis and 5 cm (2 inches) below the ASIS.

Collimation
- Adjust to 43 × 35 cm (17 × 14 inches) on the collimator.

Structures shown
This projection shows the pelvis, including both hip bones; the sacrum and coccyx; and the head, neck, trochanters, and proximal portion of the femora (Fig. 20.18).

EVALUATION CRITERIA
The optimum image obtained using correct positioning, CR-part-IR alignment, collimation, and exposure factors will demonstrate:
- The side marker placed clear of anatomy of interest
- Evidence of proper collimation
- Entire pelvis, including proximal femora and both hip bones
- No rotation
- Symmetric appearance of iliac wings and obturator foramina
- Both greater trochanters and ilia equidistant from edge of radiograph
- Lower vertebral column centered
- Femoral necks not foreshortened and greater trochanters in profile

NOTE: It is common for the patient's weight to cause the bottom edge of the grid to tilt upward. The x-ray tube may need to be angled caudally to compensate and maintain proper grid alignment, preventing grid cutoff. The exact angle needed is not always known or easy to determine. The radiographer may want to lower the foot of the bed slightly (Fowler position), shifting the patient's weight more evenly on the grid and allowing it to be flat. A rolled-up towel or blanket placed under the grid may also be useful to prevent lateral tilting. If the bed is equipped with an inflatable air mattress, the maximum inflate mode is recommended. Tilting the bottom edge of the grid downward is another possibility. Check the level of the grid carefully and compensate accordingly.

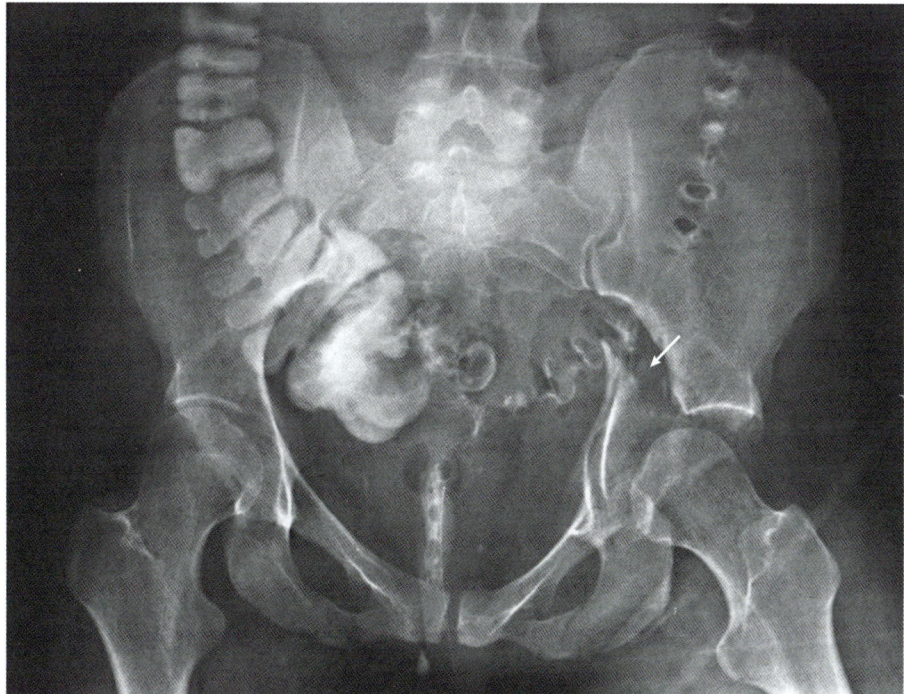

Fig. 20.18 Mobile AP of the pelvis. This patient has a comminuted fracture of the left acetabulum with medial displacement of medial acetabular wall (arrow). Residual barium is seen in the colon, sigmoid, and rectum.

Femur

AP PROJECTION[f]

Most mobile AP and lateral projections of the femur may be radiographs of the middle and distal femur taken while the patient is in traction. The anatomy demonstrated for the proximal femur would be included in an AP pelvis image, if a pelvic exam is also ordered on the same patient. If not, the technologist should include an AP proximal femur image.

Image receptor + grid: Positioned by manufacturer or department protocol for proper anatomy display orientation.

Position of patient
- The patient is in the supine position.

Position of part
- Cautiously place the grid lengthwise under the patient's femur, with the distal edge of the grid low enough to include the fracture site, pathologic region, and knee joint.
- If necessary, elevate the grid with towels, blankets, or blocks under each side to ensure proper grid alignment with the x-ray tube.
- Center the grid to the midline of the affected femur.
- Ensure that the grid is placed parallel to the plane of the femoral condyles (Fig. 20.19).

Respiration
- Suspended.

[f]The nonmobile projection is described in Chapter 7.

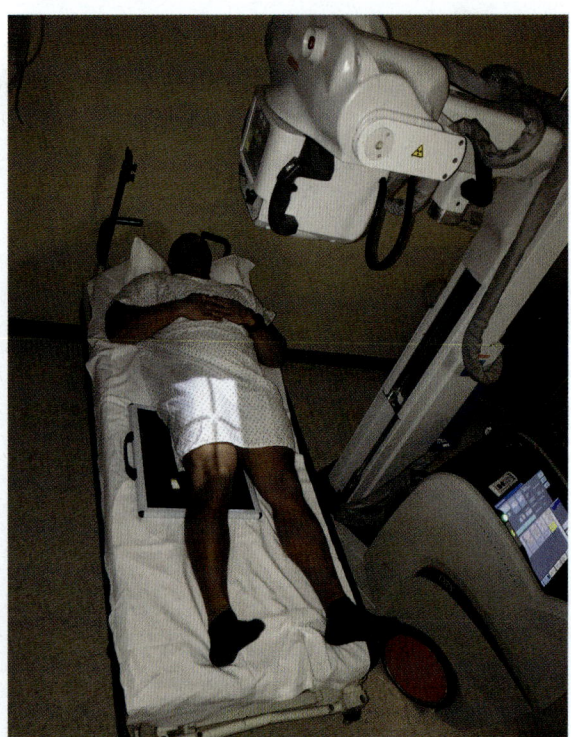

Fig. 20.19 Mobile of the AP femur.

Femur

Central ray
- Perpendicular to the long axis of the femur and centered to the grid.
- Make sure that the central ray and grid are aligned to prevent grid cutoff.

Collimation
- Adjust the top of the light field to the level of the ASIS to include hip joint for proximal anatomy, and the bottom of the light field at tibial tuberosity for knee joint for distal. Adjust light field to 2.5 cm (1 inch) beyond the sides of the femur shadows and 43 cm (17 inches) in length.

Structures shown
The distal two-thirds of the femur, including the knee joint, are shown (Fig. 20.20).

EVALUATION CRITERIA
The optimum image obtained using correct positioning, CR-part-IR alignment, collimation, and exposure factors will demonstrate:
- The side marker placed clear of anatomy of interest
- Evidence of proper collimation
- Most of femur, including knee joint for distal and hip joint for proximal
- No knee rotation
- Adequate penetration
- Any orthopedic appliance, such as plate and screw fixation

NOTE: If the entire length of the femur must be visualized, an AP projection of the proximal femur can be performed by placing a 35 × 43 cm (14 × 17 inches) grid lengthwise under the proximal femur and hip. The top of the grid is placed at the level of the ASIS to ensure that the hip joint is included. The central ray is directed to the center of the grid and long axis of the femur (see Fig. 20.4).

The thickest portion of the femur (proximal area) must be carefully measured, and an appropriate kVp must be selected to penetrate this area. The computer cannot form an image of the anatomy in this area if penetration does not occur. A light area of the entire proximal femur would result. Positioning the cathode over the proximal femur would improve image quality.

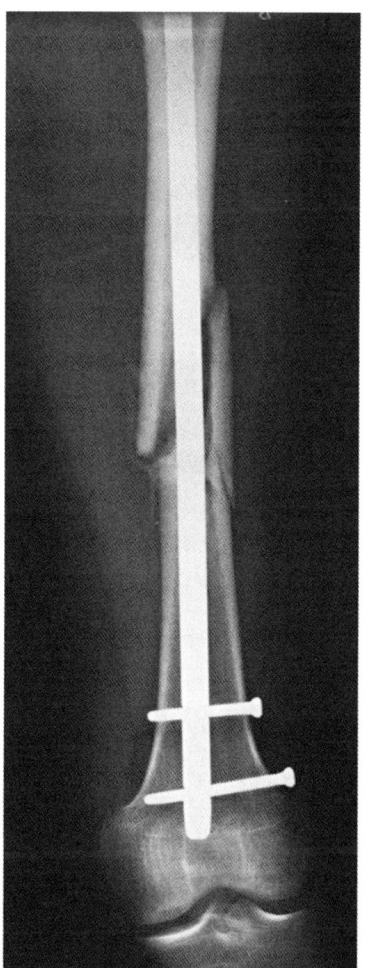

Fig. 20.20 Mobile of the AP femur showing a fracture of the midshaft with femoral rod placement. The knee joint is included on the image.

Femur

LATERAL PROJECTION[g]
Mediolateral or lateromedial projection
Dorsal decubitus position

It may not be possible to move the femur, which presents a challenge to the radiographer. The *mediolateral* projection is generally preferred because more of the proximal femur is demonstrated.

Image receptor + grid: Positioned by manufacturer or department protocol for proper anatomy display orientation.

Position of patient
- The patient is in the supine position.

Position of part
- Determine whether a mediolateral or lateromedial projection is to be performed.

  Mediolateral projection
- Visualize the optimal length of the patient's femur by placing the grid in a vertical position next to the lateral aspect of the femur.
- Place the distal edge of the grid low enough to include the patient's knee joint.
- Have the patient, if able, hold the upper corner of the grid for stabilization; otherwise, support the grid firmly in position.
- Support the unaffected leg by using the patient's support (or a trapeze bar if present) or a support block.
- Elevate the unaffected leg until the femur is nearly vertical (Fig. 20.21).

  Lateromedial projection
- Place the grid next to the medial aspect of the affected femur (between the patient's legs) and make sure that the knee joint is included (Fig. 20.22).
- Make sure that the grid is placed *perpendicular* to the epicondylar plane.

Respiration
- Suspended.

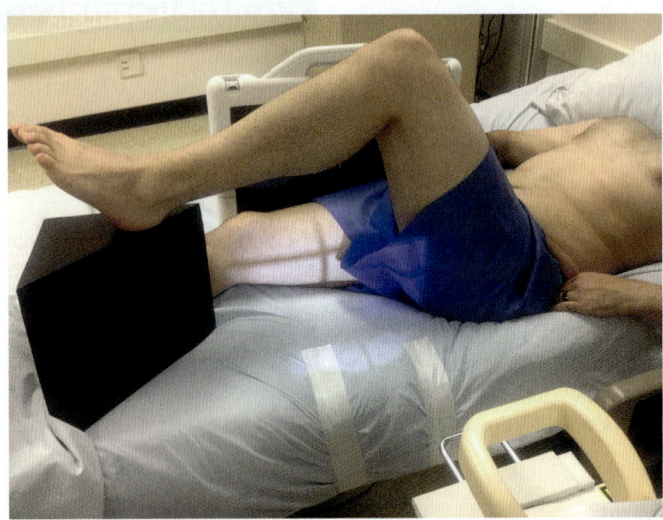

Fig. 20.21 Mobile of the mediolateral femur.

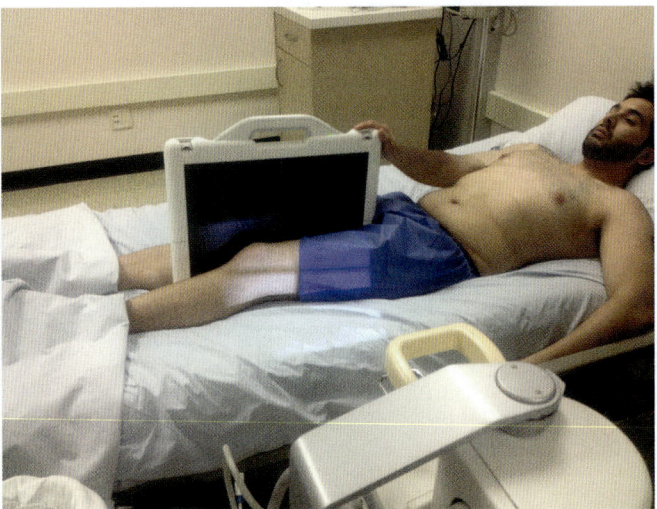

Fig. 20.22 Mobile lateromedial of the left femur. The grid is placed between the legs and steadied by the patient.

---

[g]The nonmobile projection is described in Chapter 7.

Femur

Central ray
- Perpendicular to the long axis of the femur, entering at its midpoint.
- Make sure that the central ray and grid are aligned to prevent grid cutoff; the central ray is centered to the femur and not to the center of the grid.

Collimation
- Adjust the top of the light field to the level of the ASIS to include hip joint for proximal anatomy, and the bottom of the light field at tibial tuberosity for knee joint for distal. Adjust light field to 2.5 cm (1 inch) beyond the sides of the femur shadows and 43 cm (17 inches) in length.

Structures shown
This projection shows the distal two-thirds of the femur, including the knee joint, without superimposition of the opposite thigh (Fig. 20.23).

EVALUATION CRITERIA
The optimum image obtained using correct positioning, CR-part-IR alignment, collimation, and exposure factors will demonstrate:
- The side marker placed clear of anatomy of interest
- Evidence of proper collimation
- Most of femur, including knee joint
- Patella in profile
- Superimposition of femoral condyles
- Opposite femur and soft tissue out of area of interest
- Adequate penetration of proximal portion of femur
- Orthopedic appliance (if present)

NOTE: The thickest portion of the femur (proximal area) must be measured carefully, and an appropriate kVp must be selected to penetrate this area. The computer cannot form an image of any anatomy in this area if penetration does not occur. A light area of the entire proximal femur would result. Positioning the cathode over the proximal femur would improve image quality.

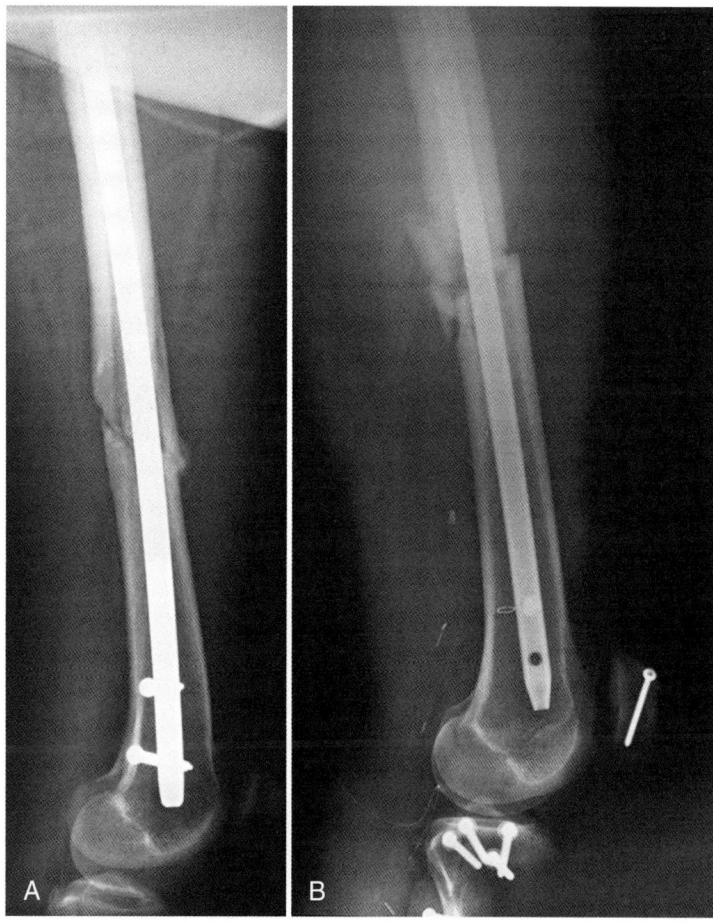

Fig. 20.23 Mobile of the lateral femur showing midshaft fractures and femoral rod placement. The knee joints are included on the image. (**A**) Mediolateral. (**B**) Lateromedial.

Cervical Spine

🔆 LATERAL PROJECTION[h]
Right or left dorsal decubitus position

Image receptor + grid: Positioned by manufacturer or department protocol for proper anatomy display orientation.

Position of patient
- Position the patient in the supine position with arms extended down along the sides of the body.
- Observe whether a cervical collar or another immobilization device is being used. *Do not remove the device without consent from the physician or authorized personnel.*

Position of part
- Ensure that the upper torso, cervical spine, and head are not rotated.
- Place the grid lengthwise on the right or left side, parallel to the neck.
- Place the top of the grid approximately 2.5 cm (1 inch) above the external acoustic meatus (EAM) so that the grid is centered to C4 (upper thyroid cartilage).
- Raise the chin slightly. If the patient has a new trauma, suspected fracture, or known fracture of the cervical region, check with the physician before elevating the chin. Improper movement of a patient's head can disrupt a fractured cervical spine.
- Immobilize the grid in a vertical position. The grid can be immobilized in multiple ways if a holding device is unavailable. Another method is to place pillows or a cushion between the side rail of the bed and the IR, holding the IR next to the patient. Tape also works well in many instances (Fig. 20.24).
- Have the patient relax the shoulders and reach for the feet if possible.

Respiration
- Full expiration to obtain maximum depression of the shoulders.

Central ray
- Horizontal and perpendicular to the center of the grid. This should place the central ray at the level of C4 (upper thyroid cartilage).
- Make sure that proper alignment of the central ray and grid is maintained in order to prevent grid cutoff.

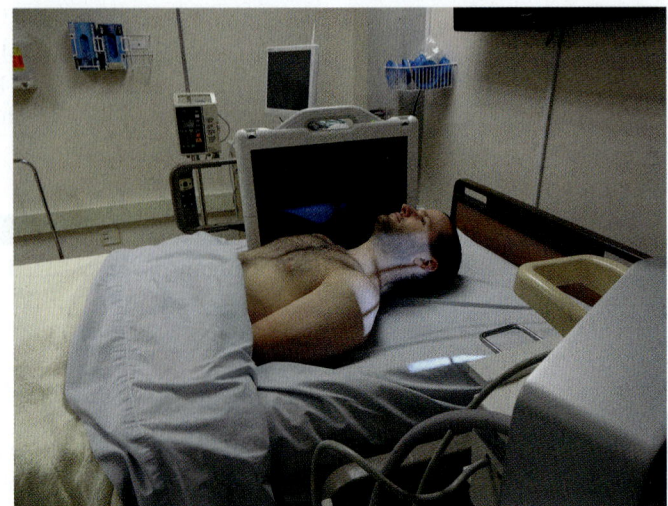

Fig. 20.24 Mobile of the lateral cervical spine.

---

[h]The nonmobile projection is described in Chapter 9.

Cervical Spine

- Because of the great object-to-image receptor distance (OID), SID of 158 to 183 cm (60–72 inches) is recommended. This also helps show C7.

Collimation
- Adjust the top of ear attachment (TEA), bottom to jugular notch, and 2.5 cm (1 inch) on the sides of the neck.

Structures shown
This projection shows the seven cervical vertebrae, including the base of the skull and the soft tissues surrounding the neck (Fig. 20.25).

EVALUATION CRITERIA

The optimum image obtained using correct positioning, CR-part-IR alignment, collimation, and exposure factors will demonstrate:
- The side marker placed clear of anatomy of interest
- Evidence of proper collimation
- All seven cervical vertebrae and at least one-third of the T1 (otherwise a separate radiograph of the cervicothoracic region is recommended)
- Neck extended when possible so that rami of mandible are not overlapping C1 or C2
- C4 in center of grid
- No rotation or tilt of the cervical spine
- Superimposed posterior margins of each vertebral body

NOTE: It is essential that C6 and C7 be included on the image. To accomplish this, the radiographer should instruct the patient to relax the shoulders toward the feet as much as possible. If the examination involves pulling down on the patient's arms, the radiographer should exercise extreme caution and evaluate the patient's condition carefully to determine whether pulling of the arms can be tolerated. Fractures or injuries of the upper limbs, including the clavicles, must be considered. Applying a strong pull to the arms of a patient in a hurried or jerking manner can disrupt a fractured cervical spine. If the lateral projection does not adequately visualize the lower cervical region, the Twining method (sometimes referred to as the "swimmer's" position), which eliminates pulling of the arms, may be recommended for patients who have experienced trauma or have a known cervical fracture. One arm must be placed above the patient's head (the Twining method is described in Chapter 9). To ensure that the lower cervical vertebrae are fully penetrated, the kVp must be set to penetrate the C7 area.

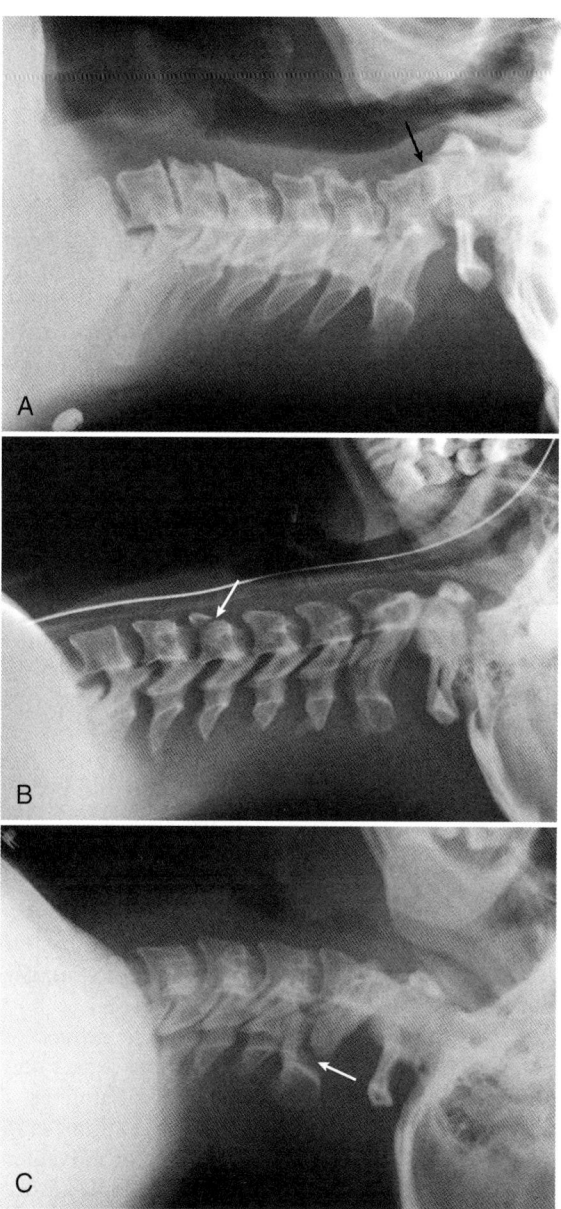

Fig. 20.25 Mobile of the lateral cervical spine obtained at the patient's bedside several weeks after trauma. (**A**) Entire cervical spine shows slight anterior subluxation of the dens on the body of C2 (arrow). (**B**) Entire cervical spine shows nearly vertical fracture through the body of C5 with slight displacement (arrow). (**C**) First five cervical vertebrae show vertical fractures through the posterior aspects of the C2 laminae (arrow) with 4-mm displacement of the fragments. Earlier radiographs showed that C6 and C7 were unaffected and did not need to be included in this follow-up radiograph.

Best Practices in Mobile Imaging

Mobile (portable) radiography enables technologists to perform standard imaging procedures in an environment outside of a dedicated radiographic exposure room. Portable radiography requires the technologist to use critical thinking skills to provide quality images. The following best practices provide some universal guidelines for performing mobile radiography.

1. *Speed:* There are many circumstances that require radiographers to produce quality images as quickly as possible. Although speed is an excellent skill set, **it is important to maintain image quality.** The quality of an image should take precedence over how quickly an exam can be performed.
2. *Knowledge:* An understanding of alternate projections to meet routine protocols while, at the same time, considering how the patient's condition might affect positioning are necessary qualities to ensure optimal production of images.
3. *Positioning accuracy:* Performing mobile radiography creates opportunities to use critical thinking skills. Tube angulation and IR placement with structures to be demonstrated must be similar to those radiographs obtained in routine exposure rooms. Most exams can be accomplished with mobile radiographic equipment while maintaining image quality in accordance with established imaging standards. Mobile radiographic images should demonstrate optimum detail of structures with only the minimum distortion of the image. The alignment of the central ray, part, and image receptor (IR) is as important with mobile radiography as it is in performing exams in departmental radiology rooms. To reduce motion, use a short exposure time to avoid blurring the image caused by involuntary patient motion.
4. *Practice standard precautions:* The risk of working in an environment where blood and body fluids are present is often a real and present danger to radiographers performing mobile radiography. The radiographer should be aware of signs posted outside the patient's room listing certain isolation attire, including gloves, mask, gown, or eye shields that the radiographer should wear to perform the radiographic procedure. Image receptors and sponges should be placed in nonporous plastic covers to prevent contamination of body fluids. Hand hygiene should be performed frequently. All equipment and accessory devices should be cleaned after each patient to ensure that everything is ready for its subsequent use.
5. *Portable placement:* Proper portable placement for different types of exams will increase exam efficiency. The technologist should plan the best maneuverability of the equipment, allowing enough room for tube adjustment. This will also help when multiple exams are ordered on the same patient.
6. *Proper body mechanics:* To improve occupational health and reduce strain on the technologist's back, technologists should adjust the height of the patient's bed or stretcher to their preferred level before placing the IR under the patient. Be mindful of the patient's equipment before and after raising and lowering the bed or stretcher. When performing a chest exam, the technologist will often lower the bed or stretcher as low as possible to maximize the recommended SID.
7. *Multiple exams:* When performing multiple exams on the same patient, the radiographer should take into consideration the order of exams to minimize movement of the patient. For example, a clavicle and shoulder exam can be performed back to back, especially with a DR mobile unit in which the IR remains under the patient between exposures. Unlike in the routine department, there is no floating table to assist with the exam.
8. *Image flow:* When there are multiple mobile exams ordered at the same time, the technologist should prioritize the level of urgency based, for example, on the patient's condition during trauma, codes, and vital signs. This also requires the technologist to develop a plan for efficiency, such as placing the requisitions in the order to be performed, either left to right or upper to lower. Remember to reduce the movement of the patient as much as possible for both patient comfort and exam efficiency.
9. *Anatomic body parts:* The technologist should remember the surface landmarks used for various radiographic procedures. For example, when performing an AP chest, 8 cm (3 inches) below the jugular notch is equivalent to the inferior angle of the scapula location at level T-7. The greater trochanters are in line with the pubic symphysis when conducting abdominal exams.
10. *Tube angles:* When performing exams that require tube angulation, the tube on a portable is highly maneuverable, and unintended double angles may result in unwanted size and shape distortions. Most mobile units have angulation scales built into the unit to help with the angulation; however, the technologist must ensure that the x-ray beam is aligned with the part to reduce distortion.
11. *Immobilization:* The radiographer must *never* remove any immobilization device without a physician's orders. The radiographer should provide proper immobilization and support to minimize patient movement. Additionally, radiographers must be cautious about moving or adjusting orthopedic devices that are attached to the patient.
12. *Equipment:* Radiology departments might have portable machines in the facility that are different models or from different manufacturers. All technologists assigned to perform mobile radiography must be proficient with various vendor types. In addition, the technologist should ensure that all the necessary positioning aids are loaded before leaving the department.
13. *Attention to detail:* Technologists should be aware of the patient's condition and continuously observe the patient during the exam. A radiographer should *never* leave a patient unattended during imaging procedures because the patient's condition could quickly change for the worse. Radiographers are also responsible for noting and reporting changes immediately to the nursing staff or attending physician.
14. *Intensive care units (ICUs):* There are numerous intensive care units, such as burn units, neuro units, pediatric units, medical units, and surgical units, to name a few. Extra precautions

are essential when performing exams in these areas. Always ask the nurse whether the patient has any medical precautions or conditions to consider before starting the exam. Many times, these patients have multiple IV lines, feeding tubes, NG tubes, cooling or heating devices, chest tubes, and wall suction. The technologist must take extreme caution when positioning these patients to avoid dislodging lifesaving devices. Extreme caution should be taken when imaging patients on extracorporeal membrane oxygenation (ECMO). Any mistakes with these patients can be fatal.

15. **Attention to department protocol and scope of practice:** Radiographers should know department protocols. The scope of practice for radiographers varies from state to state and from country to country. Radiographers should know the scope of their role when performing mobile radiographic imaging procedures. For example, a radiographer should not give a patient anything to eat or drink without first getting permission from the nursing staff or the attending physician. Many patients are fasting in case of emergency surgery.

16. **Professionalism:** Ethical conduct in all situations is a requirement for all health care professionals. All radiographers should adhere to the Code of Ethics for Radiologic Technologists (see Chapter 1) and the Radiography Practice Standards.

Reference

1. National Council on Radiation Protection. *Report 102: Medical X-Ray, Electron Beam and Gamma Ray Protection for Energies up to 50 Mev*; 1989. Bethesda, MD.

Selected bibliography

Adler AM, Carlton RR. *Introduction to Radiologic Sciences and Patient Care*. 4th ed. Philadelphia: Elsevier; 2007.

Bontrager KL. *Textbook of Radiographic Positioning and Related Anatomy*. 7th ed. St Louis: Elsevier; 2010.

Bushong SC. *Radiologic Science for Technologists*. 9th ed. St Louis: Elsevier; 2009.

Ehrlich RA, Daly JA. *Patient Care in Radiography*. 7th ed. St Louis: Elsevier; 2009.

Hall-Rollins J, Winters R. Mobile chest radiography: improving image quality. *Radiol Technol*. 2000;71(5):427–434.

Samei E, Pfeiffer DE. *Clinical Imaging Physics: Current and Emerging Practice*. Hoboken, NJ: Wiley-Blackwell; 2020.

Statkiewicz Sherer MA, Visconti PJ, Ritenour ER. *Radiation Protection in Medical Radiography*. 6th ed. St Louis: Elsevier; 2011.

Tucker DM, Souto M, Barnes GT. Scatter in computed radiography. *Radiology*. 1993;188(1):271–274.

21
SURGICAL RADIOGRAPHY
J. TYLER CARTER; GARRETT JOHNSON

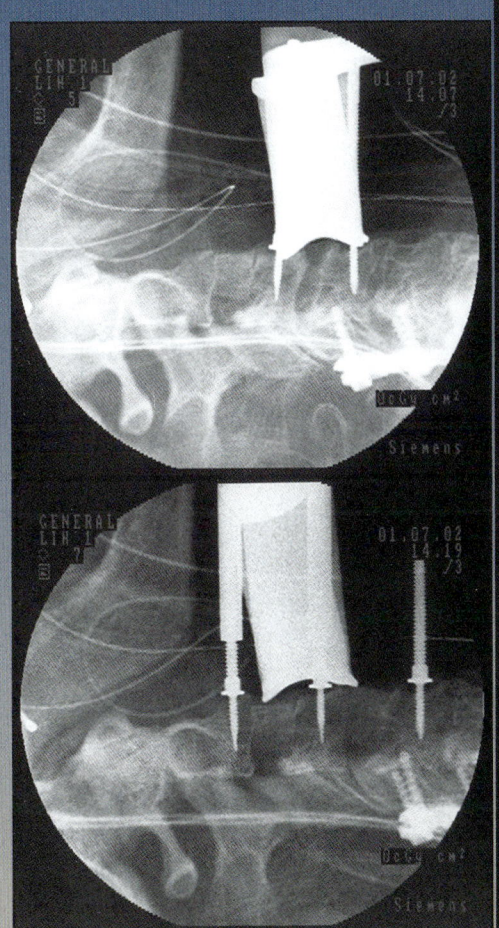
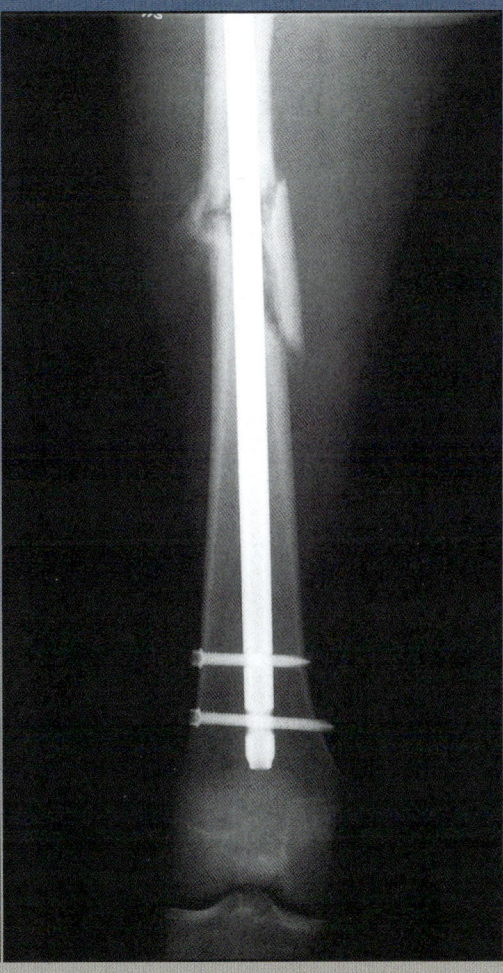

OUTLINE

Surgical Team, 30
Proper Surgical Attire, 32
Operating Room Attire, 33
Dance of the Operating Room, 34
Equipment, 37
Cleaning of Equipment, 38
Radiation Exposure
  Considerations, 39
Fluoroscopic Procedures for the
  Operating Room, 39
Mobile Radiography Procedures for
  the Operating Room, 57
O-Arm Equipment and Basics, 65
Best Practices in Surgical
  Radiography, 69
Definition of Terms, 69

Surgical radiology is a dynamic experience. The challenges that a radiographer encounters in the surgical suite are unique. Knowing the machinery and its capabilities and limitations is most important; in that regard, the radiographer can enter any operating room (OR) case, whether routine or extraordinary, and, with good communication, be able to perform all tasks well. An understanding of common procedures and familiarity with equipment enables the radiographer to perform most mobile examinations ordered by the physician. Surgical radiography can be a challenging and exciting environment for the radiographer, but can also be intimidating and stressful. Surgical radiology requires educated personnel familiar with specific equipment routinely used during common surgical procedures. Preparedness and familiarity with equipment are key. Standard health and safety protocols must be followed to avoid contamination and to ensure patient safety. These are the basics, and the pieces come together in surgical radiology in distinctive ways.

This chapter focuses on the most common procedures performed in the surgical area. The basic principles of mobile imaging are detailed, and helpful suggestions are provided for the successful completion of the examinations. This chapter is not intended to cover every possible combination of examinations or situations that a radiographer may encounter; rather, it provides an overview of the surgical setting and a summary of common examinations. The scope of radiologic examinations in a surgical setting is vast and may differ greatly among health care facilities (Box 21.1). The goals of this chapter are to (1) provide an overview of the surgical setting and explain the role of the radiographer as a vital member of the surgical team, (2) assist the radiographer in developing an understanding of the imaging equipment used in surgical situations, and (3) present common radiographic procedures performed in the OR. The radiographer should review the surgery department protocols, which vary from one institution to another.

Surgical Team

Members of the surgical team generally include a surgeon, one or two assistants, a surgical technologist, an anesthesia provider, a circulating nurse, and various support staff who surround the patient. Each member of the surgical team has a specific function to perform. The OR team has been described as a symphony orchestra. The medical staff are in unison and harmony with their colleagues for the successful accomplishment of the expected outcomes. The OR team is subdivided, according to the functions of its members, into sterile and nonsterile teams.

BOX 21.1
Scope of surgical radiography

Surgical fluoroscopic procedures
- Abdomen: cholangiogram
- Chest-line placement: bronchoscopy
- Cervical spine: anterior cervical discectomy and fusion
- Lumbar spine
- Hip: cannulated hip screws or hip pinning, decompression hip screw
- Femoral and tibial nailing
- Extremity fluoroscopy
- Humerus: shoulder in beach chair position
- Femoral/tibial arteriogram

Mobile surgical radiography procedures
- Localization examinations of cervical, thoracic, and lumbar spine
- Mobile extremity examinations in operating room

STERILE TEAM MEMBERS

Sterile team members scrub their hands and arms, don a sterile gown and gloves over proper surgical attire, and enter the sterile field. The sterile field is the area of the OR that immediately surrounds and is specially prepared for the patient. To establish a sterile field, all items necessary for the surgical procedure are sterilized. After this process, the scrubbed and sterile team members function within this limited area and only handle sterile items (Fig. 21.1). The sterile team consists of the following members:

- *Surgeon:* The surgeon is a licensed physician who is specially trained and qualified by knowledge and experience to perform surgical procedures. The surgeon's responsibilities include preoperative diagnosis and care, selection and performance of the surgical procedure, and postoperative management of care. The surgeon assumes full responsibility for all medical acts of judgment and for the management of the surgical patient.
- *Surgical assistant:* The first assistant is a qualified surgeon or resident in an accredited surgical education program. The assistant should be capable of assuming responsibility for performing the procedure for the primary surgeon. Assistants help to maintain visibility of the surgical site, control bleeding, close wounds, and apply dressings. The assistant's role varies depending on the institution and the type of procedure or surgical specialty.
- *Physician assistant:* The physician assistant is a nonphysician allied health practitioner who is qualified by academic and clinical training to perform designated procedures in the OR and in other areas of surgical patient care.
- *Scrub nurse:* The scrub nurse is a registered nurse (RN) who is specially trained to work with surgeons and the medical team in the OR.
- *Certified surgical technologist (CST):* The CST is responsible for maintaining the integrity, safety, and efficiency of the sterile field throughout the surgical procedure. The CST prepares and arranges instruments and supplies and assists the surgical procedure by providing the required sterile instruments and supplies. In some institutions, a licensed practical nurse (LPN) or RN may assume this role.

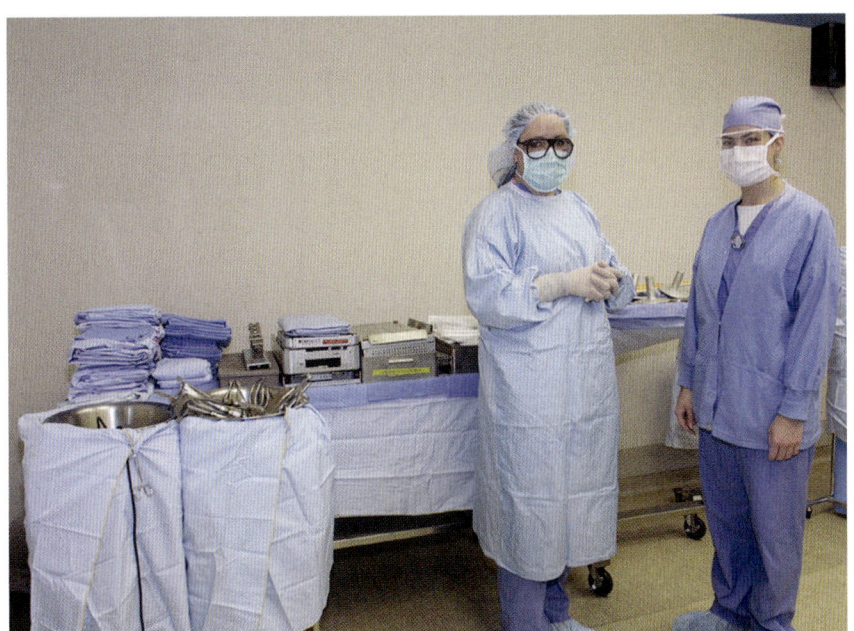

Fig. 21.1 OR staff showing sterile *(left)* and nonsterile *(right)* team members.

NONSTERILE TEAM MEMBERS

Nonsterile team members do not enter the sterile field; they function outside and around it. They assume responsibility for maintaining sterile techniques during the surgical procedure, but they handle supplies and equipment that are not considered sterile. Following the principles of aseptic technique, they keep the sterile team supplied, provide direct patient care, and respond to any requests that may arise during the surgical procedure.

- *Anesthesia provider:* The anesthesia provider is a physician (anesthesiologist) or certified RN anesthetist who specializes in administering anesthetics. Choosing and applying appropriate agents and suitable techniques of administration, monitoring physiologic functions, maintaining fluid and electrolyte balance, and performing blood replacements are essential responsibilities of the anesthesia provider during the surgical procedure.
- *Circulator:* The circulator is preferably an RN. The circulator monitors and coordinates all activities within the OR, provides supplies to the CST during the surgical procedure, and manages the care of the patient.
- *Radiographers:* The radiographer's role in the OR is to provide intraoperative imaging in a variety of examinations and with various types of equipment.
- *Others:* The OR team may also include biomedical technicians, monitoring technologists, and individuals who specialize in the equipment or monitoring devices necessary during the surgical procedure.

Proper Surgical Attire

Surgical attire protocols may change from one institution to another but should be available for review, understood, and followed by all staff members. Although small variances in protocol exist among institutions, there are common standards.

Large amounts of bacteria are present in the nose and mouth, skin, hair, and on the attire of personnel who enter the restricted areas of the surgical setting. Surgical site infections have been traced to bacteria found on surgical personnel. According to Food and Drug Administration (FDA) standards, solutions used for surgical scrub reduce microbes on the skin. In addition, wearing surgical attire limits microbial spread among the staff and patients. Proper facility design, adhering to Occupational Safety and Health Administration (OSHA) regulations, and requirements for surgical attire are important ways of preventing the transportation of microorganisms into surgical settings, where they may infect patients' open wounds.

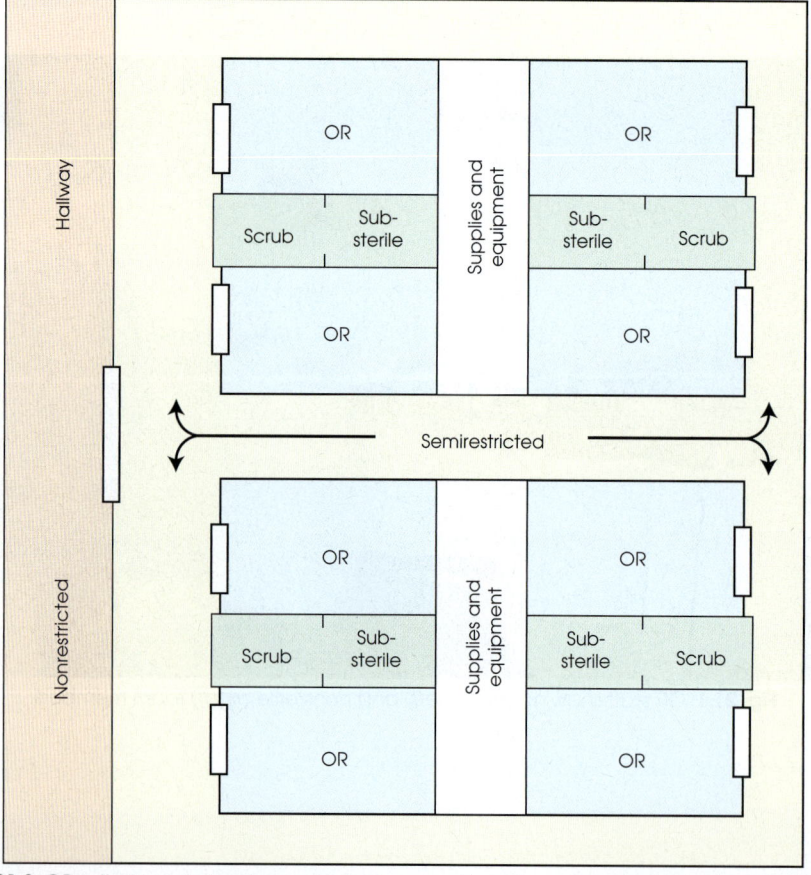

Fig. 21.2 OR suite layout showing restricted, nonrestricted, and semirestricted areas. ORs are "restricted."

Operating Room Attire

The OR should have specific written policies and procedures for proper attire to be worn within the semirestricted and restricted areas of the OR suite. The dress code should include aspects of personal hygiene important to environmental control. The protocol is strictly monitored so that everyone conforms to the established policy.

Street clothes should never be worn within semirestricted or restricted areas of the surgical suite (Fig. 21.2). Clean, fresh attire should be donned at the beginning of each shift in the OR suite and as needed if the attire becomes wet or soiled. Blood-stained or soiled attire, including shoe covers, is unattractive and can also be a source of cross-infection or contamination. Soiled attire is not worn outside of the OR suite, and steps should be taken to remove soiled clothing immediately upon exiting. OR attire should not be stored in a locker for wearing a second time. Underclothing should be clean and totally covered by the scrub suit (Fig. 21.3). Other aspects of proper attire include the following:

- *Protective eyewear:* OSHA regulations require eyewear to be worn when contamination from blood or body fluids is possible.
- *Masks:* Masks should be worn at all times in the OR but are not necessary in all semirestricted areas.
- *Shoe covers:* Shoe covers should be worn when contamination from blood or body fluids can be reasonably anticipated. Shoe covers should be changed whenever they become torn, soiled, or wet and should be removed before leaving the surgical area.
- *Caps:* Caps should be worn to cover and contain hair at all times in the restricted and semirestricted areas of the OR suite. Hoods are also available to cover hair, such as facial hair, that cannot be contained by a cap and mask.
- *Gloves:* Gloves should be worn when contact with blood or body substances is anticipated.
- *Radiation badge and identification:* A radiation badge and proper identification should be worn at all times.

PERSONAL HYGIENE

A person with an acute infection, such as a cold, open cold sore, or sore throat, is known to be a carrier of transmittable conditions and should not be permitted within the OR suite. Daily body cleanliness and clean hair are also important because good personal hygiene helps to prevent the transportation of microbial fallout that can cause open wound infections. Daily body cleanliness and clean, dandruff-free hair help prevent superficial wound infections.

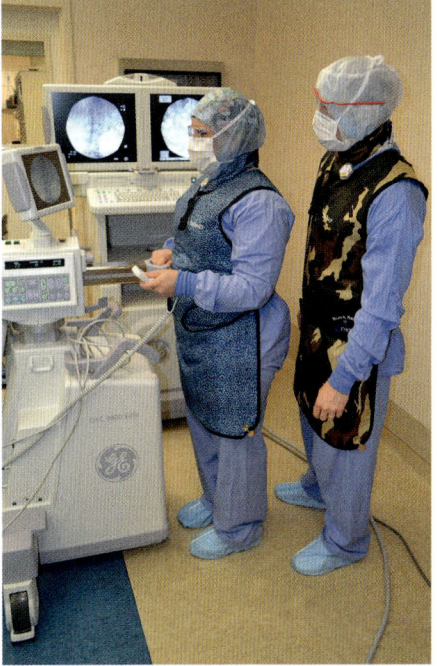

Fig. 21.3 Properly attired radiographers with protective eyewear and additional headwear to cover facial hair or long hair.

Dance of the Operating Room

The concepts of sterile and aseptic techniques date back to Hippocrates, who boiled wine and water to pour into open wounds in an attempt to prevent infection. Galen changed the technique a bit and began boiling the instruments instead, and shortly thereafter, Semmelweis noted a dramatic decline in postoperative infection by having the staff wash their hands and change gowns between surgical procedures.

Maintaining the sterile field in an OR suite can be like a well-choreographed dance when the team works well together. Certain moves and rules must be followed. Proper adherence to aseptic technique eliminates or minimizes modes and sources of contamination. Basic principles must be observed during the surgical procedure to provide the patient with a well-defined margin of safety. Everyone who cares for patients must carry out effective hospital and OR infection control programs. Infection control involves a wide variety of concepts, including methods of environmental sanitation and maintenance of facilities; cleanliness of the air and equipment in the OR suite; cleanliness of the skin and apparel of patients, surgeons, and personnel; sterility of surgical equipment; strict aseptic technique; and careful observance of procedural rules and regulations.

Up to 10,000 microbial particles can be shed from the skin per minute. Nonsterile team members should not reach over a sterile field. When working over the sterile field (e.g., performing a posteroanterior [PA] lumbar spine), the sterile field should be covered with a sterile drape to protect the field (Fig. 21.4). The technologist cannot move the radiographic equipment into position over the sterile field until after the sterile cover is in place. A sterile team member should fold over the sterile drape on itself, and then a nonsterile team member should carefully remove the covering drape, being careful not to compromise the sterile field. If a sterile field is compromised, the OR staff should be notified immediately.

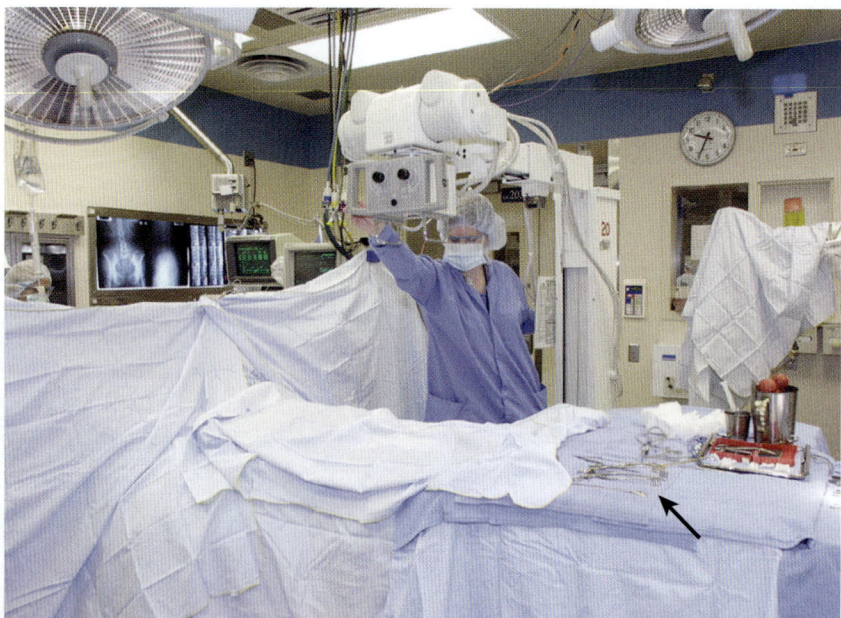

Fig. 21.4 Radiographer leaning over the sterile field while positioning the x-ray tube. The sterile incision site over which the radiographer works is properly covered to maintain a sterile field. Note the sterile instruments in the foreground (*arrow*). The radiographer should never move radiographic equipment over uncovered sterile instruments or an uncovered surgical site.

Communication is of utmost importance. As a result of the surgical sterile field, the radiographer is unable to help position the image receptor (IR) or the patient. Good professional communication is essential while using sound, basic knowledge of anatomy and positioning. The radiographer may have to instruct the surgeon or resident on the proper position to visualize the desired portion of the anatomy best.

PROPER IR HANDLING IN THE STERILE FIELD

To maintain proper universal precautions, the radiographer must follow specific steps when handling an IR in the OR.
- *Surgical technologist (CST) taking the IR:* The CST holds a sterile IR cover open toward the radiographer. The radiographer should hold one end of the IR while placing the other end of the IR into the sterile IR cover. The CST grasps the IR and wraps the protective cover securely (Fig. 21.5).

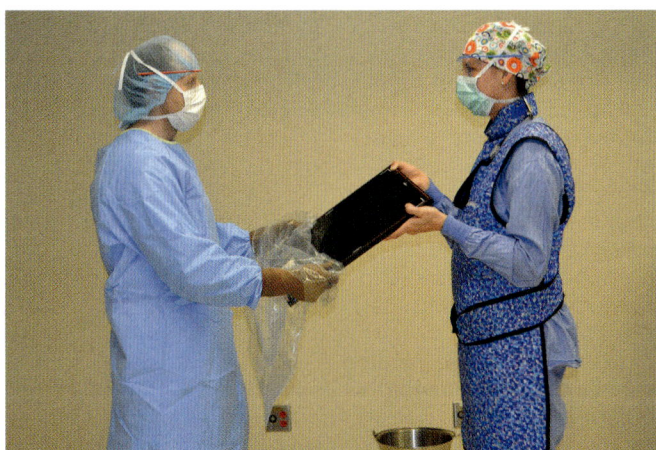

Fig. 21.5 Radiographer and CST place wireless digital radiography (DR) detector into the sterile drape.

- *Radiographer accepting the IR after exposure:* After the exposure has been made, the radiographer needs to retrieve the IR. The CST should carefully open the sterile drape, exposing the detector for the technologist to grasp (Fig. 21.6). The CST would then dispose of the drape. In the event of an urgent situation in which the CST needs to hand the IR over, the radiographer must be wearing gloves to accept a covered IR that has been in the sterile field or under an open incision. The protective cover is possibly contaminated with blood or body fluids and should be treated accordingly. The radiographer should grasp the IR, open the protective cover carefully away from himself or herself or others so as not to spread blood or body fluids, and then ask another nonsterile person to remove the IR from the cover. The radiographer should dispose of the sterile cover in a proper receptacle and remember to remove gloves before handling the IR or any other equipment because the gloves are now considered contaminated. If contamination of the IR occurs, the radiographer should use hospital-approved disinfectant for cleaning before leaving the OR (Box 21.2). Hand hygiene should be performed whenever entering or exiting the OR.

ENEMIES OF THE STERILE FIELD

Lengthy or complex procedures increase the chance of sterile field contamination. Prolonged surgical procedures increase the risk of strike-through, which refers to the penetration or perforation of a surgical drape or sterile barrier, such as a surgical gown or sterile field, by moisture or fluid. This can happen during a surgical procedure when bodily fluids, irrigation fluids, or other liquids come into contact with the sterile barrier, causing it to become compromised and potentially leading to contamination of the sterile field with bacteria and microbes.

Maintaining the integrity of the sterile field is crucial during surgery to prevent contamination and reduce the risk of surgical site infections. Surgeons and the surgical team must be vigilant in identifying and addressing any strike-through events promptly to maintain the sterility of the surgical environment. If a strike-through occurs, the affected barrier or drape should be replaced to maintain a sterile field and ensure patient safety.

Physical limitations, such as crowding, poor lighting, and under staffing, are also a consideration. The floor is always considered contaminated. The radiographer should not place IRs, lead aprons, and shields on the floor.

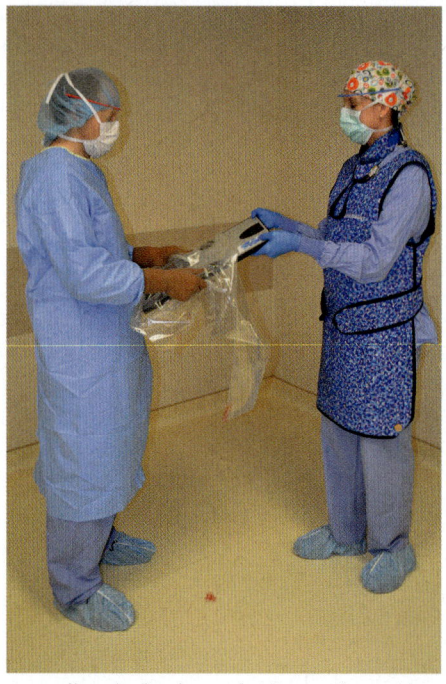

Fig. 21.6 CST correctly opens the sterile drape for the radiographer to remove the IR from the now-contaminated bag, being careful not to brush contaminants from bag onto self or others.

BOX 21.2

Principles of aseptic techniques

- Only sterile items are used within the sterile field.
- Only sterile persons handle sterile items or touch sterile areas.
- Nonsterile persons touch only nonsterile items or areas.
- Movement within or around a sterile field must not contaminate the sterile field.
- Items of doubtful sterility must be considered nonsterile.
- When a sterile barrier is permeated, it must be considered contaminated.
- Sterile gowns are considered sterile in front from the shoulder to the level of the sterile field and at the sleeves from the elbow to the cuff.
- Tables are sterile only at table level.
- Radiographers should not walk between two sterile fields if possible.
- Radiographers should avoid turning their backs toward the sterile field in compromised spaces. The radiographer should watch the front of clothing when it is necessary to be next to the patient.
- The radiographer must be aware of machinery close to the sterile field, including lead aprons hanging from the portable machine that may swing toward the sterile field.
- The lead apron needs to be secured if it is being worn next to the sterile field. The apron can easily slip forward when raising one's arms up to position the tube. A properly worn apron does not compromise the sterile field or jeopardize proper body mechanics.
- When positioning an IR under the OR table, the radiographer should not lift the sterile drapes above table level because this would compromise the sterile field.

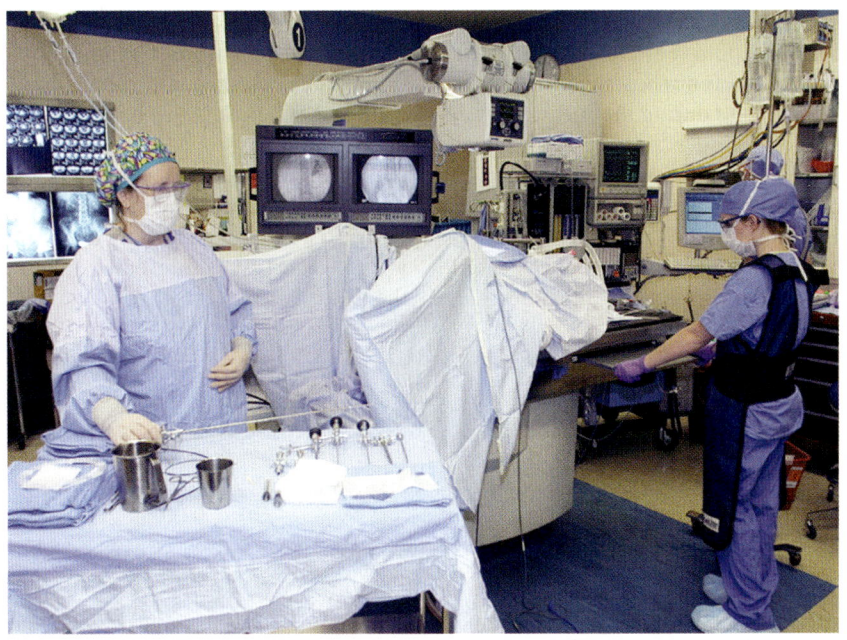

Fig. 21.7 In-room urologic radiographic equipment used for retrograde ureterograms.

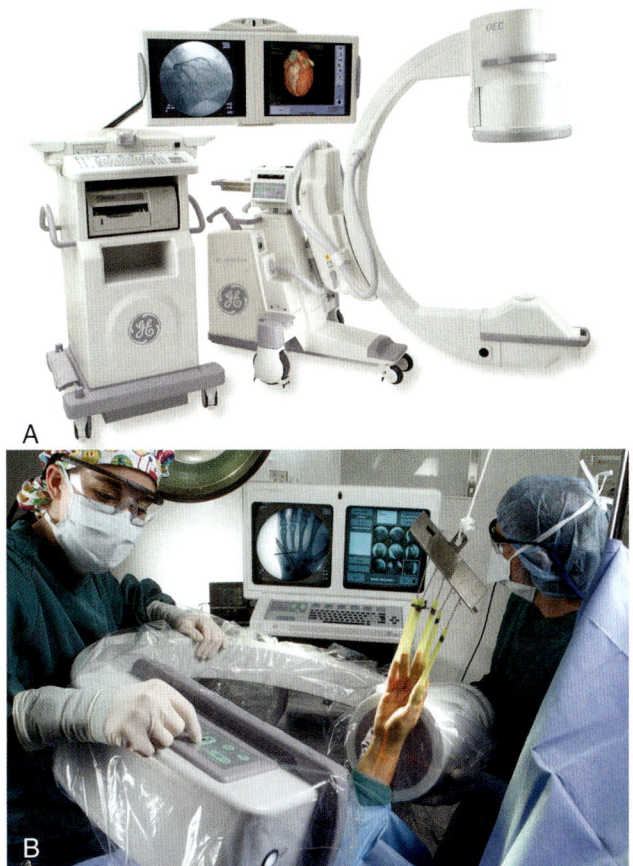

Fig. 21.8 (**A**) C-arm radiographic/fluoroscopic system used in the OR. (**B**) Mini-mobile C-arm used for extremity examinations in the OR.

Equipment

The radiographer must be well acquainted with the radiologic equipment. Some procedures may seldom occur. The radiographer should not fear a rare procedure if good communication and equipment knowledge are in place. IR holders enable the radiographer to perform cross-table projections on numerous cases and eliminate the unnecessary exposure of personnel who may volunteer to hold the IR. In mobile radiography, exposure times may increase for larger patients, and a holder eliminates the chance of motion from handheld situations.

Some OR suites, such as those used for stereotactic or urologic cases, have dedicated radiologic equipment (Fig. 21.7). Most radiographic examinations in the OR are performed with mobile equipment, however.

Mobile image machines are not as sophisticated as larger stationary machines in the radiology department. Mobile fluoroscopic units, often referred to as *C-arms* because of their shape (Fig. 21.8), are commonplace in the surgical suite. Mobile radiography is also widely used in the OR.

Good communication is imperative when providing safe and efficient imaging during a surgical case. It is important to establish a common language of terms between the surgeon and the technologist for C-arm operation (Fig. 21.9).

Cleaning of Equipment

The x-ray equipment should be cleaned after each surgical case. If possible, the radiographer should clean the mobile image machine, including the base, in the OR suite, especially when the equipment is obviously contaminated with blood or surgical scrub solution. Cleaning within the OR helps reduce the possibility of cross-contamination. The x-ray equipment must be cleaned with a hospital-approved cleaning solution. Cleaning solutions should not be sprayed in the OR suite during the surgical procedure. If cleaning is necessary during the surgical procedure, opening the cleaning container and pouring the solution on a rag for use prevents possible contamination from scattered spray. Gloves should always be worn during cleaning. The underside of the image machine should be checked to ensure contaminants that might have splashed up from the floor are removed. Cleaning the equipment after an isolation case is necessary to prevent the spread of contaminants. All equipment that is less frequently used should undergo a thorough cleaning at least once a week and just before being taken into the OR.

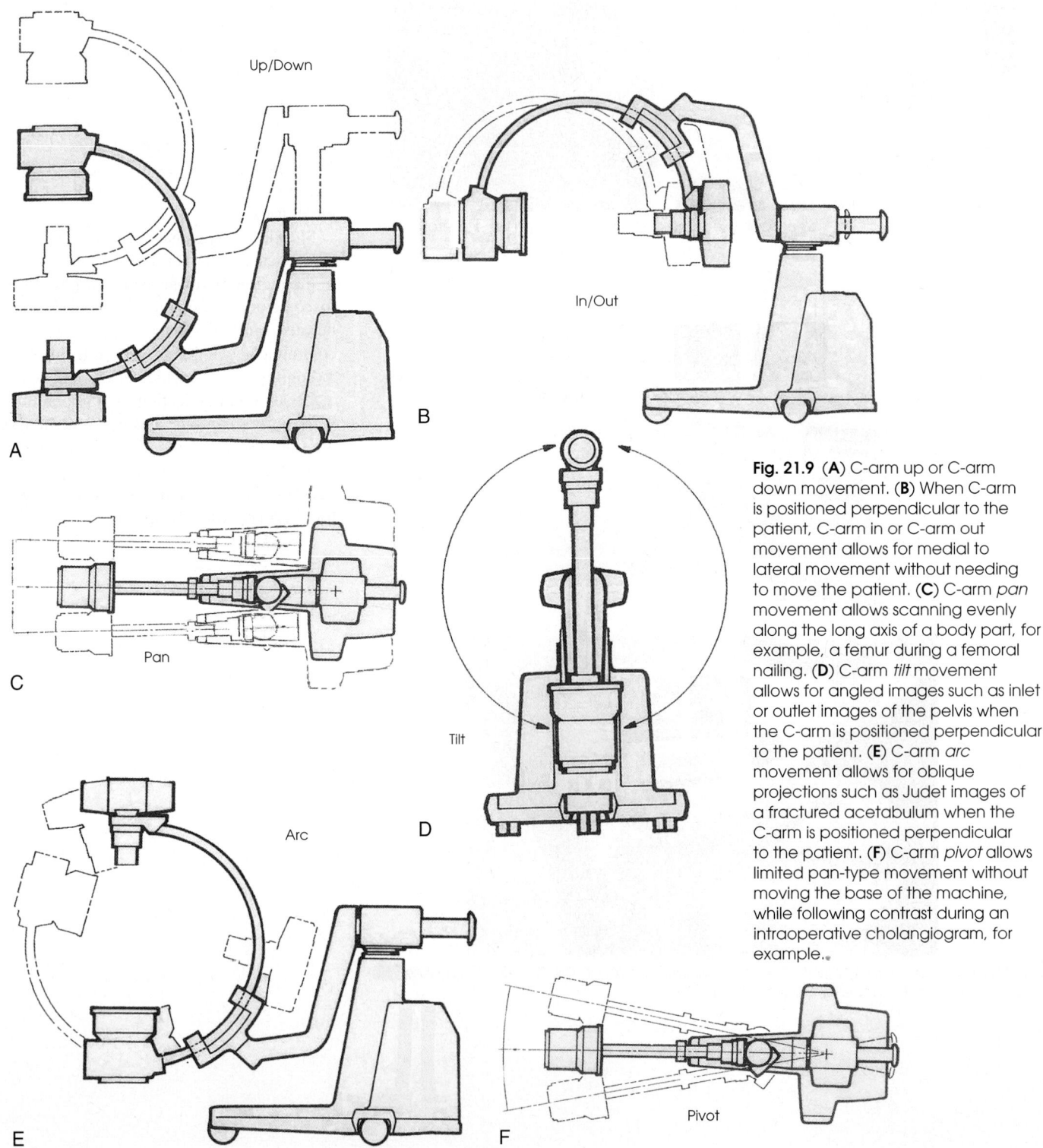

Fig. 21.9 (**A**) C-arm up or C-arm down movement. (**B**) When C-arm is positioned perpendicular to the patient, C-arm in or C-arm out movement allows for medial to lateral movement without needing to move the patient. (**C**) C-arm *pan* movement allows scanning evenly along the long axis of a body part, for example, a femur during a femoral nailing. (**D**) C-arm *tilt* movement allows for angled images such as inlet or outlet images of the pelvis when the C-arm is positioned perpendicular to the patient. (**E**) C-arm *arc* movement allows for oblique projections such as Judet images of a fractured acetabulum when the C-arm is positioned perpendicular to the patient. (**F**) C-arm *pivot* allows limited pan-type movement without moving the base of the machine, while following contrast during an intraoperative cholangiogram, for example.

Radiation Exposure Considerations

Radiation protection for the radiographer, others in the immediate area, and the patient is of paramount importance when mobile fluoroscopic examinations are performed. The radiographer should wear a lead, or lead equivalent, apron and stand as far away from the patient, x-ray tube, and useful beam as the procedure, OR, and exposure cable allow. The most effective means of radiation protection is *distance*. The recommended *minimal* distance is 2 m (6 feet). When possible, the radiographer should stand at a right angle (90 degrees) to the primary beam and the object being radiographed. The least amount of scatter radiation occurs at this position. The greatest amount of scatter radiation occurs on the tube side of the fluoroscopic machine. It is recommended that the x-ray tube should always be placed *under the patient* (Fig. 21.10). Because of the significant amount of exposure to the facial and neck region, the x-ray tube should never be placed above the patient unless absolutely necessary.

The OR may have signs posted outside the room warning of radiation in use or "lead aprons required when entering this room." Lead or lead equivalent protection should be provided for individuals who are unable to leave the room. In addition, the source-to-skin distance (SSD) should not be less than 30 cm (12 inches) when imaging the patient.

Fluoroscopic Procedures for the Operating Room

OPERATIVE (IMMEDIATE) CHOLANGIOGRAPHY

Operative cholangiography, introduced by Mirizzi in 1932, is performed during biliary tract surgery. After the bile has been drained from the ducts, and in the absence of obstruction, this technique permits the major intrahepatic ducts and the extrahepatic ducts to be filled with contrast medium.

The value of operative cholangiography is such that it has become an integral part of biliary tract surgery. It is used to investigate the patency of the bile ducts and the functional status of the sphincter of the hepatopancreatic ampulla to reveal the presence of calculi that cannot be detected by palpation. Intraoperative cholangiography can also show such conditions as small intraluminal neoplasms and stricture or dilation of the ducts. When the pancreatic duct shares a common channel with the distal common bile duct before emptying into the duodenum, it is sometimes seen on operative cholangiograms because it has been partially filled by reflux.

After exposing, draining, and exploring the biliary tract, and frequently after excising the gallbladder, the surgeon injects the contrast medium. This solution is usually introduced into the common bile duct through a needle, small catheter, or (after cholecystectomy) an inlaying T-tube. When the latter route is used, the procedure is referred to as *delayed operative* or *operative T-tube cholangiography*.

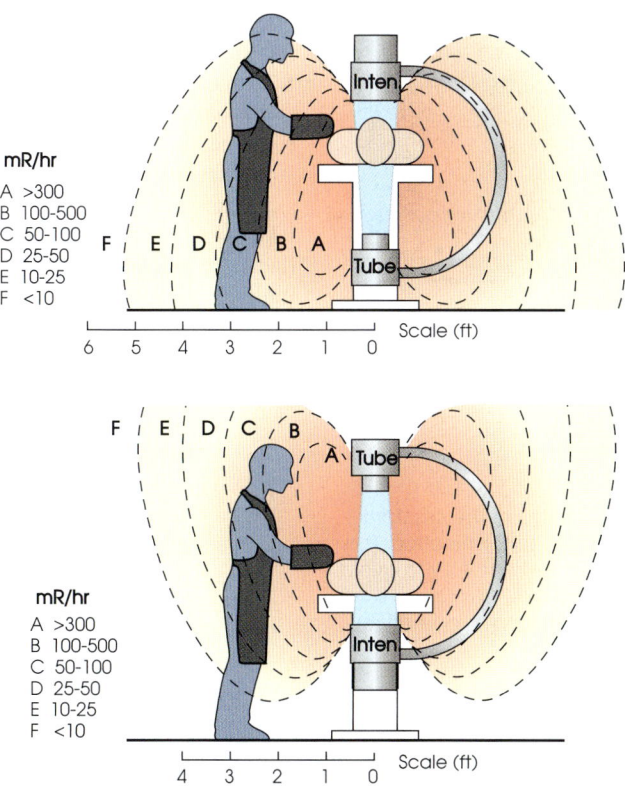

Fig. 21.10 Radiation safety with C-arm. In the *upper image*, less radiation reaches the facial and neck region when the x-ray tube is under the patient. This is the recommended position of the C-arm. In the *lower image*, there is a greater amount of radiation reaching the facial and neck regions.

(From Giese RA, Hunter DW. Personnel exposure during fluoroscopy. *Postgrad Radiol*. 1988;8:162–173.)

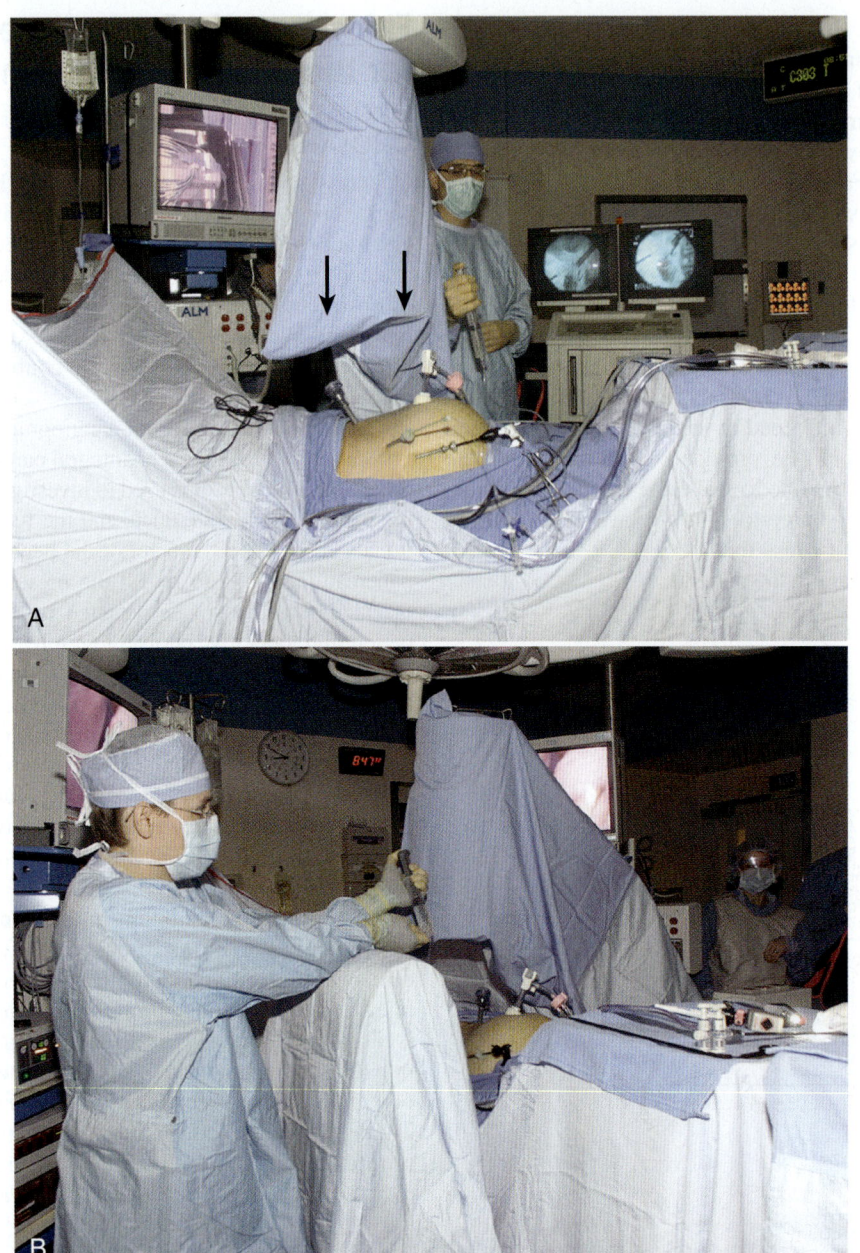

Position of patient

The patient is supine with the abdomen exposed. In laparoscopic cases, such as cholecystectomy, the abdomen is distended because air is injected into the abdominal cavity to allow adequate room for maneuvering of the camera and instruments. The radiographer should ensure that no obstacles would impede the movement of the C-arm (Fig. 21.11).

Position of C-arm

Center the C-arm in the PA projection over the right side of the abdomen below the rib line to the region of interest (ROI). The patient may be tilted to the left or in the Trendelenburg position to aid in the flow of contrast medium to the complete biliary system. The C-arm should be tilted or canted until the PA projection is achieved. The C-arm may also have to be rotated to ensure that the spine does not obscure the biliary system. When the position is obtained, the surgeon injects contrast medium into the duct system under fluoroscopy. The radiographer should do the following:

- Provide radiation protection for all persons in the room.
- Remember that examination is optimal with suspended respiration.

Because of the length of time it may take for the contrast medium to fill all ducts, respiration may be suspended at intervals throughout the examination.

Fig. 21.11 (**A**) C-arm in correct position for an abdominal cholangiogram. The assistant surgeon checks syringe for air bubbles before handing it to the surgeon for injection. The radiographer has positioned the fluoroscopic image intensifier *(arrows)* carefully to avoid hitting laparoscopic instruments protruding from the patient's abdomen. (**B**) Surgeon, standing behind a sterile draped lead shield, injecting contrast media for an operative cholangiogram.

Structures shown

This examination shows the biliary system full of contrast medium, including a portion of the cystic duct, the branches of the hepatic duct, the common bile duct, and often the pancreatic duct.

EVALUATION CRITERIA

The optimum image obtained using correct positioning, image intensifier-ROI-tube alignment, collimation, and exposure factors will demonstrate:

- Biliary system completely filled with contrast medium (Fig. 21.12)
- No extravasation of contrast medium at the injection site
- Biliary system unobscured by any extraneous anatomy or instrumentation
- Prompt emptying of contrast medium into the duodenum
- Proper radiographic technique maintained
- Sterile field maintained

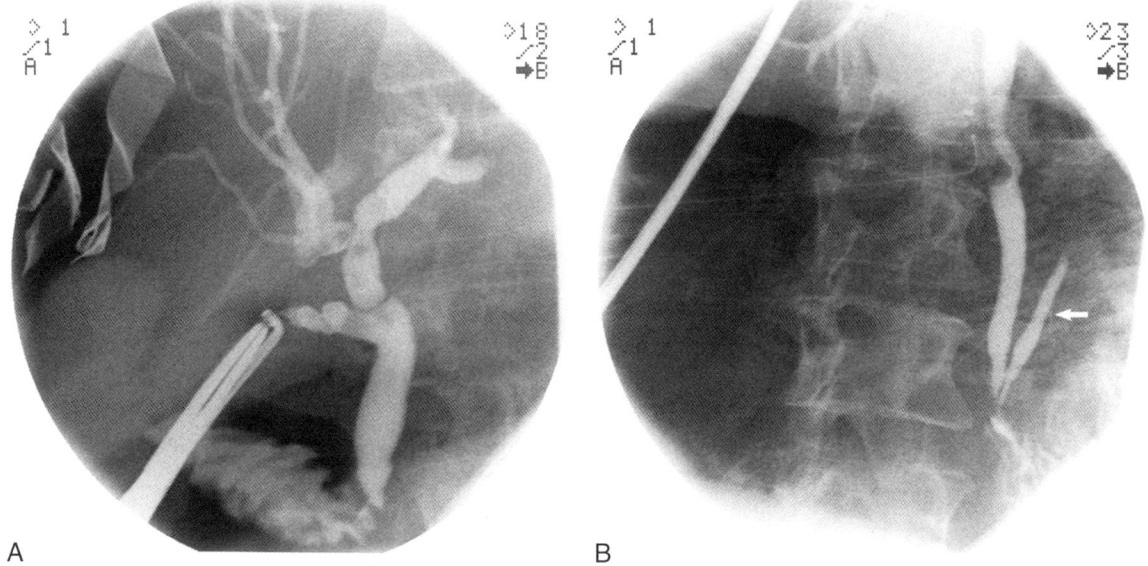

Fig. 21.12 Images of anatomy visualized during a cholangiogram using fluoroscopy. (**A**) Intraoperative cholangiogram. (**B**) Intraoperative cholangiogram showing pancreatic duct *(arrow)*.

Surgical Radiography

CHEST (LINE PLACEMENT, BRONCHOSCOPY)

Position of patient
The patient is supine with the arms secured on each side. The radiographer should ensure there are no bars or supports in the table that would obscure the view of the chest. Allow room under the table for the C-arm to maneuver.

Position of C-arm
The C-arm should be covered with a sterile drape before entering the field. The C-arm enters the sterile field perpendicular to the patient and in position for a PA projection. If the surgeon prefers, the radiographer can reverse or invert the image to obtain anatomic position. Radiation protection should be provided for all persons in the room.

- *Line placement:* Find the point of insertion and follow the catheter to its end (Fig. 21.13). This examination is done to ensure that there are no kinks in the catheter and to show that it is in proper position. Numerous catheters may be used in the OR. They are usually inserted to deliver medicines to chronically ill patients.
- *Rigid and flexible bronchoscopy:* Bronchoscopy may be done to perform biopsies, place stents, or dilate the bronchi.

Structures shown
Structures shown include all anatomy of the chest cavity, including the heart, lung fields, and ribs, and any instrumentation that may be introduced during the procedure. These instruments may include catheters, guidewires, bronchoscopes, stent devices, dilation balloons, or biopsy instruments.

EVALUATION CRITERIA

The optimum image obtained using correct positioning, image intensifier-ROI-tube alignment, collimation, and exposure factors will demonstrate:

- Pertinent parts of the chest that are easily distinguished
- Proper radiographic technique and contrast maintained on the monitor
- Image on the monitor in true anatomic position or per the physician's preference
- Sterile technique maintained

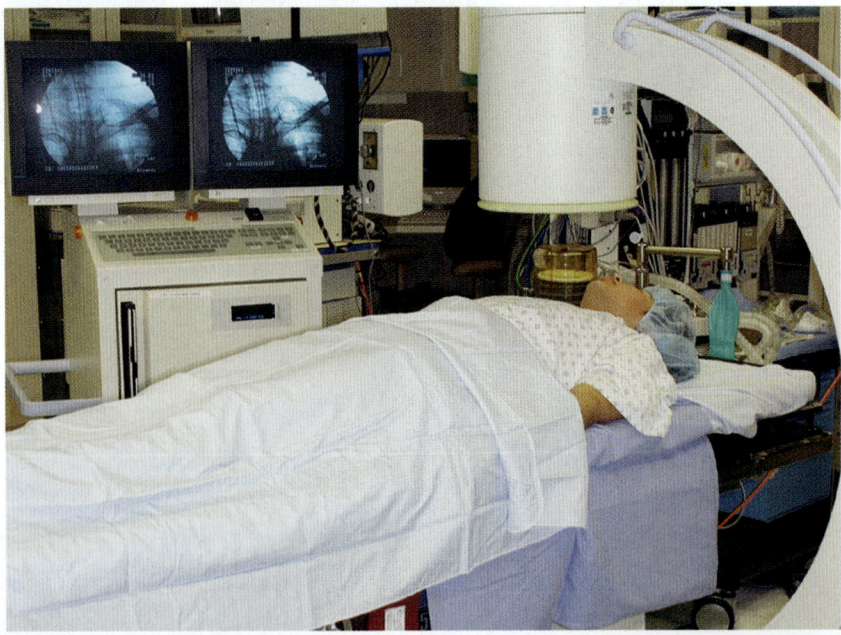

Fig. 21.13 Patient and C-arm in position for Hickman catheter placement. Introduction of catheter begins in the upper thorax and is completed with the catheter in the heart.

CERVICAL SPINE (ANTERIOR CERVICAL DISKECTOMY AND FUSION)

Position of patient
The patient is supine with the chin elevated and the neck in flexion. The patient's arms are at each side.

Position of C-arm
PA projection. Cover the C-arm with sterile drape. Enter the sterile field perpendicular to the patient. Tilt the C-arm 15 degrees cephalad and center the beam over the cervical spine. Raise the C-arm to allow the surgeon to work if necessary. Ensure that the spine is in the center of the monitor and that the top of the spine and the skull are at the top of the screen with no rotation.

Lateral projection. Rotate the C-arm under the table into lateral position with the beam parallel to the floor. Angle the C-arm either cephalad or caudal to obtain a true lateral view. Raise or lower the C-arm to bring the spine into the center of the field of view. Rotate the image on the monitor to the same plane as the patient with the spine parallel with the floor. Cases in which a PA projection is unnecessary may opt to have the C-arm positioned in "rainbow" fashion or arched over the patient (Fig. 21.14).

- Ensure that there are no obstacles under the table that impede movement of the C-arm.
- The C-arm is often positioned before the patient is draped. In this case, the surgical team drapes the C-arm into the sterile field. Ensure that the C-arm can be moved out of the way without disturbing any instrumentation.

Structures shown
These positions show the affected area of the cervical spine and any hardware that may be introduced (Fig. 21.15). Because this surgery is most often performed to repair physiologic defects, abnormalities (e.g., osteophytes, degenerated disk spaces, subluxation) may be visible, especially in the lateral view.

EVALUATION CRITERIA
The optimum image obtained using correct positioning, image intensifier-ROI-tube alignment, collimation, and exposure factors will demonstrate:
- Cervical spine and its affected part in the center of the monitor to maintain proper radiographic technique
- Image rotated in the same plane as the patient
- PA projection showing spinous processes in the center of spinous bodies
- Lateral projection showing the bodies in profile and the interarticular facets aligned
- Sterile field maintained

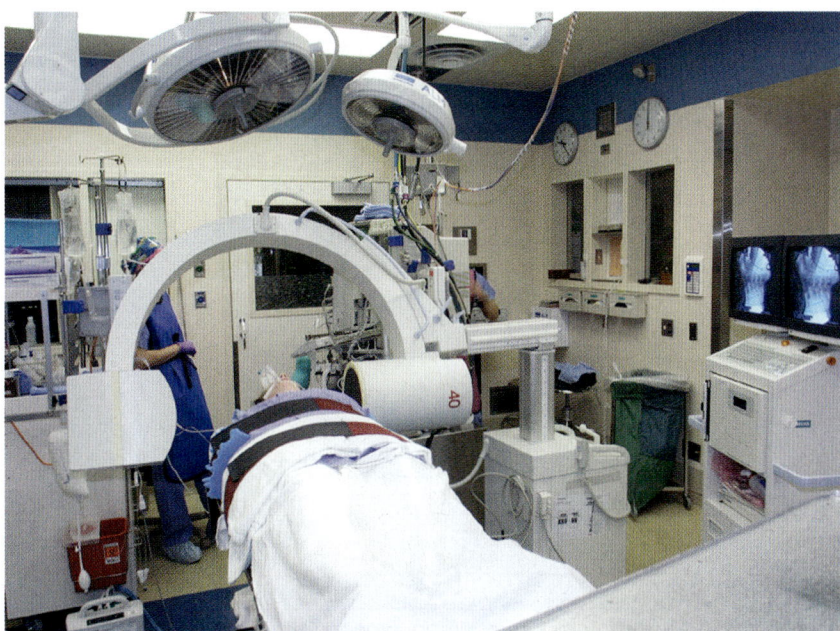

Fig. 21.14 C-arm placed in rainbow position for cervical procedures.

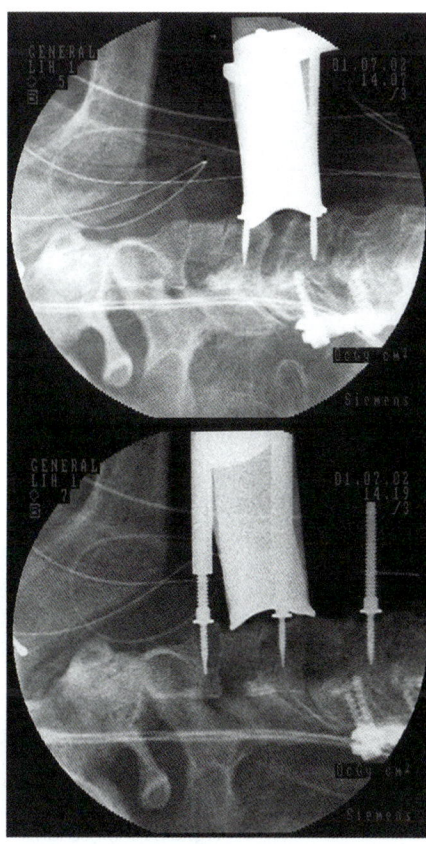

Fig. 21.15 Fluoroscopic image of cervical spine in lateral projection showing plate and screws used to fuse vertebrae.

LUMBAR SPINE

Position of patient

The patient is prone and positioned on chest rolls or a frame to flex the spine. The patient's arms are placed on arm boards and located by the head of the table to bring them out of the field of view.

Position of C-arm

AP projection. Cover the C-arm with a sterile drape. The C-arm enters the field perpendicular to the patient. Center the beam in the AP projection over the affected area of the spine. Raise the C-arm to leave enough room between the IR and the patient so that the surgeon can work without being obstructed (Fig. 21.16). Ensure that there is nothing in or under the table to impair the view of the spine.

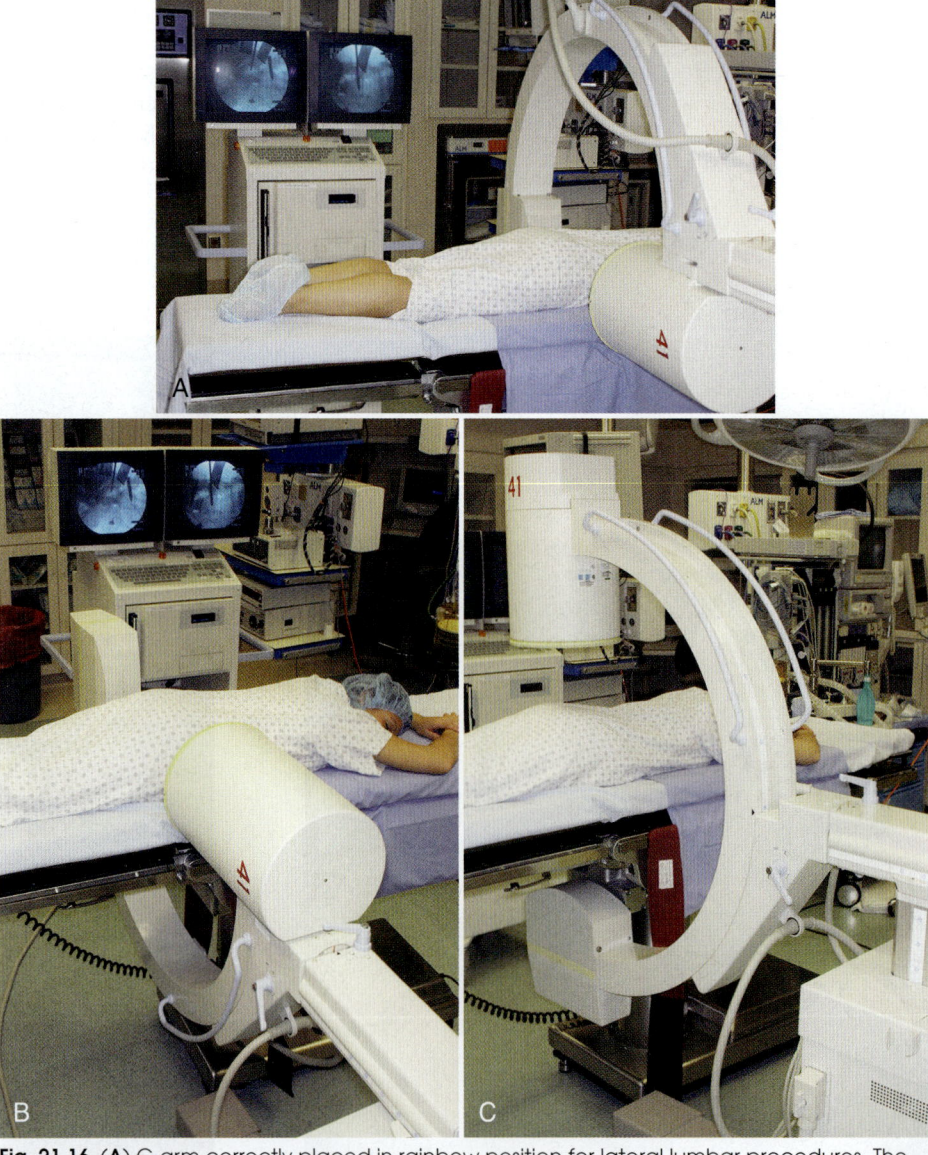

Fig. 21.16 (**A**) C-arm correctly placed in rainbow position for lateral lumbar procedures. The rainbow position is used especially for larger patients in cases in which the table size or size of the patient would not allow enough elevation of the C-arm to include the lumbar spine. (**B**) C-arm positioned under the table. (**C**) C-arm positioned for AP projection of lumbar spine.

Lateral projection

- Rotate the C-arm under the table into lateral position. Raise or lower the C-arm to bring the spine into the center of the monitor. The C-arm may need to be angled cephalad or caudal to obtain true lateral projection. Rotate the image on the monitor until the image is in same plane as the patient. The C-arm may be arched over the patient for the lateral projection, especially on hypersthenic patients, because rotating the C-arm under the table would not allow a great enough height to visualize the lumbar region.
- The surgical team members place sterile drapes over both ends of the C-arm when they drape the patient.

Structures shown

These projections show the affected area of the spine, which includes the bodies, disk spaces, spinous processes, lamina, pedicles, and facets. When the case is completed, there is hardware in the spine, such as rods, plates, and screws, to hold the spine in alignment. A bone graft or interbody fusion device may also exist in the disk space to fuse the bones together (Fig. 21.17).

EVALUATION CRITERIA

The optimum image obtained using correct positioning, image intensifier-ROI-tube alignment, collimation, and exposure factors will demonstrate:

- The affected area of the spine viewed in its entirety (Fig. 21.18)
- Spine image not rotated or angled on the monitor, showing true AP and lateral projections
- Radiographic technique maintained by properly centering the beam over the affected area
- Image of the spine, whether AP or lateral, rotated into the same plane as the patient; AP projection of the spine is in vertical axis, and lateral view of the spine is in horizontal axis
- Sterile field maintained
- Radiation protection provided for the surgical team

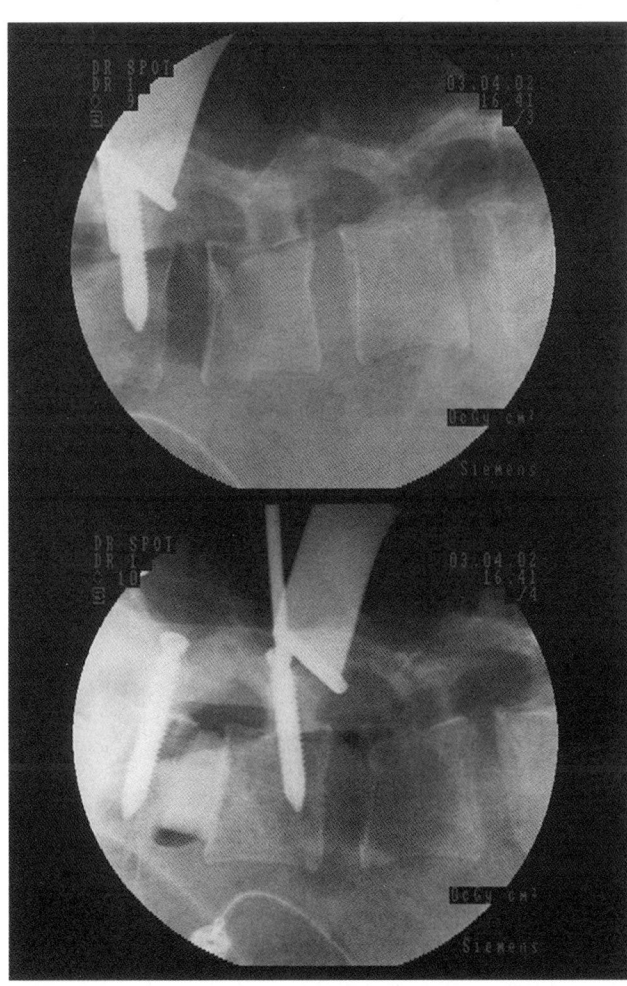

Fig. 21.17 Fluoroscopic lateral projection image of lumbar spine with instrumentation.

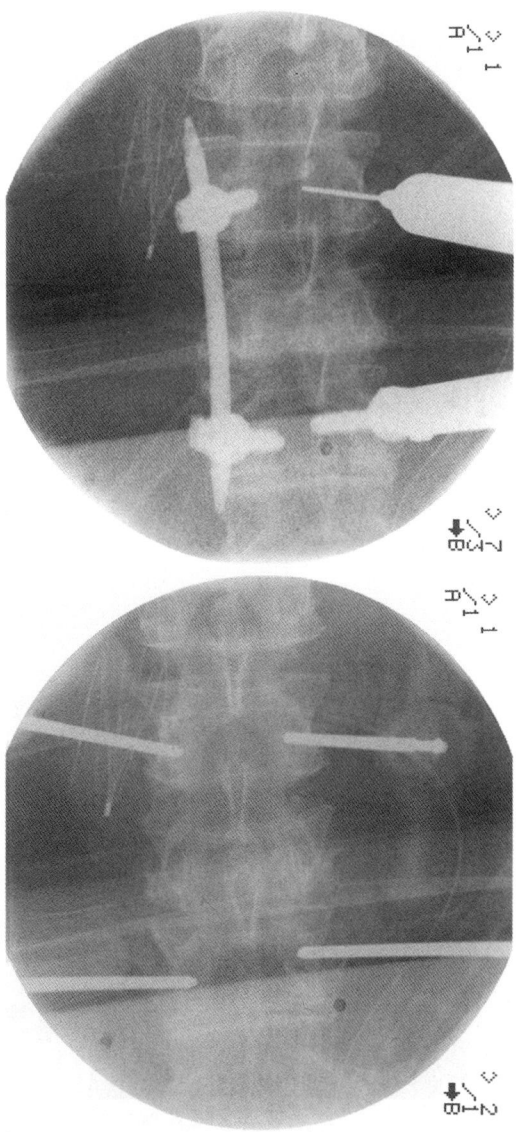

Fig. 21.18 AP projection fluoroscopic images during laparoscopic lumbar fusion.

HIP (CANNULATED HIP SCREWS OR HIP PINNING)

Position of patient
The patient is supine with the legs abducted and the affected leg held in traction. The patient's arm on the affected side is crossed over the body to be kept out of the field of view.
- These procedures are often done using an isolation drape or "shower curtain." In these cases, it is not necessary to cover the C-arm with a sterile drape; however, a nonsterile bag over the tube is recommended to prevent povidone-iodine (Betadine) staining of the C-arm.

Position of C-arm
Position the C-arm between the patient's legs, and center the beam over the affected hip (Fig. 21.19). To obtain the lateral projection, rotate the C-arm under the leg and table to a lateral position (Fig. 21.20). Do not dislodge any instrumentation when rotating the C-arm.
- Before the procedure, the surgeon manipulates the leg under fluoroscopy to reduce the fracture (Fig. 21.21).
- The C-arm may have to be manipulated to achieve projections and may not be in true PA or lateral projection. Note the position of the C-arm on PA and lateral projections to return to this angle when necessary.
- When hardware is in the hip, rotate the C-arm under fluoroscopy to ensure that no hardware is in the hip joint space.

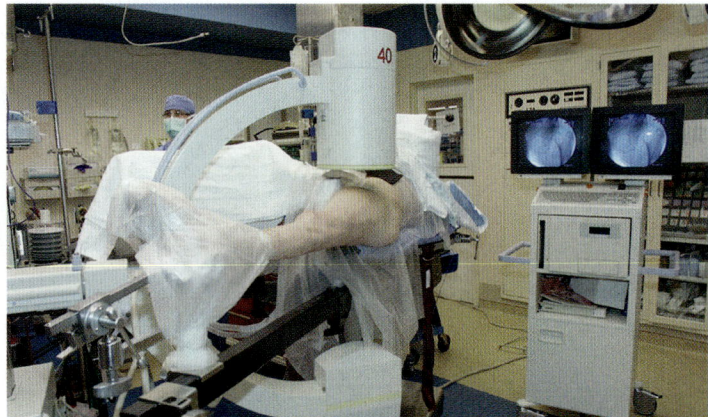

Fig. 21.19 C-arm positioned for PA projection of the hip.

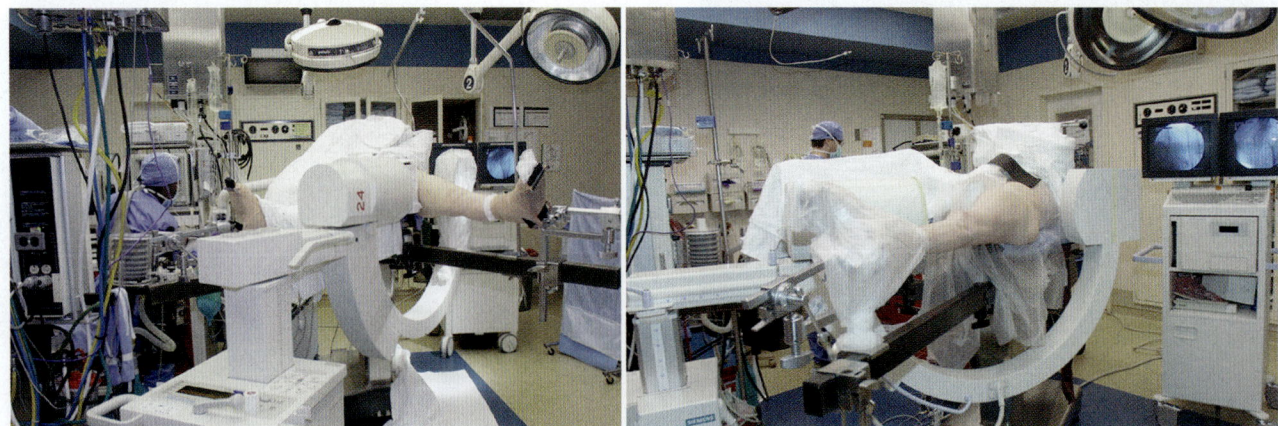

Fig. 21.20 C-arm properly positioned for lateral projection of the hip. After preliminary images are obtained, the hip is prepared for incision, and the C-arm is sterile draped.

Structures shown

This examination shows all parts of the proximal femur and hip joint, including the acetabular rim, femoral head and neck, and greater and lesser trochanters. Hardware may include cannulated screws or pins running parallel with the femoral neck used to reduce the fracture (Fig. 21.22).

EVALUATION CRITERIA

The optimum image obtained using correct positioning, image intensifier-ROI-tube alignment, collimation, and exposure factors will demonstrate:
- Hip centered on the monitor and in the correct plane
- Lateral side of femur and acetabular rim visualized to determine a starting point and to ensure that no hardware enters the joint
- The lesser trochanter visible in profile on the PA projection; the greater trochanter lies behind the femoral neck and shaft in the lateral view
- Proper radiographic technique maintained
- Sterile field maintained
- Radiation protection provided for the surgical team

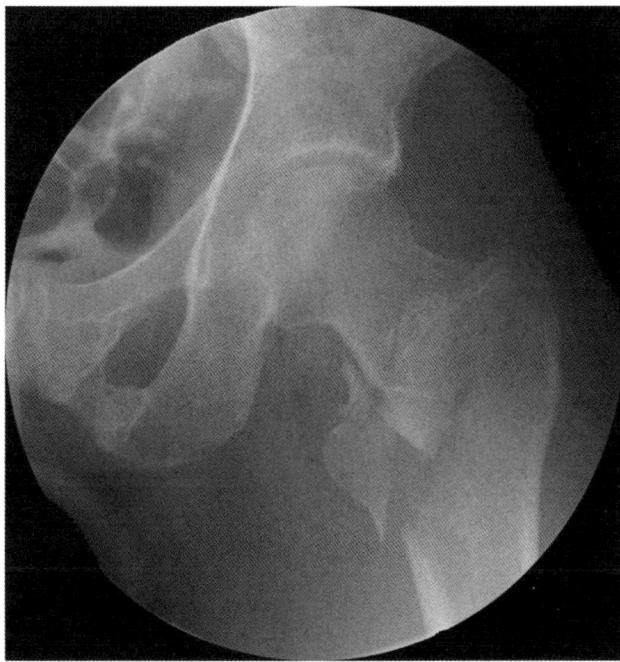

Fig. 21.21 PA projection of the hip with fracture of femoral neck.

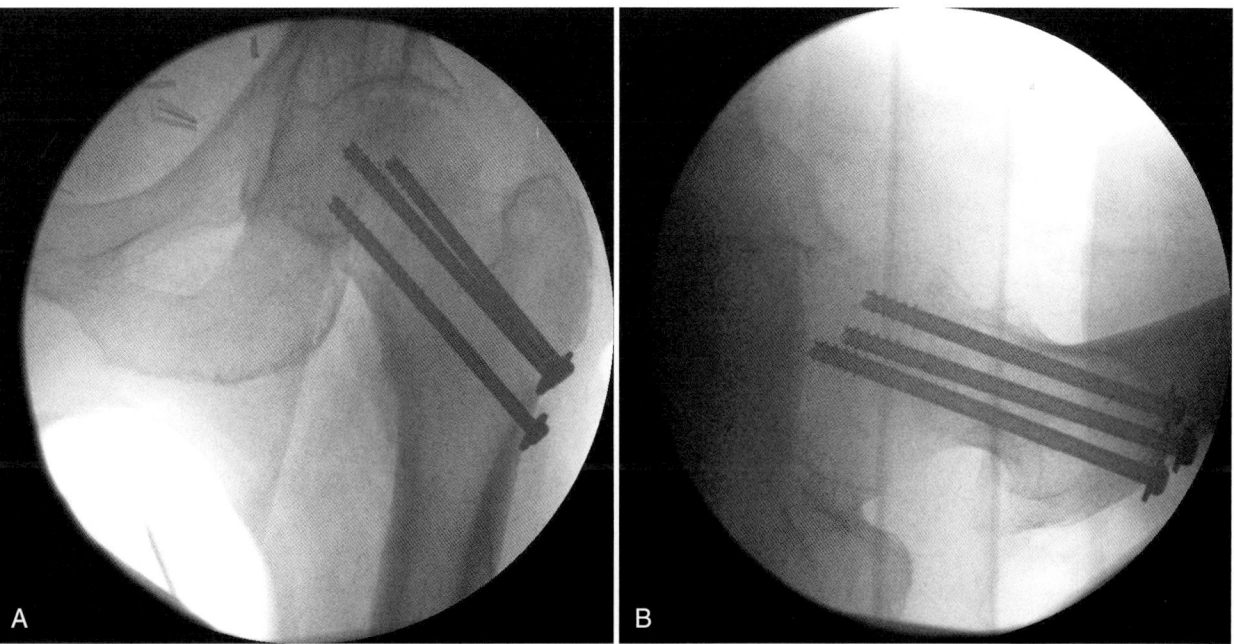

Fig. 21.22 PA projection (**A**) and lateral projection (**B**) fluoroscopic images of hip fracture reduction.

Fluoroscopic Procedures for the Operating Room

FEMUR NAIL

Position of patient and C-arm

During this procedure, a rod is inserted into the intramedullary (IM) canal to reduce a fracture of the shaft of the femur (Fig. 21.23). This rod or nail can be introduced either antegrade through the greater trochanter or retrograde through the popliteal notch.

Antegrade femoral nailing. During antegrade nailing, the patient is either supine or in the lateral position. In the supine position, the affected leg would most likely be in traction to help reduce the fracture. The legs would be abducted, and the unaffected leg would be flexed at the knee and hip and raised to allow the C-arm enough room to enter the sterile field. The patient's arm on the injured side is draped across the chest to keep it from obstructing the surgeon. The C-arm is positioned between the patient's legs, parallel to the unaffected leg, and centered over the hip. The C-arm may have to be rotated forward or backward to obtain a true PA projection. Rotate the C-arm under the table for a lateral projection.

When the patient is in the lateral position, the affected leg is extended forward to clear the opposite leg. The lateral position requires the radiographer to enter the sterile field and rotate the C-arm under the table to find a PA projection of the femur. Lateral projection is achieved with the tube starting in a true PA projection, rotating the C-arm forward 10 to 15 degrees, and tilting it 5 to 10 degrees cephalad.

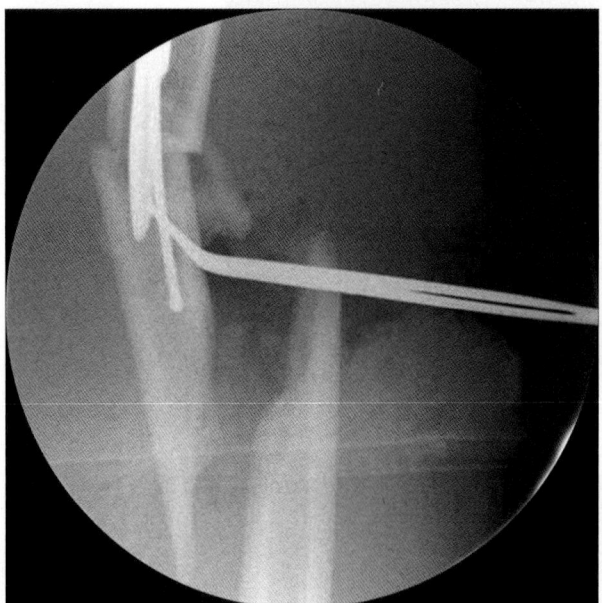

Fig. 21.23 Image of midshaft femoral fracture with guide rod being inserted to align fracture.

Retrograde femoral nailing. During the retrograde femoral nailing, the patient is supine with the injured leg exposed and the knee flexed and supported with a bump. This position allows the surgeon access to the popliteal notch without injuring the patella.

The sterile field is entered with the C-arm perpendicular to the patient. The C-arm is tilted cephalad to account for the flexed knee and to find the PA projection. The C-arm is rotated under the table for lateral position (Fig. 21.24).

Method
- Instruments or hardware may protrude from the operative site. Be sure to avoid disturbing these instruments or hardware or allowing them to puncture a sterile drape.
- Center the C-arm over the fracture site during canal reaming to ensure that the fracture remains reduced (Fig. 21.25).
- The table must allow for movement of the C-arm from the knee to the hip.
- Allow enough room between the patient and C-arm for the surgeon to work.

Screws are inserted into the femur and through the nail to fix the nail in place. When lining up the screw holes in the nail, the hole should be perfectly round and not oblong. Center the screw hole on the monitor. The magnification feature may be used to give the surgeon a better view. The C-arm may need to be tilted or rotated to obtain perfect circles. The surgeon also manipulates the leg to help align the screw holes. After the screws are inserted, check the length of the screws by placing the C-arm in PA projection. Screws should not protrude excessively from the cortical bone (Fig. 21.26).

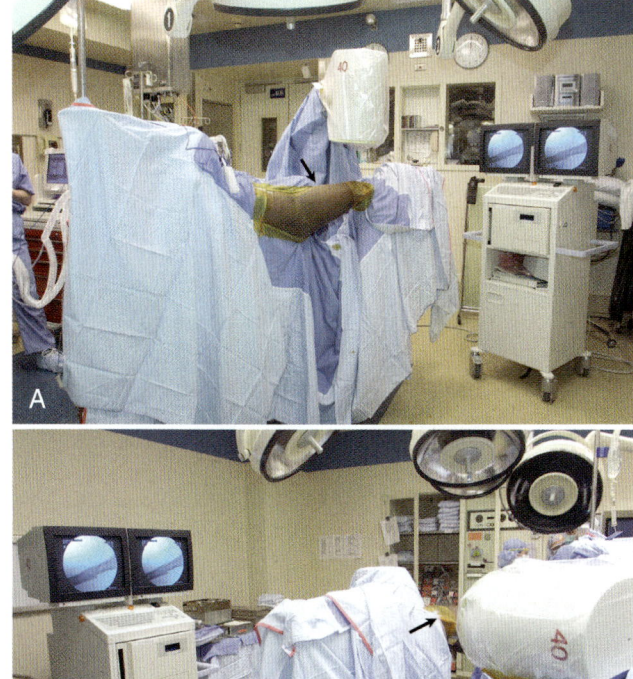

Fig. 21.24 (A) C-arm positioned between patient's legs for PA projection during femoral nailing. *Arrow* is pointing to femur. (B) C-arm rotated under femur *(arrow)* for lateral projection.

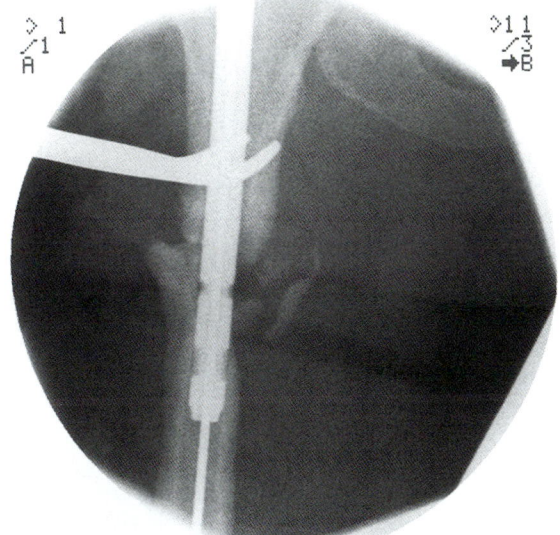

Fig. 21.25 Image of femur fracture during canal reaming.

Structures shown

All parts of the femur, including the greater and lesser trochanters, femoral neck, shaft, and condyles, are seen in the PA and lateral positions. Different instrumentation is in the IM canal, beginning with a guide rod that is used to help reduce the fracture and provide a means for the canal reamers to pass through the fracture site (Fig. 21.27). After reduction, the nail and screws are seen.

EVALUATION CRITERIA

The optimum image obtained using correct positioning, image intensifier-ROI-tube alignment, collimation, and exposure factors will demonstrate:
- Appropriate projections seen unobstructed and in the correct plane on the monitor
- Screw holes perfectly round and in the center of the monitor
- Sterile field maintained
- Proper radiographic technique maintained
- Radiation protection provided for the surgical team

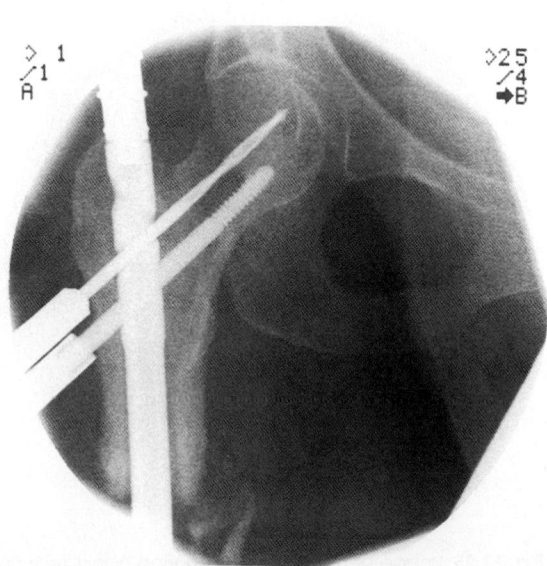

Fig. 21.26 PA projection of proximal screw in a femoral nail.

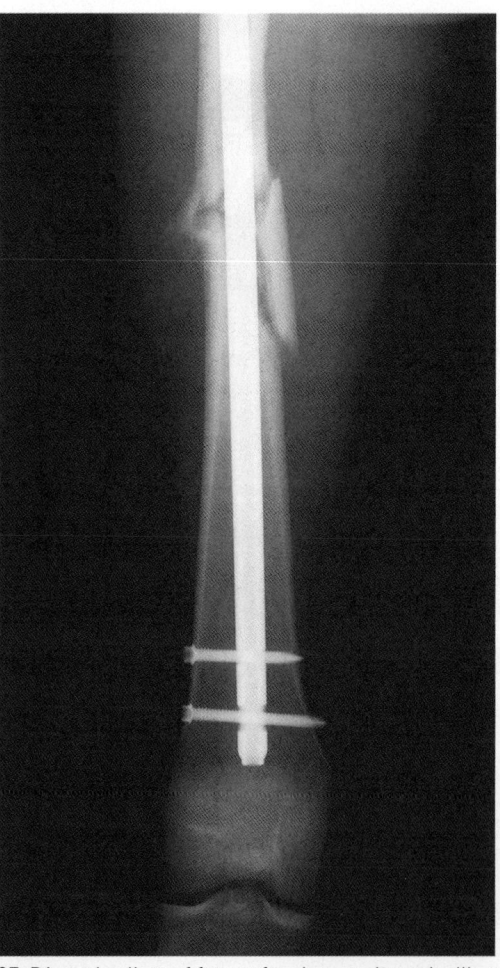

Fig. 21.27 PA projection of femur fracture reduced with guide rod and distal interlocking screws inserted.

TIBIA (NAIL)

Position of patient

The patient is supine with the affected leg exposed. The knee is flexed to allow access to the tibial tuberosity without injuring the patella. The injured leg is on the opposite side of the table so that the C-arm does not interfere with the surgical team.

Position of C-arm

Cover the C-arm with a sterile drape. Move the C-arm into the field perpendicular to the patient. Center the beam over the leg and tilt the tube to match the angle of the leg (Fig. 21.28). No obstructions should be under the table to avoid interfering with the C-arm movement. Rotate the C-arm under the table and into the lateral position, taking care not to disturb any instrumentation protruding from the operative site. Center the leg on the monitor by raising or lowering the C-arm. The surgeon manipulates the leg, and the radiographer tilts or rotates the C-arm to obtain round holes (Figs. 21.29 and 21.30). The magnification feature can be used to enlarge the image if necessary. Advance the C-arm until its tube side is far enough from the injured leg to allow the surgeon to fit the drill and drill bit into the area.

- Along its shaft the tibia is triangular, so when checking the length of the screws, the C-arm may have to be rotated forward or back to get a true length.
- Center the beam on the fracture site during canal reaming. When the leg is in the center of the monitor, turn the wheels of the C-arm horizontally to allow the machine to move longitudinally down the shaft of the leg without moving out of the field of view.

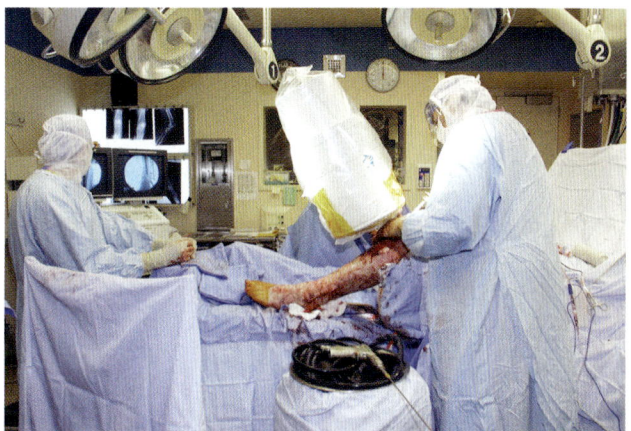

Fig. 21.28 C-arm positioned for tibial nailing. The radiographer tilted the fluoroscopic image intensifier to be parallel with the long axis of the leg.

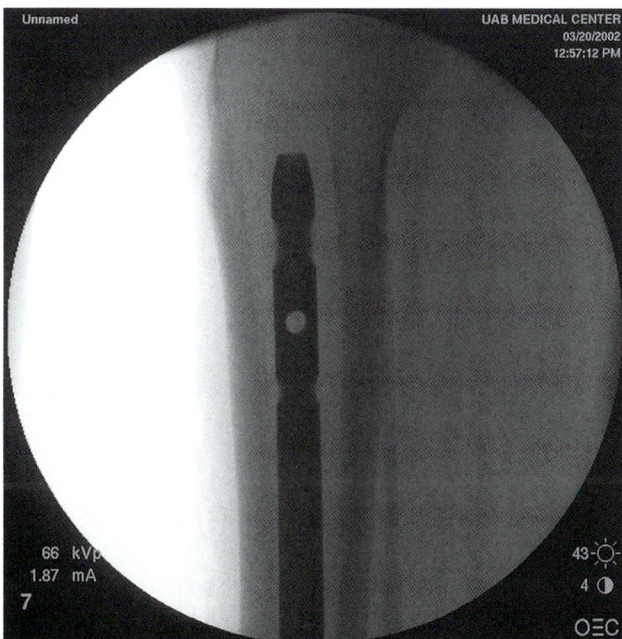

Fig. 21.29 Image of tibial nail screw holes in incorrect alignment and oblong in shape.

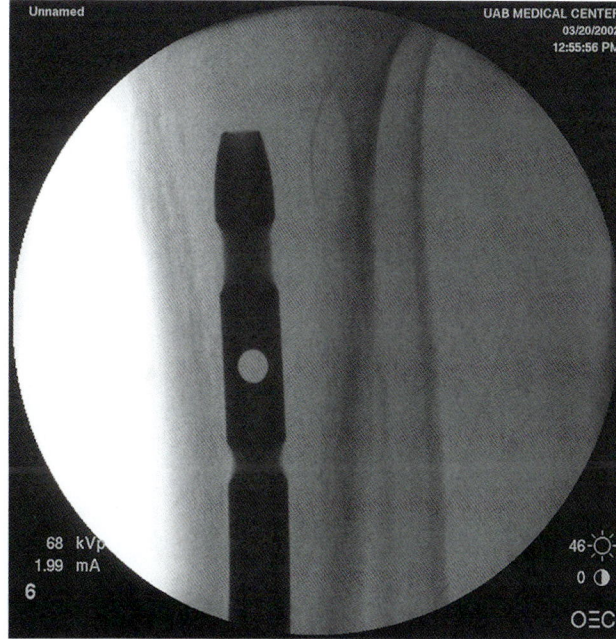

Fig. 21.30 Image of tibial nail screw holes perfectly round and magnified to assist proper alignment.

Structures shown

Structures shown include the tibia and fibula, the tibial shaft along with any fracture, the tibial plateau, tibial tuberosity, distal tibia, and ankle joint (Fig. 21.31). After hardware is inserted, the tibial nail fills the IM canal, with proximal and distal screws prominent.

EVALUATION CRITERIA

The optimum image obtained using correct positioning, image intensifier-ROI-tube alignment, collimation, and exposure factors will demonstrate:
- The tibia centered on the monitor, providing proper radiographic technique
- Appropriate projections seen unobstructed and in the correct plane on the monitor
- Sterile field maintained
- Radiation protection provided for the surgical team

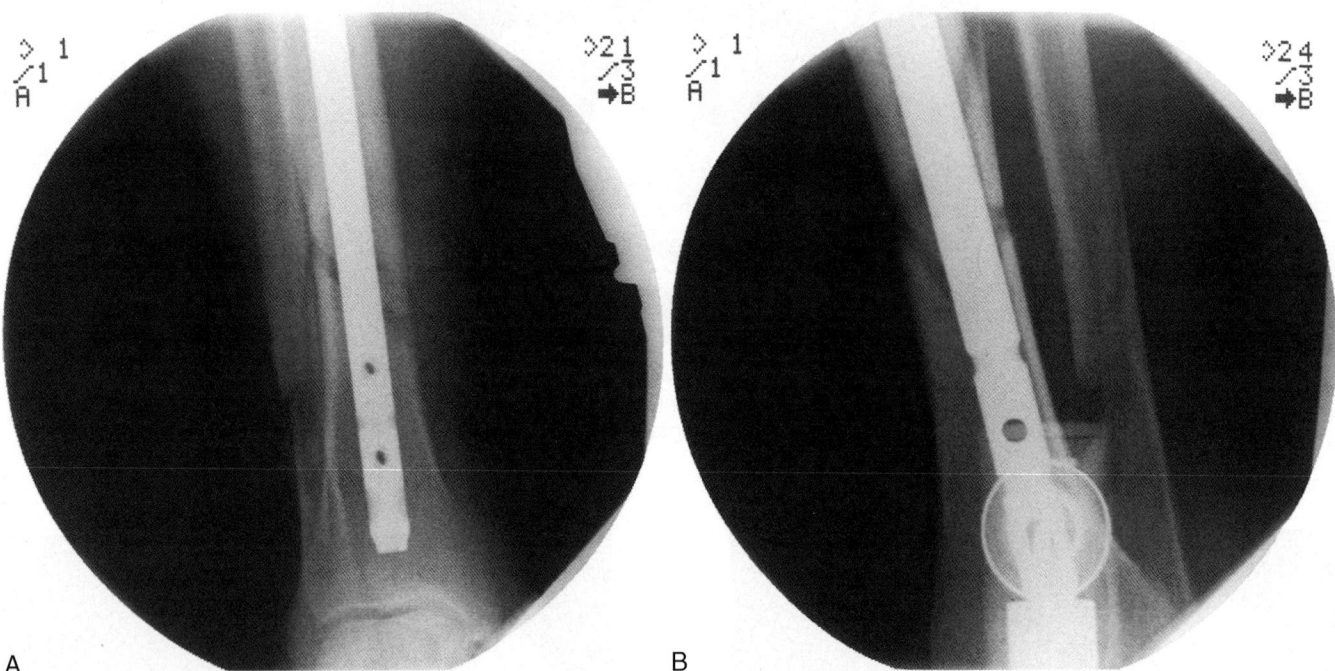

Fig. 21.31 (**A**) Improper alignment of distal screw holes. (**B**) Screw holes properly aligned with screwdriver over distal screw hole.

HUMERUS

Position of patient

The patient is supine or in a reclining or beach chair position (Fig. 21.32). The injured arm may be resting on a Mayo stand with the surgeon's assistant holding the arm to stabilize and align the humerus. The patient should be positioned with the shoulder off the side of the table. This position allows the humerus to be seen in its entirety without being obscured by the table.

Position of C-arm

Cover the C-arm with a sterile drape. Enter the field parallel to, or at a 45-degree angle to, the patient. The assistant rotates the arm medially with the elbow bent 90 degrees. The C-arm is tilted and rotated to obtain a true lateral projection, depending on the angle of patient position. The arm is held at the elbow to provide support, and the arm is rotated until the hand is pointing upward. The C-arm is tilted to obtain PA projection according to the patient's angle. Center the beam on the humerus.

- When installing a nail or rod into the humerus and trying to locate and center the distal screws, place a sterile drape over the tube or pull the sheets draping the patient over the tube. Touch only the underside of the sheets when placing them over the tube. Raise the tube to magnify the screw holes and to allow the surgeon to work.

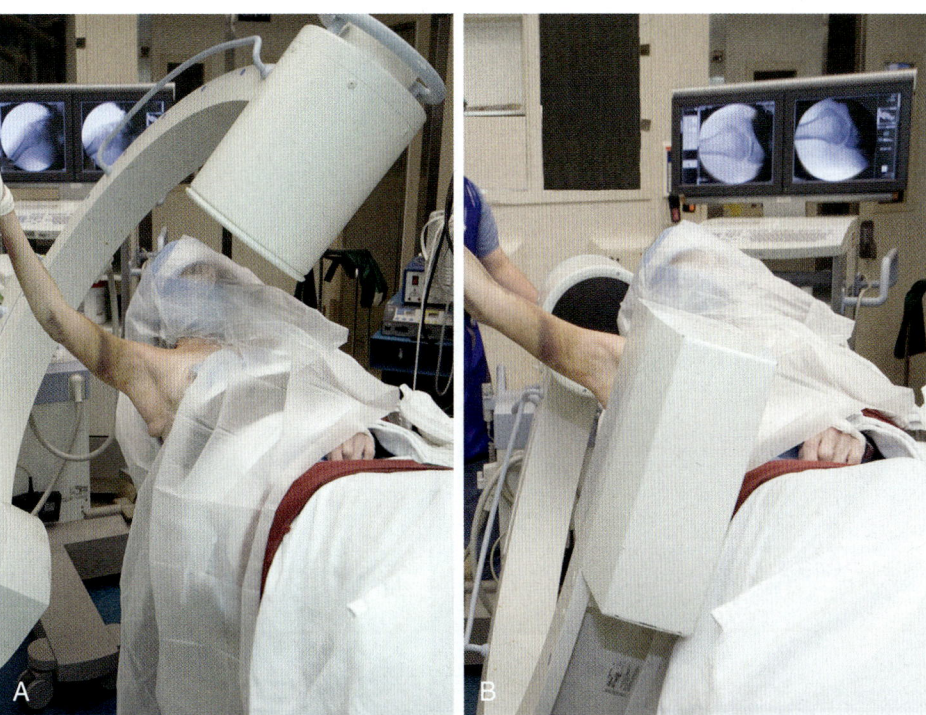

Fig. 21.32 (**A**) C-arm positioned for PA projection of the shoulder with patient in beach chair position for preliminary imaging. (**B**) C-arm positioned for axillary projection.

NOTE: Do not leave any drape over the tube for a long time to prevent unnecessary heat buildup in the tube.

- Be careful not to strike the patient's head with the image intensifier.

Structures shown

This procedure should show all parts of the humerus, including the head, neck, greater and lesser tubercles, shaft, and distal portion of the humerus. Any fractures and the hardware used for repair (Fig. 21.33) are also seen.

EVALUATION CRITERIA

The optimum image obtained using correct positioning, image intensifier-ROI-tube alignment, collimation, and exposure factors will demonstrate:

- Angle of humerus and C-arm coinciding to obtain true PA and lateral projections
- When nailing the distal screws, holes perfectly round in order to allow screws to pass through the nail
- Humerus in the center of the monitor to maintain radiographic technique
- Image rotated in the same plane as the humerus
- Sterile field maintained, especially with the proximity of possibly nonsterile portions of the tube to the sterile field
- Radiation protection provided for the surgical team

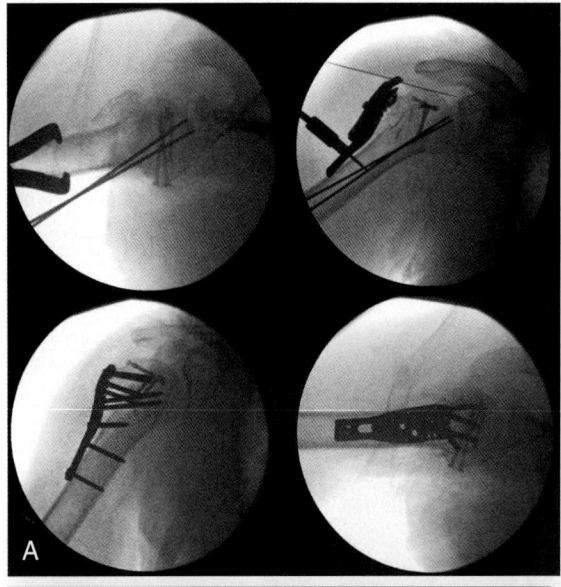

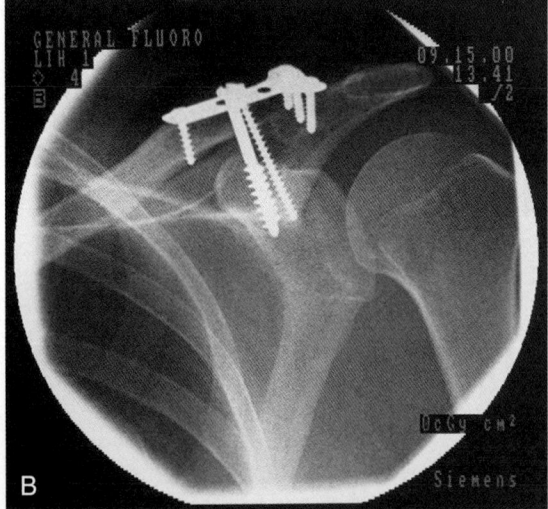

Fig. 21.33 (A) Images of humeral fracture with nails used to reduce fracture of the humeral head. **(B)** Image of clavicle fracture with plate and screw fixation.

FEMORAL/TIBIAL ARTERIOGRAM

Position of patient

The patient is supine, with the affected leg exposed from the groin area to the foot. There should be enough room under the table to allow the C-arm to move from the hip to the foot. The leg may be rotated medially or laterally to keep the femur or tibia from obscuring any vasculature (Fig. 21.34).

Position of C-arm

Cover the C-arm with a sterile drape, and enter the field perpendicular to the patient. When the leg is in the center of the monitor, turn the wheels of the C-arm horizontally to allow the machine to move to the left or right without taking the leg out of the field of view. Use the subtraction or road-mapping feature to remove all structures except the contrast medium that is injected into the artery (Fig. 21.35). This feature shows any stenoses or injuries to the artery.

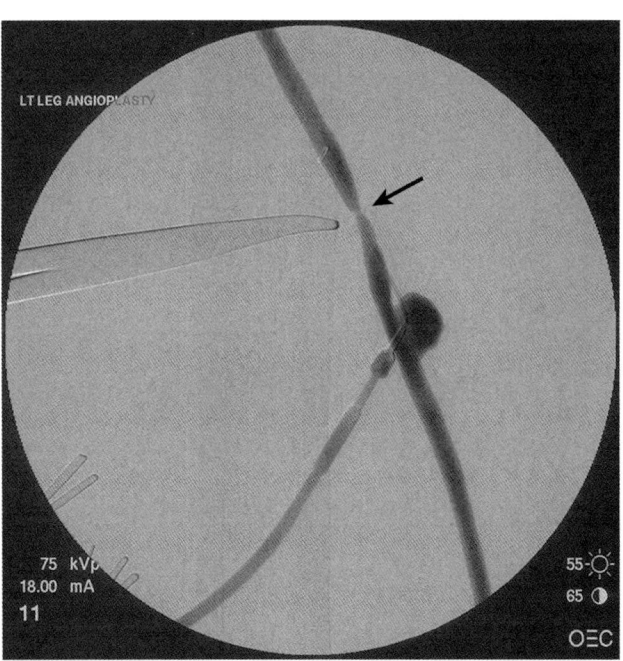

Fig. 21.34 Subtraction image of surgical femoral artery angiogram with stenosis *(arrow)*.

Structures shown

The bones of the leg are seen before subtraction. After contrast medium is introduced, the femoral artery and its branches are seen, and, following the contrast medium down the leg, the popliteal and tibial arteries are seen. The contrast images show any pathologic defects in the arterial structures.

EVALUATION CRITERIA

The optimum image obtained using correct positioning, image intensifier-ROI-tube alignment, collimation, and exposure factors will demonstrate:
- All pertinent vasculature shown without being obscured by the table or bones of the leg
- Integrity of the mask image maintained by not moving the leg or the C-arm during subtraction or road mapping
- Proper radiographic technique maintained
- Sterile field maintained
- Radiation protection provided for the surgical team

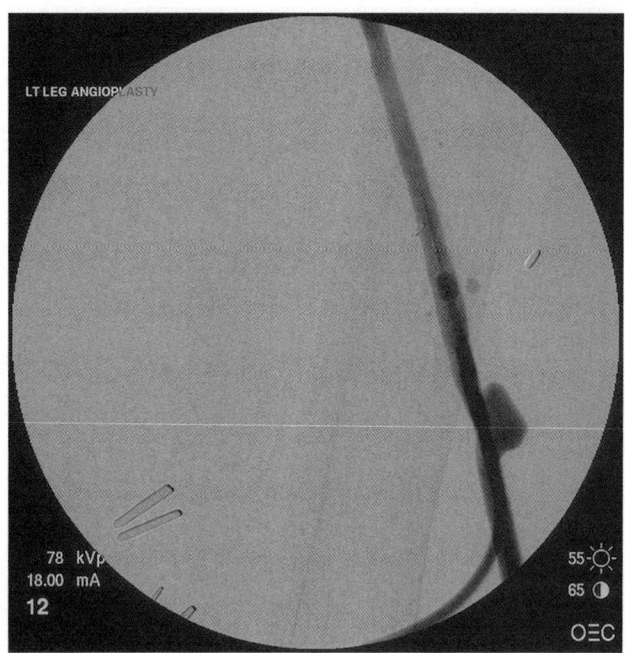

Fig. 21.35 Subtraction image of surgical femoral artery angiogram after balloon angioplasty.

Mobile Radiography Procedures for the Operating Room
CERVICAL SPINE

Image receptor: The IR should be 35 × 43 cm (14 × 17 inches) grid IR crosswise. Adjust the radiation field above the external acoustic meatus (EAM) and below T1 on the collimator.

Position of patient
The patient is upright, prone, or supine. In the upright and prone positions, the patient's head is held in a traction device to align the spine. In the supine position, the chin is elevated and held with a strap or tape.

Position of image receptor and portable machine
- Place the grid IR in the IR holder and cover with a sterile drape (Fig. 21.36).
- Position the IR holder on the opposite side of the patient. The surgical technician moves the sterile back table so that the radiographer does not compromise the sterile field.
- Direct the beam perpendicular to the IR and parallel to the floor.
- The beam enters perpendicular to the IR to eliminate grid cutoff.
- Raise or lower the tube and IR to center on the cervical spine.

Structures shown
- Cervical spine in lateral projection (Fig. 21.37).
- Degenerative or pathologic defects, such as osteophytes, fractures, or subluxation.
- Radiograph may be taken at the beginning of the case to verify the correct portion of the spine to be repaired. Instruments are placed to designate the level of the spine (Fig. 21.38).

EVALUATION CRITERIA
The optimum image obtained using correct positioning, CR-part-IR alignment, collimation, and exposure factors will demonstrate:
- The entire spine on the radiograph
- The spine in the center of the radiograph and not rotated
- The use of proper radiographic technique
- Radiation protection provided
- All hardware that may be used included
- Grid cutoff absent

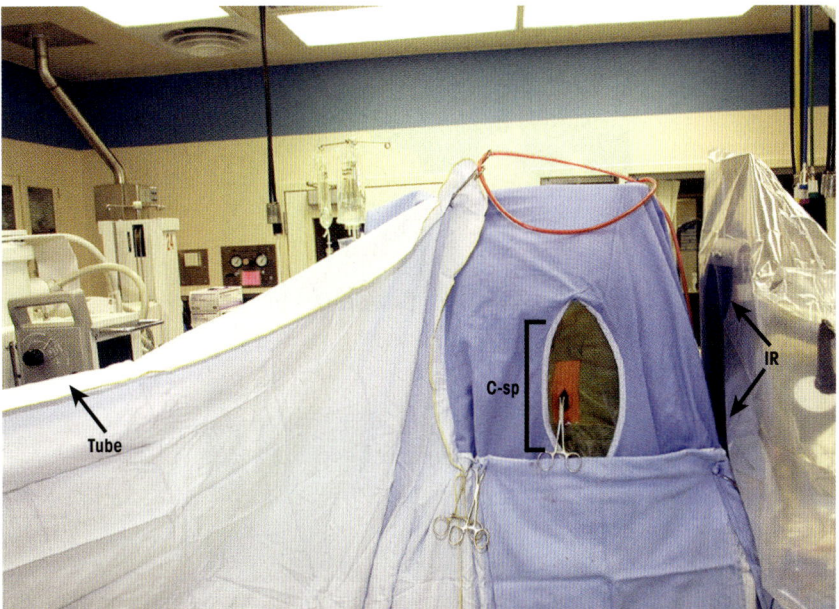

Fig. 21.36 Mobile radiographic machine *(arrow)* in position for upright lateral cervical spine. A surgical clamp, which is attached to the spinous process of interest, extends from the incision site. The IR, draped and in holder *(double arrow)*, is centered to the patient.

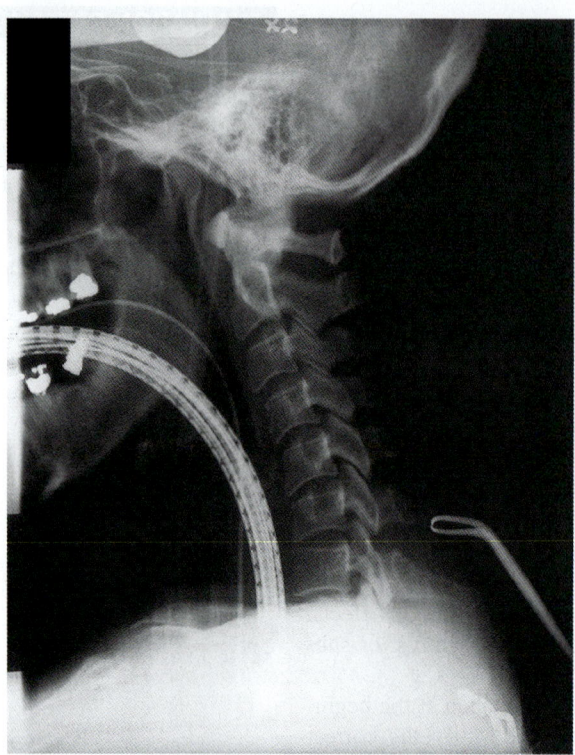

Fig. 21.37 Lateral cervical spine radiograph (patient in sitting position for surgery), showing localization marker in place on the spinous process of C6.

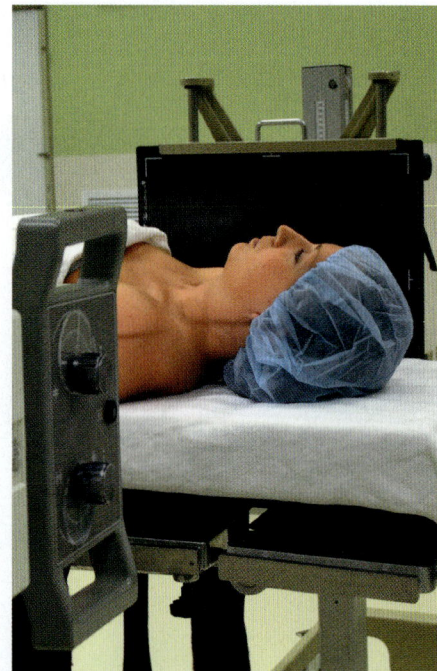

Fig. 21.38 Lateral projection of the cervical spine with patient supine. This was done to verify the correct position of instruments before continuing surgery. Often a spinal needle is placed in the disk space to show position. Note that even though a 35 × 43 cm (14 × 17 inches) wireless DR detector is used, the radiographer has properly coned to pertinent anatomy.

THORACIC OR LUMBAR SPINE

Image receptor: The IR should be 35 × 43 cm (14 × 17 inches) grid IR crosswise.

Position of patient
The patient is prone or supine with the arms placed up by the head. The chest and abdomen are supported by a frame or chest roll to flex the spine into anatomic position. A radiograph may be done to verify that the surgeon is working on the correct vertebra or to show the position of hardware (Fig. 21.39).

Lateral projection. Place grid IR in IR holder and cover with a sterile drape. Position the holder next to the patient and move the IR up or down to center on the lumbar spine. Direct the beam perpendicular to the IR and parallel to the floor (Fig. 21.40). Respiration should be suspended during exposure.

PA projection. For the PA radiograph, slide IR in the slot under the table and center on the spine. Cover field with sterile drape. Center the beam to the IR and perpendicular to the long axis of the spine.

Structures shown
- The lumbar spine in PA and lateral projections.
- Vertebral bodies, spinous processes, facets, and lamina.
- Hardware to repair any defects. Bone grafts or interbody fusion devices may be used.
- Instrumentation is often seen on radiograph.
- PA projection may be obscured by the patient support.

EVALUATION CRITERIA
The optimum image obtained using correct positioning, CR-part-IR alignment, collimation, and exposure factors will demonstrate:
- The spine in the center of the radiograph and in true PA or lateral projection
- Spine bodies seen without any rotation
- All hardware used seen on the radiograph
- All unnecessary instrumentation removed to avoid obscuring the spine
- Proper radiographic technique
- Radiation protection provided for the surgical team

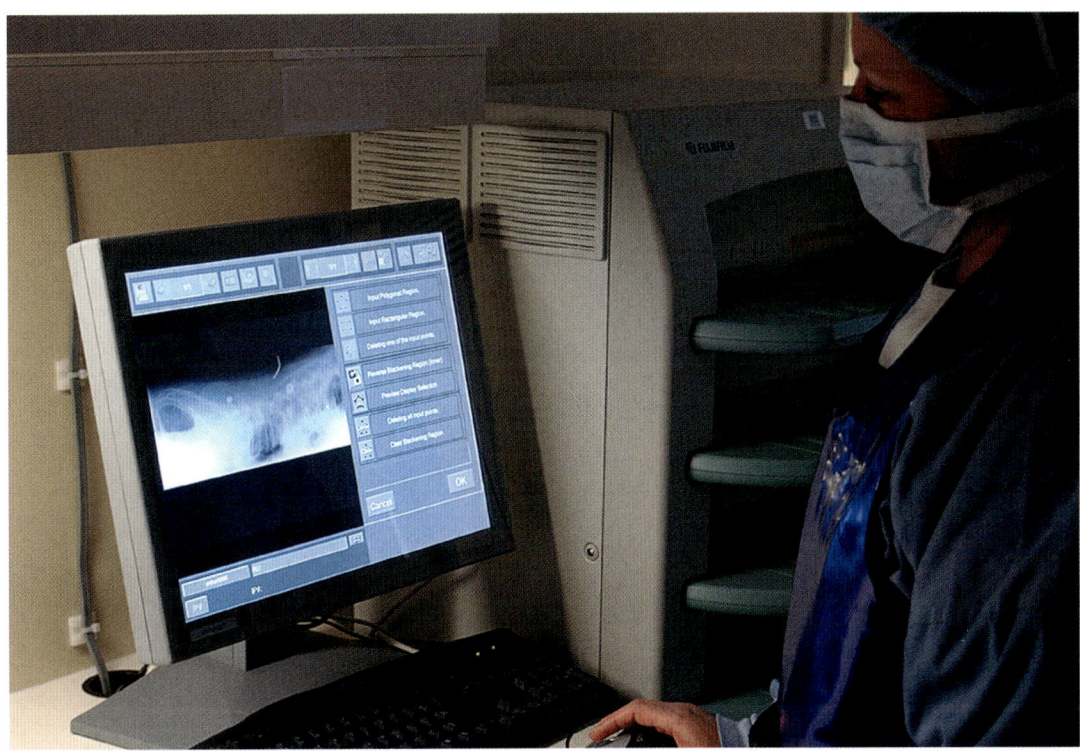

Fig. 21.39 Lateral lumbar spine with intraoperative marker to verify correct level of interest.

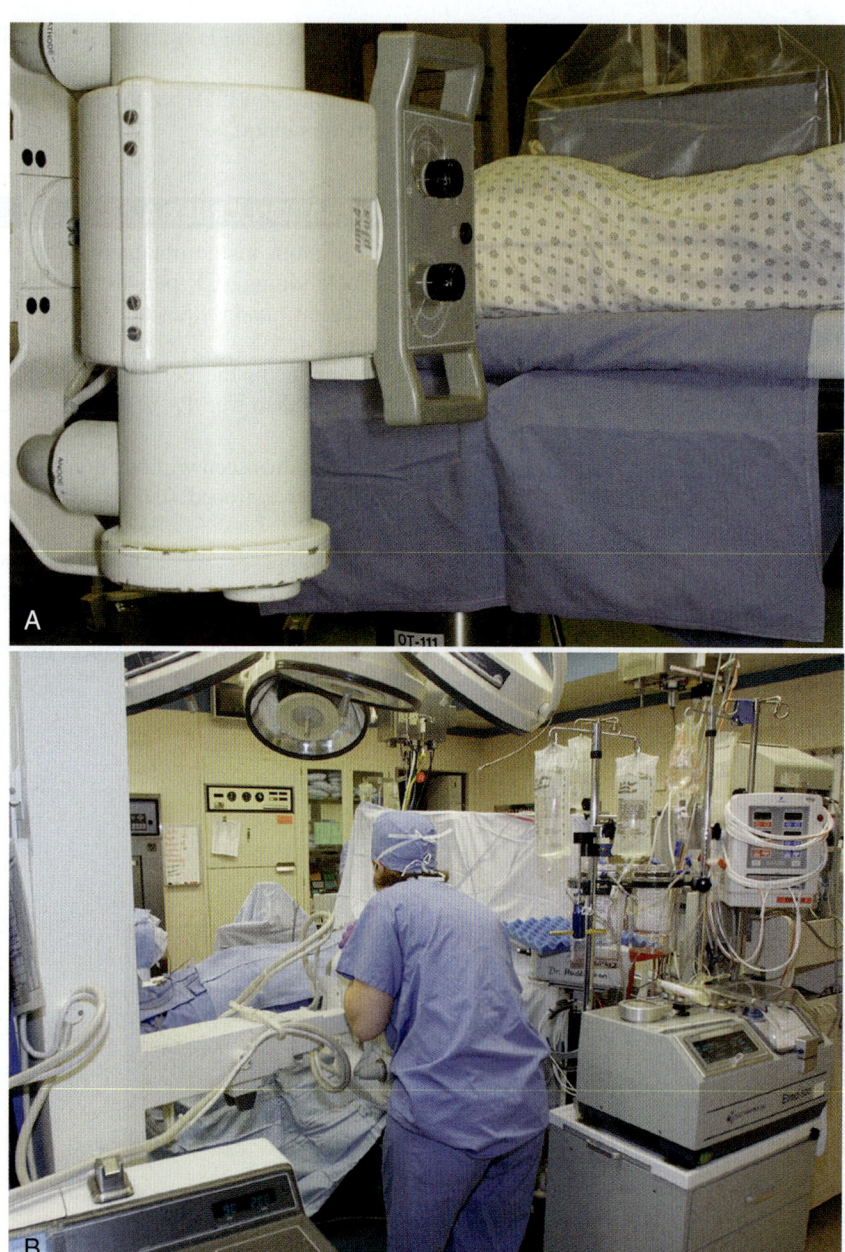

Fig. 21.40 (**A**) Mobile x-ray machine correctly positioned for cross-table lateral lumbar spine. (**B**) Radiographer positioning mobile unit intraoperatively for lateral lumbar spine procedure.

EXTREMITY EXAMINATIONS

Image receptor: Department protocol to include all appropriate anatomy and hardware.

Position of patient
The patient is supine, prone, reclining, or in the beach chair position. Portable machines approach perpendicular to the patient. Institutions may cover the tube or sterile field, or both, with a sterile drape. Angle the tube to match the IR or desired projection. The surgeon may choose to hold the patient's limb in position during the exposure. To reduce exposure to the surgeon, positioning aids, such as sterile towels, sponges, or mallets, may be used.

The surgeon may also cover the field with a cloth sterile drape rather than a plastic sterile drape. If so, the surgeon marks the location of the part to ensure proper centering. Lighting may also need to be adjusted for better visualization of the field. For crosstable examinations, the beam is directed perpendicular to the IR and parallel to the floor. Center the beam to the IR and raise or lower the tube to the center of the part.

Structures shown
- All pertinent anatomy in correct alignment.
- Hardware, including plates, wires, pins, screws, external fixation, and joint replacement components used to repair fractures or degenerative problems (Figs. 21.41 through 21.47).

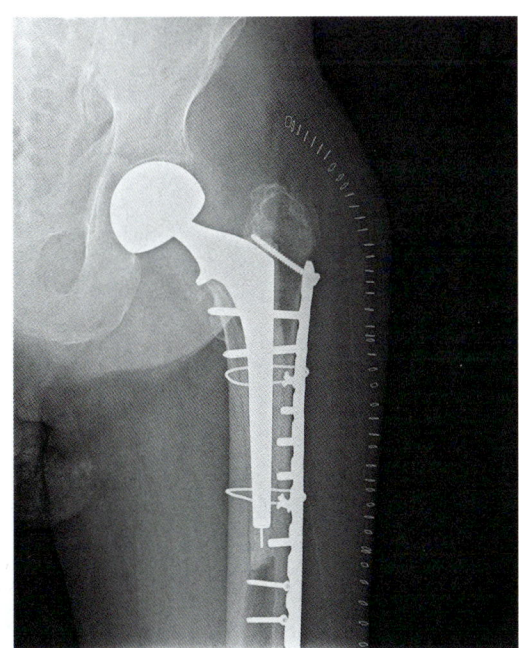

Fig. 21.41 PA projection of a hip joint replacement with plate and screw fixation following a periprosthetic femur fracture.

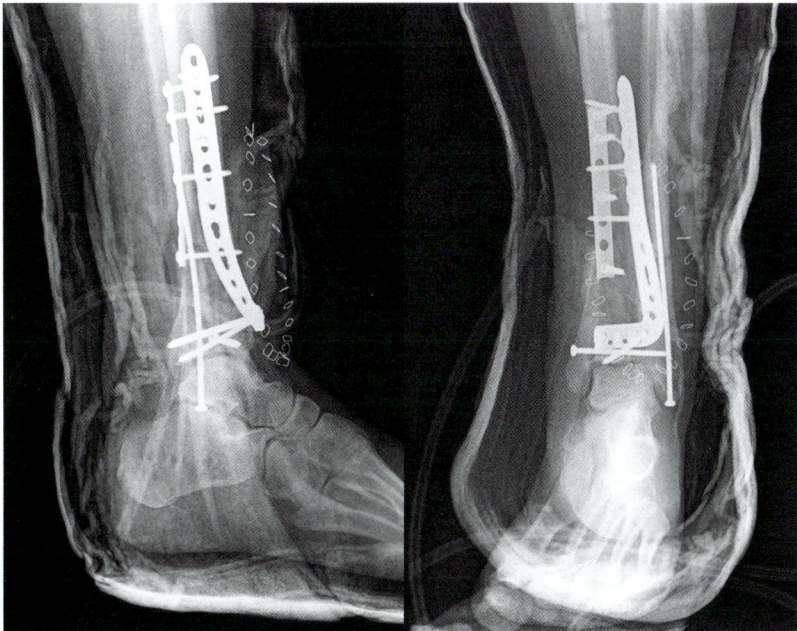

Fig. 21.42 AP and lateral postreduction images of a comminuted ankle fracture. Some casting materials require an increase in technical factors for correct penetration and image quality.

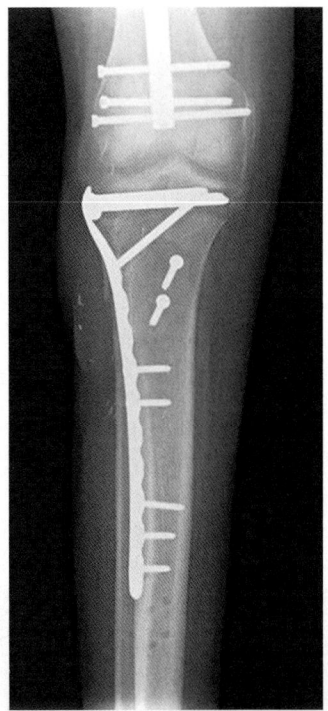

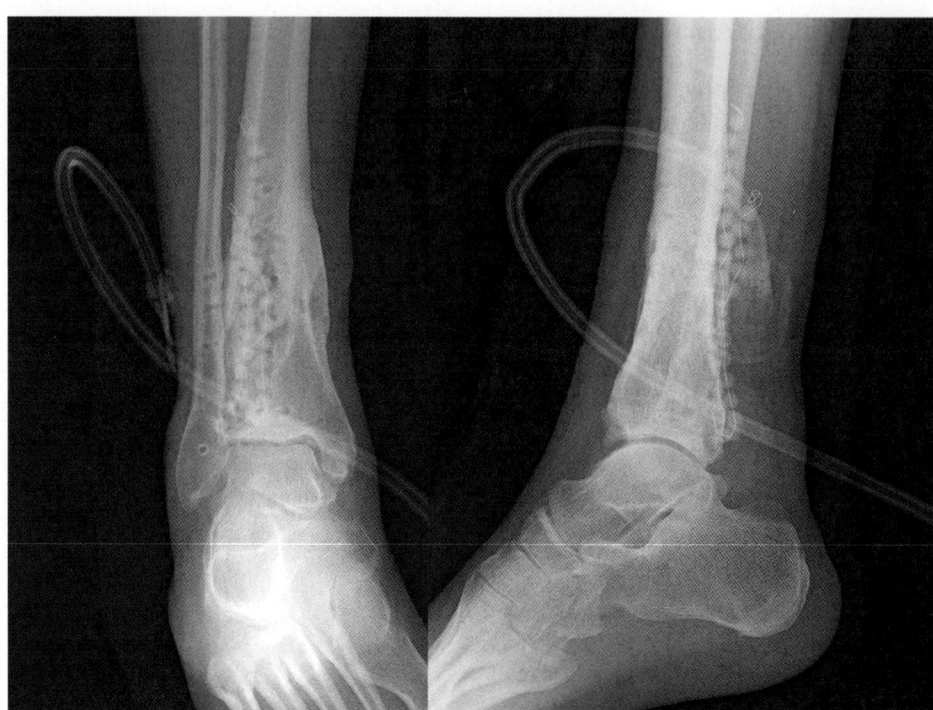

Fig. 21.43 AP and lateral image of the ankle with antibiotic beads. Antibiotic beads are placed at the site of infection to promote healing.

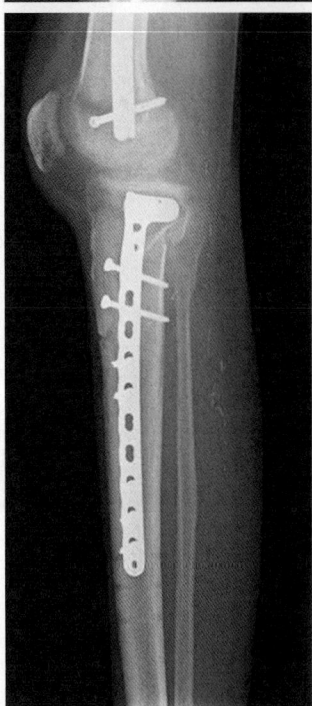

Fig. 21.44 AP and lateral projection of proximal tibia with plate and screw fixation used to repair tibial plateau fracture.

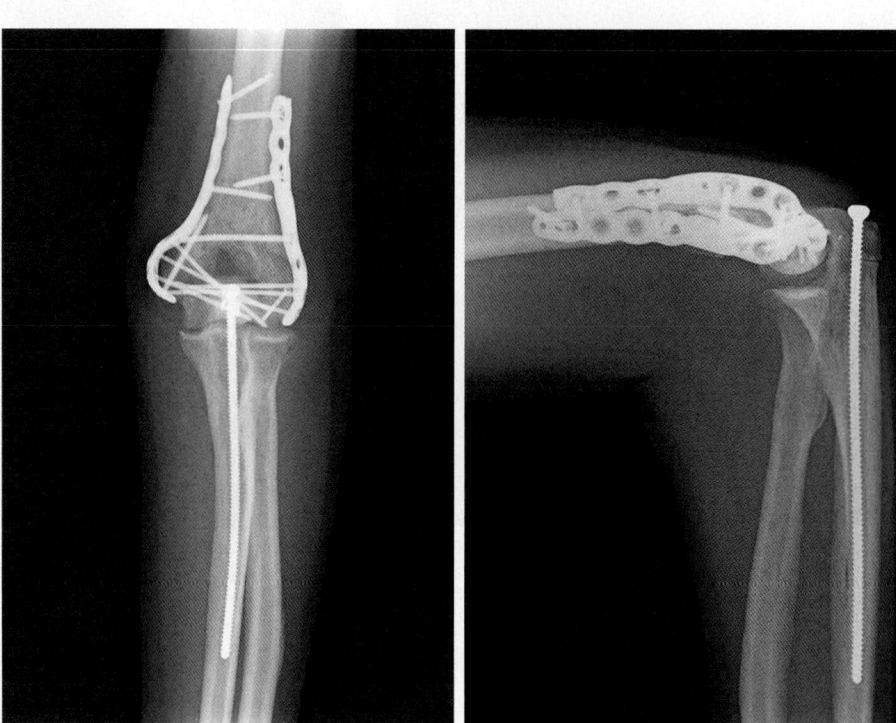

Fig. 21.45 AP and lateral projection of elbow with plate and screws used to reduce forearm fracture.

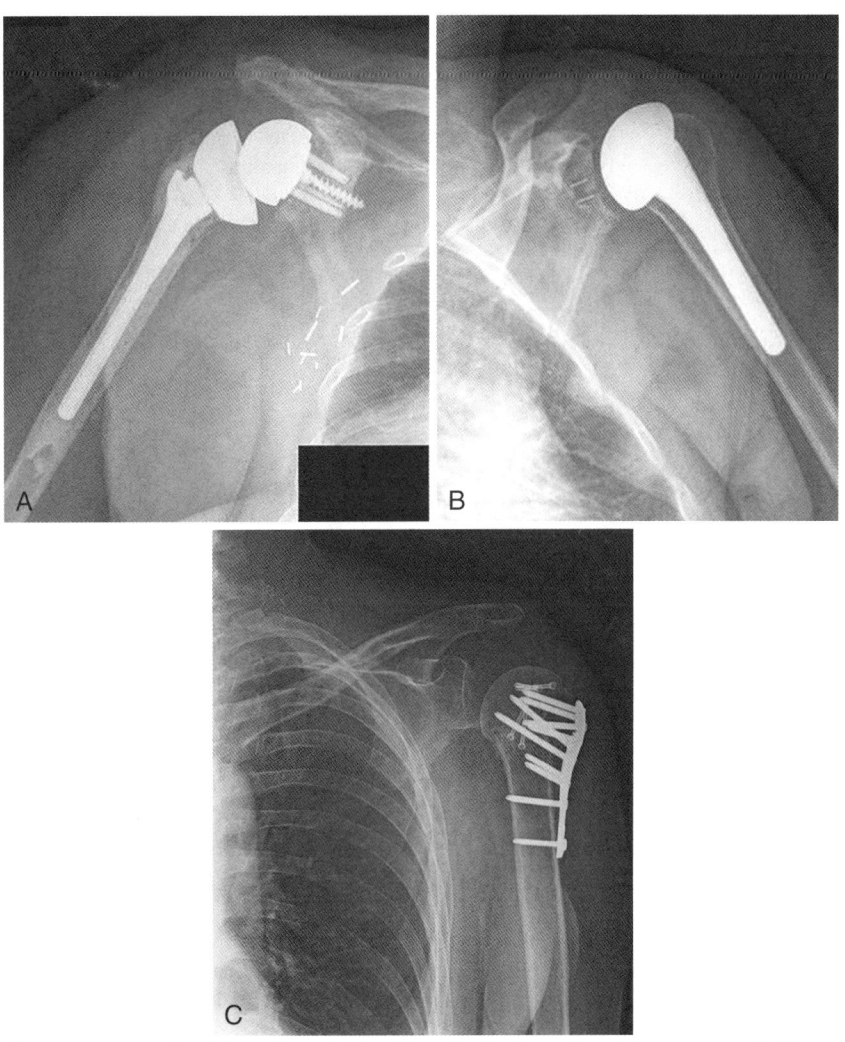

Fig. 21.46 (**A**) Total shoulder arthroplasty with polyethylene glenoid component. (**B**) Reverse total shoulder arthroplasty. (**C**) Shoulder with plate and screws fixation. Creative patient positioning or tube angulation may be necessary to achieve optimal images on complex comminuted fractures.

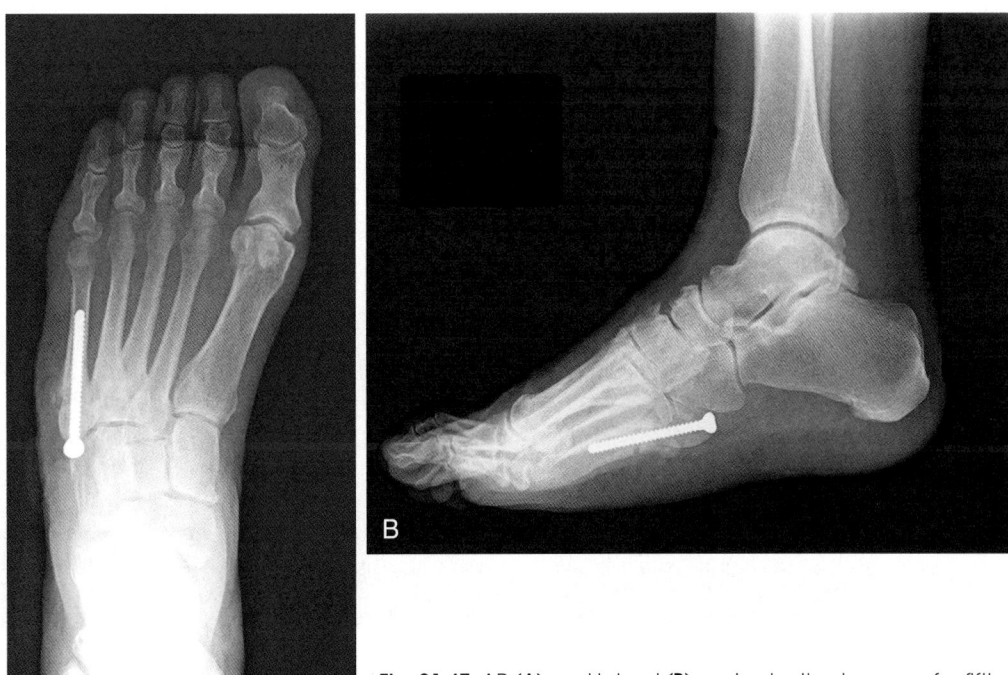

Fig. 21.47 AP (**A**) and lateral (**B**) postreduction images of a fifth metatarsal nonhealing fracture.

EVALUATION CRITERIA

The optimum image obtained using correct positioning, CR-part-IR alignment, collimation, and exposure factors will demonstrate:
- The complete joint, including all hardware, on the image
- Proper radiographic technique
- Sterile field maintained
- Radiation protection provided
- Collimation to include all hardware
- No unnecessary instruments in the field

NOTE: Many surgeons request different projections, depending on the individual case. When performing a wrist examination, the arm is positioned on one side of the imaging plate with the wrist in the AP or PA projection. Center the beam and collimate to the wrist to include all hardware. When the exposure is complete, the surgeon moves the arm to the other side of the imaging plate in the lateral position. Center the beam on the wrist and collimate (Figs. 21.48 and 21.49).

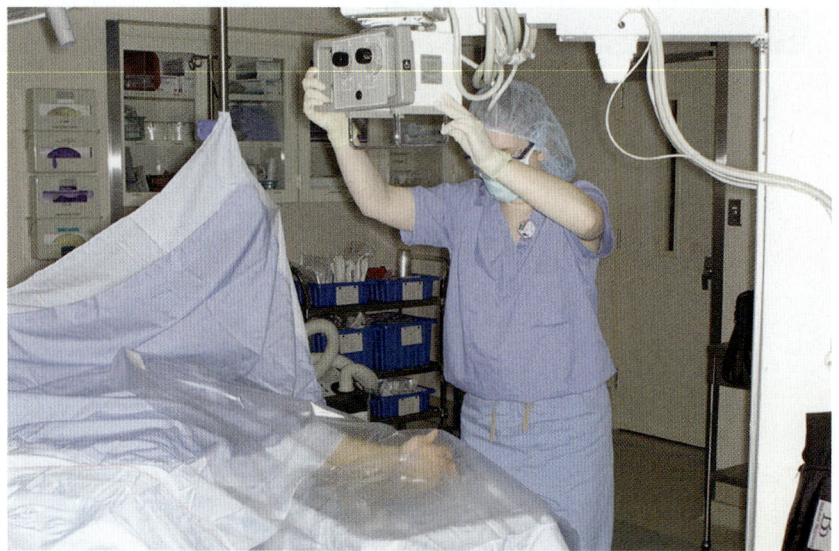

Fig. 21.48 Radiographer positioning a mobile machine for lateral projection of wrist.

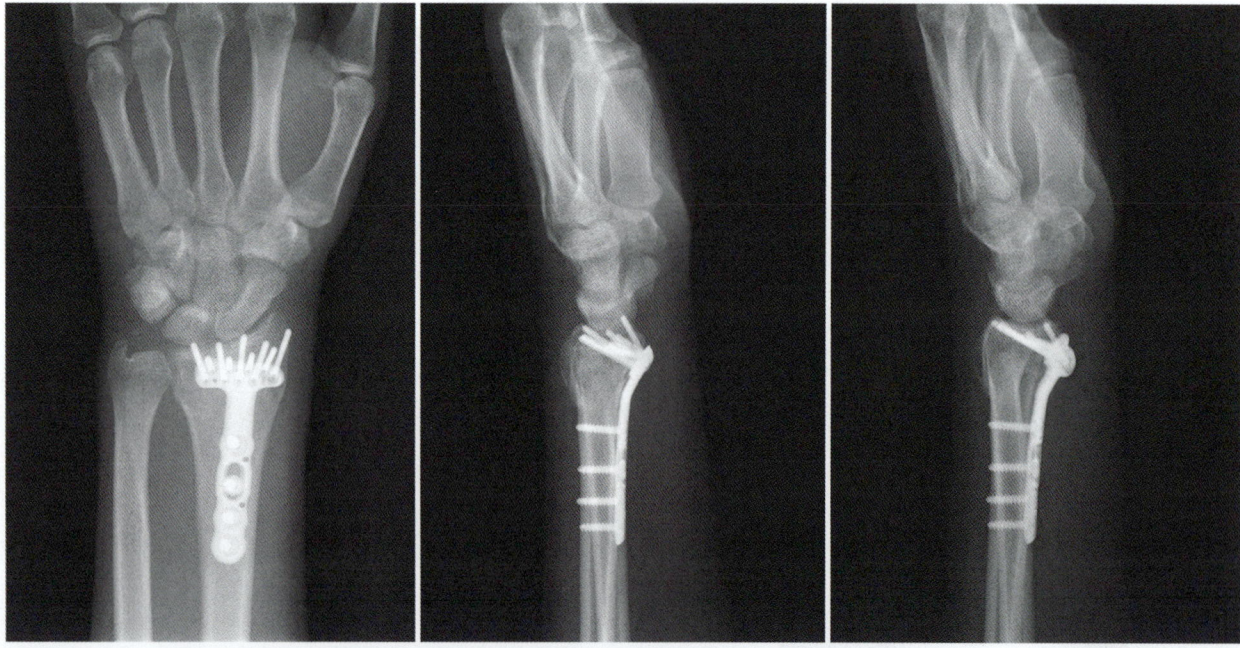

Fig. 21.49 PA, lateral, and tilt lateral projections of wrist. Note proper radial tilt of 22 degrees shows joint space clear of reduction screws.

O-Arm Equipment and Basics

Another type of imaging equipment used in the OR is known as the O-arm (Fig. 21.50). Much like the C-arm, the O-arm is given this name due to its shape. In many ways, the O-arm is similar to the C-arm in that there are two main parts: the computer console and the imaging apparatus (Fig. 21.51). The key difference is that an O-arm can obtain sectional images similar to CT. Sectional imaging can provide greater detail and spatial resolution in neurology procedures, including the spine and brain. The sectional imaging provides the ability for 3D rendering similar to computed tomography; therefore, the O-arm does not need to be moved to an oblique or lateral position. The O-arm is similar in size to a C-arm, so it is still imperative to avoid contaminating the sterile field when bringing the machine into a surgical suite. Since most O-arm equipment is not dedicated to one surgical room, the mobile device will need to have a power source such as a plug-in, which is similar to most C-arms. The O-arm must be draped with sterile covers similar to the C-arm, and the radiographer should extend the O-arm from the neutral position to the halfway extended point. This aspect ensures that the O-arm can be maneuvered in and out of the surgical area without moving the base. Once imaging is necessary, proceed to move the O-arm to the desired anatomy, using the guidance lights to ensure that the image receptor and tube are correctly aligned (Figs. 21.52 and 21.53). It is imperative for the radiographer to communicate with other team members at this point since assistance will be needed to help guide the O-arm around the sterile field. Once in position, the O-arm can be closed using the control panel (Fig. 21.54). At this point, AP and lateral images can be acquired (Fig. 21.55), and it is critical that the technologists orientate the O-arm to the patient's anatomy (Fig. 21.56). If the O-arm is not orientated early, it is difficult to reorientate later, resulting in repeat exposures. After AP and lateral images are obtained, the radiographer must reorientate the O-arm in the 3D settings (Fig. 21.57); this must be done to ensure that the 3D reconstructions are correct for the navigation. The technologist can now construct the 3D rendered images, allowing for more precise surgical processes. Before removing the O-arm from the surgical area, it must be reopened while maintaining the sterile field. Since the O-arm uses guided navigation algorithms, the 3D renderings can be uploaded into the navigational system for improved accuracy. The renderings can be used to make 3D-printed bone phantoms specific to patients with severe deformities, which will allow for safer screw placement. Advancements in surgical imaging technology show progress in reduced surgical time, increased surgical accuracy, and decreased radiation exposure to the patient and surgical team.

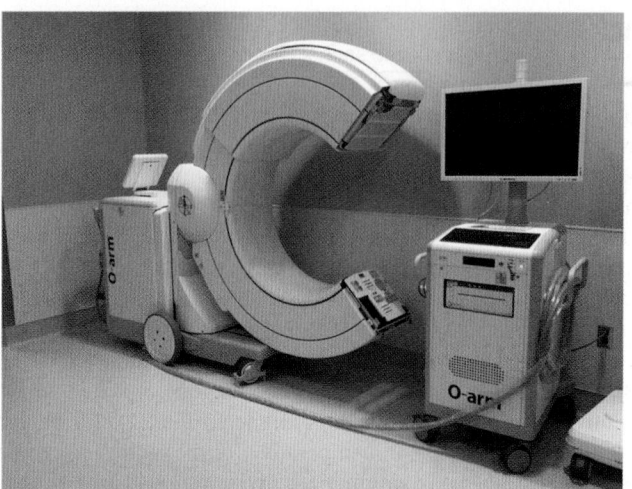

Fig. 21.50 O-arm imaging equipment and computer console.

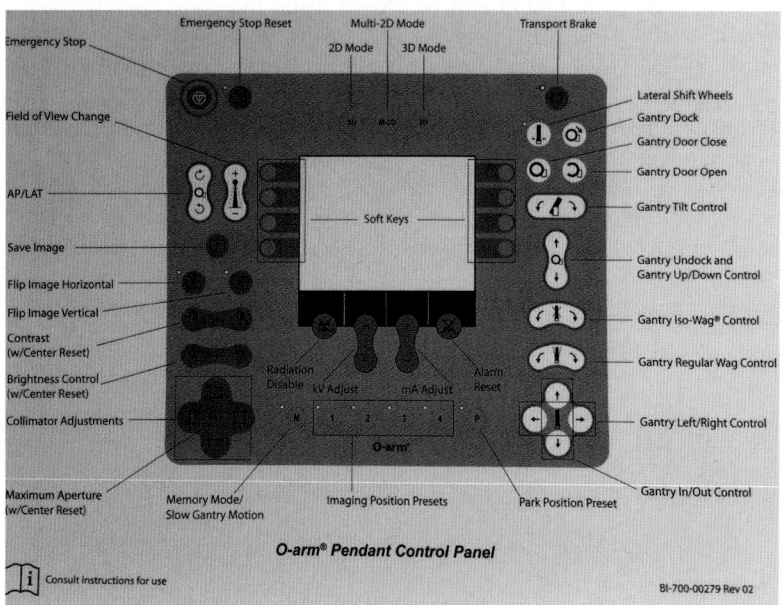

Fig. 21.51 Control panel of computer console.

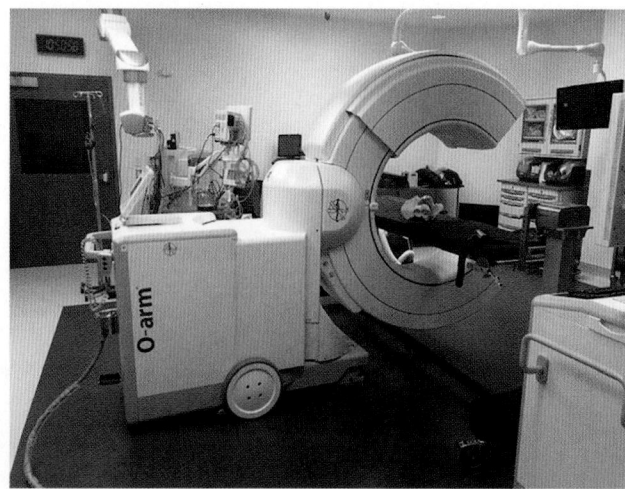

Fig. 21.52 O-arm positioned over anatomy of interest.

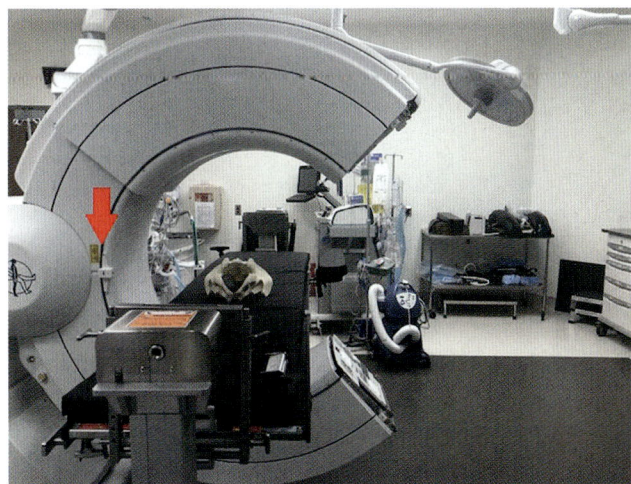

Fig. 21.53 The *red arrow* indicates one of the guidance lights used to ensure that the image receptor and tube are correctly aligned with anatomy.

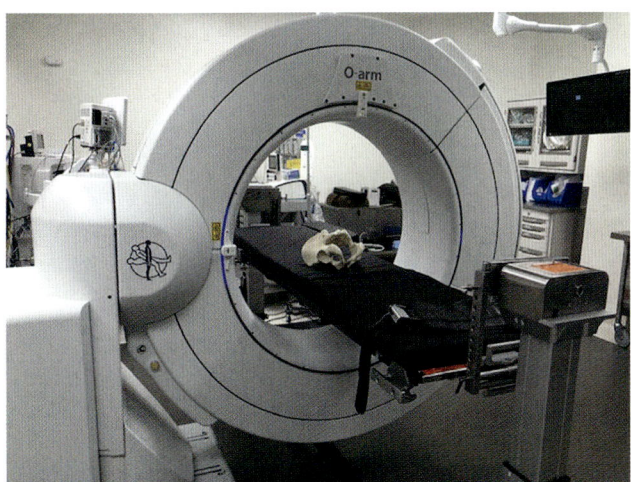

Fig. 21.54 O-arm closed in position.

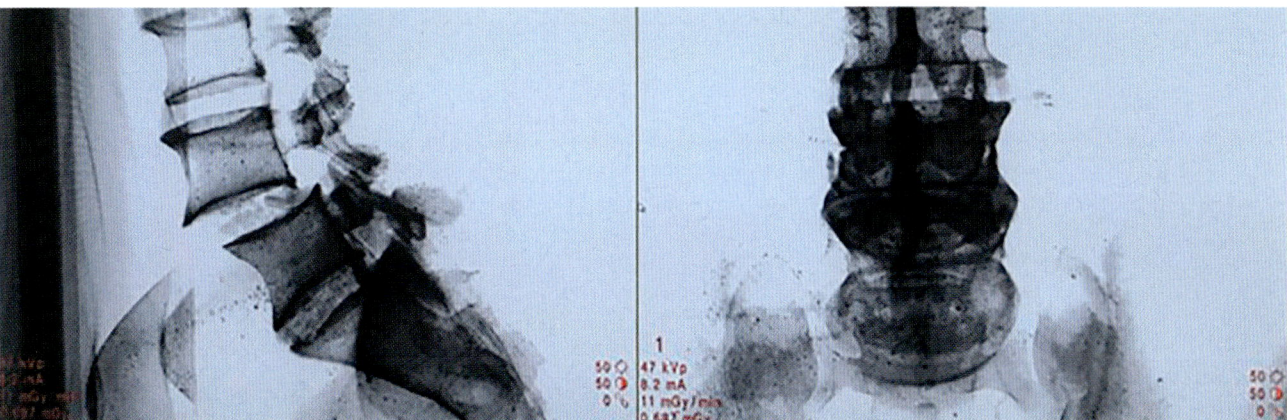

Fig. 21.55 Lateral and AP lumbar spine fusion.

O-Arm Equipment and Basics

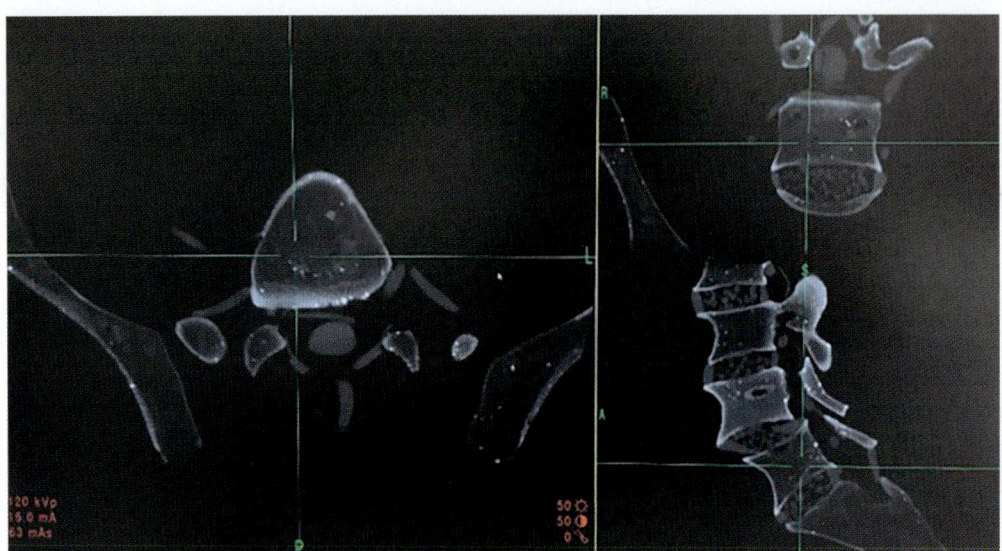

Fig. 21.56 Orientation of the O-arm to the patient anatomy of lumbar spine fusion.

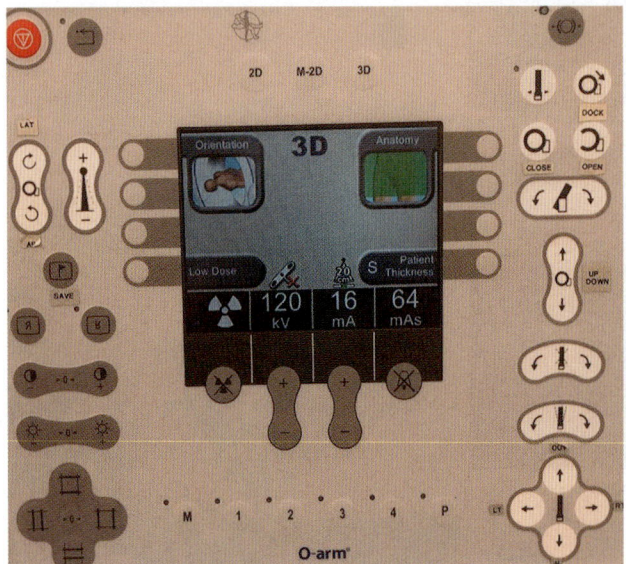

Fig. 21.57 Control panel reorientating the O-arm into the 3D settings.

Best Practices in Surgical Radiography

Performing examinations in the OR can present different challenges for the radiographer. One of the most important differences in the surgical suite is the presence of a team of individuals. Due to the team-based effort, radiation exposure and protection must become a top priority. The radiographer is responsible for all individuals in the exposure area. The uniqueness of the setting requires the radiographer to be familiar with the equipment and intraoperative examinations, which allows them to be an effective member of the surgical team.

1. *Radiation protection:* Radiation safety is essential during surgical procedures. Examinations requiring a C-arm, O-arm, or other fluoroscopic equipment can increase exposure for radiographers, patients, and other health care personnel. Proper shielding attire for the radiographer must be worn, and shielding must be available for other individuals who are in the room during procedures. During exposures, the radiographer should stand a minimum of 2 m (6 feet) from the x-ray tube, and position the x-ray tube for the beam to enter the patient PA, whenever possible, to reduce exposure.
2. *Sterile field:* Although they are part of the surgical team, radiographers are usually nonsterile; therefore, an increased effort must be made to prevent contamination of the sterile field at all times. A radiographer can contaminate the sterile field by touching or reaching over the field. Also, radiography equipment must not compromise the sterile field, surgical procedure, instruments, other personnel, or equipment. If the radiographer believes the sterile field has been contaminated, this must be communicated immediately. Radiology equipment can only be positioned over a sterile field when covered with a sterile drape.
3. *Equipment:* Surgical suites will vary by facility. Some have devoted radiography units, while others require mobile units to move from one surgical suite to another. Most C-arm units will be of similar construction and features; however, becoming familiar with the imaging equipment is the best way to be effective and efficient. Radiography equipment must be cleaned and disinfected after each procedure. Ideally, imaging equipment is cleaned before removal from the surgical suite.
4. *Communication:* Effective communication is essential to ensure that exams are performed accurately and efficiently. The surgical team must be informed before imaging equipment will be used, and the radiographer must announce an exposure before it is made. Removing obstacles, positioning equipment, maintaining the sterile field, and reducing personnel exposure are all aspects of how adequate communication between the radiographer and other team members can be beneficial.
5. *Anatomical structures:* Radiographers must possess proficient knowledge of the anatomical structures visualized in the surgical site during procedures. Understanding the structures and hardware involved in the procedure will allow proper and efficient positioning, resulting in higher-quality images and decreased radiation dose for the patient and personnel.
6. *Intraoperative examinations:* Familiarity with surgical procedures will benefit the radiographer and surgical team. Since imaging equipment is frequently used during orthopedic surgeries, the radiographer should have an understanding of applicable surgical instruments and medical hardware used for the procedure, including pins, screws, plates, and devices. Fracture repairs, spinal fusions, and laminectomies are a few common types of orthopedic surgeries that might use a C-arm. Also, anticipating which examinations require more than one projection enables the radiographer to be an integrated surgical team member.

Definition of Terms

antisepsis: Chemical disinfection of the skin.
asepsis: Absence of infection or germs or elimination of infectious agents.
aseptic technique: Principles involved with manipulation of sterile and nonsterile items to prevent or minimize microbiologic contamination.
contamination: Presence of pathogenic microorganisms.
microbial fallout: Microorganisms normally shed from skin that can contaminate sterile surfaces or areas.
restricted area: Operating rooms, clean core or sterile storage areas.
semirestricted area: Area of peripheral support, such as hallways or corridors leading to restricted areas.
sterile: Substance or object that is completely free of living microorganisms and is incapable of producing any form of organism.
strike-through contamination: Moisture from a nonsterile surface soaking through to a sterile surface, causing bacteria to reach a sterile area.
teamwork: The Association of Surgical Technologists (AST) Standards of Practice Standard I states: "Teamwork is essential for perioperative patient care and is contingent on interpersonal skills. Communication is critical to the positive attainment of expected outcomes of care. All team members should work together for the common good of the patient, for the benefit of the patient and the delivery of actions with the healthcare team, the patient and family, superiors, and peers. Personal integrity and surgical conscience are integrated into every aspect of professional behavior."
unrestricted area: Areas in which street clothes are permitted, such as outer hallways, family waiting areas, locker rooms, and employee lounges.

Selected bibliography

Anderson AC. *The Radiologic Technologist's Handbook of Surgical Procedures*. Philadelphia: CRC Press; 2000.

Fortunato N. *Berry & Kohn's Operating Room Technique*. 9th ed. St Louis: Mosby; 2000.

Huth-Meeker M, Rothrock JC. *Alexander's Care of the Patient in Surgery*. 10th ed. St Louis: Mosby; 1995.

Huth-Meeker M, Rothrock JC. *Alexander's Care of the Patient in Surgery*. 11th ed. St Louis: Mosby; 1999.

Permar JA, Wetterlin KJ. Surgical radiography. In: Frank ED, et al., eds. *Merrill's Atlas of Radiographic Positions and Radiologic Procedures*. vol. 3. St Louis: Mosby; 2007.

Tan LA, Yerneni K, Tuchman A, et al. Utilization of the 3D-printed spine model for free-hand pedicle screw placement in complex spinal deformity correction. *J Spine Surg (Hong Kong)*. 2018;4(2):319–327.

Uneri A, Zhang X, Yi T, et al. Image quality and dose characteristics for an O-arm intraoperative imaging system with model-based image reconstruction. *Med Phys*. 2018;45(11):4857–4868.

Wetterlin KJ. Mobile radiography. In: Frank ED, et al., eds. *Merrill's Atlas of Radiographic Positions and Radiologic Procedures*. vol. 3. St Louis: Mosby; 2007.

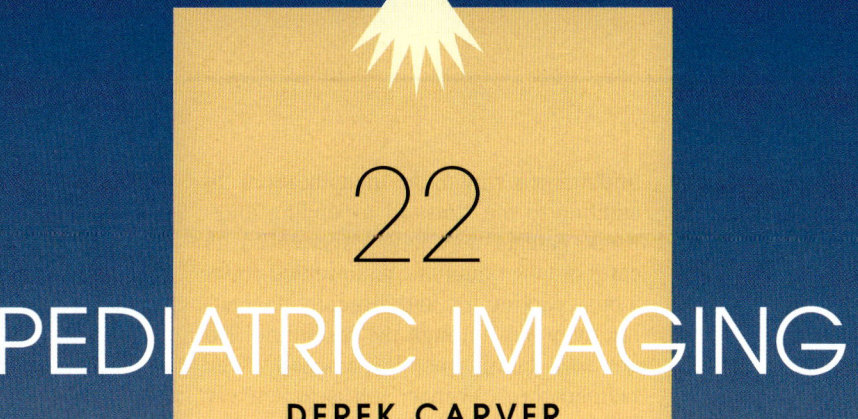

22
PEDIATRIC IMAGING
DEREK CARVER

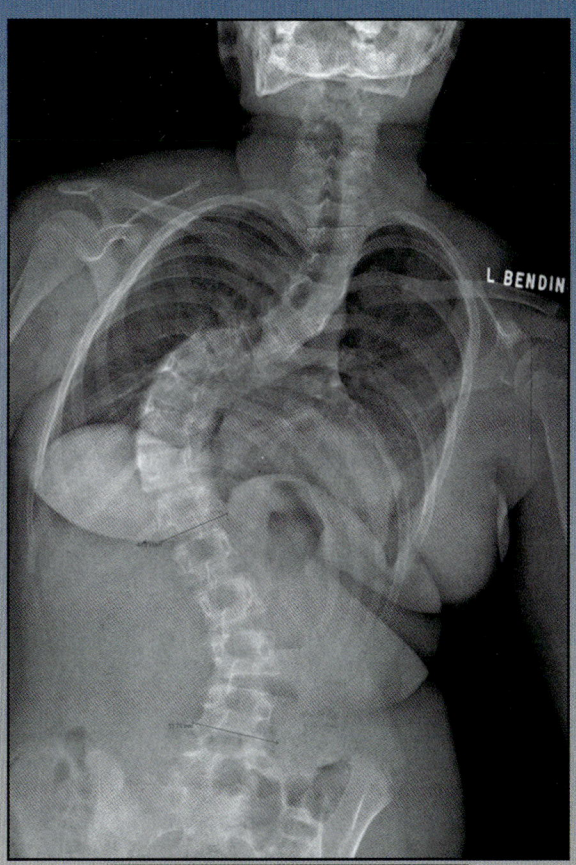

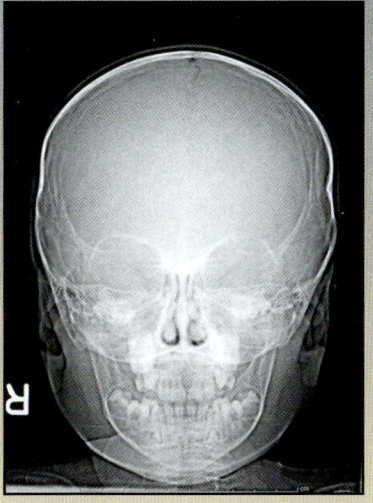

OUTLINE

Introduction to Pediatric Imaging, 72
Best Practices for Pediatric Imaging, 73
Age-Based Development, 73
Patients With Special Needs, 77
Radiation Protection, 80
Abdomen, Gastrointestinal, and Genitourinary Studies, 84
Chest, 92
Pelvis and Hips, 98
Limbs Radiography, 99
Fractures, 101
Skull and Paranasal Sinuses, 104
Soft Tissue Neck, 110
Foreign Bodies, 112
Mobile Considerations for Neonatal Intensive Care Unit (NICU), 115
Simulation: Practicing in a Safe Environment, 124
Selected Pediatric Conditions and Syndromes, 125
Nonaccidental Trauma (Child Abuse), 127
Childhood Pathologies, 134
Advances in Technology, 142

Introduction to Pediatric Imaging

Imaging children is one of the most fascinating and worthwhile specialties in radiography. To witness their cheerful resilience and the parents' acceptance of immense challenges is a privilege. At the same time, pediatric imaging can be one of the most confounding experiences. Radiographers gain skills in multitasking, such as quickly engaging and reassuring the child using an age-appropriate approach, then switching gears to gain the confidence of the parents, explaining and instructing them on immobilization techniques for the exam, all while keeping in mind that other patients are waiting. It is important to be mindful of the various stressors parents may have endured before finding their way to the imaging room. In addition to the stress of a pending diagnosis, parents may have experienced an early or long commute, an unsettled child, a busy parking lot, and difficulty navigating their way through the institution. Do not take family moods personally. The radiographer's primary job is to actively listen to, communicate with, and understand the parents and their children. This is the primary path to achieving cooperation and quality diagnostic radiography. Children take their behavioral cues from facial expressions, intonations, and body postures; an ill-at-ease parent will convey that mood to the child, making the exam more difficult to perform. This overview will present common pediatric exams, mobile considerations, and prevalent pathologies and syndromes.

WAITING ROOM

Waiting and procedure rooms that are well equipped can reduce anxiety and act as a diversion for both the parents and the children. Children are attracted to and amused by toys, thus leaving the parents free to check in, register, and ask pertinent questions. Gender-neutral toys or activities, such as coloring with crayons located at a small age-appropriate table, are most appropriate. (Children should be supervised to prevent them from putting the crayons in their mouths.) Books or magazines for older children are also good investments. The Child Life services of the hospital can provide advice and make appropriate recommendations (Figs. 22.1–22.3).

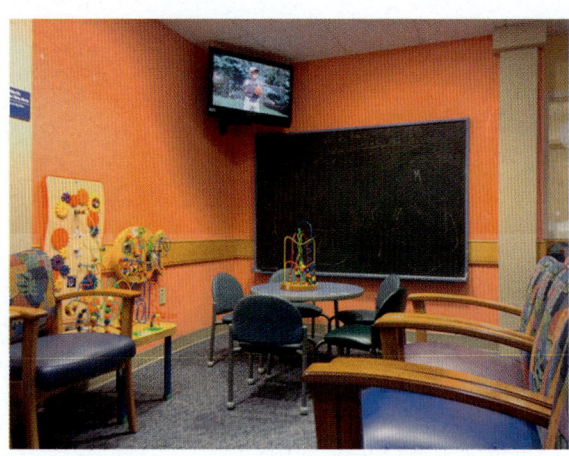

Fig. 22.2 Nuclear medicine waiting room.

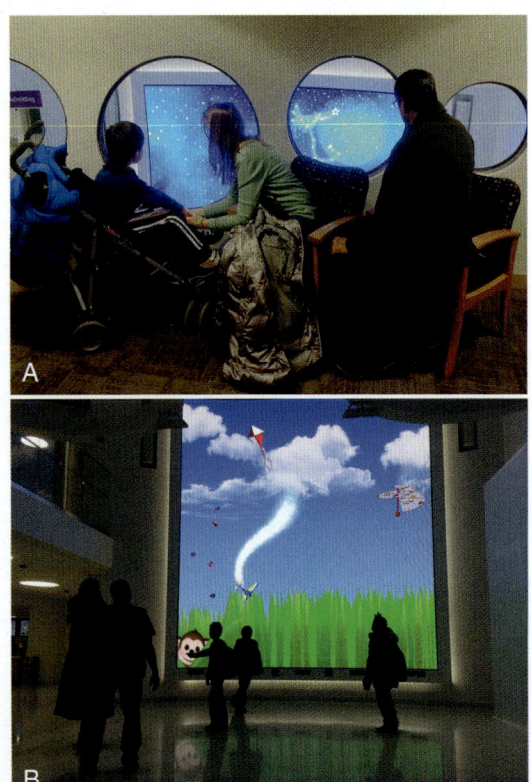

Fig. 22.1 (A) Radiology outpatient and family members viewing the interactive media wall. (B) The interactive media wall from the first-floor lobby.

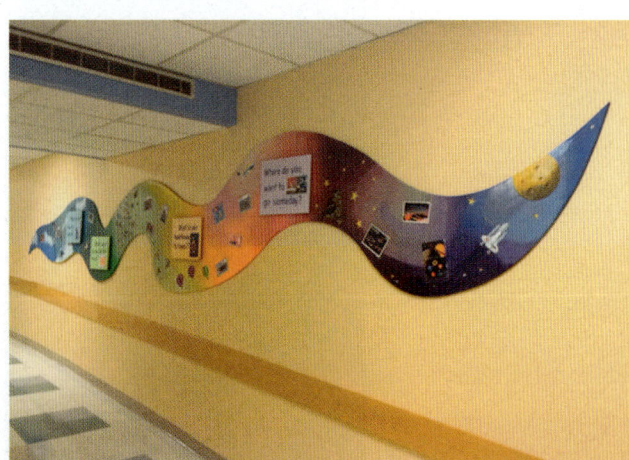

Fig. 22.3 Transition hallway from nuclear medicine to ultrasound.

Best Practices for Pediatric Imaging

SAFETY
- Never leave the patient unattended.
- Keep items that could be swallowed out of reach.

PEDIATRIC RADIOGRAPHY PROTOCOLS
- Protocols provide an easy reference for ordering physicians concerning the required projection based on the pathology indication. Protocols are helpful references for rotating resident staff or new staff radiologists.
- The use of standardized pediatric protocols clarifies the projection/pathology indication, increases image quality, and minimizes radiation (risk) to the patient and staff.

COMMUNICATION
- Introduce yourself while making eye contact with the patient and parents (if culturally appropriate).
- Always speak to a child using language appropriate for the child's developmental level.
- Explain the exam and the anticipated team approach.
- Take history (as required), and discuss pertinent medical information on a level the family can understand.
- Avoid medical jargon and unfamiliar terms. If a medical term cannot be avoided, explain it in lay terms.
- Be mindful not to engage in inappropriate conversations in the presence of the patient.
- Before beginning the exam, ask whether there are any questions or concerns.
- Use teaching sheets for the patient and family when applicable. (These are web-based outlines of your hospital's procedures.)

RESPECT FOR PATIENT/PARENT RIGHTS AND DIGNITY
- Listen to the patient's/parents' questions and concerns.
- Some patients/parents speak English as a second language, which may impede their complete understanding of the exam and the communication of exam results. To better serve the family (and for medicolegal reasons), have an interpreter present.
- Be mindful of cultural preferences and taboos. Ask your interpreter or the family or seek out resources within your institution.
- Always knock before entering, and avoid entering an imaging room while an exam is in progress.

PROVISION OF ADEQUATE CARE AND SERVICE TO THE PATIENT AND FAMILY
- Create a child-friendly environment.
- Use appropriately sized equipment.
- Remember that parents know their children best, so seek and make use of their advice.
- Utilize your child life specialist (CLS); they are invaluable for facilitating cooperation.
- If not contraindicated by the study, use a soft pad with a sheet on the exam table for patient comfort.

Age-Based Development

The pediatric patient may not always fit neatly into the following developmental stages for a variety of reasons (e.g., pathology, developmental delays, parenting, chronic illness or prolonged hospital stay, or mood at the time of exam); however, there are some universal approaches to interacting with children that will always apply (e.g., setting limits, making eye contact, and addressing their fears). Be observant, take cues from the patient and family, and tailor your approach to their interaction. Watch their eyes and body postures. Are the parents gripping things tightly? Do you need to set limits for their children? Is the child tense or clinging to a parent's leg? Listen to the child's choice of words.

With a team approach, connect with the family before the exam begins. Introductions should always be made in a slow and relaxed fashion. Cultural norms are important, and although the family might make allowances for ignorance, it is best to educate yourself on the norms and appropriate behaviors related to the family's cultural practices. Learn a few words or phrases in the languages most common to your patient's demographic. Cultural biases can also work in reverse; the family might make assumptions about you and how they treat you based on your sex or socioeconomic status in their country of origin. Consulting your interpreter for advice is the first place to start.

PREMATURE INFANTS
Generally, bedside radiography and gastrointestinal (GI) and genitourinary (GU) procedures using fluoroscopy encompass most of the contact radiographers will have with premature infants in the department. Elevate the room temperature 10 to 15 minutes prior to the patient's arrival. When these babies are in radiology for a procedure, an intensive care unit (ICU) nursing team will accompany them. The nursing team will provide care for the patient, but you will need to explain the procedure and how the nursing team can help. Obtain the current status of the patient and any special requests from the nursing staff. As with any exam, suction and oxygen must always be available and the room well stocked. Leave the patient in the incubator (warmed Isolette) until just before the procedure. Depending on the exam, you may be able to use a radiolucent cushion on the exam table for patient comfort. Discuss the patient immobilization plan (who will hold, how, what body part) with the nursing staff to ensure that you accommodate the patient's medical conditions. Have warming lights available, wash hands, wear gloves, and adhere to all isolation precautions.

NEONATE (0 TO 28 DAYS)
The neonatal period is a time of transition from the uterine environment to the outside world. During this first month, the newborn is forming attachments with caregivers. They are sensitive to the way they are held, rocked, and positioned. They love to be swaddled, which gives them a sense of security and keeps them from being disturbed by their startle reflex. Newborns are easily startled when moved quickly or upon hearing a loud noise. Bright lights cause them to blink frequently or close their eyes. Understandably, the hospital environment in particular creates stressors for neonates; these stressors should be minimized whenever possible.

Because newborns are most secure and comfortable when swaddled, keep them in this position until just before you are ready for imaging. Decrease noise and brightness levels whenever possible, maintain a warm room, and always use warming lights unless the nursing team directs otherwise. Speak soothingly and try to avoid sudden, quick movements. Let the caregivers know exactly what is expected during imaging and involve them in soothing and calming their infant. Pacifiers, oral sucrose (check with the nursing team), a personal blanket, and quiet singing can all help to soothe newborns, enabling them to feel safe and secure.

INFANT (28 DAYS TO 18 MONTHS)

During different periods of infancy, babies experience stranger and separation anxiety. When working with infants, involve the parents whenever possible; the comfort of seeing the parent's/caregiver's face, hearing that familiar voice, and feeling the caregiver's touch can be invaluable when calming the infant.

The radiographer and the CLS play important roles in establishing a relationship with the infant by talking and smiling; this will help put the parents at ease and demonstrate care and concern for their baby. The caregiver knows the infant best, so ask what soothes and comforts the baby when they are distressed. Personal objects, such as a pacifier or a blanket, can distract and soothe the infant during the exam. To ease the transition from the parent's arms to the exam table, it is advisable to decrease stimuli and eliminate loud noises. Keeping the baby swaddled or in their carrier until just prior to imaging minimizes transitions and reduces the baby's time on the exam table. The first rule of imaging infants is never to leave the infant unattended; the radiographer or parent should always have a hand on the infant. The second rule is to always cushion the exam table under the infant's skull. Be sure not to flex the head forward, which may cause respiratory difficulties.

TODDLER (18 MONTHS TO 3 YEARS)

Toddlers can be a challenge for both radiographers and staff. Toddlers are not abstract thinkers and may not understand the concept of "inside their body." They operate very much in the "here and now." They are seldom able to keep their bodies still, which can make imaging problematic, and they also have a short attention span and become overwhelmed quickly. Toddlers are fearful of medical experiences and often become unruly while they are being positioned for an exam. Unfamiliar exam positions and faces can escalate their movement.

In an effort to provide adequate care and minimize reactions, keep language brief and use concrete words. Because keeping their body still is most often an issue, efficiency is crucial. Be sure the room is organized before the patient and family enter. If the toddler has a toy or blanket, keep it within reach during the examination. Distraction techniques can be extremely helpful in keeping the toddler calm. A screaming toddler can often be distracted and calmed by being allowed to blow bubbles or use a tablet computer with an age-appropriate application.

After the imaging has been completed, let the child know they did a great job, that you are proud of them, and that they should be proud of themselves. Praise may be in the form of positive statements or a small reward, such as a sticker or balloon.

PRESCHOOLER (3 TO 5 YEARS)

New places, faces, and experiences can be overwhelming to preschoolers. Unfamiliar sights, sounds, and faces can be quite intimidating and can leave the preschooler feeling frightened. In addition, preschoolers are establishing routines and greatly benefit from structure and knowing what to expect. For preschoolers, the medical environment is unpredictable, so often these patients need time to explore and familiarize themselves with the imaging room, even if it is brief. They also need to feel comfortable with the clinicians working with them. Taking the time to establish rapport will be instrumental in making preschoolers feel comfortable, thus enhancing their coping abilities (Figs. 22.4–22.6).

Additional steps include letting them know exactly what to expect and what is expected of them. For example, mention the loud sounds of the "camera," show the movement of the "camera," let them feel the coldness of a solution or cotton ball, and most importantly, assure them that you will let them know before you do anything. These simple courtesies facilitate trust and cooperation and help the child feel more comfortable. Some preschoolers may have difficulty understanding the exam through dialogue. Therefore, when speaking with them about imaging or "taking pictures," it may be helpful to model this process using a doll or stuffed animal.

Although preschoolers are developing independence and want to establish themselves apart from their parents, they can become fearful if separated from them; utilizing parents can be instrumental to the success of the exam. If the parents are not able to remain with the child during imaging, allow the parents to pick up and comfort the child when the procedure is completed.

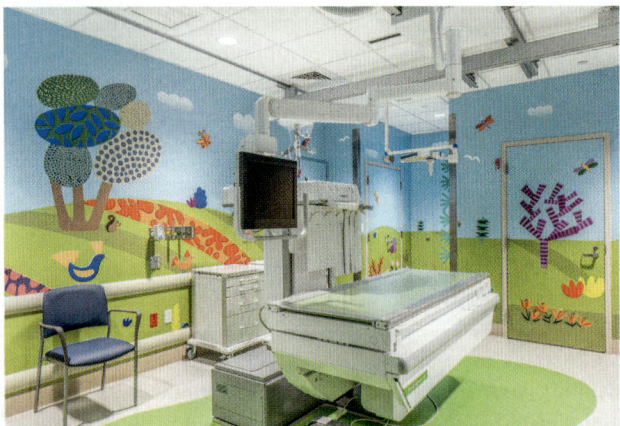

Fig. 22.4 New fluoroscopy rooms are designed with pediatric patients in mind. Imaginative décor and lighting help ease anxiety and make for an enjoyable patient and family experience.

(Courtesy Richard Gayle Photography, Boston Children's Hospital, L'Attitude Art and Lisa Houck.)

When working with patients of this age, use directive statements to facilitate cooperation; for example, "It's time to ..." or "You can help me by ..." are directive statements that will limit their response, leaving them more likely to comply. Open-ended questions that begin with "Do you want to (e.g., get on the table)?" leave preschoolers feeling as if they have a choice when, in reality, getting on the table and having the exam is not optional. Open-ended statements

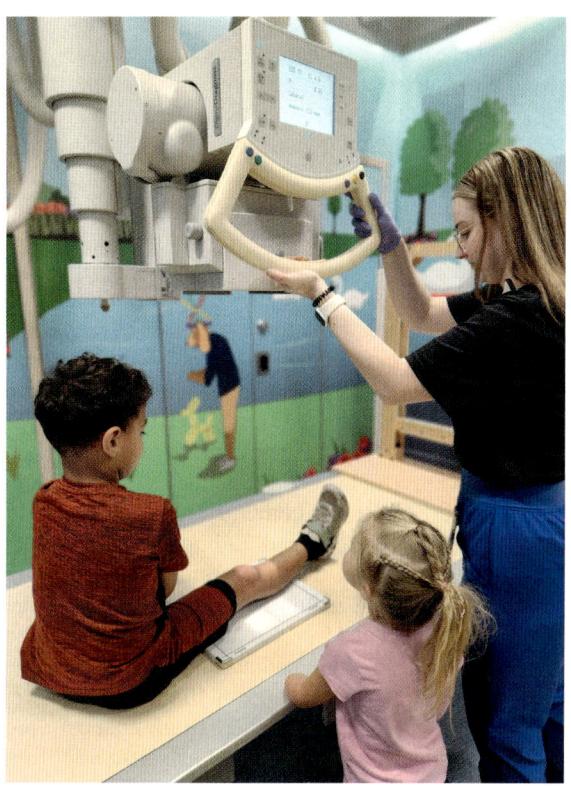

Fig. 22.5 Taking the time to establish rapport will be instrumental in making preschoolers feel comfortable in the radiography room.

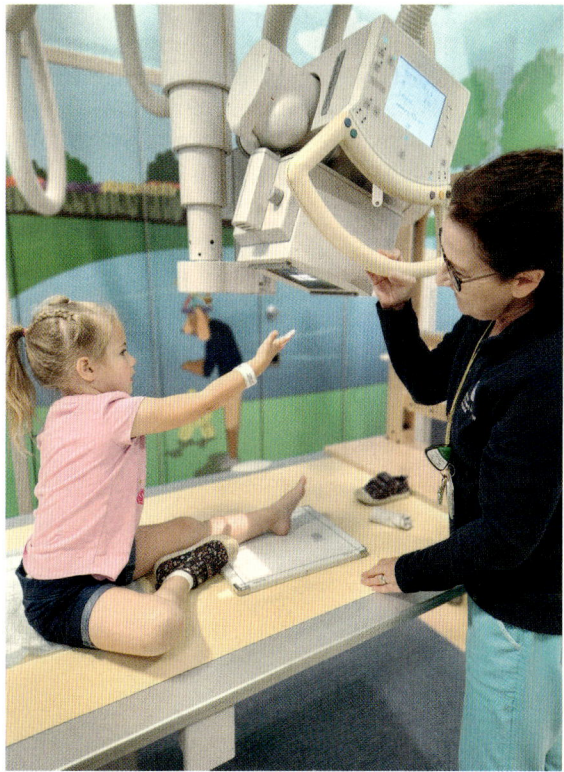

Fig. 22.6 The radiographer should make an introduction to the child and show the child how the collimator light is used.

confuse preschoolers and can leave them feeling overwhelmed. Preschoolers are constantly seeking approval from others and respond well to positive affirmations. Praise and encouragement are beneficial for this age-group, as they will create a positive experience and help boost the preschooler's confidence in future medical appointments.

SCHOOL AGE (6 TO 12 YEARS)

School-age children are becoming logical thinkers and developing a fear of failure, so positive affirmations and reassurances are extremely beneficial. They are curious and full of questions; take the opportunity to connect using age-appropriate explanations. Break down the exam into steps, let them know exactly what to expect and what is expected of them, and most importantly, let them know before you do anything. These simple courtesies will facilitate trust and cooperation and help the child feel more comfortable.

Avoid unfamiliar medical jargon, as this will only confuse school-age children and can decrease their ability to cope. Children of this age range are very literal, so it is crucial to avoid words that can be misconstrued, such as *shoot, shot,* or *dye*. School-age patients benefit from being given choices; this will give them a sense of control and entitlement, which inevitably enhances their coping abilities. However, be cautious to give only realistic choices; cajoling the child using open-ended questions could mislead the child.

It is important to make imperative or interrogative statements, such as "It's time to get changed; would you like the green gown or the blue one?" or "You need to get on the table; would you like me to help you, or would you like your mom to help you?" These choices are direct and allow for realistic decisions. Coping and distraction techniques available to patients and staff, such as taking deep breaths, blowing bubbles, listening to music, watching a movie, or playing games with a tablet, can be instrumental in helping children cope during exams.

ADOLESCENT (12 TO 18 YEARS)

When imaging adolescents, respect their need for privacy by providing a private area for changing, knocking before entering their exam room, and limiting the number of staff involved. These actions will help to alleviate stress. If you have clinicians (for GI/GU, magnetic resonance imaging [MRI], or computed tomography [CT] procedures) and radiographers of both sexes (and if time permits), ask the patient if they would feel more comfortable with a male or a female performing the exam. In many pediatric centers, girls who have reached the age of 10 to 12 years must be asked whether there is any chance they might be pregnant. You may also ask whether the girl has started menstruating. A truthful response is more probable if the parent is not present when these questions are asked. The patient's response will dictate whether further explanation is required. For example, you may need to add, "We ask these same questions of all girls because unborn babies are extremely sensitive to radiation exposure."

If it is necessary for adolescent patients to disclose their medical history, speak directly to them and their parents rather than just the parents. Radiographers tend to ask the parents this information, but it is important to remember that adolescents most often know their bodies best. As adolescents, they do not always discuss things with their parents for reasons of embarrassment or shame. In addition, before beginning the exam, ask the adolescent patient whether they would like to have a parent present during imaging. This gives adolescents a choice and lets them know it is okay to ask parents to step out.

It is not uncommon for the adolescent patient to respond negatively to having an exam. In addition to being extremely modest, they often see themselves as invincible and do not believe that anything could possibly be wrong with them. Adolescents also fear being "different" and are afraid of something happening to their bodies that would alter their appearance or make them unlike their peers. Validating their feelings and letting them know you want to help will reassure them. For example, you might say: "I understand the way you are feeling; lots of teenagers have this test done and they feel the same way" or "I am here to help you as best I can." Assisting adolescents with preparation, explaining the rationale for why the exam is taking place, and giving them tools for coping will facilitate cooperation and decrease fears. Deep breathing, listening to music, or having a conversation with a caregiver can help put the patient at ease.

Patients With Special Needs

The radiographer should consider age and behavior when approaching children with physical and mental disabilities. School-age children with disabilities strive to achieve as much autonomy and independence as possible. They are sensitive to the fact that they are less independent than their peers. The radiographer should observe the following guidelines:

- Introduce yourself and identify the patients at their level (you may have to kneel down); then briefly explain the procedure to the child and parents. All children appreciate being given the opportunity to listen and respond. As with all patients, children want to be spoken to rather than talked about.
- If this approach proves ineffective, turn to the parents. Generally, the parents of these patients are present and can be very helpful. In strange environments, younger children may trust only one person—the parent. In that case, the medical team can gain cooperation from the child by communicating through the parent. Parents often know the best way to lift and transfer the child from the wheelchair or stretcher to the table. Children with physical disabilities often have a fear of falling and may want only a parent's assistance.
- Place the wheelchair or stretcher parallel to the imaging table, taking care to explain that you have locked the wheelchair or stretcher and will be getting help for the transfer. These children often know the way they should be lifted—*ask them*. They can tell you which areas to support and which actions they prefer to do themselves.

Finally, children with spastic contractions are often frustrated by their inability to control movements counterproductive to the exam. A gentle massage or a warm blanket may be used to help relax the muscles.

Communicating with a child who has a mental disability can be difficult, depending on the severity of the disability. Some patients react to verbal stimuli, whereas loud or abrupt noises may startle or agitate them. Ask the parent or caregiver if there is anything you should know about the child to help achieve a quick and accurate exam. Limitations of psychological, behavioral, or physical impairments may not be obvious or referenced on the exam order.

AUTISM SPECTRUM DISORDERS[a]

Medical imaging of individuals with autism spectrum disorders (ASDs) can be difficult. In addition to difficulties with communication, there are also behavioral issues, medical issues, and environmental concerns that need to be considered. There are important steps that should be taken before the patient is brought into the examination room and, in some cases, before they come to the imaging facility.

According to the Centers for Disease Control and Prevention (CDC), ASDs are a group of developmental disabilities that can cause significant social, communication, and behavioral challenges. People with ASDs handle information differently than other people do. The word "spectrum" means that autism can range from very mild to severe. There are some similar symptoms across the spectrum, such as problems with social interaction; however, there are differences in time of onset, severity, and the nature of the symptoms. One popular saying within the autism community is "If you know one person with autism, then you know one person with autism." Patients with ASDs require specialized treatment plans for parents, caregivers, and physicians. What works well for one individual may not be effective for another, which makes imaging individuals with ASDs a unique challenge.

The prevalence of autism is on the rise. In 2020, the CDC estimated the prevalence of ASD among children in the United States at 1 in 36 diagnosed by age 8. Males are four times as likely to be diagnosed as females, and on average the diagnosis is earlier for those with more severe symptoms. Parents may notice the difference as early as the age of 6 months, whereas high functioning individuals, such as those with Asperger syndrome, may be diagnosed at around 6 years of age.

Occasionally patients with ASDs are identified before scheduling imaging procedures. The CDC has several publications on the diagnosis of ASDs; however, for facilitating imaging procedures, the following are commonly recognized signs of autism:

- Difficulty with social interaction.
- Problems with verbal and nonverbal communication.
- Repetitive behaviors or narrow, obsessive interests.

Special considerations for imaging

Once an ASD patient is identified, there are many things we can do to provide a successful imaging experience for both the radiographer and the patient. Whether or not the patient is in the department, we should begin by asking more questions. Box 22.1 is an example of a patient questionnaire. It might be beneficial to schedule the exam at a time when the department is not busy. Loud noises or visual overstimulation can be distracting and, in some cases, can cause severe behaviors. This can be especially true during the adolescent years. Because these children are larger, aggressive or violent behavior can be dangerous for the patient or staff. It is wise to prepare for all possibilities. A good patient questionnaire can help gather resources and prepare the environment. You can use the questionnaire to know when to eliminate noises or adjust lighting.

[a] Written by Jerry Tyree.

BOX 22.1

Autism patient questionnaire

Is your child sensitive to fluorescent lighting?
Is your child comfortable in a dimly lit room?
Is your child tactile defensive, or sensitive to touch?
  If yes, explain.
Is your child sensitive to loud noises?
  High frequencies?
  Low frequencies?
Is your child uncomfortable in cool or cold situations?
Is your child uncomfortable in warm or hot situations?
Do you have any calming objects you would like your child to have in the imaging suite?
Will your child find a video played during the procedure calming?

Try to give the patient with an ASD the first or last appointment of the day. People with ASD find waiting around for an appointment extremely stressful. Waiting in busy hospital corridors will increase the stress level of an already anxious child or adult. If possible, find a small side room the family can wait in. Alternatively, they may prefer to wait outside or in the car, and a member of staff should be identified to collect them or call their cell phone when the radiographer is ready. If the appointment is likely to be delayed, the family may wish to leave the building completely and return at a later agreed-upon time.

Temperature is often difficult to adjust, but patient dress can be modified if it is an issue. Many individuals with autism are sensitive to touch. They have difficulty habituating stimuli of any type. Some may wear socks inside out so that they cannot feel the seams on their toes. These are serious issues for individuals on the spectrum.

Sometimes we need to modify our positioning techniques for individuals who are tactile defensive, or sensitive to touch. A sensitivity to the "poking" often used to find anatomic landmarks can also be problematic. Some barbers have found that once you touch, you maintain the touch until you are finished with the haircut. One hand must remain on the head until the haircut is complete. We can use this same concept with imaging; once you begin to touch, do not remove your hand until you have all the information you need.

Videos can be a double-edged sword. Although a familiar video can be calming, if it varies in any small way from the one the child is used to, it can instead cause a severe reaction. It might be best if patients bring in videos of their own, especially if the procedure is expected to be long.

Personal space and body awareness

A crowded waiting room may be distressing for people with an ASD who may need their personal space. Similarly, close proximity to the radiographer could be uncomfortable for the patient.

Problems can also occur when trying to explain where pain is experienced. Those who have difficulty with body awareness may not be able to experience where different body parts are.

Touch

Individuals with ASDs may be hypersensitive to touch, or tactile defensive. They may find a light touch very painful. Some of these patients may prefer more deep pressure in touching, or you may not be able to touch them at all.

Patient responses

Do not be surprised if the patient does not make eye contact, especially if they are distressed. Lack of eye contact does not necessarily mean the patient is not listening to what you are saying. Allow the patient extra time to process what you have said. Do not assume that a nonverbal patient cannot understand what you are saying.

People with ASD can have a high pain threshold. Even if the child does not appear to be in pain, they may, for example, have broken a bone. ASD patients may show an unusual response to pain, including laughter, humming, singing, and clothing removal. Agitation and behavior may be the only clues that the child or adult is in pain.

Communication

Use clear, simple language with short sentences. People with ASDs tend to take everything literally. Thus, if you say, "It will only hurt for a minute," they will expect the pain to have gone within one minute.

Make your language concrete, and avoid using idioms, irony, metaphors, and words with double meanings (e.g., "It's raining cats and dogs out there," which could cause the patient to look outside for cats and dogs). Avoid using body language, gestures, or facial expressions without verbal instructions, as the patient may not understand these nonverbal messages.

Consider involving a caregiver to facilitate communication. Many individuals respond slowly, and patience is required.

Noise

Some departments use buzzers to indicate when it is a patient's turn to have an exam. They may also have music playing in the waiting room. Crying babies or children in the waiting room may also be quite noisy. For those with hypersensitive hearing, these types of noises can be magnified and become disturbing or even painful. Additionally, with this heightened volume, surrounding sounds could become distorted. This could make it difficult for the person with ASD to recognize sounds, such as a name being called. Individuals may respond by putting their fingers in their ears, whereas others may "stim" (e.g., flap hands, flick fingers, rock back and forth). This kind of behavior is calming to the individual, so do not try to stop it unless absolutely necessary. Individuals with ASDs often retreat when overstimulated.

Injections/needlesticks

If the patient needs an injection or blood test, divert their attention elsewhere. The use of pictures or a doll is a good idea to demonstrate what is going to happen. People with ASD can be either undersensitive or oversensitive to pain, such that some may feel the pain acutely and be very distressed, whereas others may not appear to react at all.

It is advisable to assume that the patient will feel pain. Use of a local anesthetic cream, such as a eutectic mixture of local anesthetics, helps to numb the site of injection. Sand timers and clocks can be used as distracters during procedures such as injections, allowing the person with autism to see a definite end.

Tips for radiographers

Relaxation techniques such as deep breathing, counting, singing favorite songs, talking about a favorite interest, or looking at favorite books or toys could also help during physical examinations or treatments. Parents may be instructed to bring a favorite toy or a video if a player is available in the procedure room.

Make sure that directions are given step by step, verbally, visually, and by providing physical support or prompts as needed by the patient. Patients with ASDs often have trouble interpreting facial expressions, body language, and tone of voice. Be as concrete and explicit as possible in your instructions and feedback to the patient. Demonstrating on others or on toys to show what will happen during a physical examination can reassure an individual with ASD.

Many children with autism fixate on routines. Most medical imaging will fall outside of their routines. To make something unfamiliar seem more routine, social stories can be used. A social story can be a written or visual guide describing various social interactions or situations. These stories can be in books, on flashcards, or provided online by the department so that the family can share with the patient what it is like to go to the x-ray department. The caregiver can revisit or practice these social stories prior to the exam. Pictures of the parking garage, waiting room, imaging room, and even the individual radiographer can be added. The more accurate these pictures are, the better they will work. It might even be helpful to take pictures from the perspective of the individual with ASD. If the patient is lying on an x-ray table, a picture taken up toward the tube or scanner might be appropriate. In this way, a social story can be used to make something the individual has never done before seem routine. Parents of many children with ASDs create social stories for vacations, plane rides, trips to the amusement park, and so on. Parents and caregivers who use these social stories will vouch for their effectiveness. In addition to social stories, allowing the patient with autism and their caregivers access to the facility before the exam may be helpful. This allows a "dry run" of the procedure, which may reduce anxiety during the actual exam.

In summation, the combination of a questionnaire, social stories, and the patient application of the aforementioned principles should greatly help when imaging individuals with ASDs. Preparation is key, but it need not be prohibitively time consuming. Creating a social story for every exam an imaging department does is ideal, but simplification is possible. Making social stories accessible online is desirable. Adding pictures and images, especially accurate ones of specific facilities, increases the comfort level of patients. These practices are also good for all patients, not just those with ASDs. Many advocates would say that better serving individuals with ASDs (or others with "different" abilities) has improved schools, social services, and the lives of all they touch. The same could be said of our imaging departments.

Radiation Protection
DOSE AND DIAGNOSTIC INFORMATION

The goal in administering radiation for a specific clinical indication is to ensure that the *diagnostic* information obtained will be of greater value than the potential risks associated with the radiation. To protect our patients, we should identify through scientific testing an acceptable level of quantum mottle for each exam that will not compromise the diagnostic goal of the image. As medical practitioners, we attempt to use the minimum radiation dose required to produce a *clinically diagnostic* image for a specific clinical indication; this is our primary goal as radiographers and radiologists. Radiographers should observe the following steps:

- Take direct efforts toward proper centering and selection of exposure factors, as well as precise collimation, which all contribute to safe practice.
- Instead of the anteroposterior (AP) projection, use the posteroanterior (PA) projection of the thorax and skull to reduce the amount of radiation reaching the breast tissue and lens of the eye, respectively.
- Use pulsed fluoroscopy with "last image hold" to reduce patient dose and length of examination.

A cautionary note: The fact that digitally acquired images can be "post-processed," thereby correcting some exposure errors, does not negate an important truth—images of diagnostic quality are achieved by proper positioning. The anatomy to be demonstrated must be in proper alignment with the automatic exposure control (AEC) detector.

Child versus adult

The possible long-term stochastic effects of a low linear energy transfer (LET) radiation dose on pediatric patients, if they exist, are much greater than the same dose to an adult because the child has a longer lifetime over which to express any long-term effects, and due to the child's smaller body volume, the potential exists to expose multiple organ systems to radiation for any given exam.

Dose reduction and gonad shielding

The AAPM, ACR, ASRT, ARRT, and several other professional imaging organizations published their position statements in early 2019, which state that gonadal shielding can negatively impact exam efficacy (see Chapter 1). Additionally, research has failed to link damage from radiation exposure to the developing fetus or reproductive organs. Shielding can also contribute to obscuring pertinent anatomy and pathology and could increase patient dose. With this in mind, males and females are not shielded for pelvic exams (Figs. 22.7 and 22.8).

Discussing radiation risks and benefits with parents

Just as you have developed exam-based routines, you should have an example-based "script" for discussing the risk/benefit equation of radiation exposure. Fortunately, most radiology departments

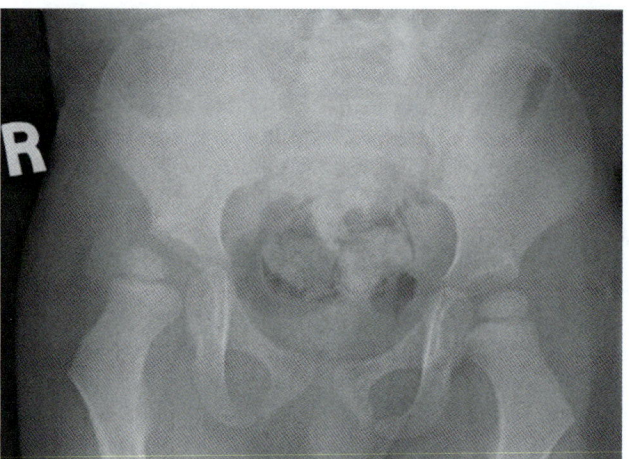

Fig. 22.7 First time AP pelvis exam for hip dysplasia (no gonad shielding).

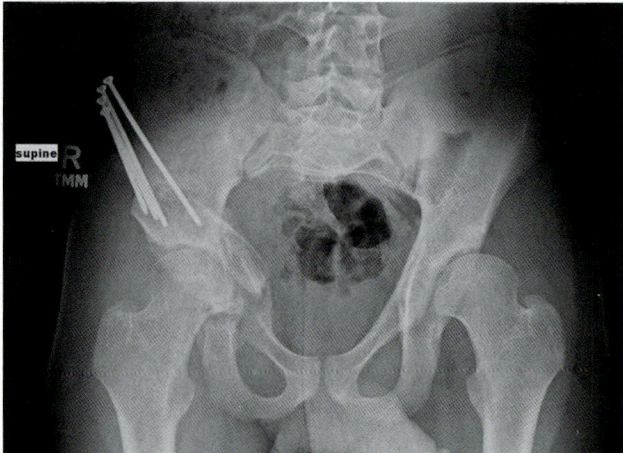

Fig. 22.8 Pelvis x-ray demonstrating a postoperative right-sided periacetabular osteotomy (PAO) for developmental dysplasia of the hip (DDH).

have developed patient information sheets of frequently asked questions (FAQ) concerning radiation dose and patients' fears, with answers that are backed up by current science and regulations. Regardless, when parents have questions, listen carefully and hear their fears (which may only be implied), and take into consideration their points of reference for understanding radiation dose (usually CT) and their educational level. Be aware that people in medical settings, especially when under stress, often hear only 50% of what is being said; additionally, they often give greater weight to negative information. Be knowledgeable and confident with your answers (e.g., through body language, tone, interest, and clarity of presentation without technical jargon); a rambling or confusing presentation will do more harm than good. "In risk perception theory, perception equals reality. This means there may be no correlation between public perceptions of risk and scientific or technical information. Therefore, you must discuss the risk based on the perception."[1]

Reframing the way patients and parents understand radiation risks (if they exist) and benefits should be your first goal. Human exposure to x-radiation is usually "understood" through the subjectivity of the lay press, the sensationalism of TV shows, and the half-truths of word of mouth. A wonderfully clear and effective, but often overlooked, approach to help place radiation exposure in perspective is to reference the dose the child will receive for any given exam to the background radiation we all receive daily. Background equivalent radiation time (BERT) equates a particular exam-based radiation dose to the equivalent amount of radiation dose received daily from our natural background (Table 22.1). The BERT method has several advantages: (1) the patient readily understands it; (2) it does not mention radiation risk, which is unknown; and (3) it educates the patient that they live in a sea of natural background radiation.

The lay public's preoccupation with the perceived risks of x-radiation often overshadows the benefits of the diagnostic imaging exam. When a physician orders a radiation-based exam, it is with confidence that the diagnostic information obtained will outweigh any potential risks (if there are any) of an image. Declining an exam based on perceived risks creates the real risk of a missed diagnosis.

TABLE 22.1
Comparison of pediatric exam dose to background radiation level

Exam	Natural background radiation equivalent[a] (time to receive equivalent background radiation)
Chest CT, high resolution (pulmonary embolism, angiogram)	730 days (6 mSv)
Abdominal CT	365 days (3 mSv)
Abdomen/pelvic radiograph	90 days (0.75 mSv)
Chest radiograph, two view	2.5 days (0.02 mSv)
Natural background radiation	1 day (0.008 mSv)

[a]Using an average background radiation level of 3 mSv/year.
Data from Peck DJ, Samei E: How to understand and communicate radiation risk. *Image Wisely* (website). 2017. https://www.imagewisely.org/imaging-modalities/computed-tomography/medical-physicists/articles/how-to-understand-and-communicate-radiation-risk. (Accessed October 2023); Colang JE, Killion JB, Vano E: Patient dose from CT: a literature review, *Radiol Technol* 79:17, 2007.

Radiographers holding for exams

Effective use of immobilization techniques must always be attempted first, which means imaging pediatric patients may require the radiographer to hold the patient. The challenge for the radiographer is to avoid repeating the exam. Contrary to the literature, the use of tape, Velcro, plexiglass, and sandbags does have limitations. Radiographers are encouraged to hold only as a last resort, but there are many challenging exams that would, even with the best of instruction, have a low chance of success using only parents to hold the patient. Avoiding repeat radiographs is the primary objective for any pediatric radiographer to align with ALARA, so in many cases, technologists will have to hold the infant or toddler when performing images of the abdomen, skull, soft tissue neck (STN), pelvis, chest, scoliosis, hips-to-ankles, or upper or lower extremities. In deciding whether to hold for an exam, radiographers seek to balance the potential stochastic risks of radiation exposure to themselves (scatter) against the possibility of having to repeat a child's x-ray (primary beam) because of a parent's unsuccessful attempt at immobilization. If our ultimate goal is to reduce the overall dose to the patient and ourselves, where is the balance?

Evaluating the parents' ability to hold their child firmly enough to prevent movement and achieve correct positioning should begin when you introduce yourself. Is the parent/guardian attentive to what you say? Are they tentative first-time parents? Are they overindulgent and unable to set limits? Are they so concerned with radiation exposure that they have difficulty listening to instructions? Are they overwhelmed with parenting? Do they come with an attitude that will prevent them from listening? Does the patient's physical condition make the patient a challenge to hold? Is the presence of social media in the exam room a distraction? An affirmative answer to any of these questions may suggest that a radiographer do the holding. Allowing a parent who is probably not capable of successfully holding the patient to do so in order to prevent a small, low LET, occupational dose (scatter) to the radiographer is not in the patient's best interest; the patient, now facing a repeat, receives twice the primary beam radiation dose, and the radiographer will still end up having to hold. Before making the decision to hold, the radiographer should make every attempt at immobilization or instruct the parent/caregiver clearly and slowly, using lay terms, while demonstrating the technique. After the parent has attempted to hold the child, the radiographer must decide whether to continue to allow the parent to hold or to step in personally, thereby assuring that a diagnostic exam is achieved on the first try. The goal of any radiographic exam is to produce an image with a radiation dose as low as diagnostically achievable while providing good patient and family care. This is a lot to juggle even for the seasoned pediatric radiographer, and it takes a lot of experience to perform well.

Artifacts

The dynamic range of digital radiography has increased the universe (number and type) of artifacts visible on images. The usual suspects are dirt, scratches, metallic or radiopaque objects on the patient, equipment errors, and motion. The following is a partial list of artifacts unique to digital radiography:

- Soap or starches in patient gowns that appear as long, slender objects of irregular densities (Fig. 22.9).
- Textured or thick hair, cornrows, dreadlocks, ponytails, bobby pins, hair clips, or any object woven into the hair.
- Clothing seams, sweatpants eyelets, silkscreen designs, appliqué or embroidery, textured t-shirts, onesies, dry or wet diapers, and sanitary pads.

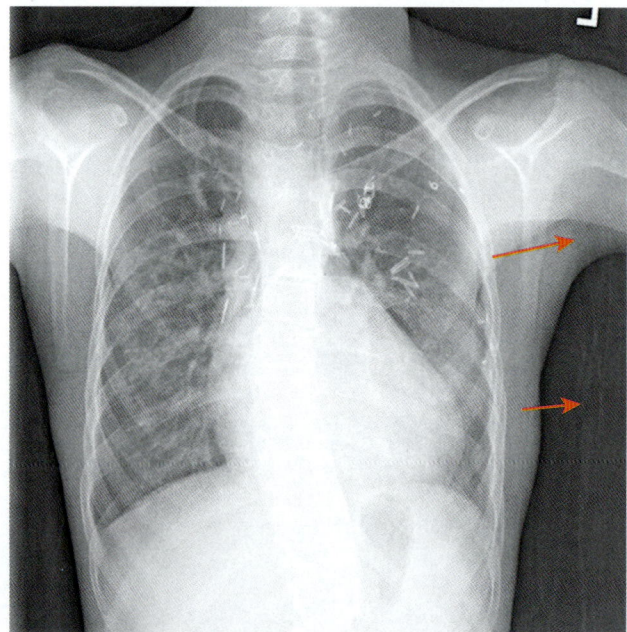

Fig. 22.9 Soap or starches in patient gowns appear as long, slender irregular densities (arrows).

- Earrings, glitter, rhinestones, pearls, belly button rings, or other piercings. You may encounter some resistance from parents concerning the removal of an infant's new ear piercing studs; assure the parent that the holes will not close during the time it takes to generate the exam images (Fig. 22.10).

The ratio of artifact size to body volume is greater in pediatric patients than adults. In other words, given two images, one of an adult and one of an infant and both of the same anatomic area, and given two artifacts of the same size, shape, and density located in the same spot within those same anatomic areas, the likelihood of detecting the artifact in the infant's image would be greater due to the artifact's size relative to the anatomy. To reduce clothing artifacts, remove any piece of clothing covering the anatomy of interest. Paper orthopedic shorts are radiolucent and can be used for pelvic and abdominal imaging. Years of experience support this approach; failure to remove clothing will result in clothing artifacts and possible repeat images. When there is a need to observe breathing patterns (chests), particularly in children who cannot hold their breath (those younger than 6 or 7 years old), a good rule of thumb is to remove clothes from the waist up so that the radiographer can observe breathing. In general, with patients who cannot follow breathing instructions and with the rotor prepped, full belly distention equals a full chest inspiration! As noted earlier, it is well documented that patients in a hospital setting hear about 50% of what is said, so when the patients/parents enter the exam room after changing, ask them again if they have removed the requested pieces of clothing. Clear communication is paramount, followed closely by checking for compliance. Trust, but verify. Do not assume.

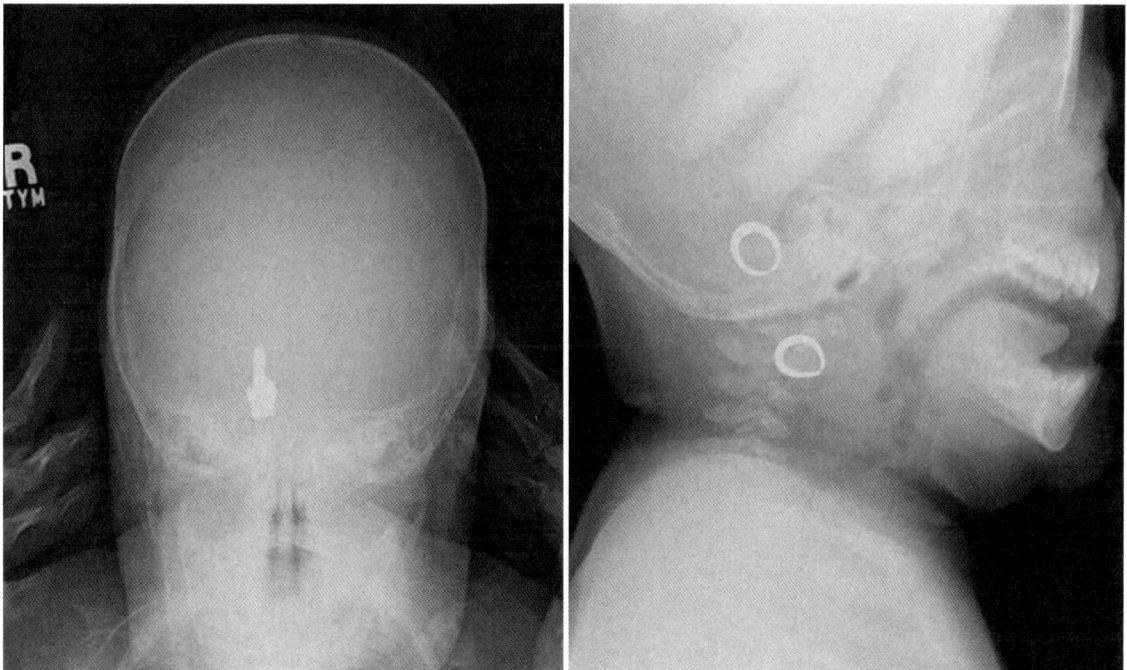

Fig. 22.10 Poor patient preparation prior to the exam can produce unwanted artifacts on the final radiographs. A zipper artifact and fingers are seen on a Towne projection skull. Earrings and fingers are seen on a lateral soft tissue neck (STN).

Abdomen, Gastrointestinal, and Genitourinary Studies

ABDOMEN, GASTROINTESTINAL, AND GENITOURINARY STUDIES

Abdomen

Abdominal radiography in children is requested for different reasons than it is for adults. Consequently, the initial procedure or protocol differs significantly. In addition to supine and upright images, the assessment for acute abdomen conditions or the abdominal series in adult radiography usually includes images obtained in the left lateral decubitus position. Often the series is not considered complete without a PA projection of the chest. To keep radiation exposure to a minimum, the pediatric abdominal series need only include two images: the supine abdomen and an image to show air-fluid levels. The left-lateral decubitus image is preferred over the upright in patients younger than 2 years old because, from an immobilization and patient-comfort perspective, it is much easier to perform. The "baby box" device can accommodate various projections with comfort to the patient, obtaining the images in a timely fashion (Figs. 22.11–22.13; see Fig. 22.22 later in the chapter). The upright image of a child over 2 years old can be obtained traditionally at the end of the table with the image plate holder or by using the upright bucky with the grid removed. As mentioned for hip radiography, the diaper should be completely removed for all abdominal and pelvic imaging to avoid artifacts.

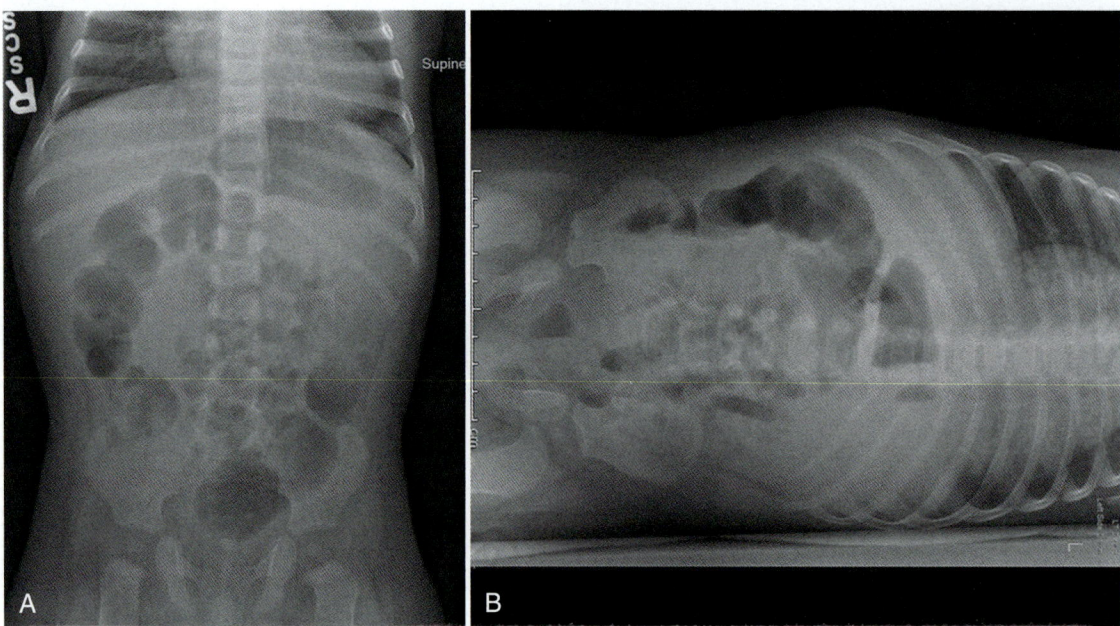

Fig. 22.11 AP (**A**) and left-lateral (**B**) abdomen radiographs obtained on an 8-month-old patient using the baby box device.

Abdomen, Gastrointestinal, and Genitourinary Studies

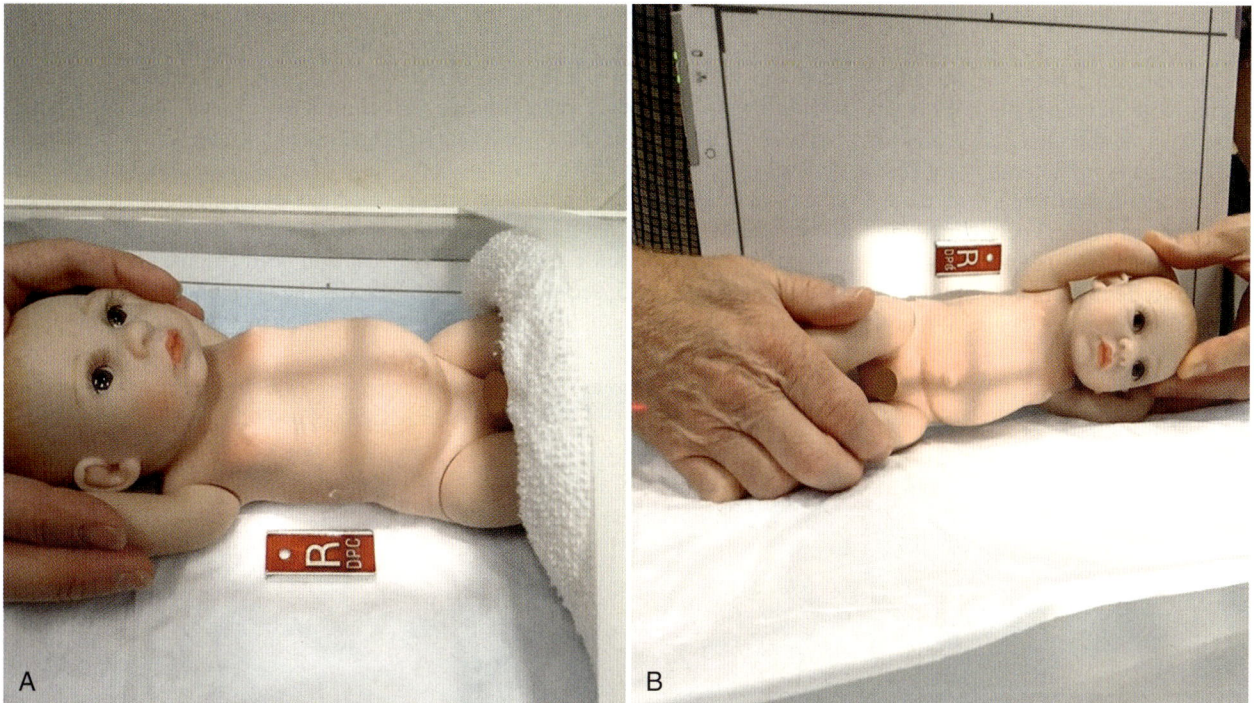

Fig. 22.12 (A) and (B) The baby box device is a valuable positioning tool with pediatric abdomen imaging up to 1 year of age. The image receptor can be adjusted accordingly underneath the plexiglass. The Velcro strap can be used to immobilize the legs and thus the parent can immobilize the head and chest to counter any rotation. The baby box can aid in performing supine and decubitus exams and more.

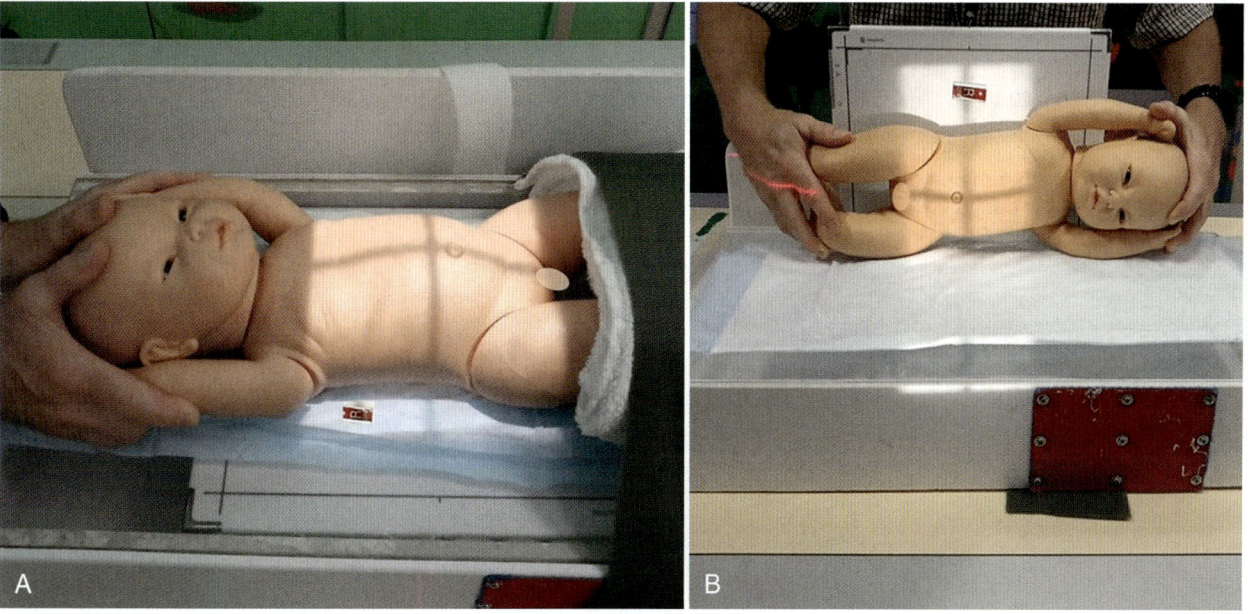

Fig. 22.13 The baby box used for positioning an infant for AP abdomen (A) and lateral decubitus abdomen (B).

Abdomen, Gastrointestinal, and Genitourinary Studies

Positioning and immobilization

Infants, toddlers, and young children can be immobilized for supine abdominal imaging with the same methods used for radiography of the hips and pelvis to facilitate the legs being internally rotated. A modification of the "bunny method" aids in performing hip and pelvic imaging when the patient's legs need to be internally rotated to demonstrate anatomy. To achieve this method, raise the infant's arms above their head. Fold a towel in half and place the towel lengthwise underneath the infant's head. Use the ends of the towel to wrap and secure each arm one at a time. Fold the ends of the towel centered under the infant's head for a cushion. This acts as a weight to immobilize the arms, thereby allowing the parent or technologist to rotate the infant's legs internally (Figs. 22.14 and 22.15; see also Fig. 22.36 later in the chapter).

Note that it is common for pediatric clinicians to request two projections of the abdomen. This should be supported by the clinical indications. A neonatal patient with necrotizing enterocolitis requires supine and left *lateral decubitus* images to rule out air-fluid levels indicative of bowel obstruction. However, the patient with an umbilical catheter needs supine and *lateral* images to verify the location and position of the catheter. *When in doubt, consult the radiologist.*

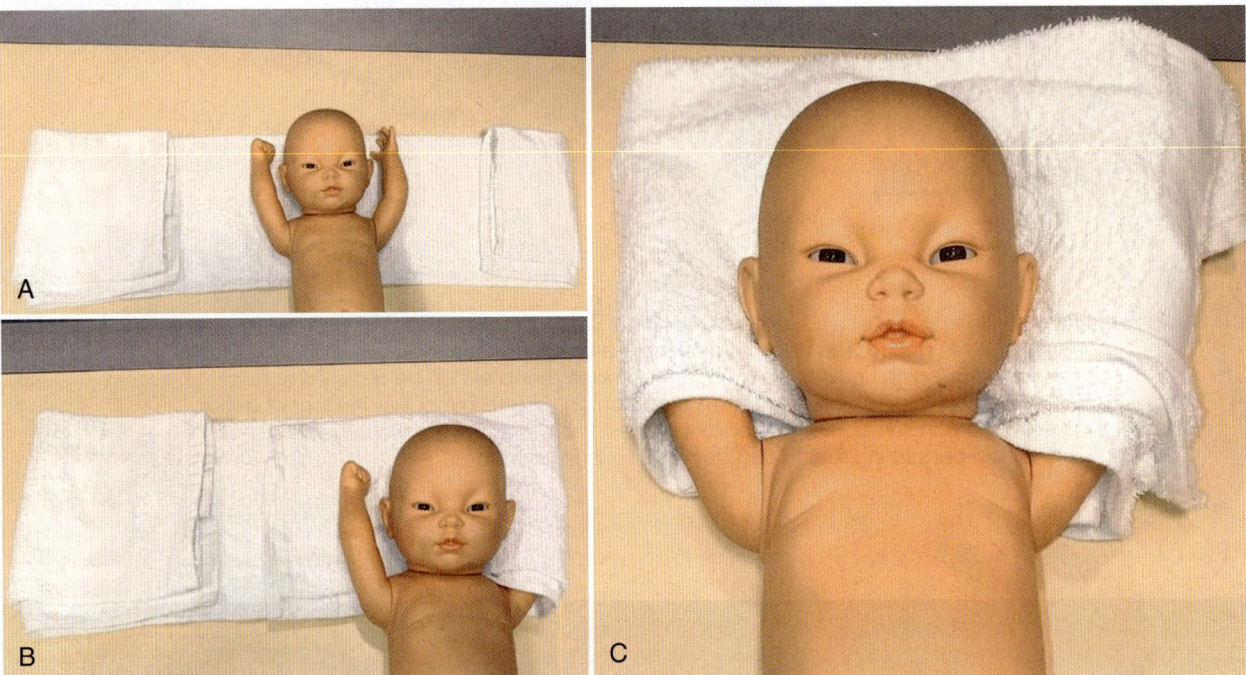

Fig. 22.14 This "modified bunny" method can be accomplished using a single towel. (**A**) Raise the infant's arms above their head. Fold a towel in half and place the towel lengthwise underneath the infant's head. Use the ends of the towel to wrap and secure each arm one at a time (**B**). Fold the ends of the towel centered under the infant's head for a cushion (**C**).

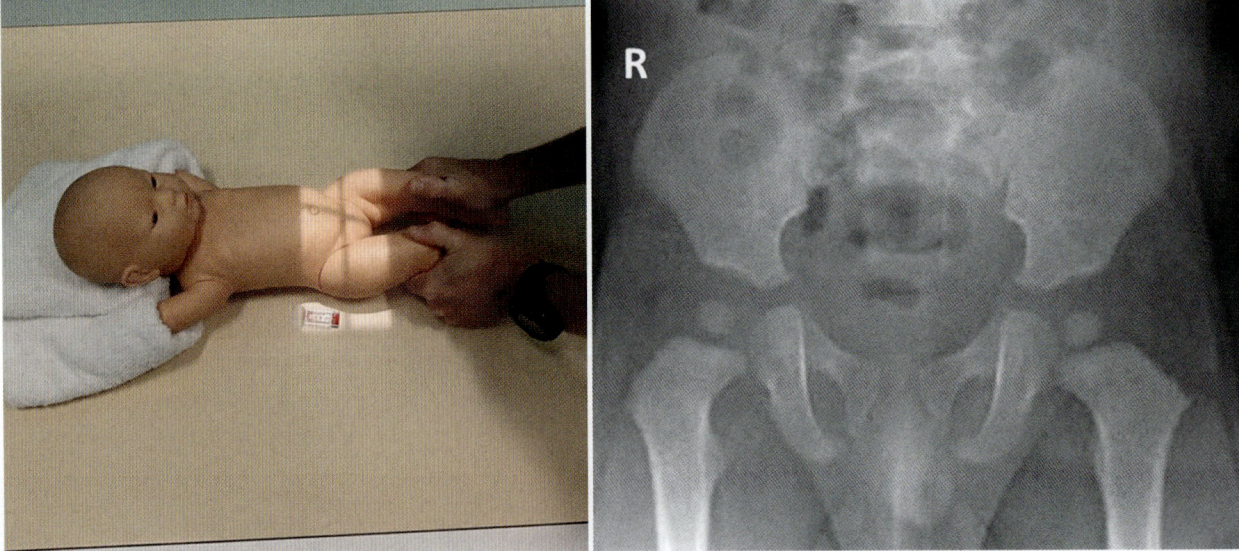

Fig. 22.15 This "modified bunny" method is effective when performing hip/pelvis imaging when the legs need to be internally rotated.

Abdomen, Gastrointestinal, and Genitourinary Studies

Pathology

Intussusception. Intussusception is the invagination or telescoping of the bowel into itself; most cases (90%) are ileocolic (Fig. 22.16). Idiopathic intussusception is most common and is the most frequent cause of small intestinal obstruction in the infant to toddler age-group, reaching peak incidence between 2 months and 3 years of age. The majority of cases (60%) occur in males. Intussusception can present with an abrupt onset of abdominal pain that becomes more frequent over time. There can be bouts of diarrhea, vomiting, and lethargy. Blood and blood clots in the stool with the consistency and color of currant jelly are highly suggestive of intussusception. No matter how high the clinical index of suspicion is for intussusception, an abdominal image is always indicated; in some patients, this supine image may be negative. Bowel perforation and degree of obstruction are ruled out with a horizontal beam image, whereas a prone or left-side-down decubitus is more likely than the supine position to demonstrate a soft tissue mass. The combination of diminished colonic stool and bowel gas, especially when accompanied by a visible soft tissue mass, indicates a high likelihood of intussusception. An abdominal physical exam by an experienced surgeon is a useful precaution before proceeding to reduction.

Although there are significant procedural variations among radiologists for the reduction of intussusceptions, many pediatric radiology departments use the pneumatic enema under fluoroscopic guidance as the treatment of choice because of its ease of use, reduced risk for peritonitis in the event of a perforation (as compared with hydrostatic), reduced time of procedure, and reduced radiation dose. The pneumatic filling of a large portion of the small bowel is usually necessary to confirm reduction. Contraindications to radiologic reduction are intestinal perforation, frank peritonitis, and hypervolemic shock.

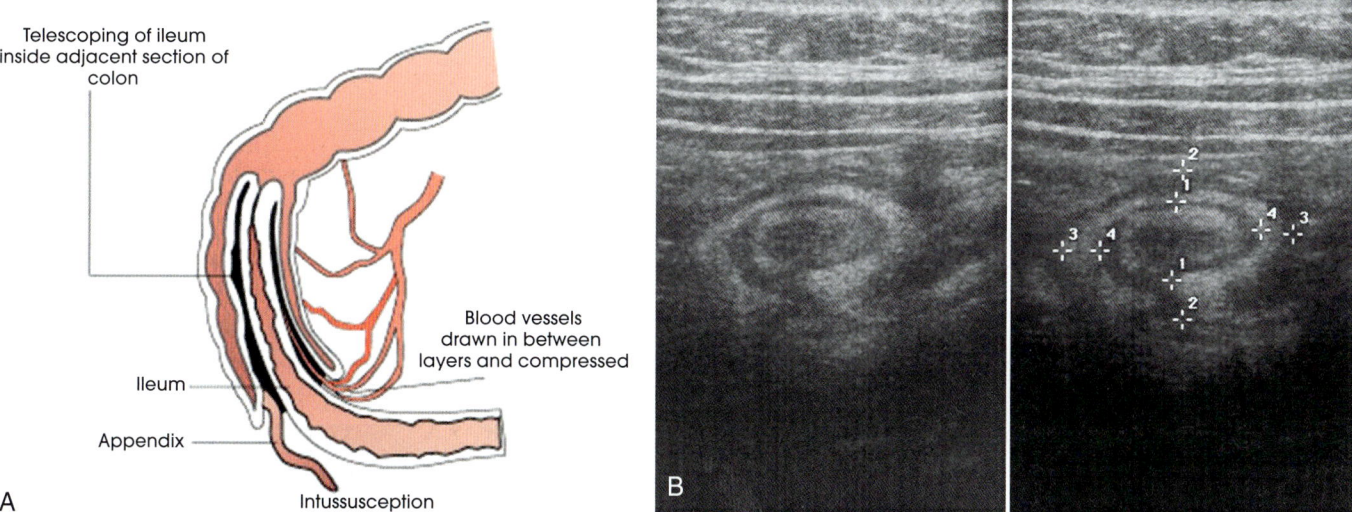

Fig. 22.16 (**A**) Intussusception. (**B**) Ultrasound image illustrates doughnut-shaped lesion marked for measurement.

(A, from Van Meter K: *Gould's Pathophysiology for the Health Professions*, ed 5, St Louis, 2014, Elsevier. B, from Eisenberg RL, Johnson NM: *Comprehensive radiographic pathology*, ed 5, St Louis, 2010, Elsevier.)

Abdomen, Gastrointestinal, and Genitourinary Studies

Pneumoperitoneum. Intraperitoneal air/gas is most commonly the result of perforation of the hollow viscera (stomach or intestines) and can be caused by surgical complications, such as abdominal drainage tubes, percutaneous gastronomy tubes, or insufflation of CO_2 or air during liver and renal biopsies or during laparoscopy (Fig. 22.17A). These causes may have the same radiologic appearances but different clinical significance. Patients normally have pneumoperitoneum following abdominal surgery, which clears more rapidly in children than adults. Studies have demonstrated clearing of free air in most postoperative children within 24 hours.

Diagnosis of pneumoperitoneum is most easily made with a cross-table decubitus projection, which is also indicated to rule out free air or intestinal obstruction. However, when small amounts of free air are suspected, the decubitus position is recommended (Fig. 22.17B). A properly positioned abdominal image, performed upright, cross-table, or decubitus, will include both the pubic symphysis and the bases of both diaphragms. In the upright image, free air is easily demonstrated under the diaphragms, displacing the liver on the right and stomach, liver, and spleen on the left. A child who is younger than 1 year or unable to stand can be examined in the left decubitus position, which allows the liver to fall away from the wall of the peritoneal cavity, revealing lucency between the abdominal wall and the liver.

The tabletop decubitus view is most successfully achieved when the patient's back is parallel and in contact with the imaging IR. Arms are on either side of the head and above the shoulders, with elbows bent on either side of the head. The patient's pelvis is perpendicular to the table with knees bent and legs stacked one atop the other. The person holding will immobilize the patient's arms and head as one unit (left hand) and hold the lower torso just below the buttocks (right hand).

The horizontal beam image may be useful in distinguishing a pneumoperitoneum caused by bowel perforation (air-fluid levels present) and a dissecting pneumomediastinum presenting with air in the peritoneal space and no fluid levels (this difference is not always present). Pneumomediastinum is usually suspected when there is a history of assisted ventilation or chest trauma and is best visualized in PA and lateral views of the chest.

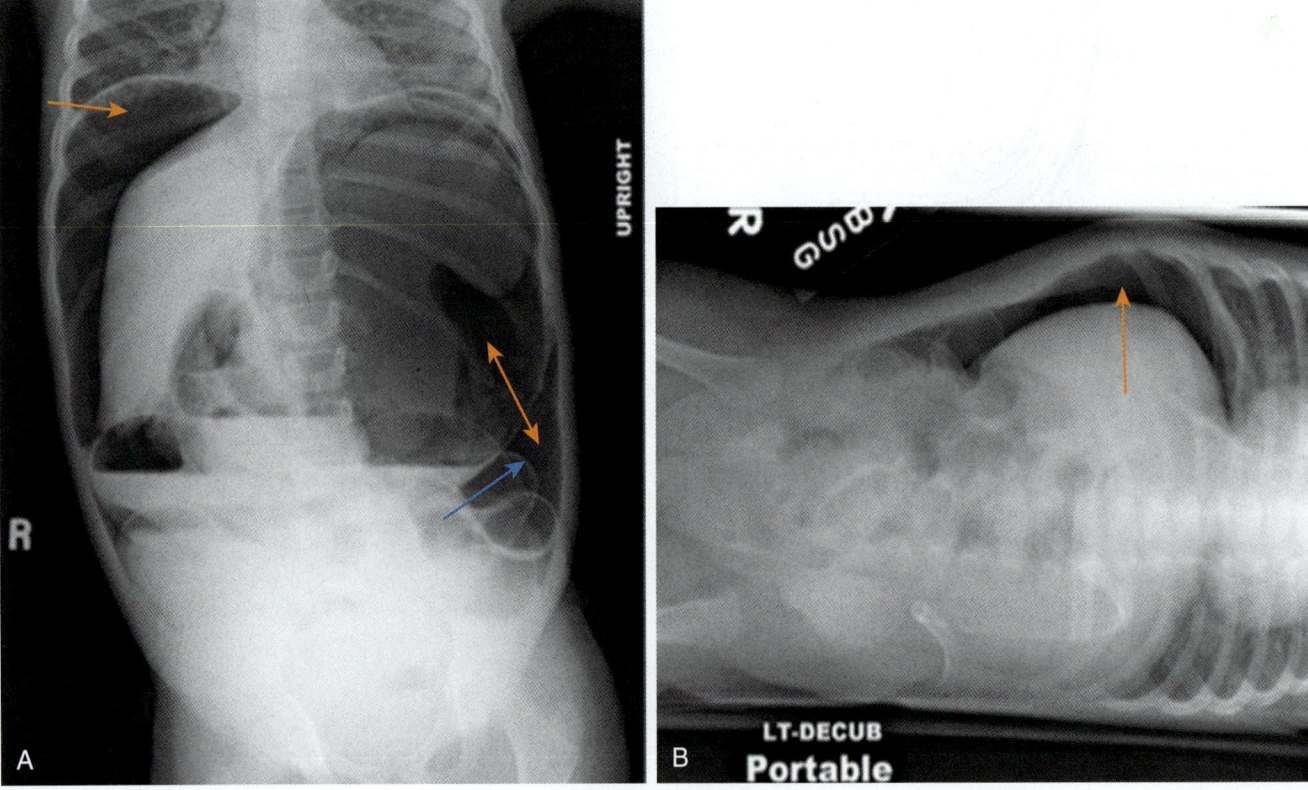

Fig. 22.17 **(A)** Pneumoperitoneum resulting from a fundoplication procedure *(orange arrows)*. Rigler's sign (air on both sides of bowel wall) is present at *blue arrow*. **(B)** Pneumoperitoneum seen *(orange arrow)* as a complication from percutaneous gastronomy tube procedure.

Abdomen, Gastrointestinal, and Genitourinary Studies

Gastrointestinal and genitourinary studies

As with any radiology procedure-based modality, a team approach to the care of the patient and family is essential. There are many procedures unique to pediatrics that fall under the headings GI/GU. Although it is beyond the scope of this chapter to delve into the specifics of each of these exams, many of which are complex, some of the most common procedures and indications are discussed. Common to each of these procedures is the use of a contrast medium, which enhances the visualization of soft tissue. These media can be either water-soluble iodine-based or non–water-soluble barium sulfate–based. The water-soluble contrast media are used for intravenous (IV) injection and non-IV excretory urography studies, for postsurgical assessments where leakage might occur, and for suspected perforations. They are characterized as being either nonionic (fewer side effects) with low osmolality (low-osmolality contrast agents [LOCAs]) or ionic (increased side effects) with high osmolality (high-osmolality contrast agents [HOCAs]). The choice of which LOCA to use is based on the desired concentration of iodine within the blood plasma and urine, the cost, and safety. Dosage is based on patient weight for IV injections; after injection of a bolus at a moderate rate, contrast excretion begins almost immediately and peaks at 10 to 20 minutes. Studies have shown that the adoption of a LOCA offers a definite improvement in patient experience and safety compared to that of a HOCA. The American College of Radiology (ACR) has specific criteria for the use of LOCAs, which include questions about previous history of contrast reactions, asthma, allergies (especially to shellfish), and cardiac issues. Adverse reactions can be life threatening. When administering a contrast agent, the trained radiographer should have a nurse present and a doctor available.

Barium sulfate–based contrast agents are not water soluble and are for oral or rectal administration to investigate esophageal problems, perform swallow studies, or rule out malrotation or Hirschsprung disease. The patient should be advised to drink plenty of liquids after the study, as the body does not break down barium. Barium is contraindicated for suspected perforations, instances of lower bowel obstructions, or attempted reduction of meconium ileus or meconium plug (Table 22.2).

TABLE 22.2
Gastrointestinal/genitourinary studies

Indications	Procedure	Contrast agent
Gastrointestinal studies		
R/O esophageal atresia	Swallow	LOMC
Dysphasia	Swallow	Barium
Stridor, R/O retropharyngeal abscess	Airway fluoroscopy	Air
R/O malrotation	UGI	Barium
R/O irritable bowel syndrome	UGISB	Barium
R/O Hirschsprung, low bowel obstruction	Contrast enema	Cysto Conray 17.2%
CF cleanout	Contrast enema	Cysto Conray 17.2% w/Gastrografin
Meconium ileus	Contrast enema	Gastrografin w/Water 1:1
Intussusception reduction	Air enema	Air
R/O swallowing dysfunction	MBSW	Barium
Genitourinary		
Febrile UTI, R/O reflux, hydronephrosis	VCUG	Cysto Conray 17.2%
Megaureter	VCUG, IVP	Cysto Conray 17.2%
Ectopic ureter	VCUG	Cysto Conray 17.2%
Ureterocele, ureteral duplication	IVP	LOMC, Optiray 320
Neurogenic bladder	VCUG	Cysto Conray 17.2%
Bladder diverticula		

Abdomen, Gastrointestinal, and Genitourinary Studies

Vesicoureteral reflux

For infants and small children experiencing first-time febrile urinary tract infections (UTIs), the goal after antibiotic treatment is to rule out the possibility of vesicoureteral reflux (VUR) (Fig. 22.18), existing renal scarring, and structural or functional abnormalities of the urinary tract that may predispose the patient to reflux and infection, particularly anomalies that may require prompt surgical treatment. This is accomplished with an ultrasound (US) and, if indicated, a voiding cystourethrogram (VCUG). Patient assessment may begin with a noninvasive US to assess the upper urinary tracts and kidneys. If the US is negative, the decision to proceed with the VCUG is made after a thorough discussion between the parents, the attending urologist, and the pediatrician. Some radiologists feel that a VCUG for a first-time nonfebrile UTI with a negative US is not indicated. The VCUG is an invasive procedure in which a Foley catheter (5–8 French) is inserted into the urethra, advanced into the bladder, and then taped to the inside of the leg in a female or to the shaft of the penis in a male. An iodinated contrast agent (see Table 22.2) designed for the lower urinary tract is instilled into the bladder by gravity. The volume used is based on the patient's age. Bilateral, oblique, pulsed fluoroscopy captures are made to check for reflux (Fig. 22.19A) and assess urinary anatomy. Fluoroscopy captures are made of voiding as the Foley is removed (Fig. 22.19B). VCUG teams often include an attending fellow or resident, a radiographer, and a CLS with access to a registered radiologist assistant (RRA) as required. The parents are encouraged to participate, as this can help soothe and calm the infant or child. Age-appropriate distraction devices are employed as required. Figure 22.20 demonstrates severe grade IV reflux with moderate bilateral ureter dilatation with loss of sharp calyceal fornices.

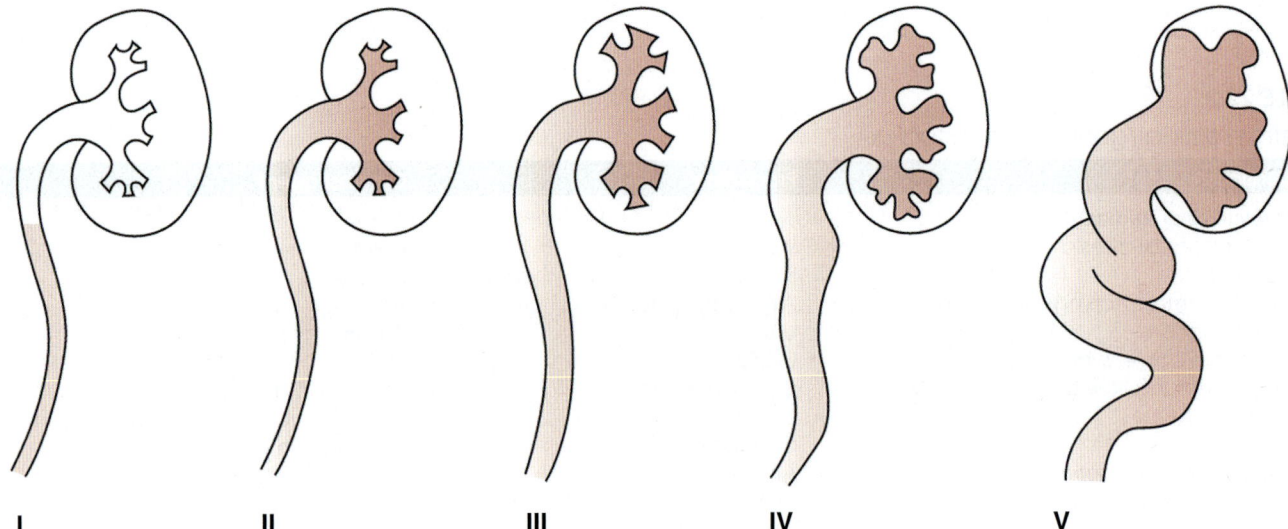

Fig. 22.18 Vesicoureteral reflux (VUR) is described according to five grades. Grade I represents no urine reflux to the renal pelvis, and Grade V is the most severe, with gross dilatation of the renal pelvis.

(Reproduced from Lebowitz RL, Olbing H, Parkkulainen KV, et al. International system of radiographic grading of vesicoureteric reflux. *Pediatr Radiol*, 1985;15(2):105–109.)

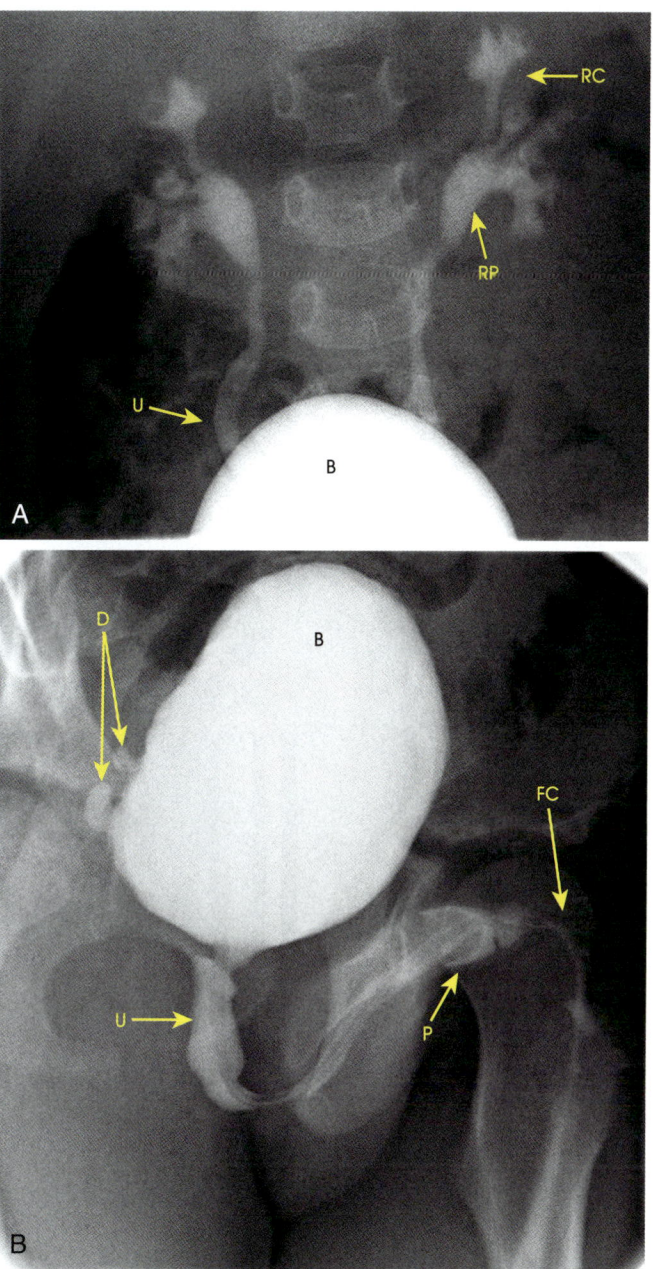

Fig. 22.19 (**A**) VCUG, 33-month-old female with bilateral grade III reflux as seen in the AP projection under fluoroscopy. *B,* Bladder; *RC,* renal calyx; *RP,* renal pelvis; *U,* ureter. (**B**) VCUG, 8-year-old male with bladder diverticula *(D)* as seen in the LPO projection. Voiding shows moderate dilatation of the posterior urethra *(U)*. *B,* bladder; *FC,* Foley catheter; *P,* uncircumcised penis.

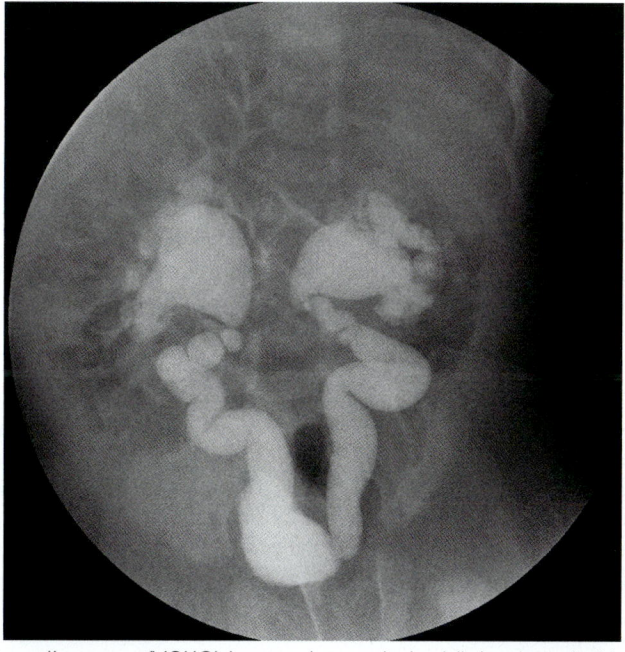

Fig. 22.20 This voiding cystourethrogram (VCUG) image demonstrates bilateral grade IV vesicoureteral reflux (VUR).

Chest

CHEST

The most frequently ordered and one of the most challenging imaging exams in pediatric imaging is the chest x-ray. Patients between 1 and 4 years can be difficult to immobilize and position because they are relatively strong and in an unfamiliar setting. The anxiety level created in this situation can be high for parents, students, and even the experienced radiographer. Take the time to adequately explain to the parents the goals of the exam and how to correctly hold the child for it. Even if you are assured the parent can hold properly, it is essential that you remain vigilant in your transition from the patient to the exposure control station, ensuring that the parents continue to immobilize correctly and effectively. If the parent is struggling and frustrated, consider using the Pigg-O-Stat (Fig. 22.21) or, as a last resort, a radiographer to hold the child. Radiation delivered to the patient must always be as low as diagnostically achievable, and every attempt must be made to acquire the image on the first attempt. Quite simply, if you think the positioning is compromised or the immobilization ineffective, do not make the exposure.

The central ray for AP, PA, and lateral projections of the chest is directed to the level of T6-7 (nipple line). Adjust the radiation field on the collimator to include the earlobes to approximately 4 cm (1.5 inches) above the umbilicus. Inclusion of the earlobes shows the upper airway; narrowed or stenotic airways are a common source of respiratory problems in pediatric patients. By collimating 4 cm (1.5 inches) above the umbilicus, the radiographer will ensure inclusion of the chest and the gastric bubble. Numerous children arrive in the imaging department with long lung fields resulting from hyperinflation (e.g., patients with cardiac disorders and asthma).

Most radiologists will agree that upright chest images yield a great deal more diagnostic information than supine images. However, it is important that you be able to achieve diagnostic quality in both positions. Infants needing supine and cross-table lateral images can be immobilized using Velcro straps around the knees and a Velcro band across the legs. The patient is supine on a radiolucent pad with the arms held above the head for both the AP and the cross-table lateral. This technique is particularly useful for patients with chest tubes, delicately positioned gastrostomy tubes, or soft tissue swellings or protrusions that may be compromised by the sleeves of the Pigg-O-Stat.

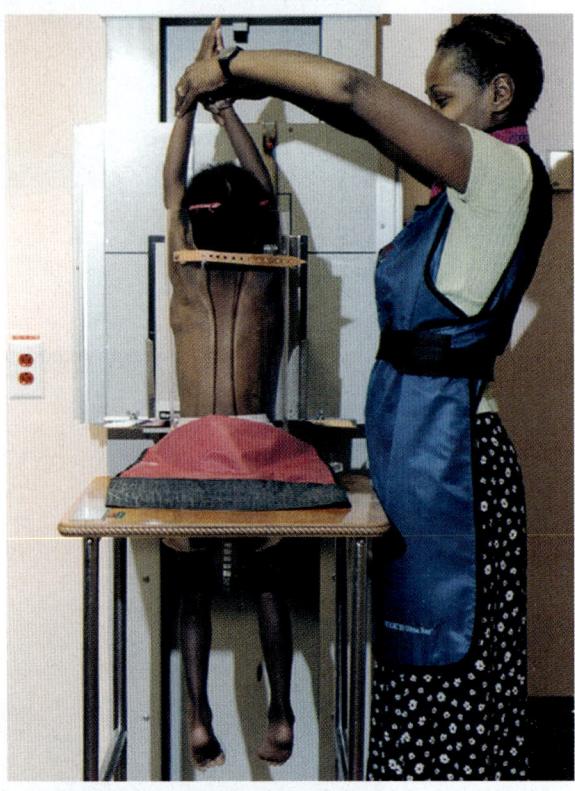

Fig. 22.21 Position for PA chest image. The Pigg-O-Stat (Modern Way Immobilizers, Clifton, TN) is a pediatric positioner and immobilization tool. The IR is held in the metal extension stand.

Chest (<1 year)

One device that has proven invaluable for immobilizing and positioning the infant with minimal discomfort and helping to ensure a diagnostic and reproducible exam in a timely manner is the baby box. All nonbedside, two-view chest exams and most decubitus projections of infants 0 to 365 days old are performed using the baby box (Figs. 22.22–22.24). The patient must be unclothed from the waist up with all heart monitor leads removed (when safe) and lines and tubes (especially nasogastric tubes) positioned away from the chest anatomy. The baby is placed supine on the box and the lower torso is immobilized with the attached Velcro strap (Velcro USA, Inc., Manchester, NH) and sandbag as necessary. The parent is directed to slowly raise the baby's arms up and alongside its head. While holding the arms at the level of the elbows, the parent places their thumbs at the sides of the head or on the forehead to ensure that the baby's head is in a true supine position (see Fig. 22.23). A small rotation of the head will cause distortion of the infant's lung fields, and if the baby arches its back the image will be rendered lordotic. Special attention should be paid to the tendency of parents to pull the arms and baby toward them rather than simply holding the arms and head together. This results in the patient being slowly pulled out from under the Velcro and off the IR, causing the lung apices to be clipped. Adjust collimation, ensure that the parent continues to immobilize effectively, and expose when the baby's belly is fully distended, indicating a full inspiration. Do not rush the exam—activate the rotor, observe the rhythm of the infant's breathing, and time the exposure. If the infant is hyperventilating, an inspiratory image will be obtained, although it may not be at full inspiration.

The left cross-table lateral projection (see Fig. 22.24) is obtained by placing the IR in the shallow groove on the left side of the baby box. Using the same holding technique, the Velcro is released and the patient is moved closer to the IR, thus minimizing object-to-image receptor distance (OID) (magnification); the Velcro is then refastened. Collimation should allow the x-ray beam to

Chest

overlap onto the side of the box closest to the x-ray tube to prevent clipping the posterior lung fields. It is imperative, especially for medicolegal reasons, that all first-time AP images and all subsequent images contain the correct marker placement.

Chest (>1 year)

This population of little patients will resist any positioning the radiographer attempts by wiggling, twisting, crying, contorting, or all of the above in what appears to be an effort to force a repeat image. The biggest reason for repeats in this age-group is the patient pulling away from the image receptor, resulting in a lordotic image. Properly positioning this age-group requires good communication between the radiographer and parents. Parents can be tentative about holding their child firmly. If the child is allowed to twist or lean away from the IR, the image will be nondiagnostic. If the parents are unsuccessful in immobilization, use the Pigg-O-Stat (if age-appropriate) or use a radiographer as a last resort.

Chest x-rays for children 1 to 6 years old can be obtained by seating the child at the end of the exam table using a custom-made frame that supports the IR and aids in the positioning of the child. The PA or AP chest x-ray is accomplished with the child's arms raised next to the head with instructions to the parent that the child's head and arms be held as a unit (Fig. 22.25). A slight upward pull on the child's body will keep a straight torso. Do not let the patient lean away from the IR, as this will produce a lordotic image; this can be prevented either by moving the patient's bottom away from the IR or by placing a 15-degree positioning sponge between the patient and the IR at the level of the patient's abdomen, with the thicker portion at the level of the pelvic ilia. Patients should be naked from the waist up in order to visualize and time the inspiration. (The medical physicist at Boston Children's Hospital has approved this position. Primary beam radiation is confined to the IR and there is no primary beam exposure to

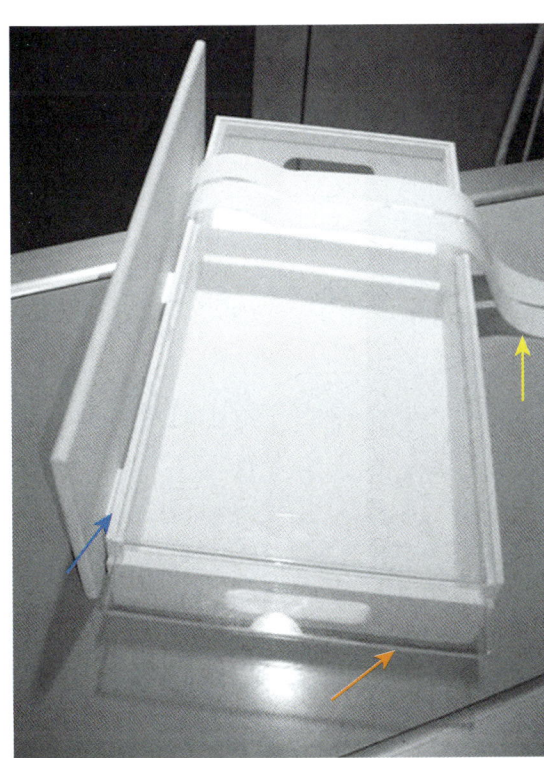

Fig. 22.22 The baby box aids in the immobilization of an infant (0–12 months) for AP and cross-table lateral chest x-rays and for soft tissue neck and C-spine imaging. There is a sliding tray *(orange arrow)* that holds the imaging plate for supine positions, a slot on the side *(blue arrow)* holds the IR for cross-table work, and Velcro straps *(yellow arrow)* are used to immobilize.

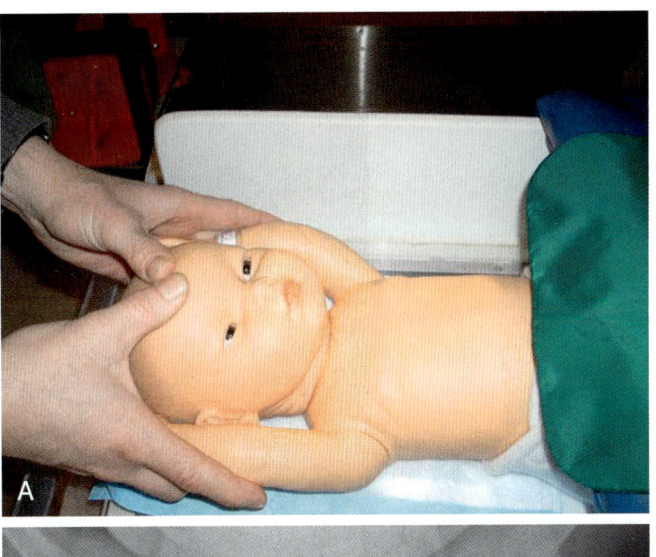

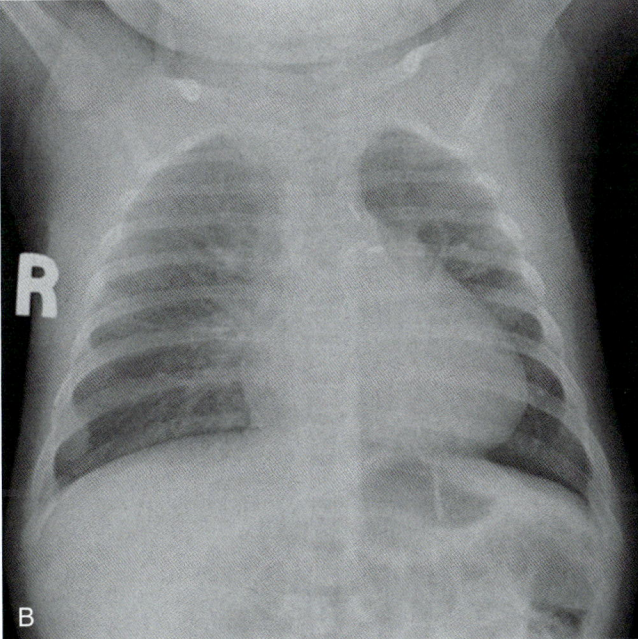

Fig. 22.23 (A) Supine AP chest x-ray for an infant younger than 12 months. Parent immobilizes at the elbows with thumbs at or on the sides of the forehead. **(B)** AP chest image of an infant younger than 12 months.

Chest

the technologist or the parent. This has been the routine standard of care at this hospital for the past 15 years).

For the sitting left lateral, patients are held from behind or the front, with arms in the same position as used for the PA (Fig. 22.26). A large, firm positioning sponge can be placed between the parent's chest and the patient's back (positioning can be done without the sponge on older children). While holding the child's head and arms as a unit, the parent is instructed to exert a slight upward pull while keeping the patient's back against the sponge and perpendicular to the IR. If the patient is unruly, a second person will be required to hold down on the child's knees. Make sure you have a clear view of the patient's belly to check for inspiration. Older patients are examined standing with an upright bucky.

Image evaluation

The criteria used to evaluate the image are inclusion of the full lung fields, airway, visibility of peripheral lung markings, rotation, inspiration, cardiac silhouette, mediastinum, and bony structures. In the PA chest image, the ideal technical factor is a selection that permits visualization of the intervertebral disk spaces through the heart (the densest area) while showing the peripheral lung markings (the least dense area). Rotation should be assessed by evaluating midline structures (e.g., sternum, trachea, and spinous processes). These anterior and posterior midline structures should be superimposed. Similar to chest radiography in adults, the visualization of eight to nine posterior ribs is a reliable indicator of an image taken with good inspiration (Table 22.3).

Chest (3 to 18 years)
Upright

Upright images of children 3 to 18 years old are easily obtained by observing the following steps:

- Help the child sit on a large wooden box, a wide-based trolley with brakes, or a stool, with the IR supported using a metal extension stand. Young children are curious and have short attention spans. By having them sit, the radiographer can prevent them from wiggling from the waist down.

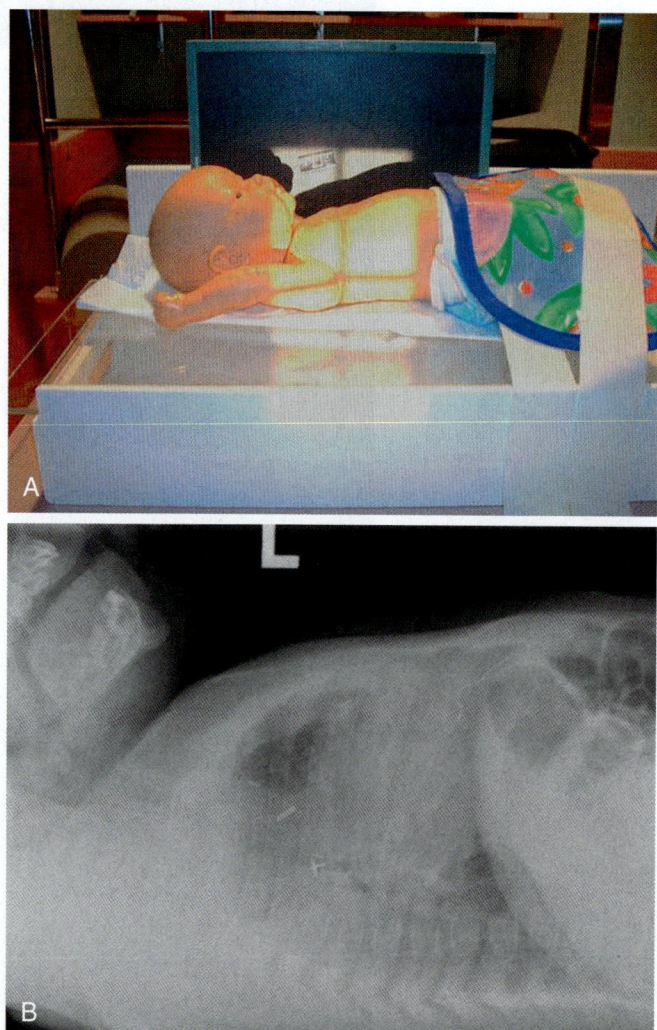

Fig. 22.24 (A) Left cross-table lateral chest projection: same immobilization as for AP, but infant must be moved closer to the IR to reduce OID and avoid clipping the spine. (B) Lateral projection chest image of an infant younger than 12 months.

Chest

- For the PA position, have the child hold onto the side supports of the extension stand with the chin on top of or next to the IR. This prevents upper body movement.
- When positioning for the lateral image, have the parent (if their presence is permitted) assist by raising the child's arms above the head and holding the head between the arms (Fig. 22.27).

Supine

Infants needing supine and cross-table lateral images can be immobilized using Velcro straps around the knees and a Velcro band across the legs (Fig. 22.28). The patient is elevated on a sponge with the arms held up, and a cross-table lateral projection is performed. This technique is particularly useful for patients with chest tubes, delicately positioned gastrostomy tubes, or soft tissue swellings or protrusions that may be compromised by the sleeves of the Pigg-O-Stat.

Image evaluation

As in adult chest radiography, the use of kVp is desirable in pediatric chest imaging; however, this is relative. In adult imaging, high kVp generally ranges from 110 to 130, but for pediatric PA projections, kVp ranges from 80 to 90. The use of higher kVp is not always possible because the corresponding mAs are too low to produce a diagnostic image.

The criteria used to evaluate recorded detail include the resolution of peripheral lung markings. Evaluating any image for adequate density involves assessing the most and least dense areas of the anatomy that is shown. In the PA chest image, the ideal technical factor is a selection that permits visualization of the intervertebral disk spaces through the heart (the densest area) while showing the peripheral lung markings (the least dense area). Rotation should be assessed by evaluating the

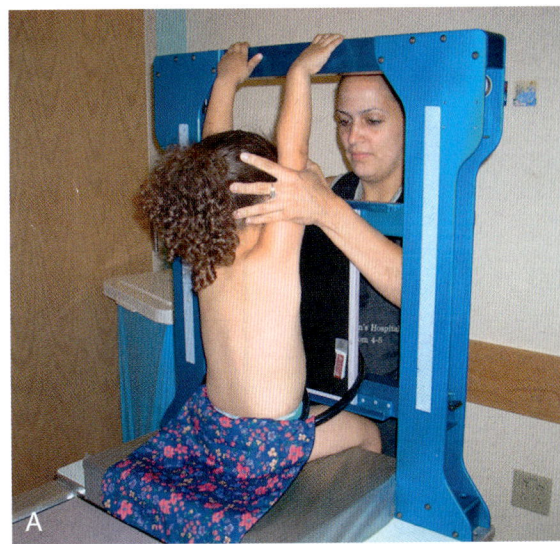
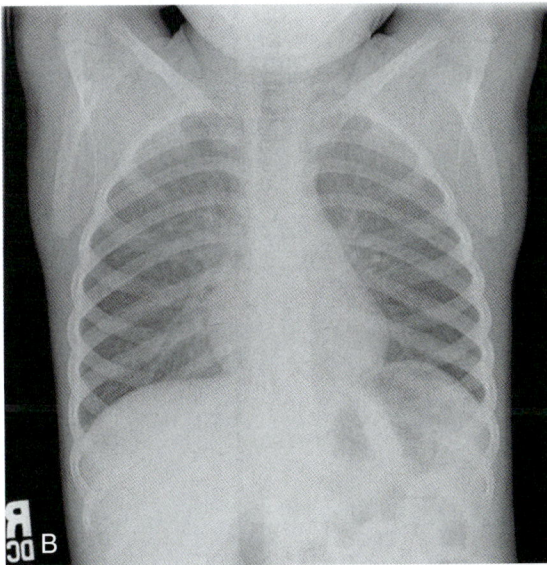

Fig. 22.25 (A) Parent holding for a PA chest on a child older than 1 year. (B) Resultant chest image. Care should be taken to tie up textured hair, as it can show as an artifact on digital images.

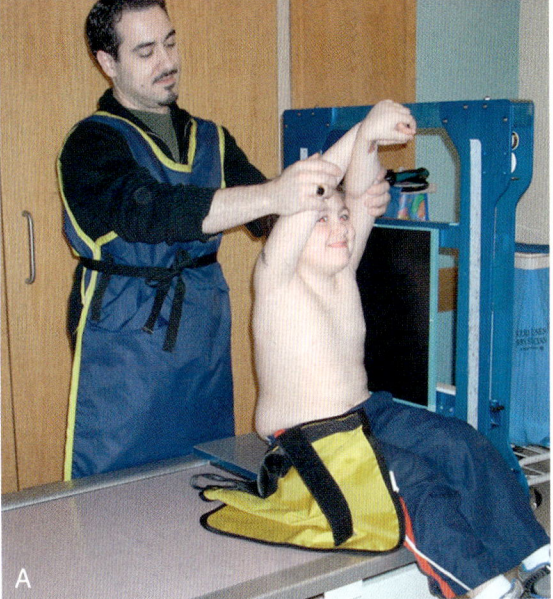
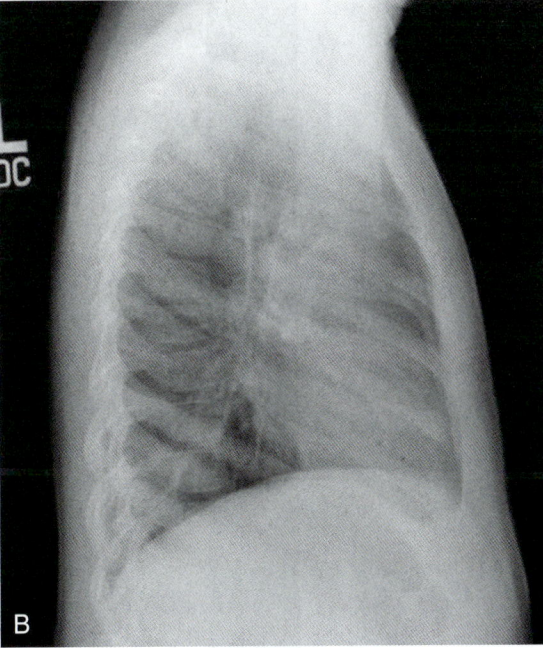

Fig. 22.26 (A) Parent holding for a lateral chest on a child older than 1 year. (B) Resultant chest image.

TABLE 22.3
Quick reference guide for image assessment

	Density		Contrast			
	Most dense	Least dense	Recorded detail	Long scale >3 shades	Short scale >3 shades	Anatomy	Rotation check
PA chest	Midline; intervertebral disk spaces, heart	Peripheral lung markings	Peripheral lung markings	Airway, heart, apices, bases, mediastinum, lung markings behind diaphragm and heart		Airway to bases	Airway position, SC joints, lung field measurement, cardiac silhouette
PA chest	Heart	Retrocardiac space	Peripheral lung markings	Airway, heart, apices, bases		Airway to bases, spinous process to sternum	Superimposition of ribs, spinous processes on profile
Abdomen	Lumbar spine	Peripheral edges, soft tissue above the iliac crests	Organ silhouettes	Diaphragm, liver, kidney, spine, gas shadows		Right and left hemidiaphragm, pubic symphysis, right and left skin edges	
Limbs	Bone	Soft tissue	Bony trabecular patterns		Bone, muscle, soft tissue	Joints above and below injury, all soft tissue	AP and lateral images must not resemble obliques
Hips	Hip joints	Iliac crests	Bony trabecular patterns		Bone, soft tissue	Iliac crests, lesser trochanter	Symmetric iliac crests
Lateral lumbar spine	L5-S1	Spinous processes	Bony trabecular patterns		Bone	T12 to coccyx, spinous processes to vertebral bodies	Alignment of posterior surfaces of vertebral bodies

Evaluating the image to determine its diagnostic quality is a practiced skill. This chart, designed as a quick reference guide, outlines the five important technical criteria and the related anatomic indicators used in critiquing images.

Chest

position of midline structures. Posterior and anterior midline structures (e.g., sternum, airway, and vertebral bodies) should be superimposed. The anatomic structures to be shown include the airway (trachea) to the costophrenic angles. Similar to chest radiography in adults, the visualization of eight to nine posterior ribs is a reliable indicator of an image taken with good inspiration (see Table 22.3).

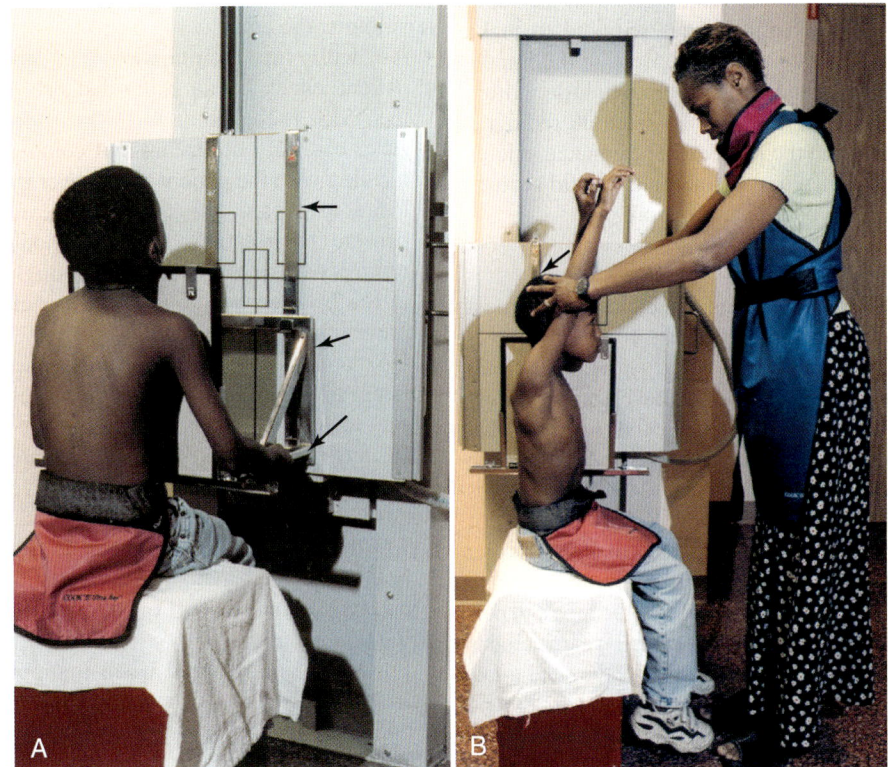

Fig. 22.27 (**A**) PA chest images should be performed on the 3 to 18 year old with the child sitting. (**B**) The parent, if present, can assist with immobilization for the lateral image by holding the child's head between the child's arms. Metal extension stands (*arrows* on A and B) are commercially available from companies that market diagnostic imaging accessories.

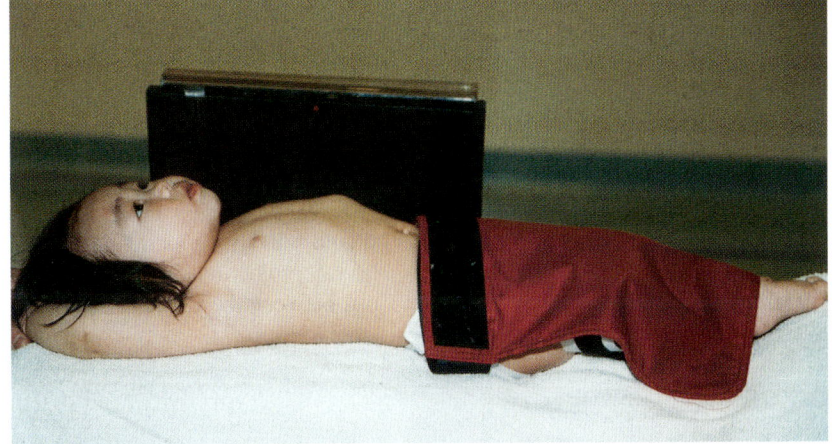

Fig. 22.28 The patient is raised on a sponge with arms up by the head, and the legs are immobilized using Velcro straps. The IR is in place for the horizontal lateral beam (cross-table lateral)

Pelvis and Hips

PELVIS AND HIPS
General principles
The initial radiography examination of the pelvis and hips is routinely done for children older than 6 months. Ultrasonography of the hips is the first modality for infants younger than 6 months. With a basic comprehension of the most common pediatric pelvic positions, pathologies, and disease processes, the radiographer can provide the radiologist with the superior diagnostic images required to make an accurate diagnosis. Despite the importance of radiation protection, little written literature is available to guide radiographers on the placement of gonadal shields and when to use shielding. Shield according to your department policy.

Initial images
Hip examinations on children are most often ordered to assess for Legg-Calvé-Perthes disease (aseptic avascular necrosis of the femoral head), developmental dysplasia of the hip (DDH), and slipped capital femoral epiphyses (SCFE) and to diagnose nonspecific hip pain. These conditions require the evaluation of the symmetry of the acetabula, joint spaces, and soft tissue; therefore, symmetric positioning is crucial. The initial examination of the hips and pelvis in children older than 1 year includes a well-collimated AP projection and a lateral projection commonly referred to as a frog lateral. This position is more correctly described as a coronal image of the pelvis with the thighs in abduction and external rotation or the Lauenstein position (see Chapter 8). This bilateral imaging serves as a baseline for future imaging and allows comparison of right and left hips.

Preparation and communication
All images of the abdomen and pelvic girdle should be performed with the child's underwear or diaper removed. Buttons, silk screening, and metal on underwear, as well as wet diapers, produce significant artifacts on images, often rendering them nondiagnostic. The radiographer should have all required positioning devices on the table prior to the patient's arrival.

Positioning and immobilization
As described previously, *symmetric positioning* is crucial. As in many examinations, the hip positions that are the most uncomfortable for the patient are often the most crucial. When a child has hip pain or dislocation, symmetric positioning is difficult to achieve because the patient often tries to compensate for the discomfort by rotating the pelvis. The radiographer should observe the following steps when positioning the patient:

- As with hip examinations in any patient, check for an equal distance of the ASISs to the table.
- After carefully observing and communicating with the patient to discover the location of pain, use sponges to compensate for rotation. Sponges should routinely be used to support the thighs in the frog-leg position. This can help prevent motion artifacts.
- Do not accept poorly positioned images. Repeat instructions as necessary to achieve optimal positioning.

Because *immobilization techniques* should vary according to the aggressiveness of the patient, the radiographer can follow these additional guidelines:

- Make every effort to use explanation and reassurance as part of the immobilization method.
- For active children and when immobilization fails, it is always best to use an additional technologist to help hold and position correctly. This reaffirms the importance of positioning and comforts the parent. This approach will facilitate completing the exam in a timely manner with less duress to the patient and reducing repeat radiographs.
- When performing supine abdominal exams, images of the pelvis, intravenous urograms (IVUs), overhead GI procedures, and spinal radiography, ask a parent to sit or stand at the head of the table and hold the child's arms above the child's head with "elbows by the ears" for AP projections to minimize rotation. Conversely, the parent should stand or sit facing the patient for lateral projections with a radiolucent pad between the knees for comfort and support. Depending on the age of the patient, sandbags are optional.
- If the radiology department is equipped, the versatile baby box can be used for abdomen, chest, and decubitus imaging on newborns (see Fig. 22.22). A towel across the knees plus the addition of a Velcro strap provide excellent immobilization and allow the parent or technologist to control the upper torso, thus minimizing rotation.

Leg-length discrepancies, which can cause hip problems, are diagnosed using a *Scanogram,* a technique in which three exposures of the lower limbs (single exposures centered over the hips, knees, and ankles) are made on a single 35 × 43 cm IR (see Chapter 7). Two radiolucent rulers with radiopaque numbers are included bilaterally and within the collimated field, making it possible for the orthopedic surgeon to then calculate the difference in leg lengths. Scanograms performed on ambulatory patients are done using the EOS and with new post-processing software; the rulers are no longer required to obtain measurements. The EOS system uses low-dose radiation to produce high-quality images. Therefore, this system is recommended for use with progressive conditions such as scoliosis and spinal deformities.

Image evaluation
Rotation or symmetry can be evaluated by ensuring that midline structures are in the midline and that the ilia appear symmetric. Depending on the degree of skeletal maturation, visualization of the trochanters can indicate the position of the legs when the image was taken. Symmetry in the skinfolds is also an important evaluation criterion for the diagnostician. The anatomy to be shown includes the crests of the ilia to the upper quarter of the femora. The image should demonstrate the bony trabecular pattern in the hip joints, which is the thickest and most dense area within the region. The visualization of the bony trabecular pattern is used as an indicator that sufficient recorded detail has been shown; this should not be at the expense of showing the soft tissues—the muscles and skinfolds (see Table 22.3).

Limb Radiography

LIMB RADIOGRAPHY

Limb radiography accounts for a high percentage of pediatric general radiographic procedures in most clinics and hospitals. Producing a series of diagnostic images will require you to assess the child's age-appropriate development, behavior, and age in order to determine which forms of immobilization you will employ. This is best accomplished in consultation with the parents; an active 3-year-old may require that you use immobilization techniques that are one or two age-groups below the patient's chronologic age-group.

Immobilization
Newborn to 2 years old

Depending on the exam, swaddling the child in a blanket, towel, or pillowcase will make the child manageable when performing upper limb radiography. When imaging small hands, a piece of plexiglass can be used to firmly hold the hand while making the exposure (Fig. 22.29). Lower extremities are best imaged with the help of swaddling, a Velcro band, or a parent holding down the abdomen with a large sandbag placed over the unaffected leg (Fig. 22.30).

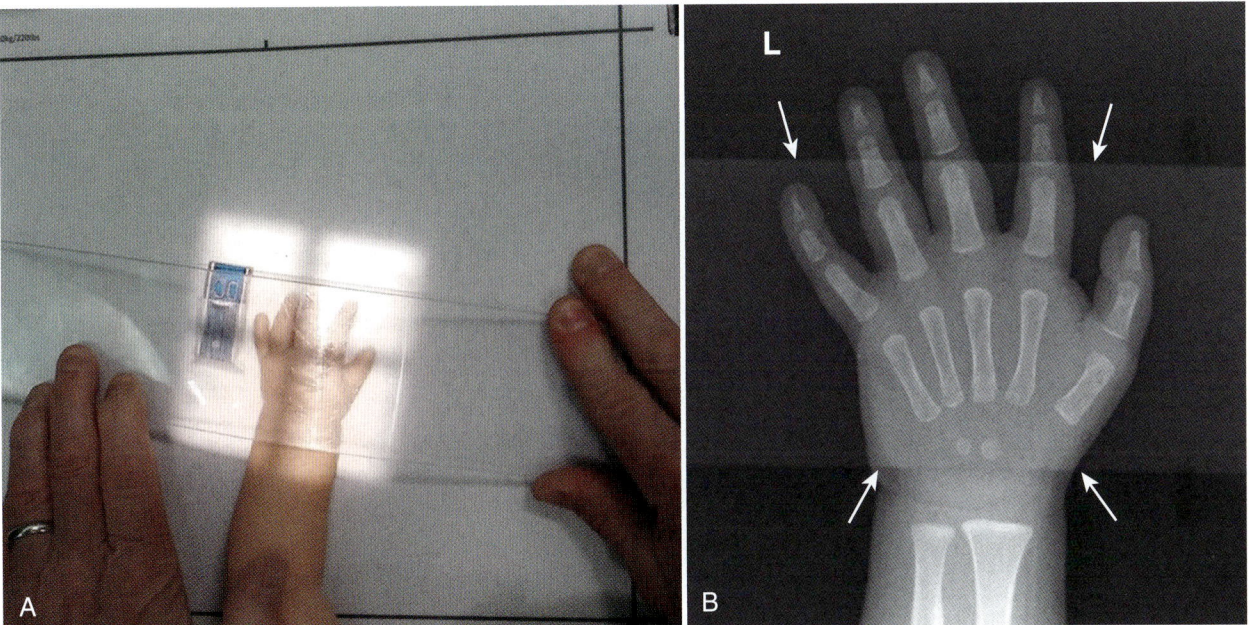

Fig. 22.29 PA left hand on an infant using a piece of plexiglass for immobilization (**A**). Note the plexiglass artifact (*arrows*) on the radiograph (**B**).

Limb Radiography

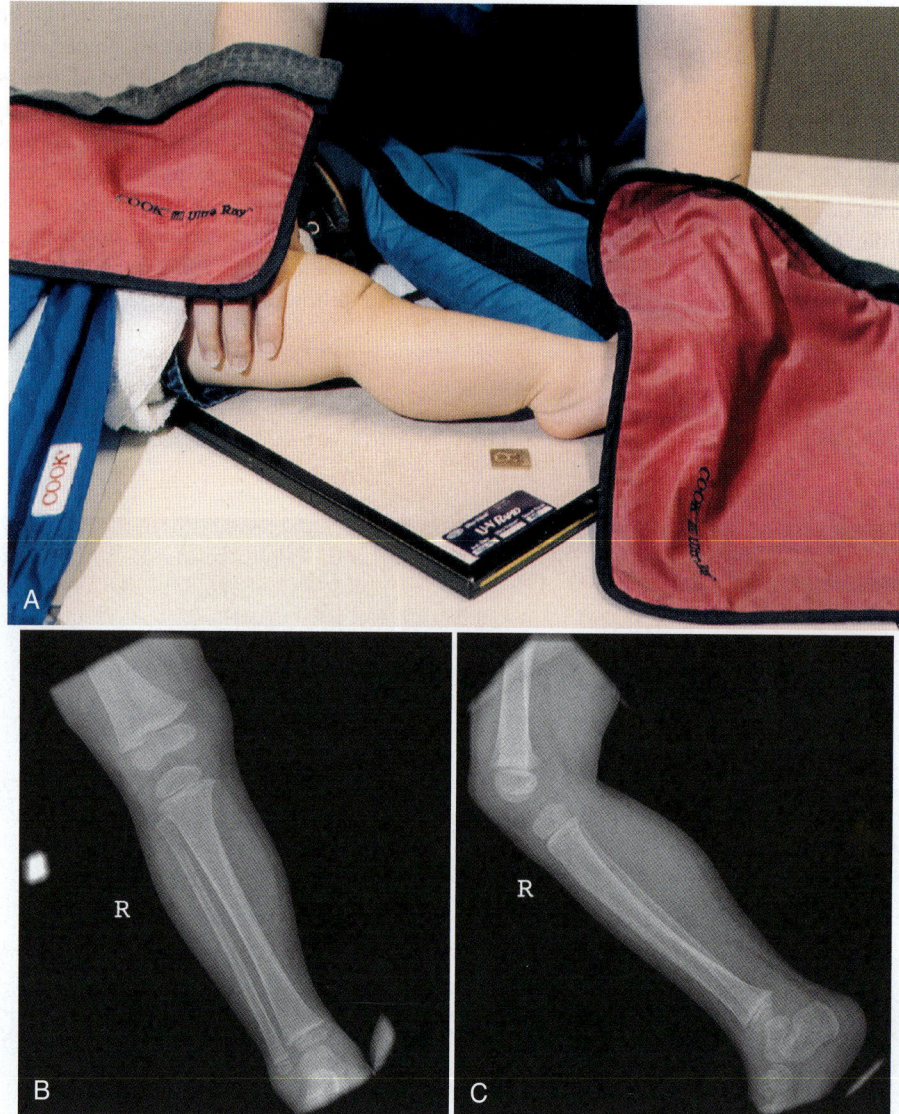

Fig. 22.30 (A) The challenges of immobilizing lower limbs are greater than those of immobilizing upper limbs. After wrapping both of the patient's arms in a towel and placing a Velcro band over the abdomen, the radiographer can place a large sandbag over the unaffected leg. With careful collimation and proper instruction, the parent can hold the limb as demonstrated. Normal 21-month-old AP (B) and lateral (C) tibia and fibula.

Fractures

Preschool age
The upper limbs of toddlers and preschoolers are sometimes best imaged with the child sitting on the parent's lap, as shown in Fig. 22.31, using a piece of plexiglass for immobilization. In many cases, the child will be reluctant to hold their hand still and will pull their hand away as the exposure is being taken. With this in mind, timing is crucial. Consider asking another technologist to help if they are available.

With parental participation, radiography of the lower limbs can be accomplished with the child sitting or lying on the table. Preventing the patient from falling from the table is always a primary concern with preschoolers. Instruct the parent to remain by the child's side if the child is seated on the table or stool. If the examination is performed with the child lying on the table, a Velcro band over the abdomen or a parent holding should be employed.

NOTE: The child's ankle should be in flexion, not extension.

School age
School-age children generally can be managed in the same way as adult patients for upper and lower limb examinations.

Radiation protection
The upper body can be protected from scatter radiation in all examinations of the upper limbs because of the proximity of the thymus, sternum, and breast tissue. Child-sized lead aprons with cartoon characters are both popular and practical (Fig. 22.32). Depending on the department protocol, technologists are advised to attempt to explain the latest AAPM research and the National Council on Radiation Protection and Measurements (NCRP) recommendations (see Chapter 1). Students and technologists should also be aware that there are some states in the United States that have specific gonadal shielding requirements. Using appropriate collimation, exposure time, and SID can minimize dosage to the patient.

Fractures
Fractures in children's bones occur under two circumstances: abnormal stresses in normal bone and normal stresses in abnormal bone. A fracture is defined as the breaking or rupture of a bone caused by mechanical forces either applied to the bone or transmitted directly along the line of the bone. Children's bone fractures differ from those of adults because growth is active and favors rapid repair and remodeling. In general, children's bones are less dense than those of adults, and the ability to visualize soft tissue and bony detail is of utmost importance; in particular, small linear fractures are difficult to discern without good soft tissue detail. Fat pad displacement and tissue swelling may be the only radiographic signs of injury. Such subtle findings can disguise an epiphyseal growth plate fracture, which could result in irregularity or cessation of growth in the affected bone if left untreated. Overriding and distraction deformities may correct without residual deformity, but rotational deformities will not. Consequently, images of the fractured bone showing the relative positions of the two ends of the bone (AP, lateral, oblique) are necessary for evaluation of rotation; preliminary assessment may require the *contralateral* side to be examined for comparison.

The earlier in a child's life this epiphyseal fracture occurs, the better the chances of spontaneous correction of angulation fractures.

Here is an abbreviated list of some of the more common pediatric extremity fractures.

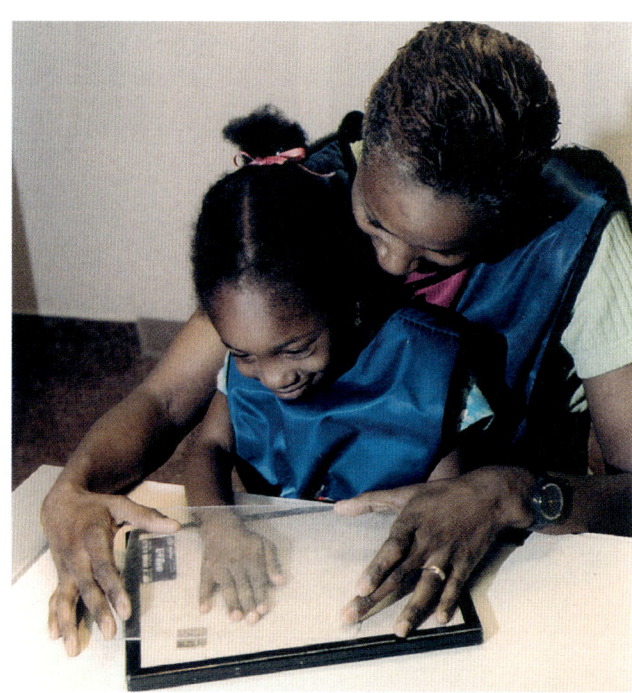

Fig. 22.31 Preschoolers are best managed sitting on a parent's lap. A lead mat is used to keep the IR from sliding. Note the use of plexiglass to immobilize fingers.

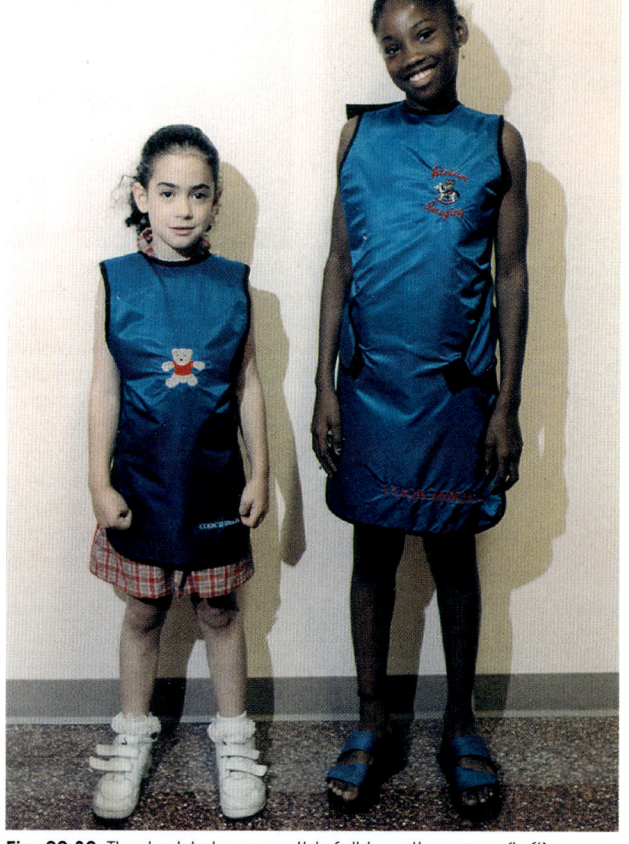

Fig. 22.32 The teddy bear on this full-length apron *(left)* makes it appropriate for young children.

Fractures

Salter-Harris
About one-third of all skeletal injuries to children are at the epiphyseal growth plates, especially in the ankle and wrist. Salter and Harris described these fractures in 1963 as Salter-Harris types I through V (Fig. 22.33).

Plastic or bow
The bones of children, compared with those of adults, can absorb and deflect more energy without breaking due to a lower bending resistance. Plastic or bowing fractures occur in children when this bending resistance is exceeded, and the bone or bones bow without breaking. The bowing fracture is a bending deformity that usually occurs in the forearm. There is no grossly visible fracture in the tubular structure of the bone; however, microfractures are visible using microscopy. The bowing is appreciable on plain images and often requires a comparison view to confirm the deformation. A bowing fracture is usually reduced under general anesthesia, as the force required to reduce the bowing is substantial.

Greenstick
A greenstick fracture occurs when one cortex of the bone's diaphysis breaks and the side remains intact.

Torus
The torus fracture is a type of greenstick fracture in which the load on the bone is in the same direction as the diaphysis, causing the cortex to fold back on itself.

Toddler's fracture
A toddler's fracture is described as a subtle, nondisplaced, oblique fracture of the distal tibia in children 9 months to 3 years of age; the fracture may only be seen on one view of the lower shaft of the tibia. If AP, lateral, and oblique projections are radiographically negative but there is strong suspicion of a toddler's fracture, a radionuclide scan may be indicated. The child's age and the presentation are significant to this diagnosis. It is important to realize that this is a common accidental injury that the parents may not have witnessed. If the onset of symptoms (e.g., pain, non–weight-bearing) is rapid and the patient's age is within the noted range, a toddler's fracture has a high index of suspicion. Remember, however, that a similar fracture in a very young infant who is not yet a "toddler" cannot be ascribed to accidental falls and, therefore, would be suspicious of abuse.

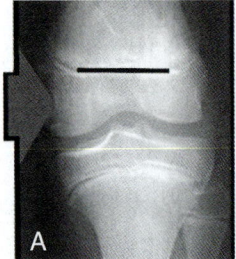 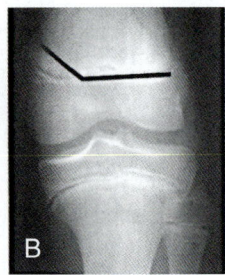 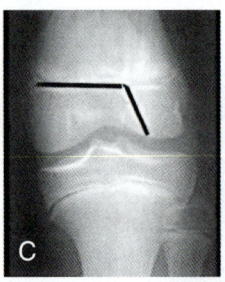 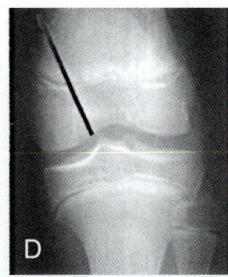 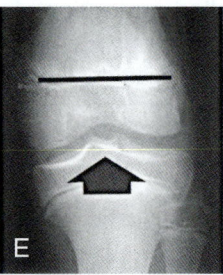

Fig. 22.33 Salter-Harris fractures. The black lines represent the fracture lines. (**A**) A type I fracture occurs directly through the growth plate. (**B**) A type II fracture extends through the growth plate and into the metaphyses. (**C**) A type III fracture line extends through the growth plate and into the epiphyses. (**D**) A type IV fracture line extends through the metaphyses, across or sometimes along the growth plate, and through the epiphyses. (**E**) A type V fracture involves a crushing of all or part of the growth plate. Fractures that occur through the epiphyses are significant injuries because they can affect growth if not recognized and treated properly. A proper radiographic technique is required for the demonstration of both soft tissue and bone. This is especially important with type I fractures, in which the growth plate is separated as a result of a lateral blow, and type V fractures, in which the growth plate has sustained a compression injury. Types I and V fractures do not occur through the bone.

Fractures

Supracondylar fracture

More severe than the toddler's fracture, the supracondylar fracture is the most common elbow fracture in children, accounting for 60% of all pediatric elbow fractures (Figs. 22.34 and 22.35). Occurring frequently in children between the ages of 3 and 10 years of age, the supracondylar fracture is caused by the child falling on an outstretched hand with hyperextension of the elbow. The most extensively displaced of these fractures can cause serious vascular and nerve damage. Great care should be taken when positioning for this fracture.

Image evaluation

Among the many striking differences in radiographic appearance between adult and pediatric patients are the bone trabeculae and the presence of epiphyseal lines or growth plates in pediatric patients. As they gain experience in evaluating pediatric images, radiographers develop a visual appreciation for these differences. For example, to the uneducated eye, a normally developing epiphysis may mimic a fracture. For this reason, and because fractures can occur through the epiphyseal plate, physicians (and, to a certain degree, radiographers) must learn to recognize epiphyseal lines and their appearance at various stages of ossification. Fractures that occur through the epiphysis are called *growth plate fractures* (Salter-Harris). Because the growth plates are composed of cartilaginous tissue, the *density* of the image must be such that soft tissue is shown in addition to bone (see Table 22.3). Visualization of the bony trabecular pattern is used as an indicator that sufficient *recorded detail* has been achieved. Because of the small size of pediatric extremities, an imaging system with superior resolution is required. Generally, the speed of the imaging system should be half that used for spines and abdomens.

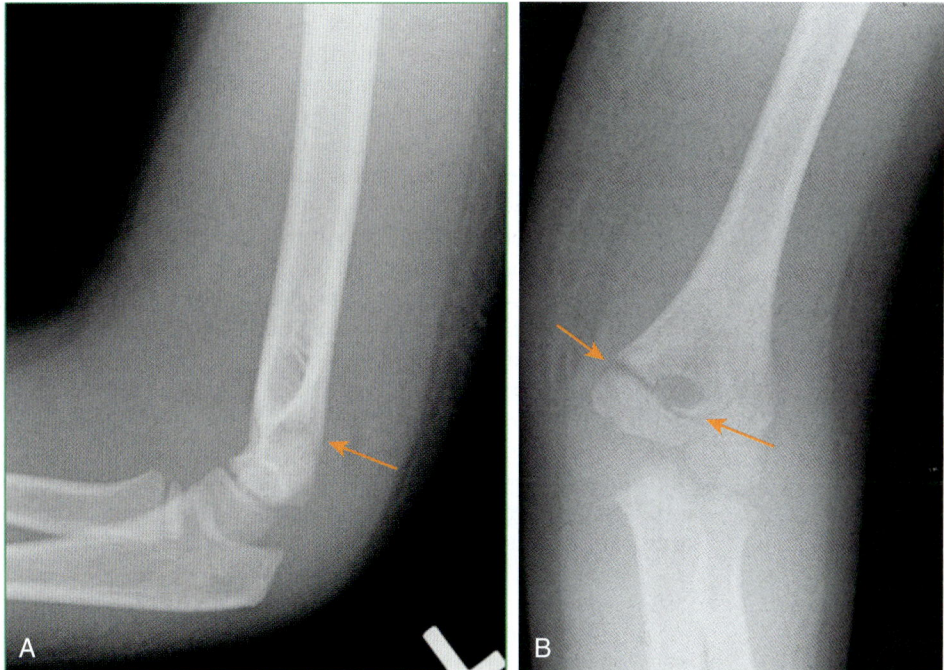

Fig. 22.34 (**A** and **B**) AP and lateral projections of a supracondylar fracture *(arrows)*.

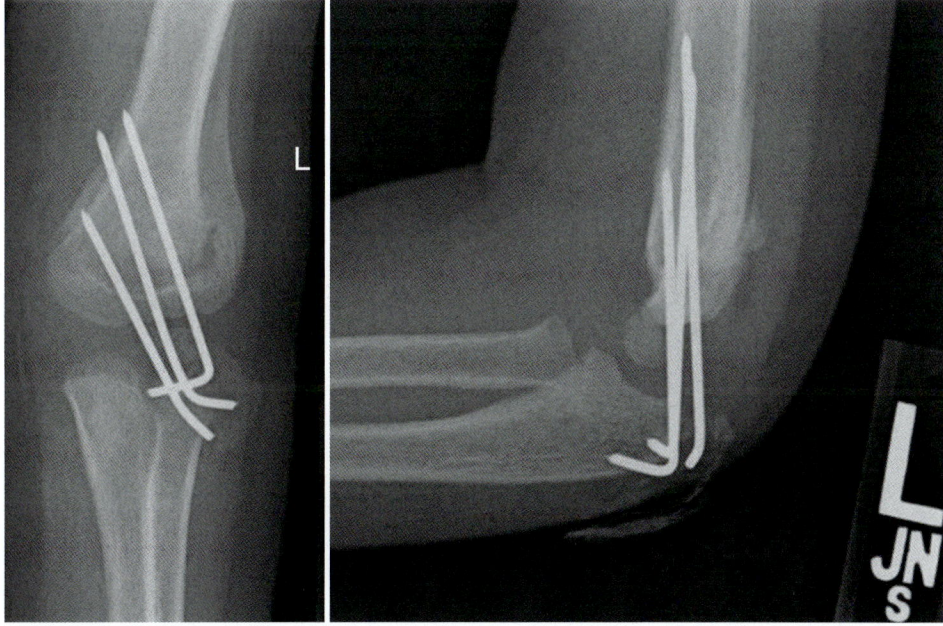

Fig. 22.35 AP and lateral elbow images of a closed reduction percutaneous pinning (CRPP) of a supracondylar fracture performed with C-arm fluoroscopic guidance in the operating room.

Skull and Paranasal Sinuses

SKULL AND PARANASAL SINUSES
Skull

The two most common indications for a pediatric radiographic skull series are to rule out craniosynostosis and fracture. Synostosis is the fusion of two bones, and it can be normal or abnormal. The term *craniosynostosis,* or *premature cranial suture synostosis,* describes the premature closure of one or more of the cranial sutures and may be isolated or part of a craniofacial syndrome; both result in the deformity of the calvaria's shape. Etiologically, abnormal synostosis is described as either primary or secondary. Primary craniosynostosis is characterized by some type of defect in one or more of the cranial sutures and can be intrinsic or familial. The familial form manifests as a component of a craniofacial syndrome (e.g., Pfeiffer, Apert, Crouzon, or Beare-Stevenson) and may be the result of one of several genetic mutations. Secondary craniosynostosis is the result of some underlying medical condition, which can be systemic or metabolic (e.g., hyperthyroidism, hypercalcemia, vitamin D deficiency, sickle cell anemia, or thalassemia). Microcephaly, encephalocele, and shunted hydrocephalus can diminish the growth stretch at sutures, which can lead to craniosynostosis secondarily.

Calvarial growth takes place perpendicular to the suture lines. The suture lines involved, time of onset, and the sequence in which individual sutures fuse will determine the nature of the deformity. When sutures fuse prematurely, calvarial growth occurs along the axis of the fused suture. The altered skull shape is diagnostic. Restoring growth is dependent on the early release of all fused sutures.

The birth prevalence of craniosynostosis ranges from approximately 3 to 5 cases per 10,000 live births. The isolated variety (only one suture affected) constitutes 80% to 90% of cases, and the sutures most commonly involved, in descending order of frequency, are sagittal, coronal, metopic, and lambdoid. The syndromic variety accounts for up to 10% to 20% of cases. Coronal synostosis is more frequently seen in females, whereas sagittal synostosis is more common in males. Most cases are diagnosed early in life. Skull images of infants are obtained in the supine position. Radiographic views include (1) a supine AP projection obtained to demonstrate the calvaria, (2) one or both lateral projections obtained to demonstrate the calvaria and skull base (both lateral projections are indicated in trauma and focal lesion evaluation), and (3) an AP axial Towne projection, but only with a 30-degree caudad angle (due to differing skull morphology in pediatric patients younger than 10 years of age), obtained to demonstrate the occipital bone and foramen magnum.

Skull fractures occurring in children are usually the result of blunt force trauma and include both accidental and nonaccidental trauma, as well as those sustained from forceps extraction at birth. Fractures can occur with minimal force in the abnormally fragile bone associated with osteogenesis imperfecta (OI). Diastatic fracture lines (breaks along the sutures) present as more lucent and linear and exhibit no interdigitations, which distinguish them from sutures. Depressed skull fractures appear dense due to the overlapping bone fragments. Skull radiography will demonstrate horizontal linear fracture lines that may not be visible on CT when the fracture is parallel to the CT axis. All skull imaging is done with a grid, a large focal spot, and using a set technique (can use AEC for AP). Clothing should be removed from the waist up as metal snaps and zipper artifacts will migrate into the finished radiograph. Immobilizing an infant for a skull series is accomplished most efficiently by using the "bunny immobilization" technique (Fig. 22.36), and in general, all three projections can be accomplished with the help of an additional technologist holding. The parents can also be drafted to immobilize the shoulders, torso, and legs (sandbags will work if the patient is younger than 2 years); however, this technique requires much more instruction and is less reliable.

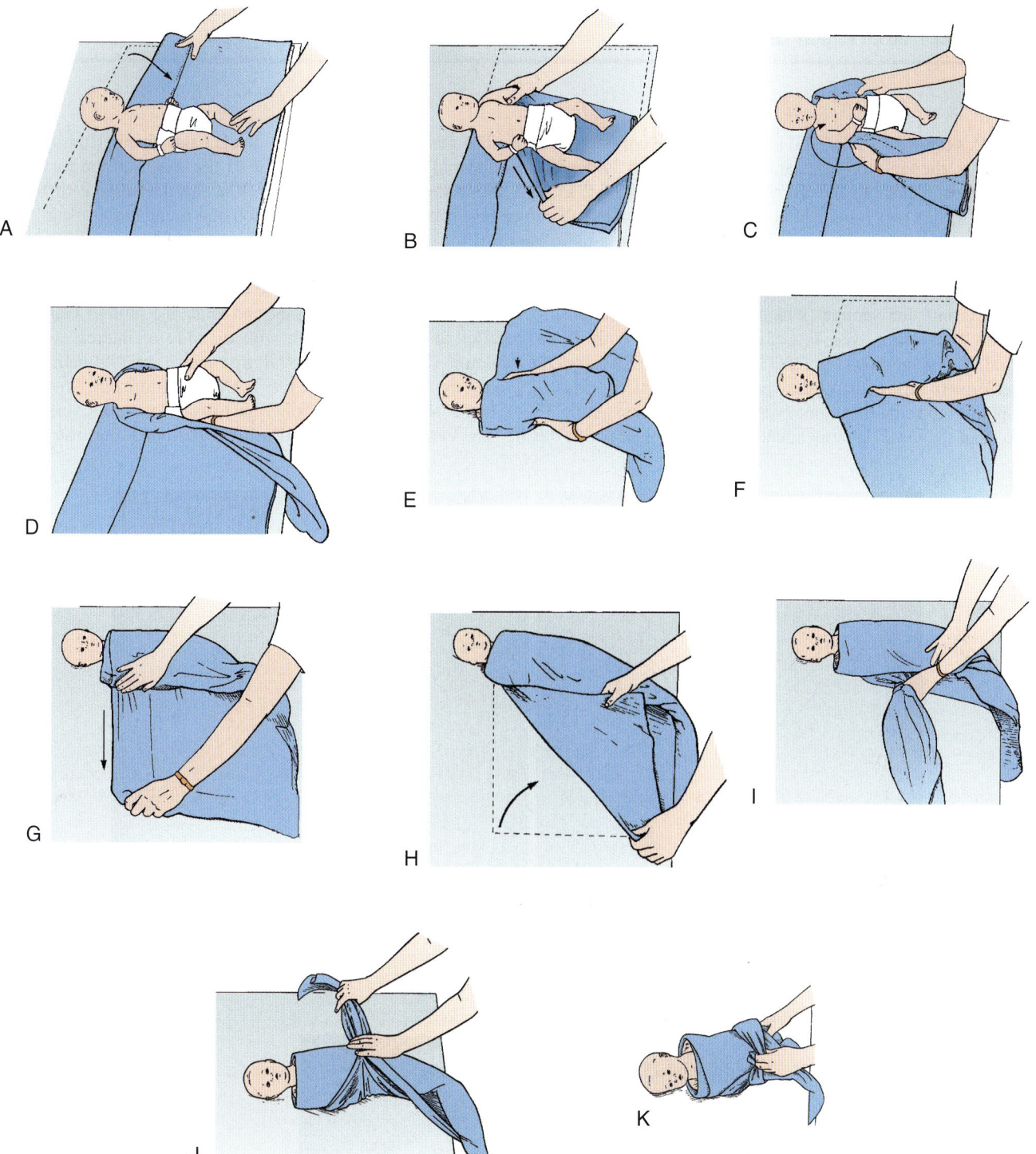

Fig. 22.36 The "bunny" method used to immobilize the patient for cranial radiography. (**A**) to (**D**) focus on immobilization of the shoulders, (**E**) to (**G**) concentrate on the humeri, and (**H**) to (**K**) illustrate the way the sheet is folded and wrapped to immobilize the legs. (**A**) Begin with a standard hospital sheet folded in half lengthwise. Make a 15-cm (6-inch) fold at the top and lay the child down about 2 feet from the end of the sheet. (**B**) Wrap the end of the sheet over the left shoulder and pass the sheet under the child. (**C**) This step makes use of the 15-cm (6-inch) fold. Reach under, undo the fold, and wrap it over the right shoulder. (Steps (**B**) and (**C**) are crucial to the success of this immobilization technique because they prevent the child from wiggling their shoulders free.) (**D**) After wrapping the right shoulder, pass the end of the sheet under the child. Pull it through to keep the right arm snug against the body. (**E**) Begin wrapping, keeping the sheet snug over the upper body to immobilize the humeri. (**F**) Lift the lower body and pass the sheet underneath, keeping the child's head on the table. Repeat steps (**E**) and (**F**) if material permits. (**G**) Make sure the material is evenly wrapped around the upper body. (Extra rolls around the shoulder and neck area produce artifacts on 30-degree fronto-occipital and submentovertical images.) (**H**) Make a diagonal fold with the remaining material (approximately 2 feet). (**I**) Roll the material together. (**J**) Snugly wrap this over the child's femora. (The tendency to misjudge the location of the femora and thus wrap too snugly around the lower legs should be avoided.) (**K**) Tuck the end of the rolled material in front. (If not enough material remains to tuck in, use a Velcro strip or tape to secure it.)

(From the Michener Institute for Applied Health Sciences, Toronto, Ontario, Canada.)

Skull and Paranasal Sinuses

The AP skull (Fig. 22.37A) is positioned with the infraorbitomeatal line (IOML) perpendicular to the IR with no tube angle, using two round, radiolucent sponges, one on either side of the head. It is important when using these sponges to use your palms rather than pressing your fingers into the sponge (which will appear on the image, see Fig. 22.10). The axial Towne method (Fig. 22.37B) is also performed supine using the "mouse ears" sponges to bring the chin toward the chest so that the OML is perpendicular to the exam table and IR. The central ray is directed 30 degrees caudad and enters 2.5 to 5 cm (1–2 inches) above the glabella. The lateral skull can be best imaged using a left cross-table lateral (Figs. 22.38 and 22.39) approach with the infant supine and elevated on a radiolucent pad or box device and positioned supine. The grid holder with IR is parallel to the skull and extends to the tabletop (below the radiolucent pad) to avoid clipping of the posterior skull. The infant's shoulder is in contact with the IR. The central ray is perpendicular and enters 1 cm (0.4 inch) superior to the external auditory meatus (EAM). Use the flat surface of the hand to position one round "mouse ear" sponge just superior to the vertex of the skull and the other hand to hold the mental protuberance of the mandible. Leave the infant supine and rotate the skull to a lateral position with the side of interest down. The central ray enters 1 cm (0.4 inch) superior to the EAM. Position one "mouse ear" sponge just posterior to the vertex of the skull using a flat hand, and use the other

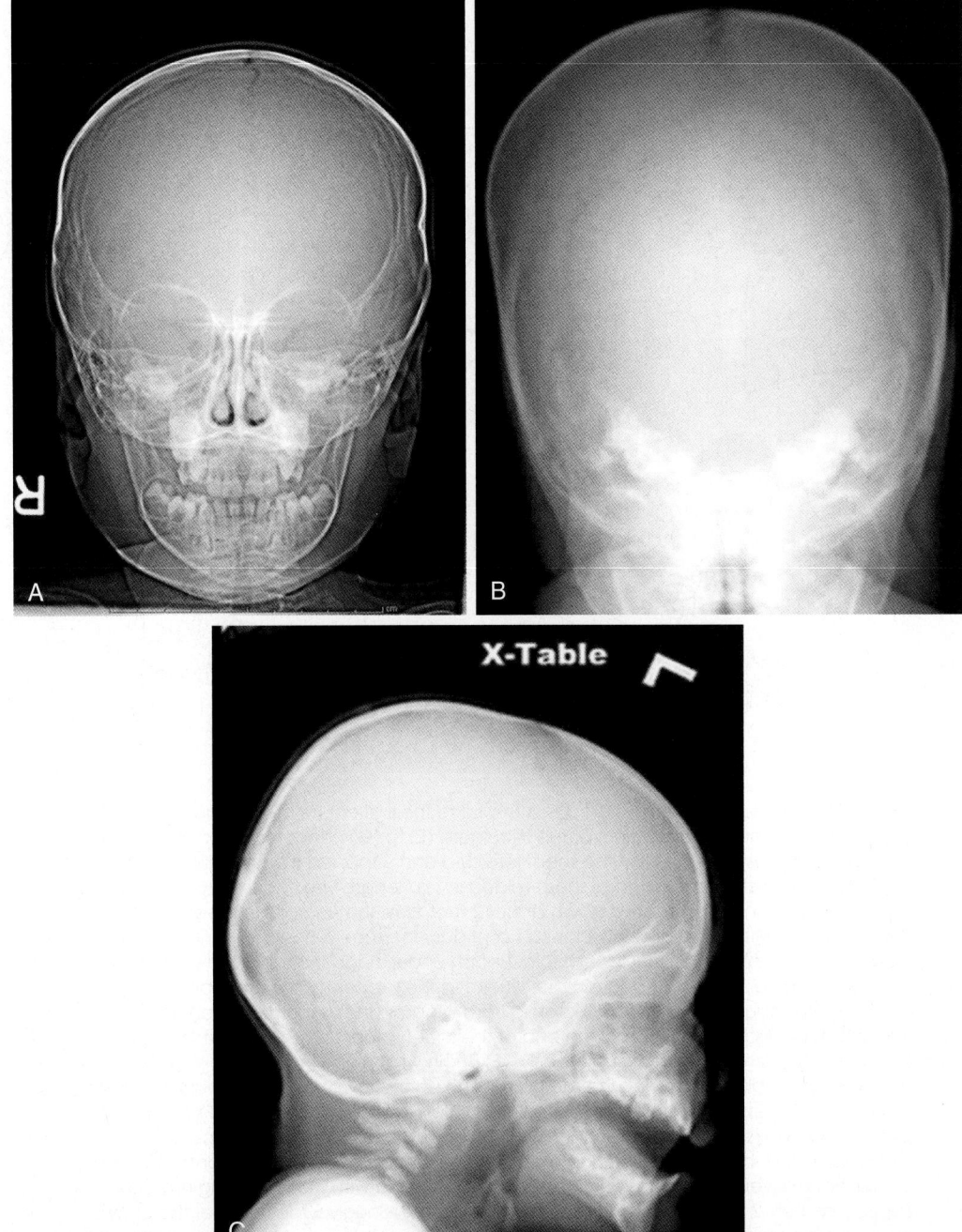

Fig. 22.37 (**A**) AP skull. (**B**) Towne 30 degrees. (**C**) Lateral.

Skull and Paranasal Sinuses

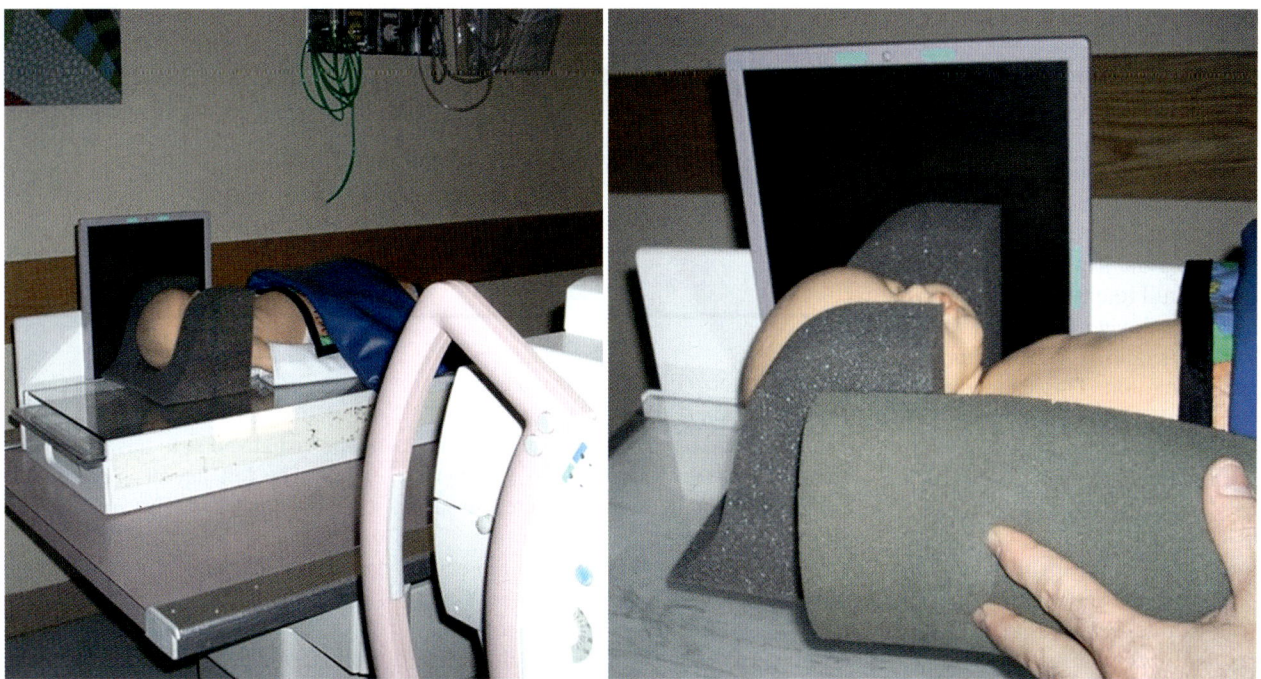

Fig. 22.38 Cross-table lateral skull positioning. Note the use of radiolucent sponges and modified "bunny wrap" immobilization. One sponge cradles the skull and elevates the back of the skull to ensure the occipital is included in the image. The other radiolucent sponge acts as a light compression to minimize motion. This technique usually requires the use of two persons.

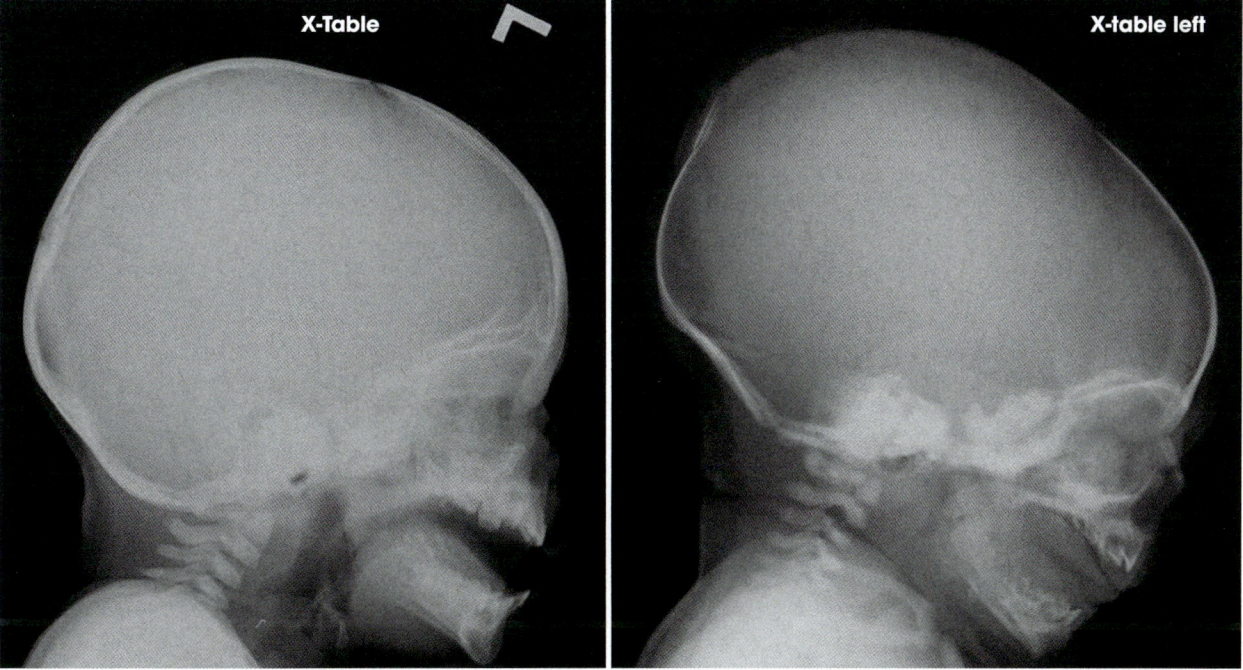

Fig. 22.39 Cross-table lateral skull imaging can be accomplished with radiolucent sponges.

Skull and Paranasal Sinuses

hand to hold the mental protuberance of the mandible. This is an awkward position for infants, so expect them to struggle (Table 22.4). A successful alternative method for lateral skull imaging is to use a cross-table technique. Note the use of radiolucent sponges and modified "bunny wrap" immobilization in Fig. 22.38. One sponge cradles the skull and elevates the back of the skull to ensure the occipital is included in the image. The other radiolucent sponge acts as a light compression to minimize motion. This technique usually requires the use of two people. Two cross-table images using this technique are shown in Fig. 22.39.

Paranasal sinuses

The main indication for performing a paranasal sinus series on the pediatric patient is to rule out sinusitis. However, radiographic opacification is not a clear indication of sinus disease; incidental findings of mucosal thickening with magnetic resonance imaging (MRI) are common in children younger than 5 years when examined for other indicated reasons. Because errors in positioning may simulate pathologic change in this age group, demonstrating air-fluid level in an upright exam with compelling clinical and laboratory support would probably warrant the diagnosis of sinusitis without resorting to CT. The maxillary, ethmoid, and sphenoid sinuses are present and aerated at birth, whereas the frontal sinuses do not usually appear until the second year.

The paranasal sinus protocol may include three views: Caldwell (Fig. 22.40), Waters (Fig. 22.41), and a left lateral projection (Fig. 22.42), which should include frontal sinus anatomy, C-spine, and airway to the thoracic inlet. Improper collimation to the area of interest is the single most common shortcoming. To preserve image quality, consider precollimating before moving the patient into position; collimate to the area of interest only. Adjusting your light field on the back of the head does not allow for the divergence of the central ray, leading to the inclusion of too much of the skull. Experience has shown that in children younger than 8 years, the Caldwell method requires no central ray angulation, orbitomeatal line (OML) perpendicular or can be accomplished with forehead and nose against the bucky. This is possible due to the immature and varying morphology of the pediatric skull (Fig. 22.43).

The central ray is horizontal and exits at the nasion for the Caldwell method. For the Waters method, the child's nose and chin touch the bucky and the central ray remains horizontal, exiting at the acanthion and projecting the petrous ridges below the maxillary sinuses. Central ray angulation may cause the sinuses to either not be visualized or to falsely appear obliterated. The left lateral is equivalent to a soft tissue neck (STN) and sinus series combination, which includes the frontal sinuses (where frontal sinuses will be seen, but not usually prior to 2 years), the nasal shadow, and the C-spine to the thoracic inlet. With both the Waters and the Caldwell methods, ask the patient to move away from the bucky or upright grid once you have determined the appropriate receptor height, precollimate to the area of interest, and then place the patient back in the light field. The image quality will be improved and radiation to the patient will be reduced. This technique takes some getting used to because the projected light field on the back of the head will appear too small, but trust science: the beam will diverge. Place your marker so that it will not appear over an area of interest. The exposure should be taken during inspiration through the nose to fill the nasopharynx with air to help evaluate for adenoid hypertrophy.

TABLE 22.4
Summary of skull projections

AP skull	No angle on central ray, which enters at the nasion with the orbitomeatal line perpendicular to the imaging plate
AP axial Towne	Central ray 30-degree caudad, enters at the nasion
Lateral 1	Dorsal decubitus projection (cross-table lateral); central ray enters superior to external auditory meatus
Lateral 2	Supine with side of interest down; central ray enters superior to external auditory meatus

Skull and Paranasal Sinuses

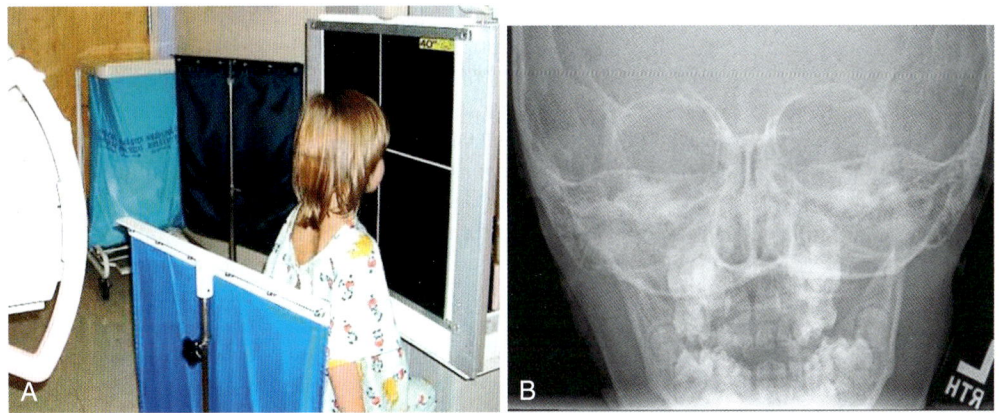

Fig. 22.40 (A) Caldwell without 15-degree angle. Note that both nose and forehead touch the grid at this age. (B) Caldwell image.

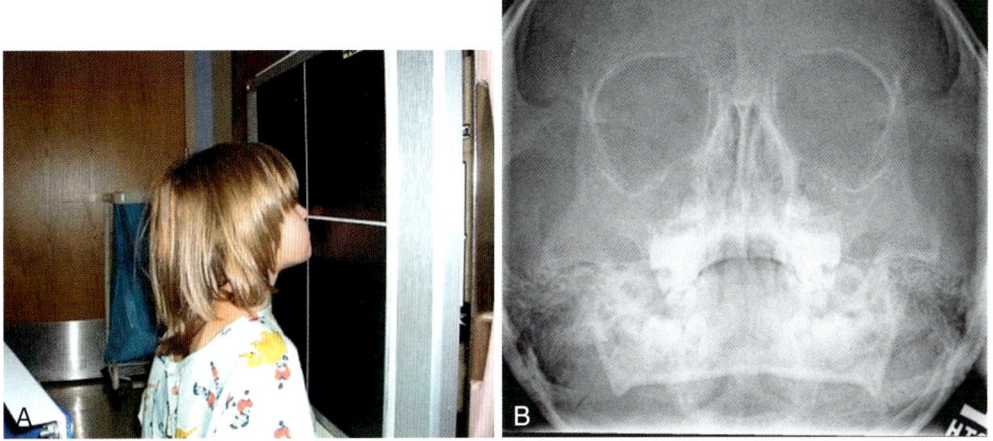

Fig. 22.41 (A) Waters method with chin and nose touching grid. (B) Waters image.

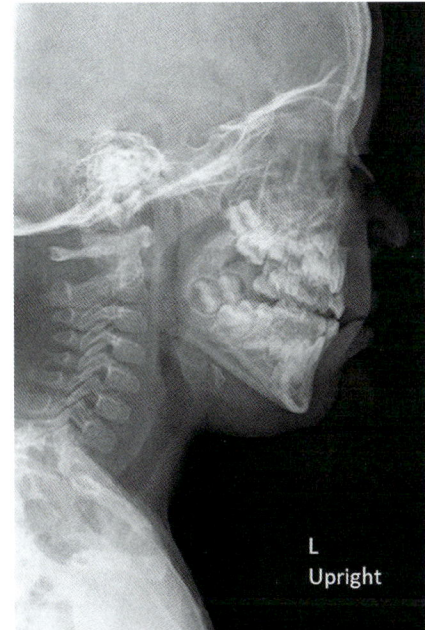

Fig. 22.42 Lateral projection for sinus series. The indication for the exam is normally noisy breathing with suspected adenoid hypertrophy. Often collimation includes from the frontal sinus to the thoracic inlet on inspiration through the nose in cases of other possible causes such as foreign bodies and retropharyngeal space anomalies (e.g., abscess). This collimation is also used for soft tissue neck for similar reasons.

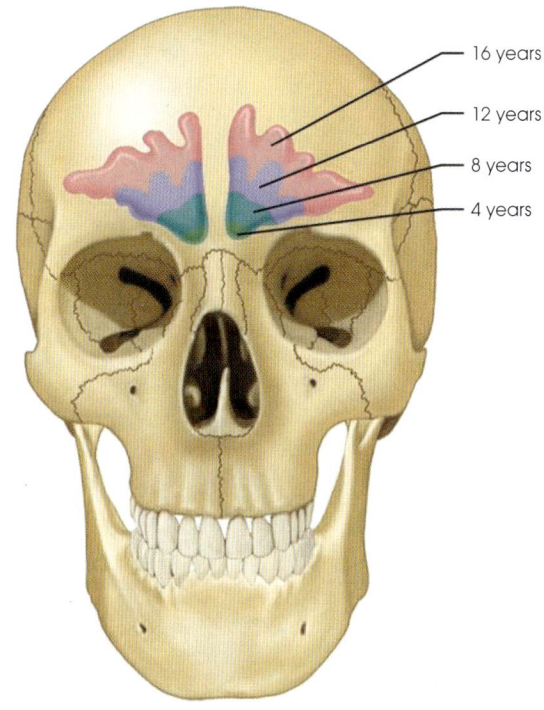

Fig. 22.43 Frontal sinus development correlated with age—*green*, 4 years; *blue*, 8 years; *purple*, 12 years; *pink*, 16 years.

(From Fonseca RJ, Barber DH, Powers M, et al.: *Oral and maxillofacial trauma*, ed 4, St Louis, 2013, Elsevier.)

Soft Tissue Neck

SOFT TISSUE NECK

Indications for the STN include foreign bodies (FBs), stridor, laryngo- and tracheomalacia, laryngotracheal bronchitis, epiglottitis, and adenoid hypertrophy. The diagnostic quality of this exam requires careful instructions, neck extension, inspiratory exposure, and complete immobilization. These requirements are more easily achieved with the infant or child in the supine position, although the exam can be done successfully with the patient in the upright position, depending on how much the child cooperates. The only contraindication to the supine position is the presence of epiglottitis (Fig. 22.44); these patients must always be imaged in the sitting or upright position. *Never place these patients in the supine position, as a swollen epiglottis can block the airway.* A baby box can be used for STN exams with infants and small children (6 months–3 years). A 15-degree radiolucent sponge is placed under the infant's/child's shoulders to achieve a slight extension of the neck and airway (shielding and immobilization are identical to the chest x-ray). STN exams require two technologists. A parent will hold the patient at the shoulders, pulling down slightly. The second technologist uses two round ear sponges (with their hands flat), one on either side of the head and above the sella turcica, to hold the head in a true lateral position in extension and without rotation (Fig. 22.45). Collimation should be from the frontal sinuses (including complete nasal passage) to the thoracic inlet, including the entire C-spine. The head in flexion or an expiratory image may cause a false positive for enlargement of the retropharyngeal soft tissues and therefore mimic pathology. The lateral projection should be done with a set technique, no grid, at an 182-cm (72-inch) SID. If possible, with a cooperative patient, take the exposure *during inspiration through the nose*. This will facilitate adequate filling of the nasopharynx to diagnose adenoid hypertrophy. Also, cooperative toddlers may achieve this by instructing them to "smell a flower." The experienced pediatric radiographer will have the rotor prepped and will take the exposure during the "smell" inspiration. It is advised to do a "smell test" practice first to adjust for timing, positioning, and collimation.

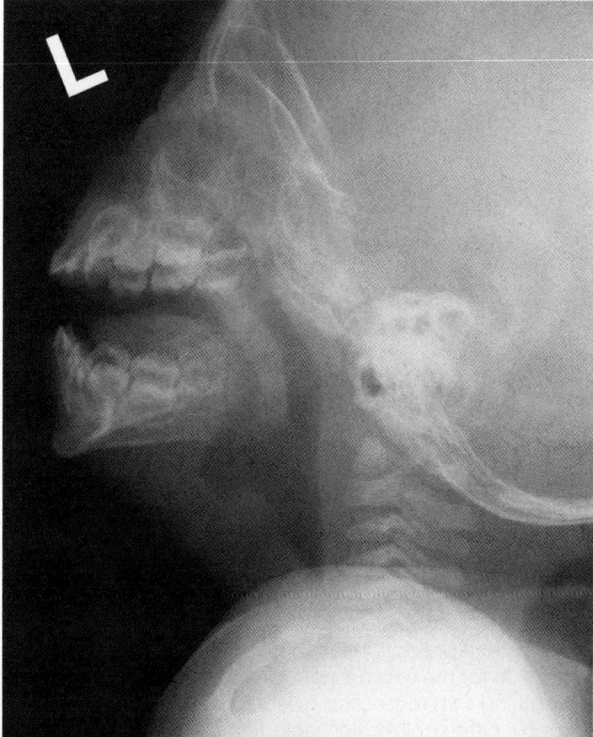

Fig. 22.44 Diffuse swelling of the epiglottis, aryepiglottic folds, and the retropharyngeal soft tissues. These findings are consistent with epiglottitis.

Soft Tissue Neck

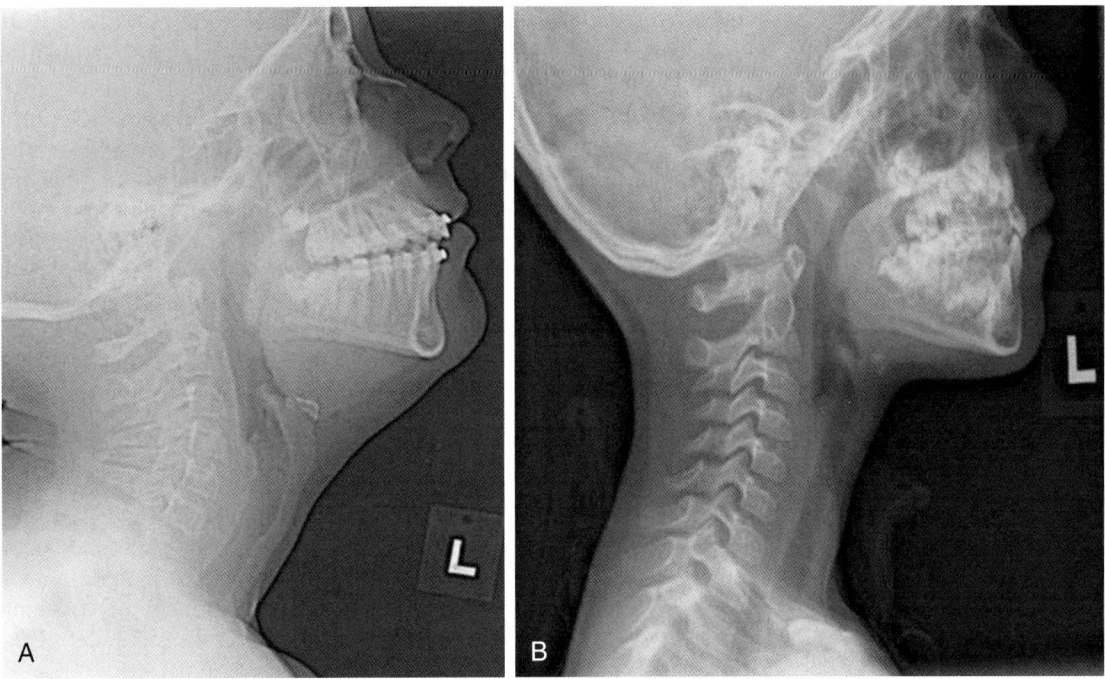

Fig. 22.45 (**A**) Soft tissue neck (STN) with a Fuji Synapse soft tissue preset. (**B**) STN without preset.

The AP axial STN projection must be performed with a 102-cm (40-inch) SID no grid technique. Patients from infants to adolescents should be positioned with the patient's occlusal plane perpendicular to the image receptor (exact positioning will vary with age) to prevent the occipital bone from superimposing the airway (overextension). Flexion will also cause superimposition of the airway. The thick part of a 15-degree radiolucent sponge placed under the patient's shoulders will help position the skull for the AP axial supine extension (Fig. 22.46) using a 15-degree extension of the skull). A small cephalad angle can also be used with the AP projection to better visualize C1 and C2.

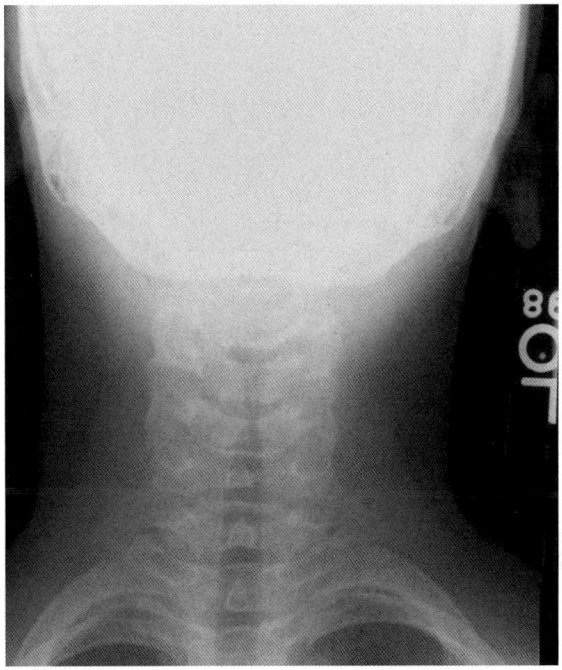

Fig. 22.46 A well-positioned and collimated AP axial projection with a 15-degree wedge radiolucent sponge placed under the patient's shoulders and a small cephalad angle.

Foreign Bodies

Foreign Bodies

AIRWAY FOREIGN BODY

Airway FBs occur frequently in children aged 6 months to 3 years and are not uncommon in teenagers. Radiolucent objects include firm vegetables, peanuts, hard candy, peas, carrots, and raisins. Round-shaped foods are the most frequently aspirated. Radiopaque FBs (Fig. 22.47) include coins (most common), hair clips, safety pins, and small toys. Splintered wood and glass have also been discovered, usually as the result of traumatic injury. Balloons are most likely to result in death. A young child with a persistent cough but without a fever carries a high index of suspicion for FB aspiration. Clinical presentations may also include stridor, a wheezing cough, recurrent pneumonia, or hemoptysis. If a radiolucent FB is in the trachea, the chest image may be normal and require a CT, or it may demonstrate bilateral overinflation or underinflation (air trapping). More commonly, the FB is found in the bronchial tree, and most frequently the right main stem bronchus, which is larger and more in line with the trachea. In images, the FB presents most commonly as a unilateral hyperlucent lung (see Fig. 22.47A).

If an FB is suspected clinically, inspiratory and expiratory images may be obtained to rule out air trapping, as younger children will be unable to cooperate with inhalation and expiration commands; right and left decubitus views would then be indicated. The hyperinflated lung will not deflate when the patient is lying on the affected side. A routine protocol for imaging FB includes an AP chest to include the full airway, an abdomen to include lung bases and pubic symphysis, and a lateral STN (frontal sinus to thoracic inlet, including C-spine). All images must overlap. This survey ensures that multiple objects are not missed and provides a complete imaging of the airway and alimentary tract. If the FB is suspected of being in the airway, then bilateral decubitus views would be indicated.

INGESTED FOREIGN BODY (PICA)

Whereas older children and parents might provide a history of FB ingestion, young children may simply present with unexplained drooling or the inability to swallow solids. The image readily demonstrates a radiopaque object, of which coins are the most common. A coin in the esophagus will usually lie in the coronal plane (Fig. 22.48B), whereas a coin in the trachea will be visualized in the sagittal plane; a nonradiopaque FB may require an esophagogram for visualization. If a contrast study is indicated, a small amount of low-osmolar, nonionic, water-soluble contrast should be used, such as Iohexol (Omnipaque 350). Pica, or the compulsive ingestion of nonfood articles, may be common in those with serious mental impairment or developmental delay (Figs. 22.49 and 22.50). Pica is the medieval Latin name for a magpie, a bird that is claimed to have a penchant for eating almost anything.

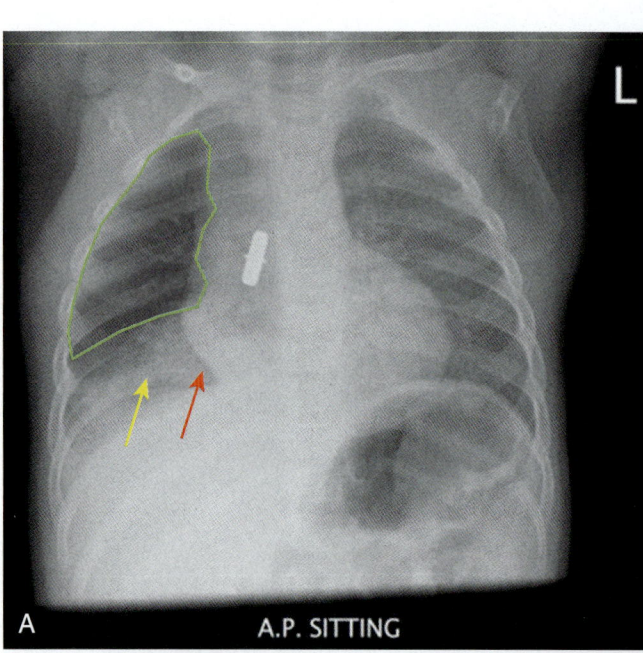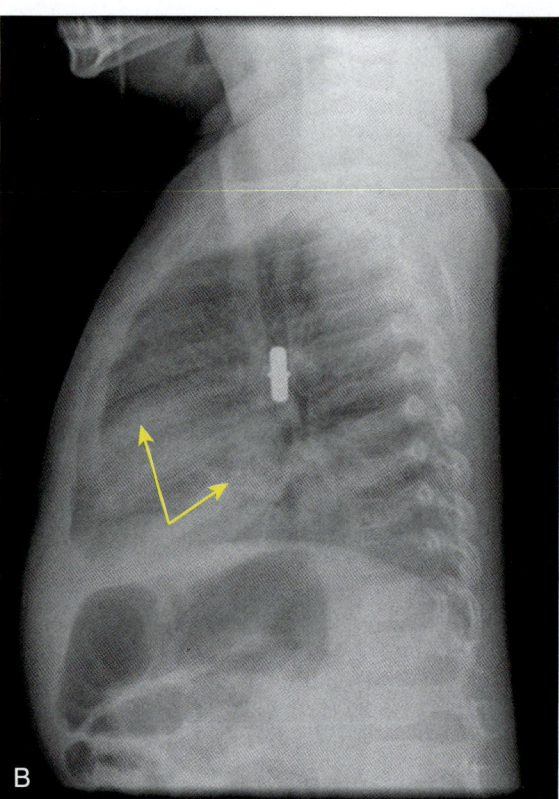

Fig. 22.47 (A) A foreign body in the right main stem bronchus. There is atelectasis (collapse) predominantly affecting the right lower lobe (yellow arrow). Note the distinct right heart border on the AP (red arrow) and unilateral hyperlucent lung (green outline). (B) Note the patchy opacities below the foreign body in the lateral view (yellow arrows).

(Used with permission from Lifeinthefastlane.com at https://litfl.com/inhalational-emergency/.)

Foreign Bodies

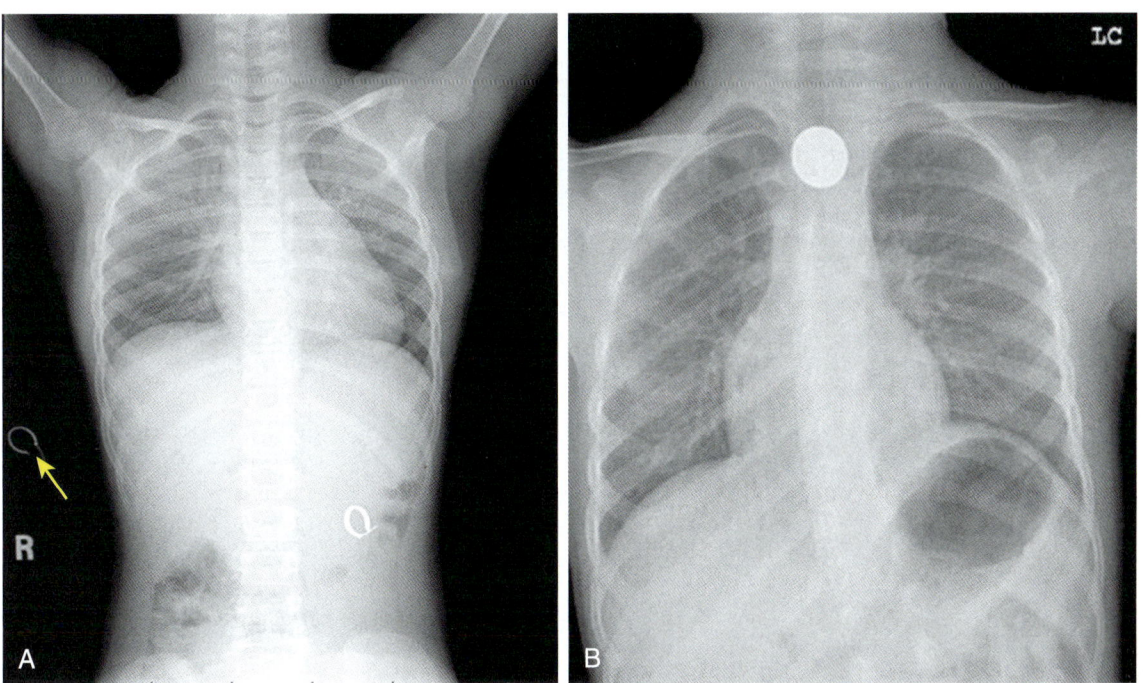

Fig. 22.48 (**A**) Ingested earring. Reference earring placed lateral to the patient *(yellow arrow)* to assist in confirmation. (**B**) Coin in the coronal plane.

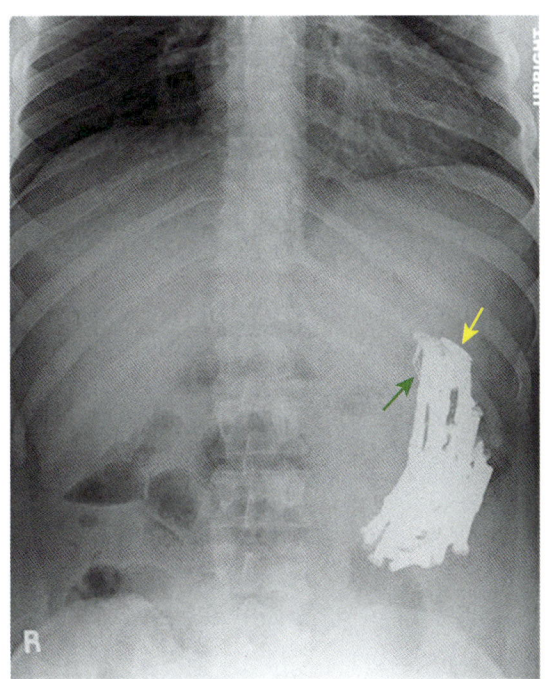

Fig. 22.49 Gastrointestinal pica with paper clip *(green arrow)* and coin *(yellow arrow)*.

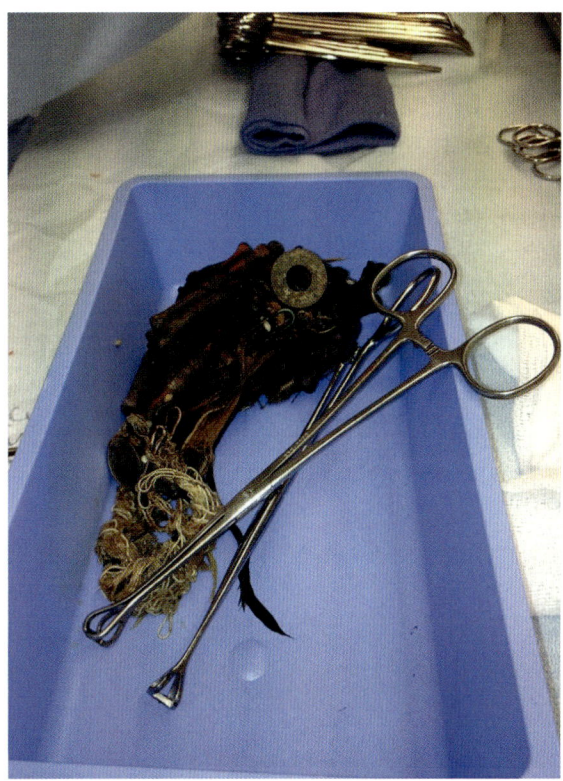

Fig. 22.50 This operating room photo shows the ingested items removed from a patient with pica seen in the radiograph in Fig. 22.49.

Foreign Bodies

INSERTED FOREIGN BODY (POLYEMBOLOKOILAMANIA)

When children *insert* radiopaque foreign objects into body cavities, it is termed *polyembolokoilamania*. The PA and lateral images seen here demonstrate a 5-year-old boy who inserted a screw into his nasal cavity (Figs. 22.51 and 22.52).

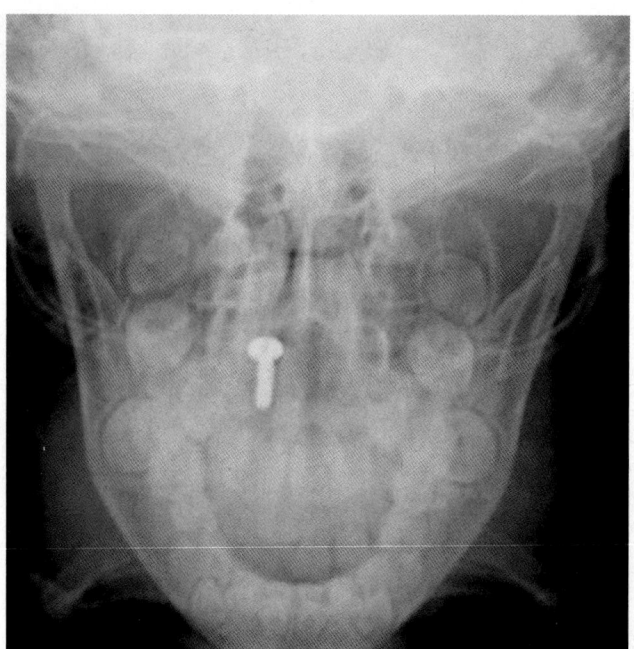

Fig. 22.51 PA facial bone projection of a 5-year-old boy with polyembolokoilamania who pushed a screw into his nasal cavity.

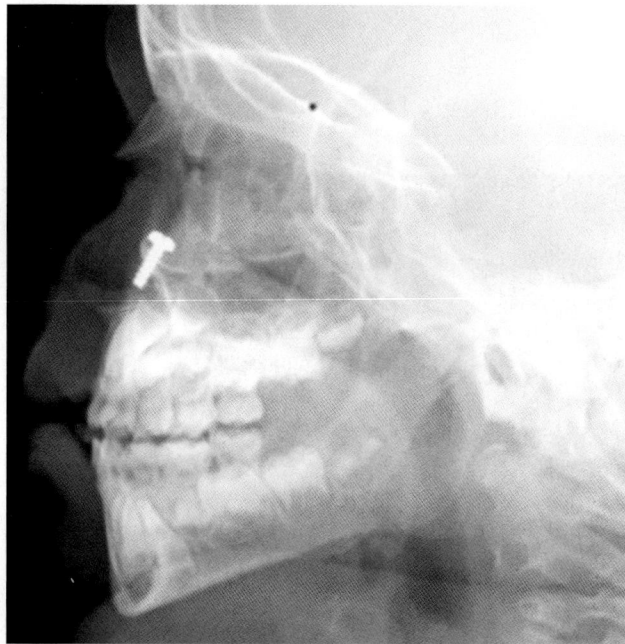

Fig. 22.52 Lateral facial bone projection of the 5-year-old patient in Fig. 22.51.

Mobile Considerations for Neonatal Intensive Care Unit (NICU)

Mobile Considerations for Neonatal Intensive Care Unit (NICU)

Neonatal mobile radiography is a specialty within itself, and assertive radiographers are imperative to producing diagnostic images. Imaging of neonates requires a systematic approach and specialized training. This section will address medical efficacy from the ordering physician to the technical and positioning challenges presented to the radiographer when performing mobile radiography in the NICU environment. Teamwork, communication, procedural considerations, soft tissue landmarks, and standardized neonatal radiography protocols are discussed. Recommendations of simulation exercises for student radiographers are presented.

TEAM-BASED APPROACH

Communication and teamwork with NICU nursing and surgical staff are critical to creating a quality radiograph of a neonate. Creating a friendly dialogue with NICU staff is essential to expediting the exam. In most cases, the NICU nurse is anticipating the arrival of the radiographer and will have the NICU patient ready for the exam (free of artifacts). Monthly meetings and opportunities to meet with the NICU physicians, charge nurses, and staff nurses can create a cohesive partnership of team-based communication and expectations.

ELEMENTS OF AN ACCEPTABLE IMAGE

The radiographer should consider specific elements when producing an acceptable or diagnostic image of a neonate. Some of the important elements include but are not limited to the following:
- Exams are performed at a standardized source-to-image receptor distance (SID) of 102 cm (40 inches).
- Radiograph includes correct marker.
- Proper exposure factors to demonstrate pathology, soft tissue, and bony detail.
- Correct positioning of structural anatomy (i.e., free from rotation).
- Removal of artifacts (e.g., diapers, ECG leads, tubes, radiopaque wires). Follow departmental protocol and request assistance.
- Proper collimation to the anatomy of interest.
- Optimal image contrast and exposure index range.

When performing a mobile neonatal exam, radiographers are presented with additional challenges. The patient's condition in the NICU is almost always compromised. The neonate is normally intubated, has central venous access devices (CVADs), feeding tubes, chest tubes, and endotracheal tubes (ETTs). Before entering the NICU, the radiographer should clean the mobile unit, disinfect markers, wash their hands, and don proper PPE. The radiographer should also wash their hands and change gloves between patients. The radiographer must always first verify patient identification and confirm the order with the nurse prior to exposure. Proceeding without the help of a nurse and moving the patient could result in desaturation of the patient, further compromising the patient's condition, and may be considered negligent. Always seek help from the NICU nurse or caretaker assigned to the patient when performing mobile exams.

NEONATE SOFT TISSUE LANDMARKS

An additional challenge to imaging neonates is to determine the anatomy to include for each exam. In nearly all cases, the radiographer has only *soft tissue* landmarks of the chest or abdomen. In general, it is good practice to avoid palpating for any bony landmarks to reduce the possibility of infection or desaturation. The (1) earlobes, (2) chest nipple line, (3) umbilicus (belly button), and (4) pubic symphysis (bottom of buttocks) are four visible soft tissue landmarks that every radiographer can identify visually (Figs. 22.53 and 22.54).

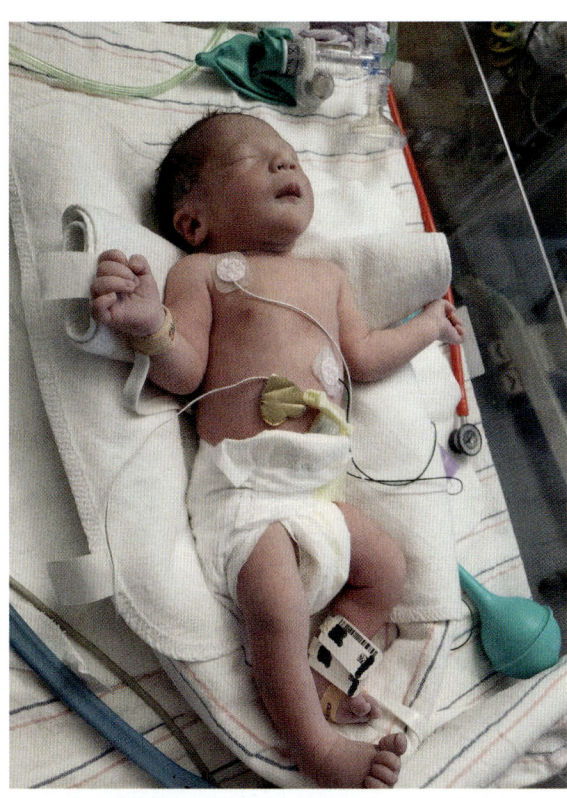

Fig. 22.53 A typical newborn seen in a NICU. (Courtesy Karlie McDaniel, RTR.)

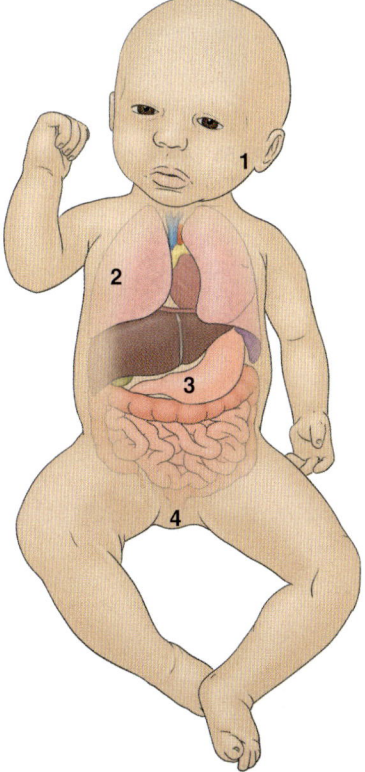

Fig. 22.54 This diagram demonstrates the four visible soft tissue landmarks used in portable and routine pediatric abdominal and chest radiography: The earlobes *(1)*, chest nipple line *(2)*, umbilicus (belly button) *(3)*, and pubic symphysis (bottom of buttocks) *(4)*.

Mobile Considerations for Neonatal Intensive Care Unit (NICU)

NEONATE NUANCES

When performing neonatal radiographs, the easiest way to determine inspiration is to observe the rise and fall of the neonate's chest and abdomen. In general, when the belly "rises" to its maximum height, this is full inspiration. Other items that may be considered prior to exposure (if negotiable) are the removal of the diaper, leads, and wires that will cause image artifacts. Check first to make sure that removing artifacts does not compromise the patient's condition and to obtain the permission of the nurse or caretaker. Be sure to check departmental protocol before removal of ECG leads, and request assistance to reduce the possibility of infection. In many institutions, there are commercially available radiolucent neonatal ECG leads (electrodes). Using radiolucent ECG leads reduces artifacts on images and frees the radiologist from "reading" through the myriad of radiopaque ECG wire leads that may obscure anatomy or mimic pathology (Figs. 22.55A and B).

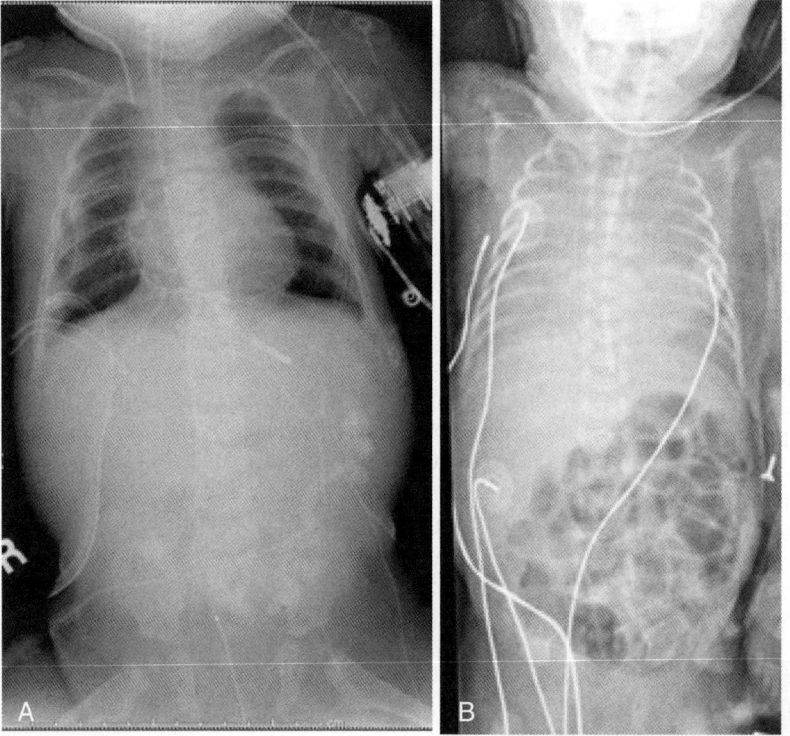

Fig. 22.55 (**A**) AP chest and abdomen with radiolucent ECG leads (electrodes). (**B**) AP chest and abdomen with radiopaque ECG leads (electrodes).

Mobile Considerations for Neonatal Intensive Care Unit (NICU)

The following are recommendations for performing neonatal imaging exams.

PORTABLE AP NEONATE CHEST
Preexposure positioning
- If the IR size allows, place it inside the tray located underneath the incubator (Fig. 22.56). If the IR does not fit, wrap or cover the IR and place it directly under the neonate. A warm blanket is recommended.
- Adjust the patient and center the chest to the IR.
- Ensure that the four borders (top, bottom, and two sides) of the IR include the anatomy of interest. (Caution: Patients tend to migrate to the edge of the image receptor.)
- Have the nurse adjust the neonate's head until the MSP is perpendicular to the IR to avoid chest rotation. Check first to make sure that moving the head will not compromise the patient's condition.
- Ask the nurse to move the patient's arms out of the chest area and to hold them if necessary. Provide the nurse with a lead apron to hold for the exposure.
- Direct the central ray perpendicular to the MSP at level T7 near the nipple line (Fig. 22.57A) with 102 cm (40 inches) SID.
- Place side marker in the collimated exposure field.
- Adjust the radiation field on the collimator to below the earlobes and approximately 4 cm (1.5 inches) above the umbilicus (Fig. 22.57B).
- With the rotor prepped and when the neonate's chest and abdomen rise to its maximum height (full inspiration), take the exposure.

EVALUATION CRITERIA
The optimum image obtained using correct positioning, CR-part-IR alignment, collimation, and exposure factors will demonstrate:
- Upper airway to the gastric bubble
- Evidence of proper collimation and presence of a side marker placed clear of anatomy of interest
- Entire lungs, from the apices to the costophrenic angles (Fig. 22.57C)
- Diaphragm visualized below or at the apex of the heart
- No rotation, as demonstrated by the sternal ends of the clavicles equidistant from the spine

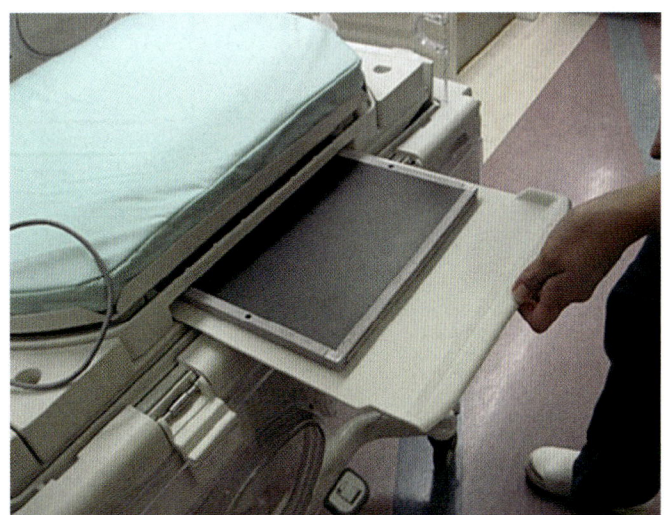

Fig. 22.56 IR placement in incubator (Isolette) tray.

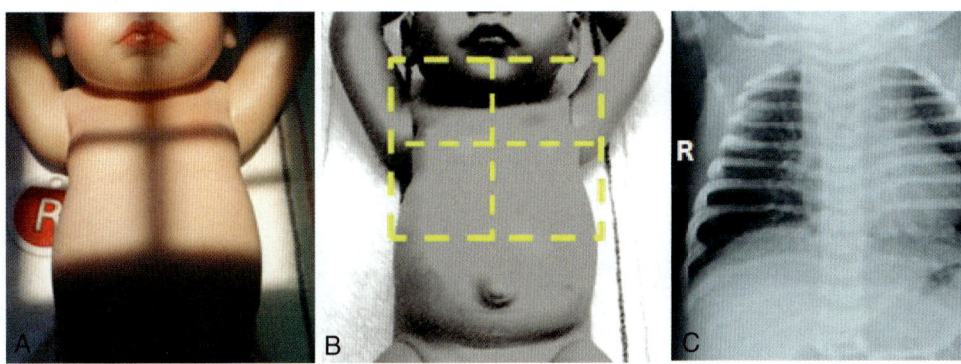

Fig. 22.57 (**A**) AP chest, central ray directed to nipple line. (**B**) AP chest, radiation light field. (**C**) AP chest radiograph.

Mobile Considerations for Neonatal Intensive Care Unit (NICU)

PORTABLE DECUBITUS NEONATE CHEST
R or L lateral recumbent
Preexposure positioning
- Place the patient in a lateral decubitus position, lying on either the affected or the unaffected side, as indicated by the existing condition. Assess the patient's condition and request assistance with positioning.
- Place the radiolucent sponge (covered) directly under the neonate patient.
- Wrap or cover the IR and ensure that the bottom edge of the vertical IR drops below the sponge to include anatomy on side down (Fig. 22.58).
- Have the nurse extend the patient's arms above the head and position the thorax in a true lateral position. Indicate the side up/down.
- Direct the central ray horizontally and perpendicular to the MSP at level T7 near the nipple line (Fig. 22.59), and ensure 102 cm (40 inches) SID.
- Place side marker in the collimated exposure field.
- Adjust the radiation field on the collimator to include the earlobes and approximately 4 cm (1.5 inches) above the umbilicus. This collimation will ensure inclusion of the upper airway and gastric bubble.
- Observe the patient's breathing, and expose on inspiration.

EVALUATION CRITERIA
The optimum image obtained using correct positioning, CR-part-IR alignment, collimation, and exposure factors will demonstrate:
- Entire lungs, from the apices to the costophrenic angles (Fig. 22.60)
- No rotation, as demonstrated by the sternal ends of the clavicles equidistant from the spine
- Evidence of proper collimation and presence of a side marker placed clear of anatomy of interest
- Fluid levels in the pleural cavity are best visualized with the affected side down. Air levels are best visualized with the affected side up

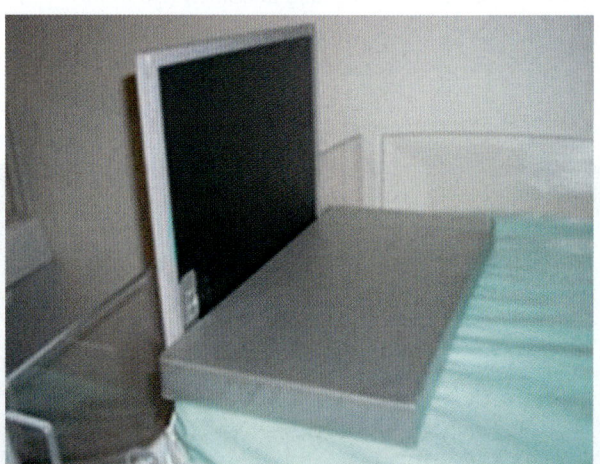

Fig. 22.58 Radiolucent sponge and IR.

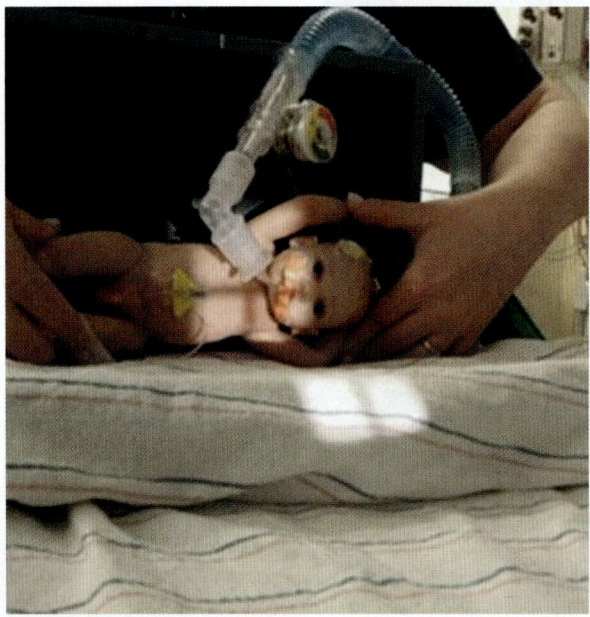

Fig. 22.59 AP left lateral decubitus chest position.

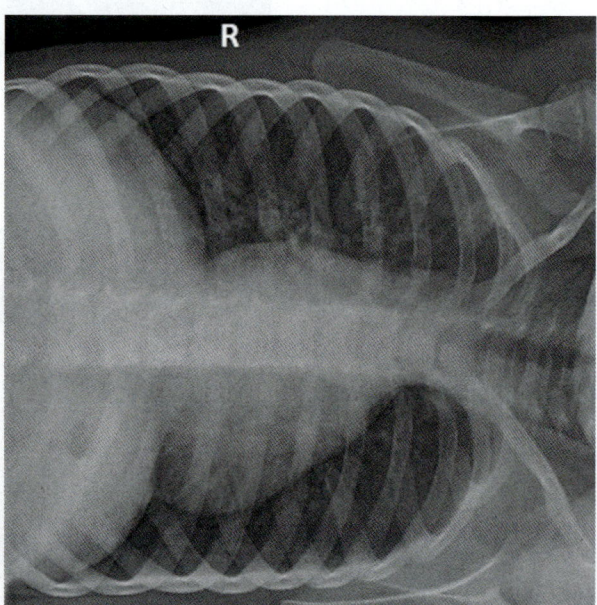

Fig. 22.60 AP left lateral decubitus chest radiograph.

Mobile Considerations for Neonatal Intensive Care Unit (NICU)

PORTABLE NEONATE ABDOMEN

Preexposure positioning

- If the IR fits, place it inside the tray located underneath the incubator. If the IR does not fit, wrap or cover the IR and place it directly under the neonate.
- Have the nurse remove the patient's diaper if possible (a soiled/wet diaper causes artifacts).
- Center the area of interest to the IR, and ensure that the four borders (top, bottom, and two sides) of the IR include the anatomy of interest.
- Have the nurse adjust the neonate's head until the MSP is perpendicular to the IR to avoid rotation. Make sure that this will not compromise the patient's condition.
- Direct the central ray perpendicular to the IR, entering the MSP at the level of the iliac crest with 102 cm (40 inches) SID (Fig. 22.61A).
- Adjust the collimator light field to include from the nipple line to the pubic symphysis (Fig. 22.61B). This collimation will ensure inclusion of the diaphragm and pubic symphysis.
- Place side marker in the collimated exposure field.
- Observe the patient's breathing, and expose at the end of expiration.

EVALUATION CRITERIA

The optimum image obtained using correct positioning, CR-part-IR alignment, collimation, and exposure factors will demonstrate:

- Diaphragm to pubic symphysis (Fig. 22.61C)
- Free from wet diaper artifacts
- No rotation of the abdomen, as demonstrated by spinous processes in the center of the lumbar vertebrae and symmetric wings of the ilia

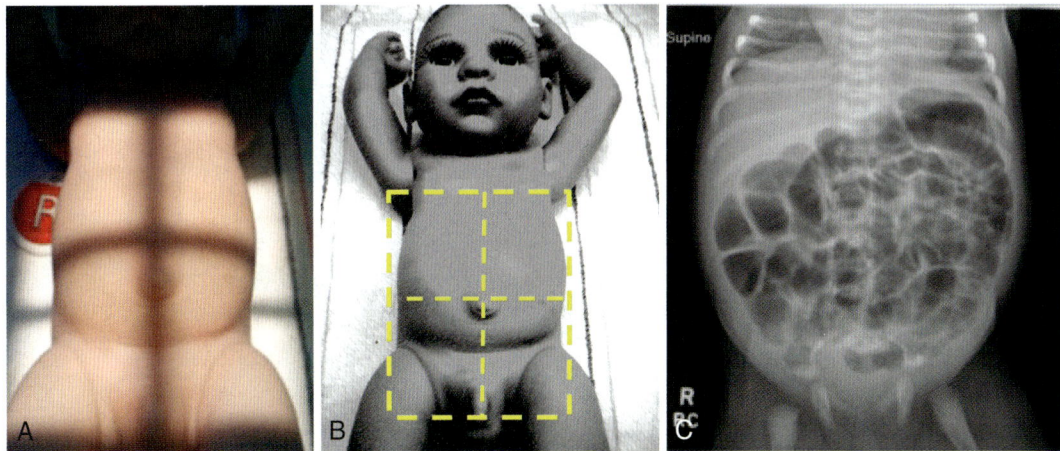

Fig. 22.61 (**A**) AP abdomen, central ray directed at level of iliac crest. (**B**) AP abdomen, radiation light field. (**C**) AP abdomen radiograph.

Mobile Considerations for Neonatal Intensive Care Unit (NICU)

PORTABLE DECUBITUS NEONATE ABDOMEN
R or L lateral recumbent
Preexposure positioning

- Have the nurse remove the patient's diaper, if possible, to reduce artifacts.
- Place the patient in a lateral decubitus position, lying on either the affected or the unaffected side, as indicated by the existing condition. Assess the patient's condition and request assistance with positioning.
- Place a radiolucent sponge (covered) directly under the neonate.
- Wrap or cover the IR, ensure that the bottom edge of the vertical IR drops below the sponge, and obtain 102 cm (40 inches) SID.
- Have the nurse raise the patient's arms above the head (Fig. 22.62).
- Adjust the radiation field on the collimator to include from the nipple line to the pubic symphysis. This collimation will ensure inclusion of the diaphragm and pubic symphysis. Place side marker in the collimated exposure field.
- Direct the central ray horizontally and perpendicular to the IR, entering the MSP at the level of the iliac crests.
- Observe the patient's breathing, and expose at the end of expiration.

EVALUATION CRITERIA
The optimum image obtained using correct positioning, CR-part-IR alignment, collimation, and exposure factors will demonstrate:
- Diaphragm to pubic symphysis (see Fig. 22.17B)
- An image free from wet diaper artifacts
- No rotation of the abdomen, as demonstrated by spinous processes in the center of the lumbar vertebrae and symmetric wings of the ilia

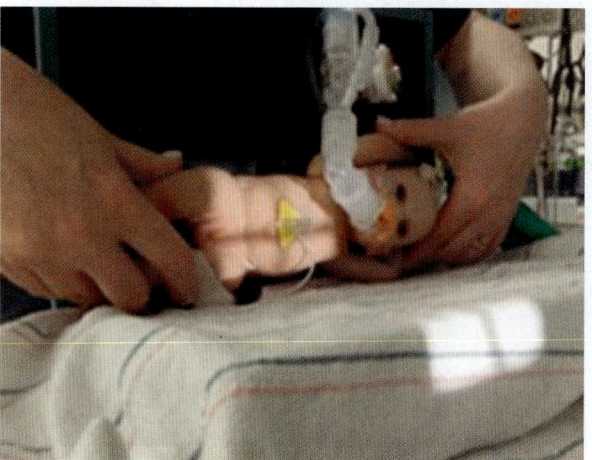

Fig. 22.62 AP left lateral decubitus abdomen position.

Mobile Considerations for Neonatal Intensive Care Unit (NICU)

PORTABLE DORSAL DECUBITUS NEONATE CHEST OR ABDOMEN

Preexposure positioning

- When the condition of the neonate will not permit the patient to roll into lateral recumbent, perform the exam with the patient supine and the central ray horizontal.
- Place a radiolucent sponge (covered) directly under the neonate. Assess the patient's condition, and request assistance with positioning.
- Ensure that the bottom edge of the vertical IR drops below the sponge, and obtain 102 cm (40 inches) SID.
- Have the nurse extend the neonate's arms above the head, and ensure that the chest and pelvis are flat.
- Adjust the collimator light field to include:
  - For chest, below the earlobes and approximately 4 cm (1.5 inches) above the umbilicus.
  - For abdomen, from the nipple line to the pubic symphysis.
- Place side marker in the collimated exposure field.
- Direct the central ray horizontally and perpendicular to the IR, entering the MCP:
  - For chest, at level T7 (see Fig. 22.24).
  - For abdomen, at the level of the iliac crests (Fig. 22.63A).
  - For a combination chest and abdomen, at the midpoint between the thorax and pubic symphysis.
- Observe the patient's breathing, and expose at the end of inspiration for chest or at expiration for abdomen.
- Gonadal shielding is used at discretion to avoid obscuring pertinent anatomy.

EVALUATION CRITERIA

The optimum image obtained using correct positioning, CR-part-IR alignment, collimation, and exposure factors will demonstrate:

- Structural anatomy:
  - For chest, from apices to costophrenic angles
  - For abdomen, from diaphragm to the pubic symphysis (Fig. 22.63B)
  - For combination chest and abdomen, from apices to pubic symphysis
- Evidence of proper collimation and presence of side marker placed clear of anatomy of interest
- No rotation, as demonstrated by sternum, ribs posteriorly, superimposed ilia, superimposed lumbar vertebrae pedicles, and open intervertebral foramina

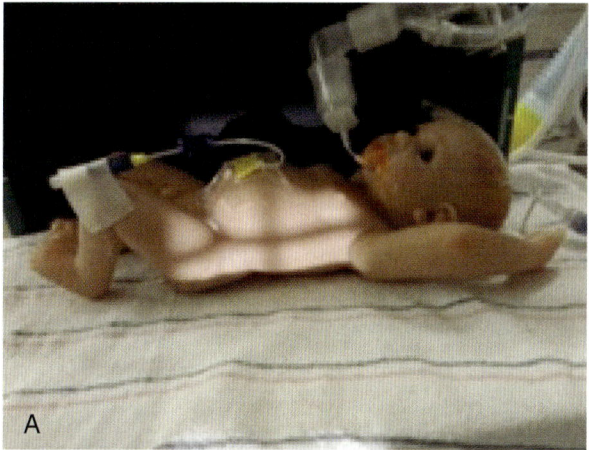

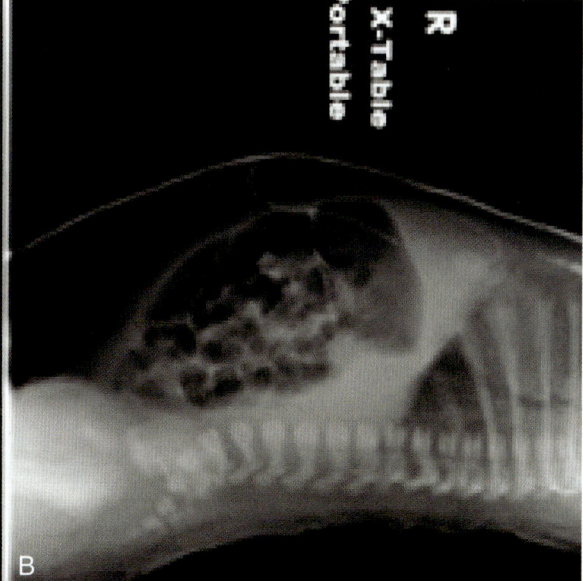

Fig. 22.63 (A) Right lateral dorsal decubitus abdomen position. (B) Right lateral dorsal decubitus abdomen radiograph.

Mobile Considerations for Neonatal Intensive Care Unit (NICU)

PORTABLE CHEST AND ABDOMEN FOR LINE PLACEMENT

The chest and abdomen combination described in this section is typically ordered for premature newborns. IV access is often necessary to provide medication and nutrition needed for growth and development. When prolonged IV support is required, maintaining access with peripheral IV catheters can reduce infection and the number of needlesticks. Peripherally inserted central catheters (PICCs) are the most common type of central line utilized in NICU patients. Although PICCs have many benefits, they also have potential complications. Confirming the position of the catheter tip is essential to decreasing complications. Physicians caring for NICU patients frequently order chest and abdomen combination views for PICC or central venous catheter (CVC) placement. In many cases, the exam is ordered STAT during or after placement under a sterile field. Chest and abdomen combination exams, sometimes referred to as "babygrams," result in a loss of radiographic detail and contrast when compared with separate images. In some instances, the radiographer may need to question the physician's order. Are both the chest and abdomen anatomy really warranted if only looking at chest pathology or for upper PICC? Is inclusion of the chest warranted for abdomen pathology or lower PICC? These are important questions. The order must reflect the pathology indication and region of interest to be demonstrated. Overuse of chest and abdomen (babygram) radiographs should be avoided. The following are recommendations for imaging the chest and abdomen combination exam.

Preexposure positioning

- If the IR size allows, place it inside the tray located underneath the incubator. If the IR does not fit, wrap or cover the IR and place it directly under the neonate.
- Adjust the patient and center the chest and abdomen to the IR.
- Ensure that the four borders (top, bottom, and two sides) of the IR include the anatomy of interest.
- Have the nurse move the infant's arms away from the body or over the head, bring the legs down and away from the abdomen, and adjust the pelvis flat to avoid rotation. The arms and legs may need to be held by a nurse, who should wear a lead apron.
- If possible, keep the head and neck of the infant straight so that the anatomy in the upper chest and airway is accurately visualized. However, straightening the head of a neonate in the supine position can inadvertently advance an ETT too far into the trachea. Sometimes it is more important to leave the head of an intubated neonatal patient rotated in the position in which the infant routinely lies to obtain an accurate representation of the position of the ETT.
- Direct the central ray perpendicular to the midpoint of the chest and abdomen along the MSP with 102 cm (40 inches) SID (Fig. 22.64A).
- Place side marker in the collimated exposure field.
- Adjust the collimator field to include the apices to the pubic symphysis (Fig. 22.64B).
- When the neonate's chest and abdomen rise to their maximum heights for full inspiration, make the exposure.
- Shield the patient accordingly.

EVALUATION CRITERIA

The optimum image obtained using correct positioning, CR-part-IR alignment, collimation, and exposure factors will demonstrate:

- Anatomy from apices to pubic symphysis in the thoracic and abdominal regions (Fig. 22.64C)
- Evidence of proper collimation and presence of side marker placed clear of anatomy of interest
- No motion
- No blurring of lungs, diaphragm, and abdominal structures
- No rotation of patient

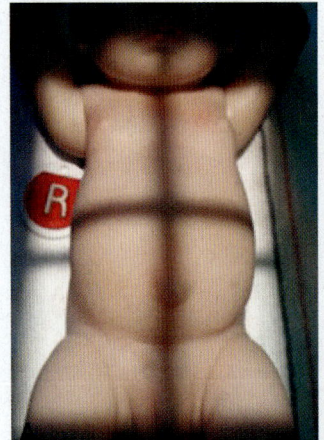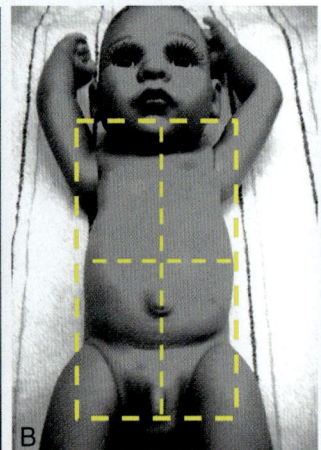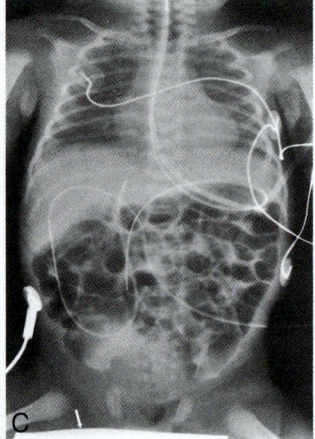

Fig. 22.64 (A) Central ray directed to midpoint of chest and abdomen. (B) AP chest and abdomen, radiation light field. (C) AP chest and abdomen radiograph.

Mobile Considerations for Neonatal Intensive Care Unit (NICU)

Tips for performing chest and abdomen line placement with sterile field

Approach the patient with caution to avoid compromising the sterile field with equipment (Fig. 22.65). Communicate with the scrub physician to request one of the following:
- Ask the neonate PICC scrub physician to mold the patient's body habitus with the sterile drape to accentuate the shape of the neonate's body (Fig. 22.66A).
- Ask the neonate PICC scrub physician to use a sterile marker and draw boundary points or region of interest (Fig. 22.66B).

Adjust technical factors to clearly demonstrate the PICC/CVC line and tip placement.

If the tip of the catheter is not in the correct location, the line is repositioned and a follow-up image is expected.

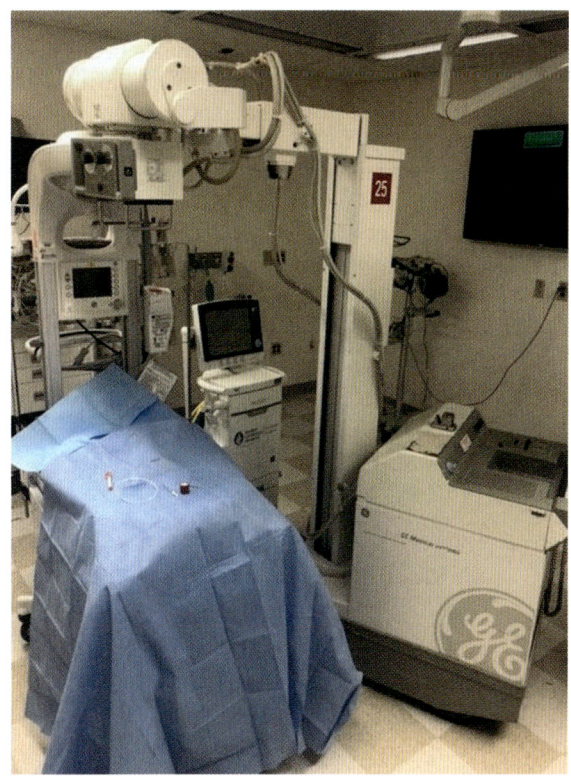

Fig. 22.65 Mobile unit positioned over sterile field.

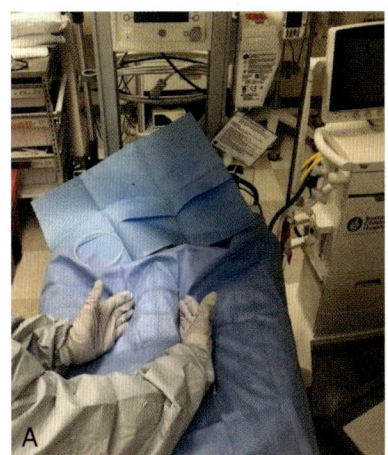 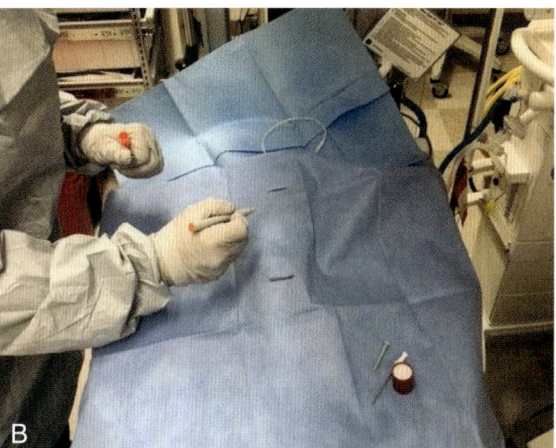

Fig. 22.66 (A) Scrub physician molding the patient's body habitus and shape with the sterile drape. (B) Scrub physician using sterile marker to draw boundary points or region of interest.

Simulation: Practicing in a Safe Environment

Radiography in the NICU at any institution can be somewhat intimidating to a new or student radiographer. Practicing simulated exams in a safe environment is an excellent way to achieve positive outcomes without the real-time environmental stressors of the NICU (e.g., phones ringing, compromised neonates, alarms, stressed clinicians, worried parents, and sterile fields). Simulation in a *safe environment* can be achieved by using a neonate doll, a portable x-ray machine, and a neonate bed (Fig. 22.67). Similar to using a phantom in adult radiography in the exposure lab, simulation is an excellent way to develop good radiography habits before heading to the NICU to perform images on the live neonate population. A simulation workshop can go a long way to improve image quality and develop technical skills to create a timely approach to any neonatal exam. A simulation lab in a safe environment can exponentially improve centering, collimation, and positional issues with neonates. According to the well-known educator Edgar Dale, who developed the *Cone of Learning* theory, "actively doing and simulating the real experience" results in a retention rate of 90% for up to 2 weeks later. Important elements to consider during simulation training include soft tissue positional landmarks, minimizing artifacts, adjusting technical factors, collimation, shielding, developing a team-based approach, verifying orders, reducing infection, and the importance of standardized protocols.

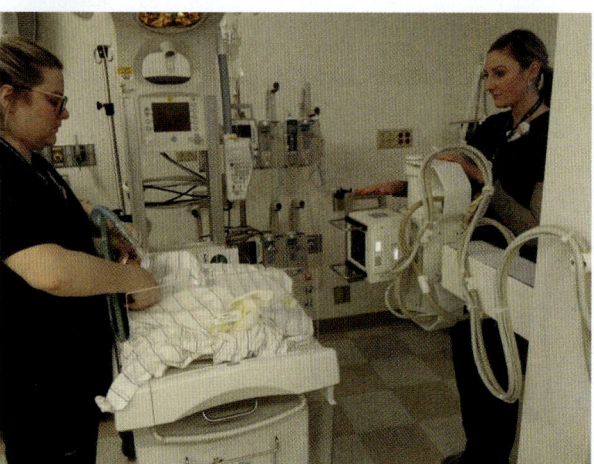

Fig. 22.67 Radiography students practicing mobile exam in NICU simulation lab.

Selected Pediatric Conditions and Syndromes

CYSTIC FIBROSIS

Cystic fibrosis (CF) is an autosomal recessive disorder of the exocrine system caused by mutations located on chromosome 7. Generally speaking, these mutations affect the sodium and chloride ion transport system, which operates at the surface level of epithelial cells, resulting in thick mucus in the lungs and pancreatic ducts that cannot be cleared. These epithelial cells line the airways, sweat glands, GI tract, and GU system. The organ systems most impacted are the lungs, sinuses, pancreas, intestines, hepatobiliary tree, and spermatic ducts in the male (vas deferens), and reduced fertility rates in the female. Most symptomatic adult CF patients present with two manifestations characteristic of the disorder—persistent cough due to mucus-infiltrated lungs and pancreatic insufficiency that inhibits their ability to gain weight). There are approximately 30,000 CF patients in the United States and 70,000 worldwide. In the United States, the median life expectancy for persons born with cystic fibrosis between 2013 and 2017 was 44 years of age or longer. As a result of current treatment strategies, 80% of CF patients should reach adulthood.

One of the earliest manifestations of CF is meconium ileus in the neonate. Most patients are diagnosed in the first year, with 50% presenting with a chronic cough by 10 months. Pulmonary complications are the leading cause of morbidity and mortality with CF. In a healthy person, the surfaces of the respiratory tract are bathed in a salty surfactant that traps and, with the help of cilia, removes pathogens and foreign substances from the lungs. This system is compromised in the CF patient, allowing microbes such as *Pseudomonas aeruginosa*, *Staphylococcus aureus*, and *Haemophilus influenza* to flourish in stagnant mucus, leading to inflammation and bronchoconstriction, ultimately causing irreversible lung damage. Due to its low radiation dose, chest radiography is the modality of choice for evaluating respiratory complications resulting from CF. The earliest sign of irreversible lung disease in these patients is bronchiectasis. Radiographic findings include bronchial thickening and dilation, peribronchial cuffing, mucoid impaction, and cystic radiolucencies (Fig. 22.68).

Nonrespiratory manifestations include a whole range of GI complications, from meconium ileus in neonates to adult gastroesophageal reflux and rectal mucosal prolapse. As the patient ages, GU complications include renal compromise, nephrolithiasis (3%–6% of patients), and diabetic nephropathy. Musculoskeletal disorders include abnormal bone mineralization of unknown etiology and metabolic bone disease due to malnutrition and decreased lung function. Reproductive manifestations include late-onset puberty (by 1–4 years), a 95% to 99% infertility rate in male patients due to blockage or absence of the spermatic ducts (vas deferens), and incomplete epididymides.

Depending on the course and severity of the disease, CF can develop into one of the most debilitating illnesses of adolescence. It is important that radiographers understand the challenges facing these teenagers.

Standard precautions for CF patients follow the Cystic Fibrosis Foundation recommendations and include the following.
1. Departments sending a CF patient for imaging must call ahead to place a room on hold.
2. Check-in sends the arriving patient immediately to the room on hold.
3. The patient is assigned a "fast pass," which pushes them to the front of the imaging queue.
4. The patient is dressed appropriately (chest or KUB).
5. The radiographer is gowned and gloved and should attempt to maintain a 3-foot separation from the patient.
6. The radiographer, in the presence of the patient, should clean all surfaces that the patient will come into contact with during the exam.
7. Gown and gloves must be replaced if the radiographer must leave the room.
8. Upon completion of the exam, the patient is sent back to the ordering department, and all horizontal surfaces that were within 6 feet of the patient, as well as surfaces the patient touched, must be disinfected.

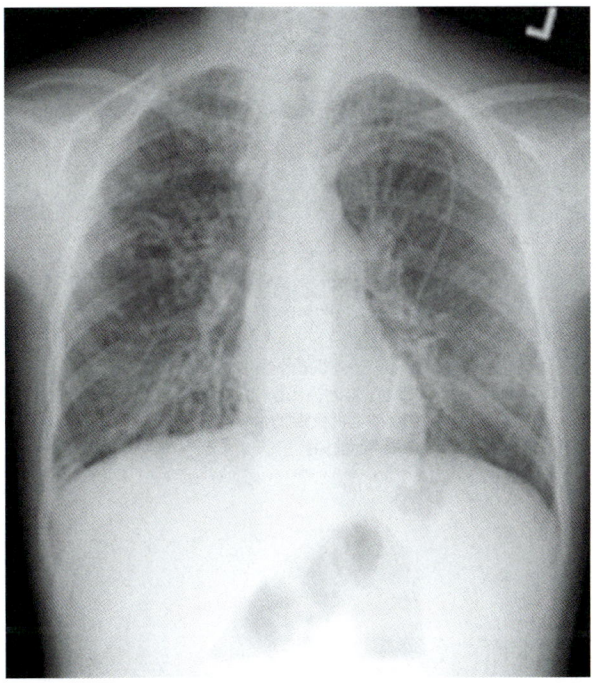

Fig. 22.68 AP chest of patient with CF.

Selected Pediatric Conditions and Syndromes

DEVELOPMENTAL DYSPLASIA OF THE HIP (DDH)

DDH is the malformation of the acetabulum in utero and is usually the result of fetal positioning or a breech birth. The acetabulum fails to form completely, and the femoral head or heads are displaced superiorly and anteriorly. The ligaments and tendons responsible for proper alignment are often affected. Females are affected at a rate five times higher than males, the left hip is involved more than the right, and 5% to 20% of cases occur bilaterally. The clinical diagnosis is made when there is partial or complete displacement of the femoral head from the acetabulum relative to the pelvis. With infants younger than 6 months of age, the modality of choice is US due to its lack of radiation and because the cartilaginous nature of the hip is better visualized at this stage of development. US is used for infant follow-up until 6 months, at which time images can be used to confirm placement of the femoral head(s).

Radiographic exams used to diagnose DDH include the frog lateral and the Von Rosen positions. There is some discussion among radiologists saying that because the frog lateral position is used to reduce the dysplasia, the Von Rosen should be the preferred position. Treatment of DDH varies with the diagnosis. Subluxation of the hip in the neonate may be stabilized in weeks if the femora are abducted in flexion, aided by double and triple diapering. A dislocated hip, or hips suspected to dislocate easily, may be stabilized and immobilized by the use of a Pavlik harness worn for 1 to 2 months; more complex cases may require surgery and a spica cast. During follow-up imaging, care should be taken when the spica cast is removed to keep the legs abducted to ensure hip stability. Adult interventions include periacetabular osteotomy (PAO) surgery to correct developmental dysplasia of the hip (DDH) (Fig. 22.69).

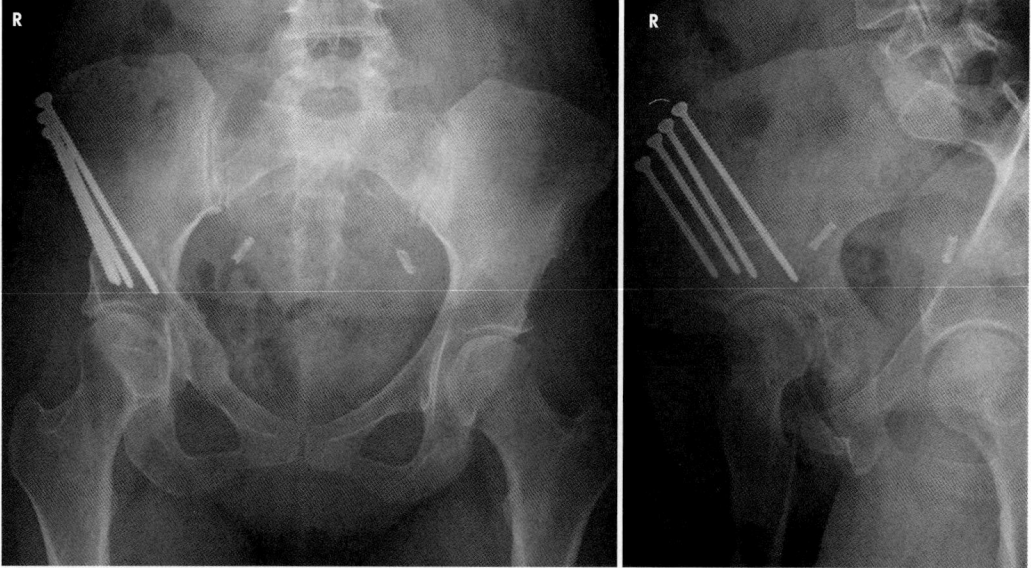

Fig. 22.69 Standing AP pelvis and right false profile hip projections for postoperative periacetabular osteotomy (PAO) on an adult female patient. Note the tubal ligation clips seen on both images.

Nonaccidental Trauma (Child Abuse)

Nonaccidental Trauma (Child Abuse)

Although no *universal* agreement exists on the definition of child abuse, the radiographer should have an appreciation of the all-encompassing nature of this problem. *Child abuse* has been described as the involvement of physical injury, sexual abuse or deprivation of nutrition, care or affection in circumstances, which indicate that injury or deprivation may not be accidental or may have occurred through neglect.[2] Although diagnostic imaging staff members are usually involved only in cases in which physical abuse is a possibility, they should realize that sexual abuse and nutritional neglect are also prevalent.

It is mandatory in all states and provinces in North America for health care professionals to *report suspected cases of abuse or neglect*. The radiographer, while preparing or positioning the patient, may be the first person to suspect abuse or neglect (Fig. 22.70). The first course of action for the radiographer should be to consult a radiologist (when available) or the attending physician. After this consultation, the radiographer may no longer have cause for suspicion because some naturally occurring skin markings mimic bruising. *If the radiographer's doubts persist, the suspicions must be reported to the proper authorities, regardless of the physician's opinion.* Recognizing the complexity of child abuse issues, many health care facilities have developed a multidisciplinary team of health care workers to respond to these issues. Radiographers working in hospitals have access to this team of physicians, social workers, and psychologists for the purpose of reporting their concerns.

The ACR defines a skeletal survey as "a systematically performed series of radiographic images that encompasses the entire skeleton or those anatomic regions appropriate for the clinical indications." There are three indications for a skeletal survey, according to the ACR: suspected nonaccidental trauma (abuse), skeletal dysplasias, and neoplasms. Fractures in the first year of life are relatively rare, so their occurrence might warrant a skeletal survey to rule out child abuse (Fig. 22.71). Although 64% of all reported cases of maltreatment with major physical injury occur in patients 0 to 5 years of age, those with radiologic evidence of healing or older fractures, will generally be younger than 2 years of age. Pediatric imaging departments have specific protocols that protect the patient when there is suspicion or evidence of child abuse. The diagnosis of abuse becomes more likely when there is a discrepant history of minor trauma in a child with multiple complex fractures. Although policies vary from institution to institution, the goal is always protection of the child. Nonaccidental traumas often present in the emergency room (ER) for other indications, and when imaged, the patients are found to have fractures of a suspicious nature. A scenario may go something like this:

1. Parent and 9-month-old infant are seen in the ER, where the infant presents with shortness of breath, wheezing, and low-grade fever for 2 days.
2. The patient is assigned to an exam room for nurse/doctor interview, assessment, and physical examination.
3. Routine standard-of-care chest x-rays are ordered to rule out pneumonia.
4. Radiographer alerts radiologist to the presence of what appears to be healing rib fractures (Figs. 22.72 and 22.73) and corner fractures (Fig. 22.74).
5. Radiologist consults with a child protection team and ER attending.
6. The hospital's social services department is called to conduct an interview with the parent.
7. The hospital's child protection team, ER attending, and social worker explain the findings to the parent. The family is then escorted, by security, to radiology for an immediate skeletal survey.

Depending on the findings, the infant may be admitted for care or removed from the home by Child Protective Services. Children presenting with emergent head trauma would be admitted and transferred to a surgical ICU. The abuse of a child is so repugnant that the urge to judge the parents will almost be reflexive; try to resist this temptation and stay focused on the very difficult and emotional task of providing medical care to the patient. Give a thorough explanation of what the skeletal survey entails: the time involved, the

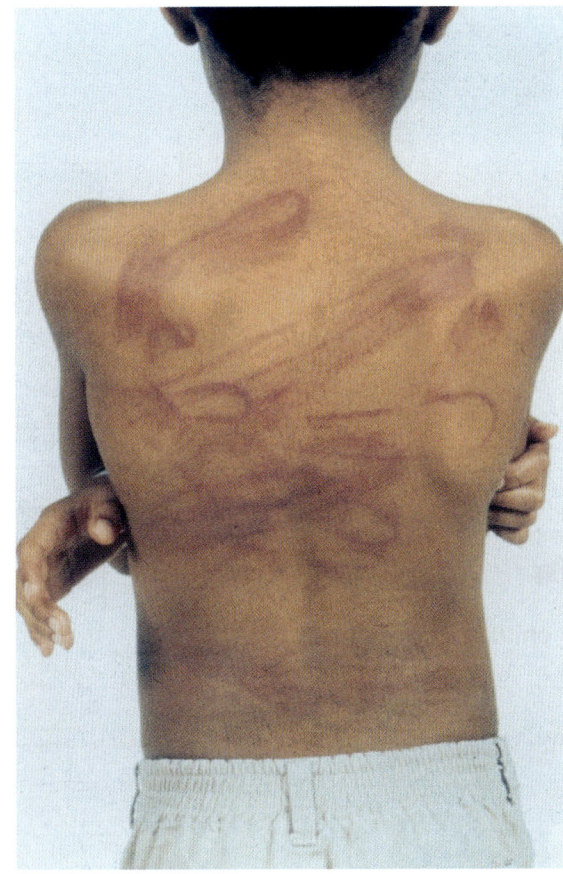

Fig. 22.70 A 7 year old with loop marks, representative of forceful blows by a looped belt.

Nonaccidental Trauma (Child Abuse)

special accommodations that are provided for their infant, and that the infant will cry. Allowing the parents to participate in the exam is a judgment call; overly emotional parents may be more of a hindrance, whereas calm parents may help to soothe their infant. The parents who will not be helping should be escorted to a nearby waiting room. The survey can be accomplished quickly and efficiently with experienced radiographers.

Due to the medicolegal sensitivity of the skeletal survey and to expedite the exam, it is always best to have three radiographers working the exam: one immobilizes and positions; the second sets technique, positions, collimates, and makes the exposure; the third supplies the two-person team with image plates (if CR) and immobilization devices, and also processes and assesses the quality of each image. The table should have a pad with sheet, chucks, positioning sponges, pacifier, and reward stickers, among other items. Have all supplies at the table or readily accessible within the room. The room should be warmed as appropriate and warming lights used as required. All images are made with the infant lying on the IR (nothing is placed between the IR and the patient). The patient can stay in a diaper, which will be removed when the abdomen/pelvis/femurs are imaged. Imaging should be timely and efficient, with repeats avoided. The radiologist accesses the images when the imaging is complete and will request additional images as needed.

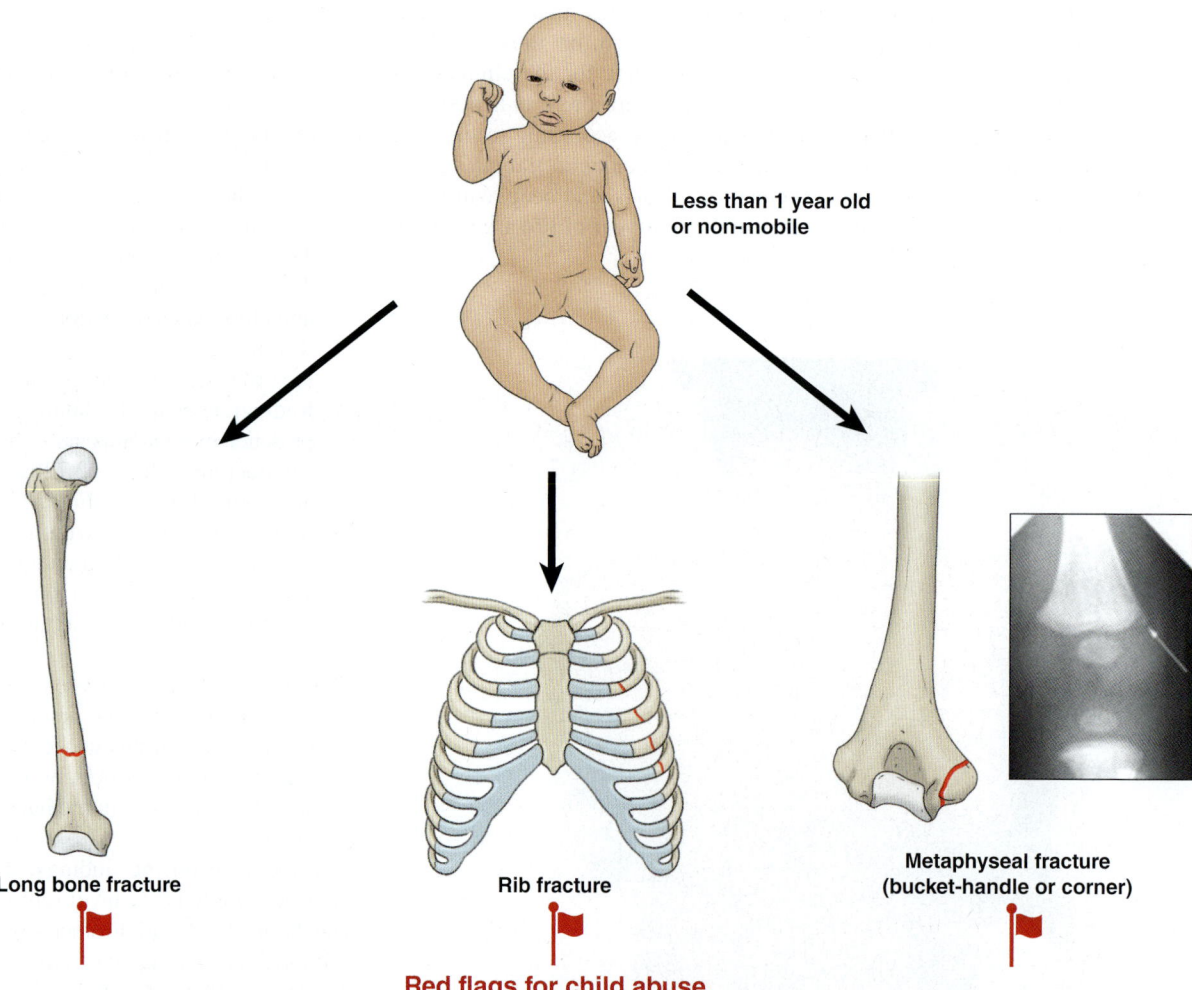

Red flags for child abuse

Fig. 22.71 Long bone, rib, and metaphyseal fractures are commonly found on abused children.

(Redrawn from Frank E, Atigapramoj N. PEM pearls: Red flags for child abuse—case 2. Academic Life in Emergency Medicine (ALiEM) (website). 2018. https://www.aliem.com/pem-pearls-child-abuse-case-2/.)

Nonaccidental Trauma (Child Abuse)

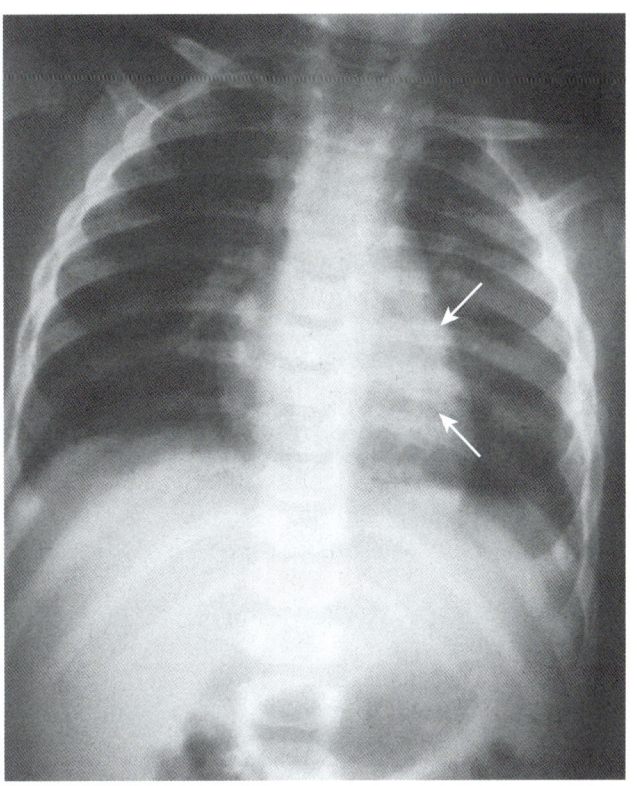

Fig. 22.72 Chest radiograph showing different stages of healing posterior rib fractures *(arrows)*.

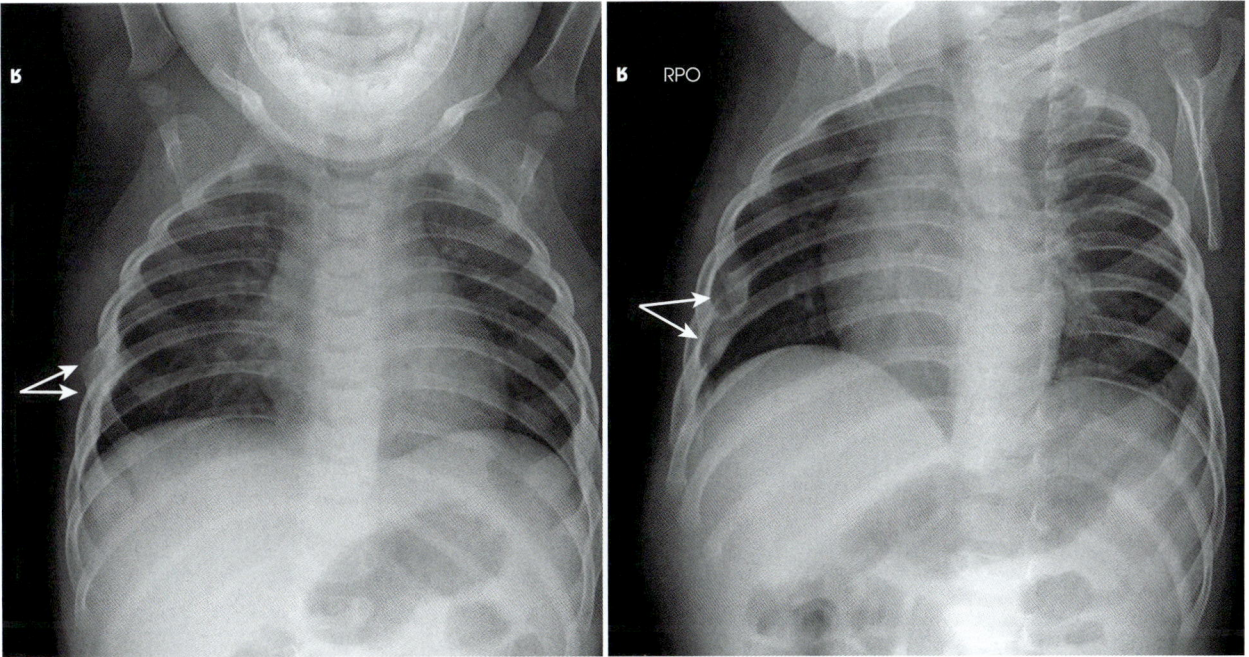

Fig. 22.73 AP and RPO rib images delineating right-sided healing rib fractures *(arrows)*.

Nonaccidental Trauma (Child Abuse)

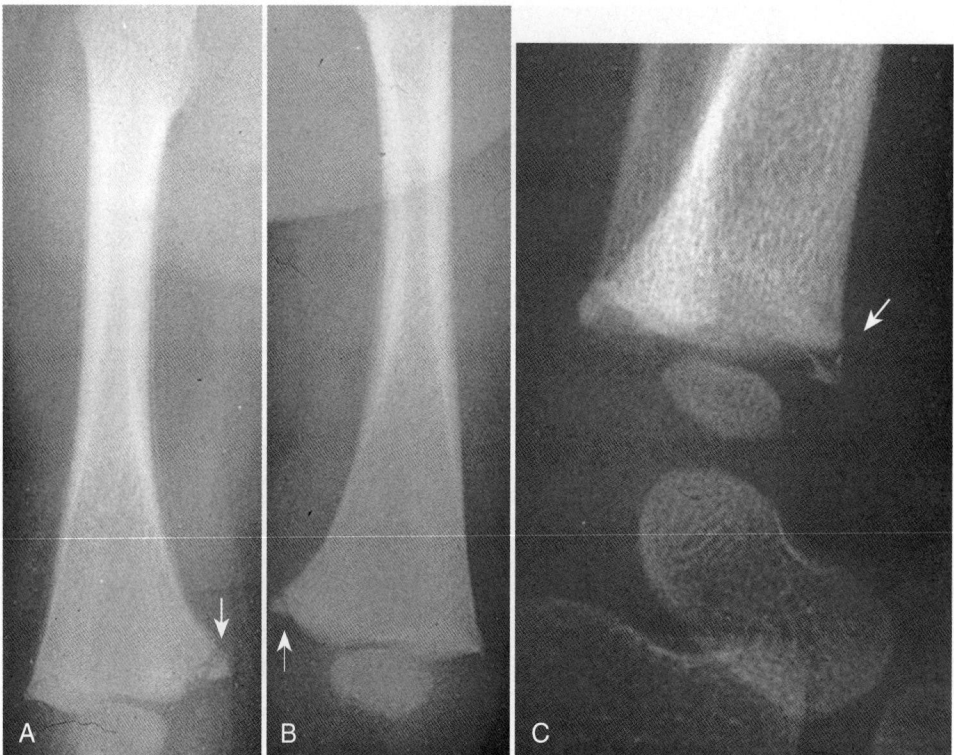

Fig. 22.74 Images demonstrating physical abuse. Left and right corner fractures (*arrows,* **A** and **B**) and bucket-handle fractures (*arrow,* **C**) are considered classic indicators of physical abuse in children. The bucket-handle appearance is subtle and demonstrated only if the "ring" is seen on profile *(arrow).*

Nonaccidental Trauma (Child Abuse)

Imaging protocol at Boston Children's Hospital

- For efficiency and for medicolegal reasons, two radiographers should be in the room when imaging.
- Only AP projections are required for long bones unless there is a positive finding (Boxes 22.2 and 22.3).
- Equivocal findings in a long bone may necessitate a lateral projection.
- Hand images should be slightly oblique rather than PA.
- All skeletal survey images should be done with 60 kVp (increased bony detail for CR-based systems).
- The 2-week follow-up exam does not require skull images.
- There should be nothing between the IR and the body part.
- Chest and abdominal images should overlap.

Box 22.2 is a skeletal survey protocol for nonaccidental traumas in infants younger than 12 months and is tabletop at 102 cm SID, using a large focal spot with bone technique. Box 22.3 lists radiologic findings. Figs. 22.75 through 22.77 are positive radiographic findings seen on the same 8-month-old patient on a skeletal survey exam for nonaccidental trauma (child abuse).

BOX 22.2
Survey skeletal projections

AP and lateral skull (a positive finding may require right and left laterals and Towne)
AP and lateral chest
Bilateral shallow obliques of chest to show ribs
Abdomen (to overlap with chest)
AP bilateral femurs
AP bilateral tibias
AP bilateral feet
AP bilateral humeri
AP bilateral forearms
Bilateral hands, oblique 20 degrees
Lateral C-spine
Lateral L-spine
A positive finding in long bones may additionally require lateral images of the extremities

---

BOX 22.3
Specificity of radiologic findings

High specificity
Metaphyseal lesions
Rib fractures, especially posterior
Scapular fractures
Spinous process fractures
Sternal fracture

Moderate specificity[a]
Multiple fractures, especially bilateral
Fractures of different ages
Epiphyseal separations
Vertebral body fractures and subluxations
Fractures of the digits
Complex skull fractures

Low specificity (but common)[a]
Clavicle fractures
Long bone shaft fractures
Linear skull fractures
Subperiosteal new bone formation

[a]Moderate- and low-specificity lesions become high specificity when history of trauma is absent or inconsistent with injuries.
Used with permission of Dr. Paul Kleinman, Boston Children's Hospital, Boston, MA.

Nonaccidental Trauma (Child Abuse)

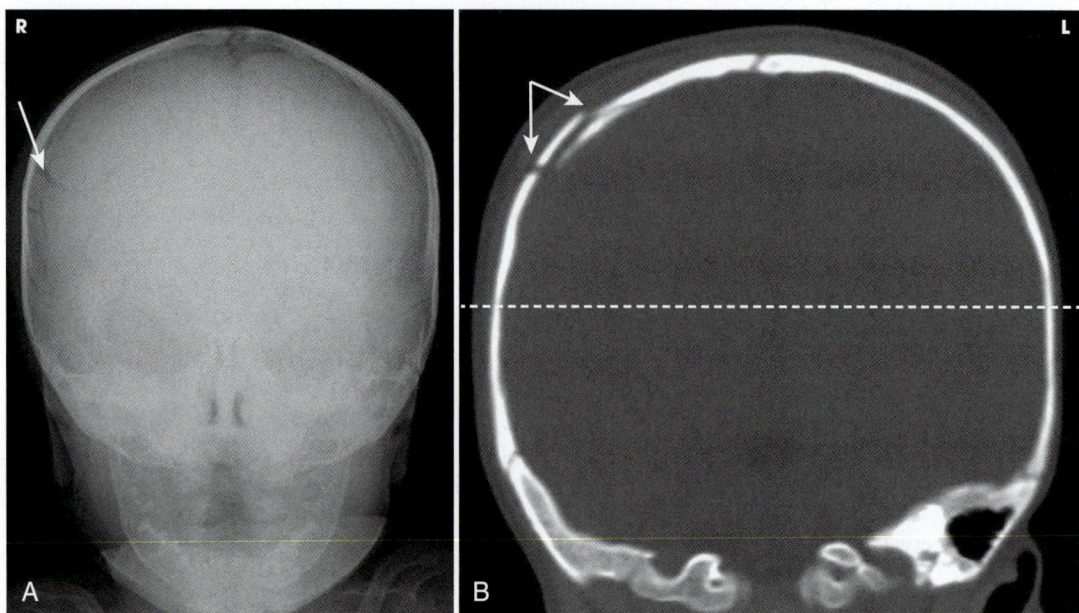

Fig. 22.75 AP skull projection (**A**) and coronal CT image (**B**) on an 8-month-old patient, demonstrating a parietal bone fracture *(arrows)*.

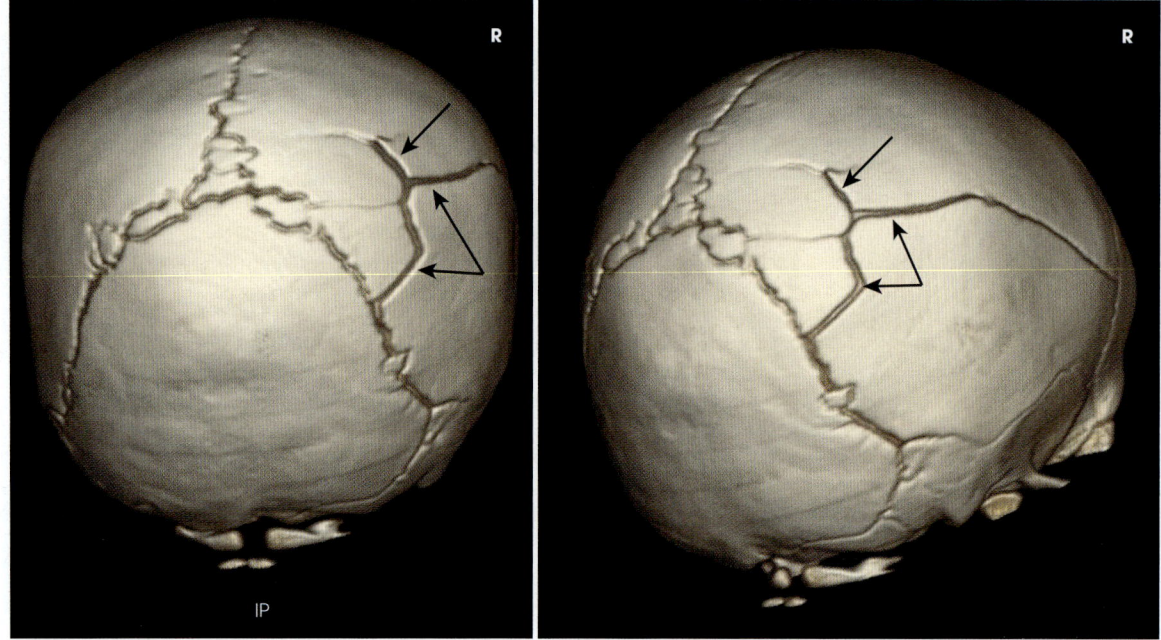

Fig. 22.76 CT 3D model post-processed images demonstrating right parietal bone fracture *(arrows)* on the same 8-month-old patient shown in Fig. 22.75.

Nonaccidental Trauma (Child Abuse)

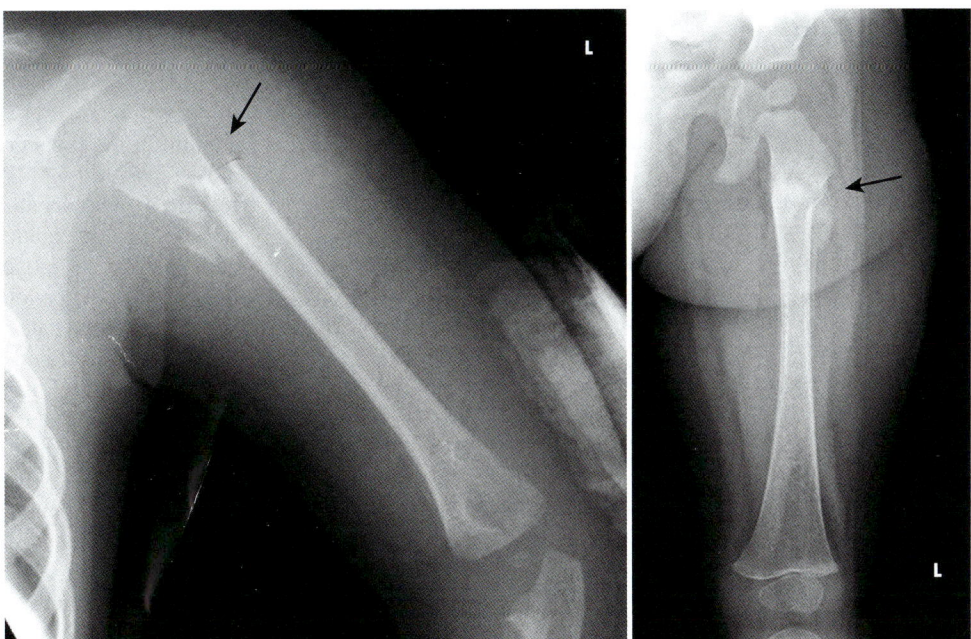

Fig. 22.77 Skeletal survey images for child abuse demonstrating a left proximal humerus fracture and a left proximal femur fracture (*arrows*) on the same 8-month-old infant as in Fig. 22.75.

Childhood Pathologies

Childhood Pathologies
OSTEOGENESIS IMPERFECTA

OI means "imperfectly formed bone." It is a serious but rare heritable or congenital disease of the skeletal system (20,000 to 50,000 cases in the United States). It results from a genetic defect in two genes that encode for type I collagen, the main collagen of osseous tissue, tendons, teeth, skin, inner ear, and sclera of the eyeballs. Although people with OI may have different combinations of symptoms, they all have weaker bones. Some common symptoms of OI include the following:
- Short stature.
- Triangular-shaped face.
- Breathing problems.
- Hearing loss.
- Brittle teeth.
- Bone deformities, such as bowed legs or scoliosis.

There are several types of OI, which vary in severity and symptoms and are classified as types I to IV.

Type I
Type I is the most common and the mildest form. In this type, the collagen is normal but is produced in reduced quantities. There is little or no bone deformity, although the bones remain fragile and easily broken. Teeth are prone to caries and are easily broken. The sclera of the eyes may have a purple, blue, or gray tint.

Type II
Type II is the most severe form of the disease, and many infants do not survive. The collagen suffers from the genetic defect, and bones may break in utero (Fig. 22.78).

Type III
Type III patients have improperly formed collagen, often with severe bone deformities, as well as other complications. The infant is often born with numerous fractures and tinting of the sclera. Children are generally shorter and have spinal deformities, respiratory complications, and brittle teeth.

Type IV
Type IV is considered a moderately severe condition marked by defective collagen formation resulting in bones that are prone to fractures with mild to moderate deformity. Some people may be shorter than average with brittle teeth.

Use verbal communication when imaging the patient with OI, being careful not to physically move or position the body. Let the patient position themselves, possibly with the help of a parent, to avoid causing new fractures. The caregiver or parent should do the transfer and changing, and aid in positioning. The exam table will require a radiolucent pad with a sheet, a pillow, or a towel under the patient's head, and radiolucent positioning devices to help support the patient. The radiographer should communicate the exact positioning required and then review the position before exposure. Positioning devices may be employed, but the family should place them. The radiographer will use their positional skills with the radiographic tube (move tube, not patient) to obtain two projections differing by 90 degrees, thereby avoiding manipulating the part of interest. It is important to ask the patient, "Is there anything I should know about your medical condition that would help me to help you?" because the patient might have OI without it being indicated on the exam requisition. Although the omission of such critical information is hard to believe, it does happen, which is why we have "time-outs" before invasive procedures.

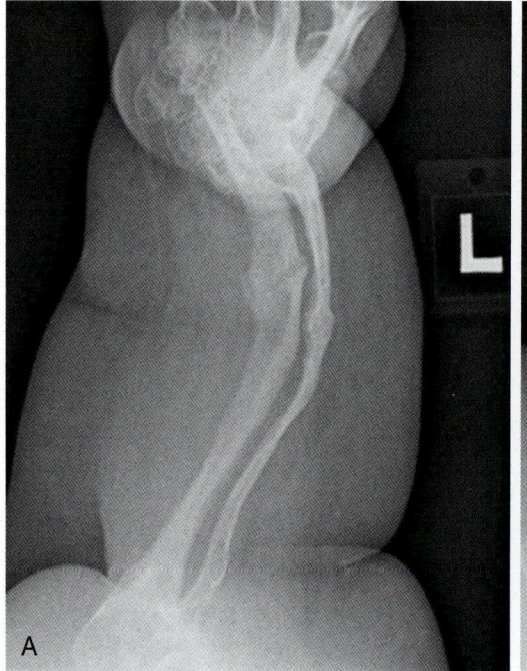 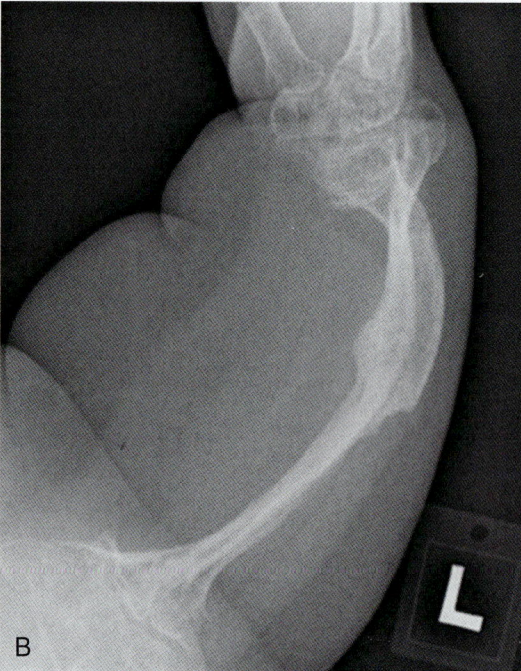

Fig. 22.78 AP (**A**) and lateral (**B**) projections of the left forearm. Patients with OI are not only fragile, but their anatomy can be misshaped, making it difficult to determine the correct position for AP and lateral projections.

Childhood Pathologies

PATHOLOGIC FRACTURES AND BENIGN AND MALIGNANT NEOPLASMS

Long bones, ribs, and facial bones are susceptible to fibrous displacement of their osseous tissue, creating a benign condition called fibrous dysplasia. As these neoplasms grow, they erode the bone, causing the cortices to thin and weaken, which may lead to pathologic fracture. These dysplasias can become filled with fluid and are then known as bone cysts, often occurring in the upper ends of the humeri, femurs, and tibias of children, which are usually located beneath the epiphysis, traveling down the metaphysis as they grow. The cysts often appear as incidental findings from another exam or following a pathologic fracture. Radiographically, they present as thin-walled lucencies with sharp boundaries.

Osteochondroma

Osteochondromas are one of three types of chondromas, also known as osteochondromas. They do not appear in the fetal skeleton and are virtually nonexistent until the second year of life. Growing from the bone's shaft, the tumor widens the bone, weakening the cortex (Figs. 22.79 and 22.80). Covered in periosteum that is continuous with the bone shaft and with its tip covered by a proliferative cartilage cap, the exostosis usually grows away from the joint, using a similar mechanism to that of the epiphysis; there is no involvement of the bone's epiphyseal ossification center. When the person reaches maturity, bone growth ceases, as it does in the tumor. There can be secondary vascular and neural manifestations; the patient can present with pain and swelling or, alternately, the patient may be asymptomatic.

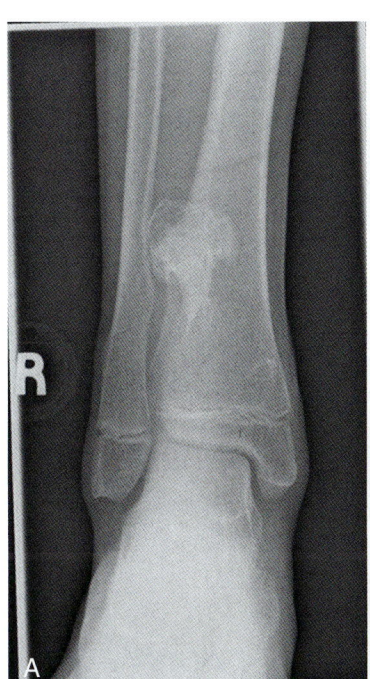
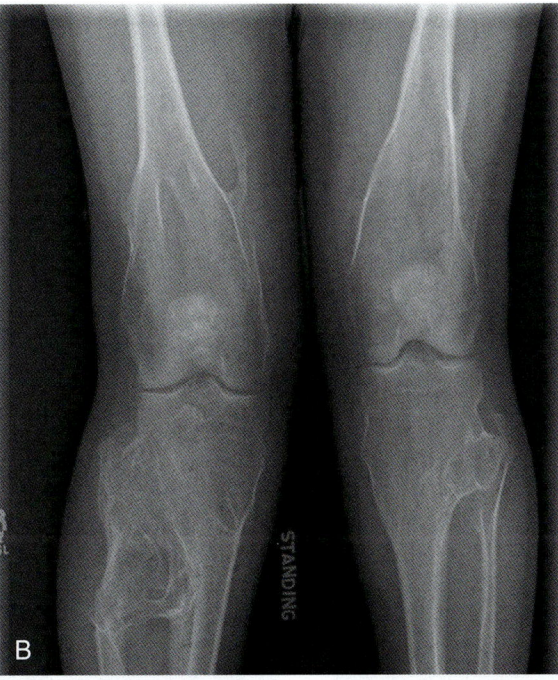

Fig. 22.79 (**A**) A 14 year old with a right distal tibial pedunculated osteochondroma and deformation of the distal fibula. (**B**) Bilateral osteochondromas.

(Courtesy Dr. George Taylor, Radiology, Boston Children's Hospital.)

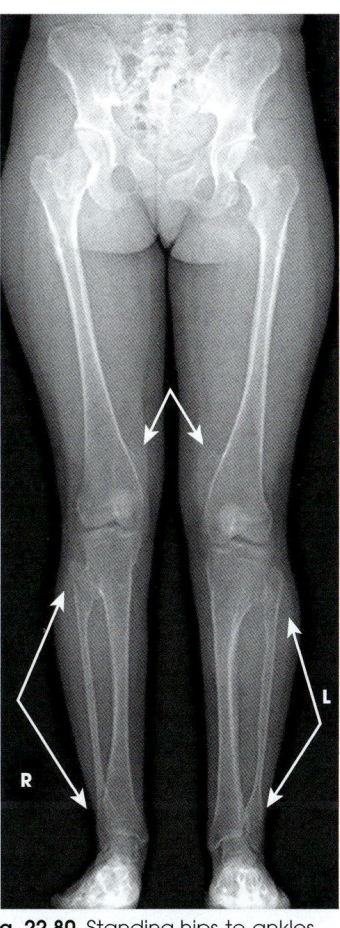

Fig. 22.80 Standing hips-to-ankles exam performed in EOS scanner that demonstrates lower leg osteochondroma multiple exostosis lesions *(arrows)*.

Childhood Pathologies

Aneurysmal bone cyst

Aneurysmal bone cysts (ABCs) occur in children and young adults and have an unknown etiology. Secondary ABCs make up about 50% of all cases, and there is a preponderance in females. The most commonly affected sites are both long and short tubular bones (Fig. 22.81A), neural arches of the vertebral bodies, and pelvic and facial bones. The cyst is composed of blood and connective tissue with connective tissue predominating as the ABC ages (Fig. 22.81B). The most characteristic radiologic finding is a thin shell of bone containing the dilated cyst. ABCs are classified into five types, I through V, and should be removed immediately due to their potential for rapid and extensive damage.

Osteoid osteoma

An osteoid osteoma is a small benign ovoid tumor, rarely exceeding 1 cm in diameter. Osteoid osteomas occur most commonly in the tibia, femur, and the tubular bones of the feet and hands (basal phalanges), including their respective epiphyses (Fig. 22.82A). About 90% of these lesions occur in the first two decades of life. Radiographically, they appear as a well-circumscribed radiolucency with a density at the center (nidus) in the midst of extensive bony thickening and sclerosis. These tumors are hard to penetrate radiographically and may require an increased technique. Although the lesion rarely exceeds 1 cm in diameter, the sclerosis that accompanies it can reach to 2 cm. A lesion larger than 2 cm is most likely an osteoblastoma. Treatment of osteoid osteomas includes, but is not limited to, tetracycline localization in the nidus. Radiofrequency (RF) ablation is another treatment option, in which an electrode tip heated to 90-degree centigrade ((194°F) is placed into the nidus for 6 minutes (Fig. 22.82B).

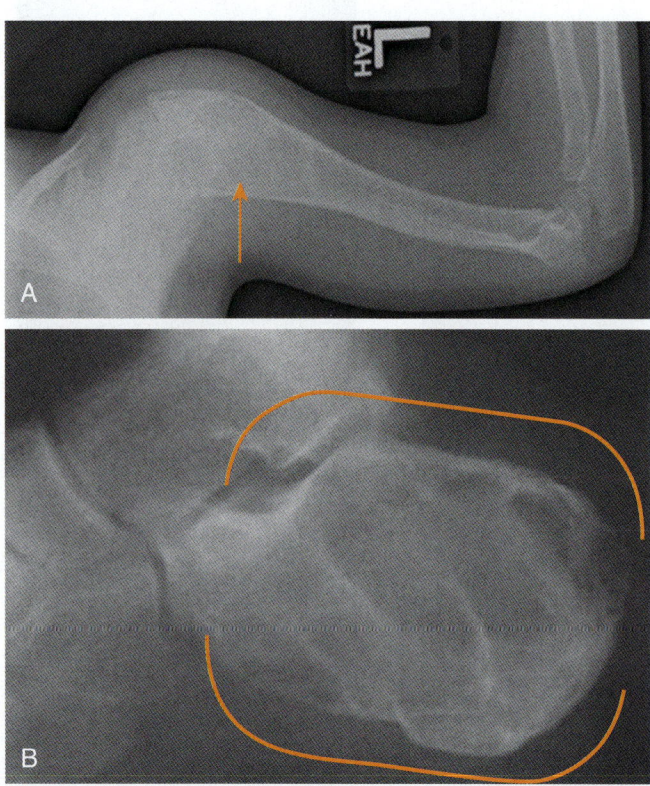

Fig. 22.81 (**A**) ABC of the left proximal humerus (*arrow*). (**B**) ABCs in the tarsus (*parentheses*).

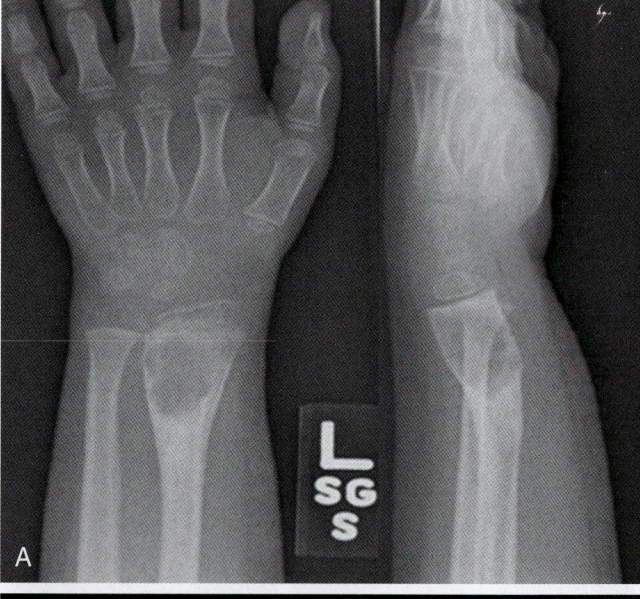

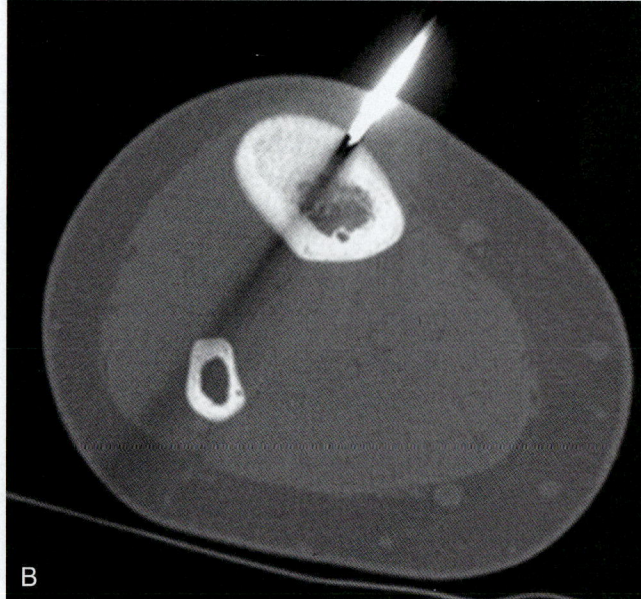

Fig. 22.82 (**A**) AP and lateral views of distal radial osteoid osteoma. (**B**) Radiofrequency ablation of an osteoid osteoma of the right tibia.

Childhood Pathologies

Malignant neoplasms
Osteosarcoma
Alternatively known as osteogenic sarcoma, osteosarcoma is the most common of the primary malignant tumors. Usually appearing in the second decade of life, it often begins in the center of the metaphysis, enlarges, and destroys the bone. Males seem to have a slight preponderance. The most common sites are the metaphysis of the proximal humeri and proximal tibias, as well as the femurs. The earliest presentations of this rapidly growing tumor are pain and swelling at the site. Pathologic fractures are not uncommon, and systemic signs attesting to its rapid growth are weight loss, anemia, and dilated surface veins at the site. The chief radiologic finding is an increase in ossification of the tumor tissue, which may present as an irregularly radiolucent, multiloculated mass. Metastases occur early, usually in the lungs, and chemotherapy increases the risk for secondary tumors, both sarcomas and osteosarcomas, after the treatment of the primary tumor. Bone sarcomas show a chromosome band that supports a recessively transmitted predisposition for this tumor and for retinoblastomas.

Ewing sarcoma
Occurring usually at the end of the first decade or at the beginning of the second, Ewing sarcoma is the second most common malignant tumor in children, and almost any bone in the body may be affected. These tumors grow most frequently in the ilium, femurs, humeri (Fig. 22.83), and tibias. Unlike most of the primary malignancies, Ewing sarcoma does present with fever, weakness, pallor, and lassitude in contrast to most of the primary malignancies. It is not an osteogenic tumor, and the distinctive radiographic findings are the normally opaque spongiosa and cortical bone replaced by more radiolucent tumor tissue with bone destruction, layered periosteal new bone (onion-skin), and overlying large and swollen soft tissue mass.

PNEUMONIA
Pneumonia is the most frequent type of lung infection, resulting in inflammation with compromised pulmonary function. It ranks sixth among the leading causes of mortality in the United States and is the most lethal nosocomial infection. Viruses are the most common cause of both upper and lower respiratory tract infections, whereas bacteria account for about 5% of all childhood pneumonias. In children younger than 2 years old, 90% of cases are viral, with the respiratory syncytial virus responsible for about one-third of these cases. Viral or interstitial pneumonias are more common, are usually less severe than bacterial pneumonia, and are frequently caused by influenza. Radiographic findings are minimal, and the infection is usually confirmed clinically or through serologic tests.

Although chest images are important in determining the location of the inflammation, they are not definitive as to whether the causative agent is viral or bacterial; some knowledge of the suspected pathogens and their radiographic appearances can offer clues (Fig. 22.84). Pneumonias appear as soft, patchy, ill-defined alveolar infiltrates or pulmonary densities. The inflammation may affect the entire lobe of a lung (lobar pneumonia), a segment of a lung (segmental pneumonia), the bronchi and associated alveoli (bronchopneumonia), or the interstitial lung tissue (interstitial pneumonia).

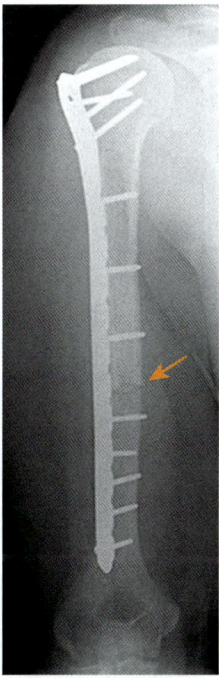

Fig. 22.83 Neutral view of right humerus postosteotomy and plating for Ewing osteosarcoma. (*Arrow* points to osteotomy site.)

Childhood Pathologies

The single most common pneumonia-producing bacterial agent in school-age children is *Mycoplasma pneumonia* (present in 40% to 60% of cases). Pneumococcal (lobar) pneumonia is the most common bacterial pneumonia, probably because the bacteria are present in our healthy throats. It presents on the image as a collection of fluid in one or more lobes; the degree of segmental involvement can usually be identified with a lateral view. Staphylococcal and streptococcal bacterial pneumonia are far less common. Staphylococcal pneumonia occurs infrequently except during epidemics of influenza, when it can be common and life-threatening, especially in infants. Streptococcal pneumonia is even rarer, accounting for less than 1% of all hospital admissions for acute bacterial pneumonia. Radiographic findings are localized around the bronchi, usually of the lower lobes.

Mycoplasma pneumonia is caused by mycoplasmas and is most common in older children and young adults. This disease appears as a fine reticular pattern in a segmental distribution, followed by patchy areas of air space consolidation. In severe cases, the radiographic appearance may mimic tuberculosis. The morbidity rate associated with mycoplasma pneumonia is very low, even when the disease is not treated. Aspiration (chemical) pneumonia or chemical pneumonitis is caused by aspirated vomitus and appears on the image as densities radiating from either hilum.

One of the most common challenges facing the radiologist is to rule out pneumonia. In most cases, the PA and lateral positions of the chest will suffice. In equivocal cases, the decubitus views are helpful in clarifying a suspected pulmonary abnormality. Images should be made with short exposure times (large focal spot) and must be inspiratory. Artifacts, possibly leading to a false positive, can be avoided with careful patient positioning, a peak inspiratory image, and ensuring that the neonate's head is midline without any rotation. Pathologic conditions, such as CF and asthma with atelectasis, will distort the lung fields and could lead to an erroneous finding of pneumonia. Comparison to earlier images is essential to rule out residual or recurrent problems that might suggest an underlying abnormality. A pneumatocele (a thin-walled, radiolucent, air-containing cyst) is the characteristic radiographic lesion and is more typically seen in children. In later stages of the disease, these can enlarge, forming empyemas.

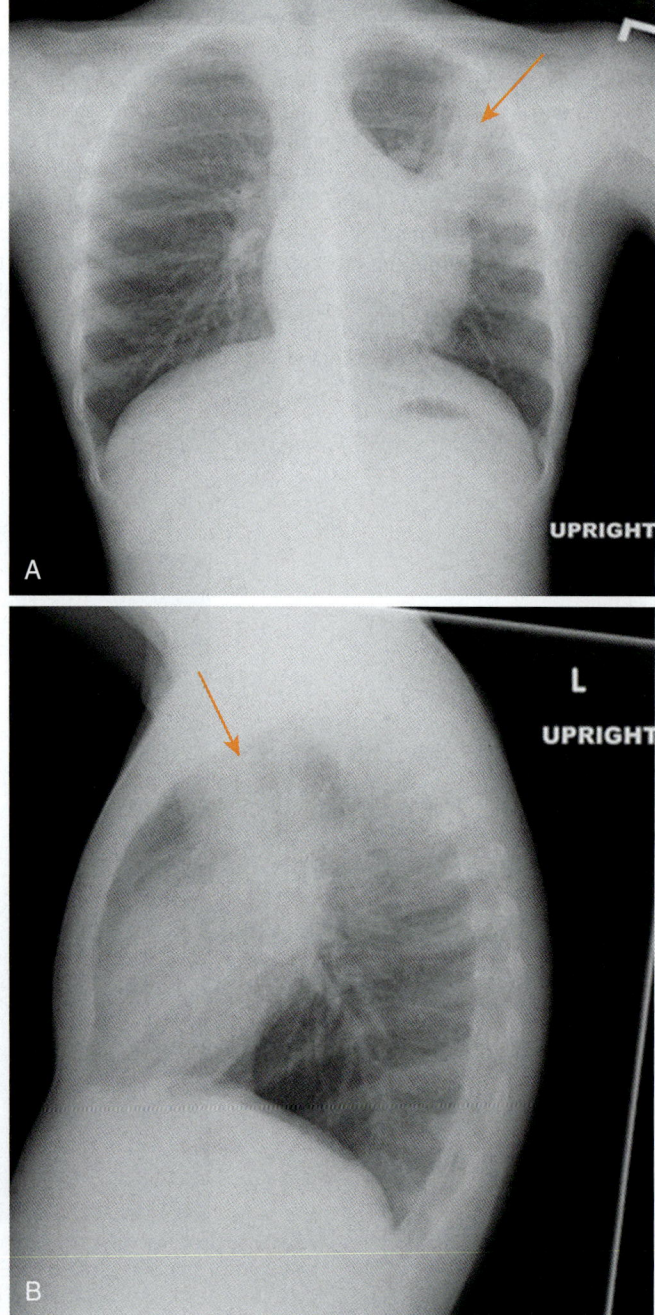

Fig. 22.84 PA (**A**) and lateral (**B**) chest images of an adolescent with pneumonia *(arrows)*.

Childhood Pathologies

PROGERIA

Progeria, or Hutchinson-Gilford progeria syndrome (HGPS), is a rare, fatal genetic condition characterized by an appearance of accelerated aging in children. The Greek word *progeria* means "prematurely old." Progeria affects every 1 in 8 million children. Progeria was named after the doctors who first described it in England—in 1886 by Dr. Jonathan Hutchinson and in 1897 by Dr. Hastings Gilford. Progeria children die of heart disease and atherosclerosis at a much younger age, just like older adult patients. Recent drug trials and research have increased the lifespan of these highly intellectual children by reducing cardiovascular disease and osteoporosis.

Progeria is probably an autosomal recessive syndrome affecting the *LMNA* gene that produces a defective lamina A protein, resulting in a weakened cell nucleus. This unstable nucleus apparently results in premature aging. There is no cure for progeria. Symptoms include scleroderma, loss of hair and subcutaneous fat, short stature (average 100 cm), low weight (12–15 kg), abnormal dentition, an increased prominence of scalp veins, coxa valga, and osteopenia (Figs. 22.85 and 22.86).

SCOLIOSIS

Scoliosis is an abnormal lateral curvature of the spine in excess of 10 degrees, which has a component of rotation, bringing the ribs anteriorly in the direction of the rotation, and affecting lung function in more serious cases (Fig. 22.87). The scoliotic curve may be simple or may involve a compensating curve that results in an "S" shape; the spinal curvature may occur on the right, the left, or both sides. In the greater population, between 3 and 5 children out of every 1000 develop a scoliosis that requires treatment. It affects girls about seven times more than boys, and idiopathic scoliosis tends to run in families, although no genetic link has been found. Scoliosis occurs, and is treated, as three main types.

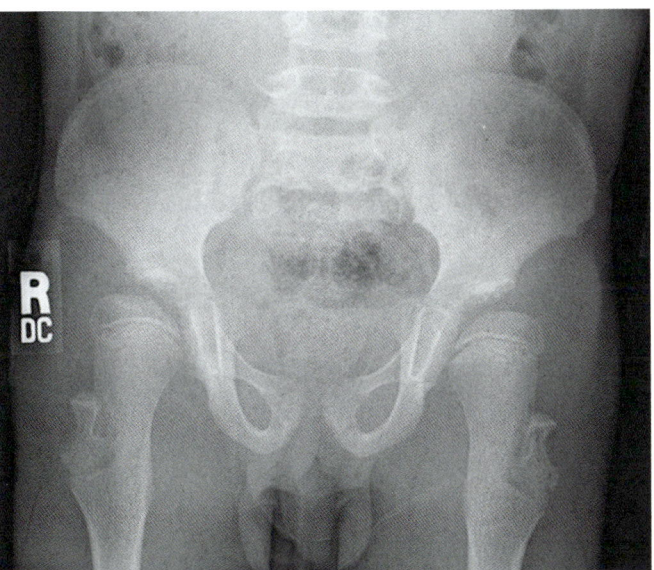

Fig. 22.85 AP pelvis radiograph of a progeria child with osteopenia and hip dysplasia (DDH).

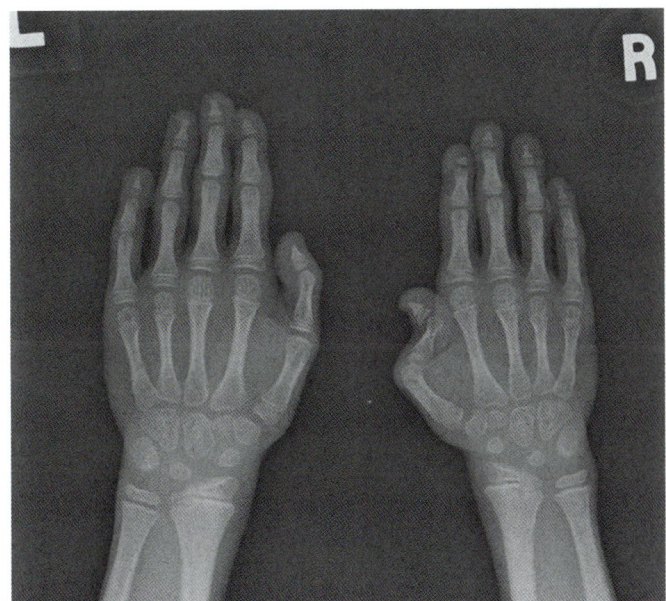

Fig. 22.86 PA radiograph of the hands of a child with progeria.

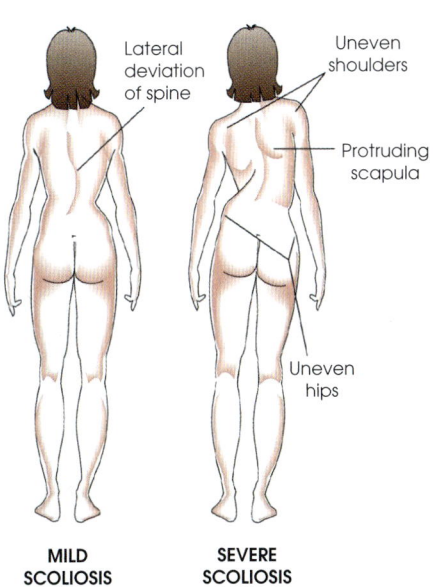

Fig. 22.87 Symptoms that suggest scoliosis.

(From VanMeter KC: *Gould's pathophysiology for the health professions*, ed 5, St Louis, 2014, Elsevier.)

Childhood Pathologies

Idiopathic
The most common type occurs mostly in preadolescent and adolescent girls; however, most cases either remain asymptomatic or the curves are too small to require treatment. Idiopathic scoliosis is comprised of three subtypes.

Adolescent. Represents the majority of cases, mostly in girls between 10 and 13 years old, and often requires no treatment.

Juvenile. Represents about 10% of cases in the age range of 3 to 9 years.

Infantile (early onset). Accounts for about 5% of cases, occurring in boys from birth to 3 years old, and is mostly self-resolving.

Neuromuscular
This refers to scoliosis that is associated with disorders of the nerve or muscular systems (e.g., cerebral palsy [CP], spina bifida, muscular dystrophy, or spinal cord injury).

Congenital
This is the least common form and occurs in utero between 3 and 6 weeks, causing partial, missing, or fused vertebrae.

Scoliosis imaging
Usually indicated are standing *erect* PA/AP and lateral images of the entire spine from the EAM to include the hips and pelvis. The first PA or AP image should allow for visualization of the ribs and spine in their entirety. The lateral view should also include from the EAM to the bottom of the pelvis (Fig. 22.88).

Patient preparation for scoliosis imaging is crucial to avoid image artifacts. The patient should remove all piercings and be undressed, wearing only underwear or boxers (check to make sure females have removed their bras), a hospital gown, and socks, with long hair placed in a bun on top of their head. Posture should be as the patient normally carries themselves and erect. Sitting images are more involved and require care in patient transfer to the special scoliosis-imaging chair. Holding help will most likely be required, and the lateral position should have a positioning sponge between the patient's back and the holder for support. The patient's pelvis should be as close to the grid or sponge as possible. This can be difficult with CP patients, as they tend to slide away from a support and may require that their knees be held so that they cannot slide forward. If the patient is in a wheelchair with removable sides, they can be imaged in their chairs, but great care should be made to maintain *erect* posture. The more advanced modality is the slot-scan EOS system (Biospace Med, Paris, France), which is covered later under the section titled Advances in Technology. In general, any patient group who is unable to stand and keep extremely still (e.g., patients with CP, ADHD, autism spectrum disorder, spastic quadriplegia, or developmental delay) should be imaged on the "Fuji Panel," where the exposure is limited to milliseconds compared to the 3- to 4-second acquisition time of the EOS slot scanner as motion will be mapped into the image.

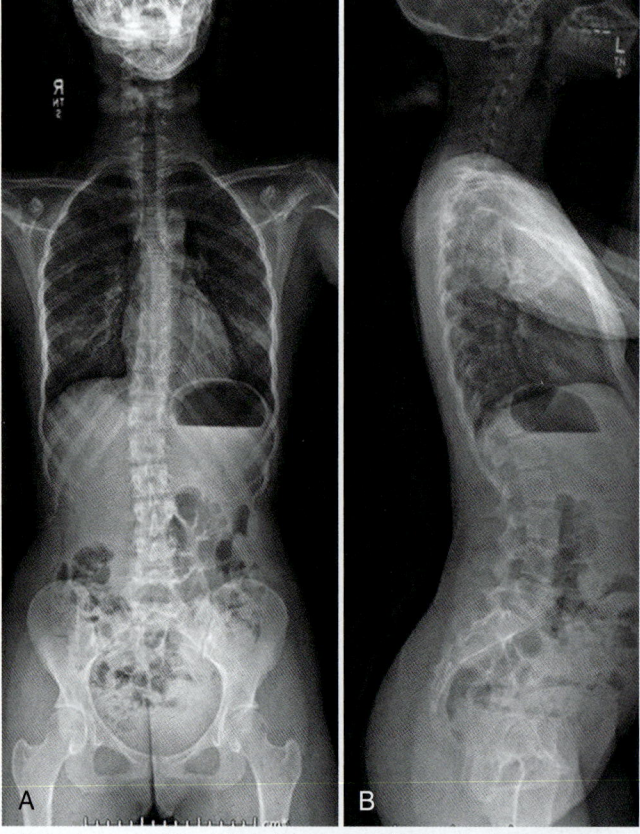

Fig. 22.88 AP (**A**) and lateral (**B**) scoliosis images performed in the EOS to include the entire ribs and pelvis.

Childhood Pathologies

Cobb angle, patterns of scoliosis, and estimation of rotation

The degree of curvature is measured from the PA view using the Cobb method. The image is examined to see what type of curve is present—acute (possible fracture?), smooth and arcuate, lumbar or thoracic, single or double—and whether there are any rib or vertebral anomalies. To measure the Cobb angle, one identifies the curve's superior and inferior end vertebrae, which are the two vertebrae that tilt most severely toward the concavity of the curve. Straight lines are then drawn across the superior and inferior end plates of the curve's upper and lower end vertebrae; the lines extend toward the concavity. These lines will intersect off the image, making the Cobb angle impossible to measure, so to the right of the spine from each end plate line, extend a perpendicular line until they both intersect. The angle superior to the intersection represents the Cobb angle. Once the Cobb angle is determined, an estimation of the degree of rotation can be determined with reference to the vertebrae at the apex of the curve. In cases when severe kyphosis, spondylolysis or spondylolisthesis is suspected, the clinician will include a lateral projection of the entire spine in addition to the PA projection (Fig. 22.89).

Lateral bends

Pediatric patients scheduled for surgery will have bending images to assess the rigidity and flexibility of the curve(s). A left thoracolumbar curve would be considered the major curve (structural) if it failed to correct with either right or left bends. The lumbar curve on the same patient would be considered a compensatory curvature (nonstructural) if it corrects on the right bend. Once the patient has reached skeletal maturity, curves of less than 30 degrees will not progress.

Skeletal maturity

In pediatric radiology, evaluation of skeletal maturity is made based on bone growth in an image of the left hand and wrist. In children with endocrine abnormalities and growth disorders, the determination of skeletal maturation (bone age) is important in their diagnosis and treatment. In clinical practice, bone age is most often obtained by comparing the image with a set of reference hand images from the atlas by Greulich and Pyle. This reference work is the result of a 1950s survey of a healthy white middle- to upper-class population. A study by Zhang[3] questioned the validity of using the Greulich and Pyle atlas for an ethnically diverse population and found that ethnic and racial differences in growth patterns exist at certain ages with both Asians and Hispanics; this was seen in both male and female subjects, especially in girls aged 10 to 13 years and boys aged 11 to 15 years. A recent paper by Tsai et al.[4] in *Pediatric Radiology* provides strong support for using fibular shaft length as a more accurate alternative to current methods for bone age estimation with infants aged less than 1 year.

Treatment options

Options for treatment of scoliosis range from observation and monitoring to physical therapy, bracing, casting, and surgery. Invasive treatments may include spinal fusion/instrumentation, dual posterior growing rods to control spinal deformity, rod lengthening for infantile scoliosis, thoracoscopic anterior spinal surgery and instrumentation, osteotomy, or a combination of surgical procedures.

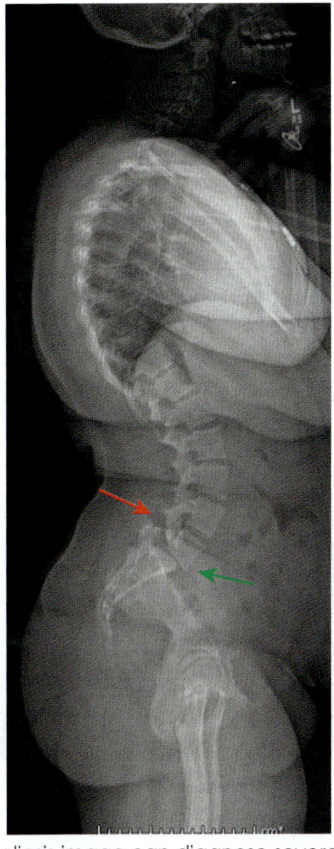

Fig. 22.89 The lateral EOS scoliosis image can diagnose severe kyphosis, seen here, plus spondylolysis *(red arrow)* and spondylolisthesis *(green arrow)*.

Advances in Technology

Advances in Technology

RADIOGRAPHY

Although this technology has been available in Europe for some time, it has been approved in North America more recently. The EOS system (Biospace Med) (Figs. 22.90 and 22.91) for orthopedic imaging has three advantages over conventional x-ray–based systems, according to the company:

1. Greatly reduces dose to patient.
2. Allows three-dimensional modeling for the evaluation of rotation, torsion, and orientation.
3. Imaging is always on-axis and distortion free.

EOS allows the slot-scan–based image to be made weight-bearing, sitting (without assistance), and without the need for stitching. The biggest disadvantage of the EOS system is that motion can be mapped into the image, mimicking long bone dysplasia in cases in which the patient cannot keep still or has tremors (Fig. 22.92). Various clinical parameters useful in evaluating and developing a patient's path to recovery are calculated automatically, including a patient report with images. Lower limb modeling is not adapted for patients younger than 15 years. Spine modeling is not adapted for patients aged 7 and younger or for the following pathologies: supernumerary vertebrae, congenital deformities, and spondylolisthesis.

MAGNETIC RESONANCE IMAGING

Many imaging centers routinely see young children before an MRI, incurring anesthesia costs; overnight admissions for infants; costs associated with sedation, anesthesia preparation, and recovery; and reduced patient and family satisfaction. To this end, BCH conducted two pilot studies during 2009 and 2010 to assess the feasibility of pediatric scans without sedation ("Try Without," unpublished); in the initial pilot, children between the ages of 5 and 7 were assessed, and in the second pilot, children from 4 to 6 years and infants 0 to 6 months were assessed. With adequate preparation and age-appropriate distractions, some children under the age of 7 remained still without sedation for 20 to 60 minutes. Results showed that 88% of children between the ages of 5 and 7 and 82% of those in the study of children 4 to 6 years old and infants 0 to 6 months completed their scans without sedation. Since 2010, 3300 children have completed their MRI scans without sedation. You will see more of this cost/benefit and patient satisfaction analysis in the future of health care.

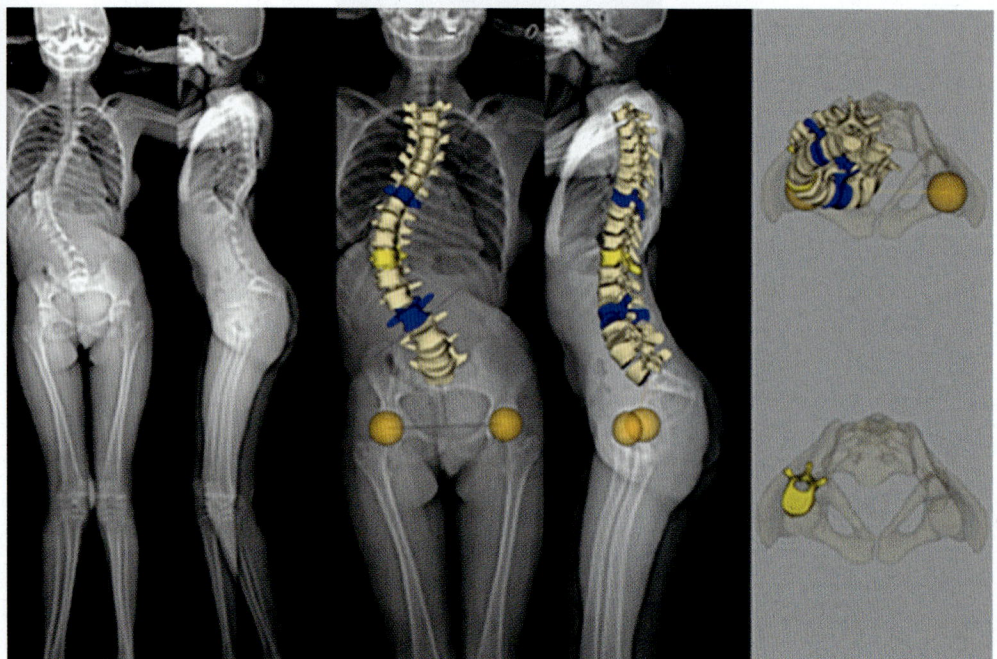

Fig. 22.90 EOS slot-scan standing scoliosis images of a 13-year-old female CP patient, with 3D remodeling showing axial rotation of individual vertebrae and large lateral ejection of the apical vertebrae.

(Courtesy EOS Imaging, Cambridge, MA.)

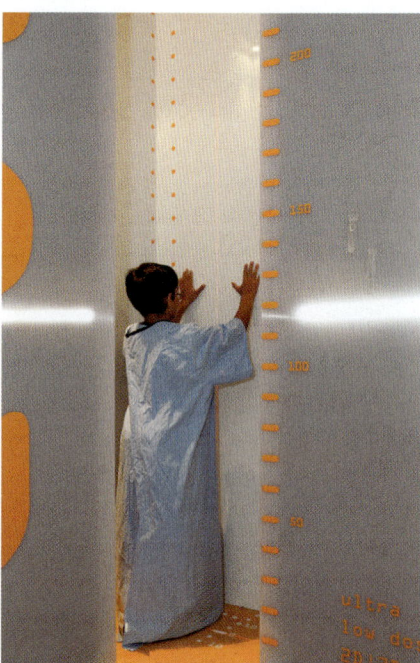

Fig. 22.91 EOS system; patient positioned for simultaneous acquisition of PA and lateral full spine views for scoliosis.

Advances in Technology

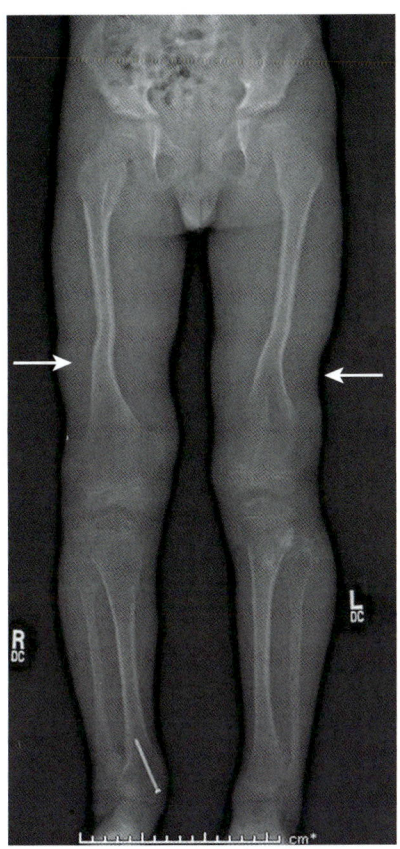

Fig. 22.92 The biggest disadvantage of the EOS system is that motion can be mapped into the image, mimicking long bone dysplasia, when the patient cannot keep still or has tremors. Note the "wobbly" distal femurs.

A "noiseless" MRI system (Silent Scan, GE Healthcare, Waukesha, Wisconsin), which scans at a noise level of about 4 dB, compared with 86 to 110 dB with current technology, is available commercially; the reduced noise is the result of 3D MR acquisition, in combination with proprietary high-fidelity gradient and RF system electronics, according to the company (Fig. 22.93). If this technology meets expectations, it could offer the potential for further reductions in sedation for younger patients.

ULTRASOUND

A wireless transducer (Siemens) is available that will transmit over a distance of 3 meters, which may assist with imaging infants and children. Called a point-of-care system, the transducer will expand the use of US in both interventional radiology and therapeutic applications. US has made huge advances through the years, but it is still largely constrained by bandwidth (0–50 MHz) and sensitivity. In a collaborative effort to overcome these limitations, Texas A&M University, King's College London, the Queen's University of Belfast, and the University of Massachusetts, Lowell, have developed a new meta-material that converts US waves into optical signals, making images with greater detail (0–150 MHz) possible, maintaining sensitivity, and allowing one to see deeper into tissues.

COMPUTED TOMOGRAPHY

In pediatric patients, CT has been useful in diagnosing congenital anomalies, assessing metastases, and diagnosing bone sarcomas and sinus disease. Young children have difficulty following the instructions needed for a diagnostic scan. Suggestions regarding approach and atmosphere are presented at the beginning of this chapter. As in the care of any pediatric patient, the role of the CT radiographer is essential to the success of the examination; the radiographer must gain the respect and confidence of the young patient and the caregiver, if present. The CT scanner itself is an imposing piece of equipment that needs careful explanation to help allay the patient's fears. One of the most significant fears is claustrophobia, which can be reduced through distraction devices such as virtual goggles, music, and creative room décor (Fig. 22.94).

Toshiba has unveiled its Aquilion One Vision 640-slice CT scanner. This new system is equipped with a gantry rotation of 0.275 seconds, a 100-kW generator, and 320 detector rows (640 unique slices) covering 16 cm in a single rotation, with the industry's thinnest slices at 500 microns (0.5 mm). The One Vision uses an alternating focal spot that allows 16-cm z-axis coverage to be sampled twice, generating 640 slices in one rotation. The system can accommodate larger patients with its 78-cm bore and fast rotation, including

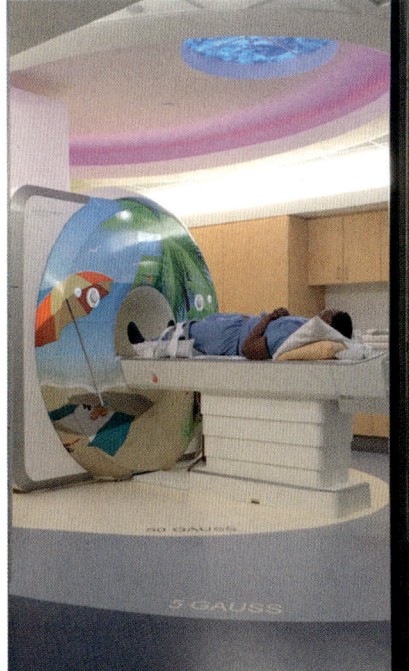

Fig. 22.93 An MRI suite with a Siemens Skyra scanner. This machine can be used for adults and children.

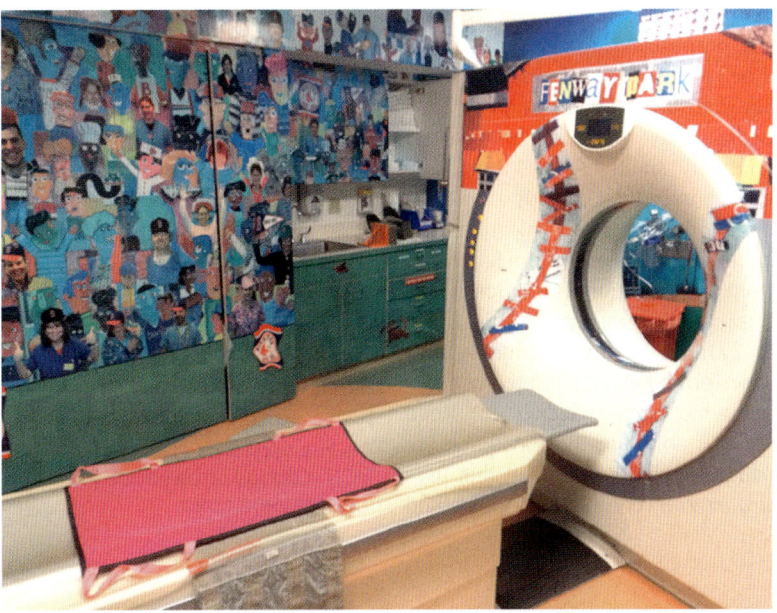

Fig. 22.94 A Siemens Sensation CT scanner decorated for children.

Advances in Technology

bariatric patients and patients with high heart rates. More slices and shorter scan times reduce the possibility of patient motion (cardiac CT) and allow for scanning bariatric patients or those with larger anatomy. The faster scan times should reduce the number of patients requiring sedation. The Image Gently campaign has suggested CT protocols for reducing CT dose to patients.

INTERVENTIONAL RADIOLOGY

Image-guided, minimally invasive IR has dramatically changed the role of the radiology department in teaching and nonteaching hospitals and clinics. In the past, the justifications and rationales for radiology departments were diagnostic ones. Radiology departments with interventional staff now offer hospitals therapeutic services in addition to diagnostic procedures. This heightened awareness has largely resulted from the nature and efficacy of interventional procedures. Therapeutic procedures performed in IR provide an attractive alternative to surgery for the patient, parent, hospital, and society. A procedure performed in IR is much less invasive and expensive than one performed in the operating room. Shortened inpatient stays for IR procedures translate into economic savings for the parents and the hospital.

For simplicity, interventional radiology can be divided into vascular and nonvascular procedures. Vascular procedures are generally performed in angiographic suites. During these therapeutic interventions, angiography and ultrasonography are also performed for diagnostic and guidance purposes. Angiography can be arterial or venous; pediatric vasculature is well suited to both. IV injection of contrast media is favored in infants because their relatively small blood volume and rapid circulation allow for good vascular imaging. In infants, hand injections are often preferred over power injections to help avoid extravasation. Intraarterial digital subtraction angiography (DSA) (see Chapter 27) has become a valuable tool. DSA is performed using a diluted contrast medium, which can reduce pain. Road mapping is a software tool, available on newer angiographic equipment, that uses the *intraarterial* contrast injection and fluoroscopy to display arterial anatomy—a useful tool for imaging tortuous vessels.

Vascular procedures can be neurologic, cardiac, or systemic in nature. Nonvascular procedures often involve the digestive and urinary systems; examples include the insertion of gastrostomy tubes to supplement the nutrition of pediatric patients and the insertion of cecostomy tubes in chronically constipated patients with spina bifida. Vascular access devices are of three types: nontunneled, tunneled, and implanted. The selection of device is often determined by a combination of factors, including the purpose of the access and estimated indwelling time. The physician or patient may choose a particular device after assessing issues of compliance or underlying clinical factors.

Nontunneled catheters are commonly referred to as *peripherally inserted central catheters (PICCs)*. They are available with single or multiple lumens. The insertion point is usually the basilic or cephalic vein at or above the antecubital space of the nondominant arm. Multiple lumens are desirable when a variety of medications (including total parenteral nutrition) are to be administered (Fig. 22.95). These devices must be strongly anchored to the skin because children often pull on and displace the catheters, resulting in damage to the line and potential risk to themselves.

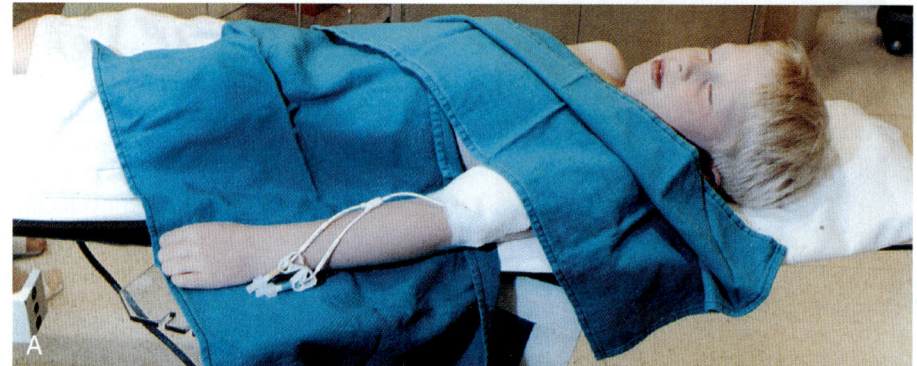

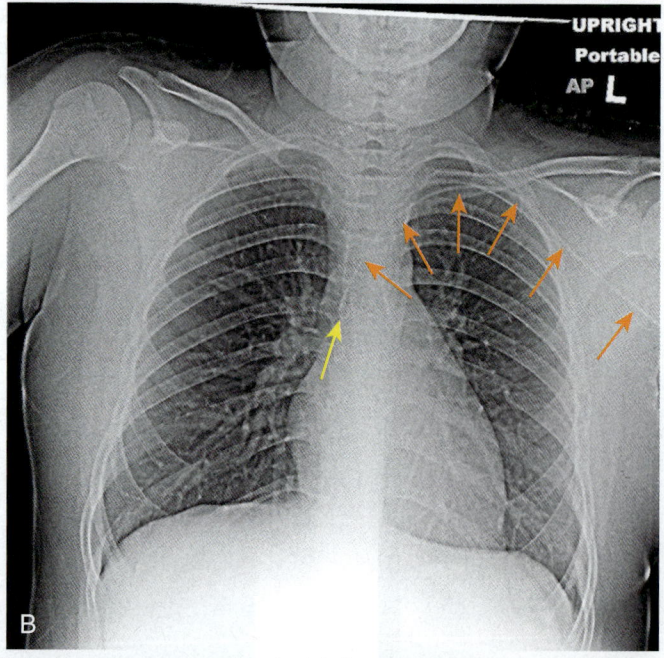

Fig. 22.95 (A) Postinsertion image of a double-lumen PICC in a 7-year-old boy (shown in the interventional suite). Conscious sedation was used for this procedure. (B) Left-sided PICC. *Orange arrows* track the double lumen PICC to its terminus *(yellow arrow)* in the superior vena cava.

Advances in Technology

Tunneled catheters, as with PICCs, can have multiple lumens. In contrast to PICCs, they are not inserted into the peripheral circulation; rather, they are inserted via a subcutaneous tunnel into the subclavian or internal jugular veins. Tunneling acts as an anchoring mechanism for the catheter to facilitate long-term placement (Fig. 22.96). Larger lumen or "French size catheters" are referred to as Hickman lines and facilitate chemotherapy, antibiotics, fluids, and hemodialysis, and when placed in subclavian or internal jugular veins.

Implanted devices are often referred to as ports. These are titanium or polysulfone devices with silicone centers attached to catheters. The whole device is implanted subcutaneously with the distal end of the catheter tip advanced to the superior vena cava or right atrium. A port is the device of choice for noncompliant patients, and children and adults who are undergoing chemotherapy, and for aesthetic purposes or long-term use, would rather not have the limb of a catheter protruding from their chest (Fig. 22.97).

Vascular access devices have dramatically changed the course of treatment for many patients in a positive way. Patients who would have previously been hospitalized for antibiotic therapy can now go home with the device in place and resume normal activity. The increased prevalence of these devices means that patients with vascular access devices are in the community and visiting radiology departments everywhere. PICCs have a smaller likelihood of introducing catheter-related infections; tunneled lines present a greater risk.

Radiographers must recognize vascular access devices and treat them with utmost care. They should report dislodged bandages and sites showing signs of infection (i.e., redness, exudate immediately). Catheter-related infections constitute the largest nosocomial source of infection; they can be life threatening and cost hospitals hundreds of thousands of dollars each year.

Postprocedural care vascular access devices currently represent a significant and ongoing challenge for all personnel who treat, manage, and come in contact with these patients.

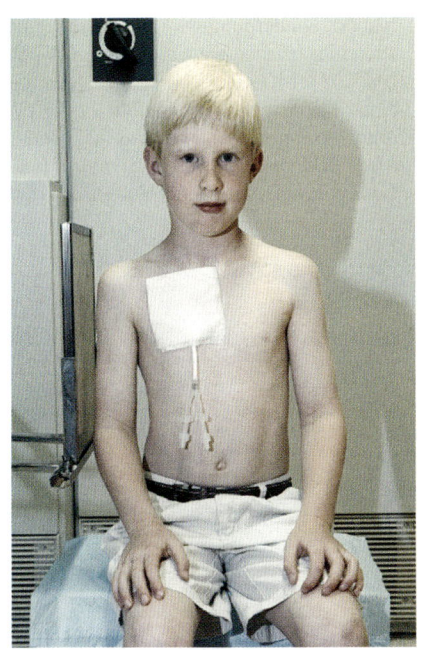

Fig. 22.96 External appearance of tunneled, double-lumen central venous access device. These catheters are used for long-term therapy. Their short track to the heart can increase the risk of infection, necessitating proper care for maintenance.

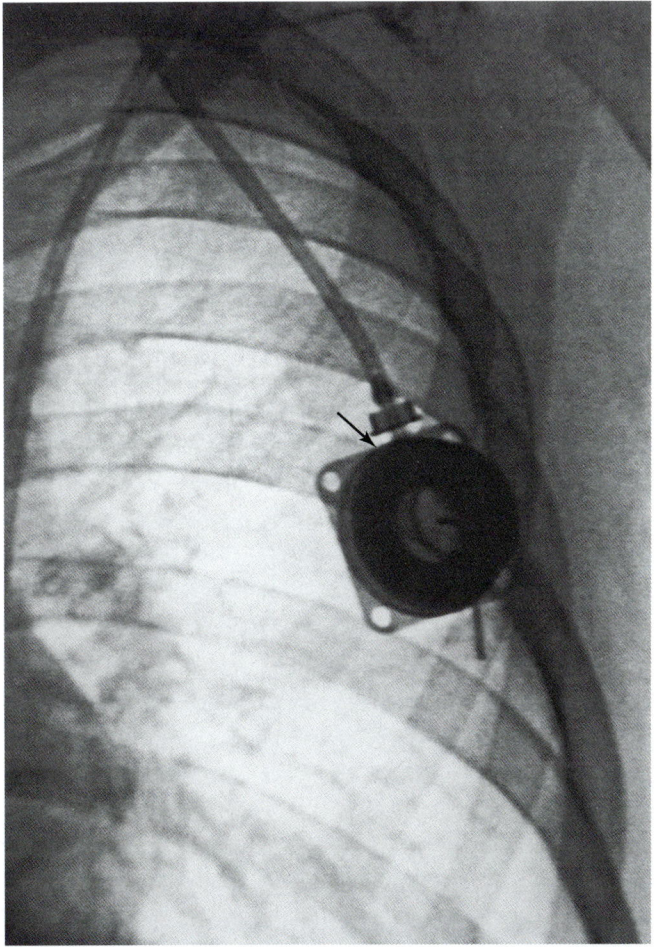

Fig. 22.97 Digital image of port (arrow). Ports are vascular devices that must be accessed subcutaneously. They are preferred for active children and for aesthetic reasons.

ACKNOWLEDGMENTS

To all who came before us and shared their knowledge and the many people who gave willingly of their time, experience, and expertise: George Taylor, MD, Department of Radiology, Boston Children's Hospital (BCH); Jeanne Chow, MD, Department of Radiology, BCH; Carol Barnewolt, MD, Department of Radiology, BCH; Alison Ames, RT(R), outpatient supervisor, Department of Radiology, BCH; Judith Santora, RT(R), inpatient supervisor, Department of Radiology, BCH; Richard Cappock, RT(R), CT, CT modality operations manager, Department of Radiology, BCH; Diane Biagiotti, BS, RT(R), MRI modality operations manager, Department of Radiology, BCH; Judy Estroff, MD (BCH); Jennifer Doran, RTR (BCH); Victoria Glassman, RTR, Brigham and Women's Hospital (BWH); Tiziana Stuto, RTR (BWH); Raymond Thies, RT(R); and Angela Franceschi, MEd, CCLS; Brielle Moorhead, RT(R); Elizabeth Minchella, RT(R); and Gina Farrell, RT (R).

References

1. Peck DJ, Samei E. How to understand and communicate radiation risk. *Image Wisely [website]*. 2017. Available at: https://www.imagewisely.org/imaging-modalities/computed-tomography/medical-physicists/articles/how-to-understand-and-communicate-radiation-risk. (Accessed July 15, 2024).
2. Centers for Disease Control and Prevention. *Autism Spectrum Disorder (ASD)*; 2023. Available at: https://www.cdc.gov/ncbddd/autism/data.html. (Accessed October 2023).
3. Zhang A, Sayre JW, Vachon L, et al. Racial differences in growth patterns of children assessed on the basis of bone age. *Radiology*. 2009;250(1):228–235.
4. Tsai A, Stamoulis C, Bixby SD, et al. Infant bone age estimation based on fibular shaft length: model development and clinical validation. *Pediatr Radiol*. 2016;46(3):342–356.

Selected bibliography

Coley BD. *Caffey's Pediatric Diagnostic Imaging*. 12th ed. St Louis: Elsevier; 2013.

Cystic Fibrosis Foundation Patient Registry. *2021 Annual Data Report*. Bethesda, Maryland: Cystic Fibrosis Foundation; 2022. Available at: https://www.cff.org/sites/default/files/2021-11/Patient-Registry-Annual-Data-Report.pdf. (Accessed July 15, 2024).

Dale E. *Audio-Visual Methods in Teaching*. 3rd ed. New York: Holt, Rinehart & Winston; 1969.

Erikson EH. *Childhood and Society*. New York: WW Norton; 1993.

Godderidge C. *Pediatric Imaging*. Philadelphia: WB Saunders; 1985.

Gray C, White AL. *My Social Stories Book*. Jessica Kingsley; 2002.

Hudson J. *Prescription for Success: Supporting Children with ASD in the Medical Environment*. Shawnee, KS: Autism Asperger Publishing Company; 2006.

Kleinman PK. *Diagnostic Imaging of Child Abuse*. Baltimore: Williams & Wilkins; 1987:2.

Kreiborg S. Postnatal growth and development of the craniofacial complex in premature craniosynostosis. In: Cohen Jr MM, MacLean RE, eds. *Craniosynostosis: Diagnosis, Evaluation and Management*. New York: Oxford University Press; 2000:158–170.

Kwan-Hoong NG, Cameron JR. Using the BERT concept to promote public understanding of radiation. International conference on the radiological protection of patients. In: *C&S Paper, Series 7*. Malaga, Spain: Organized by the International Atomic Energy Agency; 2001:784–787.

Mace JD, Kowalczyk N. *Radiographic Pathology for Technologists*. 4th ed. St Louis, MO: Mosby; 2004:23–24.

Morton-Cooper A. *Health Care and the Autism Spectrum: A Guide for Health Professionals, Parents and Careers*. Jessica Kingsley; 2004. Available from the NAS Publications Department.

Robinson MJ. *Practical Pediatrics*. 6th ed. New York: Churchill Livingstone; 2007.

Silverman F, et al. The limbs. In: *Caffey's Pediatric X-Ray Diagnosis: An Integrated Approach*. 9th ed. vol 2. St Louis: Mosby; 1993:1881–1884.

Unruh BT, Nejad SH, Stern TW, et al. Insertion of foreign bodies (polyembolokoilamania): underpinnings and management strategies. *Prim Care Companion CNS Disord*. 2012;14(1):PCC.11f01192.

Volkmar FR, Wiesner LA. *Healthcare for Children on the Autism Spectrum: A Guide to Medical, Nutritional and Behavioural Issues*. Bethesda, MD: Woodbine House; 2004.

23
GERIATRIC RADIOGRAPHY
CHERYL MORGAN-DUNCAN

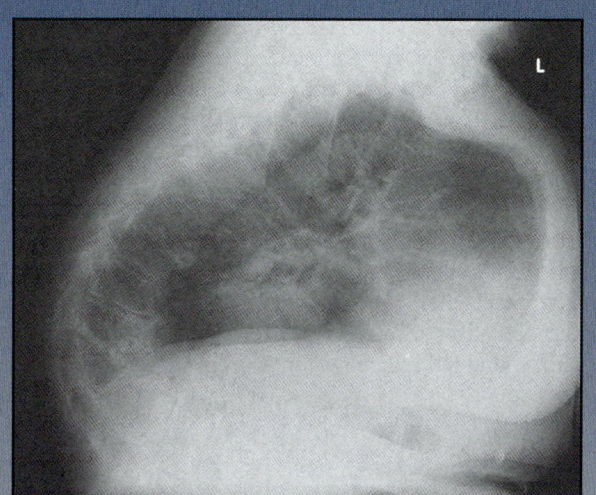

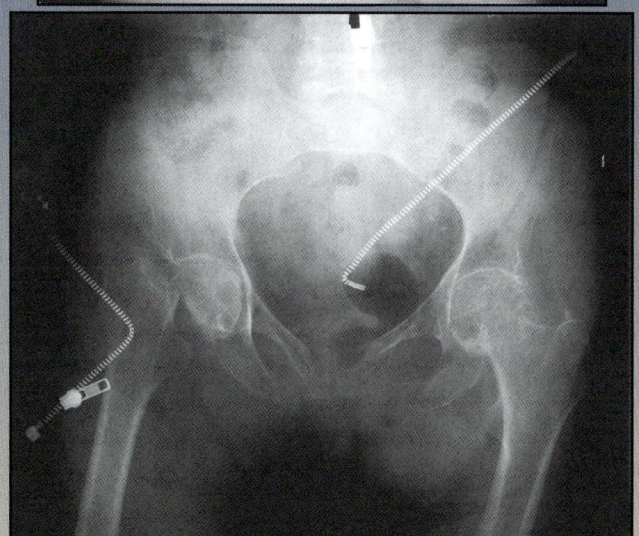

OUTLINE

Demographics and Social Effects of Aging, 148
Elder Abuse, 151
Attitudes Toward the Older Adult, 151
Physical, Cognitive, and Psychosocial Effects of Aging, 152
Physiology of Aging, 154
Summary of Pathology: Geriatric Radiography, 160
Patient Care, 161
Performing the Radiographic Procedure, 162
Radiographic Positioning for Geriatric Patients, 163
Best Practices in Geriatric Radiography, 168
Conclusion, 168

Geriatrics is the branch of medicine dealing with the aged and the problems of aging individuals. The field of *gerontology* includes illness prevention and management, health maintenance, and the promotion of quality of life for aging individuals. The ongoing increase in the number of people older than the age of 65 in the US population is well known. An even more dramatic aging trend exists among people older than 85 years. The number of people 100 years old is approximately 100,000 and increasing. Every aspect of the health care delivery system is affected by this shift in the general population. The 1993 Pew Health Commission Report noted that the "aging of the nation's society and the accompanying shift to chronic care that is occurring foretell major shifts in care needs in which allied health professionals are major providers of services." As members of the allied health professions, radiographers are an important component of the health care system. As the geriatric population increases, so does the number of medical imaging procedures performed on older adult patients. Students and practitioners must be prepared to meet the challenges that this shift in the patient population represents. An understanding of geriatrics can foster a positive interaction between the radiographer and the older adult patient.

Demographics and Social Effects of Aging

The acceleration of the "gray" American population began when individuals born from 1946 to 1964 (known as the "baby boomers") began to turn age 50 in 1996. The number in the age 65 and older cohort is expected to reach 70.2 million by 2030 (Fig. 23.1). The US experience regarding the increase in the older adult population is not unique; it is a global one. As of 1990, 28 countries had more than 2 million persons older than 65, and 12 additional countries had more than 5 million people older than 65. The entire older adult population of the world has begun a predicted dramatic increase for the period 1995–2030.

According to research studies, the aging experience has been influenced by family aspects, economic resources, delivery of long-term care, gender, race, ethnicity, and social class. The aging experience results from the interaction of physical, mental, social, and cultural factors. Aging varies across cultures. Culturally, aging and the values of an ethnic group often determine the treatment of health problems in older adults. Culture may also determine the way in which older people view the process of aging and the manner in which they adapt to growing older. The United States is a multicultural society in which a generalized view of aging would be difficult. Health care professionals need to know not only diseases and disorders common to a specific age-group but also the disorders common to a particular ethnic group. An appreciation of diverse backgrounds can help the health care professional provide a personal approach when meeting the needs of older adult patients. Many colleges and universities have incorporated cultural diversity into their curricula.

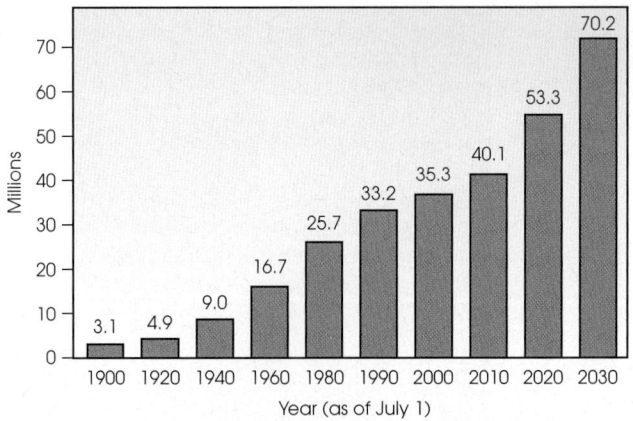

Fig. 23.1 Number of persons older than 65 years in millions, 1900–2030.

(Reprinted from US Department of Commerce, Economics and Statistics Administration: *65+ in the United States*. Washington, DC: US Bureau of the Census; 1996.)

The *economic status* of older adults varies and has an important influence on their health and well-being (Fig. 23.2). Most older adults have adequate income, but many minority patients do not. Single older adults are more likely to be below the poverty line. Economic hardships increase for single older adults, especially women. Of the population older than age 85, 60% is composed of women, making women twice as likely as men to be poor. By age 75, nearly two-thirds of women are widows. Financial security is extremely important to an older adult. Many older adults are reluctant to spend money on what others may consider necessary for their well-being. A problem facing aging Americans is health care finances. Older adults often base decisions regarding their health care not on their needs but exclusively on the cost of health care services.

Increases in both health care and the aging population go hand in hand. In the United States, heart disease, cancer, COVID-19, and stroke are the leading causes of deaths among people older than 65.[1] By 2025, an estimated two-thirds of the US health care budget will be devoted to services for older adult patients.

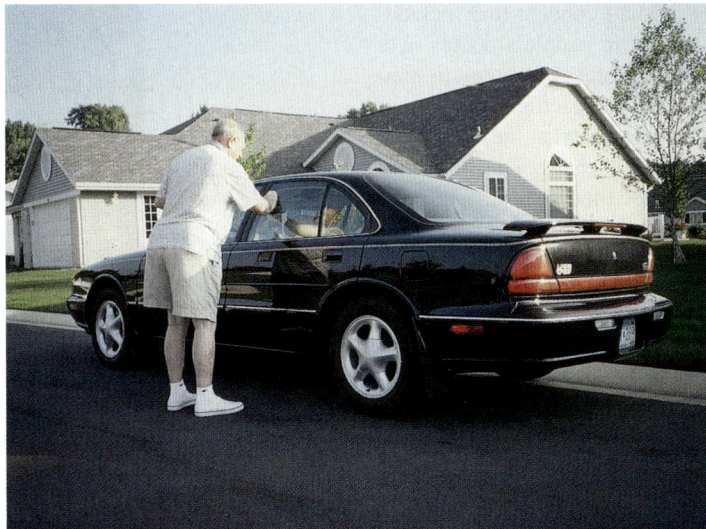
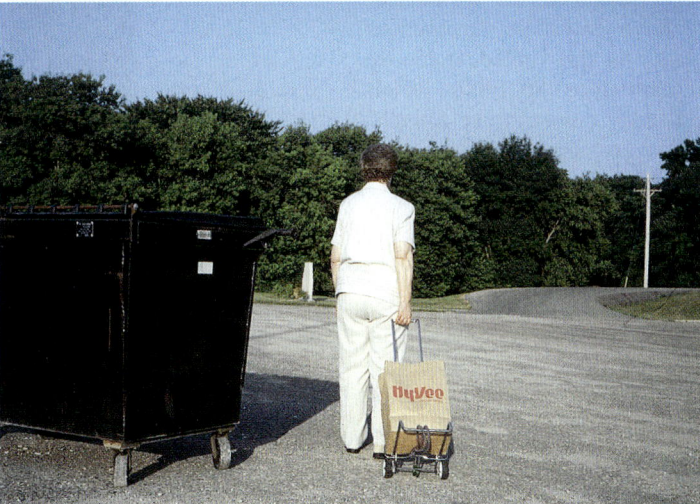

Fig. 23.2 The economic status of older adults varies and has an important influence on their health and well-being.

Aging is a broad concept that includes physical changes in people's bodies over adult life; psychological changes in their minds and mental capacities; social psychological changes in what they think and believe; and social changes in how they are viewed, what they expect, and what is expected of them. Aging is a constantly evolving concept. Notions that biologic age is more critical than chronologic age when determining the health status of the older adult are valid. Aging is an individual and extremely variable process. The functional capacity of major body organs varies with advancing age. Environmental and lifestyle factors affect the age-related functional changes in the body organs. Advancements in medical technology have extended the average life expectancy in the United States by nearly 20 years since the 1960s, which has allowed senior citizens to be actively involved in every aspect of American society. People are healthier longer today because of advanced technology, the results of health promotion and secondary disease prevention, and lifestyle factors, such as diet, exercise, and smoking cessation, which have been effective in reducing the risk of disease (Fig. 23.3). Older adult patients seen in the health care setting have been diagnosed with at least one chronic condition. Individuals who lived in the 1970s would not have survived a debilitating illness such as cancer or a heart attack. Today, individuals not only survive chronic diseases but also live for extended periods. Although age is the most consistent and strongest predictor of risk for cancer and death from cancer, management of an older adult cancer patient becomes complex because of other chronic conditions, such as osteoarthritis, diabetes, chronic obstructive pulmonary disease, and heart disease. Box 23.1 lists the top 10 chronic conditions for people older than 65 years.

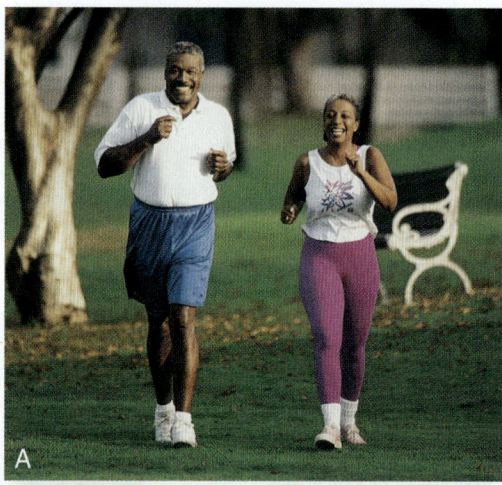
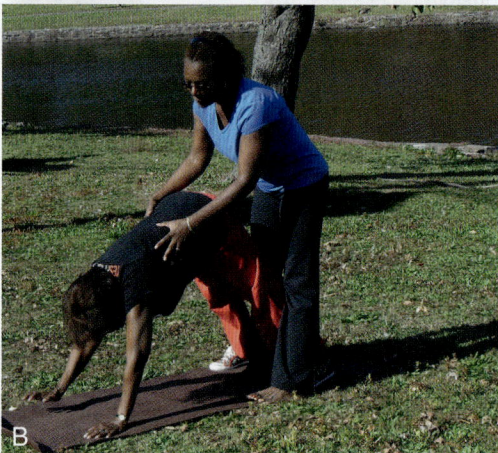

Fig. 23.3 (A) Lifestyle factors—such as diet, exercise, and smoking cessation—reduce the risk of disease and increase life span. (B) Yoga emphasizes breathing and slow, low-impact motion, which are good for those with arthritis.

BOX 23.1

Top 10 chronic conditions of people older than 65 years

Arthritis
Hypertension
Hearing impairment
Heart disease
Cataracts
Deformity or orthopedic impairment
Chronic sinusitis
Diabetes
Visual impairment
Varicose veins

Elder Abuse

Another emerging worldwide issue for older adults is elder abuse. It has been estimated that 2.1 million cases of elder abuse are reported each year. These numbers may be suspect, however, because studies estimate that only one in five cases is reported to the authorities. It is thought that elder abuse is approximately as common as child abuse. Elder abuse is defined as the knowing, intentional, or negligent act by a caregiver or any other person that causes harm or a serious risk of harm to a vulnerable adult. Box 23.2 lists the various types of abuse. The typical victim of abuse is older than 75 years. Most studies of elder abuse show the incidence to be gender neutral. Physical abuse is usually received from the victim's spouse (50%), less often from the victim's children (23%), and only in 17% of cases is the abuse from nonfamily caregivers.

The radiologic technologist should be aware that the presence of injury is not proof of abuse. It is important to be watchful for the warning signs of abuse or neglect listed in Box 23.3. The older adult is often embarrassed by the situation and may be hesitant to communicate their concerns for fear of retaliation. The technologist needs to employ excellent communication skills, accurate documentation, and quality radiographs, and the technologist should report any suspicions of neglect or abuse. Injuries sustained by older adult victims are typical to the head, face, and neck, as well as defensive injuries.

Attitudes Toward the Older Adult

The attitudes of health care providers toward older adults affect their health care. Research indicates that health care professionals have significantly more negative attitudes toward older patients than younger ones. This attitude must change if health care providers are to have positive interactions with older adult patients. These attitudes seem to be related to the pervasive stereotyping of the older adult, which serves to justify avoiding care and contact with them, as well as the older adults being reminders of one's own mortality. *Ageism* is a term used to describe the stereotyping of and discrimination against older adults and is similar to that of racism and sexism.[2] Ageism emphasizes that frequently older adults are perceived to be repulsive and that distaste for the aging process itself exists. Ageism suggests that most older adults are senile, miserable most of the time, and dependent rather than independent individuals. For example, sometimes radiologic technologists and students assume that the elderly patient in their care is unable to raise their arms for the lateral chest x-ray and proceed to perform the examination with the arms partially raised. This results in the humeri and soft tissue superimposing the apices of the lungs. To avoid this, simply ask the patient to raise their arms, and offer assistance if necessary. The media have also influenced ongoing stereotypic

---

BOX 23.2
Forms of elder abuse

Physical: inflicting physical pain or injury
Sexual: nonconsensual sexual contact of any kind
Neglect: failure by those responsible to provide food, shelter, health care, or protection
Exploitation: illegal taking, misuse, or concealment of funds, property, or assets of a senior
Emotional: inflicting mental pain, anguish, or distress through verbal or nonverbal acts
Abandonment: desertion of a vulnerable older adult by anyone who has assumed the responsibility for care or custody of that person
Self-neglect: failure of a person to perform essential self-care tasks, which threatens their personal health or safety

---

BOX 23.3
Warning signs of elder abuse

- Bruises, pressure marks, broken bones, abrasions, and burns may be an indication of physical abuse, neglect, or mistreatment.
- Unexplained withdrawal from normal activities, sudden change in alertness, or unusual depression may be indicators of emotional abuse.
- Bruises around the breasts or genital area may occur from sexual abuse.
- Sudden changes in financial situation may be the result of exploitation.
- Bedsores, unattended medical needs, poor hygiene, or unusual weight loss may be indicators of possible neglect.
- Behaviors such as belittling, threats, or other uses of power and control by a caregiver may be indicators of verbal or emotional abuse.
- Strained or tense relationships, or frequent arguments between a caregiver and older adult can be warning signs of elder abuse.

notions about older adults. Commercials target older adults as consumers of laxatives, wrinkle creams, and other products that promise to prolong the condition of being younger, more attractive, and desirable. Television sitcoms portray the older adult as stubborn and eccentric. Health care providers must learn to appreciate the positive aspects of aging so that they can assist older adult patients in having positive experiences with imaging procedures. Education would enable health care providers to adapt imaging and therapeutic procedures to accommodate mental, emotional, and physiologic alterations associated with aging and to be sensitive to cultural, economic, and social influences in the provision of care for older adult patients.

Physical, Cognitive, and Psychosocial Effects of Aging

The human body undergoes a multiplicity of physiologic changes second by second. Little consideration is given regarding these changes unless they are brought on by sudden physical, psychological, or cognitive events. Each older adult is a unique individual with distinct characteristics. These individuals have experienced a life filled with memories and accomplishments.

Young or old, the definition of quality of life is an individual and personal one. Research has shown that health status is an excellent predictor of happiness. Greater social contact, health satisfaction, low vulnerable personality traits, and fewer stressful life events have been linked to successful aging. *Self-efficacy* can be defined as the level of control one has over one's future. Many older adults feel they have no control over medical emergencies and fixed incomes. Many have fewer choices about their personal living arrangements. These environmental factors can lead to depression and decreased self-efficacy. An increase in illness usually parallels a decrease in self-efficacy.

Older adults may experience changing roles from a life of independence to dependence. The family dynamic of a parent caring for children and grandchildren may evolve into the children caring for the aging parent. Older adulthood is also a time of loss. Losses may include the death of a spouse and friends and a loss of income, owing to retirement. Loss of health may be the reason for the health care visit. The overall loss of control may lead to isolation and depression in the older adult. Death and dying are also imminent facts of life.

A positive attitude is an important aspect of aging. Many older people have the same negative stereotypes about aging that younger people do.[3] For them, feeling down and depressed becomes a common consequence of aging. One in five people older than age 65 in a community shows signs of clinical depression. However health care professionals know that depression can affect young and old. Research has shown that most older adults rate their health status as good to excellent. How older adults perceive their health status depends largely on their successful adaptation to disabilities.

Radiographers need to be sensitive to the fact that an older adult may have had to deal with many social and physical losses in a short period. More importantly, they must recognize symptoms resulting from these losses to communicate and interact effectively with these patients. The radiographer must remember that each older adult is unique and deserves respect for their personal opinions.

The aging process alone is unlikely to alter the essential core of the human being. Physical illness is not aging, and age-related changes in the body are often modest in magnitude. As one ages, the tendencies to prefer slower-paced activities, need extra time to learn new tasks, become more forgetful, and lose portions of sensory processing skills increase slowly but perceptibly. Health care professionals need to be reminded that *aging and disease are not synonymous*. The more closely a function is tied to physical capabilities, the more likely it is to decline with age, whereas the more a function depends on experience, the more likely it will increase with age. Box 23.4 lists the most common health complaints of older adults.

Joint stiffness, weight gain, fatigue, and loss of bone mass can be slowed through proper nutritional interventions and low-impact exercise. The importance of exercise cannot be overstated. Exercise has been shown to increase aerobic capacity and mental speed. Exercise programs designed for older adults should emphasize increased strength, flexibility, and endurance. One of the best predictors of good health in later years is the number and extent of healthy lifestyles that were established in earlier life.

An older adult may show decreases in attention skills during complex tasks. Balance, coordination, strength, and reaction time all decrease with age. Falls associated with balance problems are common in the older adult population, resulting in a need to concentrate on walking. *Not overwhelming older adults with instructions is helpful*. Their hesitation in following instructions may be a fear instilled from a previous fall. Sight, hearing, taste, and smell are all sensory modalities that decline with age. Older people have more difficulty with bright lights and tuning out background noise. Many older adults become adept at lip-reading to compensate for the loss of hearing. For radiographers to assume that all older adult patients are hard of hearing is not unusual, but they are not all hard of hearing. Talking in a normal tone while making volume adjustments only if necessary, is a good rule of thumb. Speaking slowly, directly, and distinctly when giving instructions allows older adults an opportunity to sort through directions and improves their ability to follow them with better accuracy (Fig. 23.4).

Cognitive impairment in older adults can be caused by disease, aging, and disuse. *Dementia* is defined as a progressive cognitive impairment that eventually interferes with daily functioning. It includes cognitive, psychological, and functional deficits, including memory impairment. With normal aging comes a slowing down and a gradual wearing out of bodily systems, but normal aging does not include dementia. Yet the prevalence of dementia increases with age. Persistent disturbances in cognitive functioning, including memory and intellectual ability, accompany dementia. Fears of cognitive loss, especially Alzheimer disease, are widespread among older people.

Alzheimer disease is the most common form of dementia. Health care professionals are more likely to encounter people with this type. Most older adults work at maintaining and keeping their mental functions by staying active through mental games and exercises and keeping engaged in regular conversation. When caring for patients with any degree of dementia, verbal conversation should be inclusive and respectful. One should never discuss these patients as though they are not in the room or are not active participants in the procedure.

BOX 23.4
Most common health complaints of older adults

Weight gain
Fatigue
Loss of bone mass
Joint stiffness
Loneliness

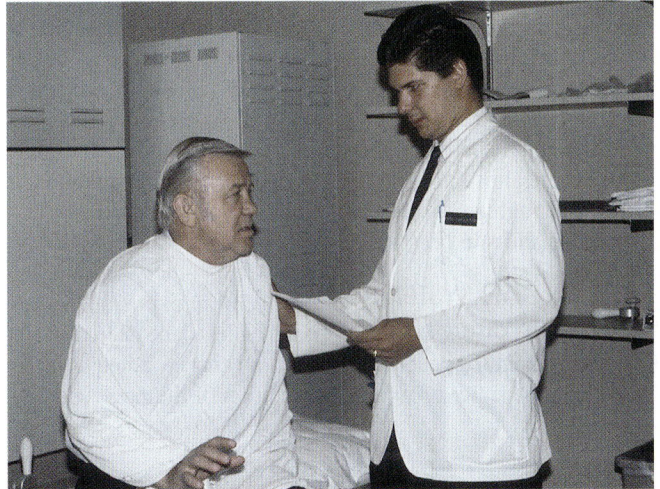

Fig. 23.4 Speaking slowly, directly, and distinctly when giving instructions allows older adults an opportunity to sort through directions and improves their ability to follow them with better accuracy.

One of the first questions asked of any patient entering a health care facility for emergency service is, "Do you know where you are and what day it is?" Health care providers need to know just how alert the patient is. Although memory does decline with age, this is experienced mostly with short-term memory tasks. Long-term memory or subconscious memory tasks show little change over time and with increasing age. There can be various reasons for confusion or disorientation. Medication, psychiatric disturbance, or retirement can confuse the individual. For some older people, retirement means creating a new set of routines and adjusting to them. Most older adults like structure in their lives and have familiar routines for approaching each day.

Physiology of Aging

Health and well-being depend largely on the degree to which organ systems can successfully work together to maintain internal stability. With age, there is apparently a gradual impairment of these homeostatic mechanisms. Older adults experience nonuniform, gradual, ongoing organ function failure in all systems. Many of the body organs gradually lose strength with advancing age. These changes place older adults at risk for disease or dysfunction, especially in the presence of stress. At some point, the likelihood of illness, disease, and death increases. Various physical diseases and disorders affect the mental and physical health of people of all ages. They are more profound among older adults because diseases and disorders among older people are more likely to be chronic in nature. Although aging is inevitable, the aging experience is highly individual and is affected by heredity, lifestyle choices, physical health, and attitude. A great portion of usual aging risks can be modified with positive shifts in lifestyle.

AGING OF THE ORGAN SYSTEMS
Integumentary system disorders
Disorders of the integumentary system are among the first apparent signs of aging. The most common skin diseases among older adults are herpes zoster (shingles), malignant tumors, and decubitus ulcers. With age comes flattening of the skin membranes, making it vulnerable to abrasions and blisters. The number of melanocytes decreases, making ultraviolet light more dangerous, and the susceptibility to skin cancer increases. Wrinkling and thinning skin are noticeable among older adults; this is attributable to decreases in collagen and elastin in the dermis. A gradual loss of functioning sweat glands and skin receptors occurs, which increases the threshold for pain stimuli, making an older adult vulnerable to heat strokes. With age comes atrophy or thinning of the subcutaneous layer of skin in the face, back of the hands, and soles of the feet. Loss of this "fat pad" can cause many foot conditions in older adults.

The most striking age-related changes to the integumentary system are the graying, thinning, and loss of hair. As a person ages, the number of hair follicles decreases, and the follicles that remain grow at a slower rate with less concentration of melanin, causing the hair to become thin and white. A major problem with aging skin is chronic exposure to sunlight. The benefits of protecting one's skin with sunscreen and protective clothing cannot be overemphasized and become more evident as one grows older. The three most common skin tumors in older adults are basal cell carcinoma, malignant melanoma, and squamous cell carcinoma.

Nervous system disorders
The nervous system is the principal regulatory system of all other systems in the body. It is probably the least understood of all body systems. Central nervous system disorders are among the most common causes of disability in older adults, accounting for almost 50% of disability in individuals older than the age of 65. Loss of myelin in axons of the nervous system contributes to the decrease in nerve impulse velocity that is noted in aging. One such condition of the nervous system decline is Alzheimer disease, which is known to be the most common form of dementia. More than 5 million Americans currently suffer from the disease, and it is estimated that this number will rise to about 13 million by 2050. Regardless of the existence of current lifestyle modification practices, drug remedies, and therapies that will stifle its progress, there is no cure for the disease.

In the healthy brain, an intricate network of billions of nerve cells communicates using electrical signals that regulate thoughts, memories, sensory perception, and movement. In an Alzheimer patient, brain cells die when genes and other factors cause the formation of an amyloid protein, which eventually breaks up and forms plaques—the hallmark of Alzheimer disease (Fig. 23.5). These plaques ultimately lead to the destruction of brain cells. Once the brain cells are destroyed, neural connections are shut down, causing decreased cognitive functions. Other known risk factors of this disease are, of course, age and family history. The greatest risk factor for this disease is increasing age. After age 65, the risk doubles every 5 years. After age 85, the risk is nearly 50%.

Although family history increases the risk for getting the disease, there are many Alzheimer patients with no family history, suggesting that there are other factors influencing the development of the disease. In addition to the Alzheimer gene, there is some evidence that some forms of the disease may be due to a "slow virus," and it is possible that the disorder is caused by an accumulation of toxic metals in the brain or by the absence of certain kinds of endogenous brain chemicals.

Health experts inarguably propose that as the baby boomers become closer to the age where they may contract the disease, Medicare will become burdened with an estimated $626 billion more in Alzheimer disease–related health care costs. There is also a considerable psychological burden that is attached to this debilitating disease. Adults are becoming more concerned that the disease will affect them or someone they know.

Current attempts to detect Alzheimer disease include imaging procedures such as structural imaging with magnetic resonance imaging (MRI) or computed tomography (CT). These tests are used to rule out other conditions that may cause symptoms similar to Alzheimer but require different treatment options. As for functional imaging of Alzheimer disease, position emission tomography (PET) scans show diminished brain cell activity in the regions affected. Molecular imaging research studies are aggressively being pursued to detect biologic cues indicating the early stage of Alzheimer before it alters the brain's structure or function and causes irreversible loss of memory or the ability to reason and think.

Like any other organ system, the nervous system is vulnerable to the effects of atherosclerosis with advancing age. When blood flow to the brain is blocked, brain tissue is damaged. Repeated episodes of cerebral infarction can eventually lead to multi-infarct dementia. The changes in the blood flow and oxygenation to the brain slow down the time to carry out motor and sensory tasks requiring speed, coordination, balance, and fine motor hand movements. This decrease in the function of motor control puts the older adult at a higher risk for falls. Healthy changes in lifestyle can reduce the risk of disease. High blood pressure is a noted risk and can be decreased with medication, weight loss, proper nutritional diet, and exercise.

Sensory system disorders

The sensory system undergoes changes with age. Beginning around age 40, the ability to focus on near objects becomes increasingly difficult. The lens of the eye becomes less pliable, starts to yellow, and becomes cloudy, resulting in farsightedness *(presbyopia)*. Distorted color perception and cataracts also occur. Changes in the retina affect the ability to adapt to changes in lighting, and the ability to tolerate glare decreases, making night vision more difficult for older adults.

Hearing impairment is common in older adults. The gradual progressive hearing loss of tone discrimination is called *presbycusis*. Men are more often affected than women, and the degree of loss is more severe for high-frequency sounds. Speech discrimination is problematic when in noisy surroundings, such as a room full of talking people.

There is a decline in sensitivity to taste and smell with age. The decline in taste is consistent with a decreased number of taste buds on the tongue, decreased saliva, and dry mouth that accompany the aging process.

Hyposmia is the impairment of the ability to smell. It accounts for much of the decreased appetite and irregular eating habits that are noted consistently in older adults. Similar to taste, the degree of impairment varies with a particular odor, and the ability to identify odors in a mixture is gradually lost with age.

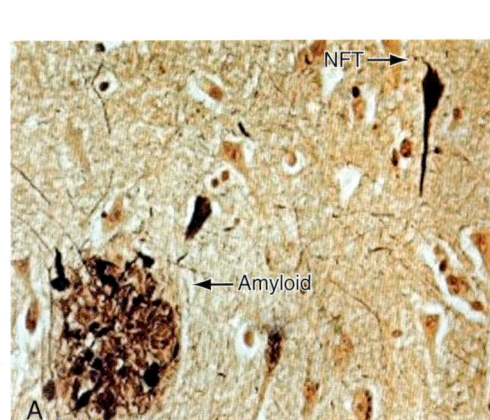
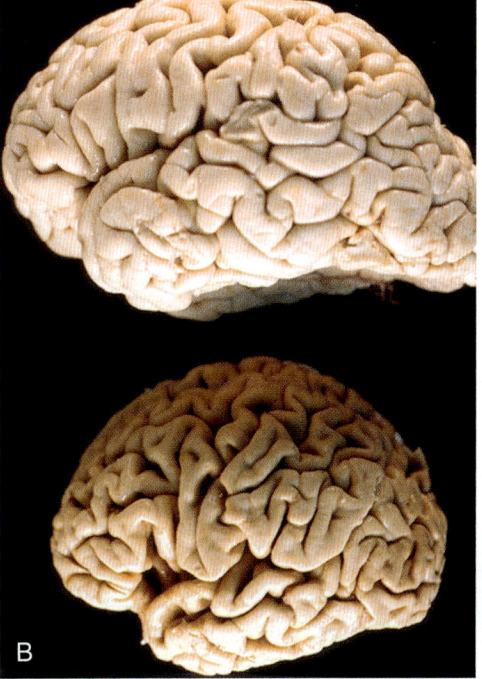

Fig. 23.5 Pathologic changes in Alzheimer disease (AD). (**A**) A mature plaque with central amyloid core next to a neurofibrillary tangle (NFT). (**B**) Comparison of normal and AD brains. Top, normal brain. Bottom, brain of a patient with Alzheimer disease. The AD brain shows gyral atrophy and sulcal widening greater than that seen in a person with no cognitive impairment.

(From Naidich TP, Castillo M, Cha S, et al. *Imaging of the brain*. 7th ed. Philadelphia: Elsevier; 2013.)

Musculoskeletal system disorders

Musculoskeletal dysfunction is the major cause of disability in older adults. Osteoporosis, the reduction in bone mass and density, is one of the most significant age-related changes. Women are four times as likely as men to develop this disease. Risk factors for osteoporosis include estrogen depletion, calcium deficiency, physical inactivity, testosterone depletion, alcoholism, and cigarette smoking. The rate of new bone resorption surpasses the rate of new bone formation at approximately age 40. This accounts for a subsequent loss of 40% of bone mass in women and 30% of bone mass in men over the course of the life span. Osteoporosis is associated with an increased risk of fractures. Common fracture sites are the vertebral bodies, distal radius, femoral neck, ribs, and pubis. Changes in the shape of the vertebral bodies can indicate the degree and severity of osteoporosis. Advanced cases may show complete compression fractures of the vertebral bodies. Compression fractures can result in severe kyphosis of the thoracic spine (Fig. 23.6).

The incidence of degenerative joint disease, osteoarthritis, increases with age. Osteoarthritis is the chronic deterioration of the joint cartilage, and the weight-bearing joints are the most affected. Obesity is probably the most important risk factor. Osteoarthritis of the joint cartilage causes pain, swelling, and a decrease in range of motion in the affected joint. Osteoarthritis is the second most common cause of disability in the United States, affecting more than 50 million Americans. At age 40, most adults have osteoarthritic changes visible on radiographic images of the cervical spine. The most progressive changes occur in weight-bearing joints and hands as age increases (Fig. 23.7).

Total joint replacement or arthroplasty procedures are common among older adult patients. Joint replacement may offer pain relief and improve joint mobility. Joint replacements can be performed on any joint, including the hip, knee, ankle, foot, shoulder, elbow, wrist, and fingers. Hip and knee replacements are the most common and the most effective (Fig. 23.8).

With age, women are more likely to store fat in their hips and thighs, whereas men store fat in their abdominal area. Without exercise, muscle mass declines, resulting in decreased strength and endurance, prolonged reaction time, and disturbed coordination. It cannot be overemphasized that regular physical training can improve muscle strength and endurance, along with cardiovascular fitness, even in the oldest individuals.

Cardiovascular system disorders

The cardiovascular system circulates the blood, which delivers oxygen and nutrients to all parts of the body and removes waste products. Damage to this system can have negative implications for the entire body. Decreased blood flow to the digestive tract, liver, and kidneys affects the absorption, distribution, and elimination of substances, such as medications and alcohol.

Cardiovascular disease is the most common cause of death worldwide. The maximum heart rate during exercise decreases with age; older adults become short of breath and tire quickly. Loss of arterial elasticity results in elevated systolic blood pressure, increasing the risk of heart disease and stroke. Another prevalent problem is postural hypertension, in which there is a decrease in systemic blood pressure when rising from a supine to a standing position. The predominant change that occurs in the blood vessels with age is atherosclerosis, which is a development of fatty plaques in the walls of the arteries. These fatty plaques within the artery wall can lead to ulcerations of the artery wall, subsequently making the artery prone to the formation of blood clots. The plaques also cause destruction of the artery wall, leading to a balloon and risk of an aneurysm. Complications can lead to an embolism, heart attack, or stroke.

Congestive heart failure is due to an inability of the heart to propel blood at a sufficient rate and volume. This pathology is more common in older adults,

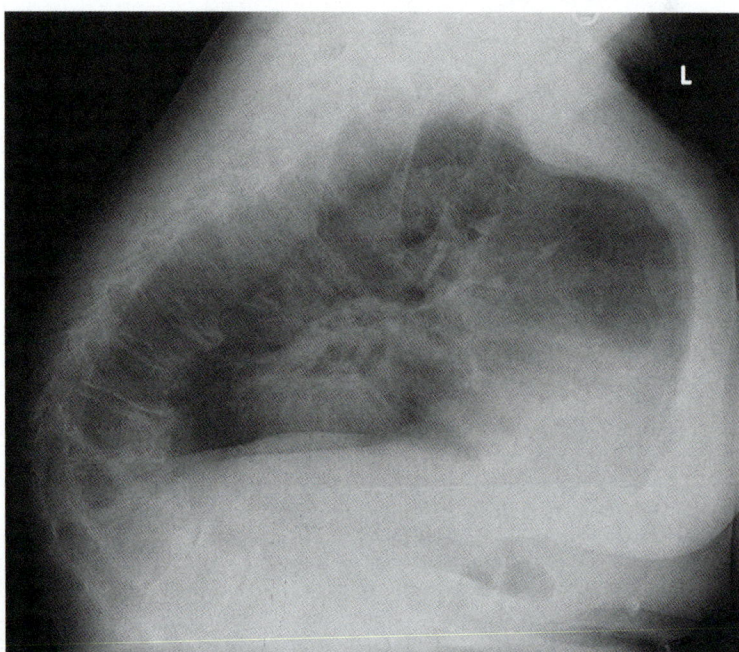

Fig. 23.6 Lateral chest radiograph of a geriatric patient with kyphosis and compression fractures.

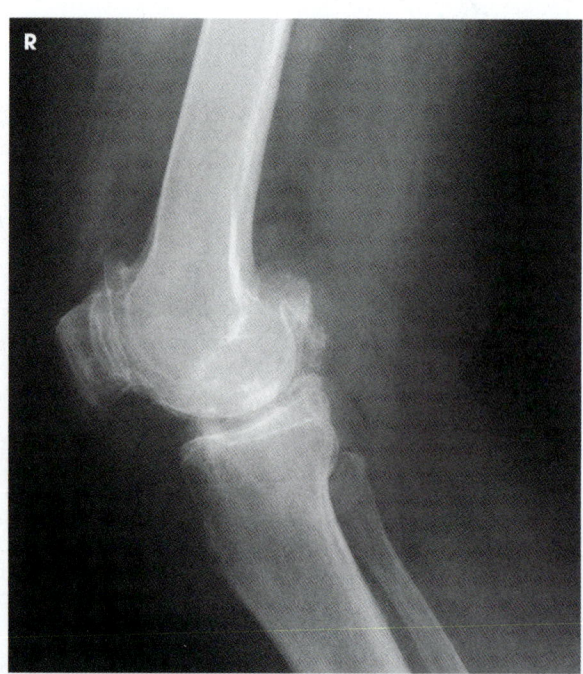

Fig. 23.7 Lateral knee radiograph showing severe arthritis.

particularly individuals 75 to 85 years old. People who are most at risk for developing congestive heart failure include individuals who have been diagnosed with coronary artery disease, heart attack, cardiomyopathy, untreated hypertension, and chronic kidney disease. Radiographically, the heart is enlarged, and the hilar region of the lungs is congested with increased vascular markings. Exposure factors must be adjusted to visualize the heart borders despite the pulmonary edema.

Preventive health measures, such as control of high blood pressure, diet, exercise, and smoking cessation, decrease the risk of cardiovascular disease. These interventions are more effective if initiated earlier in life.

Gastrointestinal system disorders

Gastrointestinal disorders in older adults include malignancies, peptic ulcer disease, gastrointestinal bleeding, pancreatitis, difficulty swallowing, diverticulitis, gastric outlet obstruction, esophageal foreign bodies, constipation, and fecal incontinence. Mouth and teeth pain, side effects of medication, decreased saliva, and dry mouth can lead to nutritional deficiencies, malnutrition, and dehydration problems. Most gastrointestinal disorders are related to an age-related decrease in the rate of gastric acid production and secretions and decreased motility of the smooth muscle in the large intestine. A decrease in acid production and secretion can lead to iron-deficiency anemia, peptic ulcers, and gastritis. Diverticulosis, a common problem in older adults, develops when the large intestine herniates through the muscle wall. Gallstone disease, hepatitis, and dehydration tend to be more common in older adults. Healthy lifestyle habits, such as smoking cessation, low alcohol intake, a high fiber–low sugar diet, and regular exercise, can decrease the risk of gastrointestinal problems. Gastrointestinal malignancies are second only to lung cancer as a cause of cancer mortality. Survival after colon and rectal cancer is increased with inexpensive early detection. Stool samples and rectal examinations are effective in detecting early cancer (Fig. 23.9).

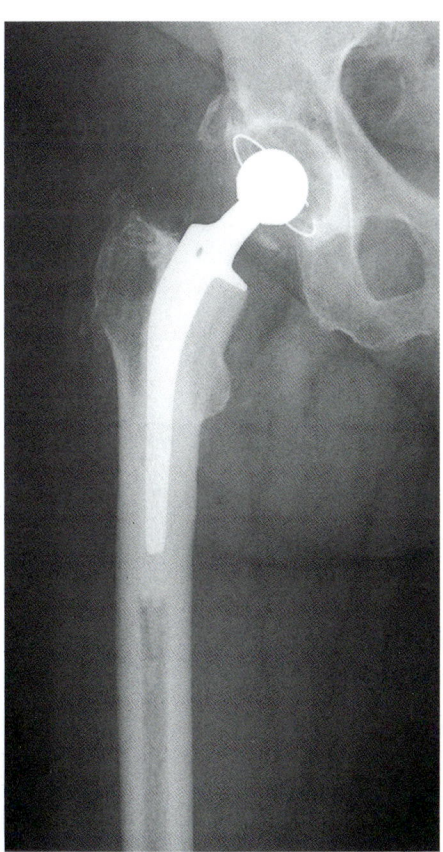

Fig. 23.8 AP proximal femur radiograph showing a total hip arthroplasty procedure.

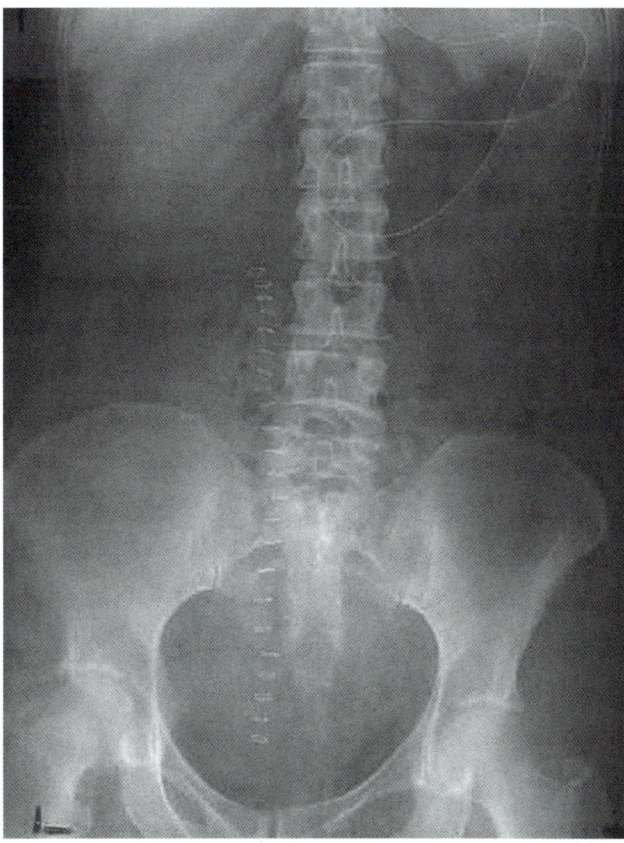

Fig. 23.9 Postoperative image of an older adult patient showing an AP abdomen with surgical staples and nasogastric tube.

Geriatric Radiography

Immune system decline

Age takes its toll on the immune system. To be immune to an infection implies protection from that infection. The ability of one's body to remain free of infections requires the immune system to distinguish healthy cells from invading microorganisms or altered cancer cells. The age-related decline of immune system function makes older adults more vulnerable to diabetes mellitus, pneumonia, and nosocomial infections. The incidence of infectious disease increases. Influenza, pneumonia, tuberculosis, meningitis, and urinary tract infections are prevalent among older adults. The three general categories of illness that preferentially affect older adults are infections, cancer, and autoimmune disease.[4]

Respiratory system disorders

Throughout the aging process, the lungs lose some of their elastic recoil, trapping air in the alveoli. This reduced elasticity decreases the rate of oxygen entering the bloodstream and the elimination of carbon dioxide. The muscles involved in breathing become a little more rigid, which can account for shortness of breath with physical stress. In the wall of the thorax, the rib cage stiffens, causing kyphotic curvature of the thoracic spine. Respiratory diseases that increase in frequency with aging include emphysema, chronic bronchitis, pneumonia, and lung cancer.

Chronic obstructive pulmonary disease refers to a variety of breathing disorders that cause a decreased ability of the lungs to perform ventilation. Emphysema is the permanent destruction and distention of the alveoli. Cigarette smoking is the most significant risk factor in the development of emphysema and is the leading cause of chronic bronchitis. Chronic bronchitis is an inflammation of the mucous membrane of the bronchial tubes. These two conditions are considered irreversible. Chest radiographs may show hyperinflation of the lungs (Fig. 23.10).

Pneumonia is the most frequent type of lung infection and among the leading causes of death in older adults. This population is also at an increased risk for aspiration pneumonia secondary to slower swallowing reflexes and other health conditions. Radiographically, pneumonia may appear as soft, patchy alveolar infiltrates or pulmonary densities (Fig. 23.11).

Lung cancer is the second most common cancer and the most common cause of cancer-related death in men and women. More Americans die each year from lung cancer than from breast, prostate, and colorectal cancers combined.

There is a strong association between low lung function and the future development of coronary heart disease. Research has shown that the total amount of air inhaled in one's deepest breath and the fastest rate at which one can exhale are powerful predictors of how many more years one will live. A sedentary lifestyle is the greatest risk factor in lung function, and lifestyle habits are the crucial factors over which one has control.

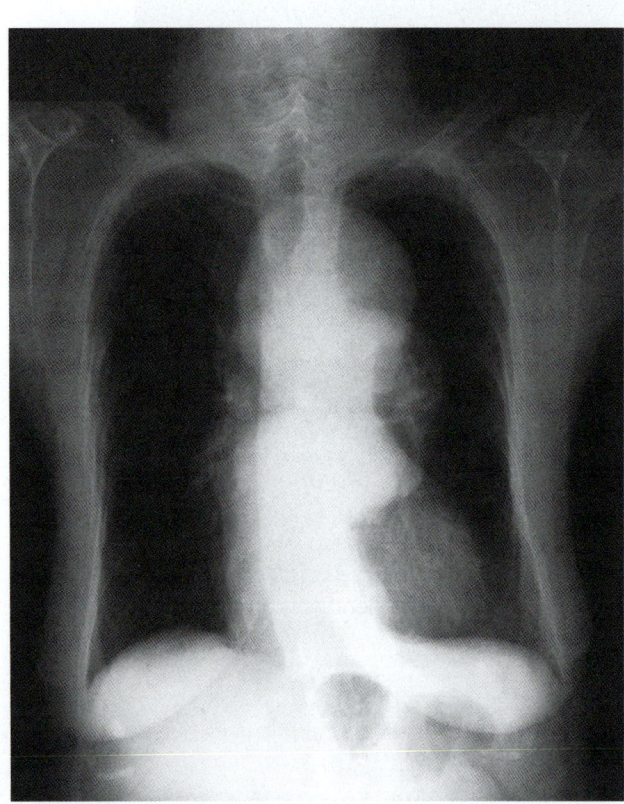

Fig. 23.10 PA chest radiograph showing emphysema.

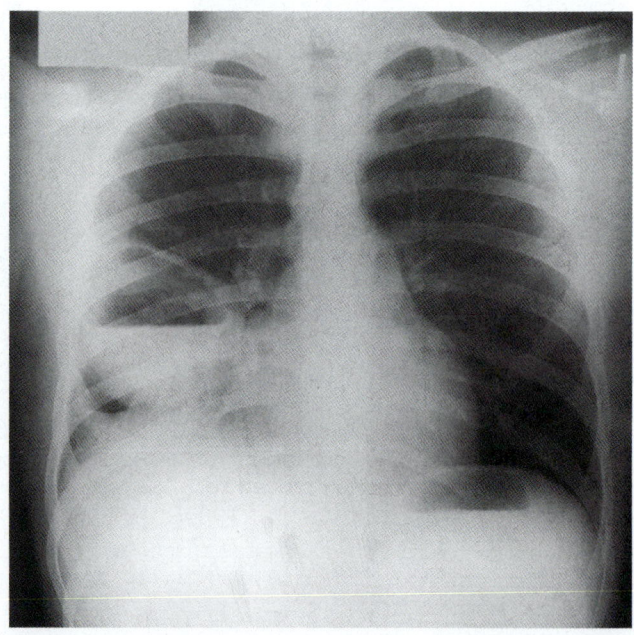

Fig. 23.11 PA chest radiograph with right middle lobe pneumonia and accompanying abscess.

Hematologic system disorders

A major hematologic concern in older adults is the high prevalence of anemia. Individuals with anemia often have pale skin and shortness of breath, and they fatigue easily. As bone ages, the marrow of the bone has a harder time maintaining blood cell production than young bone marrow when the body is stressed. The high incidence of anemia in older adults is believed to be a result not of aging per se, but rather of the high frequency of other age-related illnesses that can cause anemia. Anemia is not a single disease but a syndrome that has several causes. Insufficient dietary intake and inflammation or destruction of the gastrointestinal lining, leading to an inability to absorb vitamin B_{12}, cause a type of anemia that affects older adults. Because of other physiologic stresses affecting marrow production, older adults have an increased incidence of various blood disorders.

Genitourinary system disorders

Familiar age-related genitourinary changes are those associated with incontinence. Changes in bladder capacity and muscle structure predispose older adults to this problem. Urinary and bowel incontinence can also lead to social and hygiene concerns. Along with structural changes in the genitourinary system, the number of nephrons in the kidneys decreases dramatically after the onset of adulthood. This decreased reserve capacity of the kidneys could cause what would otherwise be a regularly prescribed dose of medication to be an overdose in an older adult. The role of the kidneys to maintain the body's water balance and regulate the concentration according to the body's need diminishes with age. Acute and chronic renal failure affects many older adults.

Benign prostatic hyperplasia can affect 70% of men older than age 70. Benign prostatic hyperplasia is an enlargement of the prostate gland, which can cause obstruction of the flow of urine. Surgical resection of the prostate may be necessary. Prostate cancer is primarily a disease of later life, and more than 80% of tumors are found in men older than 65 years. Prostate cancer is the most common cancer in men and the third most common cause of cancer deaths in men. Radiographic imaging of the male reproductive system comprises ureterograms, intravenous urography, and CT. Ultrasound is commonly used to evaluate testicular masses and prostate nodules.

Endocrine system disorders

The endocrine system is another principal regulatory system of the body. Age-related changes in thyroid function result from inadequate responses of target cells to thyroid hormone. The most common age-related disease associated with the endocrine system is diabetes mellitus. Non–insulin-dependent diabetes mellitus increases in frequency with age and accounts for about 90% of all cases. Regular exercise and weight loss can significantly reduce the risk and delay the onset of non–insulin-dependent diabetes.

SUMMARY

Aging is the one certainty in life. It starts at conception and continues throughout the life cycle. No two people age in the same way. As stated earlier, aging is individualized and is affected by heredity, lifestyle choices, physical health, and attitude. Despite the changes that occur in the body systems observed with aging, most older adults view themselves as healthy. They learn to adapt, adjust, and compensate for the disabilities secondary to aging. Older people are stereotyped into two groups: diseased and normal. The normal group is at high risk of disease but is just not there yet. By categorizing these older adults as normal, health professionals tend to underestimate their vulnerability. Modest increases in blood pressure, blood sugar, body weight, and low bone density are common among normal older adults. These risk factors promote disease, yet they can be modified. They may be age-related in industrial societies, but they are not age-determined or harmless. Positive lifestyle changes, such as diet, exercise, and smoking cessation, reduce the risk of disease and improve the quality of life. Good health cannot be left to chance, and staying healthy depends to a large degree on lifestyle choices and attitude.

SUMMARY OF PATHOLOGY: GERIATRIC RADIOGRAPHY

Condition	Definition
Alzheimer disease	Progressive, irreversible mental disorder with loss of memory, deterioration of intellectual functions, speech and gait disturbances, and disorientation
Atherosclerosis	Condition in which fibrous and fatty deposits on the luminal wall of an artery may cause obstruction of the vessel
Benign prostatic hyperplasia	Enlargement of prostate gland
Chronic obstructive pulmonary disease	Chronic condition of persistent obstruction of bronchial airflow
Compression fracture	Fracture that causes compaction of bone and decrease in length or width
Congestive heart failure	Heart is unable to propel blood at sufficient rate and volume
Contractures	Permanent contraction of a muscle because of spasm or paralysis
Dementia	Broad impairment of intellectual function that usually is progressive and interferes with normal social and occupational activities
Emphysema	Destructive and obstructive airway changes, leading to increased volume of air in the lungs
Kyphosis	Abnormally increased convexity in the thoracic curvature
Osteoarthritis	Form of arthritis marked by progressive cartilage deterioration in synovial joints and vertebrae
Osteoporosis	Loss of bone density
Renal failure	Failure of the kidney to perform essential functions
Urinary incontinence	Absence of voluntary control of urination

Patient Care

Box 23.5 lists quick tips for working with older adult patients. These tips are discussed in the following pages.

PATIENT AND FAMILY EDUCATION

Educating all patients, especially older adult patients, about imaging procedures is crucial to obtaining their confidence and compliance. More time with older adult patients may be necessary to accommodate their decreased ability to process information rapidly. Most older adults have been diagnosed with at least one chronic illness. They typically arrive at the clinical imaging environment with natural anxiety because they are likely to have little knowledge of the procedure or the highly technical modalities employed for their procedures. A fear concerning consequences resulting from the examination exacerbates their increased levels of anxiety. Taking time to educate patients and their families or significant caregivers in their support system about the procedures makes for a less stressful experience and improved patient compliance and satisfaction.

BOX 23.5
Tips for working with older adult patients

- Take time to educate the patient and the family.
- Speak lower and closer.
- Treat the patient with dignity and respect.
- Give the patient time to rest between projections and procedures.
- Avoid adhesive tape; older adult skin is thin and fragile.
- Provide warm blankets in cold examination rooms.
- Use table pads and handrails.
- Always access the patient's medical history before contrast medium is administered.

COMMUNICATION

Good communication and listening skills create a connection between the radiographer and the patient. Older people are unique and should be treated with dignity and respect. Examples of appropriate communication may include addressing the patient by their title and last name. It is inappropriate to call someone "honey" or "dear." Each older adult is a wealth of cultural and historical knowledge that becomes a learning experience for the radiographer. If it is evident that the patient cannot hear or understand verbal directions, it is appropriate to speak lower and closer. Background noise can be disruptive to an older person and should be eliminated if possible when giving precise instructions. Giving individual instruction provides the older adult time to process a request. An empathetic, warm attitude and approach to a geriatric patient result in a trusting and compliant patient.

TRANSPORTATION AND LIFTING

Balance and coordination of an older adult patient can be affected by normal aging changes. The patient's anxiety about falling can be diminished by assistance in and out of a wheelchair and to and from the examination table. Many older adult patients have decreased height perception resulting from some degree of vision impairment. Hesitation of the older adult patient may be due to previous falls. Assisting an older patient when there is a need to step up or down throughout the procedure is more than a reassuring gesture. Preventing opportunities for falls is the responsibility of the radiographer. The older adult patient often experiences vertigo and dizziness when moving from a recumbent position to a sitting position. Giving the patient time to rest between positions mitigates these disturbing, frightening, and uncomfortable sensations. The use of table handgrips and proper assistance from the radiographer create a sense of security for an older adult patient.

SKIN CARE

Acute age-related changes in the skin cause it to become thin and fragile. The skin becomes more susceptible to bruising, tears, abrasions, and blisters. All health care professionals should use caution in turning and holding an older adult patient. Excessive pressure on the skin causes it to break and tear. *Adhesive tape should be avoided because it can be irritating and can easily tear the skin of an older person.* The loss of fat pads makes it painful for an older adult patient to lie on a hard surface and can increase the possibility of developing ulcerations. Decubitus ulcers, or pressure sores, are commonly seen in bedridden people and people with decreased mobility. Bony areas such as the heels, ankles, elbow, and lateral hips are frequent sites for pressure sores. A decubitus ulcer can develop in 1 to 2 hours. Almost without exception, tables used for imaging procedures are hard surfaced and cannot be avoided. The use of a table pad can reduce the friction between the hard surface of the table and the patient's fragile skin. Sponges, blankets, and positioning aids make the procedure much more bearable and comfortable for the older adult patient.

Because skin plays a crucial role in maintaining body temperature, the thinning process associated with aging skin renders the patient less able to retain normal body heat. The regulation of body temperature of an older adult varies from that of a younger person. Older adult patients may need a blanket to prevent hypothermia, even in a room that is at comfortable temperature for the radiographer.

CONTRAST AGENT ADMINISTRATION

Because of age-related changes in kidney and liver functions, the amount, but not the type, of contrast media is varied when performing radiographic procedures on an older adult patient. The number of functioning nephrons in the kidneys steadily decreases from middle age throughout the life span. Compromised kidney function contributes to the older adult patient being more prone to electrolyte and fluid imbalance, which can create life-threatening consequences. They are also more susceptible to the effects of dehydration because of diabetes and decreased renal or adrenal function. The decision of type and amount of contrast media used for the geriatric patient usually follows some sort of routine protocol. Assessment for contrast agent administration accomplished by the imaging technologist must include age; history of liver, kidney, or thyroid disease; history of hypersensitivity reactions and previous reactions to medications or contrast agents; sensitivity to aspirin; over-the-counter and prescription drug history, including the use of acetaminophen (Tylenol); and history of diabetes and hypertension.[5]

The imaging technologist must be selective in locating an appropriate vein for contrast agent administration on the older adult patient. The technologist should consider the location and condition of the vein, decreased integrity of the skin, and duration of the therapy. Thin superficial veins, repeatedly used veins, and veins located in areas where the skin is bruised or scarred should be avoided. The patient should be assessed for any swallowing impairments, which could lead to difficulties with drinking liquid contrast agents. The patient should be instructed to drink slowly to avoid choking, and an upright position helps prevent aspiration.

THE JOINT COMMISSION CRITERIA

The Joint Commission is the accrediting and standards-setting body for hospitals, clinics, and other health care organizations in the United States. Employees in institutions accredited by the Joint Commission must demonstrate age-based communication competencies, which include the older adult. The standards were adopted as a means of demonstrating competence in meeting the physiologic and psychological needs of patients in special populations. These populations include infants, children, adolescents, and older adults.

Age-related competencies

Standard HR 01.05.03 of the Human Resources section of The Joint Commission manual states: "When appropriate, the hospital considers special needs and behaviors of specific age-groups in defining qualifications, duties, and responsibilities of staff members who do not have clinical privileges but who have regular clinical contact with patients (e.g., radiologic technologists and mental health providers)." The intent of the standard is to ensure age-specific competency in technical and clinical matters but is not limited to equipment and technical performance. Age-specific competencies address the different needs people have at different ages. Examples of age-specific care for older adults may include the following: assessing visual or hearing impairments; assessing digestive and esophageal problems, such as reflux, bladder, and bowel problems; addressing grief concerns; providing warmth; and providing safety aids. Being able to apply age-specific care also includes the use of age-appropriate communication skills. Clear communication with the patient can be the key to providing age-specific care. Knowledge of age-related changes and disease processes assists all health care professionals, including those in the radiation sciences, in providing care that meets the needs of the older adult patient.

Performing the Radiographic Procedure
RADIOGRAPHER'S ROLE

The role of the radiographer is no different from that of all other health professionals. The whole person must be treated, not just the manifested symptoms of an illness or injury. Medical imaging and therapeutic procedures reflect the impact of ongoing systemic aging in documentable and visual forms. Adapting procedures to accommodate disabilities and diseases of geriatric patients is a crucial responsibility and a challenge based almost exclusively on the radiographer's knowledge, abilities, and skills. An understanding of the physiology and pathology of aging and an awareness of the social, psychological, cognitive, and economic aspects of aging are required to meet the needs of older adult patients. Conditions typically associated with older adult patients invariably require adaptations or modifications of routine imaging procedures. The radiographer must be able to differentiate between age-related changes and disease processes. Production of diagnostic images requiring professional decision making to compensate for physiologic changes while maintaining the compliance, safety, and comfort of the patient is the foundation of the contract between the older adult patient and the radiographer.

To better care for individuals with Alzheimer disease, it is important to become familiar with some simple facts about the disease and behaviors that are associated with it. Alzheimer disease is a progressive disease with no known cure. There are five stages: preclinical stage, mild cognitive impairment, mild dementia, moderate dementia, and severe dementia. The disease is often diagnosed in the mild stage of dementia. Table 23.1 lists these stages and a brief description of each.

The rate of progression of Alzheimer disease varies widely. On average, people with this disease live 8 to 10 years after diagnosis; however, some will live as long as 25 years after diagnosis. Pneumonia is a common cause of death because impaired swallowing allows food or beverages to enter the lungs, where an infection can begin. Other common causes of death include complications from urinary tract infections and falls.

It is important that the radiologic technologist become aware of and understand the various types of physical and cognitive impairments associated with Alzheimer disease. Dealing with this patient group requires patience, compassion, and attentiveness. Patients who are at risk of falling must never be left alone, whether in the radiology waiting room or the examination room. Caregivers should be encouraged to accompany the patient to appointments whenever possible. It may be more comforting for the patient to have a familiar person with them in an unfamiliar setting. In addition, depending on the stage of the disease, some patients may tend to wander, often wanting to go home. Home sometimes is their native town, state, or even country. Confused elderly patients can travel considerable distances before they are found. There have been cases in which patients have wandered off never to be found, or never to be found alive. For that reason, the patient should never be left alone. Whenever possible, and whenever a caregiver has not accompanied the patient, a two-technologist team should be available to care for the patient while in the diagnostic radiology suite—one acquiring the images and one in the role of companion to the patient while the images are being reviewed. The patient should be then handed off to the unit or responsible party upon completion of the exam.

It is not uncommon for persons with Alzheimer disease to ask repetitive questions or to become accusatory. The technologist should exercise a great deal of patience and use distraction techniques to eliminate the frustration this may cause. Simply changing the subject or asking an unrelated question may reduce the repetitive questioning or conversation. There may be occasions when the patient requires restraints to complete the exam. Note, however, that restraints should be applied only in cases in which the patient can potentially cause harm to themselves or to others.

Working quietly and smoothly around the patient and maintaining calm, relaxing, and noise-free surroundings is the preferred situation for the Alzheimer patient in the radiology department. The music, if any, should be soothing and relaxing. This will potentially benefit all types of patients.

Radiographic Positioning for Geriatric Patients

The preceding discussions and understanding of the physical, cognitive, and psychosocial effects of aging can help radiographers adapt to the positioning challenges of the geriatric patient. In some cases, routine examinations need to be modified to accommodate the limitations, safety, and comfort of the patient. Communicating clear instructions with the patient is important. The following discussion addresses positioning suggestions for various structures.

CHEST

The position of choice for the chest radiograph is the upright position; however, an older adult patient may be unable to stand without assistance for this examination. When performing a PA projection of the lungs, the patient places the back of their hands on their hips. This may be difficult for someone with impaired balance and flexibility. The radiographer can allow the patient to wrap their arms around the wall bucky as a means of support and security (Fig. 23.12). The patient may not be able to maintain their arms over the head for the lateral projection of the chest. The radiographer should provide extra security and stability while the patient is moving the arms up and forward to grasp overhead handgrips or an IV pole.

TABLE 23.1

Stages and symptoms of Alzheimer disease

Stages of Alzheimer disease	Description of behaviors/symptoms
Preclinical stage	Symptoms usually go unnoticed during this stage. This stage of Alzheimer disease can last for years, possibly even decades. Diagnostic imaging technologies can now identify deposits of the amyloidal beta substance that have been associated with the disease.
Mild cognitive impairment	Memory lapses, interrupted thought processes. Trouble with time management. Trouble making sound decisions.
Mild dementia	Memory loss of recent events. Difficulty with problem solving. Difficulty completing complex tasks and making sound judgments. Changes in personality—may become subdued or may withdraw from certain social situations. Difficulty organizing or expressing thoughts. Gets lost or wanders away from home. Misplaces belongings.
Moderate dementia	Displays increasingly poor judgment. Confusion deepens. Memory loss increases. Needs assistance with daily routine activities. Becomes suspicious or paranoid and accusatory to caregivers or family members. Rummaging, tapping feet, rubbing hands, banging. Outbursts of physical aggression.
Severe dementia (late stage)	Inability to hold coherent conversations. Inability to recognize some or all family members. Requires assistance with personal care. Decline in physical abilities—needs assistance walking or may experience uncontrollable bladder and bowel functions. Inability to swallow; rigid muscles; abnormal reflexes.

When the patient cannot stand, the examination may be performed AP with the patient seated in a wheelchair or stretcher (Fig. 23.13), but some issues affect the radiographic quality. Hyperkyphosis can result in the lung apices being obscured. The abdomen may also obscure the lung bases. In a sitting position, respiration may be compromised, and the patient should be instructed on the importance of deep inspiration. Any alteration of the exam should be noted in the patient's recorded history.

Positioning of the image receptor (IR) for a kyphotic patient should be higher than normal because the shoulders and apices are in a higher position. Radiographic landmarks may change with age, and the centering may need to be lower if the patient is extremely kyphotic. When positioning the patient for the sitting lateral chest projection, the radiographer should place a large sponge behind the patient to lean the patient forward (Fig. 23.14).

SPINE

Radiographic spine examinations may be painful for a patient with osteoporosis who is lying on the x-ray table. Positioning aids such as radiolucent sponges, sandbags, and a mattress may be used as long as the quality of the image is not compromised (Fig. 23.15). Performing upright radiographic examinations may also be appropriate if a patient can safely tolerate this position. The combination of cervical lordosis and thoracic kyphosis can make positioning and visualization of the cervical and thoracic spine difficult. Lateral cervical projections can be performed with the patient standing, sitting, or lying supine. The AP projection in the sitting position may not visualize the upper cervical vertebrae because the chin may obscure this anatomy. In the supine position, the head may not reach the table and result in magnification. The AP and open-mouth projections are difficult to do in a wheelchair.

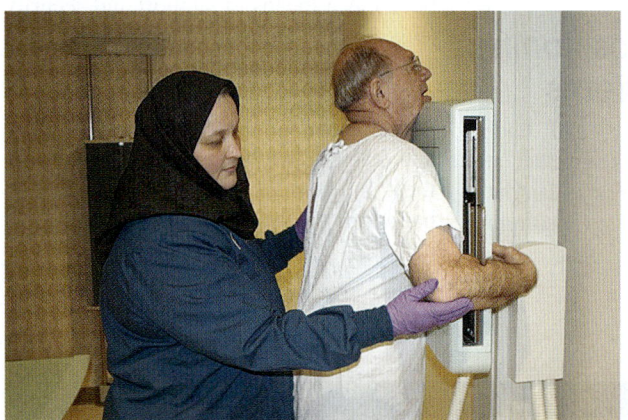

Fig. 23.12 Radiographer positioning patient's arms around the chest stand for a PA chest radiograph. Having the patient hold on in this way provides stability.

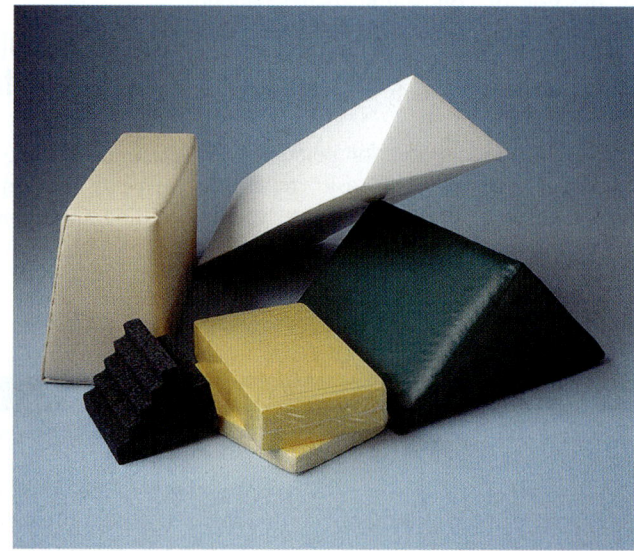

Fig. 23.14 Positioning sponges and sandbags are commonly used as immobilization devices.

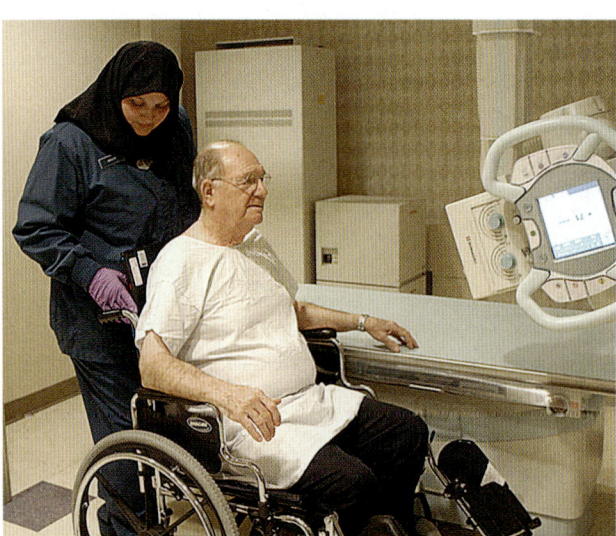

Fig. 23.13 Radiographer placing the IR behind a patient who is unable to stand. With careful positioning of the IR and x-ray tube, a quality image of the chest can be obtained.

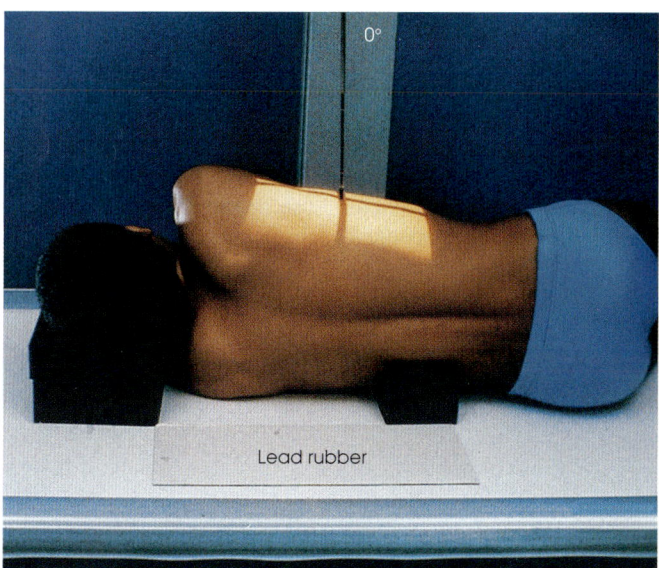

Fig. 23.15 Recumbent lateral thoracic spine. Support placed under lower thoracic region; perpendicular central ray.

The thoracic and lumbar spines are sites for compression fractures. The use of positioning blocks may be necessary to help the patient remain in position. For the lateral projection, a lead blocker or shield behind the spine should be used to absorb as much scatter radiation as possible (see Fig. 23.15).

PELVIS AND HIP

Osteoarthritis, osteoporosis, and injuries as the result of falls contribute to hip pathologies. A common fracture in older adults is to the femoral neck. An AP projection of the pelvis should be performed to examine the hip. If the indication is trauma, the radiographer should *not attempt to rotate the limbs*. The second view taken should be a cross-table lateral of the affected hip. If hip pain is the indication, assist the patient with internal rotation of the legs with the use of sandbags if necessary (Figs. 23.16 and 23.17).

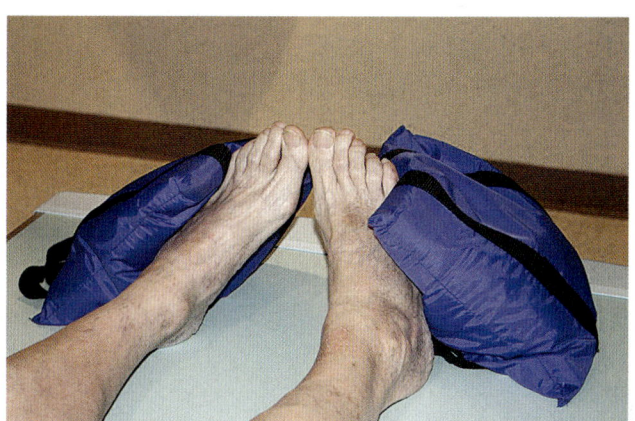

Fig. 23.16 Legs inverted for AP projection of the pelvis. Wrapping flexible sandbags around the feet can help geriatric patients hold their legs in this position.

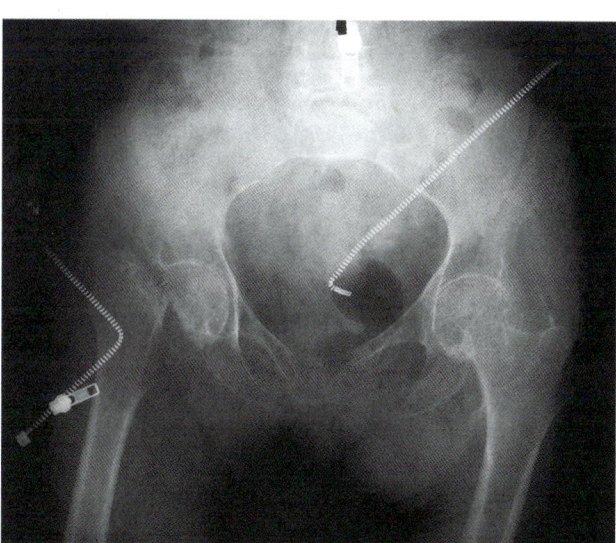

Fig. 23.17 An older adult patient with Alzheimer disease was brought to the emergency department because he could not walk. The patient did not complain of pain. Note fracture of the right hip. Trauma radiograph was made with patient's pants on, and the zipper is shown.

UPPER EXTREMITY

Positioning the geriatric patient for projections of the upper extremities can present its own challenges. Often the upper extremities have limited flexibility and mobility. A cerebrovascular accident or stroke may cause contractures of the affected limb. Contracted limbs cannot be forced into position, and cross-table views may need to be done. The inability of the patient to move their limb should not be interpreted as a lack of cooperation. Supination is often a problem in patients with contractures, fractures, and paralysis. The routine AP and lateral projections can be supported with the use of sponges, sandbags, and blocks to raise and support the extremity being imaged. The shoulder is also a site of decreased mobility, dislocation, and fractures. The therapist should assess how much movement the patient can do before attempting to move the arm. The use of finger sponges may also help with the contractures of the fingers (Fig. 23.18).

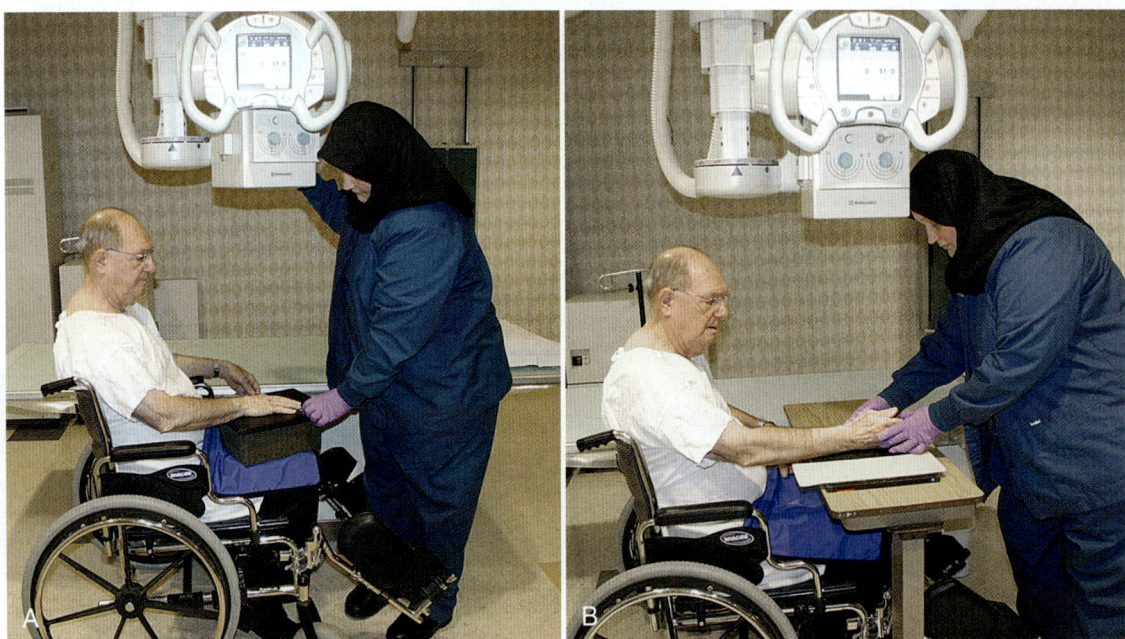

Fig. 23.18 Most projections of the upper limb can be obtained with the patient in a wheelchair and with some creativity. (**A**) Patient being positioned for an AP hand radiograph. Note use of a 10 cm (4-inch) sponge to raise the IR. (**B**) Patient being positioned for a lateral wrist radiograph. A hospital food tray table provides a base for the IR and eases positioning.

LOWER EXTREMITY

The lower extremities may have limited flexibility and mobility. The ability to dorsiflex the ankle may be reduced as a result of neurologic disorders. Imaging on the x-ray table may need to be modified when a patient cannot turn on their side. Flexion of the knee may be impaired and require a cross-table lateral projection. If a tangential projection of the patella, such as the Settegast method, is necessary, and the patient can turn on their side, the radiographer can place the IR superior to the knee and direct the central ray perpendicular through the patellofemoral joint. Projections of the feet and ankles may be obtained with the patient sitting in the wheelchair. Positioning sponges and sandbags support and maintain the position of the body part being imaged (Fig. 23.19). Whenever possible, the technologist should keep the patient in the wheelchair or stretcher to perform upper and lower extremity exams. This will minimize the stress (to both patient and technologist) of transferring the patient to and from the examination table.

TECHNICAL FACTORS

Exposure factors also need to be taken into consideration when imaging the geriatric patient. The loss of bone mass and atrophy of tissues often require a lower kilovoltage (kVp) to maintain proper image quality. The kVp is also a factor in chest radiographs when there may be a large heart and pleural fluid to penetrate. Patients with emphysema require a reduction in technical factors to prevent overexposure of the lung field. Patient assessment can help with the appropriate exposure adjustments.

Exposure time may also be a major factor. Geriatric patients may have problems maintaining the positions necessary for the examinations. A short exposure time helps reduce voluntary and involuntary motion and breathing. The radiographer should ensure that the geriatric patient clearly hears and understands the breathing instructions.

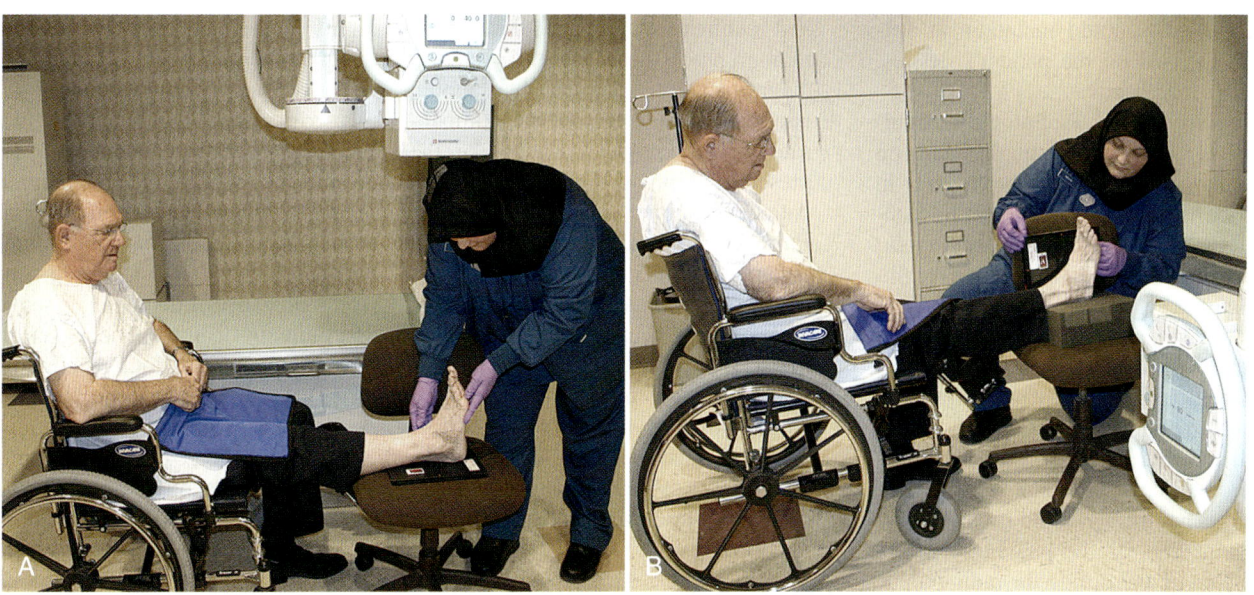

Fig. 23.19 Projections of the lower limb, especially from the knee and lower, can be obtained with the patient in a wheelchair. (**A**) AP projection of the ankle with the patient's leg and foot resting on a chair. (**B**) Lateral projection of the ankle performed by using a chair as a rest and a sponge to raise the IR.

Best Practices in Geriatric Radiography

There is no cookie-cutter approach to imaging the elderly patient. Each patient comes with a personal set of challenges. Elderly patients of advanced age often present with some form of physical or cognitive impairment, and the radiographer must be able to mitigate those challenges by applying problem-solving skills to adapt routine procedures to the patients' condition while maintaining quality images. The following are basic guidelines to the imaging approach for challenging elderly patients.

1. *Comfort:* Comfort is at the top of the list of needs for elderly patients. It is imperative that the caregiver value unique situations and provide the appropriate care for the patient. To comfort the elderly patient, the technologist should maintain an attitude focused on the patient's desires, wishes, and needs.[6]

2. *Communication:* Radiologic technology is a people-oriented, hands-on profession that requires proficiency in a wide variety of communication techniques.[7] Establishing a good rapport with the elderly patient at the beginning of the exam is a good approach to a successful procedure. Verbal communication should be clear and concise. Instructions should be given slowly and systematically so that the patient will be able to process the information and carry out the instructions. The technologist should provide clear explanations of the procedure before the start of and during the radiographic exam. Effective communication will ensure maximum cooperation from the patient.

3. *Safety:* A fall can be devastating to elderly patients, not only because of physical injuries but also because of the potential psychological effect, including the development of a fear of falling.[8] Close attention must be paid to the patient's fall risk assessment, and care must be taken that every move is supervised. The radiographer must review the fall assessment documentation for each patient and adhere to the policies and procedures established by the facility regarding falls.

4. *Speed:* Speed does not necessarily mean sacrificing image quality. The radiographer will plan and strategize the best approach to each projection, arranging the order so that the patient is spared the discomfort caused by being moved or turned multiple times. All like projections should be grouped together (e.g., perform all anteroposterior projections first, then axials, then obliques, then laterals).

5. *Positioning:* The technologist must adhere to the cardinal radiographic rule of producing orthogonal and oblique projections. Deviation from the routine protocol will be necessary at times in order to adapt to the patient's condition and limitations.

6. *Accuracy/image quality:* Chest radiography remains the initial exam of choice for diagnosing respiratory symptoms. Pulmonary fibrosis, pneumonia, and lung cancer can be detected with reasonable sensitivity and specificity. Because it is readily available and requires low radiation dose, chest radiography is usually the first step in diagnosis.[9] The radiographer should adjust technical factors to compensate for pathological changes or the presence of prosthetic devices in the patient's anatomy.

7. *Patience:* The advanced elderly and patients with dementia are sometimes confused, combative, and disagreeable, especially in unfamiliar environments and around unfamiliar people. Radiographers may experience their verbal or physical abuse. Great patience must be exercised in these situations. Resilient radiographers will develop a "thick skin" as they advance in the profession.

Conclusion

Imaging professionals will continue to see a change in the health care delivery system with a shift in the population of people older than age 65. This shift in the general population is resulting in an ongoing increase in the number of medical imaging procedures performed on older adult patients. Demographic and social effects of aging determine the way in which older adults adapt to and view the process of aging. An individual's family size and perceptions of aging, economic resources, gender, race, ethnicity, social class, and availability and delivery of health care affect the quality of the aging experience. Biologic age is much more critical than chronological age when determining the health status of the older adult.

Healthier lifestyles and advancements in medical treatment are creating a generation of successfully aging adults, which should decrease the negative stereotyping of older adults. Attitudes of all health care professionals, whether positive or negative, affect the care provided to the growing older adult population. Education about the mental and physiologic alterations associated with aging, along with the cultural, economic, and social influences accompanying aging, enables the radiographer to adapt imaging and therapeutic procedures to the older adult patient's disabilities resulting from age-related changes.

The human body undergoes a multiplicity of physiologic changes and failure in all organ systems. The aging experience is affected by heredity, lifestyle choices, physical health, and attitude, making it highly individualized. No individual's aging process is the same. Radiologic technologists must use their knowledge, abilities, critical thinking, and skills to adjust imaging procedures to accommodate for disabilities and diseases encountered with geriatric patients. Safety and comfort of the patient are essential in maintaining compliance throughout imaging procedures. Communication, listening, sensitivity, and empathy lead to patient compliance. The Joint Commission, recognizing the importance of age-based communication competencies for older adults, requires the employees of accredited health care organizations to document their achievement of these skills. Knowledge of age-related changes and disease processes enhances the radiographer's ability to provide care that meets the needs of the increasing older adult patient population.

References

1. Centers for Disease Control and Prevention. WISQARS. *10 leading causes of death, United States*. Available at https://wisqars.cdc.gov/data/lcd/home. (Accessed July 15, 2024).
2. Boswell SS. Predicting trainee ageism using knowledge, anxiety, compassion, and contact with older adults. *Educ Gerontol*. 2012;38(11):733–741.
3. Rowe JW, Kahn RL. *Successful Aging*. New York: Dell; 1999.
4. Chop WC, Robnett RH. *Gerontology for the Health Care Professional*. 2nd ed. Philadelphia: FA Davis; 2009.
5. Norris TG. Special needs of geriatric patients. *ASRT Homestudy Series*. 1999;4(5).

6. Sousa Valente Ribeiro PCP, Dourado Marques RM, Pontífice Ribeiro M. Geriatric care: ways and means of providing comfort. *Rev Bras Enferm.* 2017;70(4):830–837.
7. Adler A, Carlton R. *Introduction to Radiologic and Imaging Sciences and Patient Care.* 7th ed. St Louis: Elsevier; 2019.
8. Abujudeh H, Kaewlai R, Shah B, et al. Characteristics of falls in a large academic radiology department: occurrence, associated factors, outcomes, and quality improvement strategies. *AJR Am J Roentgenol.* 2021;197(1):154–159.
9. O'Brien J, Baerlocher MO, Asch M, et al. Role of radiology in geriatric care: a primer for family physicians. *Can Fam Physician.* 2009;55(1):32–37.

Selected bibliography

Administration for Community Living (ACL). *What is Elder Abuse?*; 2019. Available at: https://www.acl.gov/programs/elder-justice/what-elder-abuse. (Accessed July 14, 2024).

Alzheimer's Association. *Early-Stage Caregiving.* n.d. Available at: http://www.alz.org/care/alzheimers-early-mild-stage-caregiving.asp. (Accessed September 2023).

Alzheimer's Association. *Earlier Diagnosis.* n.d. Available at: https://www.alz.org/alzheimers-dementia/research_progress/earlier-diagnosis#age. (Accessed September 2023).

Campbell PR. *U.S. Population Projections by Age, Sex, Race and Hispanic Origin: 1995 to 2025.* Washington, DC: US Bureau of the Census; 1996. Population Division. PPL-47.

Chop WC, Robnett RH. *Gerontology for the Health Care Professional.* 2nd ed. Philadelphia: FA Davis; 2009.

Damjanov I. *Pathology for the Health Professions.* 5th ed. St Louis: Elsevier; 2017.

Ferrara MH. *Alzheimer's Disease: Human Diseases and Conditions,* vol 1. 2nd ed. Detroit: Charles Scribner's Sons; 2010:70–76.

Garfein AJ, Herzog AR. Robust aging among the young-old, old-old, and oldest-old. *J Gerontol B Psychol Sci Soc Sci.* 1995;50(2):S77–S87.

Health Professions in Service to the Nation. San Francisco: Pew Health Professions Commission; 1993.

Hobbs FB, Danion BL. *65+ in the United States.* Washington, DC: US Department of Commerce and US Department of Health and Human Services; 1996:23–190.

Kudlas M, Odle T, Kisner L. *The State of Forensic Radiography in the United States.* American Society of Radiologic Technologists (ASRT); 2010. Available at https://www.asrt.org/docs/default-source/publications/whitepapers/forensic_radiography_white_paperfin.pdf. (Accessed September 2023).

Mayo Clinic. *Alzheimer's Stages: How the Disease Progresses*; 2023. Available at: https://www.mayoclinic.org/diseases-conditions/alzheimers-disease/in-depth/alzheimers-stages/art-20048448. (Accessed July 15, 2024).

Mazess RB. On aging bone loss. *Clin Orthop Relat Res.* 1982;(165):239–252.

National Committee for the Prevention of Elder Abuse (NCPEA). *What Role do Health and Medical Professionals Play in Elder Abuse Prevention?*; 2008. Available at https://www.allaboutseniors.org/listing/national-committee-for-the-prevention-of-elder-abuse. (Accessed November 2017).

Norris T. Special needs of geriatric patients. *American Society of Radiologic Technologists Homestudy Series.* 1999;4(5).

Park A. Alzheimer's unlocked. *Time [serial online].* 2010;176(17):53–59.

Rimer BK, Resch N, King E, et al. Multistrategy health education program to increase mammography use among women ages 65 and older. *Public Health Rep.* 1992;107(4):369–380.

Spencer G. *What are the Demographic Implications of an Aging U.S. Population from 1990 to 2030?.* Washington, DC: American Association of Retired Persons and Resources for the Future; 1993.

Thali MJ, Viner MD, Brogdon BG. *Brogdon's Forensic Radiology.* 2nd ed. Boca Raton, FL: CRC Press; 2011:287–288.

Thibodeau GA, Patton KT. *Anatomy & Physiology.* 8th ed. St Louis: Elsevier; 2013.

Turkington C, Harris JR. Alzheimer's disease. In: *The Encyclopedia of the Brain and Brain Disorders.* 3rd ed. New York: Facts on File; 2010:16–22.

US Department of Commerce. *Economics and Statistics Administration: 65+ in the United States.* Washington, DC: US Bureau of the Census; 2000.

University of Pittsburgh Schools of the Health Sciences. New compound identifies Alzheimer's disease brain toxins, study shows. *Science Daily.* 2008. Available at https://www.sciencedaily.com/releases/2008/03/080326114855.htm. (Accessed July 15, 2024).

VanMeter KC, Hubert RJ. *Gould's Pathophysiology for the Health Professions.* 5th ed. St Louis: Elsevier; 2014.

24
SECTIONAL ANATOMY FOR RADIOGRAPHERS

REX T. CHRISTENSEN

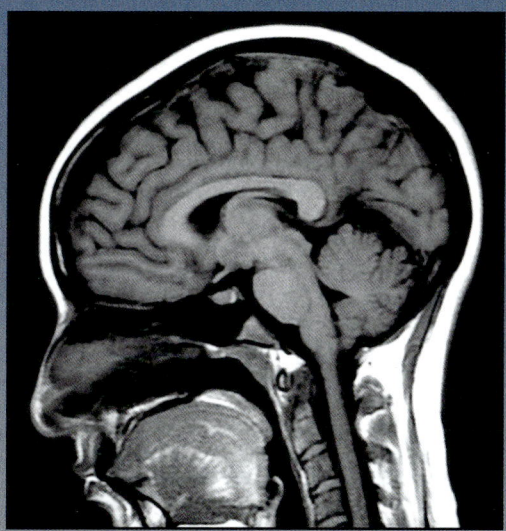

OUTLINE

Overview, 172
Cranial Region, 174
Thoracic Region, 191
Abdominopelvic Region, 204
Advanced Visualization, 222
3D Printing, 224

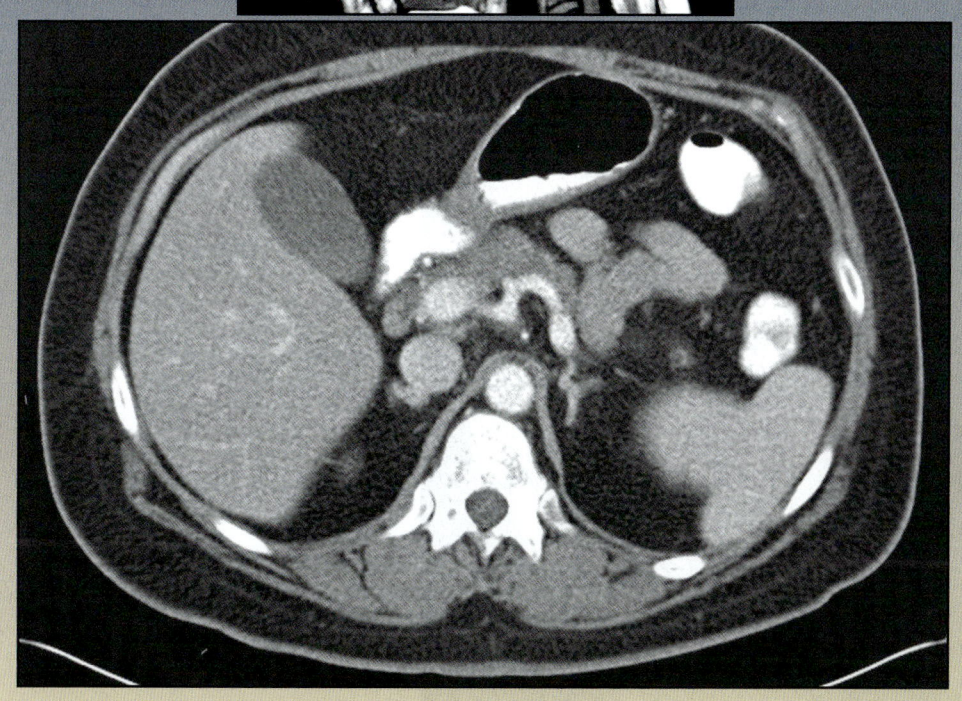

Overview

Imaging modalities, such as computed tomography (CT), magnetic resonance imaging (MRI), and diagnostic medical sonography, require the technologist to look at anatomy images in a different way than they are used to with general radiographs. These technologies create cross-sectional imaging planes, visualizing a slice through the body. The advantage of visualizing cross-sectional anatomic structures is that images can be viewed without the superimposition of other anatomic parts. Images are generated in various orientations, such as axial, sagittal, coronal, and oblique planes. These planes make it crucial for the technologists working within these modalities to have a clear and complete understanding of general anatomic principles. Without a clear understanding of general anatomy, it is difficult to feel confident identifying normal and abnormal structures in cross section. This chapter provides the radiographer who possesses a background in general anatomy with an orientation to sectional anatomy and correlates that anatomy with structures shown on images from the various computer-generated imaging modalities.

There are three major imaging planes: axial, sagittal, and coronal. Images that are off-axis from these planes are termed *oblique*. Axial planes (sometimes referred to as *transverse planes* or *transaxial*) transect the body from anterior to posterior and from side to side. In effect, this type of horizontal plane divides the body into superior and inferior portions. Most images generated by CT are examples of axial or transverse planes. When looking at an axial image, it is helpful to imagine standing at the patient's feet and looking up toward the head. With this orientation, the patient's right side is to the viewer's left and vice versa. The anterior aspect of the patient is usually at the top of the image. Coronal planes divide the body into anterior and posterior portions. Coronal planes pass from superior to inferior and from side to side. Images viewed in the coronal plane are similar to radiographs in that the patient's right side is on the technologist's left (one can imagine facing the patient while viewing this type of image). Sagittal planes divide the body into right and left portions. These planes pass from superior to inferior and from anterior to posterior. MRI images frequently use the coronal and sagittal planes to present the desired anatomy. CT images in the sagittal and coronal planes are reformatted data from axial images to display anatomy in these planes. Imaging planes that are generated from a single source are termed multiplanar reformat (MPR) images. Any plane that does not fit the previous descriptions is referred to as an *oblique plane*. Oblique planes are useful when imaging complicated structures, such as the heart. Source images obtained from the imaging modality can be compiled to produce not only MPR images but also three-dimensional images (Fig. 24.1). The CT three-dimensional images displayed in Fig. 24.1 help the physician with surgical and oncology treatment planning and patient instruction and education.

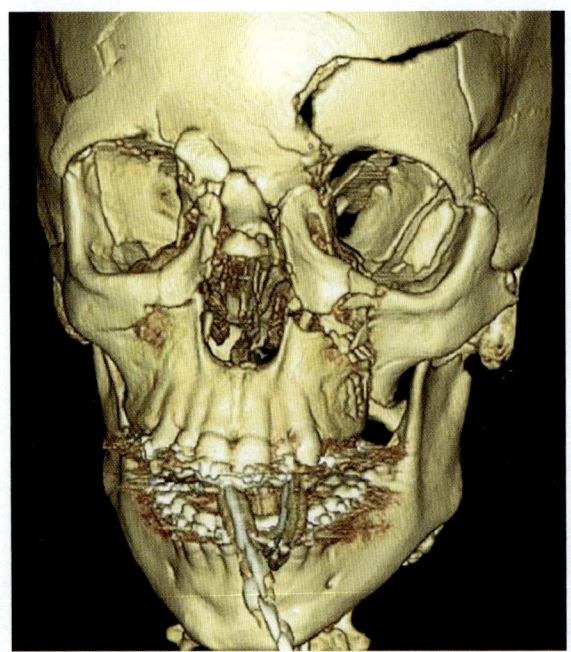

Fig. 24.1 Three-dimensional reconstructed CT image of the head.

CT uses x-rays to generate images, so the various shades on the images correspond to the gray scale that radiographers are accustomed to seeing. Bones and other dense materials are white, whereas air and lower-density materials are closer to black. Fat, muscle, and organs are represented with various shades of gray. Hounsfield units or CT numbers represent the scale of white to black that is used in CT imaging. Lower numbers represent anatomic structures that are more easily penetrated by the x-ray and appear closer to black on the image. Higher numbers are related to more radiopaque structures and are lighter gray or white on the image. Similar to routine radiographs, blood vessels and organs of the digestive system are not easily distinguishable from other structures. Tissue contrast limitations require these structures to be identified more accurately. Therefore, patients are frequently given a radiopaque contrast medium. Intravascular contrast medium highlights vessels, making them appear radiopaque and whiter on the image. To visualize the gastrointestinal system, patients may be given a contrast agent by mouth or via the rectum. A full description of CT fundamentals is presented in Chapter 25.

MRI uses magnetic fields and radiofrequencies to generate images. Anatomic structures are represented on the image regarding the signal generated from their protons. Structures that produce a strong signal are generally lighter gray or white on the image, and structures that do not generate a strong signal tend to be darker on the image. The signal generated by these structures depends on many things, including the strength of the magnetic fields, relaxation times of tissues, and the radiofrequency characteristics of anatomic structures. Contrast medium may also be used when performing MRI to change the signal intensity of particular anatomic structures. Gadolinium, air, and fluid may be used as contrast agents, depending on the organ of interest and the imaging sequences employed. MRI is discussed in depth in Chapter 26.

The cadaveric sections depicted in this chapter are representative of major organ structures for each of the body regions and *are depicted from the inferior surface to correspond to the images*. All relational terms are used in relation to the body in the anatomic position. (When a structure is described as being to the right of something, this refers to the *patient's* right, not the *viewer's* right.) The major anatomic structures normally seen when using current imaging modalities are labeled. For each region of the body, a cadaveric section is presented, and representative images are included to provide an orientation to anatomic structures normally seen using the available imaging modalities. The cadaveric sections and diagnostic images do not match exactly; some structures are seen on only one of the illustrations for each body region. Major anatomic structures in each region of the body are reviewed in the following sections to make it easier to identify the images provided. A systematic review of the bones, vessels, major organs, and muscles begins each section. Selected images are presented in axial, sagittal, and coronal planes to show these structures. In practice, images should be examined collectively because the size, shape, and placement of these structures vary from slice to slice. Scrolling through the various slices of a structure is frequently the ideal way to identify the size and characteristics of that structure.

Cranial Region

Fig. 24.2 is a cadaveric image that can be used to distinguish bone, muscle, and other soft tissue structures. Referring to this image is helpful in identifying the occasionally confusing shadows on the images. The head can be thought of systematically as being composed of the skull, central nervous system structures, various sensory organs, cranial blood supply, and associated cranial and facial muscles. The bones of the skull are categorized as the eight cranial bones and the 14 facial bones. The cranial bones include the frontal, occipital, and two parietal bones that surround and protect the external surface of the brain. The other four cranial bones include the ethmoid, sphenoid, and two temporal bones. The frontal bone forms the anterior surface of the skull, with a vertical portion that corresponds to the forehead and a horizontal portion that forms the roof of the orbits. Between the inner and outer layers of the vertical portion of the frontal bone—just superior to the level of the eyes—are the paired frontal paranasal sinuses. The vertex is the most superior portion of the skull and is formed by the paired parietal bones. These roughly square-shaped bones articulate with the frontal bone at the coronal suture, with the temporal bones at the squamosal sutures, with the occipital bone at the lambdoidal suture, and with each other at the sagittal suture.

The posterior aspect of the skull is formed by the occipital bone, which is composed of a squamous (vertical) portion and a basilar portion. The foramen magnum is a large opening within the squamous portion that allows passage of the spinal cord into the brain. The external occipital protuberance is a large prominence on the posterior surface of this bone. Roughly corresponding in position to this landmark is the internal occipital protuberance. The ethmoid bone is found within the cranium and forms the medial walls of the orbits and part of the lateral walls of the nasal cavity. The ethmoid bone is divided into a horizontal portion called the *cribriform plate* and vertical portions called the *perpendicular plate* and *two labyrinths* or *lateral masses*.

The cribriform plate lies between the orbital plates of the frontal bone and supports the olfactory bulbs (cranial nerve I). The cribriform plate is perforated by many small foramina, which transmit nerves from the nose to this cranial nerve. Projecting superiorly from the cribriform plate is a small ridge of bone called the *crista galli*, which serves as the anterior attachment for the falx cerebri. Projecting inferiorly from the center of the cribriform plate is the perpendicular plate. This thin strip of bone forms the superior part of the bony nasal septum. Extending inferiorly from the lateral edges of the cribriform plate are the labyrinths or lateral masses. These are perforated by multiple air spaces, which are collectively called the *ethmoidal paranasal sinuses*. From the medial surface of each labyrinth, two scroll-shaped ridges of bone project into the nasal cavity. These are the superior and middle nasal conchae.

In the center of the base of the skull is the sphenoid bone. This bone is sometimes referred to as the *anchor bone of the cranium* because it articulates with all

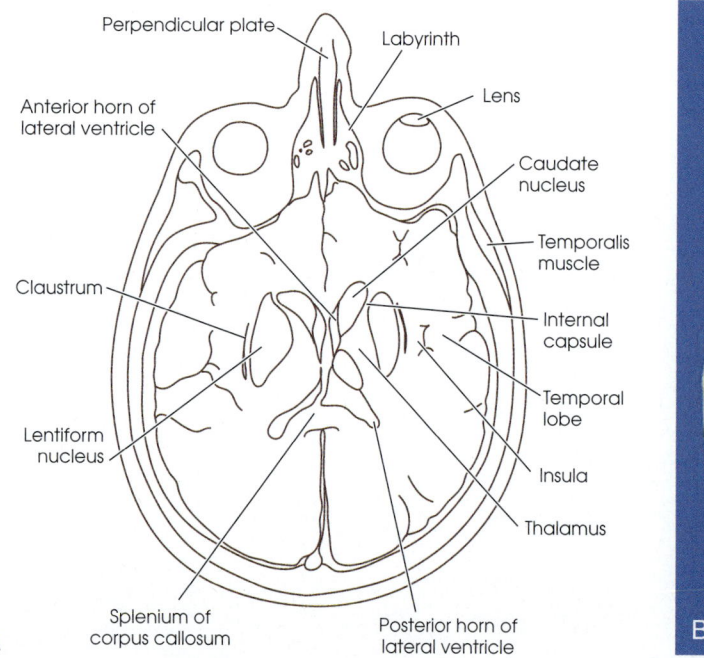
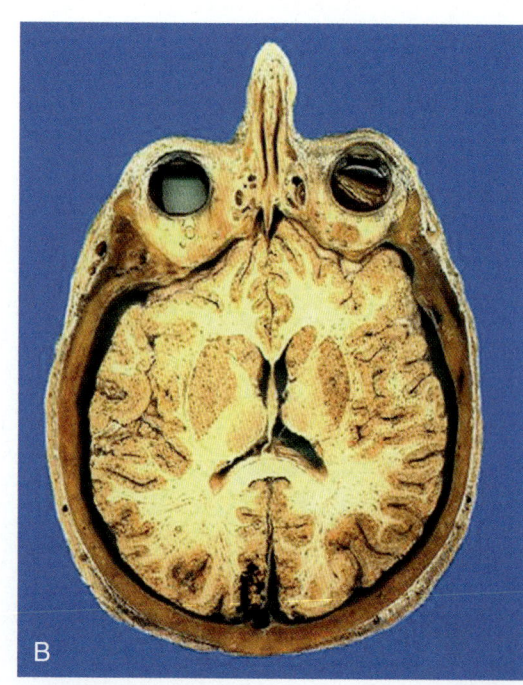

Fig. 24.2 (**A**) Line drawing of gross anatomic section. (**B**) Cadaveric image of skull.

the cranial bones. Visualizing this bone as being composed of a body, two sets of wings, and a pterygoid portion is helpful. The body is the central portion of the bone and contains the easily identifiable landmark known as the *sella turcica*. The sella turcica forms a cup-shaped depression that surrounds and protects the pituitary gland. The anterior surface of the sella is called the *tuberculum sellae*, and the posterior portion is called the *dorsum sellae*. Two posterior clinoid processes project from the superior edge of the dorsum sellae and are attachments for dura mater partitions. Within the body of the sphenoid and inferior to the sella turcica are the paired sphenoidal paranasal sinuses. The lesser wings of the sphenoid are triangular ridges of bone found posterior to the orbital plates of the frontal bone. Directly inferior to the medial edge of each lesser wing is the optic canal, which transmits the optic nerve (cranial nerve II). The larger, greater wings support the temporal lobes of the cerebrum and extend from the body to the external surface of the skull. The pterygoid processes project inferiorly from the body of the sphenoid and form the posterior walls of the nasal cavity.

The temporal bones form part of the lateral walls of the cranium and extend internally to meet the sphenoid and the basilar portion of the occipital bone. Parts of the temporal bone include the squamous, tympanic, mastoid, and petrous portions. The squamous portion is the thin, fan-shaped external part of the bone superior to the external ear. It articulates with the parietal and several other cranial bones. Its articulation with the parietal bone is called the *squamous suture*. The tympanic portion is the area of the bone surrounding the external ear canal. The zygomatic process arches anteriorly from just superior to the external ear canal. Just inferior to the origin of the zygomatic process is the mandibular fossa, in which the condyle of the mandible is found. On the inferior surface of the tympanic portion of the bone is the styloid process, which serves as an attachment for muscles. Posterior to the ear is the mastoid portion, which is perforated by many small, air-filled cavities. The mastoid portion extends inferiorly to form the cone-shaped mastoid process. The petrous portion of the bone lies within the cranium, normally forming an angle of approximately 45 degrees to the median sagittal plane. This dense ridge of bone surrounds and protects the organs of hearing and balance, the facial and vestibulocochlear nerves, and the internal carotid artery.

The organs associated with the face are surrounded and protected by 14 bones. Each of these bones is paired, with the exception of the vomer and the mandible. The lacrimal bones are about the size of a fingernail and are found in the medial wall of the orbit between the maxilla and the labyrinth of the ethmoid bones. The nasal bones form the bridge of the nose and articulate superiorly with the frontal bone, laterally with the maxilla, and with each other in the midline. The zygomatic bones form the inferolateral walls of the orbits. Each of these bones articulates superiorly with the frontal bone, medially with the maxilla, and laterally with the zygomatic process of the temporal bone. The maxilla originates as two separate bones, which ultimately fuse along the midsagittal plane. This large bone forms the inferior surface of each orbit, the lateral walls of the nasal cavity, and the anterior portion of the roof of the mouth. On either side of the nasal cavity, large air-filled maxillary paranasal sinuses are embedded within the bone. The upper teeth are rooted within the alveolar process at the anteroinferior surface of the bone. The maxilla articulates with the nasal bones, the lacrimal bones, the frontal bone, the zygomatic bones, and the palatine bones. The inferior nasal conchae are scroll-shaped facial bones found in the nasal cavity, just inferior to the middle nasal conchae of the ethmoid bone. The L-shaped palatine bones form the posterior portion of the hard palate. The vertical portions of the palatines extend superiorly along the posterior nasal cavity to form a small part of the posterior orbit.

The vomer is an unpaired facial bone that rests on the hard palate and articulates with the inferior surface of the perpendicular plate of the ethmoid. It forms the inferior portion of the bony nasal septum. The mandible, which is also an unpaired facial bone, is formed by a body and two rami. The body comprises the anterior portion of the bone and presents an alveolar ridge in which the lower teeth are embedded. The rami extend superiorly from the body and end in anterior and posterior bony processes. The anterior process at the superior end of the ramus is the coronoid process, where muscles of mastication attach. The posterior process is the condyloid process, which rests in the mandibular fossa of the temporal bone. This articulation—the temporomandibular joint—is the only movable articulation associated with the skull. (Refer to Chapter 11 for review of skull anatomy.)

The brain is surrounded by three layers of protective membranes called the *meninges*. From internal to external, they are the pia mater, arachnoid, and dura mater. The pia mater adheres directly to the brain and is composed of a fine network of capillaries and supporting tissue. The arachnoid is a delicate membrane that resembles a cobweb. The subarachnoid space lies between the arachnoid and pia mater. Cerebrospinal fluid (CSF) circulates in this space. The arachnoid does not closely adhere to cerebral structures. As it bridges the gap between various parts of the brain, enlarged regions—or cisterns—are formed in the subarachnoid space. Some of the more crucial cisterns include the cisterna magna, pontine, interpeduncular, and superior or *quadrigeminal cistern*. The cisterna magna is the largest of these and is found just inside the foramen magnum, between the cerebellum and the medulla oblongata. This cistern receives CSF from the fourth ventricle. The pontine cistern lies anterior to the pons and contains the basilar artery. The interpeduncular cistern is anterior to the midbrain. The infundibulum (stalk) of the pituitary and the vessels of the circle of Willis are seen here. The cistern found posterior to the midbrain is the superior cistern. It surrounds the pineal gland and the great cerebral vein. Ambient cisterns communicate with the superior cistern and extend laterally around the midbrain. The most external of the meninges is the double-layered dura mater. The outer layer of dura is attached to the inner surface of the cranial bones. The inner layer can be seen between cerebral structures and in large fissures. Dural sinuses are venous drainage channels formed where the inner dural layers separate from the outer layer. One of the largest dural flaps, the falx cerebri, is found in the longitudinal fissure between the cerebral hemispheres. It extends from the crista galli of the ethmoid to the occipital bone. The tentorium cerebelli extends between the cerebrum and the cerebellum. It attaches to the sella turcica and the internal surface of the occipital bones.

The structures of the central nervous system within the skull include the cerebrum, brain stem, and cerebellum. The cerebrum is the largest of these structures and is divided by the longitudinal fissure into two hemispheres. The hemispheres are connected to each other via a white matter tract called the *corpus callosum*. This arch-shaped structure is divided into the anterior genu, central body, and posterior splenium. Each cerebral hemisphere is divided into lobes that are named for the most adjacent cranial bone: frontal, parietal, temporal, or occipital. An additional lobe called the insula is located deep within the lateral sulcus of each hemisphere, below the frontal, parietal, and temporal lobes. The cerebrum is thrown into numerous folds called *gyri*, which are separated by small fissures called *sulci*. The outer surface of the cerebrum consists of a thin layer of gray matter. The central portion of this part of the brain is mainly white matter (formed by myelinated nerve fibers). These fibers, referred to as the *corona radiata*, connect the gray matter of the cortex to deeper gray matter nuclei deep within each hemisphere. The buried gray matter centers are called *basal nuclei* or *basal ganglia* and include the claustrum, putamen, globus pallidus, and caudate nucleus. White matter tracts—or capsules—are found between these gray matter structures. Other gray matter structures found within the central cerebrum include the thalamus and hypothalamus. The medial aspects of the thalamus and the hypothalamus form the lateral walls of the third ventricle. Many of these gray and white matter structures are seen in the cadaveric section in Fig. 24.2.

The brain stem is formed by the midbrain, pons, and medulla oblongata. It lies between the cerebrum and cerebellum and serves as a relay for nerve impulses between the spinal cord and these two structures. The midbrain is the most superior of the three. White matter tracts called the cerebral peduncles extend from the anterior midbrain to the cerebrum. Toward the posterior aspect of the midbrain are the corpora quadrigemina, which are formed by two superior and two inferior colliculi that lie just inferior to the splenium of the corpus callosum. The cerebral aqueduct drains CSF from the third ventricle to the fourth ventricle and passes through the posterior portion of the midbrain. The central portion of the brain stem is formed by the pons. It communicates with the medulla, with the midbrain, and via white matter cerebellar peduncles to the cerebellum. The most inferior of the brain stem structures is the medulla oblongata, which is continuous with the spinal cord as it passes through the foramen magnum.

The cerebellum lies in the posteroinferior region of the cranium. Although smaller in size, it is similar in composition to the cerebrum. A midline fissure divides the cerebellum into hemispheres that are connected by a midline vermis. It is also thrown into numerous small folds, here called folia, which are separated by numerous small fissures. The outer surface of the cerebellum is composed of gray matter, with white matter constituting most of the central portion of this part of the brain. Gray matter nuclei can be found here also, although they are difficult to distinguish on images and are not discussed in this chapter.

Four large cavities called *ventricles* are found in the brain. The ventricles' major function is to produce and store CSF; this is accomplished as blood is filtered through capillary networks called *choroid plexuses* in each of the ventricles. The largest of these chambers are the lateral ventricles, one of which is found in each cerebral hemisphere. The lateral ventricles are divided into a body and anterior, posterior, and inferior horns. CSF from these chambers passes into the midline third ventricle through the interventricular foramina. The third ventricle is found between the cerebral hemispheres inferior to the lateral ventricles. The cerebral aqueduct drains CSF from the third ventricle to the fourth ventricle. The fourth ventricle is found between the cerebellum and the brain stem. Its walls are formed by white matter tracts called *cerebellar peduncles*, which connect the brain stem and cerebellum. A central aperture and two lateral apertures allow CSF to pass from the fourth ventricle into the subarachnoid space.

The brain is a highly metabolic organ and needs a rich blood supply to function well. Four major arteries supply the brain and its related structures: the two internal carotid arteries and the two vertebral arteries. The internal carotid arteries supply the anterior structures of the brain. After passing superiorly through the neck, these arteries enter the skull via the carotid canals in the petrous portion of the temporal bones. After exiting the petrous portion, the internal carotid arteries pass along the lateral aspect of the sella turcica, ultimately dividing into the anterior and middle cerebral arteries. The posterior communicating artery arises from the internal carotid just before this bifurcation. The anterior cerebral arteries pass anteriorly and superiorly to the longitudinal fissure, where they curl around the external aspect of the corpus callosum and supply the anterior portion of the brain. The middle cerebral arteries pass laterally to the lateral fissures, where their branches supply the middle portion of the brain. The posterior communicating arteries pass posteriorly to join with the branches from the vertebrobasilar arterial system. The vertebral arteries traverse the neck in the transverse foramina of the cervical spine and enter the posterior skull via the foramen magnum. These arteries pass superiorly along the anterior aspect of the medulla and at the base of the pons join to form the basilar artery. At the superior aspect of the pons, the basilar artery splits to form the posterior cerebral arteries. A unique arterial anastomosis exists in the brain to protect it from sudden loss of blood supply. This vascular connection is called the *circle of Willis*. The blood supply to the anterior brain is connected to the blood supply for the posterior brain as the posterior communicating arteries extend from the internal carotid arteries to the posterior cerebral arteries. This communication lies in the interpeduncular cistern, just anterior to the midbrain.

Venous drainage in the cranium is accomplished by two systems: cerebral veins and dural venous sinuses. The dural sinuses are created by gaps formed between the inner and outer layers of the dura mater. These gaps are found in the areas where the dura invaginates between the various structures of the brain. The superior sagittal sinus is found in the superior border of the falx cerebri, and the inferior sagittal sinus is found in its inferior margin. The channel formed where the falx cerebri meets the tentorium cerebelli is the straight sinus (Fig. 24.3). This sinus is a continuation of the inferior sagittal sinus as it joins with the great cerebral vein. The great cerebral vein, also known as the vein of Galen, continues under the corpus callosum to form the internal cerebral vein. The transverse or lateral sinuses are found along the lateral aspect of the tentorium cerebelli as it meets the occipital bone. At the level of the petrous portions of the temporal bones, the transverse sinuses curl medially and inferiorly and become known as the *sigmoid sinuses*. As the sigmoid sinuses pass out of the cranium via the jugular foramina, these vessels change names again and become the internal jugular veins. One of the major veins within the skull is the great cerebral vein. This large venous structure is found in the superior cistern, and there, it joins the inferior sagittal sinus to form the straight sinus.

Many muscles are associated with the face, only a few of which are referred to in the following sections. The temporalis muscle is found on the external surface of the squamous portion of the temporal bone. Its inferior attachment is to the coronoid process of the mandible. On the external surface of the mandibular rami are the masseter muscles, and on the internal surface of the rami are the pterygoid muscles. These muscles are associated with moving the mandible and with swallowing (Fig. 24.4).

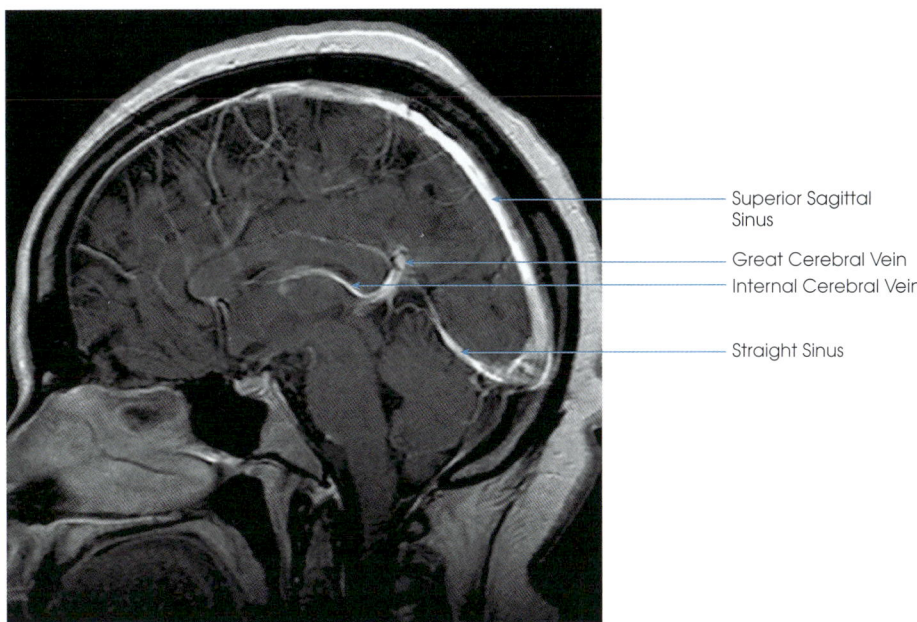

Fig. 24.3 Midsagittal contrast-enhanced MRI image of the brain.

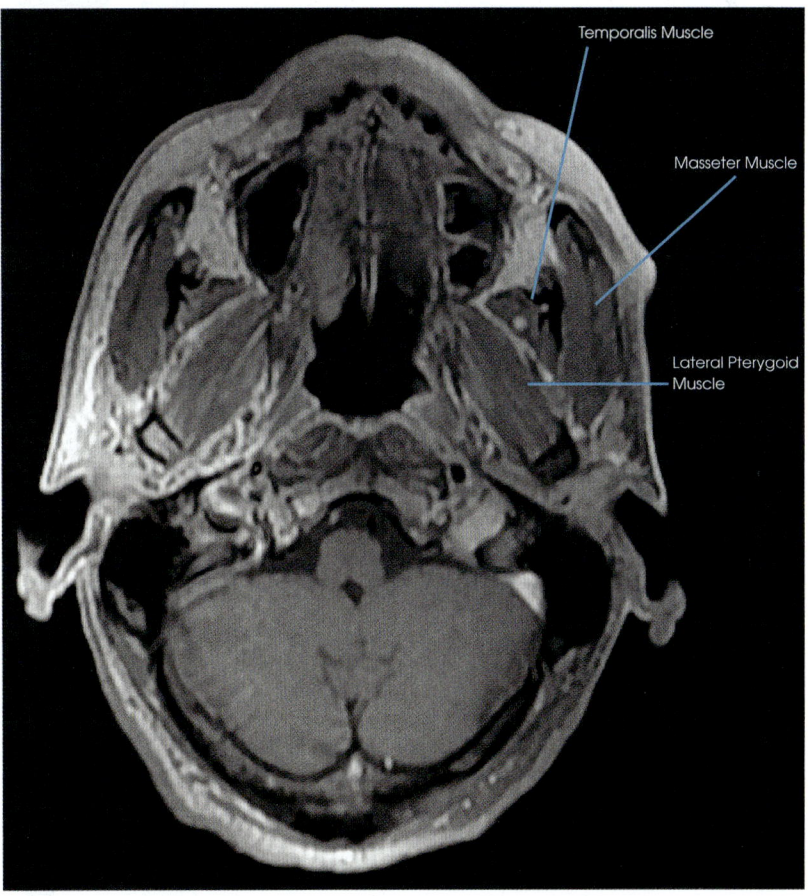

Fig. 24.4 Axial T1-weighted MRI image of the brain.

A lateral skull radiograph is used here for localization of the imaging plane in this section (Fig. 24.5A), and a sagittal MRI image (Fig. 24.5B) is used for localization of MRI cross sections of the brain. CT imaging for the cranium may be performed with the gantry parallel to or angled 15 to 20 degrees to the orbitomeatal line. Angling the gantry of the CT scanner allows for imaging of the brain without excess radiation to the eyes. MRI of the cranium generally results in images that are parallel to the orbitomeatal or infraorbitomeatal plane. More details on patient positioning for CT are provided in Chapter 25, and information on patient positioning for MRI is provided in Chapter 26. Because the imaging planes may be different for CT and MRI, some variation exists in the anatomic structures visualized in corresponding illustrations in this section. Seven identifying lines represent the approximate levels for each of the labeled images for this region.

The cranial CT image seen in Fig. 24.6 represents a CT slice obtained through the frontal and parietal bones, and Fig. 24.7 is a corresponding T1-weighted contrast-enhanced MRI image. The *cortex*—or outer layer of gray matter—can be differentiated from the deeper *white matter*. The numerous *gyri*—or *convolutions*—and *sulci* are shown and are surrounded by the darker-appearing CSF in the subarachnoid space. The *cerebral hemispheres* are separated by the *longitudinal cerebral fissure*. Invaginated in this fissure is a fold of *dura mater* called the *falx cerebri*. The *superior sagittal sinus*, which passes through the superior margin of the falx cerebri, follows the contour of the superior skull margin. In cross section, the anterior and posterior aspects of this sinus can normally be seen in the midline deep to the bony plates when the patient has been given an intravenous contrast agent and appear as triangular expansions near the bones on both CT and MRI images. Two

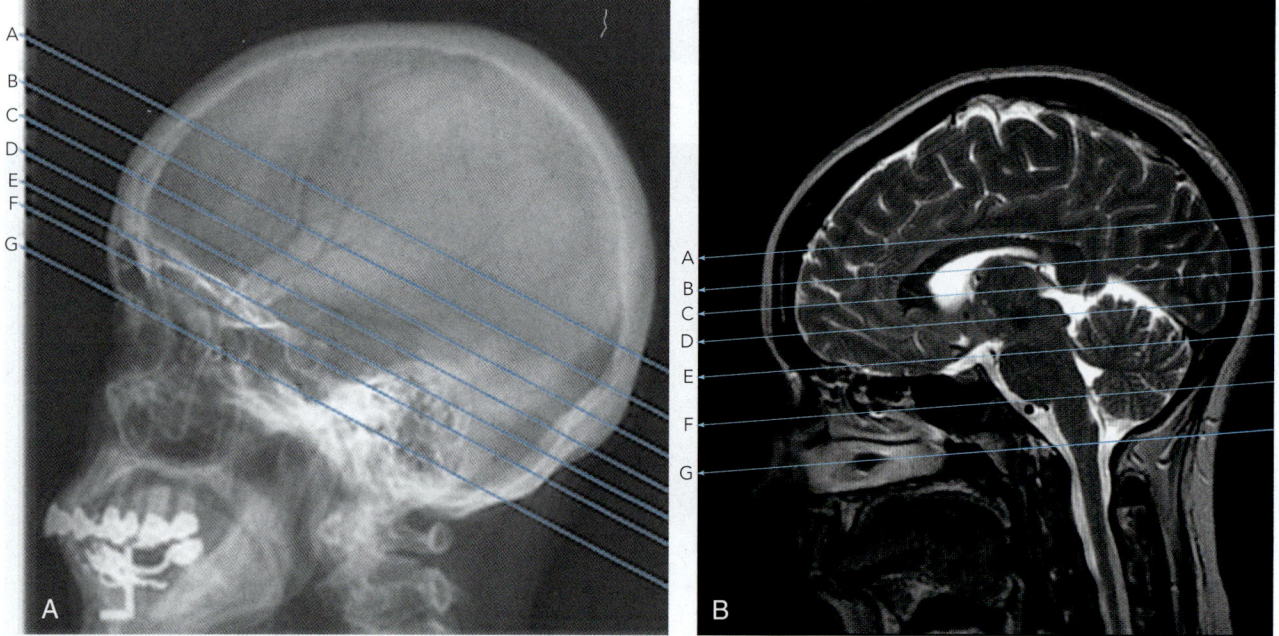

Fig. 24.5 (**A**) CT localizer (scout) image of skull. (**B**) Sagittal localizer for MRI of the brain.

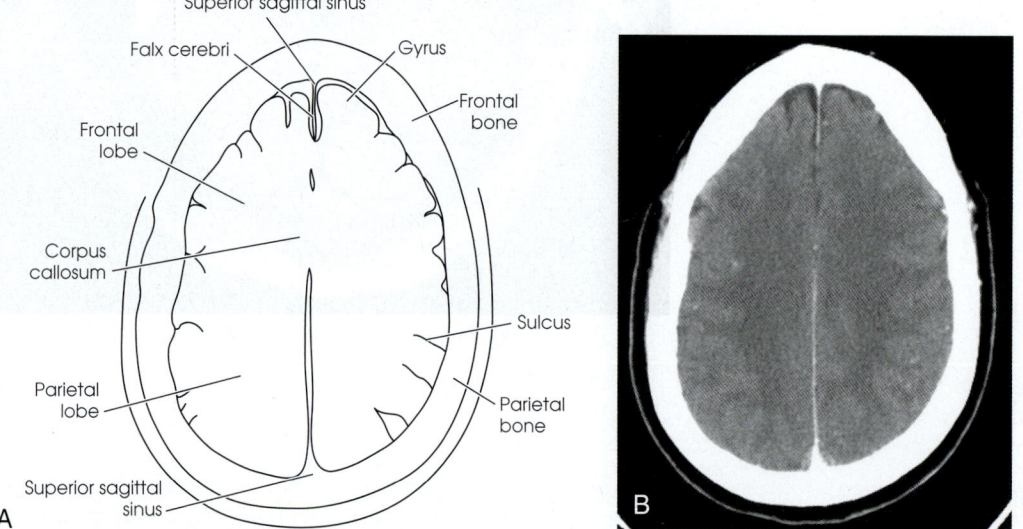

Fig. 24.6 (**A**) Line drawing of CT section. (**B**) CT image representing anatomic structures located at level A in Fig. 24.5A.

of the five *cerebral lobes* are seen (frontal and parietal). The *corona radiata* is the central tract of white matter in the cerebrum and is darker than the cortex on the CT image; the white matter is lighter than the gray matter on the MRI image. These sections were obtained at a level that passes through the superiormost portion of the *corpus callosum*, which separates the anterior and posterior portions of the falx cerebri.

Fig. 24.8 is an axial CT slice through the superior portions of the lateral ventricles; Fig. 24.9 is the corresponding T1-weighted contrast-enhanced MRI image. Visualized bony structures on the CT scan include the *frontal bone* and the two *parietal bones*. The falx cerebri is seen within the *longitudinal fissure*. The *frontal lobes* and *parietal lobes* of the cerebrum are shown. In the center of each image, the *lateral ventricles* are easily seen because of the dark appearance of the CSF circulating within each. In the posterior portions of the ventricles, the contrast-filled capillary network of the *choroid plexuses* also is visualized. A thin membrane called the *septum pellucidum* can be seen separating the ventricles. The corpus callosum is an arch-shaped structure; in cross section at this level, only the anterior *genu* and the posterior *splenium* can be seen. The *caudate nuclei* lie along the lateral surfaces of the ventricles and tend to follow their curves. Because these nuclei are composed of gray matter, they are the same shade of gray as the cortex on MRI images (see Fig. 24.9). Several contrast-filled

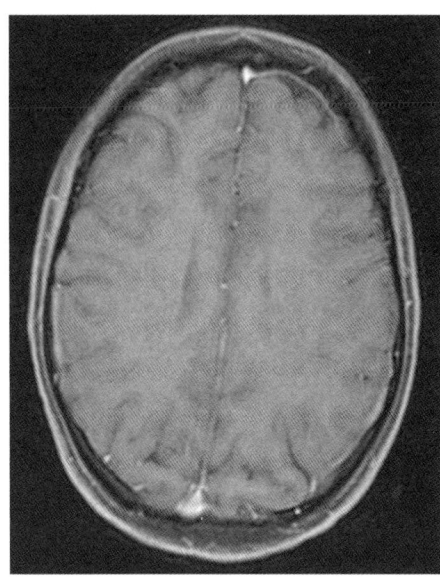

Fig. 24.7 MRI corresponding to level *A* in Fig. 24.5B.

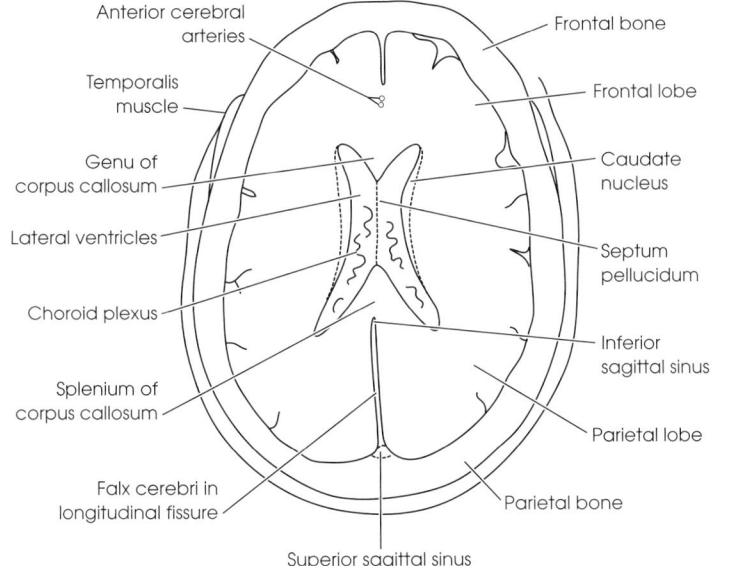

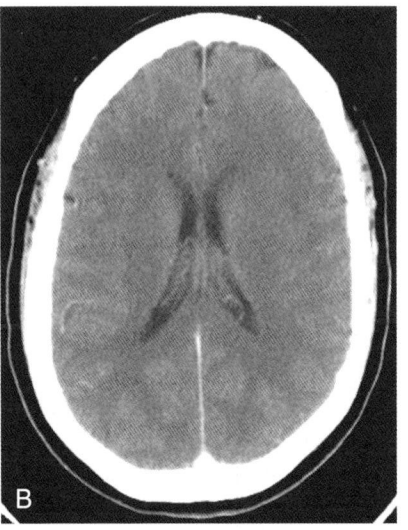

Fig. 24.8 (**A**) Line drawing of CT section. (**B**) CT image representing structures located at level *B* in Fig. 24.5A.

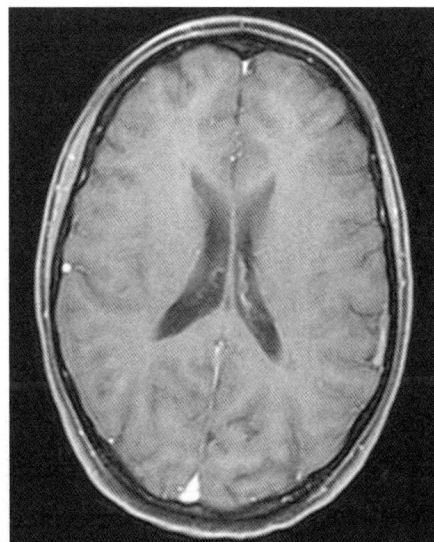

Fig. 24.9 MRI corresponding to level *B* in Fig. 24.5B.

vascular structures are visible. The *anterior cerebral arteries* lie within the longitudinal fissure just anterior to the genu of the corpus callosum. A few branches of the *middle cerebral arteries* are seen near the lateral aspect of the skull on the CT scan. The anterior and posterior portions of the superior sagittal sinus are seen in the periphery of the falx cerebri. The *inferior sagittal sinus* lies in the internal edges of the falx. The thin strips of muscle seen on the external surface of the frontal bone correspond to the superior edges of the *temporalis muscles*.

The axial sections through the midportion of the cerebrum show many of the central structures of the cerebral hemispheres. (Fig. 24.10 is a CT image, and Fig. 24.11 is a T1-weighted contrast-enhanced image.) Images at this level pass through the frontal bone, greater wing of the *sphenoid*, and squamous portion of the *temporal bones*. The posterior portion of the skull comprises the top portion (squamous portion) of the *occipital bone* at this level. The falx cerebri is shown within the longitudinal fissure, with the superior sagittal sinus best shown in the midline of the anterior and posterior margins of this membrane. In the CT image, the genu of the corpus callosum is found between the anterior horns of the lateral ventricles; however, the posterior portion of this slice is inferior to the level of the splenium. The MRI image shows the genu and the splenium. At this level, the MRI image shows the *frontal, temporal*, and *occipital lobes* along with the *insula* (fifth lobe or island of Reil), which is deep to the temporal lobe at the lateral fissure. Because of its orientation, the CT image shows the insula, frontal, and temporal lobes; the

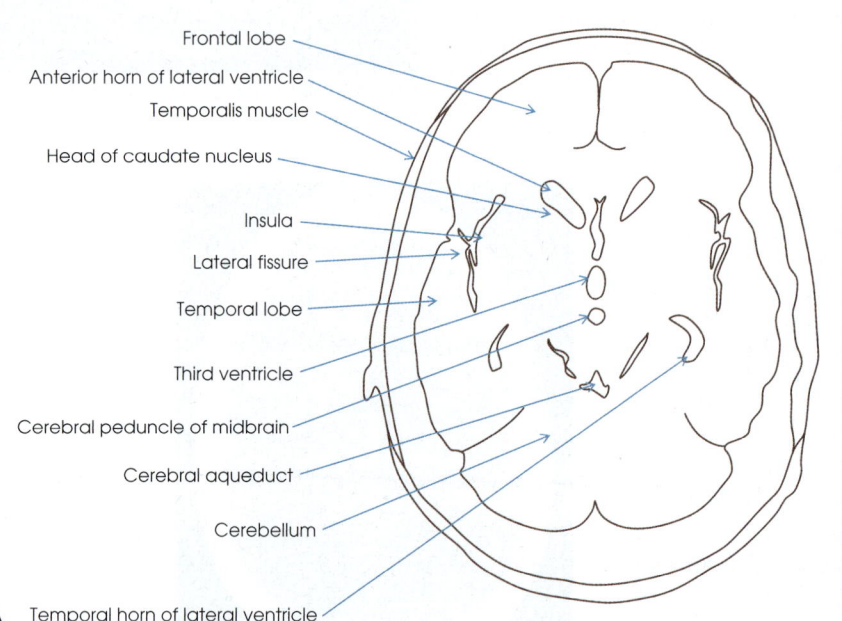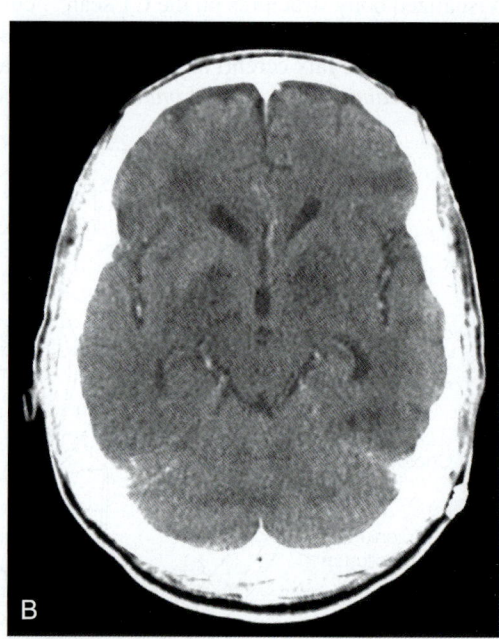

Fig. 24.10 (A) Line drawing of CT section. (B) CT image representing anatomic structures located at level C in Fig. 24.5A.

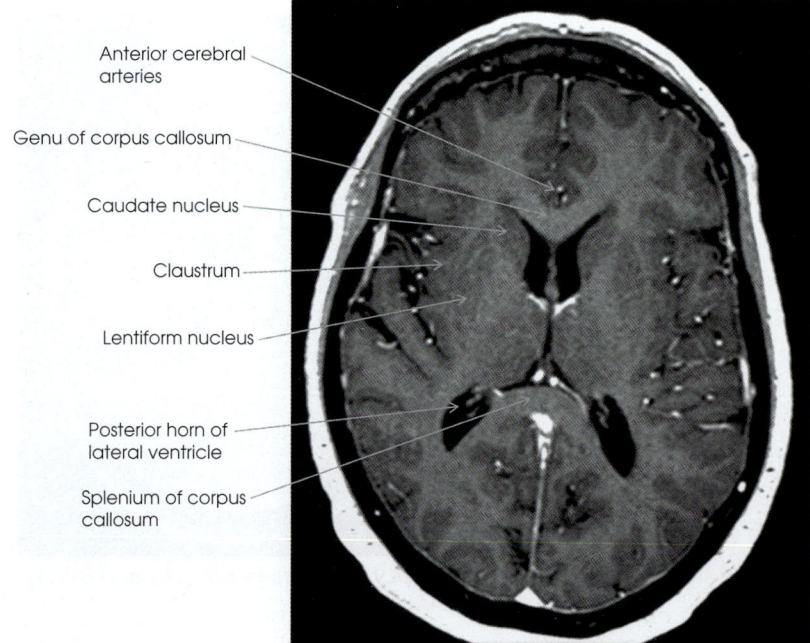

Fig. 24.11 MRI representing anatomic structures located at level C in Fig. 24.5B.

cerebellum occupies the posterior aspect of the skull in this image.

The anterior and temporal horns of the lateral ventricles are seen on the CT scan, whereas the anterior and posterior horns are visible on the MRI image. Within each posterior horn is a portion of the choroid plexus, which appears bright due to the presence of contrast medium in the capillaries. The heads of the caudate nuclei lie along the external surfaces of the anterior horns of each lateral ventricle. Several areas of gray matter can be seen faintly on the CT image deep within the white matter of the cerebrum and constitute the basal nuclei. The addition of MRI contrast provides enhancement so that the deep gray matter structures can be seen. The major components of the basal nuclei seen at this level are (from lateral to medial) the *claustrum*, *lentiform nucleus* (composed of the putamen and globus pallidus), and *caudate nucleus*. The lentiform nucleus is separated from the caudate nucleus and thalamus by a tract of white matter known as the *internal capsule*. These sections pass through the superior portion of the midline *third ventricle*. The *thalamus*, which serves as a central relay station for sensory impulses to the cerebral cortex, forms its lateral walls. The plane of the CT image passes through the structures of the midbrain. The anterior portions of the midbrain include the cerebral peduncles (white matter tracts that connect the cerebrum and the midbrain). The dark circular area at the posterior edge of the midbrain is the CSF-filled cerebral aqueduct. This passage connects the third and fourth ventricles and allows the circulation of CSF. A contrast-enhanced vessel, the great cerebral vein, is found just posterior to the third ventricle and the splenium of the corpus callosum on the MRI image. It passes through the upper portion of the *superior cistern*. The pineal gland is also found in this cistern but is not clearly visualized in either image. This is an important radiographic landmark because of its tendency to calcify in adults. Branches of the middle cerebral artery are visible within the lateral fissures, and the anterior cerebral arteries can be seen in the anterior portion of the longitudinal fissure on the MRI image.

Fig. 24.12 is a CT image that passes through the frontal lobe, pons, and cerebellum. Fig. 24.13 is the T2-weighted

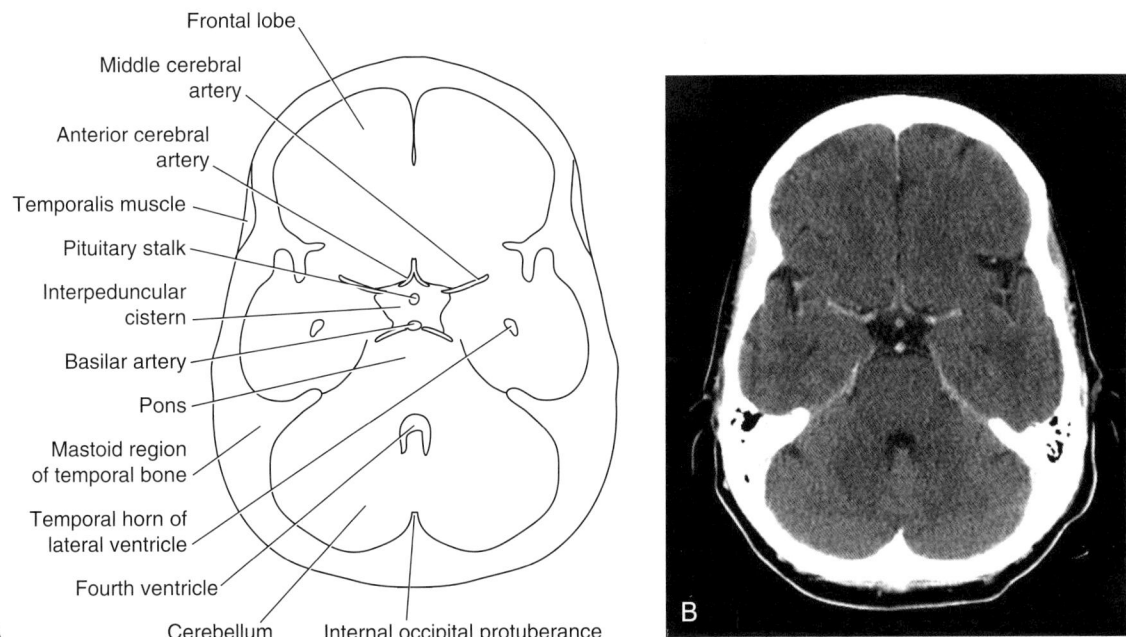

Fig. 24.12 (**A**) Line drawing of CT section. (**B**) CT image representing anatomic structures located at level *D* in Fig. 24.5A.

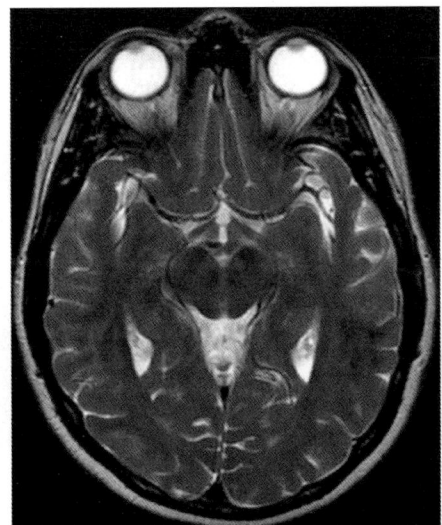

Fig. 24.13 MRI through circle of Willis, corresponding to level *D* in Fig. 24.5B.

MRI image, which passes through the orbits, the midbrain, and the occipital lobes. Bony structures visible in the CT image include the frontal bone, the temporal bones, and the occipital bone. Within the temporal bones, the black air-filled structures represent the mastoid air cells. The internal protrusion of bone in the center of the occipital bone is the internal occipital protuberance. The darker area between the eyes on the MRI image corresponds to the lower portion of the frontal sinuses. Frontal and temporal lobes of the cerebrum are shown on the CT image, whereas the frontal, temporal, and occipital lobes of the cerebrum are shown on the MRI image. The CT scan passes just inferior to the midbrain, and the MRI image passes through the level of the midbrain. The large dark area in the center of the CT image is the interpeduncular cistern. This is an enlarged area in the subarachnoid space containing CSF. The optic chiasm and the circle of Willis normally lie within the interpeduncular cistern. The pituitary stalk, also known as the infundibulum or infundibular stalk, and some of the vessels that contribute to the circle of Willis are visible in this image. The pons lies posterior to the cistern. The cerebellum lies within the posterior fossa of the skull between the pons and the occipital bone. The large dark region between the pons and cerebellum is the CSF-filled fourth ventricle. The temporalis muscles are seen on the external surfaces on either side of the cranium. On the MRI image, the *cerebral peduncles* form the anterior portions of the midbrain, and the *corpora quadrigemina* forms the posterior portion. The small light gray circle anterior to the colliculi is the CSF-filled *cerebral aqueduct*. Posterior to the midbrain is the *cerebellum*, which is surrounded by the *tentorium cerebelli*. The dark region anterior to the midbrain is the *interpeduncular cistern*, and the region posterior to the midbrain is the superior cistern. On the MRI image, within and around the interpeduncular cistern the *optic tracts* are visualized along with the *hypothalamus*, the inferior portion of the third ventricle, and *mammillary bodies*.

The CT image is just superior to the internal carotid arteries and shows the origins of the left anterior and middle cerebral arteries, at the anterior edge of the interpeduncular cistern. The anterior cerebral arteries pass from their origin toward the longitudinal fissure in the midline of the brain, and the middle cerebral arteries course from their origins toward the lateral fissures. The CT image also shows the bifurcation of the basilar artery into the two posterior cerebral arteries. These vessels can be seen just anterior to the pons. The MRI image shows the posterior portion of the superior sagittal sinus located near the internal occipital protuberance; the *straight sinus* can be seen at the edge of the tentorium cerebelli, just posterior to the cerebellum on the MRI image.

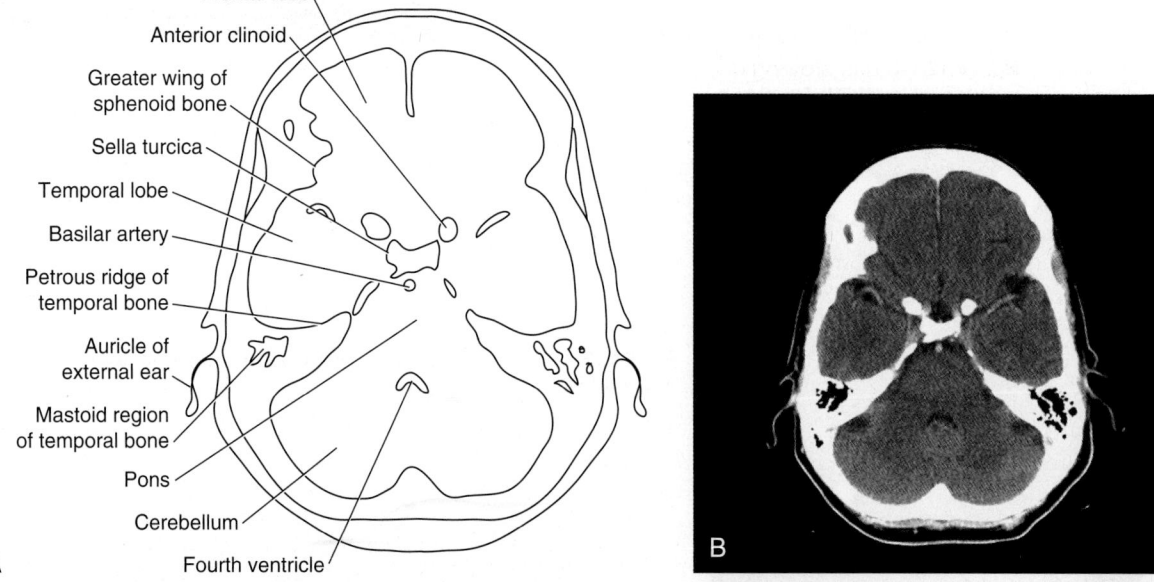

Fig. 24.14 (**A**) Line drawing of CT section. (**B**) CT image representing anatomic structures located at level *E* in Fig. 24.5A.

Fig. 24.14 is a CT image through the sella turcica and the posterior fossa. The T2-weighted MRI image (Fig. 24.15) passes through the center of the orbits, the tops of the ears, the pituitary and center of the sella turcica, and the cerebellum. The MRI image shows the *nasal bones*, visible in the anterior skull. Between the eyes, the *ethmoidal sinuses* and the *cribriform plate* of the ethmoid bone are seen. The *sella turcica* and *dorsum sellae* are seen surrounding the *pituitary gland*. Several cranial bones are visible on the CT scan. The anterior clinoids of the sella turcica and the greater wings of the sphenoid are seen. The roof of the sella is formed by the lesser wings, anterior clinoids, and posterior clinoids. The temporal bone constitutes most of the lateral portions of the skull, and the *petrous ridges* can be seen on the CT image, extending toward the median sagittal plane. The black air spaces near the lateral aspect of the petrous portions of these bones correspond to *mastoid air cells*, and the air spaces farther medial are associated with the internal structures of the ear. On the CT image, the frontal and temporal lobes of the cerebrum are visible, along with the pons and cerebellum. The dark region between the sella turcica and the pons is the pontine cistern, filled with CSF. The lower region of the fourth ventricle is seen between the pons and the cerebellum. On the MRI image, both *globes* are visible within the orbits. Rectus muscles lie along the medial and lateral walls of each. The *optic nerves* are seen in the centers of the posterior orbits passing from the eyes toward the brain via the optic canal. The temporal lobes are found lateral to the sella turcica, resting in the middle cranial fossa. The *pons* lies posterior to the sella, and the cerebellum is seen filling the posterior cranial fossa. The edges of the tentorium cerebelli can be seen faintly between the temporal lobes and the cerebellum. The dark region anterior to the pons corresponds to the CSF-filled *pontine cistern,* in which the contrast-filled *basilar artery* is easily visualized on both the CT and MRI images. The dark region between the pons and the cerebellum is the superior region of the *fourth ventricle*. On the CT image, the contrast-filled basilar artery lies between the sella and the pons. At this level in the MRI image, the *internal carotid arteries* lie lateral to the body of the sphenoid bone in an almost horizontal orientation. The *confluence of sinuses* can be seen just anterior to the internal occipital protuberance on the MRI image. The confluence is the region where the superior sagittal sinus and the straight sinus meet the transverse sinuses. The *transverse sinuses* are seen on the MRI image at this level, lying just internal to the occipital bone. On the external surface of the skull in both images, the temporalis muscles lie along the temporal bones. The *auricle*—or cartilaginous portion of each ear—lies external to the temporal bone.

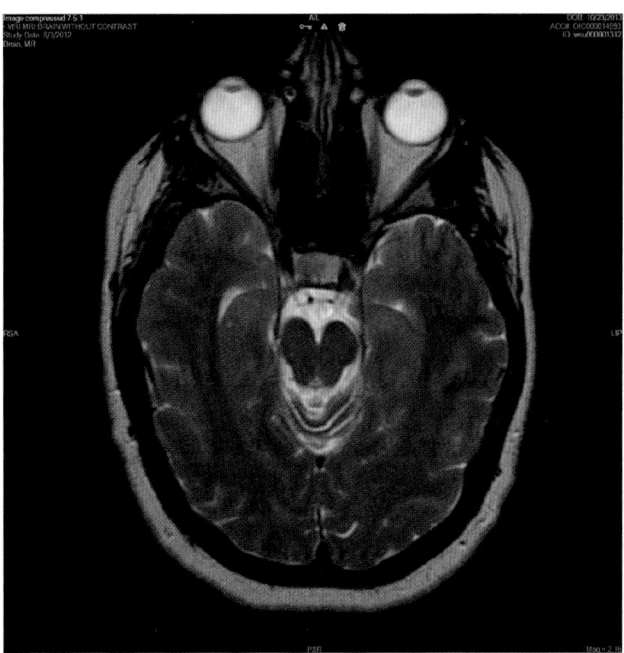

Fig. 24.15 T2-weighted MRI corresponding to the level of *E* in Fig. 24.5B.

The sectional images through the lower cranium show the inferior portions of the cerebrum, brain stem, cerebellum, and associated major skeletal structures. (Fig. 24.16 is a CT image, and Fig. 24.17 is a T1-weighted contrast-enhanced MRI image.) The CT image shows the frontal sinuses and the roofs of the orbits. The greater and lesser wings of the sphenoid bone are shown. The optic foramina (canals) can be seen between the greater and lesser wings. The optic chiasm and cavernous sinus can be seen posterior to the optic foramen. The petrous and mastoid portions of the temporal bones are shown dividing the middle and posterior cranial fossae. The maxilla, *maxillary sinuses*, and nasal bones are seen in the anterior skull on the MRI image (note the mass within the right maxillary sinus). The *zygomatic bones* form the lateral walls of the orbits, and the *maxillae* form the medial walls. The *perpendicular plate* and *vomer* form the bony nasal septum seen in the center of the nasal cavity. Posterior to the nasal cavity, the sphenoidal sinuses are seen between the lower aspects of the greater wings. Both petrous ridges extend toward the midline; these are seen as dark areas on the MRI image because of the lack of signal from this dense region of bone. Extending into the right petrous ridge is the *external auditory canal*. Just anterior to the canal is the *condyle of the mandible,* resting in the mandibular fossa. Mastoid air cells lie posterior to the external acoustic meatus.

In the center of the skull, the greater wings of the sphenoid, petrous ridges, and basilar portion of the occipital bone meet. The CT image shows the lower portions of the frontal lobes and temporal lobes, along with the lower margin of the pons and the cerebellum. On the MRI image, the most inferior folds of the temporal lobes are found in the middle cranial fossae, resting on the greater wings of the sphenoid. The *medulla oblongata* lies posterior to the basilar portion of the occipital bone.

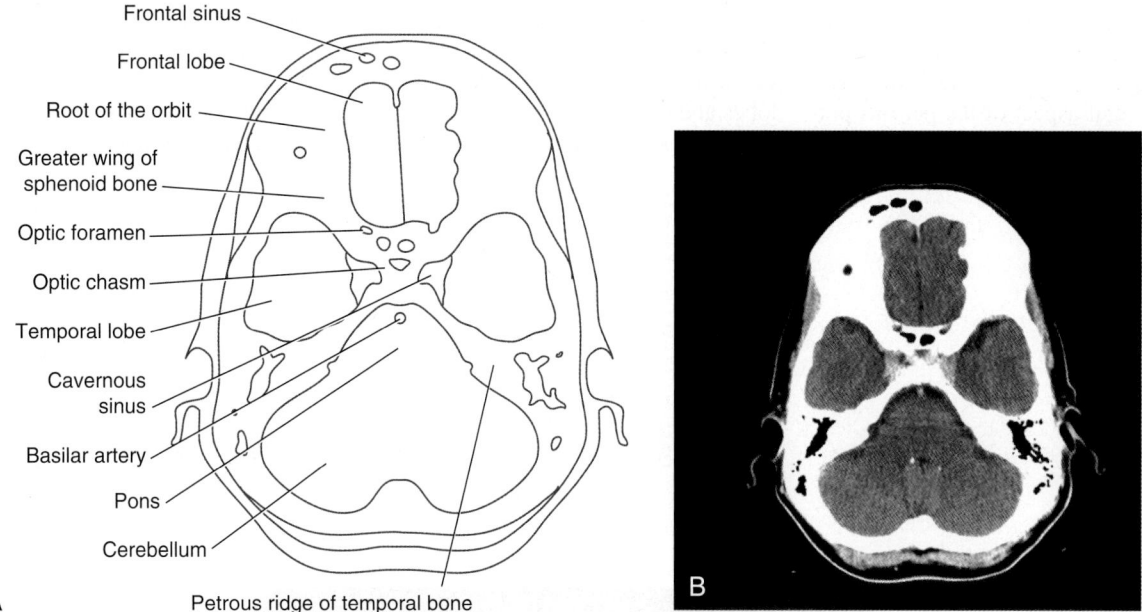

Fig. 24.16 (**A**) Line drawing of CT section. (**B**) CT image representing anatomic structures located at level *F* in Fig. 24.5A.

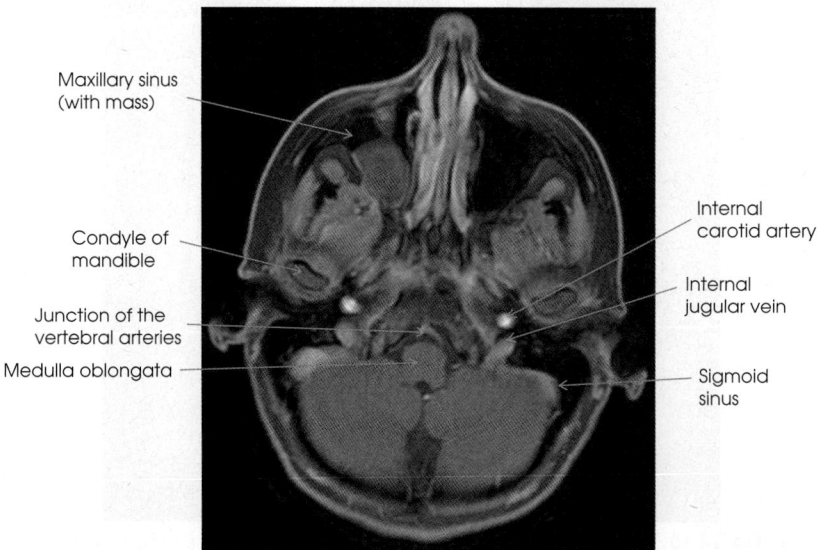

Fig. 24.17 MRI representing anatomic structures located at level *F* in Fig. 24.5B.

The cerebellum is seen within the posterior fossa. The small, dark space between the medulla and the cerebellum is the lower extent of the fourth ventricle. CSF in the *cisterna magna* circulates around the anterior and lateral reaches of the medulla. At the level of this image, the internal carotid arteries are found just posterior to the optic foramina, within the cavernous sinuses, on the CT scan. Both are clearly visible as bright circles on the MRI image. The *internal jugular veins* can also be seen on the MRI image just posterior to the internal carotid arteries. The two *vertebral arteries* join and lie anterior to the medulla on the MRI image. The CT image (see Fig. 24.16) is just superior to the junction of the vertebral arteries and shows the lower part of the basilar artery. The transverse venous sinuses have passed anteriorly to the level of the petrous ridges and are seen on the MRI image (see Fig. 24.17). At this point, they change position and change names to become the *sigmoid sinuses*.

Fig. 24.18 is a CT image, and Fig. 24.19 is a T1-weighted contrast-enhanced MRI image through the lower part of the skull. The plane of the CT image passes through the upper orbit, the sphenoidal sinuses, and the lower portion of the occipital bone. The frontal sinuses lie along the anterior skull. The crista galli is just posterior to these sinuses. This structure is a superior projection of bone from the cribriform plate of the ethmoid bone; it functions as an attachment for the falx cerebri. On either side of the crista galli, the lowermost portions of the frontal lobes can be seen resting on the cribriform plate. The sphenoidal sinuses lie

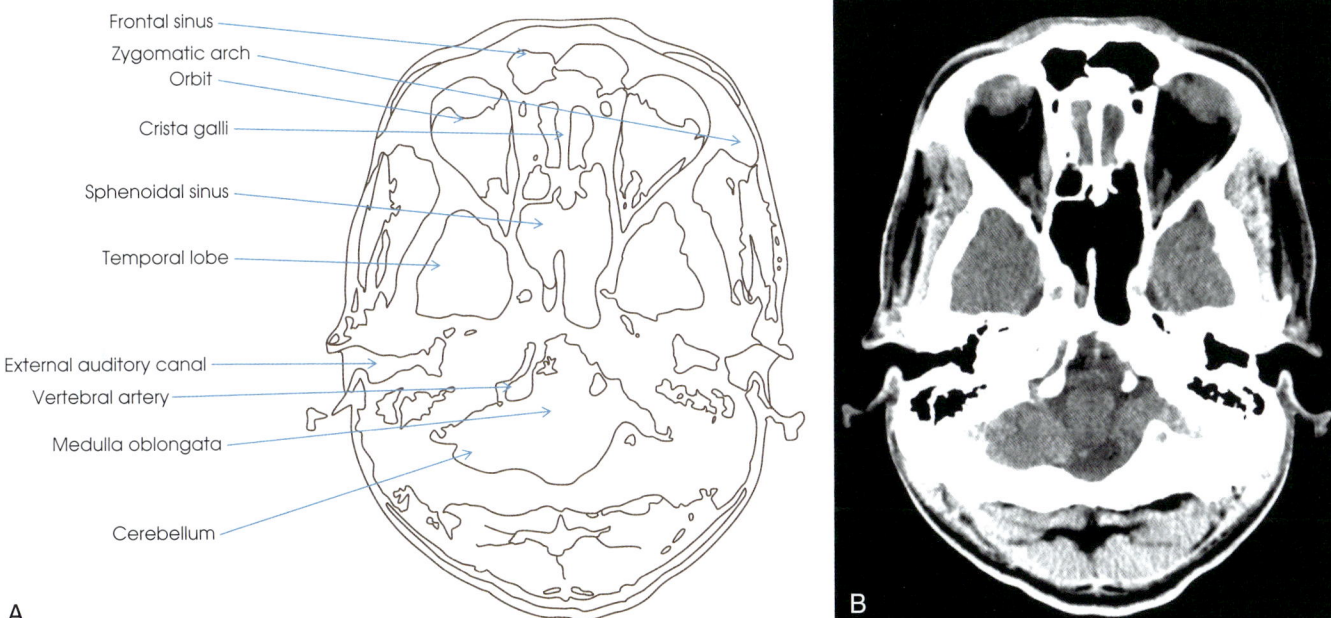

Fig. 24.18 (**A**) Line drawing of CT section. (**B**) CT image representing anatomic structures located at level *G* in Fig. 24.5A.

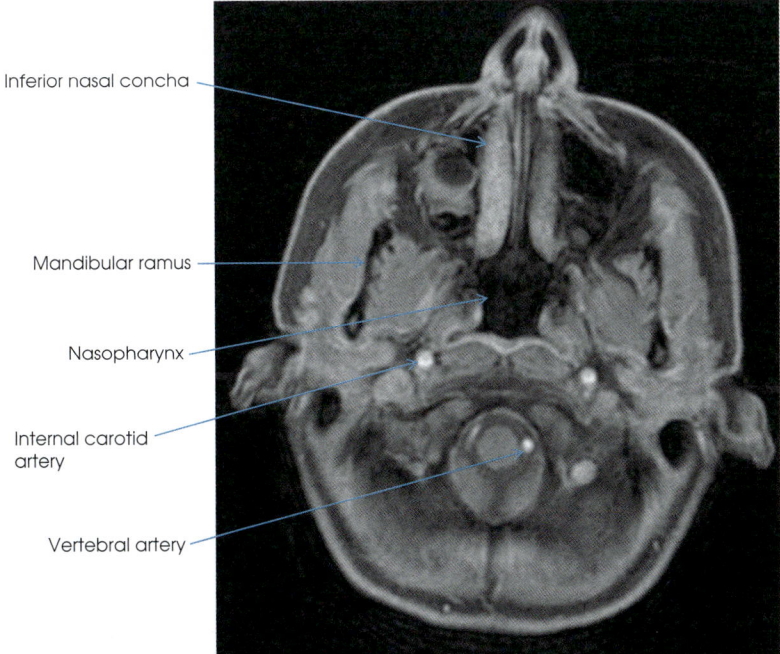

Fig. 24.19 MRI corresponding to level *G* in Fig. 24.5B.

posterior to the crista galli, and the greater wings of the sphenoid extend laterally from the region of the sinuses. The external auditory canals extend into the petrous portions of the temporal bones, and mastoid air cells are visible posterior to the canals. The lower portion of the occipital bone forms the most posterior region of the skull on this image.

The MRI image plane passes through the nose and the base of the skull. On the MRI image, air-filled maxillary sinuses lie on either side of the nose. The *inferior nasal conchae* and the vomer are seen within the nasal cavity. Posterior to the nasal cavity, the nasopharynx is seen on the MRI image. Portions of the zygomatic arches are seen extending posteriorly from the sides of the sinuses on CT. The MRI image is slightly inferior to the mandibular condyles and shows the rami of the mandible. The MRI image passes through the mastoid processes and the top of the vertebral column. The CT shows the lower temporal lobes of the cerebrum, the *cerebellar tonsils*, and the medulla oblongata. The MRI image shows the spinal cord because the structures in this image lie inferior to the foramen magnum. The contrast-filled internal carotid arteries lie anterior and lateral to the foramen magnum and spinal cord on the MRI image but are not visible on the CT image. As the sigmoid venous sinuses pass through the jugular foramina, they become the internal jugular veins. These veins are visible on the MRI image posterior and lateral to the internal carotid arteries. The contrast-filled vertebral arteries are seen along the anterolateral aspects of the medulla and spinal cord. Muscular structures on the external surface of the mandible are the *masseters*, and the structures on the internal surface are the *pterygoids*.

Images in sagittal, coronal, and oblique planes are becoming increasingly more common. CT scanners have the capability to generate images in the axial and coronal planes and to reconstruct the information in alternate planes. Magnetic resonance is capable of direct axial, sagittal, oblique, and coronal imaging. Representative images have been selected in the sagittal and coronal planes to help interpret the anatomy shown.

Fig. 24.20 is a PA skull (Caldwell method) image used to represent the locations of the following sagittal images of the brain. Fig. 24.21 is a midsagittal T1-weighted MRI image of the cranium. The relationship among the cerebral hemisphere, cerebellum, and brain stem is shown. In this image, the frontal, parietal, and occipital lobes of the cerebrum are seen and correspond to the cranial bones. The corpus callosum is a white matter tract that connects the hemispheres and is found at the inferior aspect of the frontal and parietal lobes. CSF appears dark on this T1-weighted image, making it easy to trace the ventricular system. The anterior horn of the lateral ventricle is inferior to the genu of the corpus callosum. The third ventricle lies in the midline between the two lateral ventricles. The lateral ventricles produce a great deal of CSF, which is transported to the third ventricle by way of the *intraventricular foramina (of Monro)*. The third ventricle is not optimally visualized in this image. What is seen is the thalamus, which forms the lateral wall of the third ventricle. CSF drains from the third ventricle via the *cerebral aqueduct (of Sylvius)*, which can be found within the midbrain (between the *corpora quadrigemina* and the *cerebral peduncles*). The *fourth ventricle* is also a triangular-shaped midline structure that is situated between the pons and cerebellum. The large air-filled sphenoidal sinus is located anterior to the pons. Superior to this sinus, the pituitary gland rests within hypophyseal fossa formed by the sella turcica. Directly superior to the pituitary gland is the optic chiasm.

Several vascular structures are well shown in Fig. 24.21. The basilar artery appears between the clivus and pons. Portions of the superior sagittal sinus can be seen between the cerebrum and the cranial

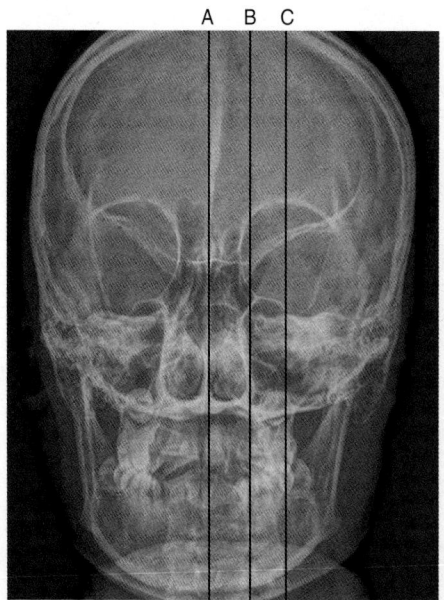

Fig. 24.20 PA projection of skull for localization of sagittal images.

bones. Between the cerebrum and cerebellum, the *straight sinus* (one of the dural venous sinuses) is noted within the tentorium cerebelli. This vessel is formed by the junction of the inferior sagittal sinus and the great cerebral vein (of Galen).

Fig. 24.22 is a sagittal T2-weighted MRI image through the medial wall of the orbit. The bright, fluid-filled lateral ventricle is seen in the center of the cerebral hemisphere. Just inferior to it are the caudate nucleus and the thalamus. Because this image was obtained in a plane lateral to the midline, one of the cerebral peduncles is seen at the inferior border of the thalamus, and one of the cerebellar peduncles can be seen connecting the pons to the cerebellum. At the floor of the cranium, a dark circle is seen that represents the internal carotid artery. Cerebral vertebral bodies and arches can be seen in the neck on either side of the vertebral canal. In the face, the ethmoid sinus and tongue can be easily identified.

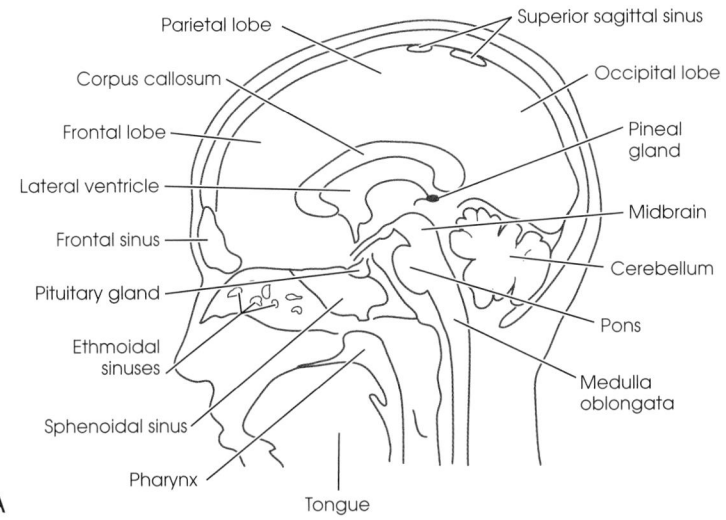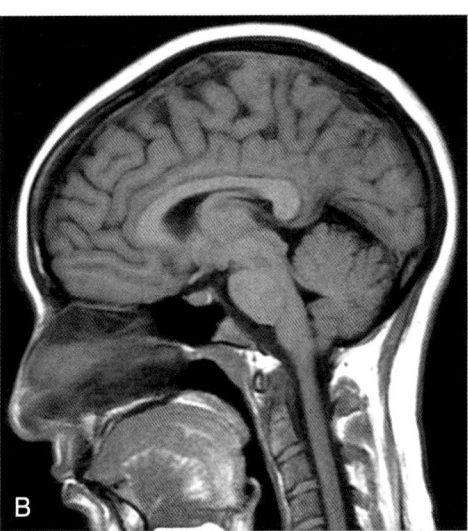

Fig. 24.21 (**A**) Line drawing of MRI section. (**B**) MRI through midsagittal plane, corresponding to level *A* in Fig. 24.20.

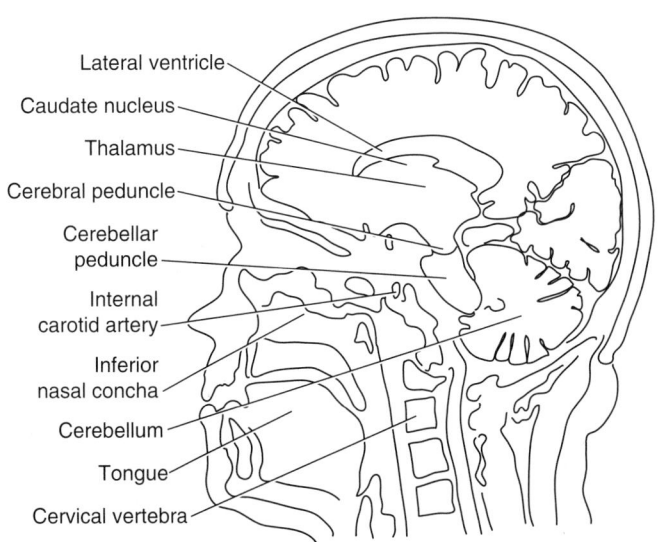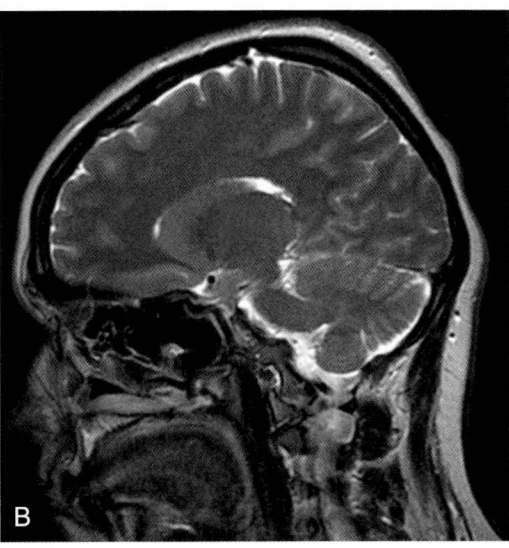

Fig. 24.22 (**A**) Line drawing of MRI section. (**B**) Sagittal MRI through medial wall of orbit corresponding to level *B* in Fig. 24.20.

The sagittal T2-weighted MRI image in Fig. 24.23 is sectioned through the center of the orbit. The frontal, parietal, occipital, and temporal lobes of the cerebrum all are visible. Within the cerebrum, CSF is seen within the temporal and posterior horns of the lateral ventricle (the fluid appears bright in this T2-weighted image). The cerebellum lies within the posterior fossa and is separated from the cerebrum by the tentorium cerebelli. Anterior to the cerebellum, the lateral aspect of the fourth ventricle can be seen. Within the orbit, several structures associated with the eye can be seen: the globe and the inferior rectus muscle. The dark area inferior to the orbit is the air-filled maxillary sinus. The medial pterygoid muscle, which lies on the internal aspect of the mandibular ramus, is visible inferior and posterior to the maxillary sinus.

A CT localizer—or scout—image (Fig. 24.24) is included as a reference for the next three coronal images. Fig. 24.25 is a coronal T2-weighted MRI image through the anterior horns of the lateral ventricles and the pharyngeal structures. The anterior portions of the cerebral hemispheres are joined by the corpus callosum, which is immediately superior to the lateral ventricles. The membrane between the anterior horns of the lateral ventricles is the *septum pellucidum*. On the lateral aspect

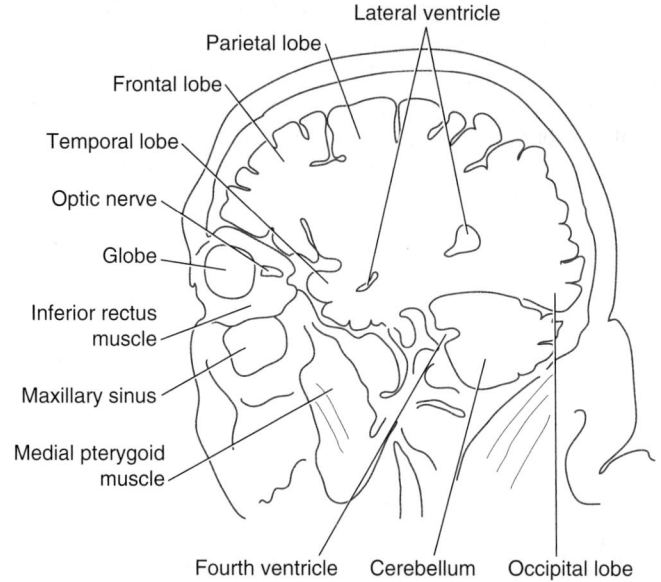

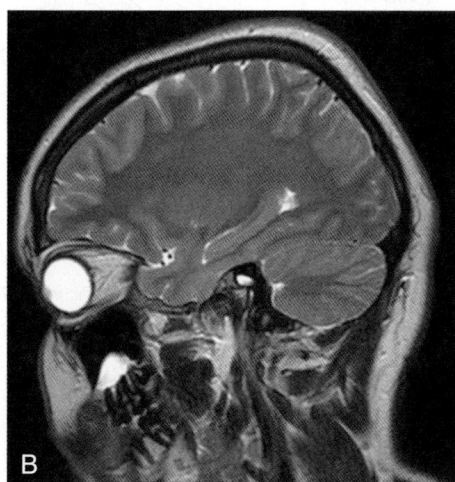

Fig. 24.23 (**A**) Line drawing of MRI section. (**B**) Sagittal MRI through midorbit corresponding to level *C* in Fig. 24.20.

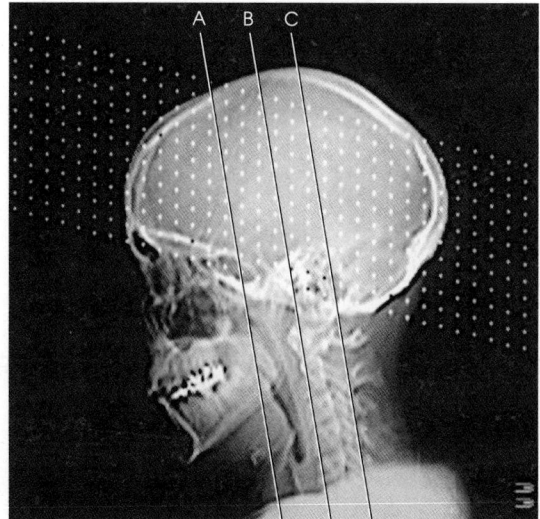

Fig. 24.24 CT localizer (scout) image of skull.

of each cerebral hemisphere is the *lateral fissure*, which divides the frontal lobe from the temporal lobe. The insula lies deep to this fissure.

Structures of the basal nuclei can be faintly identified. The caudate nucleus is lateral to the anterior horns. Inferolateral to the caudate nuclei are the internal capsules—white matter tracts that connect the cortex to deeper gray matter structures. The anterior portion of the third ventricle is found in the midline inferior to the lateral ventricles. Inferior to the third ventricle are the optic chiasm and pituitary gland (hypophysis cerebri). The *superior* and *inferior sagittal sinuses* occupy the margins of the falx cerebri in the longitudinal fissure between the hemispheres of the cerebrum. The internal carotid arteries occupy the *cavernous sinuses* along with several cranial nerves and are found lateral to the pituitary gland and sella turcica. Branches of the middle cerebral arteries occupy the lateral fissures of the cerebrum. Fig. 24.26 is a coronal T2-weighted MRI image through the bodies of the lateral ventricles, brain stem, and bodies of the cervical vertebrae. The third ventricle is well shown and bordered laterally by the thalamus. The dark region (low signal return) medial to the external acoustic canal corresponds to the *petrous portion of the temporal bone*. The first two

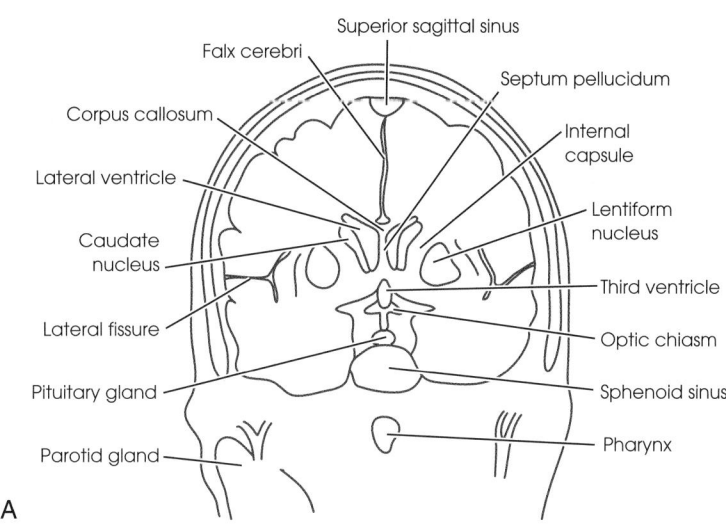

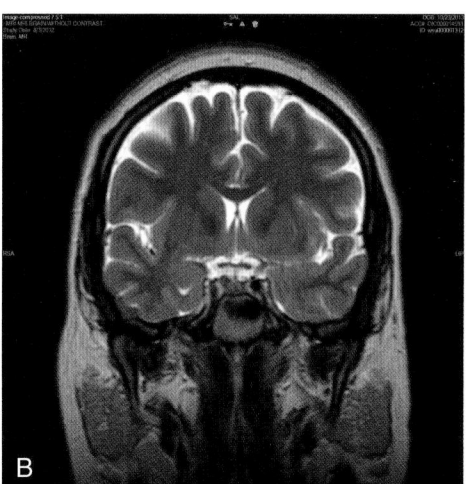

Fig. 24.25 (**A**) Line drawing of MRI section. (**B**) Coronal MRI corresponding to level *A* in Fig. 24.24.

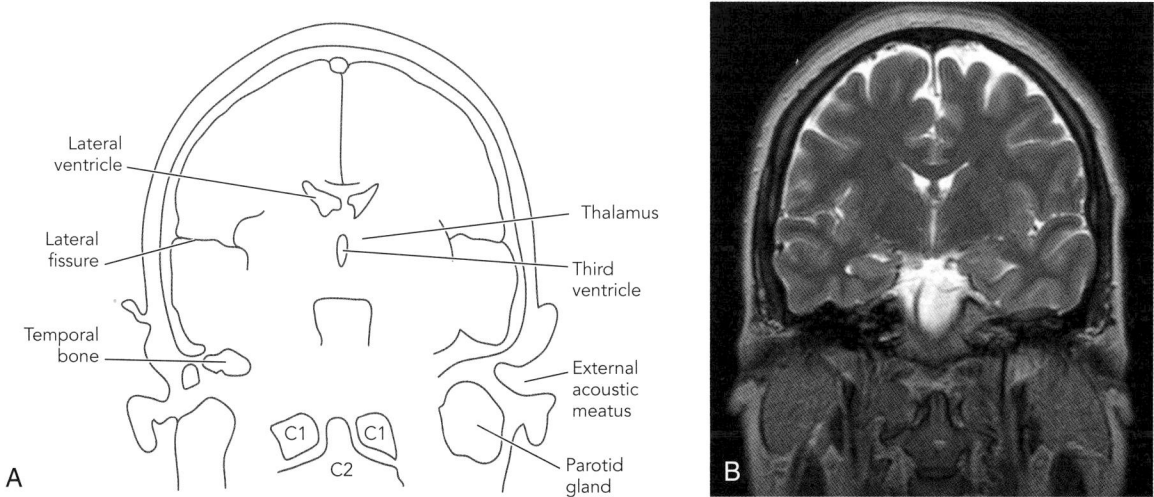

Fig. 24.26 (**A**) Line drawing of gross anatomic section. (**B**) MRI corresponding to bodies of the lateral ventricles, brain stem, and cervical vertebrae.

cervical vertebrae are detailed in this section with the *dens* of the *axis* (C2) seen between the lateral masses of the *atlas* (C1). The large, intermediate gray masses inferior to the external acoustic canals are the *parotid glands*.

Fig. 24.27 shows a coronal T2-weighted MRI image through the posterior lateral ventricles and cerebellum. The splenium of the corpus callosum is found between the lateral ventricles. Inferior to the splenium is the superior cistern. Portions of the cerebellum are visualized superior and inferior to the middle cerebellar peduncles. The large, bright area near the center of the cerebellum is the fourth ventricle. The bright line between the cerebellum and cerebrum represents the tentorium cerebelli. The large, dark areas (low signal) lateral to the cerebellum correspond to the bony mastoid portions of the temporal bone.

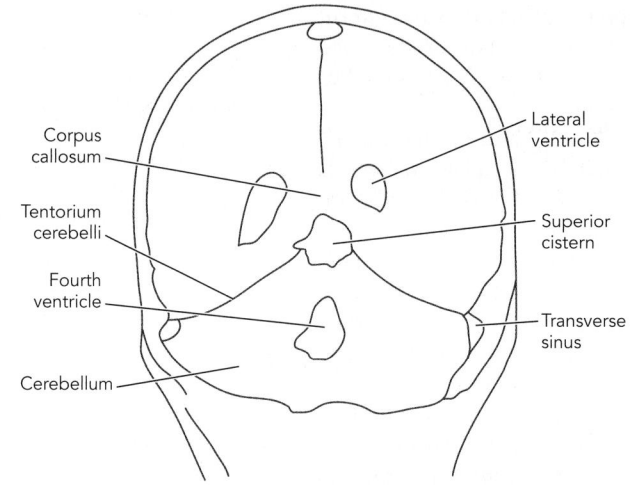

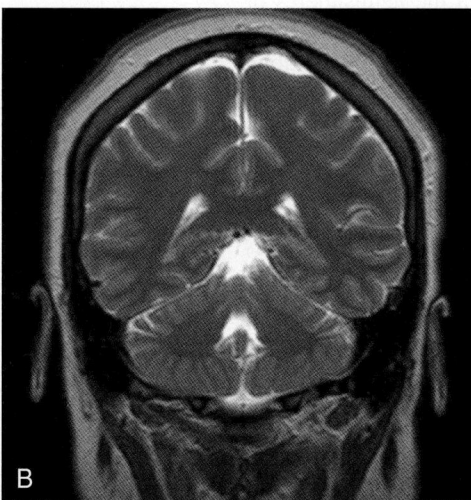

Fig. 24.27 (**A**) Line drawing of gross anatomic section. (**B**) MRI corresponding to lateral ventricles and cerebellum.

Thoracic Region

The thorax extends from the thoracic inlet to the diaphragm. The inlet is an imaginary plane through the first thoracic vertebra and the top of the manubrium. Sectional images of the thorax are obtained to include all structures between these boundaries. Two cadaveric images are included to assist in identifying some of the structures of the thorax. Fig. 24.28 is a cadaveric image that corresponds to a level just superior to the sternoclavicular joints. Fig. 24.33 (presented later in the chapter) lies near the level of the sixth thoracic vertebra and shows the chambers of the heart and other surrounding structures.

The bones of the thorax include the thoracic vertebrae, ribs, sternum, clavicles, and scapulae. Each of the 12 thoracic vertebrae is subdivided into a body and a vertebral arch. The opening formed between these divisions is the vertebral foramen, through which the spinal cord travels. Two pedicles, two laminae, two transverse processes, and one spinous process constitute the arch. The pedicles are more anterior and unite with the body of the vertebra; the laminae form the posterior part of the arch and unite to give rise to the spinous process. Transverse processes arise from the lateral arch where pedicles and laminae meet. Two superior articular processes arise from the superior arch, and two inferior articular processes arise from the inferior arch. Superior and inferior articular processes from adjacent vertebrae articulate to form zygapophyseal joints. Notches between succeeding arches form the intervertebral foramina. These foramina transmit spinal nerves. Articular disks are found between the vertebral bodies. These disks are composed of a dense cartilaginous outer rim called the *annulus fibrosus* and a gelatinous central core called the *nucleus pulposus*. Twelve pairs of ribs curl around the lateral thorax to protect the lungs and heart. The head of each rib is posterior and articulates with the body of a thoracic vertebra. These joints are called *costovertebral joints*. Tubercles of the ribs are lateral to the heads and articulate with transverse processes of the vertebrae, forming costotransverse joints. Anteriorly, the first 10 pairs of ribs articulate with the sternum either directly or indirectly via costal cartilage. The sternum lies in the midline of the anterior chest wall. From superior to inferior, the parts are the manubrium, body, and xiphoid process. An indentation

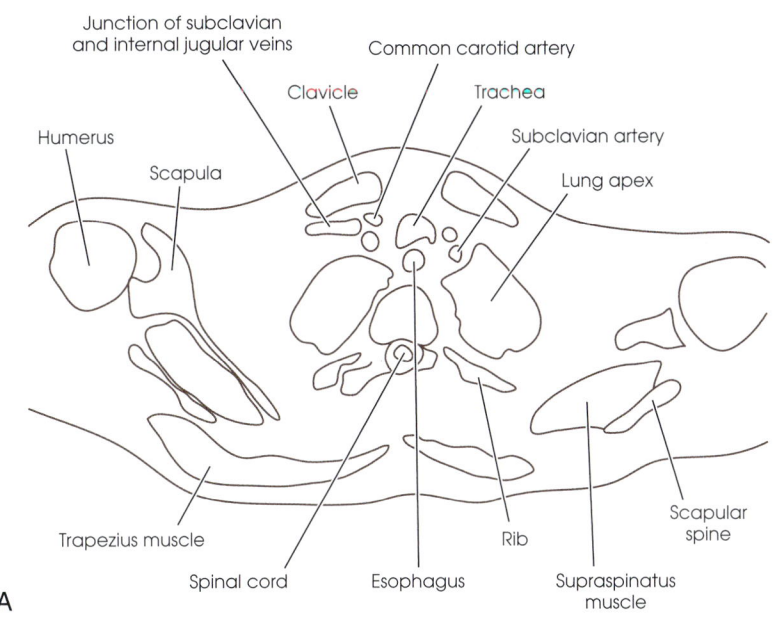

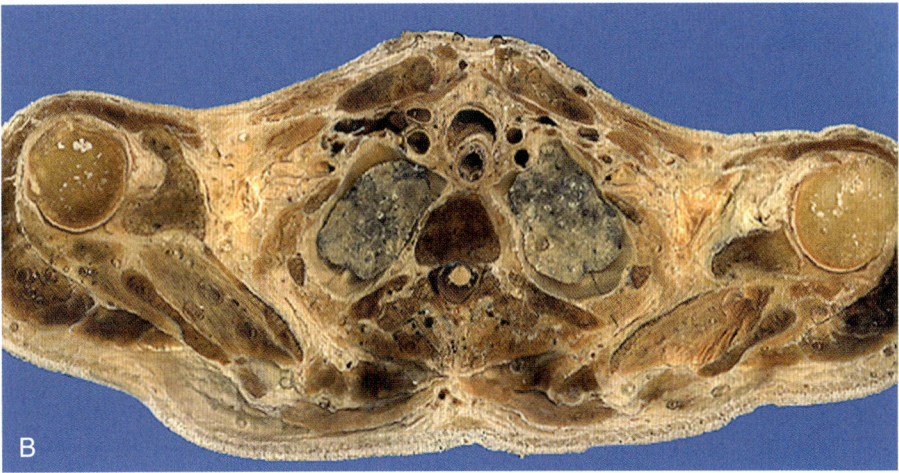

Fig. 24.28 (**A**) Line drawing of gross anatomic section. (**B**) Cadaveric image of superior thorax.

at the superior edge of the sternum, the jugular or sternal notch, lies at the level of the interspace between the second and third thoracic vertebrae. The manubrium joins the body of the sternum at the sternal angle, which corresponds to the interspace between the fourth and fifth thoracic vertebrae. The xiphoid process lies at approximately the level of the 10th thoracic vertebra. Familiarity with these vertebral levels can be helpful in orienting oneself when looking at thoracic sectional images.

The clavicles are slender, S-shaped bones that extend across the upper anterior thorax. The medial end of each clavicle articulates with the superolateral edge of the manubrium to form sternoclavicular joints. Acromioclavicular joints are formed where the lateral extremity of the clavicle articulates with the acromion process of the scapula. The scapulae are triangular bones in the superior posterior thorax. Thinking of the scapula as having two surfaces (anterior and posterior), three borders (superior, medial, and lateral), and three angles (superior, lateral, and inferior) is helpful. The posterior surface is divided into a superior fossa and an inferior fossa by the scapular spine. This bony ridge extends laterally and superiorly to end as the acromion process. The coracoid process projects from the superoanterior surface near the glenoid. The lateral angle is formed by the glenoid cavity, which articulates with the humeral head. Many of these bony structures are identifiable in Fig. 24.28.

Major components of the respiratory system are seen in the thorax. The trachea originates at the level of the sixth cervical vertebra (near the bottom of the thyroid cartilage). The trachea is formed by incomplete cartilage rings, which are open along its posterior surface. The trachea passes into the thorax and bifurcates into the right and left main bronchi near the level of the sternal angle (T4–5). The carina is the last cartilage ring of the trachea. The main bronchi pass through the hila of the lungs and branch to secondary bronchi, one for each lobe. The lungs are triangular organs enclosed in the thoracic cavity by the double-walled pleural membrane. The portion of the lung that lies superior to the clavicle is the apex; the part that rests on the diaphragm is the base. The most inferior and posterior reaches of the base constitute a region called the *costophrenic angle*. The bronchi and vascular structures enter and exit the center of the medial aspect of the lung at the hilum. Each lung is divided into superior and inferior lobes by an oblique fissure. The upper lobe of the right lung is divided further by a horizontal fissure to form a middle lobe that lies lateral to the heart. The portion of the left lung that corresponds in position to the right middle lobe is called the *lingula*.

The area between the lungs is the mediastinum. Within this cavity are the heart, trachea and bronchi, esophagus, major blood vessels, nerves, and lymphatic structures. The heart lies obliquely oriented in the lower mediastinum, surrounded by a double-walled fibrous sac called the *pericardium*. It rests on the diaphragm between the sternum and the thoracic spine. The superior surface is the base, and the inferior portion is the apex. The heart is divided into four chambers: two atria and two ventricles. The atria receive blood, and the ventricles pump blood away from the heart. The right atrium forms the right border of the heart and receives blood from the superior vena cava, inferior vena cava, and coronary sinus (the venous drainage channel for the heart muscle). Blood passes from here through the tricuspid (right atrioventricular) valve into the right ventricle. This chamber forms most of the anterior surface of the heart. As this ventricle contracts, blood passes through the right ventricular outflow tract, through the pulmonary semilunar valve, and into the main pulmonary artery toward the lungs. The left atrium forms the posterior border of the heart and receives blood from four pulmonary veins. Blood passes through the mitral (bicuspid or left atrioventricular) valve into the left ventricle. The most muscular of the chambers—the left ventricle—forms the left side and inferiormost portion of the heart. Blood is pumped out of the left ventricle through the left ventricular outflow tract through the aortic semilunar valve and into the aorta. A muscular wall—the interventricular septum—can be seen between the ventricles. Chambers of the heart are seen in Fig. 24.29.

One portion of the digestive system is typically found in the thorax. The esophagus originates at the level of the sixth cervical vertebra as the posterior continuation of the pharynx. It continues into the thorax, at first posterior to the trachea, and then posterior to the left atrium and ventricle of the heart. At the lower thorax, the esophagus pierces the diaphragm to continue into the abdomen.

The vascular system in the upper thorax can be confusing. To identify these structures, one must clearly understand the vascular anatomy. Tracing the paths of vessels through the scan can help alleviate some of the confusion. This discussion follows the path of circulation through the vessels. The discussion of arterial structures starts at the heart and follows the vessels toward the periphery. Veins are discussed from their peripheral origins and followed as they travel toward the heart.

The aorta originates from the left ventricle of the heart. Just distal to the aortic semilunar valve are the origins of the right and left coronary arteries, which supply the heart muscle. The aorta ascends along the posterior sternum, arches posterior and toward the left behind the sternal angle, and turns inferiorly to become the descending aorta. The descending aorta passes down the posterior thorax, resting against the left anterolateral surfaces of the vertebral bodies. The major vessels that supply the head and upper limbs arise from the aortic arch. From anterior to posterior, these are the brachiocephalic, left common carotid, and left subclavian arteries. The brachiocephalic artery passes superiorly and bifurcates into the right subclavian and right common carotid arteries posterior to the sternoclavicular joint. The right and left common carotid arteries ascend the neck along the lateral surface of the trachea. At approximately the level of the third cervical vertebra, each common carotid artery exhibits a dilation called the *carotid sinus* just proximal to bifurcating into internal and external carotid arteries. The subclavian arteries pass laterally across the upper thorax, just deep to the clavicles. At the outer edges of the first ribs, the subclavian arteries become the axillary arteries.

Venous drainage from the head is mainly through the jugular veins. The internal jugular veins accompany the carotid arteries down through the neck, lateral to the trachea. The subclavian veins are continuations of the axillary veins draining the upper limbs. These veins pass toward the midline, deep to the clavicles. At the sternoclavicular joints, the internal jugular veins and the subclavian veins unite to form the brachiocephalic veins. The right brachiocephalic vein passes vertically downward; the left passes obliquely down, posterior to the manubrium. These two vessels unite to form the superior vena cava. The superior vena cava lies posterior to the right border of the sternum and enters the right atrium just below the level of the sternal angle. Venous drainage from the lower body is via the inferior vena cava. This vessel is found along the right anterior surface of the vertebral bodies and empties into the inferior aspect of the right atrium. The azygos vein is a small vessel that passes up the posterior thorax along the right anterior aspect of the vertebral bodies. It arches anteriorly (near the level of the aortic arch) to drain into the superior vena cava.

The pulmonary vascular system transports blood between the lungs and heart. The main pulmonary artery receives deoxygenated blood from the right ventricle. At the level of the sternal angle, this vessel gives rise to the right and left pulmonary arteries, which pass laterally toward the hila of the lungs. The bifurcation of the main pulmonary artery is just inferior to the aortic arch. Four pulmonary veins exit the hila, two from each lung, and pass medially to enter the superolateral aspect of the left atrium.

Many muscles can be seen in the thorax, especially in the shoulder region. The pectoralis major is a large, fan-shaped muscle superficially located along the anterior chest wall. The pectoralis minor lies just deep to the pectoralis major. The trapezius is the most superficial of the posterior thoracic muscles. The rhomboid major and minor muscles are deep to the trapezius and lie between the medial scapular borders and the spinous processes of the upper thoracic spine. The serratus anterior muscles attach to the medial side of the anterior scapula and blanket the external surface of the rib cage. Several muscles are associated with the scapula; many of these also attach to the humerus. The subscapularis muscle lines the anterior surface. Supraspinatus and infraspinatus muscles lie in the supraspinous and infraspinous fossae. The teres major and teres minor also lie along the infraspinous fossa. Four of these muscles are collectively known as the rotator cuff: subscapularis, supraspinatus, infraspinatus, and teres minor.

The CT localizer—or scout—image represents an AP projection of the thoracic region with identifying lines (Fig. 24.30). These lines show the approximate levels for each of the labeled images for this region. Most of the images for this region are CT scans. When performing scans of the thorax, the patient's arms are extended above the head. This fact must be kept in mind when looking at upper thoracic scans because some anatomic structures do not correspond to the normal anatomic position. MRI images are frequently degraded by motion artifact in the thorax, so only a few representative images are included.

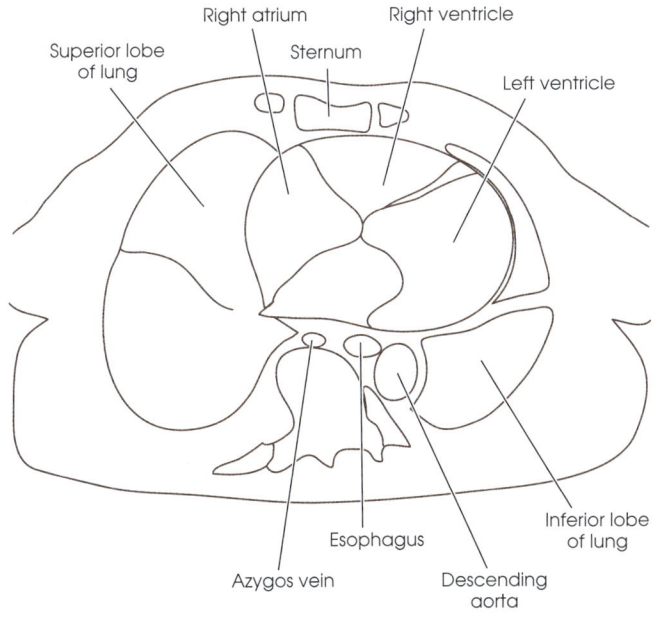
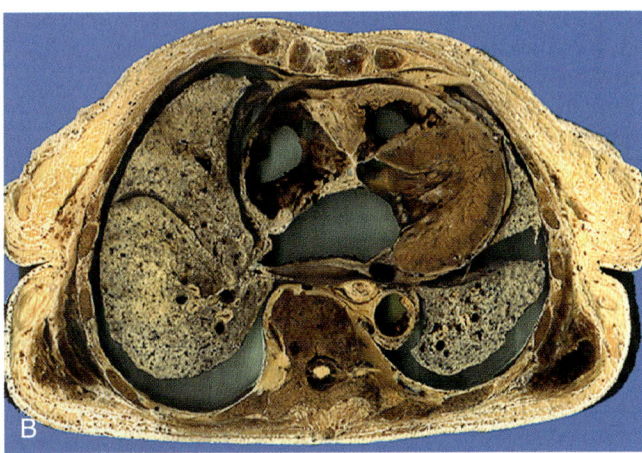

Fig. 24.29 (**A**) Line drawing of gross anatomic section. (**B**) Cadaveric image of central thorax.

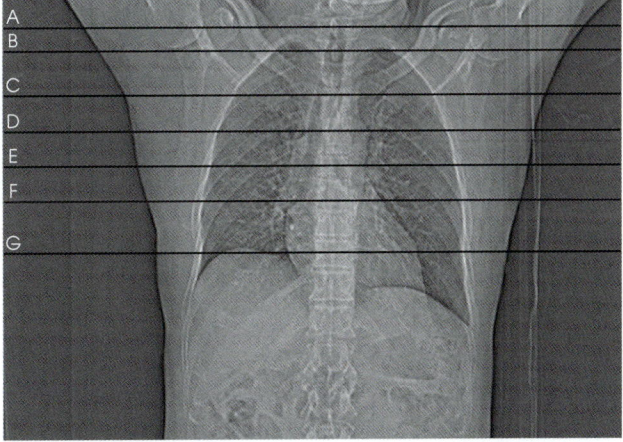

Fig. 24.30 CT localizer (scout) image of thorax.

Figs. 24.31B and C show a CT and T2-weighted MRI images at the level of T1 and show the relationship between the vertebral column, esophagus, and trachea. The body and *vertebral arch* of the first thoracic vertebra can be identified, and the spinal cord is seen in the vertebral foramen. The *costotransverse joint* between the first rib and the transverse process of the first thoracic vertebra is seen on the patient's left. Because the patient's arms are raised on the CT image, the scan passes through the surgical neck of the humerus. The inferior portion of the *thyroid gland*, which extends from C6 to T1, is positioned lateral to the *trachea*. The soft tissue shadow immediately posterior to the trachea is the *esophagus*. The outer esophageal lining is well demonstrated on the MRI image. The *vertebral arteries* are positioned lateral to the vertebral column, and the *common carotid arteries* are found lateral to the trachea. At this level, the *internal jugular veins* are positioned to the lateral aspect of the carotid arteries. The CT image demonstrates the contrast-filled axillary arteries in the medial aspect of the arms. The *sternocleidomastoid muscles* are found lateral to the thyroid gland. The *trapezius* is the most superficial muscle of the posterior thorax, with the levator scapulae muscles lying just anterior.

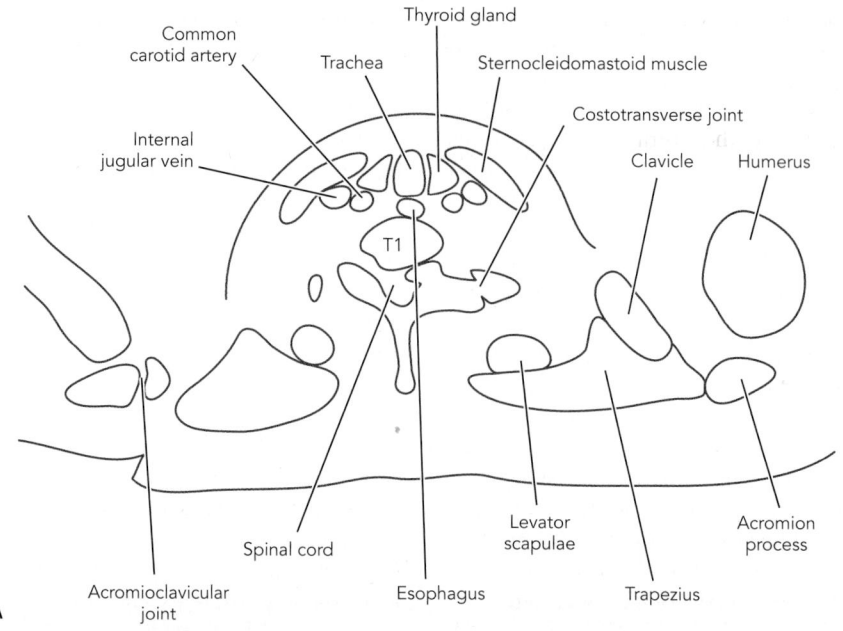

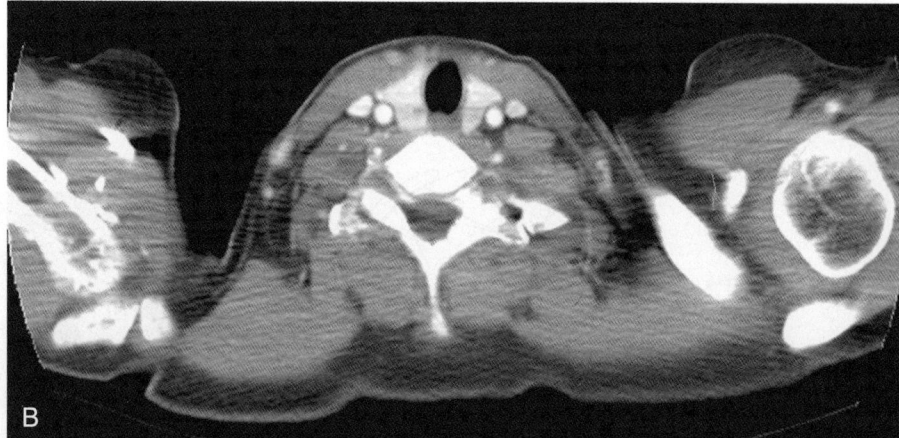

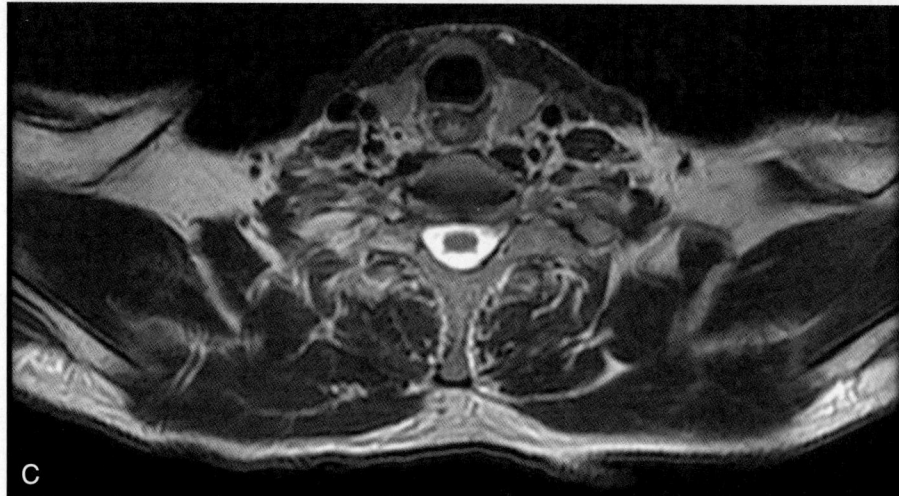

Fig. 24.31 (**A**) Line drawing of CT section. (**B**) CT image, and (**C**) MRI image corresponding to level A in Fig. 24.30 through first thoracic vertebra.

Figs. 24.32B and C show a CT and T2-weighted MRI images through the lower edge of T2. These scans pass through the *jugular notch* of the sternum and are just superior to the sternoclavicular joints. The CT image demonstrates the costovertebral and costotransverse joints that are seen between the ribs and the spine. On the right, the glenoid portion and the acromion process of the scapula are seen. The humerus is visible where it articulates with the glenoid cavity. On the left, the spine and the body of the scapula are seen. Both images demonstrate the *trachea* and esophagus located anterior to the vertebral body. The major vessels of the superior thorax are visualized posterior to the clavicles. The right and left *brachiocephalic veins* are formed by the junction of the *subclavian veins* and the internal jugular veins. Because contrast medium was injected for the CT scan, the axillary and most of the right subclavian vein are filled with contrast medium. Posterior to the right clavicle, the right subclavian vein and internal jugular vein have joined. Because the CT image is slightly more inferior on the left, the image plane passes through the left brachiocephalic vein (below the junction of these two vessels). The brachiocephalic veins unite and form the *superior vena cava* at a more inferior level. The arterial branches to the head and upper limb are also well visualized on the CT image. From the patient's right to left, they are situated as the *right subclavian artery*, *right common carotid artery*, *left common carotid artery*, and *left subclavian artery*. The brachiocephalic artery gives rise to the right subclavian and right common carotid arteries and is inferior to this level. The *pectoralis major* and *pectoralis minor* lie along the anterior thoracic wall. The trapezius is the most superficial of the posterior muscles and is seen between the scapula and the spine on each side. The *subscapularis muscle* lines the left anterior scapula, the *infraspinatus* and *teres minor* line the posterior portion of this bone, and the *supraspinatus* is seen between the body and the scapular spine.

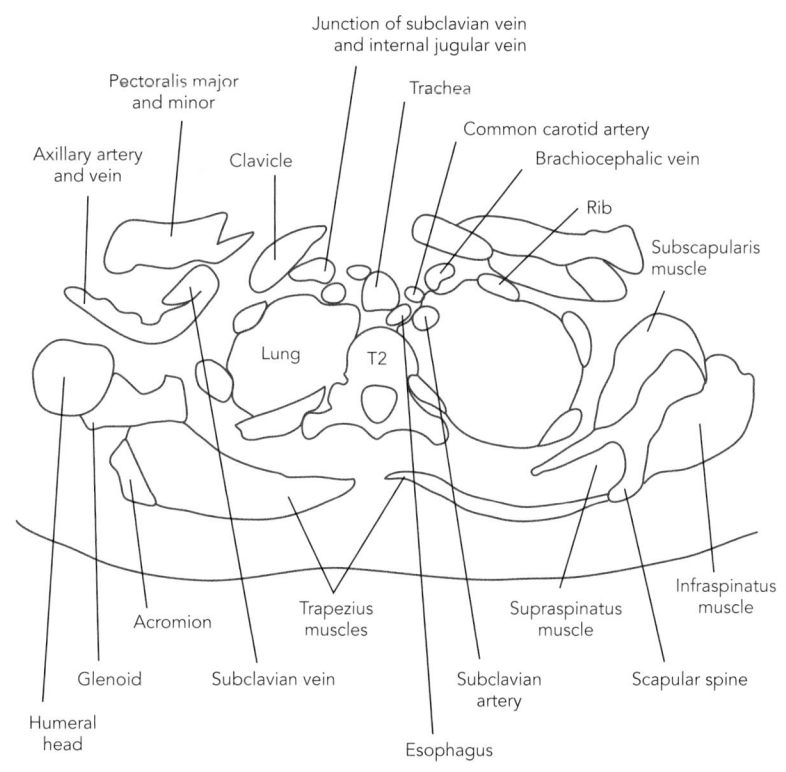

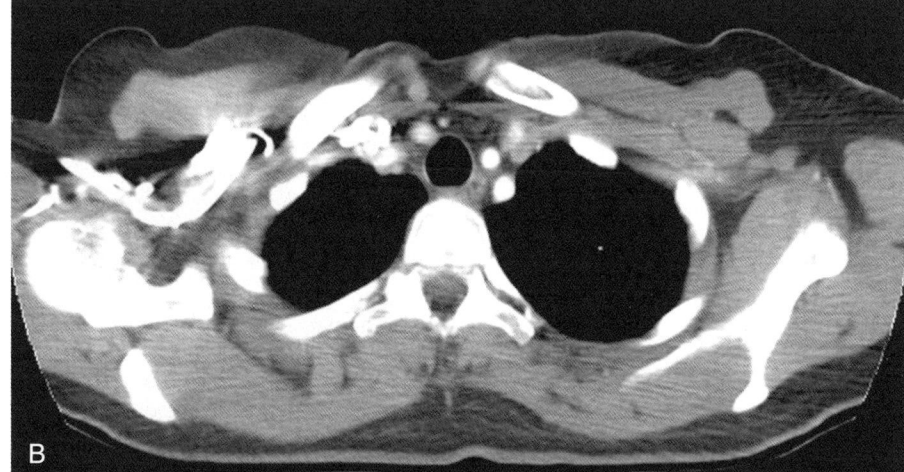

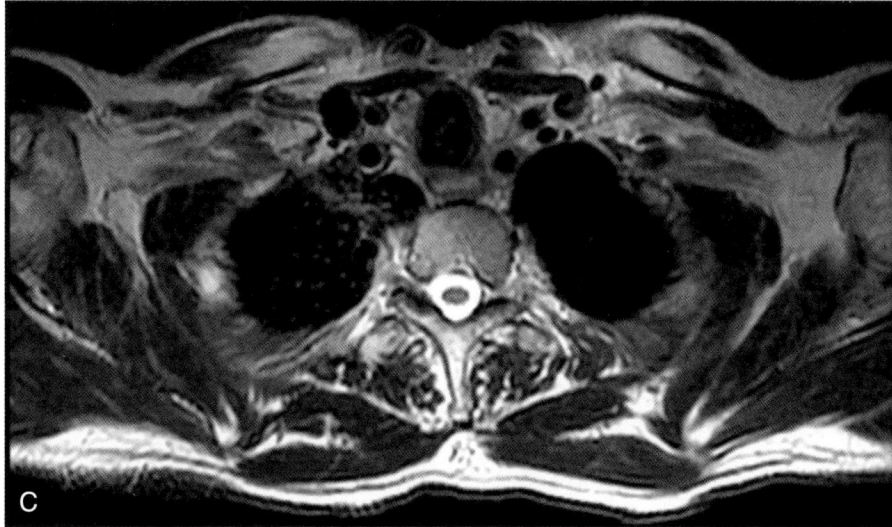

Fig. 24.32 (**A**) Line drawing of CT section. (**B**) CT image, and (**C**) MRI image corresponding to level *B* in Fig. 24.30 through jugular notch.

Fig. 24.33 is a CT image through the level of T3. Bony structures depicted in this image include the *manubrium* and sternoclavicular joints anteriorly, the ribs laterally, and the scapulae and vertebra posteriorly. The spine and the body of the right scapula are visible at this level. Costovertebral and costotransverse joints are noted along the right side of the vertebra. Several vascular structures, highlighted with contrast medium, are visible posterior to the manubrium. The right and left brachiocephalic veins are seen just posterior to the right sternoclavicular joint. This level is just superior to where the vessels join to form the superior vena cava. The brachiocephalic artery, left common carotid artery, and left subclavian artery curl around the left side of the trachea. This scan is just superior to the arch of the aorta and visualizes the origins of these three vessels. Posterior to the vessels are the trachea and esophagus. The upper lobes of each lung lie lateral to the mediastinal structures. The pectoralis major and

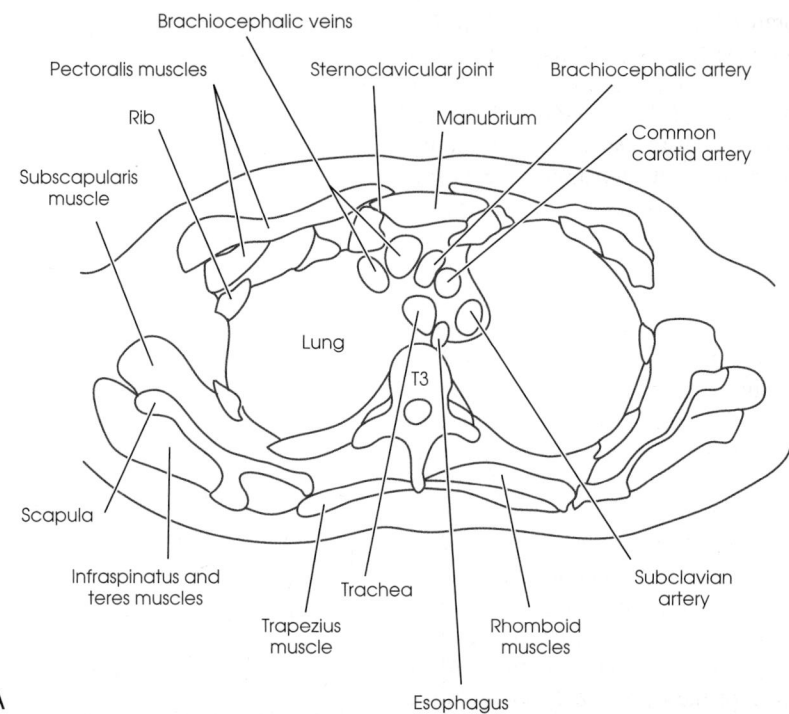

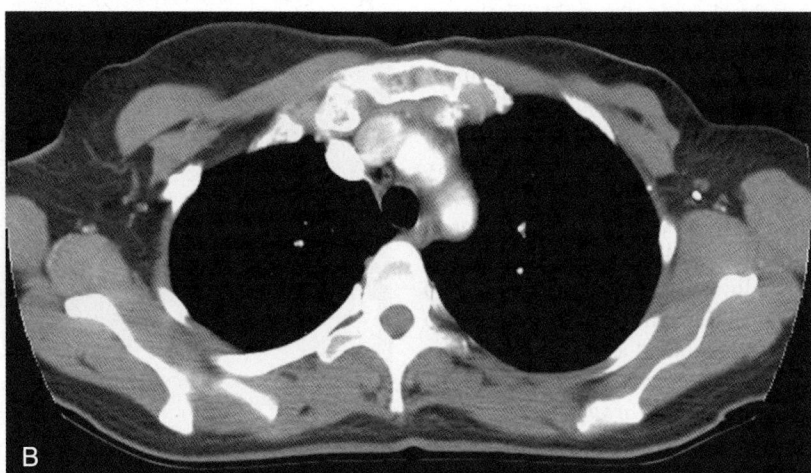

Fig. 24.33 (**A**) Line drawing of CT section. (**B**) CT image corresponding to level *C* in Fig. 24.30 just superior to aortic arch.

pectoralis minor lie external to the anterior ribs. Rotator cuff muscles (subscapularis, infraspinatus, and teres minor) are shown anterior and posterior to the scapulae. The trapezius and *rhomboid muscles* lie between the scapulae and the spinous process of the vertebra in this image.

Fig. 24.34 is a CT scan obtained through the lower edge of T4. At this level, the brachiocephalic veins have joined to form the *superior vena cava*. The large contrast-filled structure in the left anterolateral mediastinum is the *aortic arch*.

Fig. 24.35 is a CT image at the level of T5 and shows the great vessels superior to the heart. (The heart is normally positioned between T7 and T11, with most of the organ lying left of the midline). The *ascending aorta* is found anteriorly in the midline; the *descending aorta* is related to the left anterolateral surface of the vertebral bodies. (This relationship between the descending aorta and vertebral column is continuous through the thorax and abdomen.)

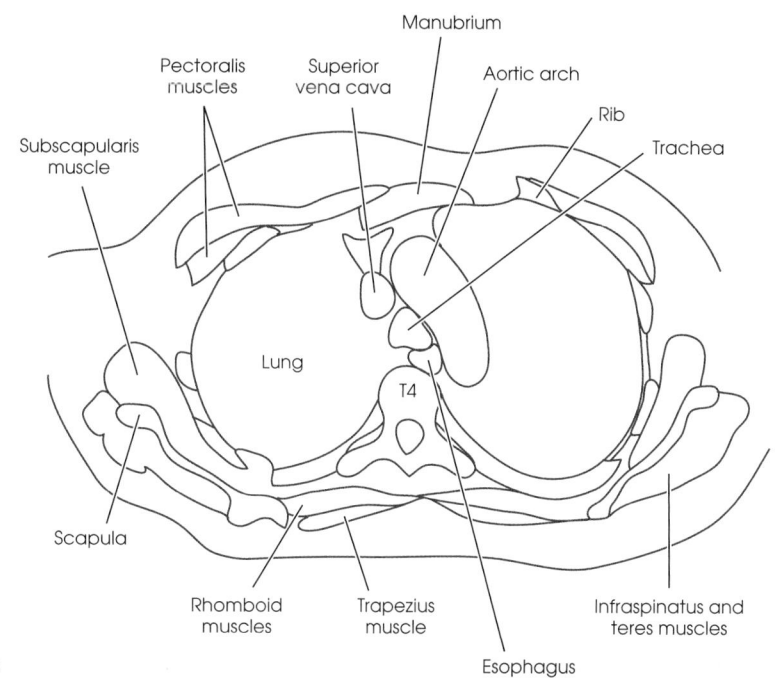

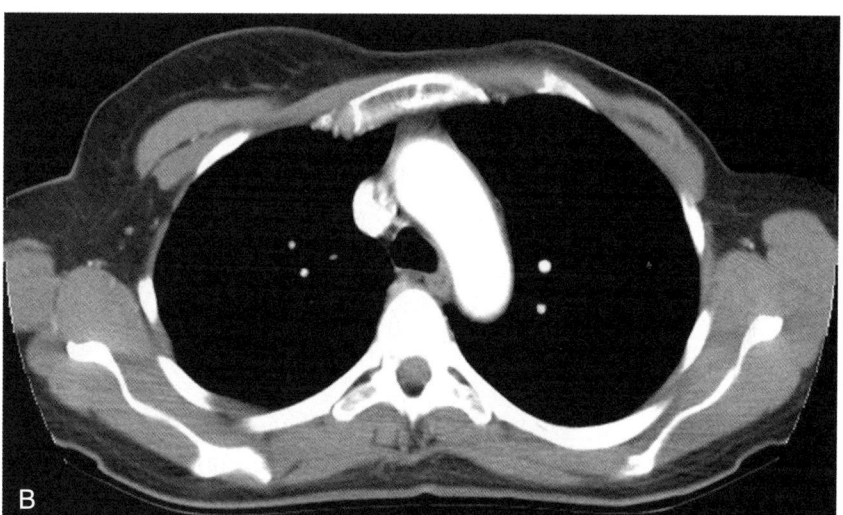

Fig. 24.34 (**A**) Line drawing of CT section. (**B**) CT image corresponding to level *D* in Fig. 24.30 through aortic arch.

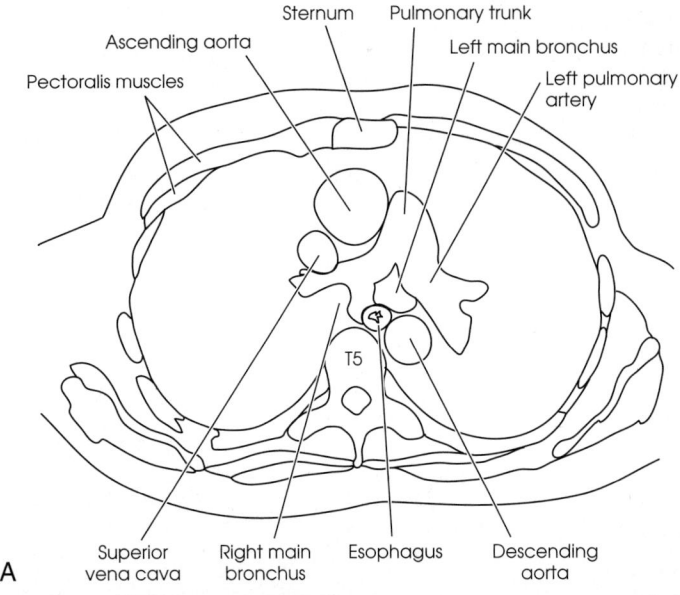

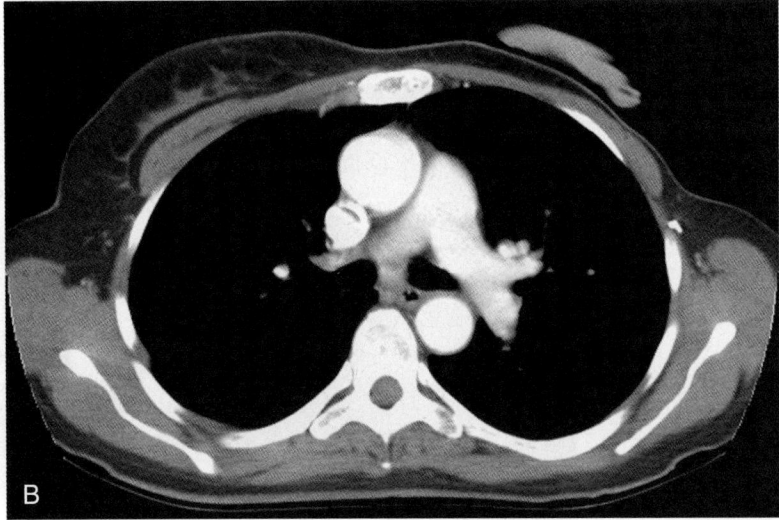

Fig. 24.35 (**A**) Line drawing of CT section. (**B**) CT image corresponding to level *E* in Fig. 24.30 through pulmonary trunk.

Note the normal difference in caliber between the ascending and descending aorta. The superior vena cava is located to the right of the ascending aorta, and the pulmonary trunk and left and right pulmonary arteries are located to the left of the ascending aorta at this level. The *pulmonary trunk* originates from the right ventricle of the heart and divides into the right and left *pulmonary arteries*, which carry deoxygenated blood to the lungs. The left pulmonary artery is seen bifurcating into the two lobar branches at the hilum of the left lung. Near the T5 level, the trachea divides into the left and right *primary bronchi*. The esophagus (in which a small amount of air is seen) is found just posterior to the left main bronchus. Fig. 24.36 is a T2-weighted MRI image that corresponds in position to the previous CT image. The main pulmonary artery and the left pulmonary artery are seen on this image, although the right pulmonary artery is not visible. Muscular structures are easily differentiated. The spinal cord is seen within the vertebral canal, where it is surrounded by CSF.

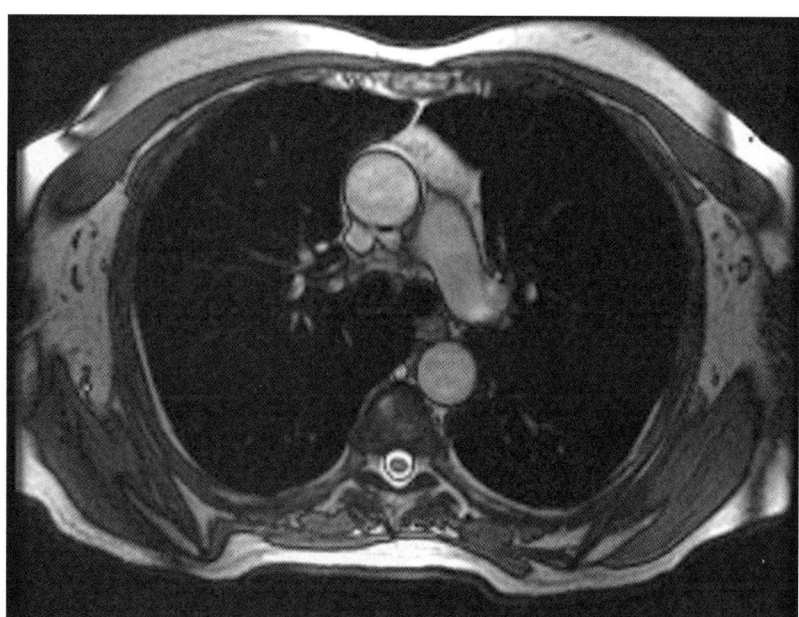

Fig. 24.36 MRI corresponding to level *E* in Fig. 24.30.

The CT image depicted in Fig. 24.37 shows the *lungs* and the base of the *heart*. In general, when the heart is imaged in cross section, the *left atrium* is the superiormost structure encountered, and the *pulmonary veins* are seen emptying into it (one of the right pulmonary veins can be seen here). The *right atrium* is seen lying the farthest toward the right side of the body, anterior and inferior to the left atrium. The superior vena cava may be seen at this level as it enters the right atrium. The *right ventricle* lies to the left of the right atrium and anterior to the more muscular *left ventricle*. Contrast-enhanced blood is seen here as blood exits the left ventricle to enter the root of the aorta. The *interventricular septum* can be seen between the ventricles.

The lungs are divided into superior and inferior lobes by the diagonally oriented *oblique fissure*. The *superior lobes* lie superior and anterior to the inferior lobes. The superior lobe of the right lung is divided further by the *horizontal fissure*, with the lower portion termed the *middle lobe*. The left lung has no horizontal fissure. The inferior and anterior portion of the left lung (corresponding to the right middle lobe) is termed the *lingula*. Although the fissures are not seen, the approximate locations of these lobes are identified here.

Muscular structures that can be seen at this level include the inferior insertions of the trapezius, the *latissimus dorsi*, and the *serratus anterior muscles*. The esophagus lies between the left atrium and the vertebral column at this level.

The CT image depicted in Fig. 24.38 lies at approximately T9 and shows the lower sternum and ribs. The descending aorta normally lies along the left anterolateral surface of the vertebral column, and the *azygos vein* is normally on the right anterolateral surface. Because this scan is inferior to the right ventricle, the *inferior vena cava* is seen between the heart and the liver. The superior portion of the liver is bulging against the base of the right lung, and the superiormost portion of the left hemidiaphragm is seen at the base of the left lung. The right and left ventricles of the heart and the interventricular septum can be seen surrounded by pericardium. The major muscle structures that are visible are the serratus anterior, latissimus dorsi, and the deep back muscles.

Fig. 24.39 is a frontal CT localizer image representing the sagittal levels of the thorax presented here. Fig. 24.40 is a

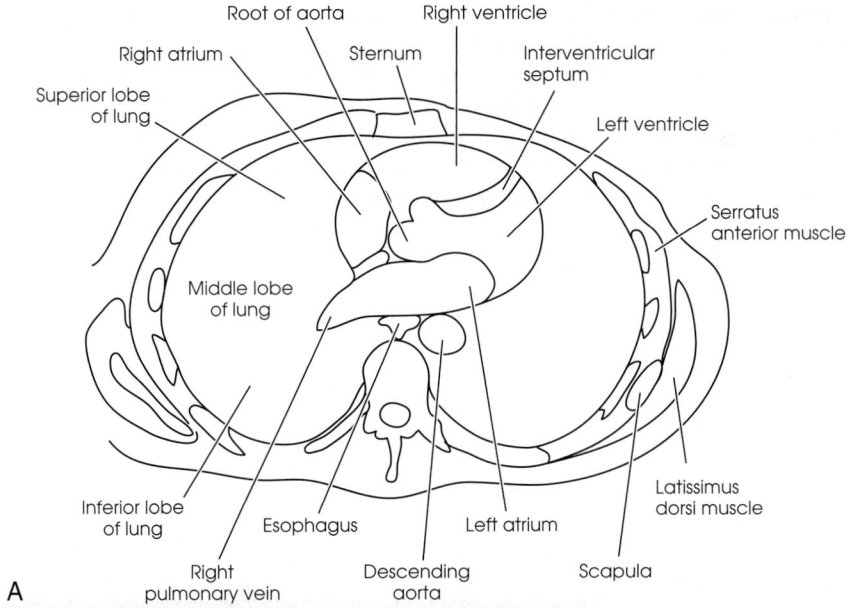

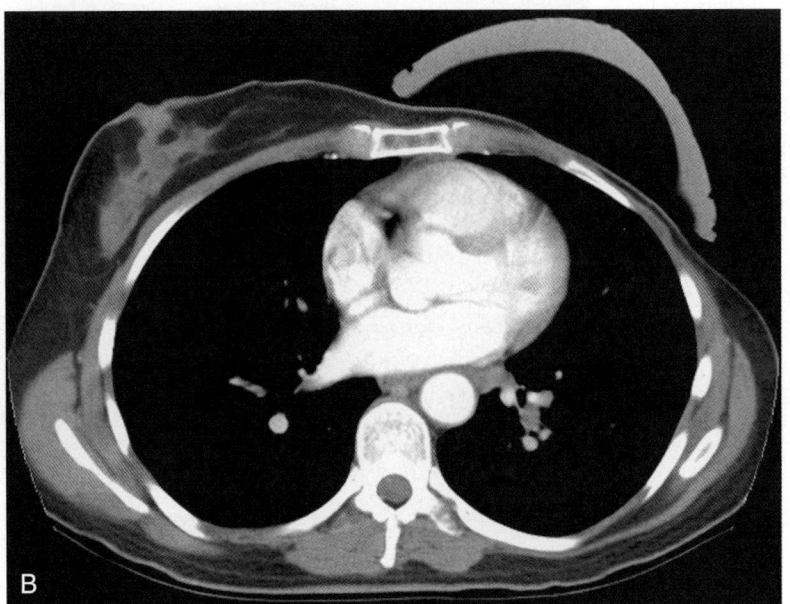

Fig. 24.37 (**A**) Line drawing of CT section. (**B**) CT image corresponding to level *F* in Fig. 24.30 through base of the heart.

CT image located near the median sagittal plane of the chest. In this image, the central portion of the manubrium can be seen in the anterior thorax. The sternal angle is represented as a dark line separating the manubrium and the body of the sternum. Thoracic vertebral bodies, spinous processes, zygapophyseal joints, and intervertebral foramina border the posterior thorax. Because the body has a slight degree of curvature in the spine, different structures are seen in the spinal column at different levels. Within the upper thorax, the cartilage rings of the trachea can be observed. The soft tissue structure posterior to the trachea is the esophagus. The heart and great vessels lie near the center of the thorax. In this image, the superior-most vascular structure is the arch of the aorta. At this level, the origin of the left common carotid artery is present. The left ventricle is the largest chamber of the heart and is seen here filled with contrast medium. It also empties into the aorta. The origin and ascending aorta can be seen just superior to the left ventricle. The left pulmonary artery lies immediately inferior to the aortic arch. This vessel is a branch of the pulmonary artery and originates from the right ventricle of the heart, which is anterior to the left ventricle. The left atrium of the heart is the most posterior chamber and is seen here posterior to the pulmonary trunk and left ventricle. The diaphragm is located inferior to the heart and separates the thoracic cavity from the abdomen.

Fig. 24.41 is a CT image that passes just medial to the left sternoclavicular joint. In this image, the entire aorta is present, from the root, through the arch, and continuing as the descending portion. The origins of the left common carotid and the left subclavian arteries are seen at the superior border of the arch. The left common carotid artery courses from its origin superiorly into the neck near the trachea. The upper portion of the esophagus is posterior to the trachea. The left pulmonary artery is visible just inferior to the arch, and the air-filled structure posterior to this vessel is the left main bronchus.

The CT image depicted in Fig. 24.42 represents a sagittal section through the left sternoclavicular joint. Anteriorly, the bony structures include the clavicle, the upper-outer corner of the manubrium, and the costosternal articulations. The posterior bony anatomy includes the thoracic spine and the upper ribs. Within the

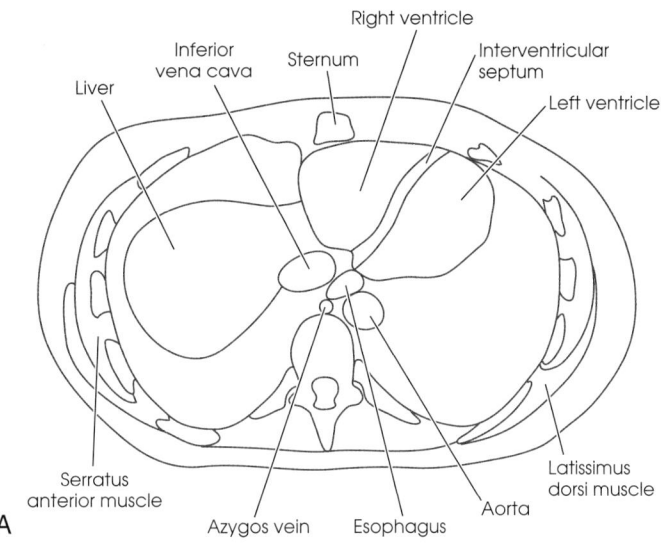

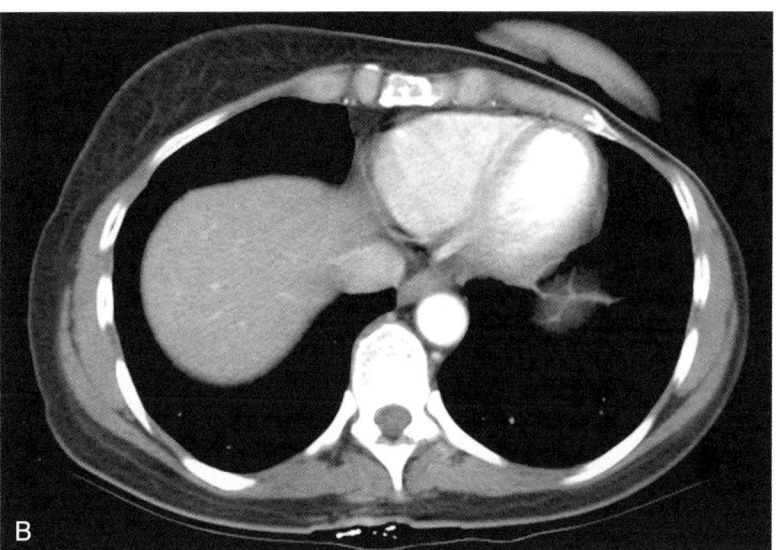

Fig. 24.38 **(A)** Line drawing of CT section. **(B)** CT image corresponding to level *G* in Fig. 24.30 through right hemidiaphragm.

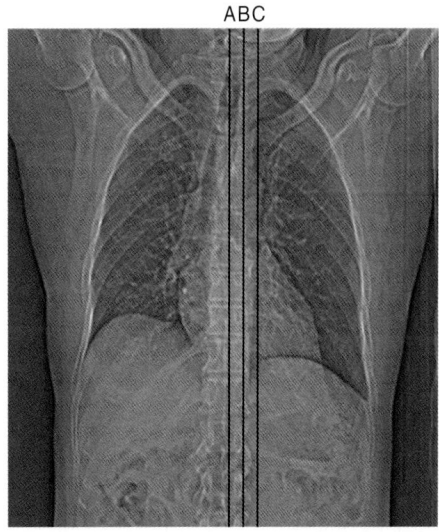

Fig. 24.39 CT localizer image representing levels of sagittal sections through thorax.

thorax, the arch and descending aorta are present. The left subclavian artery is the third branch from the aortic arch. This vessel passes superiorly to arch over the apex of the left lung. In this image, the proximal portion of this vessel is seen just superior to the aortic arch. In the anterior mediastinum, the contrast-filled right ventricle is pumping blood into the main pulmonary artery. The left pulmonary veins return blood from the lungs to the left atrium. The left ventricle lies between the right ventricle and the left atrium in this image.

Fig. 24.43 is a lateral chest x-ray to be used to localize the coronal sections of the thorax presented here. The CT image depicted in Fig. 24.44 is a coronal image passing through the anterior mediastinum. The clavicles, manubrium, and sternoclavicular joints are visible at the entrance into the thorax. Sections through the ribs line both lateral walls of the thoracic cavity. The setting for this image shows the lungs as black structures with a few vascular shadows visible within each. The mediastinum in the center of the thoracic cavity is occupied by the heart and great vessels. This scan passes through the anterior mediastinum, so the ascending portion of the aorta is visible. It lies between the pulmonary artery and the superior vena cava. In this slice, the superior vena cava is discernible at its entrance into the right atrium. The right ventricle is the most anterior chamber of the heart and is seen here lateral to the right atrium.

The CT coronal thoracic section seen in Fig. 24.45 passes through a plane near the median coronal plane of the thorax. Clavicles and ribs can be seen surrounding the superior and lateral thorax. The cartilage rings of the trachea lie in the median sagittal plane at the superior end of the thorax. The left lung is specked with several light gray vascular structures. The right lung shows infiltrates and central scar tissue from an old resection. This scan was performed with contrast enhancement, and the right axillary vein and superior vena cava are visible as bright white. The aortic arch gives rise to the vessels that supply the head and neck. In this image, the brachiocephalic artery and the origin of the left common carotid artery can be seen. The brachiocephalic veins are formed by the internal jugular and subclavian veins. The left brachiocephalic vein is located just to the left of the brachiocephalic artery and superior to the origin of the common carotid artery in this image. The main pulmonary artery is visible inferior

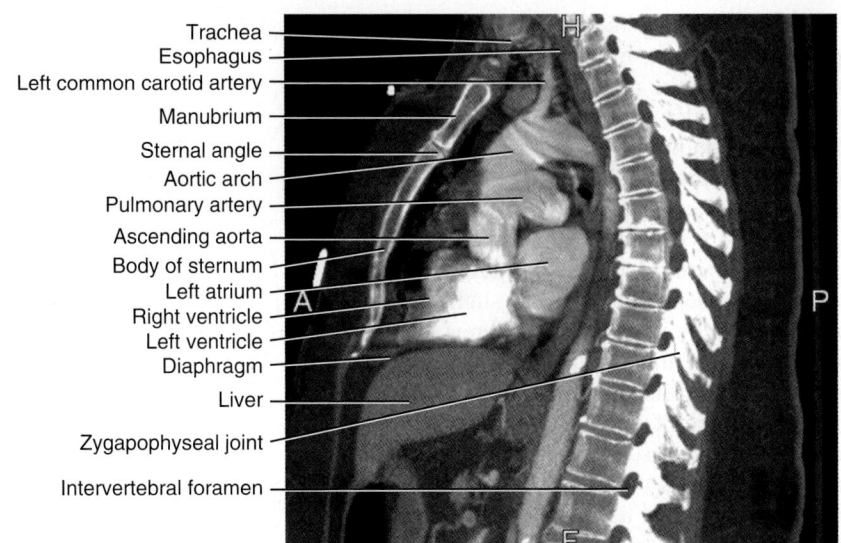

Fig. 24.40 Sagittal CT image of thorax corresponding to level A in Fig. 24.39.

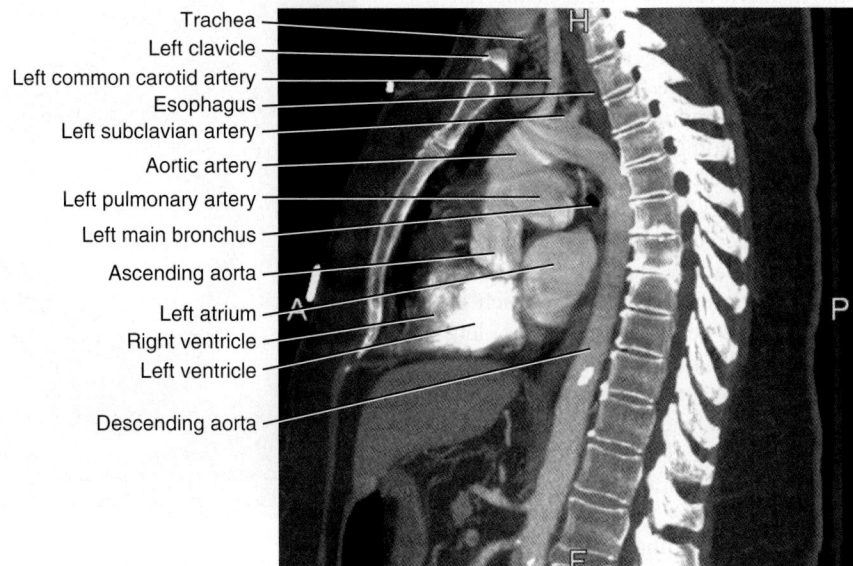

Fig. 24.41 Sagittal CT image of thorax corresponding to level B in Fig. 24.39.

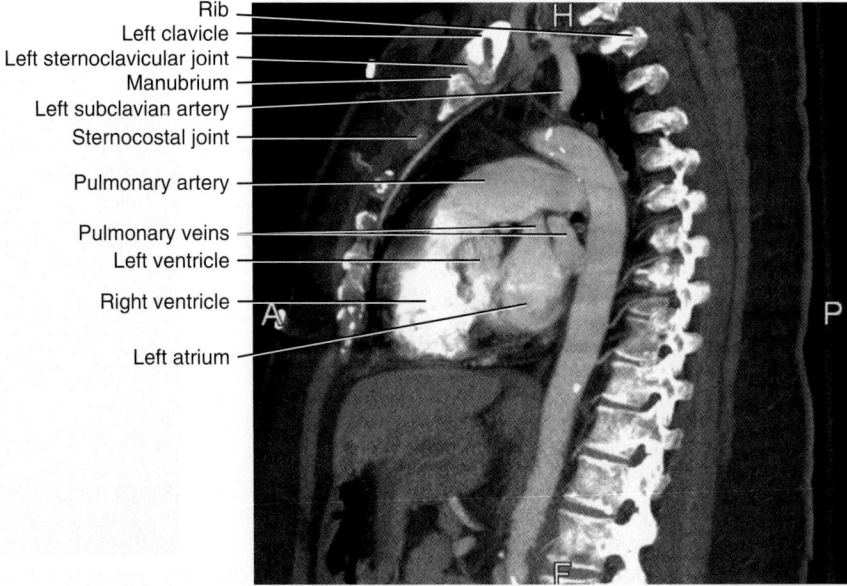

Fig. 24.42 Sagittal CT image of thorax corresponding to level C in Fig. 24.39.

to the aorta. A small portion of the left atrium and the right atrium and ventricle can be seen.

Fig. 24.46 shows anatomy in a posterior plane through the mediastinum. Because of the curve of the spine, the lower cervical and thoracic vertebrae are visible, but most of the thoracic spine is posterior to this imaging plane. Near the level of the fourth or fifth thoracic vertebrae, the trachea bifurcates into the right and left main bronchi. In this image, the lower trachea, its bifurcation, and the main bronchi are visible. On the right, the main bronchus is dividing into lobar bronchi. The soft tissue structure detectable near the top of the visible portion of the trachea is the esophagus. On the left side of the esophagus, the left subclavian artery, filled with contrast medium, is seen as it starts its arch over the apex of the lung. The round contrast-filled vessels that lie on the left side of the trachea are the aortic arch (superior) and the left pulmonary artery (inferior). Inferior to the trachea, the left atrium is detectable, filled with contrast medium. One of the four pulmonary veins is visible, filled with contrast medium and to the right of the left atrium. Because this image is relatively posterior in the mediastinum, no other chambers of the heart can be seen; however, a section of the descending aorta, filled with contrast medium, lies inferior to the left atrium.

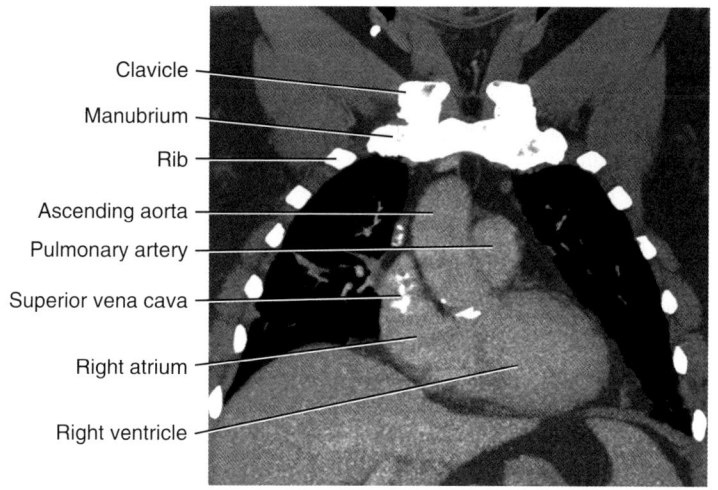

Fig. 24.44 Coronal CT image of thorax corresponding to level A in Fig. 24.43.

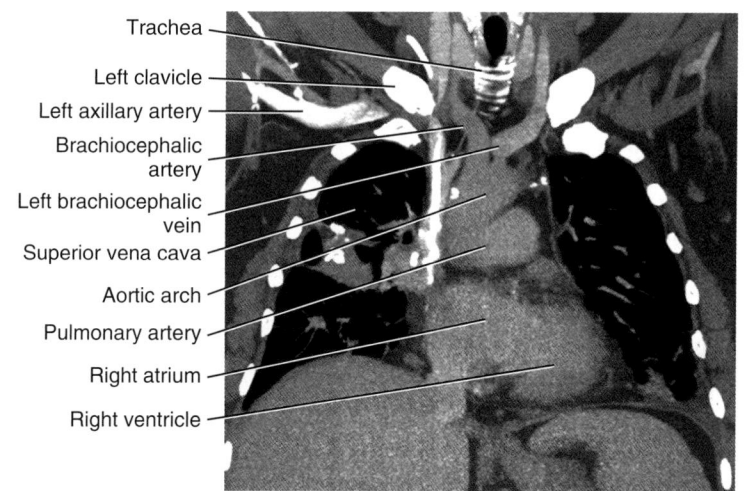

Fig. 24.45 Coronal CT image of thorax corresponding to level B in Fig. 24.43.

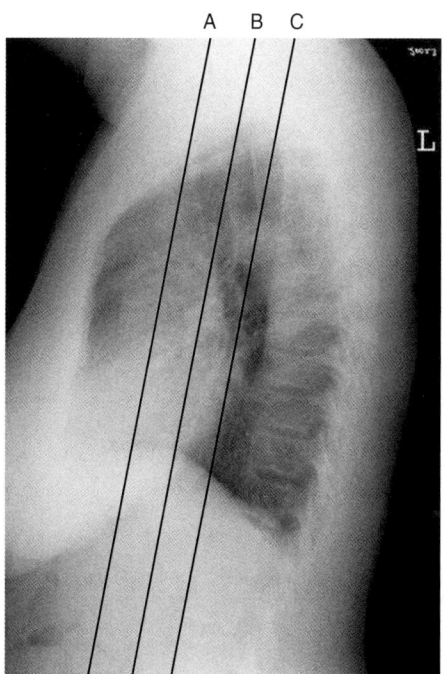

Fig. 24.43 Lateral chest x-ray representing levels of coronal sections through thorax.

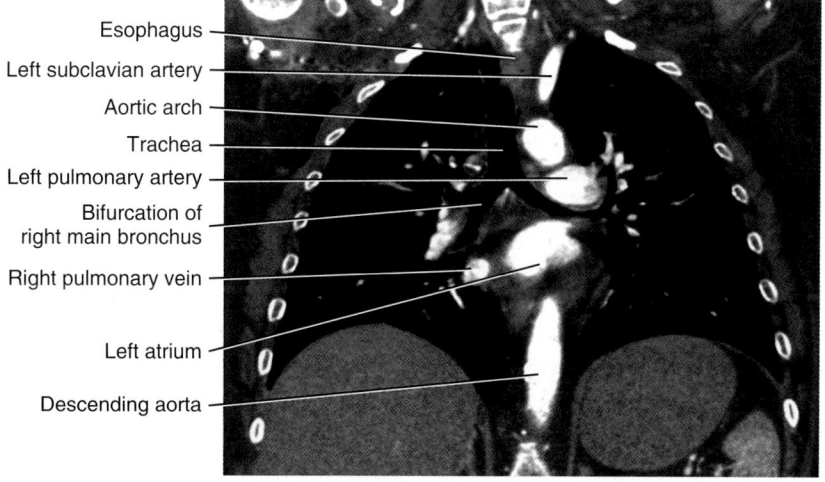

Fig. 24.46 Coronal CT image of thorax corresponding to level C in Fig. 24.43.

Abdominopelvic Region

The abdominopelvic region includes the diaphragm and everything inferior to it. Fig. 24.47 is a cadaveric image at the level of the second lumbar vertebra. Major abdominal organs and vascular structures can be identified in this image. In the abdomen, five lumbar vertebrae are visible. Although these vertebrae are slightly larger than the vertebrae in the thorax, the anatomic components are roughly the same. In the pelvis, the lower spine and hip bones (os coxae or innominate) form an attachment for the lower limbs and support for the trunk. The lower spine comprises the sacrum and coccyx. These are triangular bones with their broad bases oriented superiorly. Each os coxae lies obliquely situated in the pelvis, articulating with the sacrum (sacroiliac joint) posteriorly and with the opposite os coxae anteriorly (symphysis pubis). At birth, this bone consists of three components: the ilium, ischium, and pubis. These three ultimately fuse at the acetabulum. The superior, wing-shaped portion of the os coxae is the ilium. The superior edge is the crest, which lies at the level of the lower fourth lumbar vertebra. The anterior superior and anterior inferior iliac spines lie along the anterior surface of the ilium. At the posterior ilium, posterior superior and posterior inferior iliac spines are found at the top and bottom of the sacral articular surface. Below the posterior inferior iliac spine, the greater sciatic notch curves sharply toward the front of the bone. The inferior and anterior os coxae are composed of the pubis. The pubic bone extends from the acetabulum toward the midline and then curves inferiorly. The pubic bones articulate with each other at the symphysis pubis. The posterior inferior os coxae is formed by the ischium. This portion extends inferiorly from the acetabulum and then curls forward to meet the lower part of the pubis. The obturator foramen is a circular opening formed by the junction of the pubis and ischium.

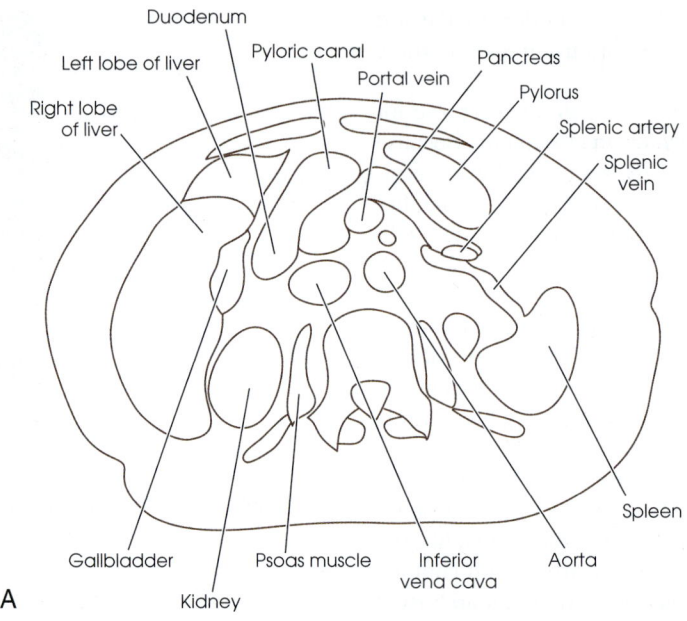

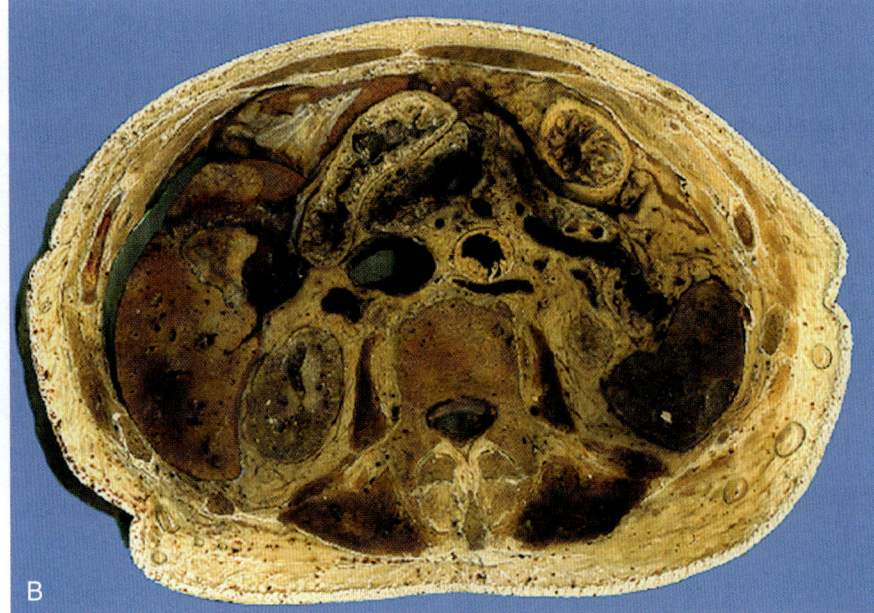

Fig. 24.47 (**A**) Line drawing of gross anatomic section. (**B**) Cadaveric section through central abdomen at the level of L2.

The abdominal cavity is lined by a double-walled membrane called the *peritoneum*. Some organs develop posterior to the peritoneum and are referred to as *retroperitoneal*. Others invaginate into the peritoneum and are referred to as *intraperitoneal*. Several large folds of the peritoneum are identifiable on sectional images because of the large amount of fat found within it. The greater omentum extends from the greater curvature of the stomach and the transverse colon to blanket the anterior surface of the abdominal organs, especially the digestive organs. The small intestines invaginate into the peritoneum as they develop, and a large flap of peritoneum—the mesentery—anchors this part of the digestive system to the posterior abdominal wall.

The spleen is an organ belonging to the lymphatic system. It lies inferior to the left hemidiaphragm and posterior to the fundus of the stomach. On the medial surface of the spleen, blood vessels enter and exit at the hilum.

The organs of the alimentary tract include the esophagus, stomach, small intestine, and large intestine. The esophagus lies anterior to the spine and passes through the diaphragm to enter the abdomen at about the level of T10. In the abdomen, the esophagus passes toward the left to enter the stomach. The opening into the stomach is the cardiac orifice, and the junction is the esophagogastric junction. The stomach is a J-shaped pouch in the left upper quadrant. The region above the level of the esophagogastric junction is the fundus, the central region is the body, and the distal part is the pyloric antrum. This last portion normally lies at about the level of the second lumbar vertebra. The medial and lateral borders are referred to as the *lesser and greater curvatures*. Internally, the stomach is thrown into multiple folds termed *rugae*. Food passes from the distal stomach through the pyloric canal into the small intestine. A muscle called the *pyloric sphincter* controls passage through the canal. The small intestine consists of the duodenum, jejunum, and ileum. The first portion, or duodenum, extends from the stomach laterally to the liver, where the remainder curls inferiorly and medially to form a C-shaped loop around the head of the pancreas. The duodenum is approximately 25 to 30 cm (10 to 12 inches) long, and at the ligament of Treitz it continues as the jejunum. The jejunum is approximately 2.4 m (8 feet) long and mainly occupies the left upper abdomen. It continues as the ileum. This distalmost part of the small bowel is about 3 m (10 feet) long and occupies the right inferior abdominal cavity and the pelvis. The large intestine is about 1.8 m (6 feet) long. It frames the periphery of the abdominal cavity and comprises the cecum, colon (ascending, transverse, descending, and sigmoid portions), rectum, and anus. The ileum empties into the saclike cecum in the right lower quadrant via the ileocecal valve. The vermiform appendix can frequently be seen projecting off the cecum. From the cecum, the ascending portion of the colon passes superiorly. Just below the liver, this portion curves anteriorly and medially at the hepatic (right colic) flexure. The transverse portion passes from here across the anterior abdomen. This portion dips inferiorly into the abdomen to a variable degree, depending on the body habitus of the patient. As the colon reaches the spleen, it turns posteriorly and inferiorly at the splenic (left colic) flexure to become the descending colon. This portion passes down the posterior aspect of the left side of the abdomen toward the pelvis, where it continues as the sigmoid colon. The sigmoid colon curls medially and posteriorly in the pelvis, and at the midsacrum it curves inferiorly as the rectum. The rectum lies anterior to and follows the curve of the sacrum to become the anal canal as the large intestine exits the pelvis.

Several accessory organs of the digestive system are located in the upper abdomen. The liver occupies most of the right upper quadrant. This triangular organ is divided anatomically into a large right lobe and a much smaller left lobe. The falciform ligament is located along the division between these lobes on the anterior surface, and the ligamentum venosum and ligamentum teres are found along the division on the posterior surface of the liver. On the posteroinferior surface of the right lobe are two smaller lobes: the caudate (superior) and the quadrate (inferior). These two lobes are separated by the porta hepatis (hilum) of the liver. The hepatic artery, portal vein, and hepatic bile ducts enter and exit the liver here. The gallbladder rests against the undersurface of the liver. This organ functions as a storage vessel for bile, which is produced in the liver. Bile drains from the liver through the right and left hepatic ducts. These ducts unite to form the common hepatic duct, which meets the cystic duct from the gallbladder. Distal to this junction, the continuation of this duct is known as the *common bile duct*. Bile passes through this duct to empty into the second part of the duodenum at the hepatopancreatic ampulla (ampulla of Vater). The pancreas, which functions as an endocrine and exocrine gland, lies transversely across the abdomen near the level of the second lumbar vertebra. The divisions of this retroperitoneal organ, from right to left, are the head, neck, body, and tail. The head is the most inferior portion and is encircled by the duodenum. The tail is located near the hilum of the spleen. The pancreatic duct traverses the length of the organ and enters the second part of the duodenum at or near the common bile duct.

The urinary system includes the two kidneys and ureters, the bladder, and the urethra. The kidneys are retroperitoneal and lie between the 12th thoracic and 3rd lumbar vertebrae. The center or hilar region is normally near the interspace between L1 and L2. Suprarenal (adrenal) glands are perched on the upper surface of each kidney. The right adrenal gland can be seen between the liver and the right diaphragmatic crus, and the left lies between the left crus and the pancreatic tail and spleen. Each kidney is surrounded by a dense membrane (the renal fasciae) and a layer of fat (the perirenal fat). Urine is formed in the parenchyma of the kidney and collects in the calyceal system. The calyces unite to form the renal pelvis, which is continuous with the ureter. The ureters are musculomembranous tubes that extend down the posterior abdomen, resting along the anterior surface of the psoas muscles. They are difficult to visualize unless filled with radiopaque contrast medium. In the pelvis, the ureters empty into the posteroinferior region of the bladder. The bladder is a collapsible muscular sac that serves as a reservoir for urine until it is expelled from the body. The bladder rests on or near the pelvic floor, posterior to the symphysis pubis and anterior to the rectum in males or the vagina in females. The urethra is the muscular passageway that originates from the apex (inferior surface) of the bladder and by which urine is expelled. The urethra is relatively short in females, passing through the floor of the pelvis. The urethra is much longer in males because it passes through the prostate gland and the membranous and cavernous portions of the penis.

The internal organs of the male reproductive system include the ductus deferens, seminal vesicles, and prostate. Internal and external reproductive structures are connected by the spermatic cord, which includes the ductus deferens, testicular vessels, nerves, and lymphatic structures. The spermatic cord is seen anterior and medial to the femoral artery and vein and anterior and lateral to the pubis. The ductus deferens enters the pelvis through the spermatic cord and then arches over the anterior and lateral aspect of the bladder. It passes down the posterior surface of the bladder and enters the superior prostate. The seminal vesicles are found on the posterior and inferior surface of the bladder near the insertion of the ureters. The prostate gland lies inferior to the bladder, between the symphysis pubis and the rectum. The prostatic portion of the urethra passes through the prostate.

The organs of the female reproductive system include the uterus, uterine (fallopian) tubes, ovaries, and vagina. The uterus, which normally lies superior and posterior to the urinary bladder, is divided into a fundus, body, isthmus, and cervix. The fundus is the upper, rounded portion of the organ, superior to the orifices of the uterine tubes. The central portion is the body, which narrows at its lower end to become the isthmus. The narrowed lower 2 cm (.75 inch) of the uterus is the cervix, which is continuous with the vagina. The uterus is suspended in the pelvis by folds of peritoneum called the *broad ligaments*. The ovaries lie lateral to the body of the uterus within the broad ligament. They are normally found near the lateral pelvic wall at or slightly below the level of the anterior superior iliac spine. Extending between the ovaries and uterus, in the superior rim of the broad ligament, are the uterine tubes. The medial ends open into the upper body of the uterus. The lateral end of each tube—the infundibulum—is expanded and terminates in multiple fingerlike projections called *fimbriae*. This end of the tube is superior to the ovary but not attached. The inferiormost part of the internal female reproductive system is the vagina. This muscular tube lies between the rectum and the bladder and opens to the external body surface posterior to the urethral meatus.

Three vascular systems can be described in the abdomen: arterial, venous, and portal. The descending—or abdominal—aorta is the main conduit for arterial blood and passes through the diaphragm at approximately the level of T11 and extends to the pelvis along the left anterolateral surface of the vertebral bodies. Just below the diaphragm, at approximately the level of the 12th thoracic vertebra, the celiac artery originates from the anterior aorta. This fairly short vessel divides into the splenic, common hepatic, and left gastric arteries. The splenic artery passes toward the left to enter the hilum of the spleen. The common hepatic artery extends to the right to the porta hepatis. The superior mesenteric artery arises from the left anterior aorta near the first lumbar vertebra. The origin of this vessel is posterior to the neck of the pancreas. It extends anteriorly for a short distance and then turns inferiorly as it sends its branches to supply the small intestine and the proximal half of the large intestine. Near the level of the second lumbar vertebra, the renal arteries arise from the lateral surface of the aorta. The renal arteries pass laterally to enter the hila of the kidneys. The right renal artery is longer than the left because it must cross the spine to reach the right kidney. The inferior mesenteric artery arises from the abdominal aorta at L3 and supplies the distal half of the large bowel. At the fourth lumbar vertebra, the abdominal aorta bifurcates to form the right and left common iliac arteries. Each common iliac artery divides into internal and external iliac arteries near the top of the sacrum. Internal iliac arteries divide rapidly and send branches to various structures within the pelvis. The external iliac arteries pass anteriorly and inferiorly through the pelvis. These vessels pass deep to the inguinal ligaments and become the femoral arteries.

The femoral veins carry venous blood from the lower limbs toward the pelvis. The femoral vein becomes the external iliac vein as it passes deep to the inguinal ligament. It is joined within the pelvis by the internal iliac vein to form the common iliac vein. The two common iliac veins unite at the level of the fifth lumbar vertebra to form the inferior vena cava. The inferior vena cava passes up the right anterolateral surface of the vertebral bodies, pierces the diaphragm, and empties into the inferior surface of the right atrium. The major tributaries of the inferior vena cava are the renal veins and the hepatic veins. The renal veins enter the lateral inferior vena cava near L2; the three hepatic veins enter near the top of the liver.

The vessels that drain the spleen and digestive system form the portal venous system. The major tributaries of this system are the superior and inferior mesenteric veins and the splenic vein. The inferior mesenteric vein empties into the splenic vein, which meets the superior mesenteric vein just posterior to the head of the pancreas. The junction of these two vessels forms the portal vein. These

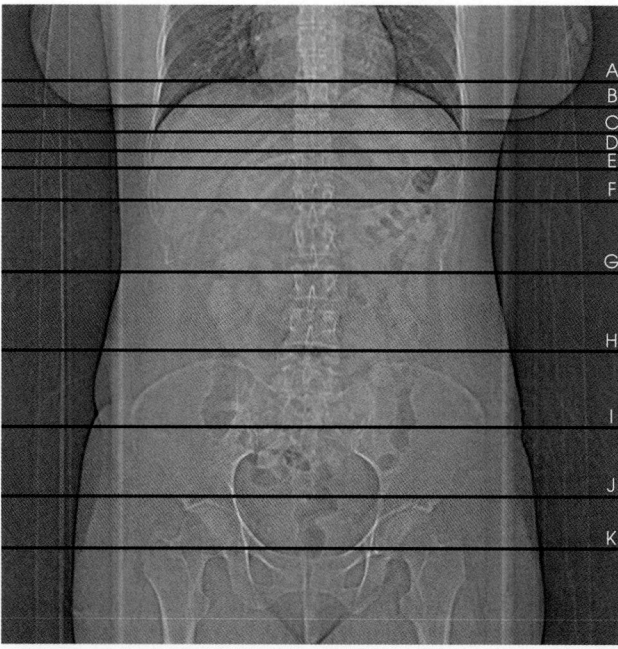

Fig. 24.48 CT localizer (scout) image of abdominopelvic region.

vessels extend superiorly to enter the porta hepatis of the liver.

Fig. 24.48 is a CT localizer—or scout—image representing an AP projection of the abdominopelvic region. See Fig. 24.48 for 11 identifying lines that show the levels for each of the labeled images for this region.

Fig. 24.49 represents structures seen at the T9 level. The tip of the xiphoid process and lower ribs are seen. The image shows the *right hemidiaphragm* surrounding the superior portion of the *liver* and the *left hemidiaphragm* encircling the pericardial fat surrounding the apex of the heart and the *fundus* of the stomach. A small amount of oral contrast agent can be seen in the dependent portion of the stomach in this image. The *esophagus*, posterior to the liver, has migrated toward the patient's left as it nears its entrance into the stomach. The lower lobes of each lung are seen external to the diaphragm. The *aorta* is in its normal position, anterior and slightly left of the vertebral body; the azygos vein lies to the right of the aorta. The inferior vena cava appears embedded within the liver. Three *hepatic veins* drain into the inferior vena cava at this level. Serratus anterior muscles are seen external to the lateral aspects of the ribs; latissimus dorsi muscles extend superficially across the posterior abdomen.

Fig. 24.50 is a CT image at the level of the 10th thoracic vertebra. It shows the aorta and inferior vena cava and contrast-enhanced vessels within the liver. These represent branches of the hepatic and portal venous circulation. The right, left, and *caudate lobes* of the liver are visible. On the patient's left, the contrast-filled body of the stomach and the *spleen* can be identified. This is normally the level at which the esophagus enters the cardiac portion of the stomach. The *greater omentum* (a large fold of peritoneum) lies along the greater curvature of the stomach. Fig. 24.50 shows the greater omentum anterior and lateral to the stomach. The inferior lobes of the lungs are seen posterior to the liver and the spleen. The *crura of the diaphragm* are the lower tendinous insertions of this muscle. They can be seen extending around the anterior aorta and the posterior liver and spleen. This scan shows the latissimus dorsi and the lower reaches of the serratus anterior. The upper portions of the anterior abdominal muscles (rectus abdominis, external oblique) can also be seen.

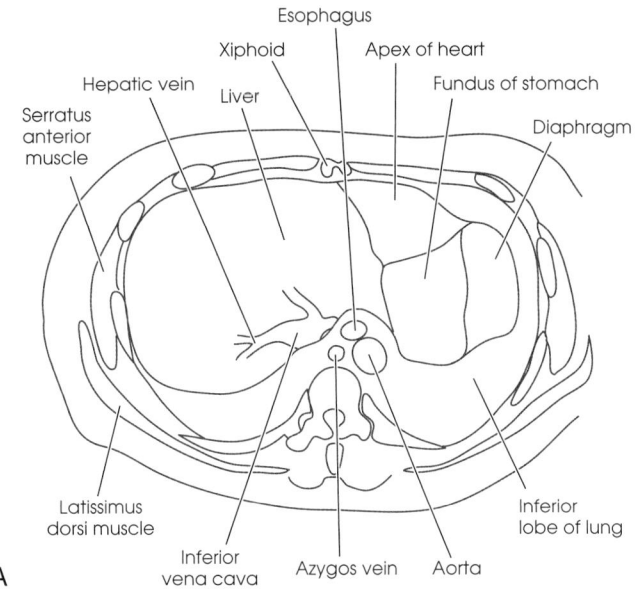
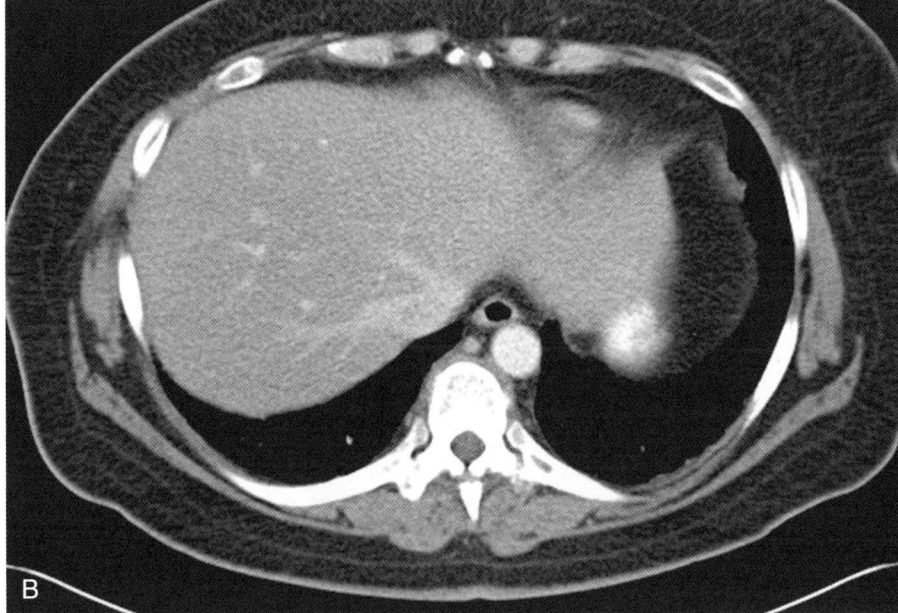

Fig. 24.49 (**A**) Line drawing of CT section. (**B**) CT image corresponding to level *A* in Fig. 24.48.

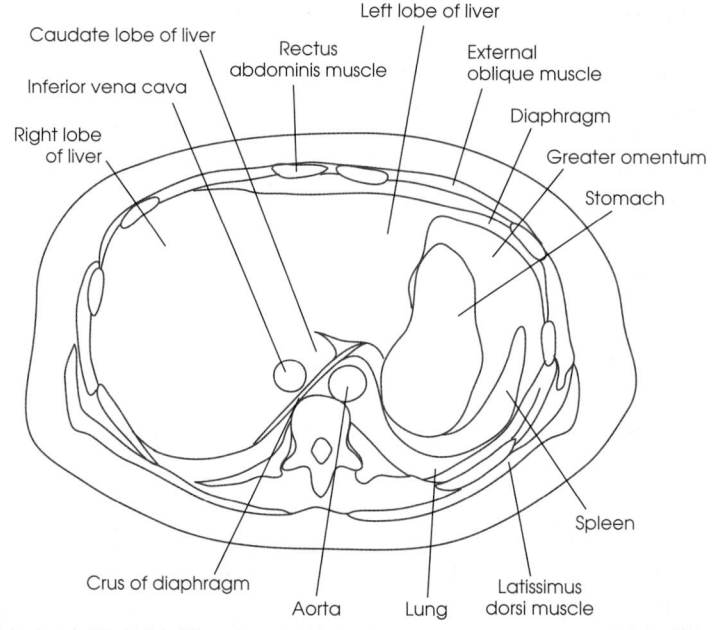

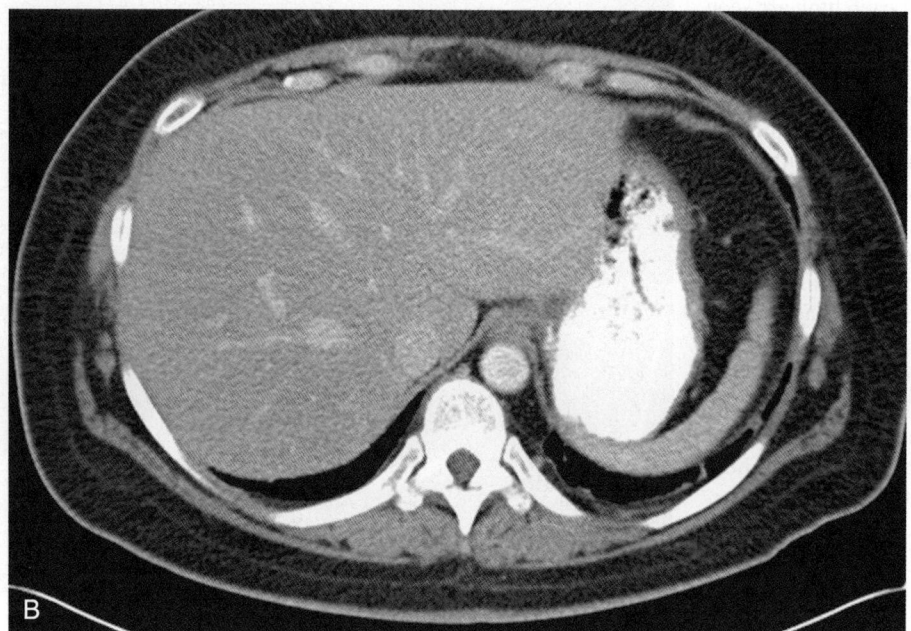

Fig. 24.50 (**A**) Line drawing of CT section. (**B**) CT image corresponding to level *B* in Fig. 24.48.

A CT image at the level of T11 (Fig. 24.51) shows the relationships among the liver, stomach, and spleen. The cardiac portion of the stomach is located at approximately the T10–11 level in the anterior aspect of the left upper quadrant, and the *pyloric portion* normally lies anterior to L2. This scan passes through the center or body of the stomach. An air-fluid level exists between the gas in the anterior stomach and the contrast medium in the posterior stomach. The spleen, located between the levels of T12 and L1, is in the posterolateral aspect of the left upper quadrant posterior to the fundus and body of the stomach. Contrast medium in the patient's colon is seen at the *splenic flexure*, seen here between the body of the stomach and the spleen. The liver is generally found between T11 and L3 and occupies the entire right upper quadrant. The right lobe of the liver has two small subdivisions, the caudate and *quadrate lobes*, which are bounded by the *gallbladder*, *ligamentum teres*, and inferior vena cava. The left lobe of the liver stretches across the midline and into the left upper quadrant. The *porta hepatis*, or hilum of the liver, is visible between the right and left lobes at this level. The inferior vena cava is found between the right and caudate lobes of the liver. In this image, it is nearly isodense with liver tissue. Large branches of the portal vein are seen at the porta hepatis.

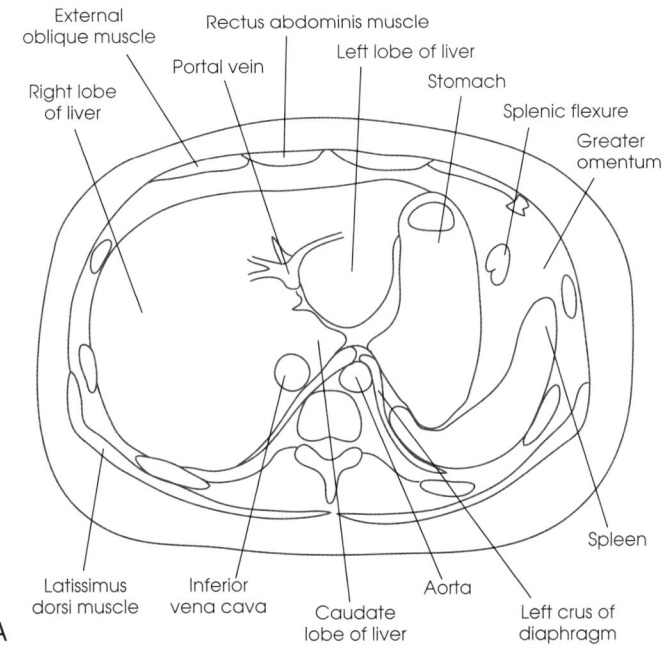

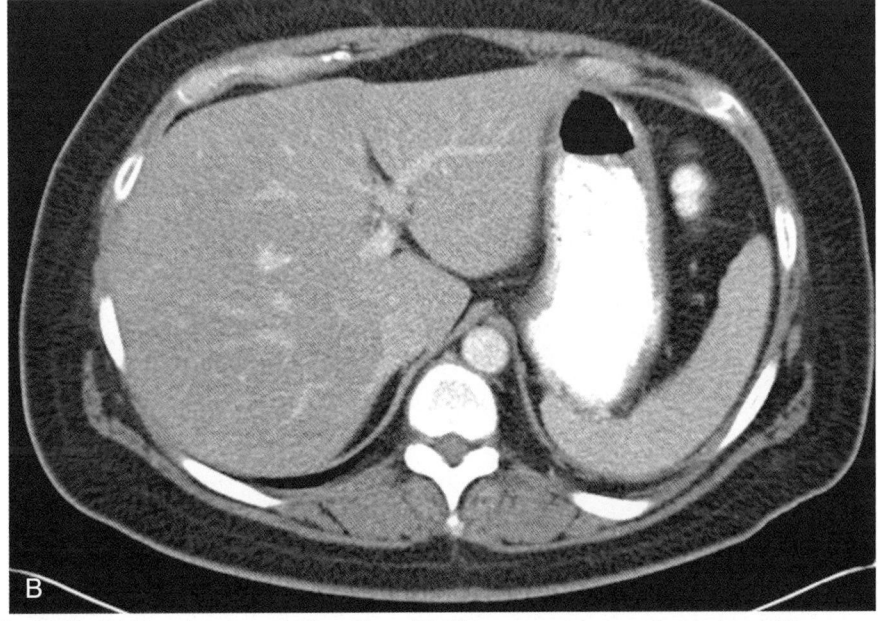

Fig. 24.51 (**A**) Line drawing of CT section. (**B**) CT image corresponding to level *C* in Fig. 24.48.

Fig. 24.52 lies at the inferior edge of T11. It shows the right, left, and caudate lobes of the liver and the porta hepatis. Anteriorly, the falciform ligament lies near the fissure between the right and left lobes (not seen on this image). The pyloric antrum of the stomach lies near the left lobe of the liver. This scan is inferior to the splenic flexure, so the *transverse and descending portions of the colon* can be differentiated. The spleen lies along the left posterior abdominal wall. This scan lies near the hilum, and vascular structures are seen in this region. The tail of the pancreas normally lies near the spleen and can be seen here between the stomach and spleen. The *suprarenal glands* are normally located superior to the kidney. The right suprarenal gland is found at this level between the liver and the right diaphragmatic crus. The left suprarenal gland is medial to the pancreas and spleen. The abdominal aorta is positioned anterior and to the left of the vertebral column; the inferior vena cava is between the right and caudate lobes of the liver. The portal vein is seen within the porta hepatis, along with branches of the hepatic artery. The splenic artery is normally tortuous and not seen in its entirety. At this level, the bright circles along the posterior pancreas most likely represent portions of the contrast-filled *splenic artery*.

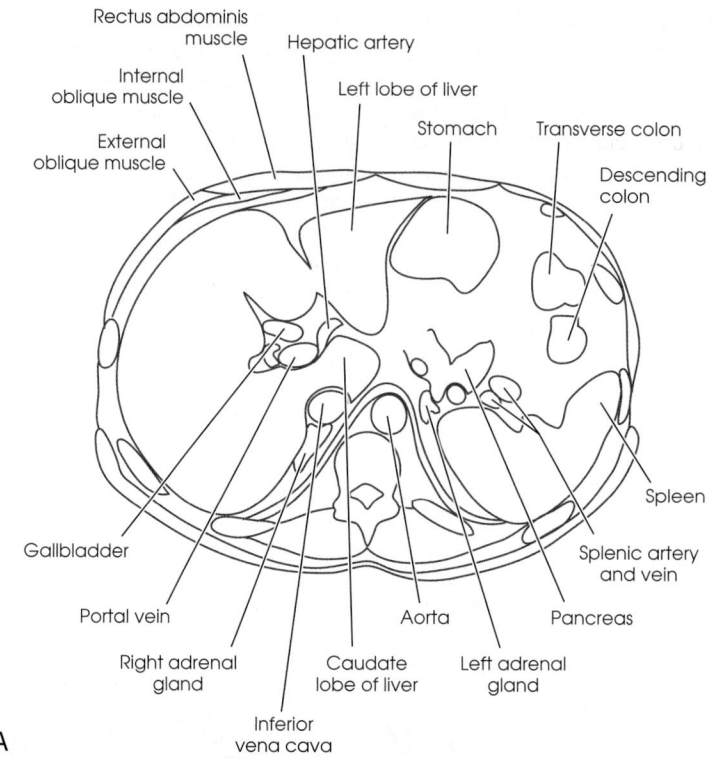

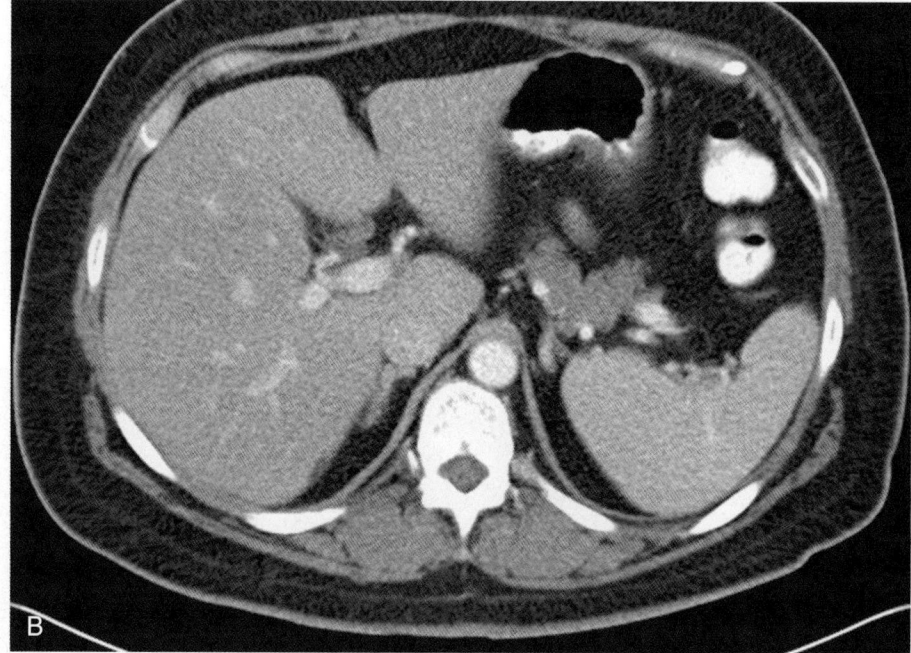

Fig. 24.52 (**A**) Line drawing of CT section. (**B**) CT image corresponding to level *D* in Fig. 24.48.

The CT scan in Fig. 24.53 passes through the upper portion of T12. The difference in density between the liver tissue and the bile-filled *gallbladder* makes these organs easy to differentiate. The antrum of the stomach, pyloric canal, and bulb (first portion) of the *duodenum* are seen in the anterior abdomen. The neck of the pancreas is posterior to the pyloric canal of the stomach in this image. The transverse and descending colon lie in the anterior left abdomen. The spleen is posterior to the descending colon. Loops of *jejunum*—the second part of the small bowel—are posterior to the antrum of the stomach. The left adrenal gland is lateral to the aorta and left diaphragmatic crus. The right adrenal gland is posterior to the IVC. The three branches of the *celiac trunk* (hepatic, splenic, left gastric arteries) supply the liver, spleen, pancreas, and stomach with oxygen-rich blood. In this image, the celiac trunk is seen as it divides into the *common hepatic artery* and the splenic artery. The left gastric artery is not seen. The splenic artery runs a tortuous course and normally cannot be visualized in its entirety in axial sections. Here, branches of the splenic artery and vein lie in close proximity and are difficult to differentiate. The inferior vena cava can be seen in its normal position anterior and to the right of the vertebral column. The main portion of the portal vein is just posterior to the duodenal bulb.

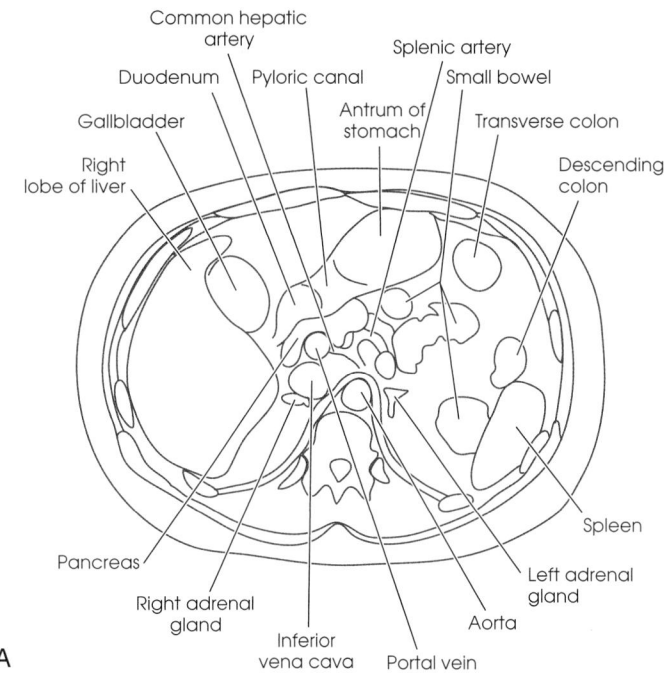

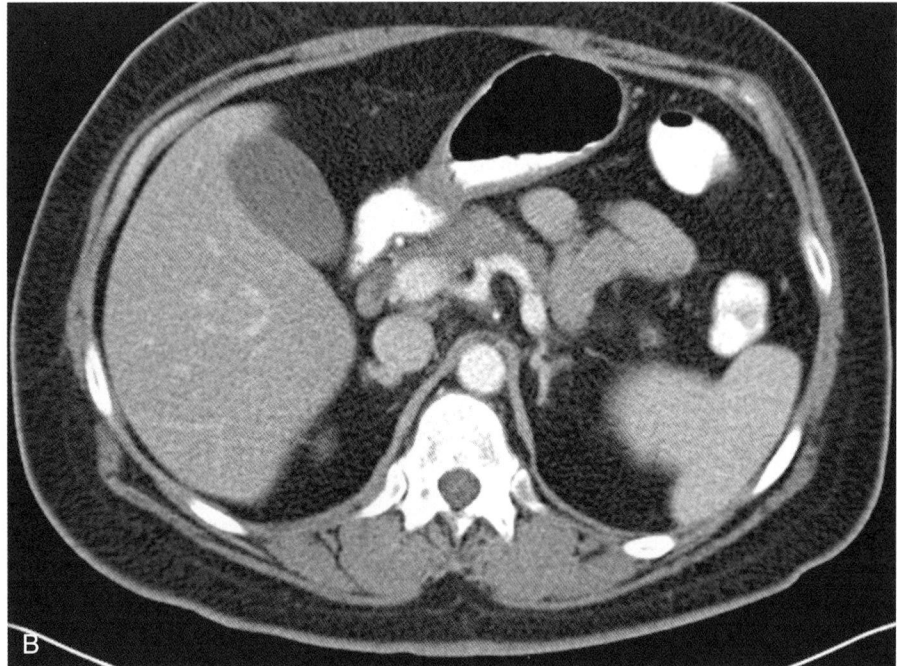

Fig. 24.53 (**A**) Line drawing of CT section. (**B**) CT image corresponding to level *E* in Fig. 24.48.

The muscles of the abdomen are located between the lower rib cage and the iliac crests. This group of muscles includes the *external oblique*, *internal oblique*, and *transverse abdominal muscles*. The two *rectus abdominis muscles* are located on the anterior aspect of the abdomen on either side of the midline and extend from the *pubic symphysis* to the xiphoid process.

The CT image in Fig. 24.54 is through the level of the first lumbar vertebra. The lower right lobe of the liver lies along the right side of the abdomen. The hepatic (right colic) flexure lies just medial to the liver. The duodenum forms a C-shaped loop around the head of the pancreas. In this scan, the head of the pancreas is seen between the duodenum (second portion) and the superior mesenteric vein. On the left side of the abdomen, loops of small bowel and the transverse and descending colon are seen. Folds of *mesentery* can be seen connecting some of the small bowel loops. The most inferior edge of the spleen lies along the left posterior abdomen. The upper poles of the kidneys appear on either side of the vertebral body. At this level, the *superior mesenteric artery* is seen as it originates from the anterior aorta. The *left renal vein* can also be seen as it empties into the lateral aspect of the inferior vena cava.

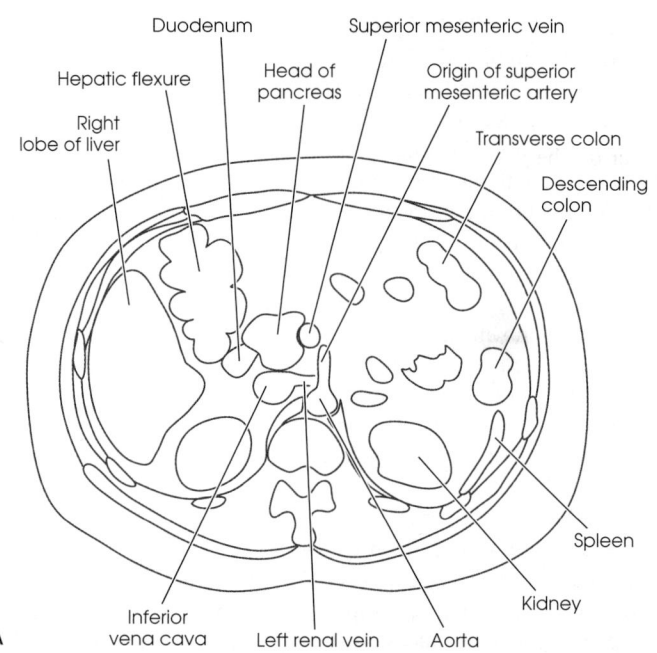

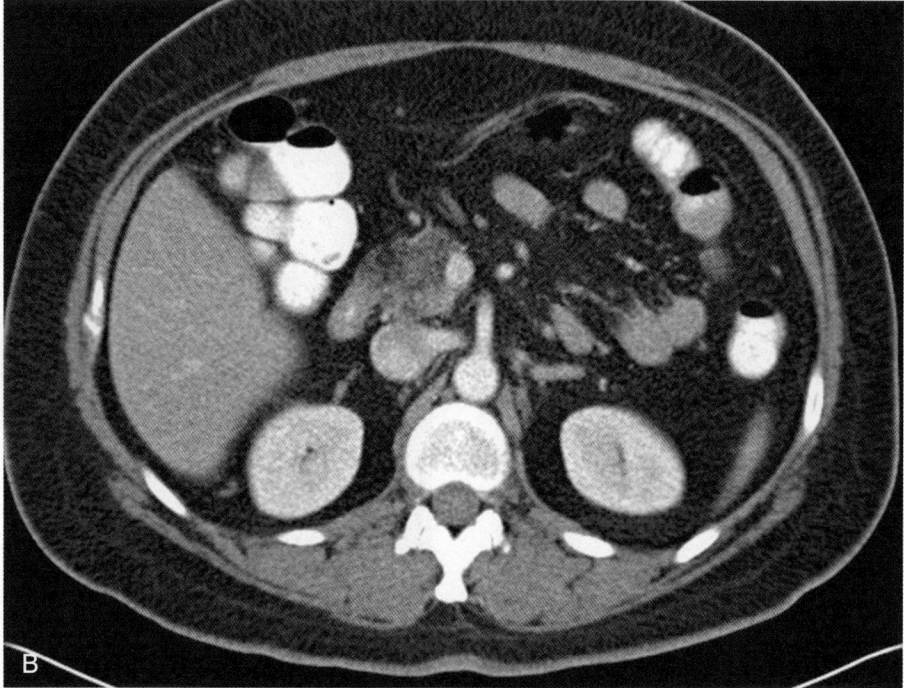

Fig. 24.54 (A) Line drawing of CT section. (B) CT image corresponding to level *F* in Fig. 24.48.

Fig. 24.55 is a CT scan through the third lumbar vertebra. The ascending colon is found on the right side of the abdomen. In this image, most of the transverse colon can be seen across the anterior abdomen. The descending colon lies along the posterior left abdomen. Loops of small bowel are found in the central portion of the abdomen. Ileal loops are filled with contrast medium that has refluxed through the ileocecal valve from the colon. This level is just below the hila of the kidneys, and some of the central collecting system can be observed. The inferior vena cava and contrast-filled aorta lie anterior to the vertebral body. The rectus abdominis muscles lie on either side of the midline in the anterior abdomen. The three layers of the lateral abdominal muscles (external oblique, internal oblique, and transverse abdominis) are separated by fat and can plainly be seen in this scan. The *psoas muscles* originate from the body of T12 and the transverse processes of the lumbar vertebrae and descend the abdomen lateral to the vertebral bodies. The *quadratus lumborum muscles* are located posterolateral to the psoas muscles through the abdomen. These muscles can be seen on either side of the vertebra. The *spinal cord* normally terminates at the level of L1. Inferior to L1, the *spinal nerves*—known as *cauda equina*—are seen within the spinal canal.

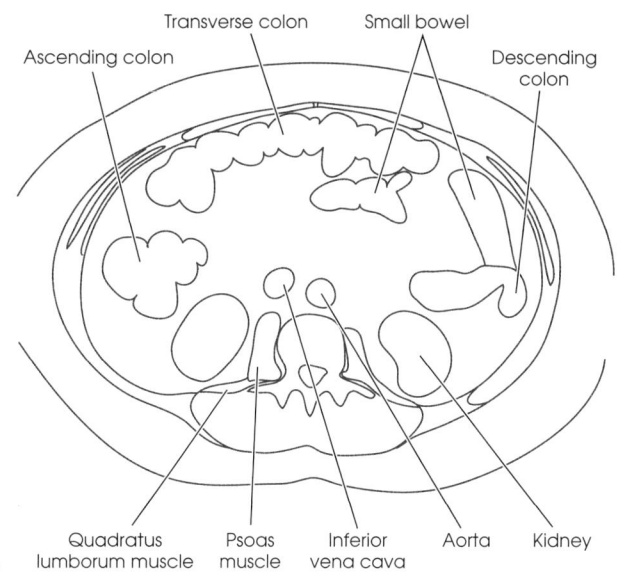

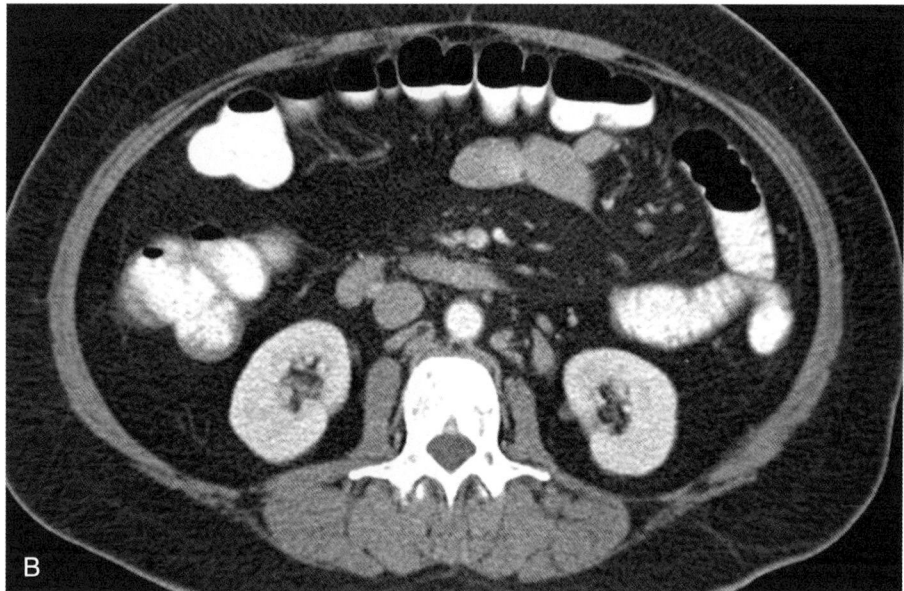

Fig. 24.55 (**A**) Line drawing of CT section. (**B**) CT image corresponding to level G in Fig. 24.48.

The CT scan in Fig. 24.56 lies near the interspace between the fourth and fifth lumbar vertebrae. The superior edge of the right *iliac crest* is visible in this image. The inferior portion of the cecum and the descending colon lie in the posterior abdomen on the right and left sides. Loops of small bowel are seen more anteriorly in the abdomen. The ureters normally lie just anterior to the psoas muscles. Because of peristalsis, no contrast medium is seen in the ureters on this image. At this level, the aorta has bifurcated to form the right and left *common iliac vessels*. The common iliac veins are fairly close to each other, indicating that this scan is just inferior to their junction (which forms the inferior vena cava).

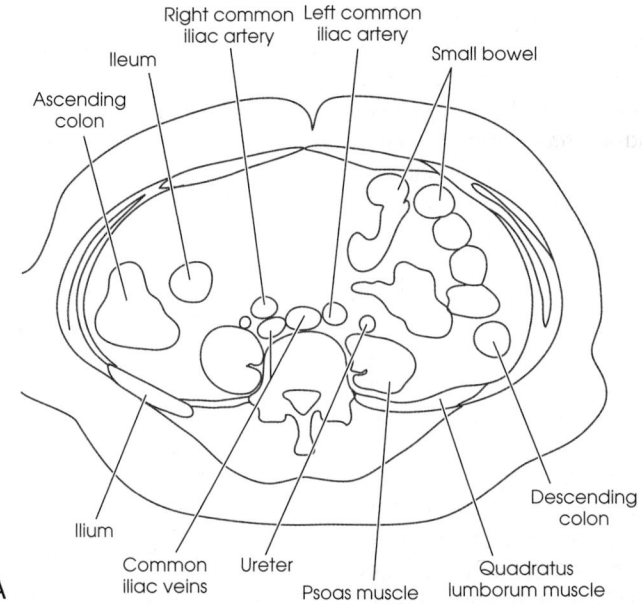

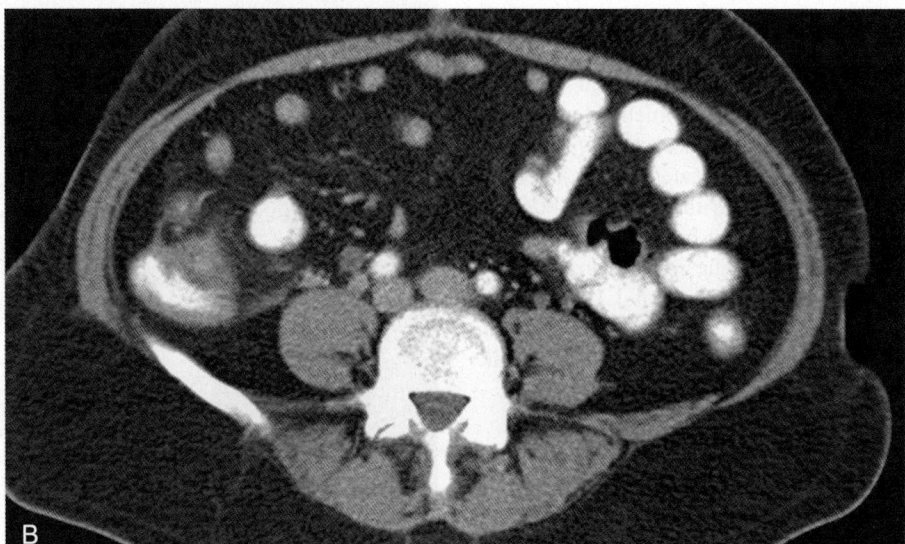

Fig. 24.56 (**A**) Line drawing of CT section. (**B**) CT image corresponding to level *H* in Fig. 24.48.

The CT image seen in Fig. 24.57 is of a female patient and was obtained at the upper sacral level. It shows the *wings of the ilia*, the right *anterior superior iliac spine*, and the *sacroiliac joints*. The descending colon is seen at the left lateral aspect of the pelvis, and multiple loops of *small intestine* are found throughout this level in the images. Three muscles lie posterior to the wings of the ilia: the gluteus minimus, gluteus medius, and gluteus maximus. The gluteus medius normally extends the farthest superiorly and is the first muscle visible as scans progress down through the pelvis. At the posterolateral aspect of the right ilium, two of the three *gluteal muscles* are visible—the gluteus medius and a small amount of the gluteus maximus—whereas on the left, only the gluteus medius is visible. The *iliacus muscle* is seen lining the internal aspect of the iliac wings near the psoas muscles. The two rectus abdominis muscles are found in the anterior abdomen on both sides of the midline. The external oblique, internal oblique, and transverse abdominis are seen extending anteriorly from the ilium on each side. The abdominal aorta bifurcates at L4 into the *common iliac arteries*. Each common iliac artery divides at the level of the anterior superior iliac spine into *internal* and *external iliac arteries*. The *internal iliac arteries* tend to be located in the posterior pelvis and branch to feed the pelvic structures. The *external iliac vessels* are found progressively anterior in succeeding inferior sections to become the femoral vessels at the superior aspect of the thigh. The internal and external iliac veins unite inferior to the anterior superior iliac spine to form the common iliac veins, and the inferior vena cava is formed anterior to L5 by the junction of the common iliac veins. This scan shows the internal and external iliac arteries. At this level, the internal and external iliac veins have joined to form the common iliac veins. The common iliac veins are positioned at the anterior aspects of the sacrum, with the internal and external iliac arteries anterior and medial to the veins in these images.

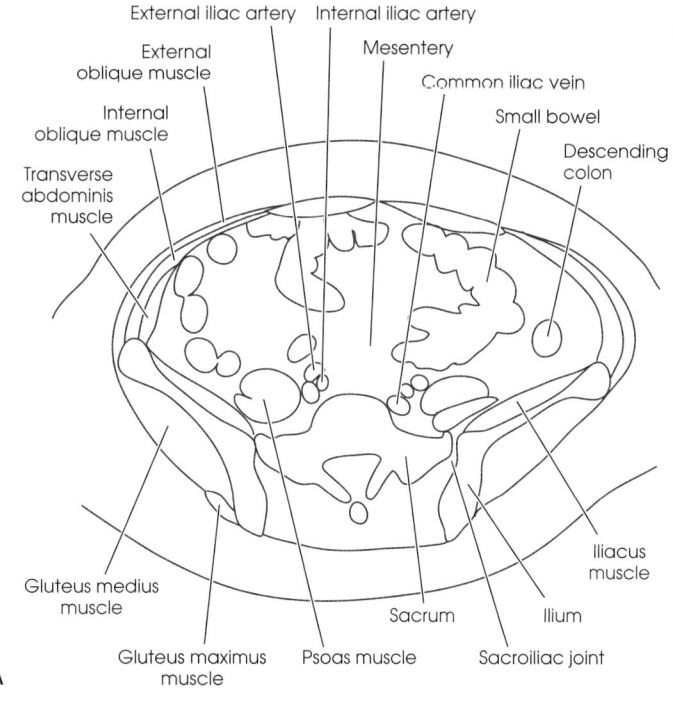

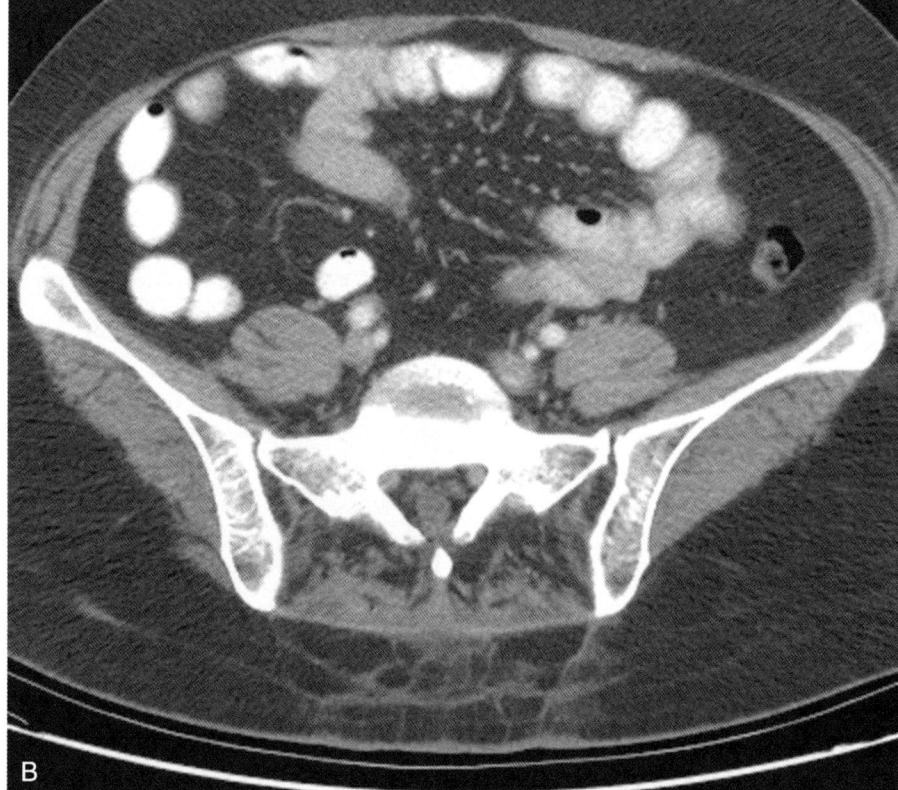

Fig. 24.57 (**A**) Line drawing of CT section. (**B**) CT image corresponding to level *I* in Fig. 24.48.

Fig. 24.58 is a CT image obtained just superior to the level of the *acetabulum*. In this image, the inferior sacrum is visible, and the junction of the *ilium*, *ischium*, and *pubis* lies near the upper part of the acetabulum. Loops of ileum filled with contrast medium are seen in the anterior right pelvis. The *haustral folds* of the *sigmoid colon* are found in the center of the pelvis as this part of the large intestine curls toward the sacrum. A portion of the rectum is seen just anterior to the sacrum in this image. The fundus of the *uterus* lies medial to the right acetabulum and posterior to the ileal folds. The ureters are filled with contrast medium in this image and are easily identifiable in the posterior and lateral regions of the pelvic cavity. The external iliac arteries and veins run a diagonal course through the pelvis, lying near the sacrum in the upper part of the pelvis and passing anteriorly as they pass down through the pelvis toward the lower extremities. In this scan, the external iliac vessels are seen just medial to the anterior edges of the acetabula. Multiple muscular structures are found at this level. The rectus abdominis muscles lie on either side of the midline in the anterior abdomen. The gluteal muscles (maximus, medius, and minimus) lie along the external surface of the posterior pelvis. Other muscles of the lower limbs are found just anterior to the acetabula. The large sciatic nerve can be plainly seen on the left between the gluteus maximus and medius muscles.

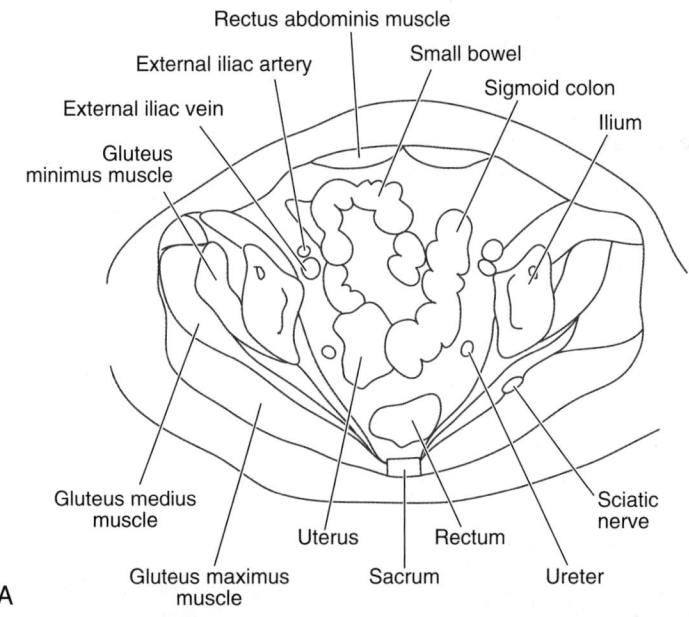

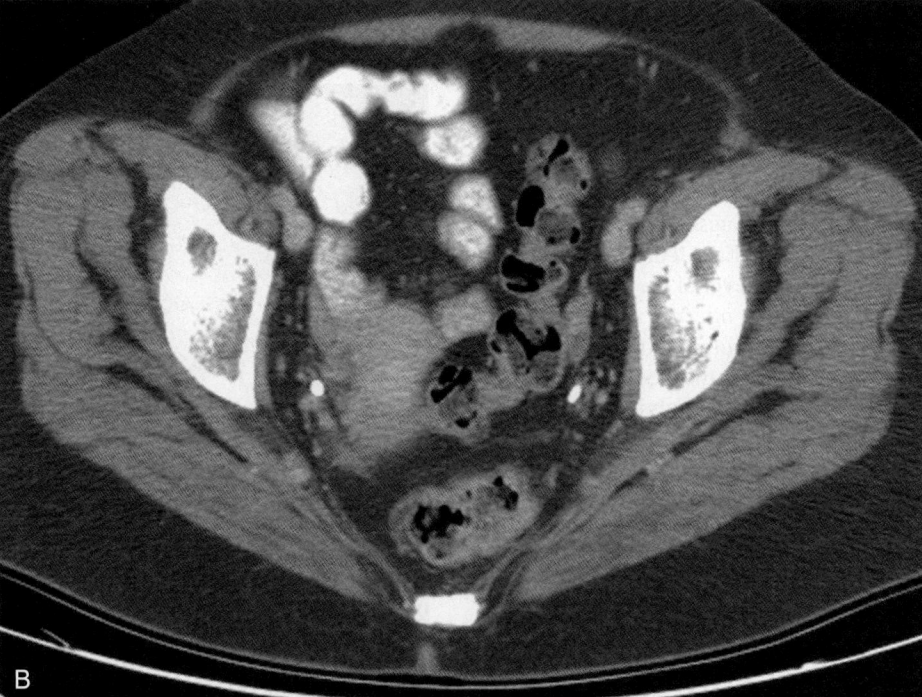

Fig. 24.58 (**A**) Line drawing of CT section. (**B**) CT image of female pelvis corresponding to level *J* in Fig. 24.48.

The CT scan in Fig. 24.59 is of a female patient and is at a level just superior to the pubic symphysis. The pubic bones, *ischia*, *acetabula*, *femoral heads*, and *greater trochanters* are visualized. The relationship between the *rectum*, *cervix*, and wall of the *bladder* is shown from posterior to anterior in the pelvic region. The ureters entered the bladder just superior to this scan and so are no longer visible. The external iliac vessels are now referred to as the *femoral vessels*, with the name change occurring at the inguinal ligament, which is found between the pubic symphysis and the anterior superior iliac spine. The *iliopsoas muscles* (formed by the junction of the psoas and iliacus muscles) are found anterior to the femoral heads; the *obturator internus muscle*, with its characteristic right-angle bend, is found medial to the acetabulum.

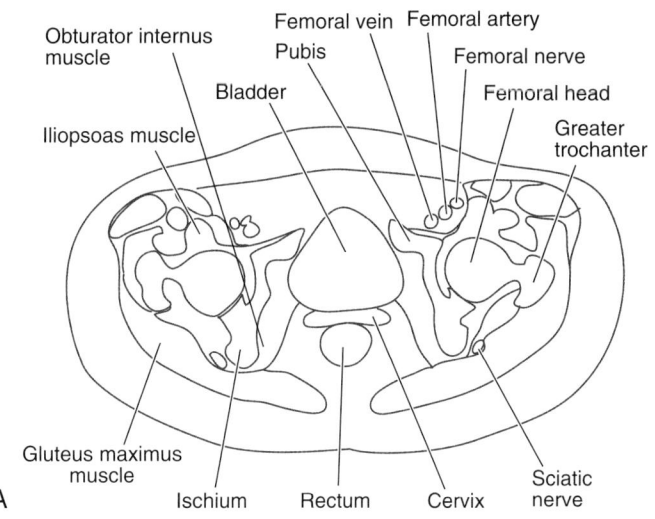

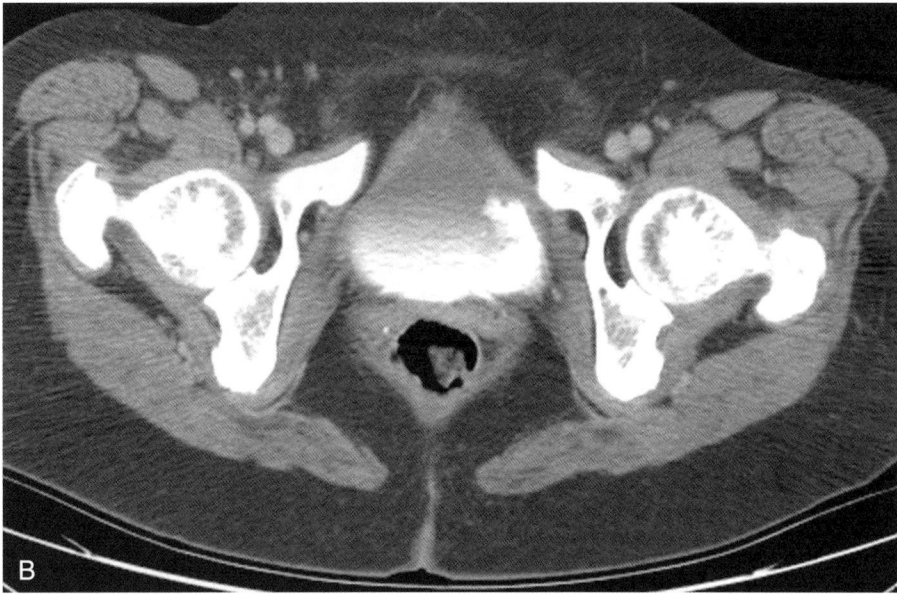

Fig. 24.59 (**A**) Line drawing of CT section. (**B**) CT image of female pelvis corresponding to level *K* in Fig. 24.48.

Fig. 24.60 is a CT scan through the lower pelvis of a male patient. This scan is at a slightly more inferior level than the previous scan. The symphysis pubis is seen here, along with the acetabula, *ischial spines*, and *femoral heads* and *greater trochanters*. The tip of the *coccyx* is visible in the posterior pelvis. In the male pelvis, the prostate gland lies inferior to the bladder and is traversed by the *urethra*. In this image, the prostate gland, seminal vesicles, and rectum occupy the pelvic cavity from anterior to posterior. The bright spot within the prostate gland is the contrast-filled urethra. The *spermatic cords* transmit the ductus deferens and vascular structures between the pelvis and the testicular structures and are found on either side of the midline just anterior to the symphysis pubis.

Fig. 24.61 is a sagittal T2-weighted MRI image of the female pelvis near the midline. The fourth and fifth lumbar vertebrae, the sacrum, and the coccyx are visualized. The cauda equina is seen descending the spinal canal. The areas of signal void anterior to the sacrum represent the rectum. The musculature and cavity of the uterus are visible anterior to the rectum. In the anterior pelvis, the bladder is seen posterior and superior to the symphysis pubis. Multiple loops of small bowel fill the upper anterior region of the pelvis but are blurry, owing to peristaltic motion. The rectus abdominis muscle extends superiorly from the pubis in the anterior abdominal wall. Fig. 24.62 is a sagittal T1-weighted MRI image of a male patient. Note the prostate gland lying inferior to the bladder. A portion of the urethra can be seen passing through the prostate in this image.

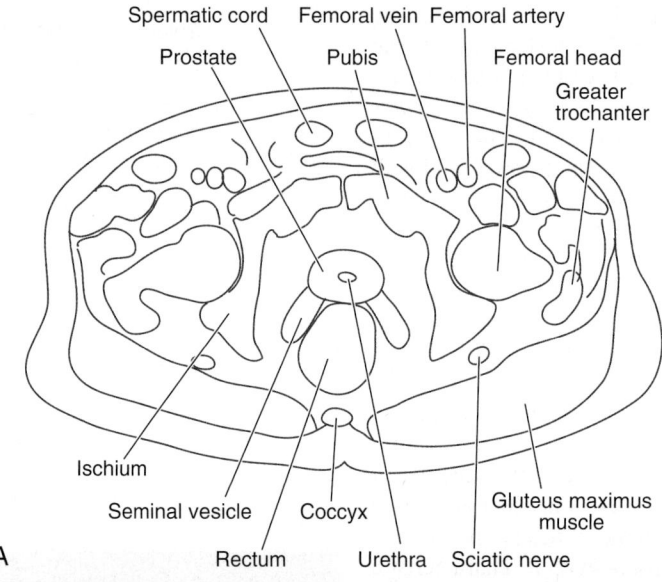
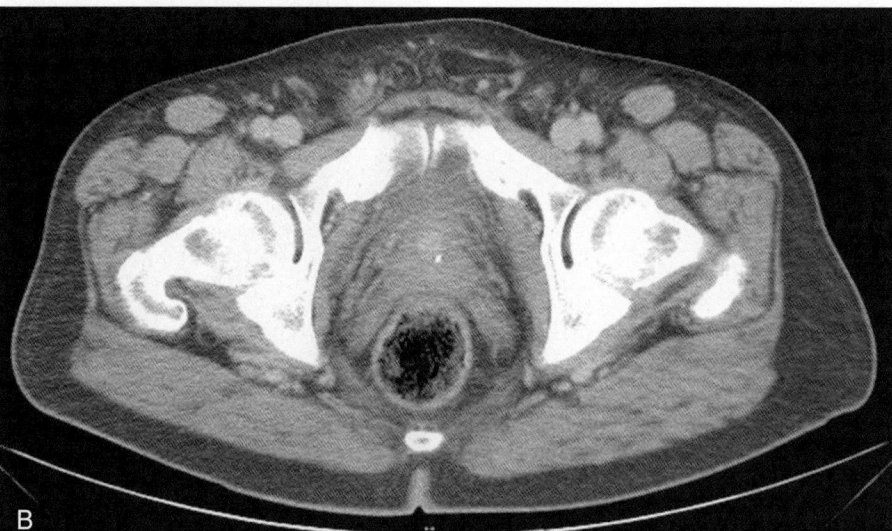

Fig. 24.60 (**A**) Line drawing of CT section. (**B**) CT image of male pelvis corresponding to level *K* in Fig. 24.48.

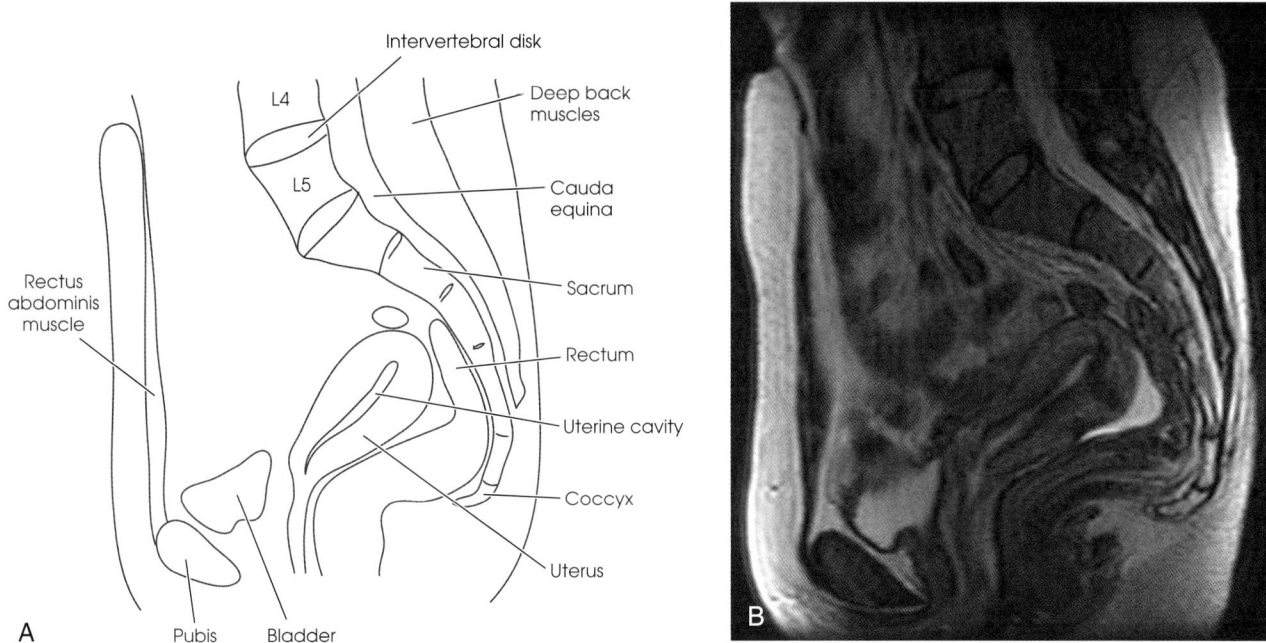

Fig. 24.61 (A) Line drawing of MRI section. **(B)** MRI of female abdominopelvic region at midsagittal plane.

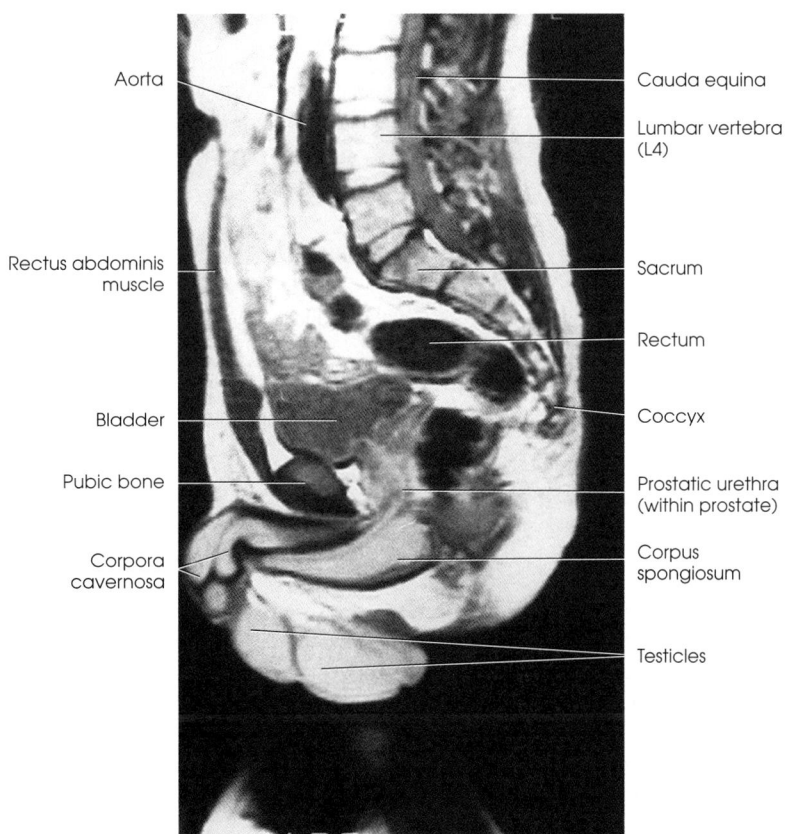

Fig. 24.62 MRI of male abdominopelvic region at midsagittal plane.

Fig. 24.63 is a coronal CT image through the abdomen and pelvis. The only bony structures visible are the lower ribs. At the top of the abdomen, the diaphragm separates the heart and lungs from the liver and gastrointestinal structures. The right lobe of the liver occupies most of the right upper quadrant. On the inferolateral surface of the liver is a fluid-filled circle, which represents the gallbladder. Several structures of the gastrointestinal system are visible in this image. Near the midline, inferior to the liver, are contrast-filled structures, which represent the proximal duodenum and the stomach. The right (hepatic) and left (splenic) flexures of the large intestine are visible. The hepatic flexure is just inferior to the liver and gallbladder; the splenic flexure is just inferior to the left hemidiaphragm. The ascending colon lies along the right lateral abdominal wall, and multiple loops of small bowel with and without contrast enhancement can be seen within the central portion of the abdomen. The urinary bladder occupies the center of the pelvis.

Fig. 24.64 lies near the median coronal plane. At this level, the right and left lobes of the liver and a small portion of the gallbladder are apparent. The porta hepatis is the region of the liver where vascular structures enter and leave the organ. It is sometimes referred to as the hilum of the liver and is seen here on the inferior surface near the center. The contrast-filled body of the stomach lies near the left lobe of the liver. Several loops of small bowel are visible in the central abdomen, and the hepatic flexure and descending portion of the colon are along the lateral walls. The aorta and inferior vena cava are found anterior to the vertebral column within the abdomen. The aorta lies on the left, and the vena cava lies on the right. Major visceral branches of the abdominal aorta are (from superior to inferior) the celiac artery (sometimes called the celiac trunk), which originates from the anterior aorta near the level of T12; the superior mesenteric artery, which originates from the anterior aorta near the level of L1; the right and left renal arteries, which originate from the lateral aorta near the level of L2; the inferior mesenteric artery, which originates

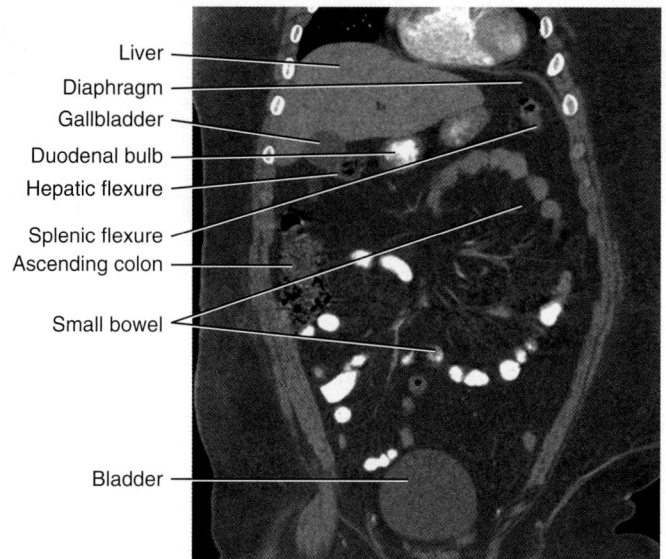

Fig. 24.63 Coronal CT image through anterior abdomen.

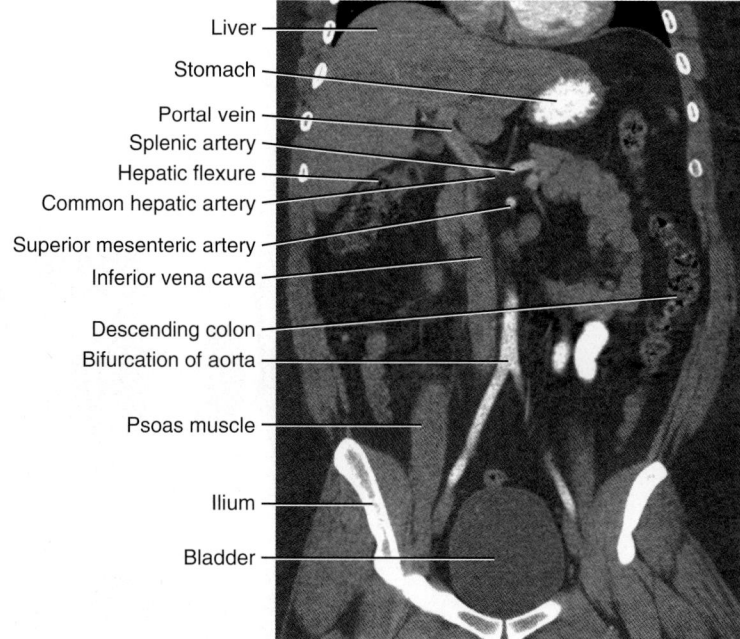

Fig. 24.64 Coronal CT image through central abdomen.

between the lateral and anterior surface of the aorta near the level of L3; and the common iliac arteries, which result when the aorta bifurcates near the level of L4. In this image, the aorta is bright because of contrast enhancement. The celiac trunk is a short vessel that almost immediately bifurcates into the common hepatic, splenic, and left gastric arteries. This image shows the common hepatic artery, which passes right to supply the liver, and the splenic artery, which branches toward the left to supply the spleen. Just below these vessels, the origin of the superior mesenteric artery is also apparent. The image clearly shows the lower abdominal aorta, its bifurcation, and the common iliac arteries. The portal system drains blood from the digestive system and carries nutrients to the liver. The portal vein is formed by the junction of the superior mesenteric vein and the splenic vein and can be seen within the porta hepatis.

Fig. 24.65 is a coronal CT image that represents a plane just posterior to the median coronal plane. Ribs are seen on the superior lateral aspect of the lower thorax and upper abdomen. Several lumbar vertebral bodies are visible in the center of the abdomen, and the iliac wings, acetabuli, femoral heads, and symphysis pubis are discernible in the pelvis. The right lobe of the liver lies in the right upper quadrant, and the spleen is found in the left upper quadrant, where it is positioned lateral to the stomach and inferior to the diaphragm. The pancreas is a long, thin organ that lies horizontally across the center of the abdomen. In this scan, the tail of the pancreas can be found near the hilum of the spleen. The stomach, filled with contrast medium, rests inferior to the left hemidiaphragm, superior to the pancreatic tail, and between the liver and spleen. The right and left kidneys are retroperitoneal organs. Most of the right kidney is visible on this image; the anterior surface of the left kidney can also be seen. The central abdominal portions of the aorta and inferior vena cava are present in the center of the abdomen. The aorta is brighter, owing to contrast enhancement. The left renal artery is visible at its origin from the aorta, and a small segment of the right renal artery is seen near the hilum of the right kidney.

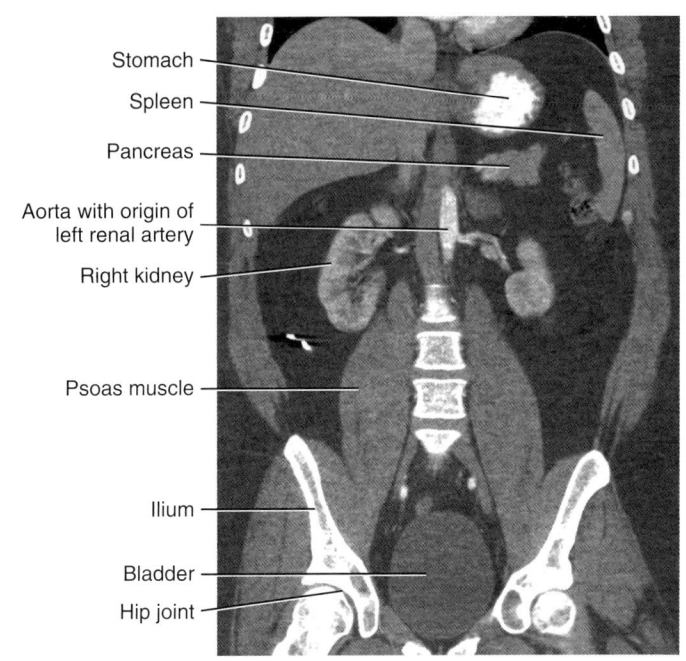

Fig. 24.65 Coronal CT image of abdomen posterior to midcoronal plane.

Advanced Visualization

The discussion of sectional anatomy in medical imaging would be incomplete without including three-dimensional (3D) advanced visualization. This section will discuss three-dimensional imaging related particularly to CT and MRI imaging.

In the early years of radiology there was a need for 3D imaging; however, there were no computers with advanced software to support the technology. Instead, there were special stereotactic devices that displayed two images, one for each eye. The two images had a minimal change of 5 degrees in the view angles between the two studies. The radiologist would use a handheld stereotactic viewer to bring the two images together to make one three-dimensional image.

The introduction of spiral CT created a change in the way three-dimensional images were viewed. In 1993, Elscint Inc. introduced the first multidetector row CT (MDRCT), which allowed for two spiral slices to be acquired simultaneously. Other manufacturers soon followed, introducing four rows of detectors, which evolved to eight, 16, 40, 64, and 128 rows. This number continues to increase as technology advances and becomes more sophisticated.

The acquisition of multiple slices over a shorter period of time helped in the evolution of three-dimensional imaging. A series of CT images creates a volumetric dataset, or a more simple "dataset" that can be manipulated by the computer to produce additional images in different planes or three-dimensional images. The thickness of these individual slices and the associated matrix size contributes to the size of the volume element or voxel. The voxel is like a pixel but with a third-dimensional element, thus creating a 3D "box" or "volume." The matrix is the number of voxels in each slice. A larger number in the size of a matrix (e.g., 512 × 512) results in smaller voxels, while a smaller matrix (e.g., 256 × 256) results in larger voxels. The shape of each individual voxel is important in the 3D reconstruction process. Voxels that are symmetric in all three dimensions are considered to be isotropic. Voxels that are not symmetric in all three dimensions are considered to be anisotropic. Having isotropic voxels, thin slices, and a large matrix size are key in the successful reconstruction of multiplanar reformatting (MPR) and 3D images. This is because the volumetric dataset, when post-processed, provides the radiologist better spatial resolution in the reconstructed planes. As mentioned previously in this chapter, source images obtained from the imaging modalities can be compiled to produce MPR images and 3D images. Three-dimensional and MPR images provide the clinician a more detailed look at complex anatomy.

The following are some of the 3D reconstruction techniques.

MULTIPLANAR REFORMATTING (MPR)

The MPR technique enables the clinician to see other planes that were not acquired directly during the acquisition stage of the imaging study. The post-processing of the acquired volumetric dataset (usually in the axial plane in CT) can be reformatted into sagittal, coronal, and oblique cross-sectional images (Fig. 24.66). This post-processing technique might be useful to adjust a particular slice to the orientation that may be relevant to a specific anatomic structure. Some vendors provide software that automatically reconstructs MPR slices after the data-set has been acquired. For example, in CT a number of axial images are acquired of the abdomen/pelvis and then automatically reconstructed in the sagittal and coronal planes. Curved MPR can be used for the analysis of patients with scoliosis or to visualize blood vessels by cutting the plane parallel to the spine or blood vessel. MPR is one of the most widely used post-processing three-dimensional imaging techniques.

CINE MODE

The cine mode technique is often used when the data-set has anisotropic voxels. The cine visualization is mostly used along the slice orientation; the clinician is able to view individual slices in a continuous movie loop. This provides better visualization of adjacent anatomic structures. The cine mode technique can be slowed down or sped up, depending on the individual user.

MAXIMUM INTENSITY PROJECTION (MIP) AND MINIMUM INTENSITY PROJECTION (MINIP)

The MIP technique is frequently used in order to see voxels with maximum intensity (bright), which represents voxels that have a hyperdense signal in MRI, or a hyperintense signal in CT (high CT number). Higher CT numbers are related to more radiopaque structures and are lighter gray or white on the image. The MIP technique is particularly helpful in the assessment and diagnosis of vascular structures (Fig. 24.67). The MIP reconstruction method is also used in positron emission tomography (PET) exams to provide greater visibility of lesions. The MinIP technique is used to show voxels with a minimum intensity (dark), which represent voxels that have a hypodense signal in MRI, or a hypointense signal in CT (low CT number). Lower CT numbers represent anatomic

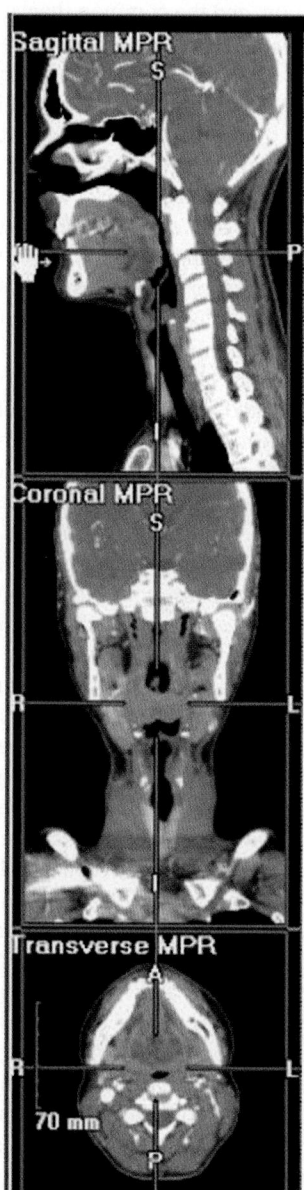

Fig. 24.66 CT multiplanar reformatting (MPR) of the head and neck.

(From Weber State University, School of Radiologic Sciences.)

structures that are more easily penetrated by x-ray and appear closer to black on the image. This type of post-processing is used to demonstrate organs filled with air in CT examinations, such as the trachea, lungs, and sinuses.

SHADED SURFACE DISPLAY (SSD)

SSD is an indirect post-processing technique by which surfaces of the object are determined within a volumetric data-set, and the resulting surface is displayed. The SSD technique is generated by applying a boundary of voxels that have the same or similar intensity values. The surface on these voxels is called an isosurface. The SSD technique applies a threshold to the data-set. Surface contours are created by generating polygonal meshes that connect adjacent voxels within the given threshold value. The user can apply a virtual lighting source in different orientations to produce shaded visualizations, which help display depth relations (Fig. 24.68).

VOLUME RENDERING (VR)

Volume rendering (VR) is a direct post-processing technique that takes the entire data-set and calculates the contributions of each voxel along a line from the viewer's eye through the data-set, displaying the resulting value for each pixel of the display. In other words, volume rendering involves the formation of a red green blue alpha (RGBA) volumetric image from the data-set. *RGB* represents the colors of the image, while the *A* (alpha) represents the opacity of the image. The opacity values range from 0 to 1. Zero is represented as totally transparent, while 1 is represented as totally opaque. The surfaces of the image can be improved by using shading techniques, which form the RGB mapping. Adjusting the opacity is helpful to see the interior structures of the data-set. Volume rendering is widely used to visualize vascular structures, as well as applications in cardiac and orthopedic imaging (Fig. 24.69).

VIRTUAL COLONOSCOPY

Virtual colonoscopy is a post-processing function similar to SSD. This post-processing method visualizes internal organs, vessels, and gastrointestinal structures using data-sets from MRI and CT. The method is similar to an endoscopy exam. The post-processing technique allows a virtual journey along a path inside a vessel or specific organ, such as the stomach, small intestine, or colon. A predefined camera path through the respective anatomic structure uses a software feature known as planned navigation. This camera path specifies camera positions and view directions (orientations) of the virtual camera. A fly-through movie is then created based on this predetermined path.

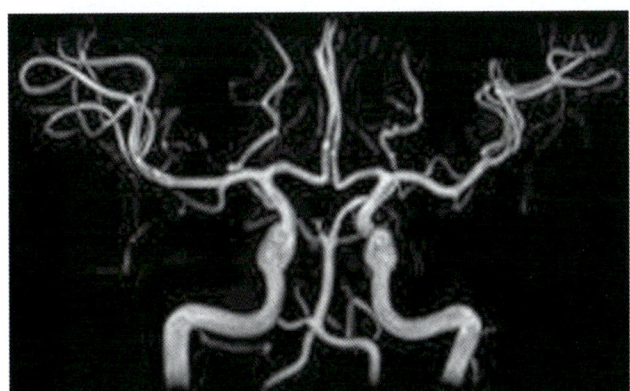

Fig. 24.67 MRI maximum intensity projection (MIP) of the circle of Willis (COW).

(From Weber State University, School of Radiologic Sciences.)

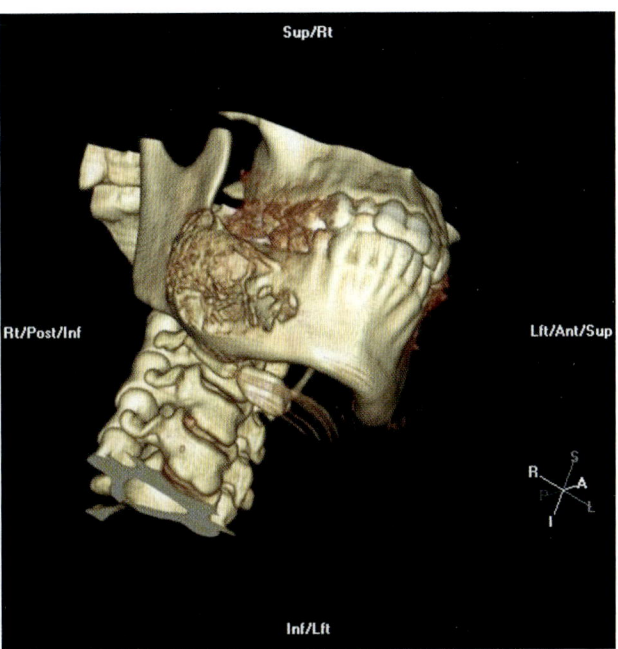

Fig. 24.68 CT shaded surface display (SSD) with anterior lighting effects.

(From Weber State University, School of Radiologic Sciences.)

3D Printing

In 1984, Charles Hull was the first to introduce 3D printing technology. Three-dimensional printing is widely known by other terms, such as additive manufacturing (AM), layered manufacturing, solid free-form fabrication, or rapid prototyping (RP). Traditional manufacturing techniques, known as subtractive manufacturing, involve the removal of material from a solid block using a milling technique to produce the final physical object. Three-dimensional printing adds different materials to the build platform until a 3D object is completed. The basic components of 3D printing can be divided into three groups: (1) hardware (the 3D printer); (2) software (which communicates instructions to the hardware); and (3) the physical materials used to print objects. Many different materials are used for 3D printing, including plastic, silicone, nylon, metal, and biomaterials. These materials are further subdivided according to such characteristics as rigid versus soft and rubberlike, single color versus multicolored, and opaque versus transparent. The workflow for 3D printing comprises five steps: (1) 3D data acquisition, (2) segmentation, (3) conversion of a Digital Imaging and Communication in Medicine (DICOM) file to a 3D mesh file format, (4) computer-aided design (CAD), and (5) 3D printing.

DATA ACQUISITION

The acquisition of images, usually from CT and MRI, is the first step in the 3D printing process. This is the most crucial step due to the fact that poor image quality can lead to poor quality in the 3D-printed model. Therefore, the acquisition of high-resolution isotropic 3D volumetric datasets with excellent image quality is a prerequisite for creating a high-quality 3D-printed model. The volumetric data should also contain sufficient signal intensity and contrast to differentiate the anatomy of interest from other surrounding structures. Acquisition protocols with different imaging modalities should be adjusted to provide the best volumetric dataset for 3D printing. In CT imaging, the risk versus benefit of the increased radiation dose and the quality of the volumetric dataset must be considered.

SEGMENTATION

DICOM is the most common medical imaging format. DICOM is a standard for distributing and viewing any kind of medical image. The process of transforming DICOM images into a 3D model is referred to as segmentation. The process of segmentation separates anatomic structures from adjacent structures (Fig. 24.70). Thresholding, region growing, and other manual operations are used to segment (cut) the anatomic structure of interest away from adjacent anatomic structures. Artificial intelligence (AI) software will be instrumental in improving the segmentation process.

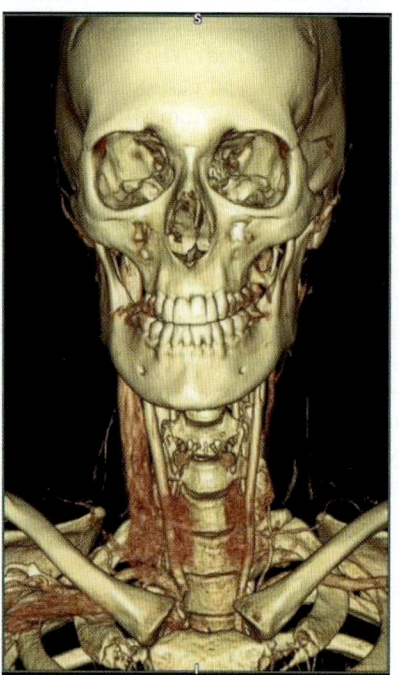

Fig. 24.69 CT 3D volume-rendered study of the head and neck.

(From Weber State University, School of Radiologic Sciences.)

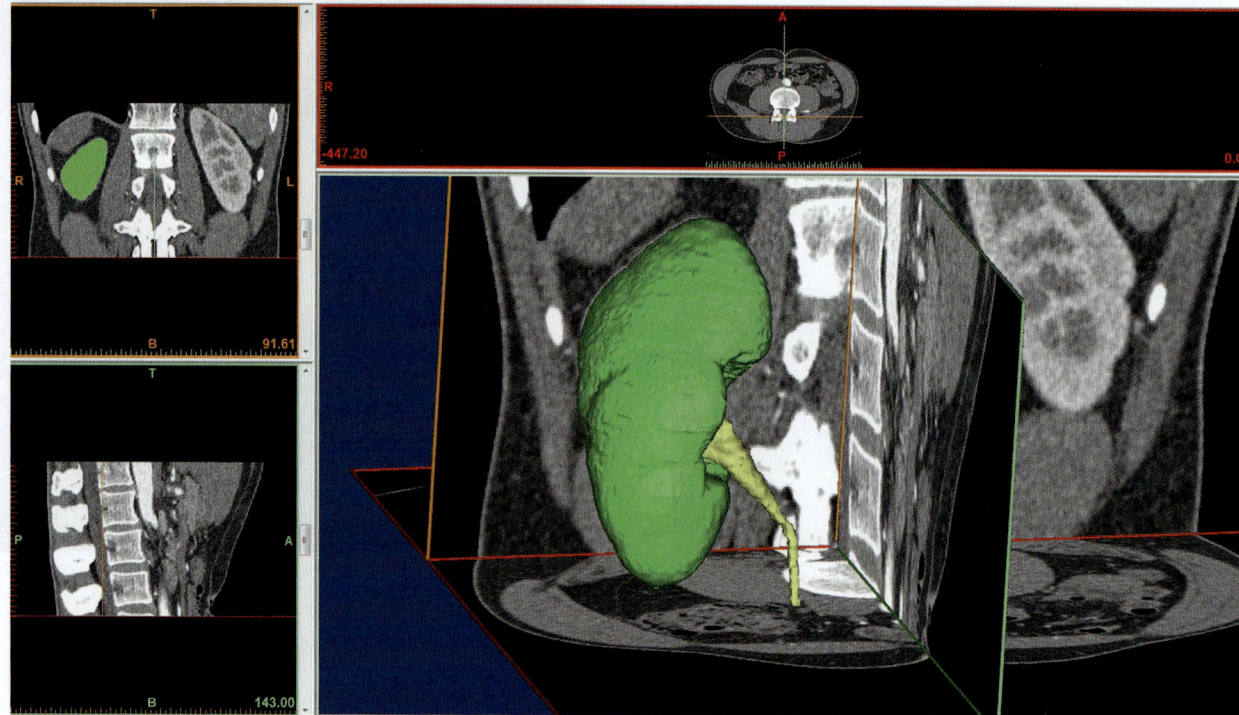

Fig. 24.70 CT structural segmentation of the right kidney.

(From Weber State University, School of Radiologic Sciences.)

DICOM FILE CONVERSION TO 3D MESH FILE

The conversion of a DICOM file to a 3D mesh file can be accomplished by a wide range of different software. Some of the software is open source (free), while other software products must be purchased from specific vendors. The software converts the DICOM image into a Standard Tessellation Language (STL) or various alternate file types, such as 3D manufacturing format (3FM), object file (OBJ), and virtual reality modeling language (VRML). The most common file types that are converted from DICOM are STL and OBJ. In addition to converting DICOM files into a different file type, the software divides the surface of the image into small triangles that compose it into a mesh.

COMPUTER-AIDED DESIGN (CAD)

CAD is the final step before sending a completed file to the 3D printer. Some of the most commonly used CAD software products are Mimics (Materialise), 3-matic (Materialise), SolidWorks (Dassault Systemes), and Creo (PTC). Most CAD software combines the DICOM conversion and mesh formation together with the CAD functions. These two functions are listed as separate steps in this chapter, but they are usually combined with the CAD software. The CAD software performs an additional step of mesh post-processing. This step refines the triangulated surfaces to repair any edges or structures that may affect the final result of the printed object. The process basically "wraps" the 3D object to repair any holes and makes the surface smooth and even. The CAD process involves design processes such as local smoothing, cuts, change of spatial orientation, and adding additional parts to the object so that other anatomic structures can be attached. Adjustments can be made to the wall thickness to provide structural integrity to the printed object.

3D PRINTERS

Printers come in various shapes and sizes. The cost can range from hundreds to thousands of dollars. Different 3D printer types can help facilitate the speed, resolution, choice of colors, and material composition of the 3D printed object. Three-dimensional printers fall into four different types: (1) liquid-based, (2) powder-based, (3) solid-based, and (4) paper-based. The following are descriptions of various types of 3D printers.

Stereolithography (SLA)

In 1988, 3D Systems Inc. introduced the first rapid prototype of the SLA 3D printer based on the work by inventor Charles Hull. SLA is a liquid-based 3D printer that builds a plastic 3D object one layer at a time by tracing a laser beam on the surface of a vat filled with a liquid photopolymer. The photopolymer solidifies when the laser beam strikes the surface of the liquid. The platform is then lowered to a distance equal to the layer thickness (typically 0.003 to 0.002 inch), and a subsequent layer is formed on top of each previous layer. The photopolymer has self-adhesive properties that allow the previous layer to bond to subsequent layers. The 3D-printed object is a result of all of these combined layers. Complex 3D objects add structural supports to provide stability to the object (Fig. 24.71). When the object is completed, it is cleaned and cured to harden the object before structural supports are removed and the object is sanded and polished.

Fused deposition modeling (FDM)

FDM was developed by Stratasys in Eden Prairie, Minnesota, and is considered a solid-based printer. The FDM process uses a solid plastic or wax material that is extruded through a nozzle to form a three-dimensional object layer by layer. The heated plastic or wax hardens very rapidly after it has left the printer nozzle. A second extrusion nozzle is used for support material. The object is built on a mechanical platform that moves vertically downward as each layer is formed. The entire object is contained in a chamber that has a temperature just below the melting point of the plastic. The FDM printer can use a wide range of materials, including ABS, polycarbonate, polypropylene, polyamide, polyethylene, and investment casting wax.

Selective laser sintering

Carl Deckard and colleagues at the University of Texas in Austin developed the selective laser sintering (SLS) technique. The SLS printer is a powder-based 3D printer that uses a thermoplastic powder that is spread over the top of the build platform. A laser beam moves over the surface of the tightly compacted powder to selectively melt and fuse the powder together to form one layer of the object. The build platform moves down one object layer thickness to accommodate the next layer of powder, and the process repeats itself. Different types of thermoplastic powder materials are used, including nylon, polyamide, polystyrene, elastomers, and composites. One of the unique things about the SLS technique is that no building supports are required. The overhangs and complex geometric shapes are supported by the residual solid powder bed surrounding the object. This process does require a considerable amount of time for the object to cool down before it can be removed from the machine.

Direct metal laser sintering (DMLS)

The DMLS technique was developed jointly by Rapid Product Innovations (RPI) and EOS GmbH, starting in 1994. The DMLS printer is a powder-based process that is similar to the SLS method. However, in the DMLS process, no binder or fluxing agents are included in the metal powder. This results in a 95% density steel final object compared with a 70% density in the SLS final object. The metal powder used in the DMLS process is 20 microns in diameter. The metal powder is completely melted by a high-powered laser beam. The size of the metal powder and the hardening of the metal powder using a high-powered laser create thinner layers, resulting in

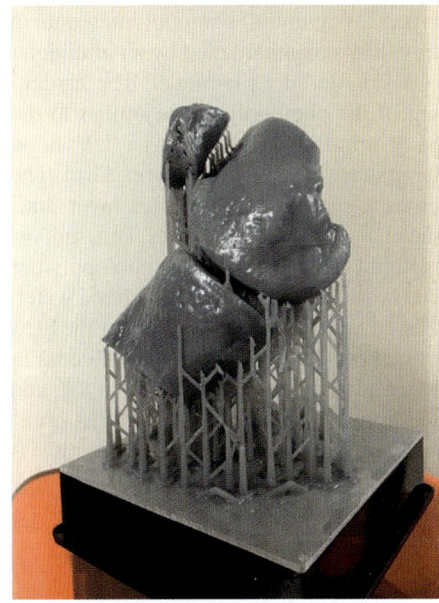

Fig. 24.71 3D-printed model of the knee with structural supports still in place.

(From Weber State University, School of Radiologic Sciences.)

higher detail resolution. Higher detail resolution results in more intricate part shapes. Material options for this process include alloy steel, stainless steel, tool steel, aluminum, bronze, cobalt-chrome, and titanium.

Inkjet printing

The inkjet 3D printing process uses liquid plastic for the build material and wax for the support material. The liquids are held in reservoirs until they are fed to the individual jet heads. The liquids are squirted in tiny droplets onto the build platform to form a layer of the 3D object. The liquid hardens by the rapidly dropping temperature as it moves along the build platform. Once the droplets have been deposited and hardened, a sharp blade is passed over the layer to make the thickness uniform. The excess particles are vacuumed away and captured in a filter. After the 3D object is completed, the wax for the support material is dissolved or melted away. The inkjet printing process produces extremely high resolution (0.0005 inch) and excellent surface finishes. The downside is that it is rather slow for large 3D objects.

Polyjet printing

In early 2000, the first polyjet technology was introduced by Objet Geometries Ltd., an Israeli company. The polyjet technology is similar to the inkjet 3D printing technique in that it has individual jet heads. However, the polyjet printer squirts layers of a liquid photopolymer onto a tray that is then hardened by an ultraviolet (UV) ray to cure the model. The hardening of the photopolymer is similar to the SLA printing technique. The UV flood lamp is mounted onto the print head. The process continues layer after layer until the 3D object is complete. The support material is also made of a photopolymer and washed away with pressurized water. The advantage of the polyjet over the SLA printer is that the photopolymers come in a cartridge rather than stored in a vat, and multiple colors can be used. Polyjet printers are also very clean and quiet, with less post-processing cleanup on parts.

Laminated object manufacturing (LOM)

LOM was developed by Helisys of Torrance, California. Three-dimensional objects are created by stacking, bonding, and cutting layers of adhesive-coated sheet material on top of each other. The outline of each sheet layer is cut by a laser. After the laser cuts the outline of the layer, another sheet is advanced on top of the previously deposited layers. A heated roller applies pressure to bond the new layer, and the process repeats until the final 3D object is complete. The LOM process can use a variety of different colors. The sheets are composed of paper and various types of plastics.

USES OF 3D PRINTING IN MEDICINE

Interactive 3D advanced visualization and 3D printing have many applications in medicine. These post-processing techniques aid clinicians in visualizing anatomic and pathologic structures that can be beneficial in the planning of radiation therapy treatment, surgical procedures, and minimally invasive interventions. Advanced post-processing imaging using these techniques provides a clearer view of anatomic structures and pathology, which aids the radiologist in making a diagnosis. Advanced visualization and the use of 3D printable models and cutting guides can help surgeons in pretreatment planning, which can result in reduced time for surgical procedures. Clinicians can use 3D models to educate patients regarding pathology, treatment options, and surgical approaches, thus giving the patient a better understanding of their disease, surgical approaches, and therapeutic options. Three-dimensional printers continue to find novel ways to improve patient outcomes and provide better continuity of care for the patient. In the future, as the cost of 3D printers declines and more physicians and technologists become familiar with the technology, there is likely to be an increase in its usage in the health care marketplace.

Selected bibliography

Anderson MW, Fox MG. *Sectional Anatomy by MRI and CT*. 4th ed. St Louis: Elsevier; 2016.

Applegate EJ. *The Sectional Anatomy Learning System*. 3rd ed. Philadelphia: Elsevier; 2010.

Bo WJ, Carr JJ, Krueger WA, et al. *Basic atlas of Sectional Anatomy with Correlated Imaging*. 4th ed. Philadelphia: Elsevier; 2007.

Calhoun PS, Kuszyk BS, Heath DG, et al. Three-dimensional volume rendering of spiral CT data: theory and method. *Radiographics*. 1999;19(3):745–764.

El-Khoury GY, Bergman RA, Montgomery WJ. *Sectional Anatomy by MRI and CT*. 3rd ed. New York: Churchill Livingstone; 2007.

Ellis H, Logan BM, Dixon AK. *Human Sectional Anatomy: Pocket Atlas of Body Sections, CT and MRI Images*. 3rd ed. London: Hodder Arnold; 2009.

Flohr TG, Schaller S, Stierstorfer K, et al. Multi-detector row CT systems and image reconstruction techniques. *Radiology*. 2005;235(3):756–773.

Goo HW, Park SJ, Yoo SJ. Advanced medical use of three-dimensional imaging in congenital heart disease: Augmented reality, mixed reality, virtual reality, and three-dimensional printing. *Korean J Radiol*. 2020;21(2):133–145.

Kalaskar DM. *3D Printing in Medicine*. St Louis: Elsevier; 2017.

Kelley LL, Petersen CM. *Sectional Anatomy for Imaging Professionals*. 4th ed. St Louis: Elsevier; 2018.

Madden ME. *Introduction to Sectional Anatomy*. 3rd ed. Philadelphia: Lippincott Williams & Wilkins; 2012.

National Institutes of HealthNational Library of Medicine. *The Visible Human Project*; 2023. Available at: www.nlm.nih.gov/research/visible/visible_human.html (Accessed July 15, 2024.)

Preim B, Bartz D. *Visualization in Medicine: Theory, Algorithms, and Applications. (The Morgan Kaufmann Series in Computer Graphics)*. Burlington: Morgan Kaufmann; 2007.

Ramya A, Vanapalli S. 3D printing technologies in various applications. *Int J Mech Eng Technol*. 2016;7(3):396–409.

Spratt JD, Salkowski LR, Loukas M, et al. *Weir & Abrahams' Imaging Atlas of Human Anatomy*. 5th ed. London: Elsevier; 2016.

Weber EC, Vilensky JA, Carmichael SW. *Netter's Concise Radiologic Anatomy*. Philadelphia: Elsevier; 2009.

25

COMPUTED TOMOGRAPHY

MEGAN WEDGEWORTH

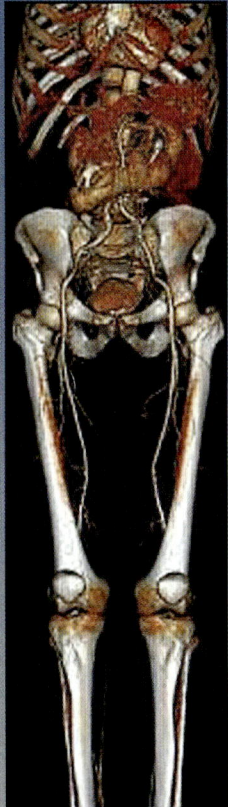
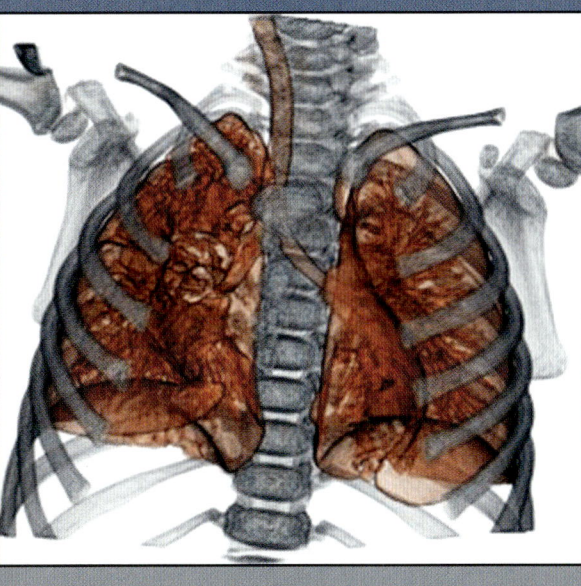

OUTLINE

Principles of Computed Tomography, 228
Computed Tomography Versus Conventional Radiography, 228
Historical Development, 231
Classifications of Computed Tomography Scanner Generation, 231
Technical Aspects, 234
System Components, 235
Diagnostic Applications, 239
Contrast Media, 242
Factors Affecting Image Quality, 244
Special Features, 247
Radiation Dose, 255
Factors That Affect Dose, 257
Radiation Dose Reduction and Safety, 259
Artificial Intelligence in Computed Tomography, 259
Advancements, 259
New Technologies, 260
Basic Computed Tomography Examination Protocols, 262
Best Practices in Computed Tomography, 265
Definition of Terms, 265

Principles of Computed Tomography

Computed tomography (CT) is the process of creating a cross-sectional tomographic plane of any part of the body (Fig. 25.1). In CT, a patient is scanned by an x-ray tube rotating around the body part being examined. A detector assembly measures the radiation exiting the patient and feeds back the information to the host computer. This is referred to as *primary data*. After the computer has compiled and calculated the data according to a preselected *algorithm*, it assembles the data in a *matrix* to form an *axial* image. Each image, or *slice*, is displayed in a cross-sectional format.

In the early 1970s, CT scanning was used clinically only for imaging the brain. The first CT scanners were capable of producing only axial images and were called *computed axial tomography (CAT)* units; this term is no longer accurate because images can now be created in multiple planes. Dramatic technical advancements have led to the development of CT scanners that can be used to image virtually every structure within the human body. Improvements in the scanner design and computer science have produced CT units with new imaging capabilities and reconstruction techniques. The reprocessing of images into three-dimensional reconstructions of internal structures is used for surgical planning, CT angiography (CTA), radiation therapy planning, and virtual reality imaging.

Interventional procedures such as CT-guided biopsies and fluid drainage offer an alternative to surgery for some patients. Although these procedures are considered invasive, they offer shorter recovery periods and lower risk of infection.

Computed Tomography Versus Conventional Radiography

When a conventional x-ray exposure is made, the radiation passes through the patient and produces an image of the body part where body structures are superimposed (Fig. 25.2). Visualizing specific structures requires the use of contrast media, varied positions, and usually more than one exposure. For example, the localization of masses or foreign bodies on an x-ray image often requires at least two exposures and a ruler calibrated for magnification.

During the CT examination, a tightly collimated x-ray beam is directed through the patient from many different angles, resulting in an image that represents a cross section of the area scanned. This imaging technique essentially eliminates the superimposition of body structures. The CT technologist controls the method of acquisition, the slice thickness, the reconstruction algorithm, and other factors related to image quality.

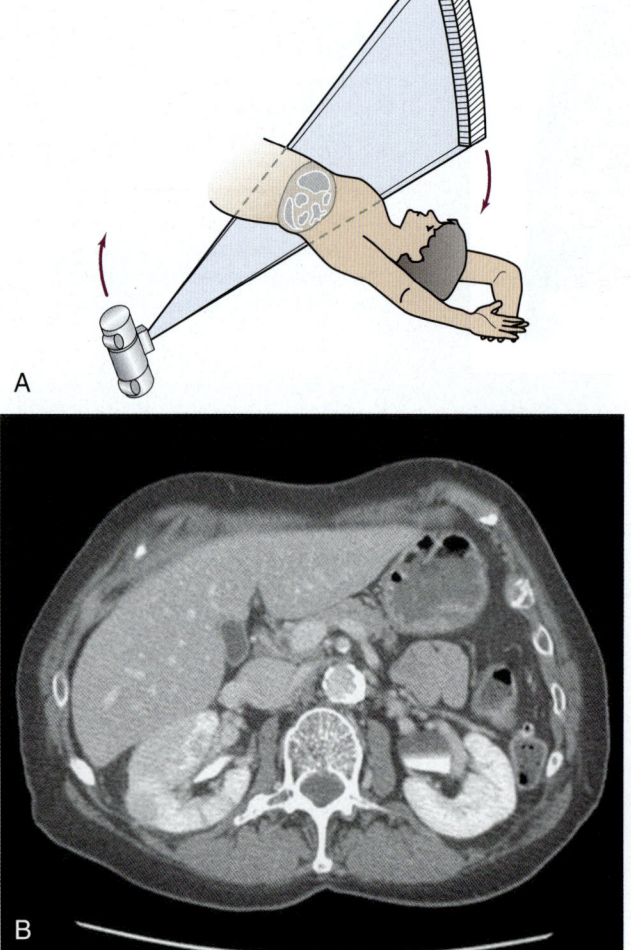

Fig. 25.1 (**A**) CT scanner provides cross-sectional images by rotating around the patient. (**B**) Axial CT showing right renal enlargement.

(B, from Zagoria RJ, Dyer R, Brady C: *Genitourinary imaging: the requisites*, ed 3. Philadelphia, 2016, Elsevier.)

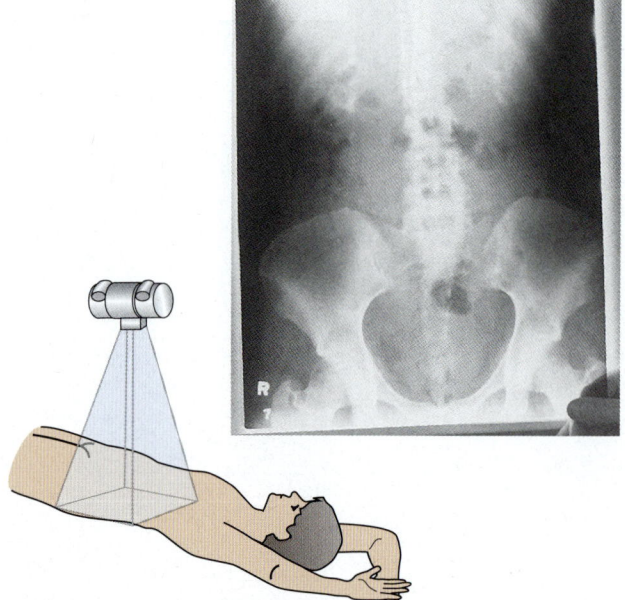

Fig. 25.2 Conventional radiograph superimposes anatomy and yields one diagnostic image with fixed density and contrast.

The digital radiograph of the abdomen illustrated in Fig. 25.3 shows high-density bone and low-density gas, but many soft tissue structures, such as the kidneys and intestines, are not clearly identified. A contrast medium is needed to visualize these structures. A CT examination of the abdomen demonstrates all of the structures that lie within a slice. In Fig. 25.4A, the liver, stomach, kidneys, spleen, and aorta can be identified. In addition to eliminating superimposition, CT is capable of differentiating tissues with similar densities. This differentiation of densities is referred to as *contrast resolution*. CT provides improved contrast resolution as compared with conventional radiography. This is due to a reduction in the amount of scattered radiation.

Fig. 25.4B is an axial image of the brain that differentiates the gray matter from the white matter and shows bony structures and cerebrospinal fluid within the ventricles. CT can show subtle differences in various tissues, as in Fig. 25.4B. This allows radiologists to diagnose pathologic conditions more accurately than if they were to rely on radiographs alone. A CT image is digitized by the computer with numerous image manipulation techniques that can be used to enhance and optimize the diagnostic information available to physicians (Fig. 25.5).

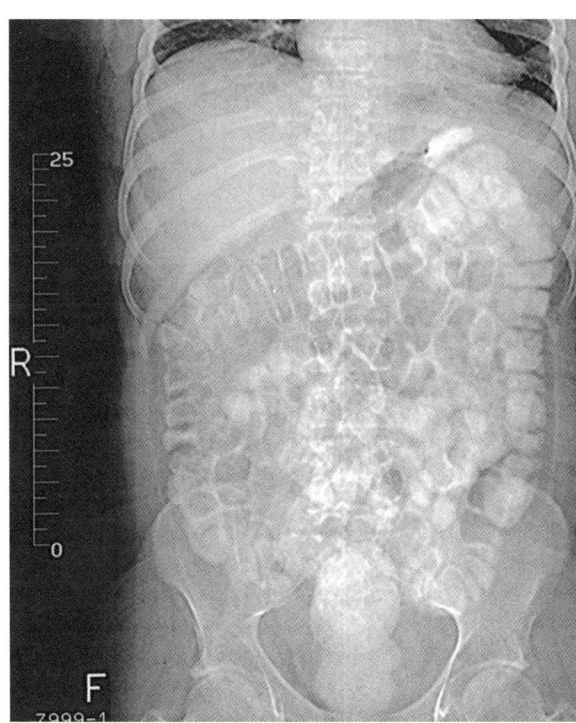

Fig. 25.3 Digital kidney, ureter, and bladder (KUB).

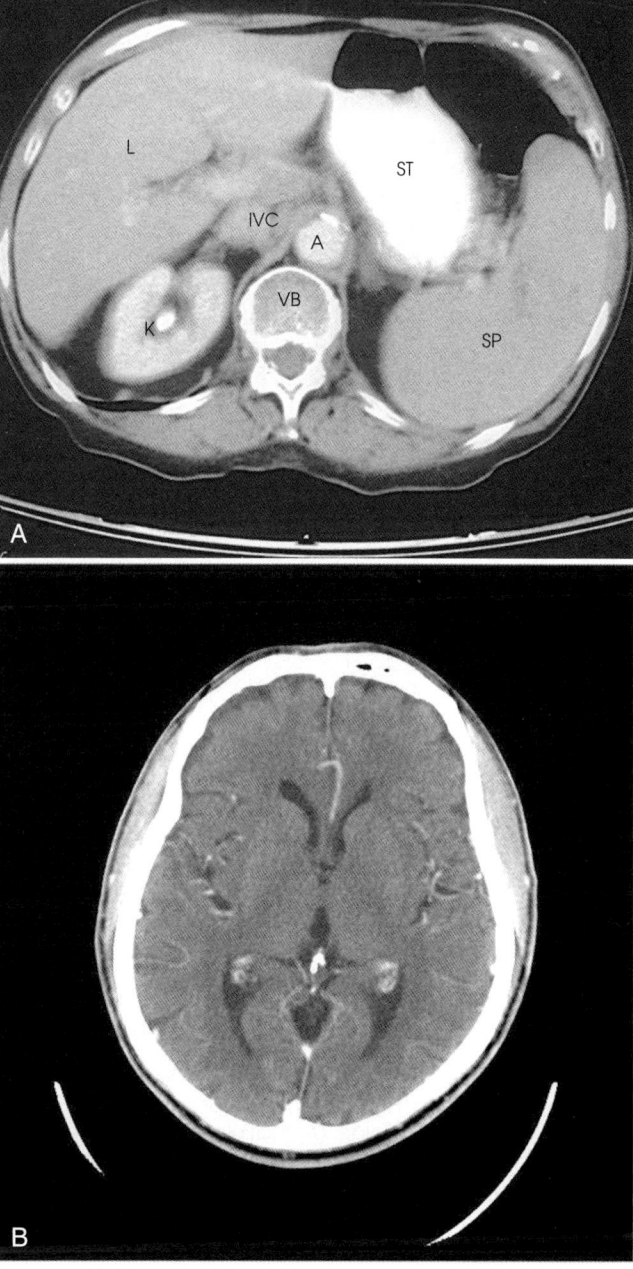

Fig. 25.4 (**A**) Axial image of abdomen showing liver *(L)*, stomach *(ST)*, spleen *(SP)*, aorta *(A)*, inferior vena cava *(IVC)*, vertebral body of thoracic spine *(VB)*, and kidney *(K)*. (**B**) Axial CT of brain.

(B, from Kelley LL, Peterson CM: *Sectional anatomy for imaging professionals*, ed 2, St Louis, 2007, Elsevier.)

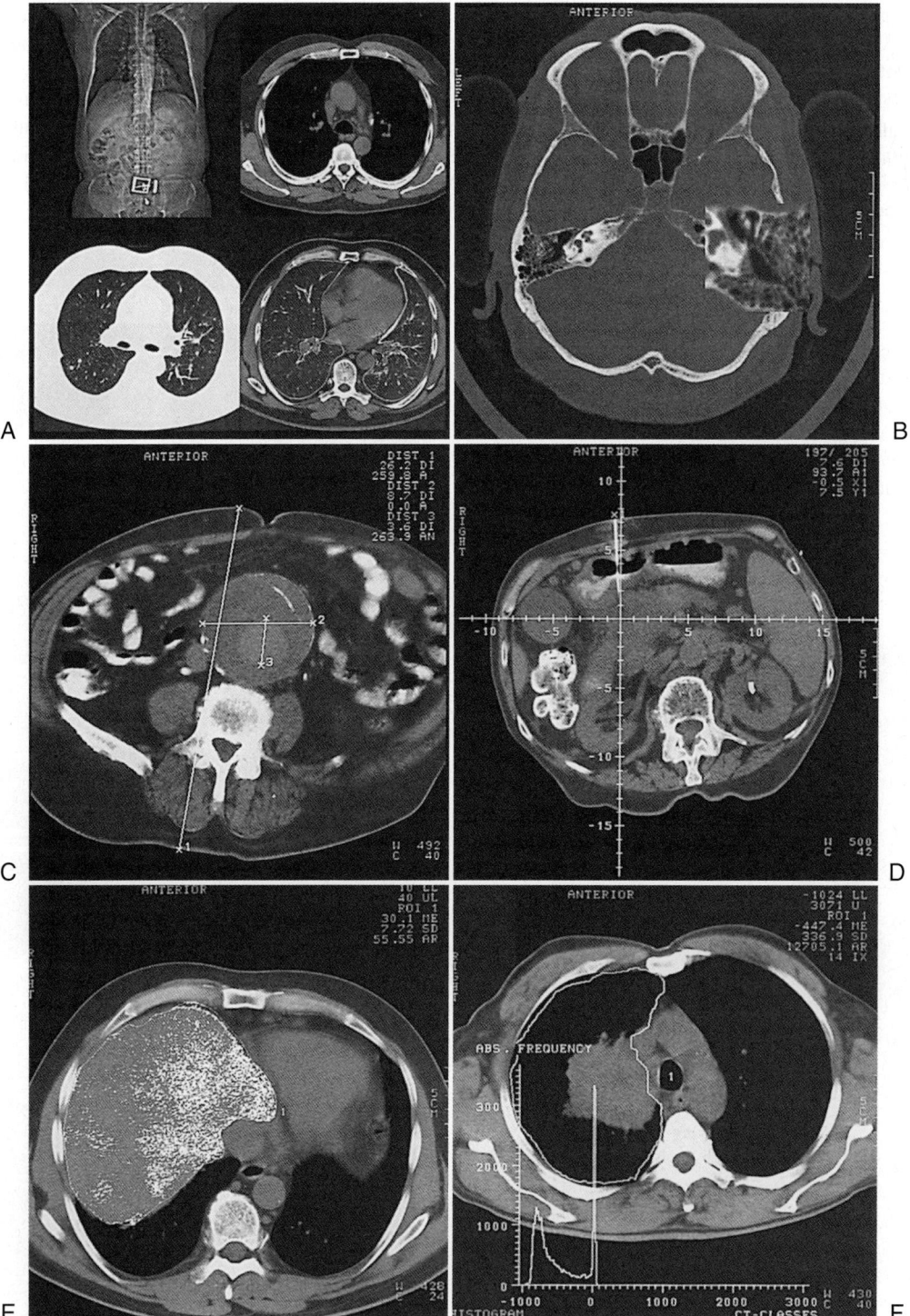

Fig. 25.5 Image manipulation techniques used to enhance diagnostic information in CT image. (**A**) Multiple imaging windows. (**B**) Image magnification. (**C**) Measurement of distances. (**D**) Superimposition of coordinates on the image. (**E**) Highlighting. (**F**) Histogram.

(Courtesy Siemens Medical Systems, Iselin, NJ.)

Historical Development

CT was first performed successfully in 1970 in England at the Central Research Laboratory of EMI, Ltd. Hounsfield, an engineer for EMI, and Cormack, a nuclear physicist from Johannesburg, South Africa, are generally given credit for the development of CT. They were awarded the Nobel Prize in Physiology or Medicine in 1979 for their research. After CT was shown to be a useful clinical imaging modality, the first full-scale commercial unit, referred to as a *brain tissue scanner*, was installed in Atkinson Morley Hospital in 1971. An early dedicated head CT scanner is shown in Fig. 25.6. Physicians recognized its value for providing diagnostic neurologic information, and its use was accepted rapidly. The first CT scanners in the United States were installed in June 1973 at the Mayo Clinic, Rochester, Minnesota, and later that year at Massachusetts General Hospital, Boston. These early units were dedicated head CT scanners. In 1974, Ledley at Georgetown University Medical Center, Washington, DC, developed the first whole-body scanner, which greatly expanded the diagnostic capabilities of CT.

After physicians accepted CT as a diagnostic modality, numerous companies, in addition to EMI, began to manufacture scanners. Although the units differed in design, the basic principles of operation were the same.

Classifications of Computed Tomography Scanner Generation

CT scanners have historically been categorized by *generation*, which is a reference to the level of technologic advancement of the tube and detector assembly. The original "generation" classification of scanners was a clear distinction of tube movement versus detector rotational path. As scanner technology has progressed, the tube movement and detector rotation relationship have remained relatively constant, but the tube power source and the detector configurations have changed.

The *first-generation scanners* worked by a process known as *translate/rotate*. The tube produced a finely collimated beam, or pencil beam. Depending on the manufacturer, one to three *detectors* were placed opposite the tube for radiation detection. The linear tube movement (translation) was followed by a rotation of 1 degree. Scan time was usually 3 to 5 minutes per scan, which required the patient to hold still for extended periods. Because of the slow scanning and reconstruction time, the use of CT was limited almost exclusively to neurologic examinations because of the

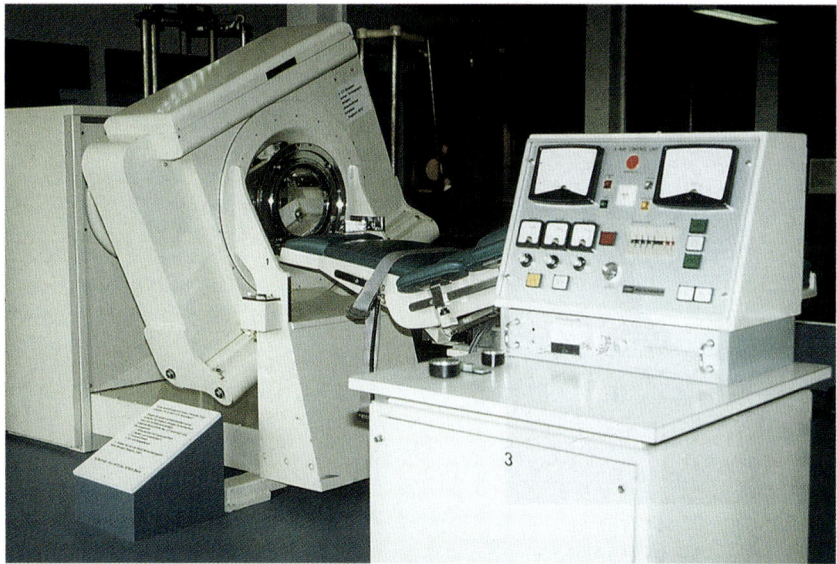

Fig. 25.6 First-generation EMI CT unit: dedicated head scanner.

(Photograph taken at Röentgen Museum, Lennep, Germany.)

aperture size and the water bag construction. A CT image from a first-generation scanner is shown in Fig. 25.7.

The *second-generation scanners* were considered a significant improvement over the first-generation scanners. The x-ray tube emitted a fan-shaped beam that was measured by approximately 30 detectors placed closely together in a *detector array*. Tube and detector movement was still *translate/rotate*; however, the gantry rotated 10 degrees between each translation. These changes improved overall image quality and decreased scan time to about 20 seconds for a single slice. The time required to complete one CT examination remained relatively long.

The *third-generation scanners* introduced a *rotate/rotate movement*, in which the x-ray tube and detector array rotate simultaneously around the patient. An increase in the number of detectors (>750) and their arrangement in a "curved" detector array considerably improved image quality (Fig. 25.8). Scan times were decreased to 0.35 to 1 second per slice, which made the CT examination much easier for patients and helped decrease motion artifact. Advancements in computer technology also decreased image reconstruction time, substantially reducing examination time.

The *fourth-generation scanners* introduced the *rotate-only movement*, in which the tube rotated around the patient but the detectors were in fixed positions, forming a complete circle within the gantry (Fig. 25.9). The use of stationary detectors required greater numbers of detectors to be

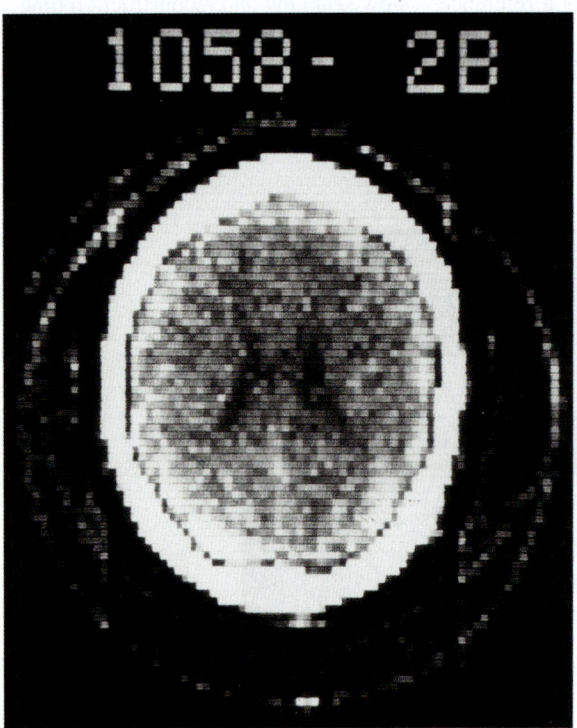

Fig. 25.7 Axial brain image from the first CT scanner in operation in the United States: Mayo Clinic, Rochester, Minnesota. The 80 × 80 matrix produced a noisy image. The examination was performed in July 1973.

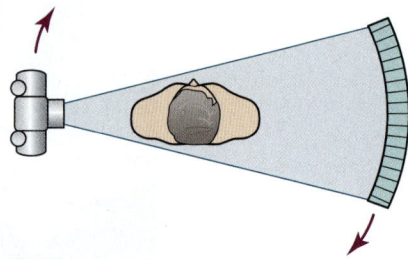

Fig. 25.8 Rotate/rotate movement: tube and detector movement of a third-generation scanner.

installed in a scanner. Fourth-generation scanners tended to yield a higher patient dose per scan than previous generations of CT scanners because the CT tube was closer to the patient.

The *fifth-generation scanners* are classified as high-speed CT scanners because of millisecond acquisition times. These scanners are electron-beam scanners (EBCT), in which x-rays are produced from an electron beam in a fan beam configuration that strikes stationary tungsten target rings (Fig. 25.10). The detector rings are in a ±210-degree arc. These scanners were primarily used for cardiac studies because of the improved temporal resolution; however, they are no longer in practice.

The *sixth-generation scanners* are dual-energy sources (two x-ray tubes; DSCT, DE-CT) with two sets of detectors that are offset by 90 degrees. These DSCT scanners provide improved temporal resolution needed for imaging moving structures such as the heart (Fig. 25.11). The latest dual source/dual detector (DSDD) CT scanners offer dual-energy capabilities, typically 80 and 120 kVp, between the two CT tubes. Using Flash Spiral scanning offered by Siemens, the dual source spiral scanning allows for gapless volume coverage using a pitch of 3.4, which increases the temporal resolution to one-quarter of the rotation time. This technology allows a marked decrease in patient radiation dose, as no overlapping scanning occurs.

The *seventh-generation scanner* allows the x-ray tube to move continuously around the gantry to allow for a faster scan time. There is no start-stop process because the cable wraparound process within the gantry does not exist. This type of scanner uses a cone-shaped beam, which allows for less patient artifact due to movement and an increase in x-ray tube efficiency. The flat-panel digital detectors use cesium iodide (CsI), which produces excellent spatial resolution but needs improvement in contrast resolution. The seventh-generation scanners are still in the prototype phase and are unavailable for clinical use at this time.

Most scanners today are either third- or fourth-generation configurations with one of the following technical variations:

- *Helical CT, single-slice helical CT (SSHCT)*. Slip-ring technology allows 360-degree continuous rotation of tube and detector. Reduces scan times to sub-second per slice.
- *Multislice detectors (MSHCT or MDCT)*. The increase in the number of detector rows allows multiple slices to be produced in one rotation. As detector rows have increased, the fan beam geometry of the x-ray beam has been adapted, the beginning of cone-beam configuration. Began with two-slice scanners and quickly moved to four slices and more.
- *Volume CT (VCT)*. Multislice scanners with 64 detector rows or more. The x-ray beam geometry must be a cone-beam configuration to accommodate the increased length of the scanning field.
- *Flat-panel CT (FP-CT or FD-CT)*. A detector plate similar to plates used in digital radiography (DR) replaces the typical detector configuration. In dedicated breast units, the tube and detector travel a full 360 degrees. In other applications, interventional and intraoperative, the unit functions more like a C-arm fluoroscopy unit, in which the tube and detector do not travel in a full 360 degrees. These scanners provide excellent spatial resolution but slightly lower contrast resolution.

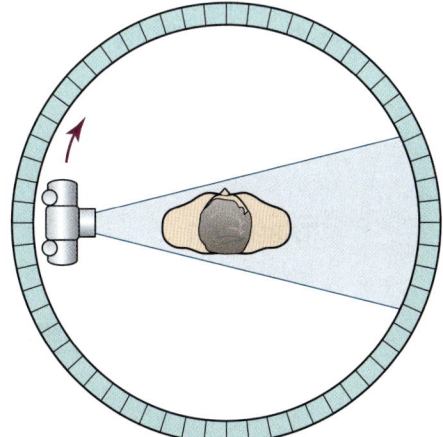

Fig. 25.9 Rotate-only movement: tube movement with stationary detectors of a fourth-generation scanner.

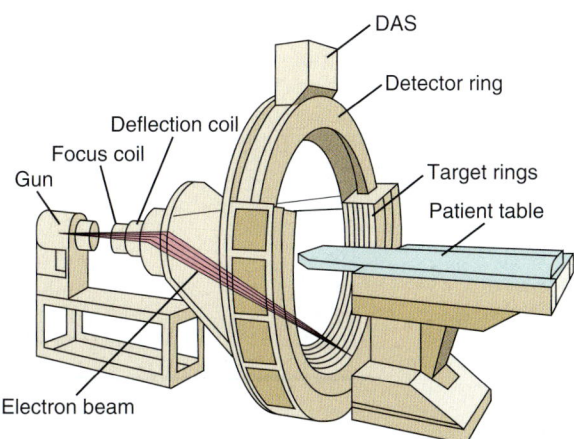

Fig. 25.10 Electron beam CT scanner configuration. X-rays, produced from electron beam, strike four target rings.

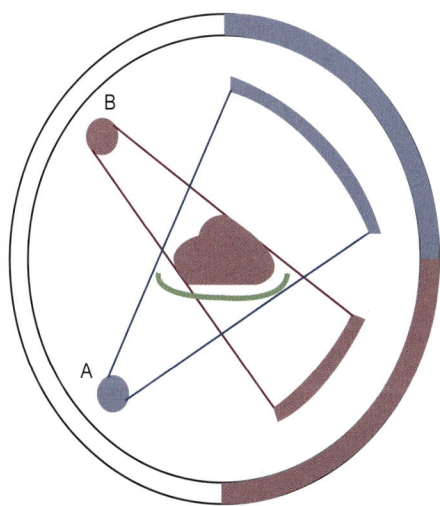

Fig. 25.11 Dual-source CT scanner (DSCT) configuration with tubes A and B rotating at a 90-degree relationship simultaneously. This is considered a sixth-generation scanner.

- *Dual-energy (DECT)/Dual-source (DSCT)/ Spectral CT.* Uses two x-ray tubes that operate at different kV values. This type of scanner delivers detailed, diagnostic cardiac images for all heart rates.

The third-generation scanners are used most commonly, but with different variations which have 4 to 320 rows of detectors in a single array. This increase in numbers of detector rows has increased the length of the scanning field, which requires the x-ray beam to be cone-shaped to encompass the full detector array. This is a change from the original third-generation fan beam. The flat-panel detector also requires cone-beam geometry. The increased detector size and the cone-beam geometry pose various challenges in maintaining image quality, but this discussion is too involved for the purpose of this chapter.

Technical Aspects

The axial images acquired by CT scanning provide information about the positional relationships and tissue characteristics of structures within the section of interest.

The computer performs a series of steps to generate one axial image. With the patient and gantry perpendicular to each other, the tube rotates around the patient, irradiating the area of interest. For every position of the x-ray tube, the detectors measure the transmitted x-ray values, convert them into an electrical signal, and relay the signal to the computer. The measured x-ray transmission values are called *projections (scan profiles)*, or *raw data*. When collected, the electrical signals are digitized, a process that assigns a whole number to each signal. The value of each number is directly proportional to the strength of the signal.

The digital image is an array of numbers arranged in a grid of rows and columns called a *matrix*. A single square, or picture element, within the matrix is called a *pixel*. The slice thickness gives the pixel an added dimension called the *volume element*, or *voxel*. Each pixel in the image corresponds to the volume of tissue in the body section being imaged. The voxel volume is a product of the pixel area and slice thickness (Fig. 25.12). The *field of view* (FOV) determines the amount of data to be displayed on the monitor.

Each pixel within the matrix is assigned a number that is related to the linear attenuation coefficient of the tissue within each voxel. These numbers are called *CT numbers* or *Hounsfield units (HU)*. CT numbers are defined as a relative comparison of x-ray attenuation of a voxel of tissue with an equal volume of water. Water is used as reference material because it is abundant in the body and has a uniform density; water is assigned an arbitrary value of 0. Tissues that are denser than water are given positive CT numbers, and tissues with lower density than water are assigned negative CT numbers. The scale of CT numbers ranges from –1000 (air/gas) to +1000 (dense bone). Average CT numbers for various tissues are listed in Table 25.1.

To display the digital image, each pixel within the image is assigned a level of gray. The gray level assigned to each pixel corresponds to the CT number for that pixel. The bit depth determines the number of shades of gray that can be assigned to a pixel. A bit depth of 8 would have 256 shades of gray available, whereas a bit depth of 12 would have 4096 shades.

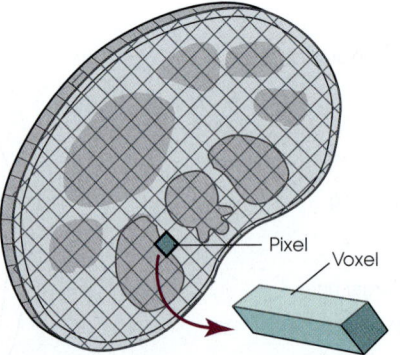

Fig. 25.12 CT image is composed of a matrix of pixels, with each pixel representing a volume of tissue (voxel).

TABLE 25.1

Average Hounsfield units (HU) for selected substances

Substance	HU
Air	–1000
Lungs	–250 to –850
Fat	–100
Orbit	–25
Water	0
Cyst	–5 to +10
Fluid	0 to +25
Tumor	+25 to +100
Blood (fluid)	+20 to +50
Blood (clotted)	+50 to +75
Blood (old)	+10 to +15
Brain	+20 to +40
Muscle	+35 to +50
Gallbladder	+5 to +30
Liver	+40 to +70
Aorta	+35 to +50
Bone	+150 to +1000
Metal	+2000 to +4000

System Components

The three major components of the CT scanner are shown in Fig. 25.13. Because each component has several subsystems, the following sections provide only a brief description of their main functions.

COMPUTER

The computer provides the link between the CT technologist and the other components of the imaging system. The computer system used in CT has four basic functions: control of data acquisition, image reconstruction, storage of image data, and image display.

Data acquisition is the method by which enough data are captured when the patient is scanned to accomplish image reconstruction. The technologist must select numerous parameters, for example, scanning in either conventional or helical mode, before the initiation of each scan. The *data acquisition system (DAS)* is involved in sequencing the generation of x-rays, turning the detectors on and off at appropriate intervals, transferring data, and monitoring the system operation.

The *reconstruction* of a CT image depends on the millions of mathematical operations required to digitize and reconstruct the raw data. The image reconstruction is accomplished using an array processor that acts as a specialized computer to perform mathematic calculations rapidly and efficiently, freeing the host computer for the next patient or other activities. Currently, CT units can acquire scans in less than 1 second and require only a few seconds more for image reconstruction.

The *host computer* in CT has limited storage capacity, so image data can be stored only temporarily. Other storage mechanisms are necessary to allow for long-term *data storage* and *retrieval*. After reconstruction, the CT image data can be transferred to another storage medium, such as an optical disk. CT studies can be removed from the limited memory of the host computer and stored independently, a process termed *archiving*.

The reconstructed images are displayed on a monitor. At this point, the technologist or physician can communicate with the host computer to view specific images, post images on a scout, or implement image manipulation techniques, such as zoom, contrast and brightness, and image analysis.

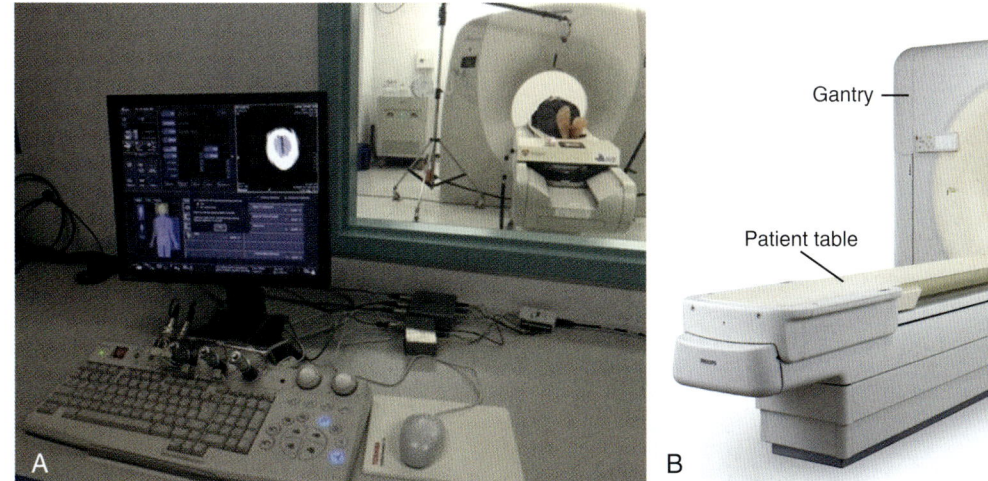

Fig. 25.13 Components of a CT scanner. **(A)** Computer and operator's console. **(B)** Gantry, gantry aperture, and patient table.

(A, From Lee K, Baird M, Lewis S, et al.: Computed tomography learning via high-fidelity simulation for undergraduate radiography students. *Radiography*, 2020;26(1):49–56; B, Courtesy Philips Medical Systems.)

GANTRY AND TABLE

The *gantry* is a circular device that houses the x-ray tube, DAS, detector array, high-voltage generator, and collimators. The components housed in the gantry collect the necessary attenuation measurements to be sent to the computer for image reconstruction.

The x-ray tube used in CT is similar in design to the tubes used in conventional radiography; however, it is specially designed to handle and dissipate excessive heat created during a CT examination. The newest CT x-ray tubes consist of a rotating anode to increase heat dissipation, a large metal anode, and a metal housing. CT x-ray tubes can handle an average of 5 million heat units (MHU), a multislice CT tube heat capacity is about 8 MHU, and the advanced CT units can tolerate up to 20 MHU.

The detectors in CT function as image receptors. A detector measures the amount of radiation transmitted through the body and converts the measurement into an electrical signal proportional to the radiation intensity. Types of detectors that are used in CT are *scintillation* or *gas-ionization chambers*. Current scintillation detectors are made of gadolinium oxysulfide (GOS) ceramic scintillation (solid-state) detectors. Gas-ionization chambers are not regularly used anymore.

The gantry can be tilted forward or backward up to 30 degrees to compensate for body part angulation. The opening within the center of the gantry is termed the *aperture*. Most apertures are about 70 cm (27.56 inches) wide to accommodate patient sizes as the patient table advances through the gantry. To accommodate larger patients and for interventional applications, an 85-cm (34-inch) aperture is available.

The *table* is an automated device linked to the computer and gantry. It is designed to move in increments *(index)* according to the scan program. Indexing must be accurate and reliable, especially when thin slices (1 or 2 mm) are taken through the area of interest. Most CT tables can be programmed to move in or out of the gantry, depending on the examination protocol and the patient.

CT tables are made of a low-density carbon fiber composite, which supports the patient without causing image artifacts. The table must be very strong and rigid to handle patient weight and at the same time maintain consistent indexing. All CT tables have a maximum patient weight limit; this limit varies by manufacturer from 450 to 650 lb (204–295 kg). Exceeding the weight limit can cause inaccurate indexing, damage to the table motor, and even breakage of the tabletop, which could cause serious injury to the patient.

Accessory devices can be attached to the table for various uses. A special device called a *cradle* is used for head CT examinations. The head cradle helps hold the head still; because the device extends beyond the tabletop, it minimizes artifacts or attenuation from the table while the brain is being scanned.

OPERATOR'S CONSOLE

The *operator's console* (Fig. 25.14) is the area in which the technologist controls the scanner. A typical console is equipped with a keyboard for entering patient data, a graphic monitor for viewing the images, a display screen, and a computer mouse. The operator's console allows the technologist to control and monitor numerous scan parameters, such as imaging technique factors, slice thickness, table index, and reconstruction algorithm.

Before starting an examination, the technologist must enter the patient's information. Usually, the first scan program selected is the scout program, from which the radiographer plans the sequence of helical scans. An example of a typical scout image is shown in Fig. 25.3. The operator's console is also the location of the monitor, where image manipulation takes place. Most scanners display the image on the monitor in a 1024 matrix interpolated by the computer from the 512 reconstructed images.

One of the most important functions of the operator's console is to initiate the process to store or archive the images for future viewing. Most modern imaging departments now have picture archiving and communications systems (PACS) that are used to store and retrieve soft copy (digital) images.

OTHER COMPONENTS
Display monitor

For the CT image to be displayed on a monitor in a recognizable form, the digital CT data must be converted into a *grayscale image*. This process is achieved by the conversion of each digital CT number in the matrix to an analog voltage. The brightness values of the grayscale image correspond to the pixels and CT numbers of the digital data they represent.

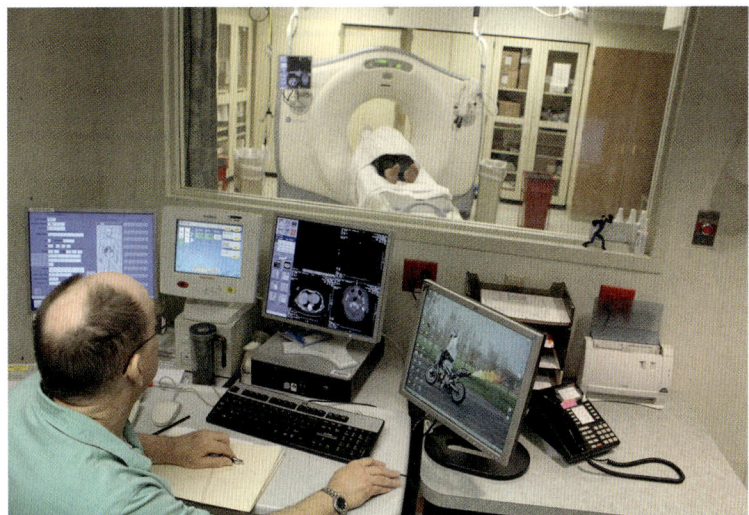

Fig. 25.14 CT scan room layout. Technologist operates CT scanner and monitors patient from control console.

(From Ehrlich RA, Coakes DM: Patient care in radiography with an introduction to medical imaging, ed 10. St Louis, 2021, Elsevier.)

Because of the digital nature of the CT image data, image manipulation can be performed to enhance the appearance of the image. One of the most common image processing techniques is called *windowing*, or *gray-level mapping*. This technique allows the technologist to alter the contrast of the displayed image by adjusting the window width (WW) and window level (WL). The *window width* is the range of CT numbers that are used to map signals into shades of gray. Basically, the WW determines the number of gray levels to be displayed in the image, controlling contrast resolution. A narrow WW means that there are fewer shades of gray, resulting in higher contrast. Likewise, a WW width results in more shades of gray in the image, or a longer gray scale. The *window level* determines the midpoint of the range of gray levels to be displayed on the monitor. It is used to set the center CT number within the range of gray levels being used to display the image, and it controls image brightness. The WL should be set to the CT number of the tissue of interest, and the WW should be set with a range of values that would optimize the contrast among the tissues in the image. Fig. 25.15 shows an axial image seen in two different windows: a standard abdomen window and a bone window adjusted for the spine.

The gray level of any image can be adjusted on the monitor to compensate for differences in patient size and tissue densities, or to display the image as desired for the examination protocol. Examples of typical WW and WL settings are listed in Table 25.2. These settings are averages and usually vary by vendor and radiologist's preference. The level, although an average, is approximately the same as the CT numbers expected for the tissue densities.

TABLE 25.2
Typical window settings

CT examination	Width	Center (level)
Brain	190	50
Skull	3500	500
Orbits	1200	50
Abdomen	400	35
Liver	175	45
Mediastinum	325	50
Lung	2000	−500
Spinal cord	400	50
Spine	2200	400

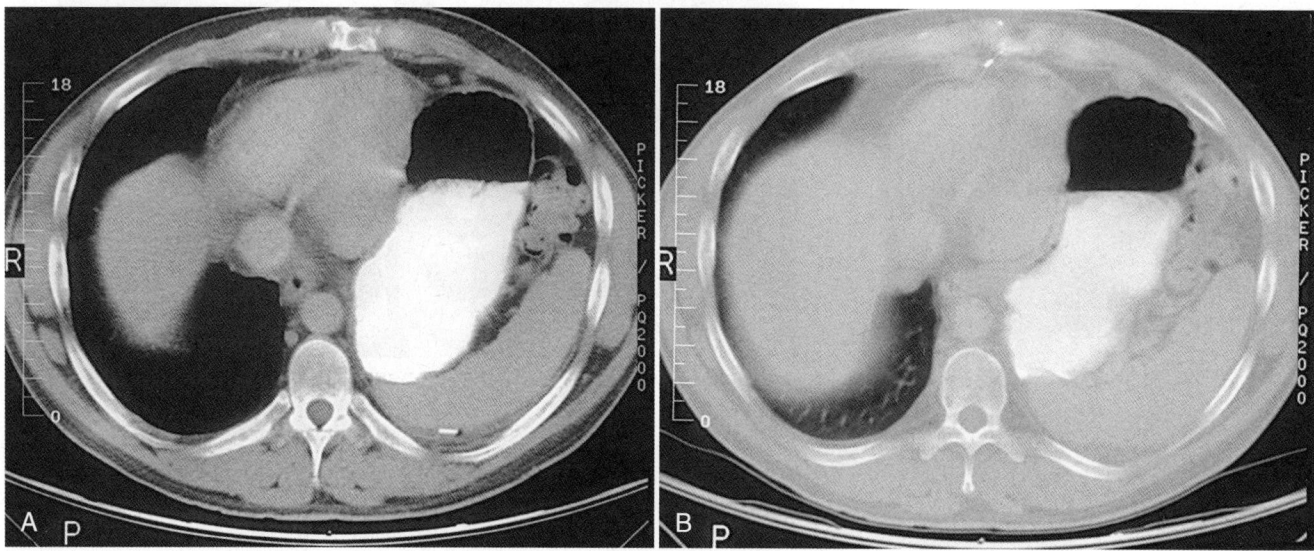

Fig. 25.15 (**A**) Abdominal image, soft tissue window. (**B**) Abdominal image, bone window.

Workstation for image manipulation and multiplanar reconstruction

Another advantage of the digital nature of the CT image is the ability to reformat the image data into coronal, sagittal, or oblique body planes without additional radiation to the patient. Image reformation in various planes is accomplished by stacking multiple contiguous axial images, creating a volume of data. Because the CT numbers of the image data within the volume are already known, a sectional image can be generated in any desired plane by selecting a particular plane of data. This post-processing technique is termed *multiplanar reconstruction* (MPR). Coronal reformations from image data are shown in Figs. 25.16 and 25.17. Fig. 25.16 shows a coronal image of the abdomen (note the liver lesion), and Fig. 25.17 shows coronal images of the lungs displayed with a lung WW and WL. MPRs may also be performed in what is referred to as *curved planar reformations* to visualize structures better. Fig. 25.18 shows an axial image and oblique reformation of the mandible from the axial images. Other post-processing techniques used today are three-dimensional imaging, surface rendering, and volume rendering (VR).

Diagnostic Applications

The original CT studies were used primarily for diagnosing neurologic disorders. As scanner technology advanced, the range of applications was extended to other areas of the body. The most requested procedures involve the head, chest, abdomen, and pelvis. CT is the examination of choice for head trauma; it clearly shows skull fractures and associated subdural

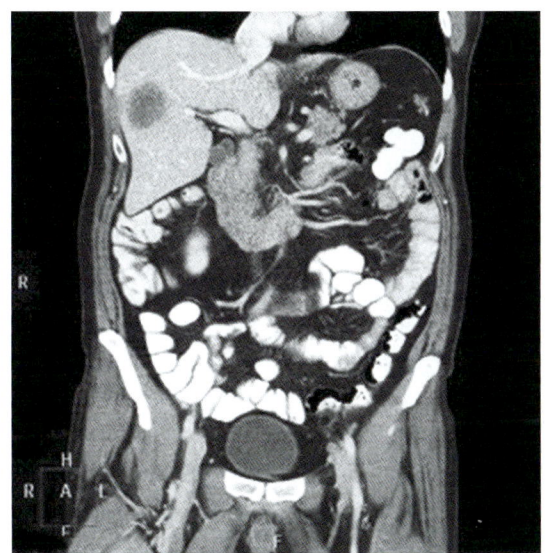

Fig. 25.16 Coronal reformatted image produced from axial images of abdomen and pelvis.

(Courtesy Philips Medical Systems.)

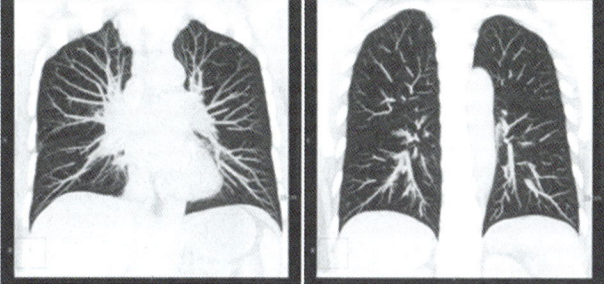

Fig. 25.17 Coronal reformatted images produced from axial low-dose lung nodule study of the chest. Scans produced with Philips Brilliance iCT.

(Courtesy Philips Medical Systems.)

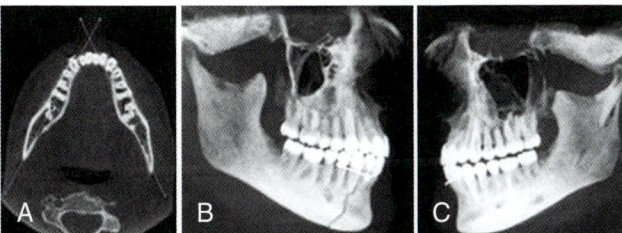

Fig. 25.18 (**A**) Axial mandible showing reformatted planes. (**B**) Oblique MPR of left mandible (note fracture). (**C**) Oblique MPR of right mandible.

(Courtesy Philips Medical Systems.)

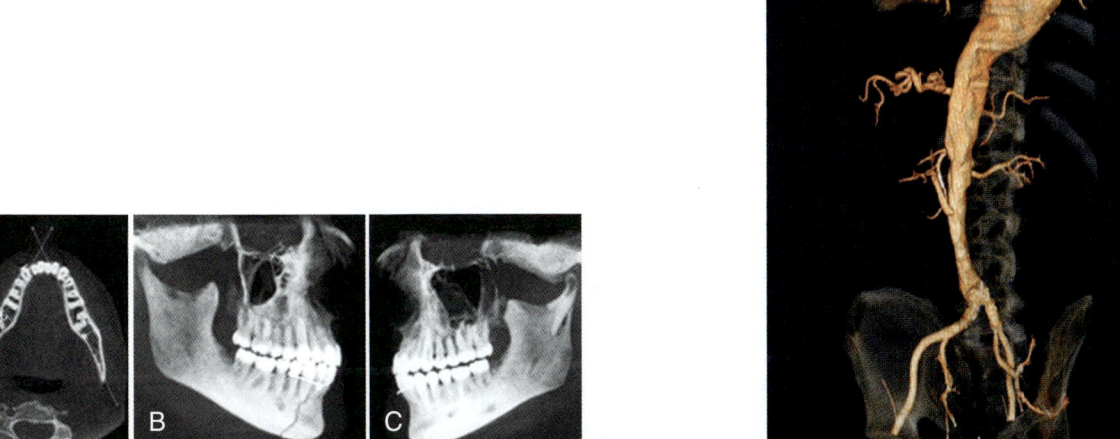

Fig. 25.19 Three-dimensional abdominal aortic aneurysm (AAA).

hematomas. CT examinations of the head are one of the first exams performed on patients being evaluated for stroke or cerebrovascular accidents where evidence of hemorrhage must be ruled out. CT imaging of the central nervous system can show infarctions, hemorrhage, disk herniations, craniofacial and spinal fractures, tumors, and cancers. CT imaging of the body excels at differentiating or distinguishing soft tissue structures within the chest, abdomen, and pelvis. Included in the numerous abnormalities shown in this region are metastatic lesions, aneurysms (Fig. 25.19), abscesses, and fluid collections from blunt trauma.

CT is also used for numerous interventional procedures, such as abscess drainage, tissue biopsy (Fig. 25.20), and cyst aspiration. In addition, CT is used during radiofrequency ablations and cryoablations of tumors. Fig. 25.21 shows numerous structures and pathologic conditions identified by CT. Fig. 25.22 shows a liver lesion before radiofrequency ablation, during the procedure, and after ablation.

For any procedure, a protocol is required to maximize the amount of diagnostic information available. Specific examination protocols vary according to the needs of different medical facilities and physicians.

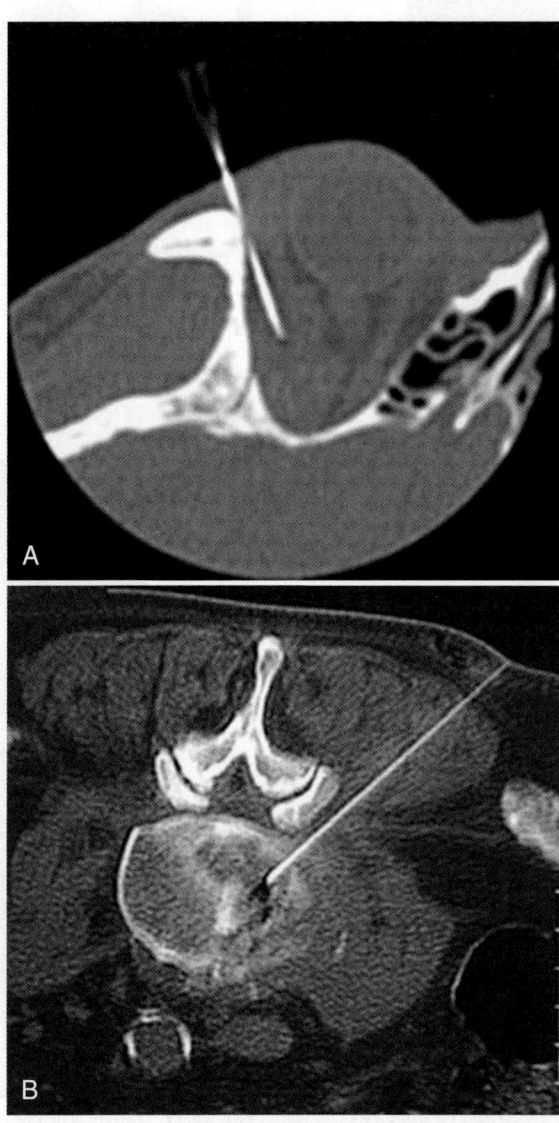

Fig. 25.20 (**A**) Needle biopsy of orbital mass. (**B**) Needle biopsy of infectious spondylitis of lumbar vertebral body.

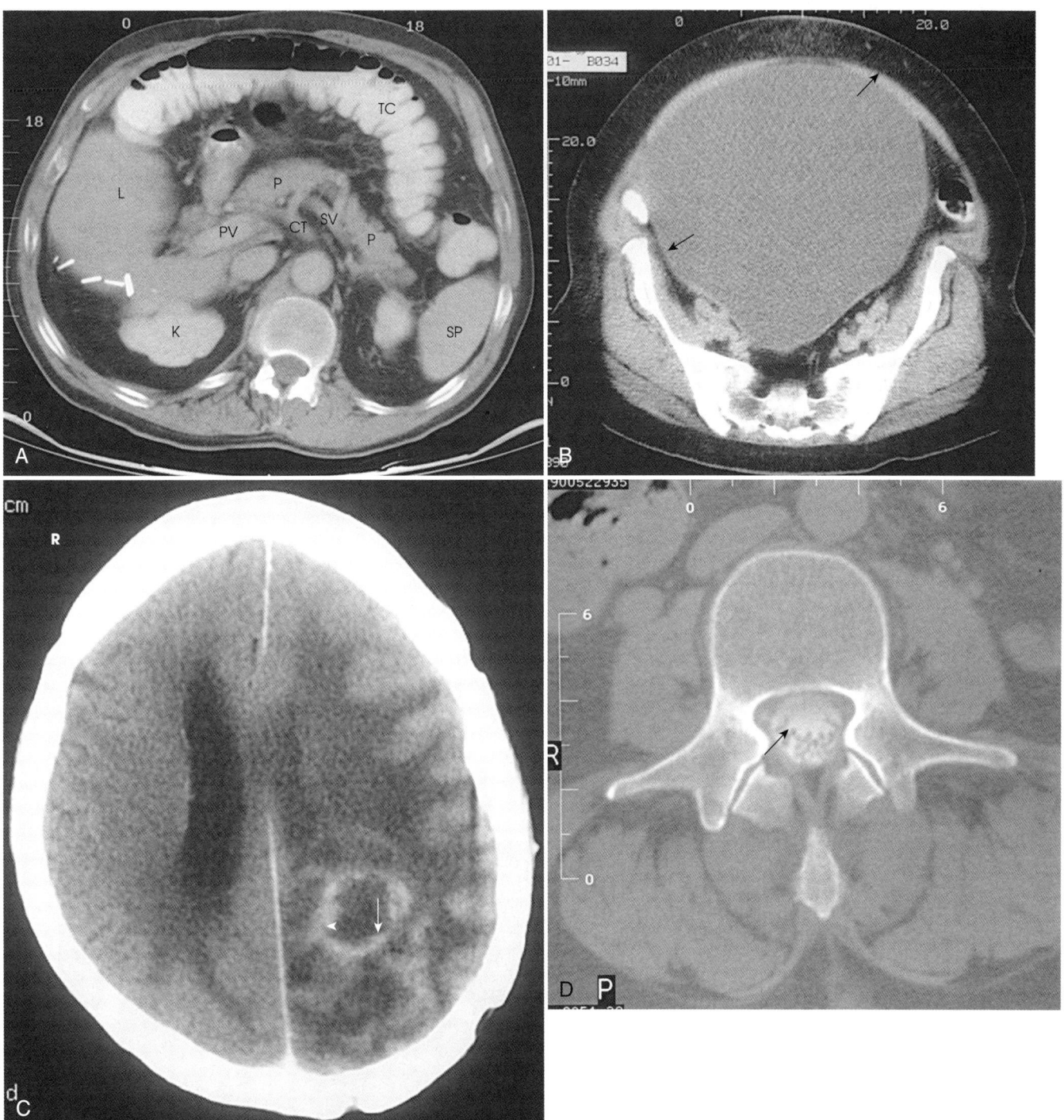

Fig. 25.21 (**A**) Abdominal image showing transverse colon *(TC)* with air-fluid levels; liver *(L)*, pancreas *(P)*, spleen *(SP)*, kidney *(K)*, portal vein *(PV)*, celiac trunk *(CT)*, and splenic veins *(SV)* are shown with contrast medium. Surgical clips are seen in posterior liver. (**B**) Abdominal image showing extremely large ovarian cyst *(arrows)*. (**C**) Brain image showing parietooccipital mass *(arrow)* with characteristic IV contrast ring enhancement *(arrowhead)*. (**D**) Image of L3 after myelography showing contrast material in thecal sac *(arrow)*.

Contrast Media

A contrast medium is used in CT examinations to help distinguish normal anatomy from pathology and to make various disease processes more visible. A contrast agent can be administered intravenously, orally, or rectally. In general, intravenous (IV) contrast media are the same media used for excretory urograms. Most facilities use nonionic contrast material versus ionic contrast material for these studies because of the low incidence of reaction and known safety factors associated with nonionic contrast material. IV contrast agents are useful for demonstrating tumors within the head; Fig. 25.23 shows a brain scan with and without contrast media. The anterior lesion is evident in the scan without contrast media, an unenhanced scan. In the enhanced scan, with contrast media, the tumor shows a characteristic ring enhancement typical of specific tumors seen in CT scans. IV contrast media are also used to visualize vascular structures in the body.

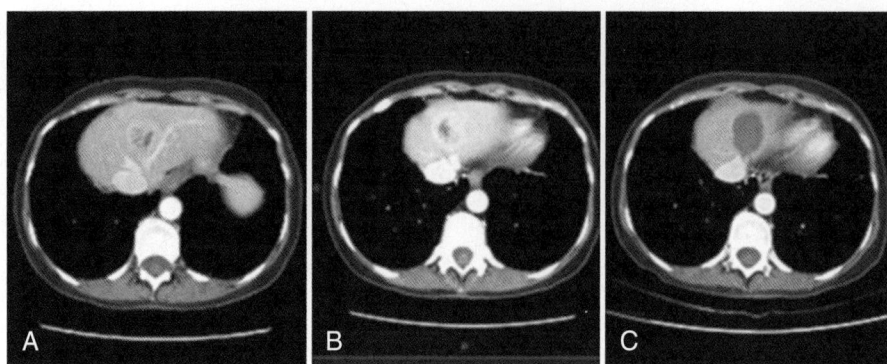

Fig. 25.22 Low-dose axial CT images from radiofrequency ablation study. Scans are before study (**A**), during study (**B**), and after study (**C**).

(Courtesy Philips Medical Systems.)

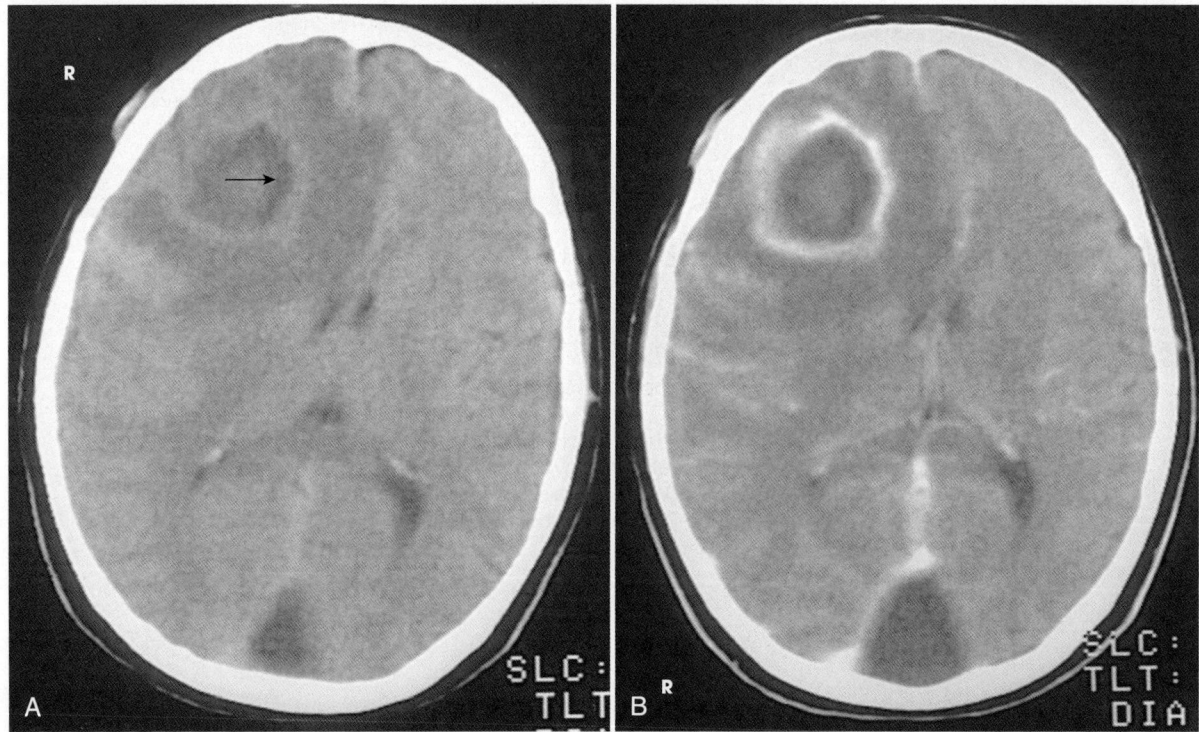

Fig. 25.23 (**A**) Brain image without IV contrast agent showing a low-density lesion *(arrow)*. (**B**) Brain image with IV contrast agent demonstrating ring enhancement.

IV contrast media should be used only with the radiologist's approval and after careful consideration of the patient's medical and allergy history. The patient's renal function must be evaluated before iodinated contrast material is given. Creatinine (Cr) level, blood urea nitrogen (BUN), and glomerular filtration rate (GFR) are the most common laboratory values used to determine renal function (Table 25.3). Many CT examinations can be performed without IV contrast media if necessary, but the amount of diagnostic information available may be limited.

Oral contrast media can be used for imaging the abdomen or pelvic region. When given orally, the contrast material travels through the gastrointestinal tract to help differentiate between loops of bowel, as well as other structures within the abdominal cavity. An oral contrast medium is a 2% barium mixture or a water-soluble iodinated medium. The low concentration barium mixture prevents contrast artifacts but allows good visualization of the stomach and intestinal tract. A water-soluble iodinated contrast agent, such as oral Hypaque diatrizoate meglumine or iohexol, can be used, but it must be mixed at low concentrations to prevent contrast artifacts. A rectal contrast medium can be requested as part of an abdominal or a pelvic protocol when considering specific pathology. Usually mixed in the same concentration as the oral contrast medium, the rectal contrast material is useful for showing the distal colon relative to the bladder and other structures of the pelvic cavity. Water may also be given orally as a contrast medium, depending on the area of interest and pathologic indications.

POWER INJECTOR USE FOR ADMINISTERING INTRAVENOUS CONTRAST MEDIA

Power injector use in CT examinations became mandatory when the first helical CT scanners were introduced. Faster delivery of IV contrast media became necessary with the reduced scan times used in helical CT. The advantage of power injector use is that a bolus injection of contrast media can be delivered quickly, which provides for better contrast enhancement of structures and better opacification of the blood vessels. The use of power injectors also provides a means to reproduce examination parameters and allows different vascular phases to be captured.

EQUIPMENT

Power injector equipment includes an injector assembly that is either ceiling mounted next to the scanner or on a movable stand. The injector head typically has two syringes, but some models may have only a single-syringe delivery system. If the injector head is a double-syringe system, each of the syringe controls is color-coded. The same color-coding system is shown on the injector control module that is next to the CT scan console. The injector must be programmed at the control module, but operational buttons are located on the injector head as well.

The control module for the system is typically placed on or near the operator console of the scanner. Each injector system has controls for the flow rate of injection, pounds per square inch (psi) of pressure used for the injection, amount of contrast media delivered, and time delays. Dual-head systems have dual sets of controls for each syringe.

Special pressure syringes and pressure tubing must be used when injecting. The pressure injections must be closely monitored, and care must be taken that no air is in the syringe or tubing. The pressure syringes have oval etchings on the side of the syringe as a safety feature. If the syringe is full of contrast media, the oval etchings appear round when viewed through the syringe, due to light refraction. If no fluid is present, the etchings remain oval in shape (Fig. 25.24).

Correct IV catheter size and placement are vital to the success of the CT examination. Catheters are typically placed in the arm veins in the antecubital fossa, but veins lower in the forearm can also be used. Small veins should be avoided

TABLE 25.3
Normal range values for a patient to receive IV contrast media

Laboratory test	Approximate normal range
Blood urine nitrogen (BUN)	7–25 mg/dL
Serum creatinine	0.6–1.7 mg/dL
Estimated glomerular filtration rate	>60 mL/min/1.73 m^2

These range values can vary depending on the laboratory, as well as for men, women, and children. Refer to the laboratory report for indication of a specific laboratory range.

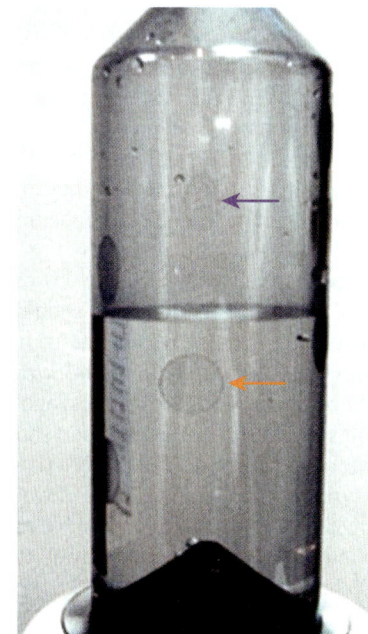

Fig. 25.24 CT pressure syringe partially filled with contrast material. Note oval etching (*purple arrow*) above fluid level and round etching (*orange arrow*) below fluid level.

because of the pressures used when injecting. Catheter size depends on the type of CT examination being performed. A routine, non-CTA examination typically uses a 22-gauge IV catheter with an injection rate of 2 mL/s. A CTA study with an injection rate of 4 to 7 mL/s requires a much larger bore, either an 18-gauge or 20-gauge IV catheter.

PATIENT CARE AND INJECTION SAFETY

Patient positioning should be considered when placing the IV line. For many CT examinations, patients must keep their arms resting above the head on a pillow or sponge during the examination. Care should be taken to make the patients as comfortable as possible while keeping their arms as straight as possible. The IV catheter should not be placed in a site that would be bent when the patient elevates the arms above the head.

Proper placement of the IV catheter should always be confirmed with a hand test injection of saline that mimics the injection rate of the examination. The ease of injection and the injection site should be observed and palpated during the test injection to confirm patency of the vein. Patients should be instructed to notify the CT technologist immediately if they experience any pain or discomfort at the injection site during the procedure.

All connections between the IV catheter injector tubing and syringe should be checked and tightened to prevent air from entering the IV line. The pressure syringe should be checked for air bubbles, and the etchings on the side of the syringe should be confirmed as round. The injected head and syringe should be pointed down to ensure that any potential air bubbles rise back into the syringe base and away from the IV line.

The patient should be instructed about the timing of the scan, the injection, and sensations of warmth and an odd taste caused by the dilation of the blood vessels. These sensations should be discussed with the patient, and the patient should be reassured that these are normal and fade quickly. The intensity of warmth and taste intensifies as the injection amount and rate increase, so these are more intense for a patient having a CTA study.

If the patient complains of discomfort at or near the injection site, the injection should be terminated, and the patient should be checked for contrast media *extravasation*. If there are any changes in the appearance of the patient's arm (swelling, discoloration), the radiologist should be notified immediately. The CT technologist should be familiar with the department policy for the treatment of extravasation, which typically includes alternating hot and cold compresses and elevation of the arm.

Factors Affecting Image Quality

In CT, the technologist has access to numerous scan parameters that can have a dramatic effect on image quality. The five main factors contributing to image quality are spatial resolution, contrast resolution, temporal resolution, noise, and artifacts.

SPATIAL RESOLUTION

Spatial resolution is determined by the degree of blur or the ability to see the difference between two objects that are close together. The method most used to evaluate spatial resolution is the number of line pairs per centimeter (lp/cm). The scan parameters that affect spatial resolution include scanning section thickness, display FOV, matrix, reconstruction slice thickness, and algorithm/kernel. The detector aperture width is the most significant geometric factor that contributes to spatial resolution.

CONTRAST RESOLUTION

Contrast resolution is the ability to differentiate between small differences in density within the image. Tissues with density differences of 0.25% to 0.5% can be detected with a CT scan. The scan parameters that affect contrast resolution are slice thickness, reconstruction algorithm, image display (window width), and x-ray beam energy. The size of the patient and the detector sensitivity also have a direct effect on contrast resolution.

TEMPORAL RESOLUTION

Temporal resolution is the ability of the CT system to freeze any motion of a scanned object. It is the shortest amount of time needed to acquire a complete dataset. The use of CT in cardiac imaging requires high (shortest time) temporal resolution to decrease heart motion. Factors that improve temporal resolution include multidetector CT (i.e., 64-, 128-, 256-, 320-slice), tube/gantry rotation time, and the development of dual-source CT.

NOISE

The most common cause of *noise* in CT is *quantum noise*. Quantum noise arises from the random variation in photon detection. Noise in a CT image primarily affects contrast resolution. As noise increases in an image, contrast resolution decreases. Noise gives an image a grainy quality or a mottled appearance. The following scan parameters may influence noise: matrix size, slice thickness, x-ray beam energy, and reconstruction algorithm. Scattered radiation and patient size also contribute to the noise of an image. New technology is available to prevent scatter radiation from hitting the detector.

ARTIFACTS

Metallic objects, such as dental fillings, pacemakers, and artificial joints, can cause starburst or *streak artifacts*, which can obscure diagnostic information. Dense residual barium from fluoroscopy examinations can cause *artifacts* similar to those caused by metallic objects. Many CT departments do not perform a CT examination on a patient until several days after a barium study. This is to allow the body to eliminate any residual barium from the area of interest. Large differences in tissue densities of adjoining structures can cause artifacts that detract from image quality. Bone-soft tissue interfaces, for example, the skull and brain, often cause streak or shadow artifacts on CT images; these artifacts are referred to as *beam hardening* (Fig. 25.25).

New software developments have greatly improved image quality and reduced artifacts. For example, interactive reconstruction methods, dual energy, metal artifact reduction algorithms, and artificial intelligence deep learning have greatly improved image quality not only at a lower dose but also with improved image resolution. Fig. 25.26 is an example of a metal artifact reduction algorithm in a tool used on Philips Medical CT systems referred to as orthopedic metal artifact reduction (OMAR).

OTHER FACTORS
Patient factors

Patient factors also contribute to the quality of an image. If a patient cannot or will not hold still, the scan is more than likely nondiagnostic. Body size also can influence image quality. Large patients attenuate more radiation than small patients; this can increase image noise, detracting from overall image quality. An increase in milliampere-seconds (mAs) is usually required to compensate for large body size. This increase results in a higher radiation dose to the patient. Image quality factors

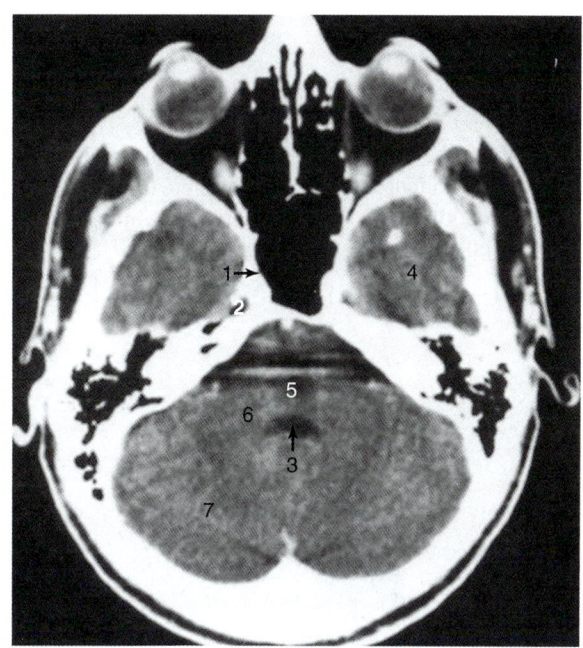

Fig. 25.25 Streaking through the posterior fossa represents beam-hardening artifact. Normal appearance of the brain. *1*, Sphenoid sinus; *2*, trigeminal ganglion; *3*, fourth ventricle; *4*, temporal lobe; *5*, pons; *6*, middle cerebellar peduncle; *7*, cerebellar hemisphere.

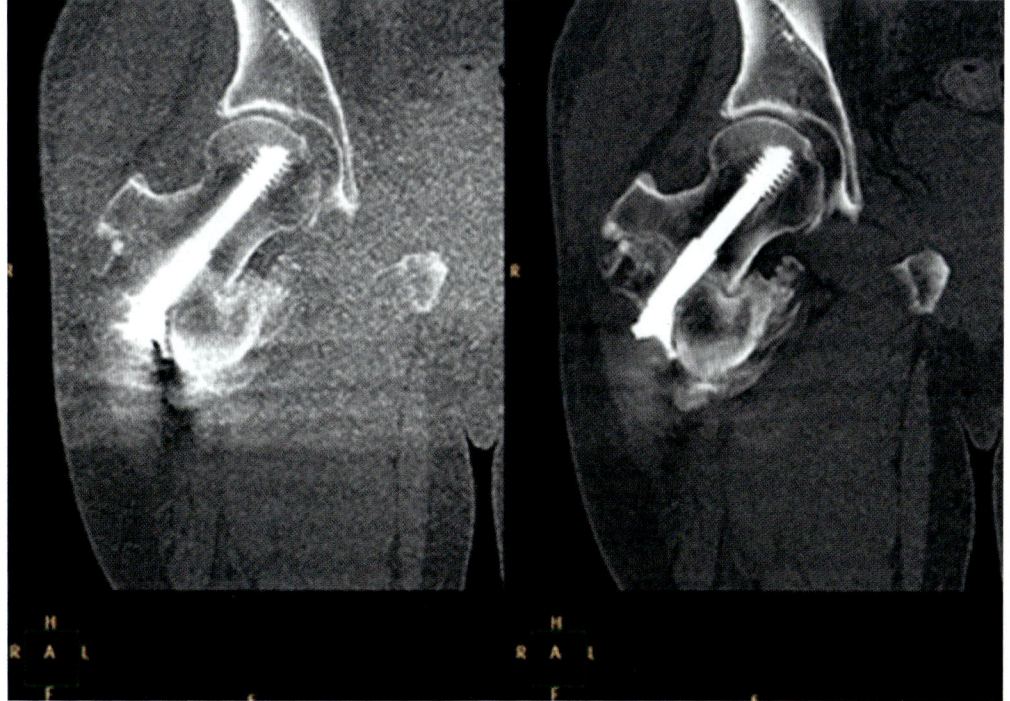

Fig. 25.26 Philips Medical Systems iDos4 and OMAR techniques to reduce noise and artifacts on patient with a hip pinning.

(Courtesy Philips Medical Systems.)

that are under the technologist's control include slice thickness, *scan time*, *scan diameter*, and patient instructions. Slice thickness is usually dictated by image *protocol*. As in tomography, the thinner the slice thickness, the better the image-recorded detail. Thin-section CT scans, often referred to as *high-resolution scans*, are used to show structures better (Fig. 25.27). However, thinner slices require more mA, which increases patient dose.

As in conventional radiography, patient instructions are a crucial part of a diagnostic examination. Describing the procedure in layman's terms helps the patient understand what to expect during the exam and increases the level of compliance.

Scan times

Scan times are usually preselected by the computer as part of the scan protocol, but they can be altered by the technologist. When selecting a scan time, the technologist must consider possible patient motion, such as involuntary body movements, breathing, or peristalsis. A good guideline is to choose a scan time that would minimize patient motion while providing the best quality diagnostic image. When it is necessary to scan an uncooperative patient quickly, using the shortest scan time possible may allow the technologist to complete the examination, although the quality of the images obtained is likely to be compromised.

Scan diameter

The amount of the detector utilized for imaging is referred to as the scan FOV (SFOV). When imaging a pediatric patient, the entire detector does not have to be active for such a small patient. The image that appears on the monitor depends on the *display FOV (DFOV)*. The technologist can adjust the DFOV to include the entire cross section of the body part being scanned or to include only a specified region within the part. For most head, chest, and abdominal examinations, the selected scan diameter includes all anatomy of the body part to just outside the skin borders. Certain examinations may require the DFOV to be reduced to include specific anatomy, such as the sella turcica, sinuses, one lung, mediastinal vessels, suprarenal glands, one kidney, or the prostate.

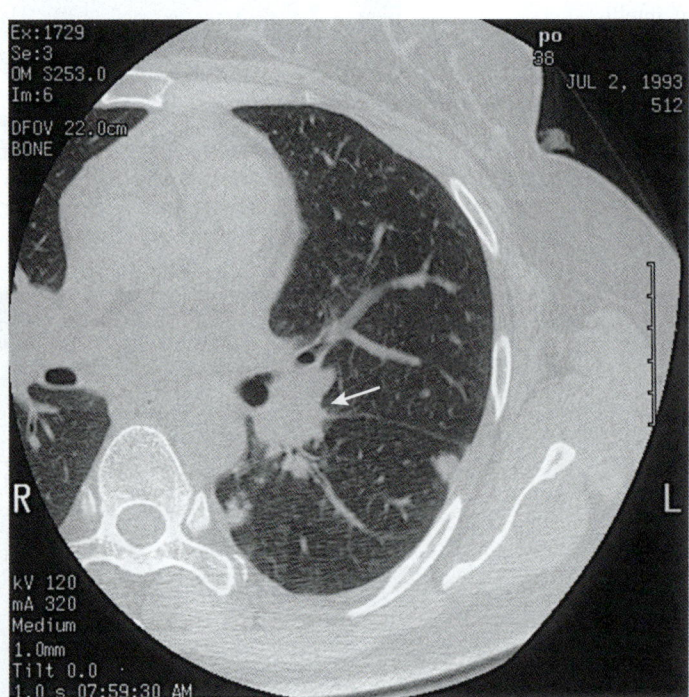

Fig. 25.27 High-resolution 1-mm slice using edge enhancement algorithm, showing nodule in left lung *(arrow)*.

Special Features

DYNAMIC SCANNING

One advantage of CT is that data can be obtained for image reconstruction by the computer at a later time. The scanner can be programmed to scan through an area rapidly. In this situation, raw data is saved, but image reconstruction after each scan is bypassed to shorten scan time.

Dynamic scanning is based on the principle that after contrast agent administration, different structures enhance at different rates. Dynamic scanning can consist of rapid sequential scanning at the same level to observe contrast material filling within a structure, such as is performed when evaluating enhancement within a tumor. Another form is incremental dynamic scanning, which consists of rapid serial scanning at consecutive levels during the bolus injection of a contrast media, such as is performed when evaluating the patient for aortic aneurysm or perfusion imaging on stroke patients.

SINGLE SLICE SPIRAL OR HELICAL COMPUTED TOMOGRAPHY

Single slice *spiral CT* (SSCT) and *helical CT* are terms used to describe a method of data acquisition in CT. During spiral CT, the gantry is rotating continuously while the table moves through the gantry aperture. The continuous gantry rotation combined with the continuous table movement forms the spiral path from which raw data are obtained one slice per revolution (Fig. 25.28). Slip-ring technology has made continuous rotation of the x-ray tube possible by eliminating the large high-voltage cables between the x-ray tube and the generators.

One of the unique features of spiral CT is that it scans a volume of tissue rather than a group of individual slices. This method makes it extremely useful for the detection of small lesions because an arbitrary slice can be reconstructed along any position within the volume of raw data. In addition, because a volume of tissue is scanned in a single breath, respiratory motion can be minimized. For a volume scan of the chest, such as shown in Fig. 25.29, the patient is instructed to hold the breath, and a tissue volume of 24 mm is obtained in a 5-second spiral scan. Two of the resulting images show a small lung nodule without breathing interference of *image misregistration;* a three-dimensional reconstruction of the lung clearly shows the pathologic condition. Spiral CT is especially useful when scanning uncooperative or combative patients, patients who cannot tolerate lying down for long periods, and patients who cannot hold still, such as pediatric patients

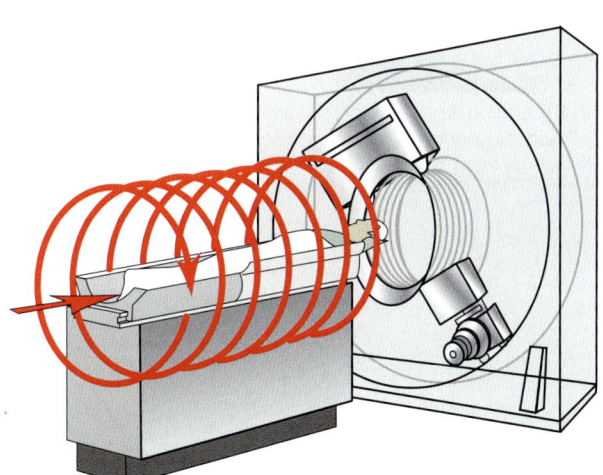

Fig. 25.28 Continuous gantry rotation combined with continuous table rotation, forming a spiral path of data.

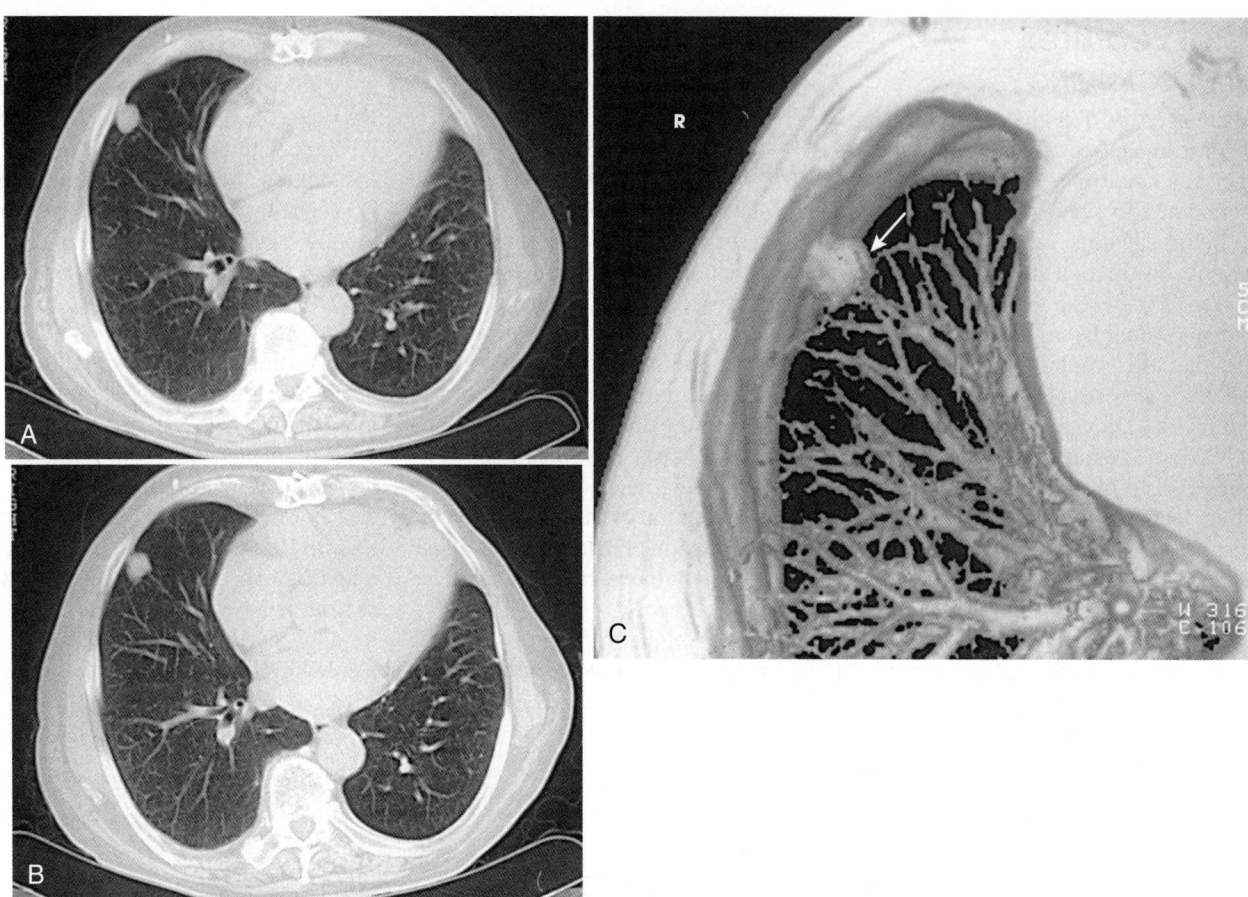

Fig. 25.29 (**A** and **B**) Spiral images of lung showing lung nodule and associated vasculature. (**C**) Three-dimensional reconstruction of lung nodule *(arrow)* after spiral scan.

(Courtesy Siemens Medical Systems, Iselin, NJ.)

or trauma patients. The use of spiral CT may decrease the amount of contrast media necessary to visualize structures, making the examination safer and more cost-effective.

MULTISLICE SPIRAL OR HELICAL COMPUTED TOMOGRAPHY

Multislice helical CT (MSHCT) or *multidetector CT (MDCT)* systems incorporate a detector array that contains multiple rows of detectors (channels) along the *z*-axis compared with the single row of detectors in conventional spiral CT (SSCT). Each channel comprises numerous elements. In a "four-row" scanner, the detector array is connected to four DASs that generate four channels of data (Fig. 25.30). This type of detector array would allow a scan four times faster than the conventional single row spiral/helical scanner. Current technology detector arrays have 4, 8, 16, 32, 64, 128, 256, and 320 rows or channels. The increased width of the detector now requires the x-ray beam to be a cone-beam configuration compared with the fan beam used for SSCT. The 64-, 128-, 256-, and 320-row scanners are referred to as volume CT (VCT) systems because of the amount of body section coverage in a single tube rotation. Figs. 25.31 and 25.32 were acquired on the Toshiba 320-row scanner in a single revolution. Fig. 25.31 is a three-dimensional volume-rendered (VR) pediatric chest image acquired in 0.035 seconds. Fig. 25.32 shows a 16-cm volume coverage that allows for whole-brain perfusion imaging for evaluation of stroke. Cardiac imaging using VCT is a rapidly growing component of CT imaging. The advantages of MSHCT/MDCT include isotropic

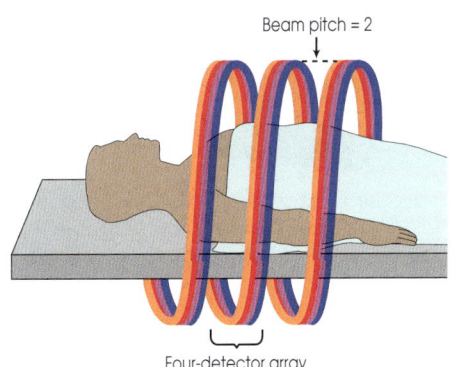

Fig. 25.30 Four-detector array with a beam pitch of 2 covers eight times the tissue volume of a single-slice spiral CT scan.

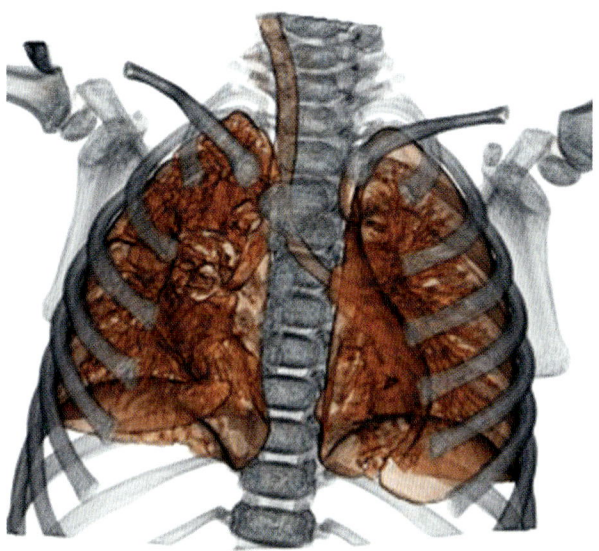

Fig. 25.31 Technology employing 320 detector rows makes it possible to scan an infant's chest with fine detail, low radiation dose, and fast acquisition times. This image is a three-dimensional VR acquired in a single rotation completed in 0.035 seconds.

(Courtesy Toshiba America Medical Systems.)

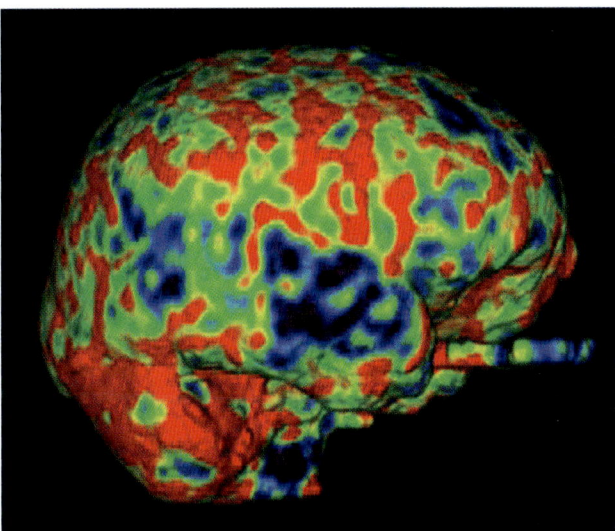

Fig. 25.32 Whole-brain imaging is possible with 16 cm of volume coverage. This three-dimensional VR whole-brain perfusion study shows evidence of acute stroke.

(Courtesy Toshiba America Medical Systems.)

imaging and post-processing, greater anatomic coverage, multiphase studies, faster examination times, and improved spatial resolution. The advancement of VCT, with increasingly larger detector arrays, has provided unique clinical opportunities in diagnostic medicine. Fig. 25.33 compares the z-axis coverage of 64-, 128-, and 320-row detectors.

COMPUTED TOMOGRAPHY ANGIOGRAPHY

CTA is an application of spiral CT that uses three-dimensional imaging techniques. With CTA, the vascular system can be viewed in three dimensions. The three basic steps required to generate CTA images are as follows:

1. Choice of parameters for IV administration of the *bolus* of contrast medium (i.e., injection rate, injection duration, and delay between bolus initiation and the start of the scan sequence)
2. Choice of spiral parameters to maximize the contrast medium in the target vessel (i.e., *scan duration*, collimation, and *table speed*)
3. Reconstruction of two-dimensional image data into three-dimensional image data

CTA has several advantages over conventional angiography. CTA uses spiral technology; an arbitrary image within the volume of data can be retrospectively reconstructed without exposing the patient to additional IV contrast media or radiation. During post-processing of the image data, overlying structures can be eliminated so that only the vascular anatomy is reconstructed. Finally, because CTA is an IV procedure that does not require arterial puncture, only minimal post-procedure observation is necessary.

Currently, CTA is replacing angiography as a diagnostic tool for some studies. This is especially true in departments using multirow detectors that allow significantly faster scanning. Fig. 25.34 shows the vessels of the brain, whereas Fig. 25.35 shows the renal vessels in a three-dimensional format. The heart and coronary vessels are shown in Fig. 25.36, and a graft is shown

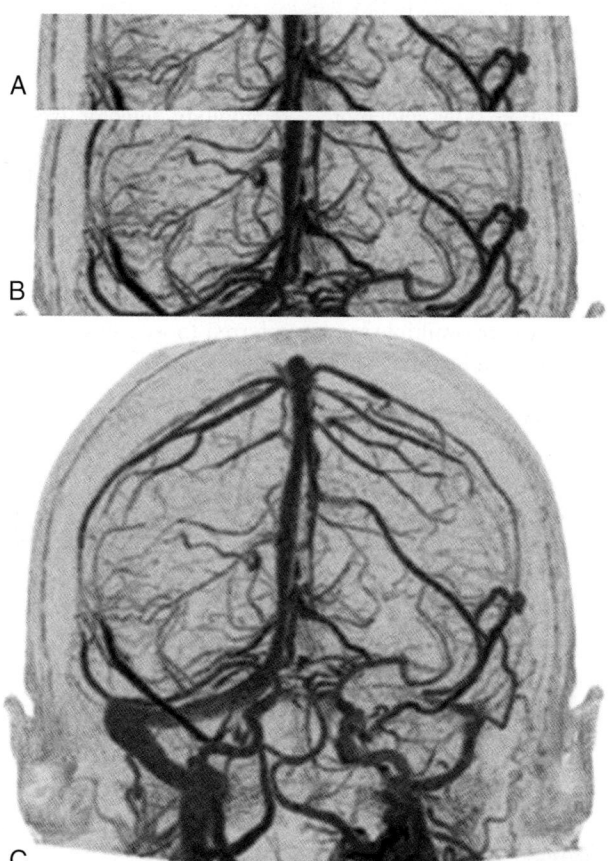

Fig. 25.33 Images show scan range for various row scanners. (**A**) 64-row scanner. (**B**) 128-row scanner. (**C**) 320-row scanner. The 320-row scanner allows complete imaging of the cranial vessels with one table location.

(Courtesy Toshiba America Medical Systems.)

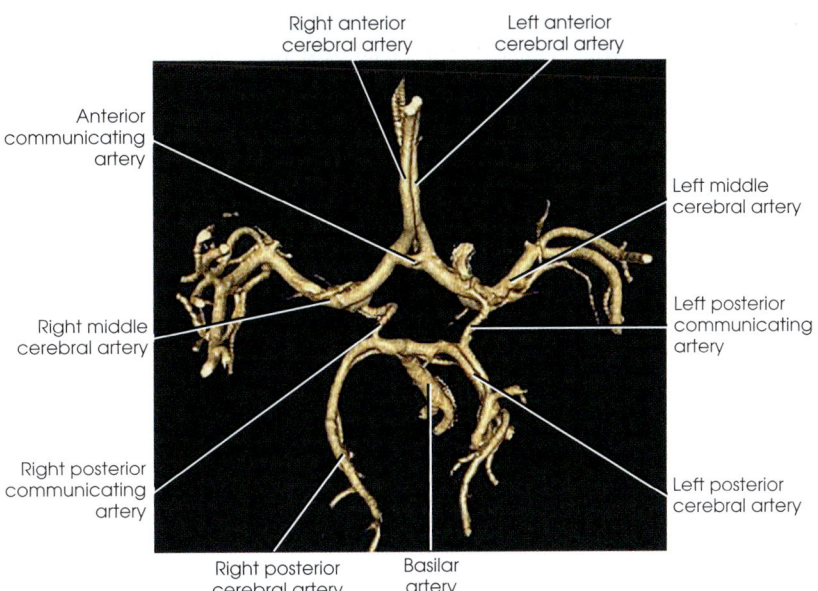

Fig. 25.34 Color CT angiography of circle of Willis.

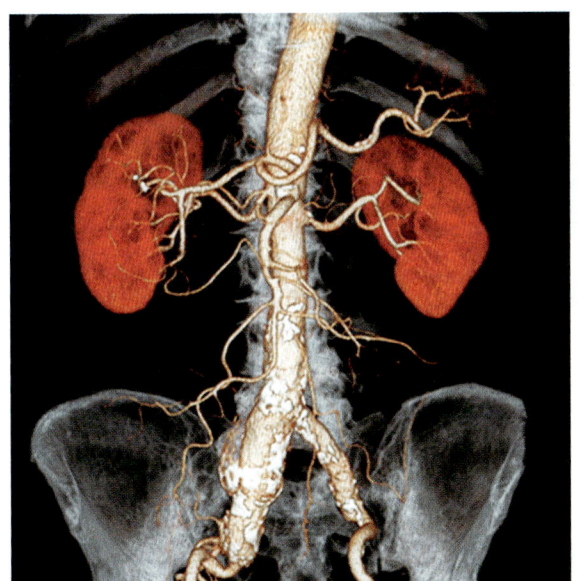

Fig. 25.35 Color CT angiography in three-dimensional format.
(Courtesy Toshiba America Medical Systems.)

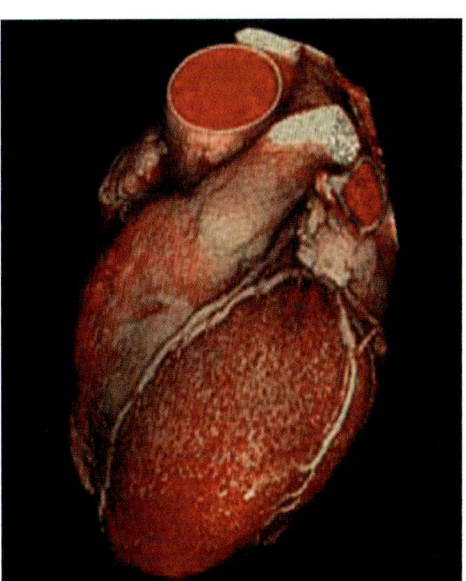

Fig. 25.36 Color three-dimensional cardiac CTA.

in Fig. 25.37. Fig. 25.38 shows multiple reformations from a cardiac gated dose reduction method performed on a Philips Medical 256-row scanner. Fig. 25.39 is a brain perfusion study showing significant vascular changes in a patient with an acute stroke.

THREE-DIMENSIONAL (3D) IMAGING

A rapidly expanding area of CT is three-dimensional imaging. This is a *post-processing* technique that is applied to raw data to create realistic images of the surface anatomy to be visualized. The introduction of advanced computers and faster software programs has dramatically increased the applications of three-dimensional imaging. The common techniques used in creating three-dimensional images include *maximum intensity projection* (MIP), *shaded surface display* (SSD), and volume rendering *(VR)*. All techniques use three initial steps to create the three-dimensional images from the original CT data:

1. *Construction* of a volume of three-dimensional data from the original two-dimensional CT image data. This same process is used in MPR.
2. *Segmentation* to crop or edit the target objects from the reconstructed data. This step eliminates unwanted information from the CT data.
3. *Rendering* or *shading* to provide depth perception to the final image.

Maximum intensity projection (MIP)

MIP consists of reconstructing the brightest pixels from a stack of two-dimensional or three-dimensional image data into a three-dimensional image. The data are rotated on an arbitrary axis, and an imaginary ray is passed through the data in specific increments. The brightest pixel found along each ray is *mapped* into a grayscale image. MIP is commonly used for CTAs.

Shaded surface display (SSD)

SSD provides a three-dimensional image of the surface of a particular structure. After the original two-dimensional data are reconstructed into three-dimensional data, the different tissue types within the image need to be separated. This process, called *segmentation*, can be performed by drawing a line around the tissue of interest or by setting *threshold values*. A threshold value can be set for a particular CT number. Any pixel that has an equal or greater CT number than the threshold value would be selected for the three-dimensional image. When the threshold value is set and the data are reconstructed into a three-dimensional image, a shading technique is applied. The shading or rendering technique provides depth perception in the reconstructed image.

Volume rendering (VR)

VR techniques incorporate the entire volume of data into a three-dimensional image by summing the contributions of each voxel along a line from the viewer's eye through the dataset. This results in a three-dimensional image in which the dynamic range throughout the image is preserved. Rather than being limited to surface data, a VR image can display a wide range of tissues that accurately depict the anatomic relationships between vasculature and viscera. Because VR incorporates and processes the entire dataset, much more powerful computers are required to reconstruct three-dimensional VR images at a reasonable speed.

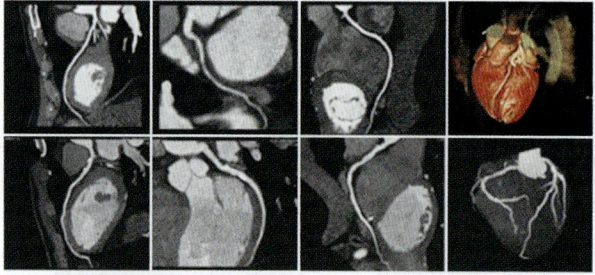

Fig. 25.38 Prospectively gated CT angiograms. Low-dose studies performed with Philips Step and Shoot Cardiac software, which has arrhythmia detection that stops scans until ECG stabilizes.

(Courtesy Philips Medical Systems.)

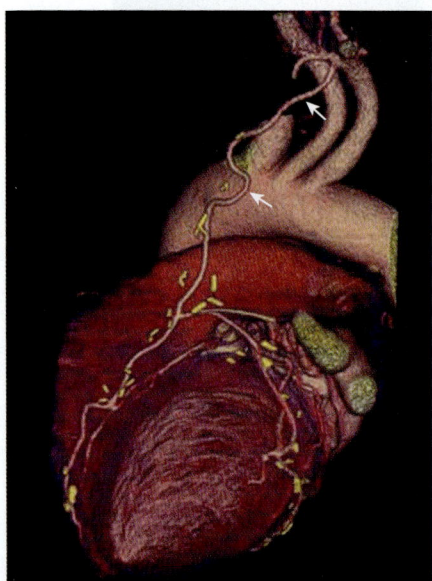

Fig. 25.37 Color three-dimensional cardiac CTA with graft *(arrows)*.

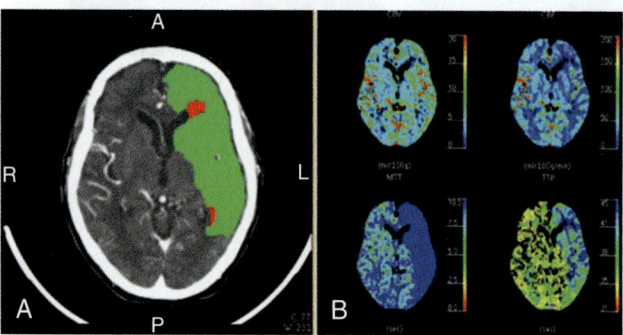

Fig. 25.39 CT brain perfusion study with brain perfusion parameter maps (**B**) and summary map overlays (**A**) showing areas of ischemic penumbra *(green)* and infarct *(red)*. Images were acquired using a lower dose protocol on a Philips Brilliance CT scanner.

(Courtesy Philips Medical Systems.)

Referring physicians and surgeons use three-dimensional images to correlate CT images clinically to the actual anatomic contours of their patients (Fig. 25.40). These reconstructions are especially useful in surgical procedures. Three-dimensional reconstructions are often requested as part of patient evaluation after trauma or for presurgical planning. Fig. 25.41 shows examples of the three common three-dimensional rendering techniques.

RADIATION TREATMENT PLANNING

Radiation therapy has been used for nearly as long as radiology has been in existence. The introduction of CT has had a major impact on radiation treatment planning. The use of spiral CT in conjunction with MPR provides a three-dimensional approach to radiation treatment planning. This method helps the dosimetrist plan the patient's treatment so that the radiation dose to the target is maximized and the dose to normal tissue is minimized. The three-dimensional simulation software offers the following: volumetric, high-precision localization; calculation of the geometric center of the defined target; patient marking systems; and virtual simulators capable of producing digitally reconstructed radiographs in *real time*. With the new, specially designed software, a single CT simulation procedure can replace a total of three procedures (one conventional CT scan and two conventional simulations) for radiation treatment planning (Fig. 25.42).

If the CT system is being used for radiation treatment planning, the standard curved couch cannot be used. Instead, a flat, firm board should be placed on the couch. A flat patient couch is substituted on the dedicated therapy units. In this way, the actual therapy delivery can be simulated more accurately. Fig. 25.43 shows the external skin markers and structures that would be in the beam's path. Most radiation therapy departments have their own CT units today.

PET/CT SCANNERS

When a CT scanner is coupled with a positron emission tomography (PET) scanner, it is referred to as a PET/CT scanner. The PET/CT scanner comprises two scanners in close proximity to one another, with a single patient couch that travels between the two scanners. In some scanner configurations, there is a small gap between the

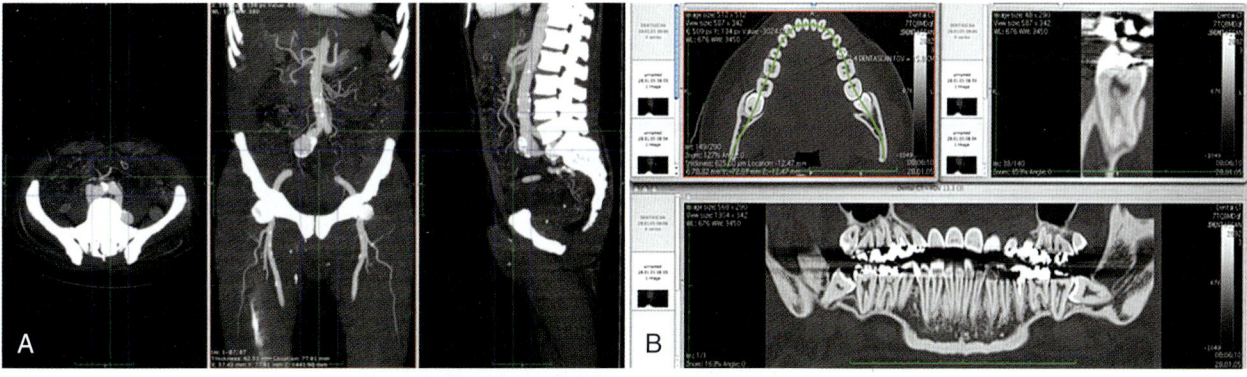

Fig. 25.40 (**A**) MPR of abdominal aorta. (**B**) Curved MPR of mandible.

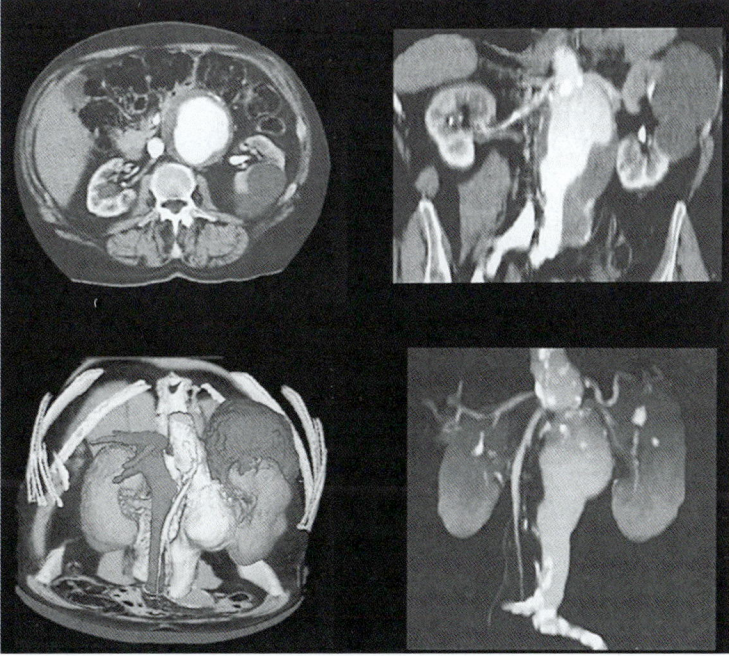

Fig. 25.41 Common three-dimensional rendering techniques used in CT.

(Courtesy Elicit, Hackensack, NJ.)

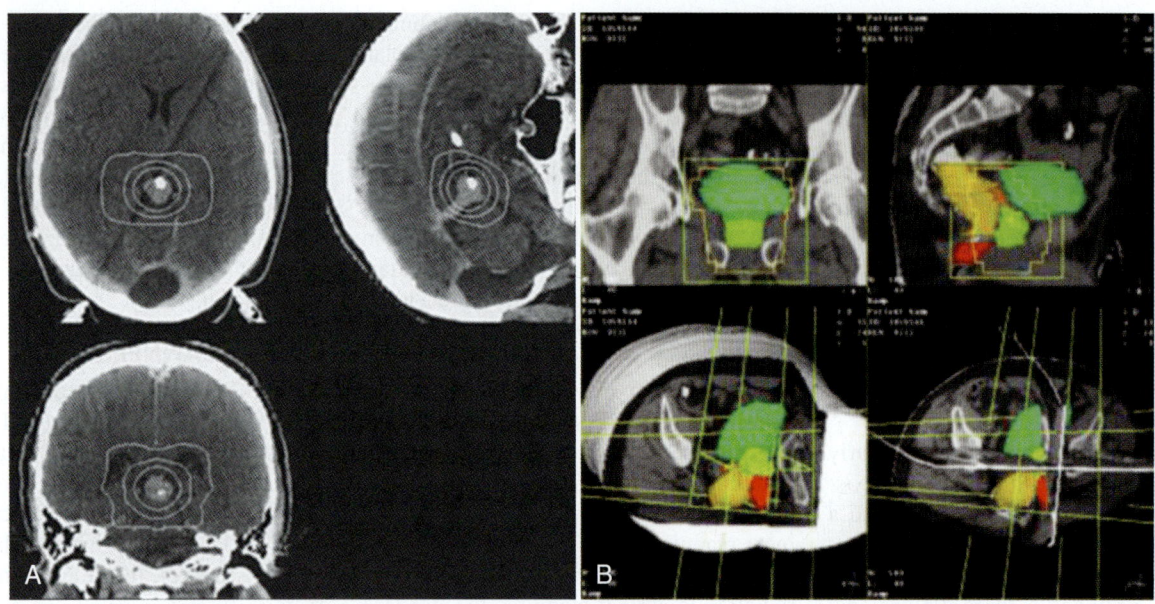

Fig. 25.42 (**A**) Brain localization in three planes. (**B**) Three-dimensional prostate therapy localization.

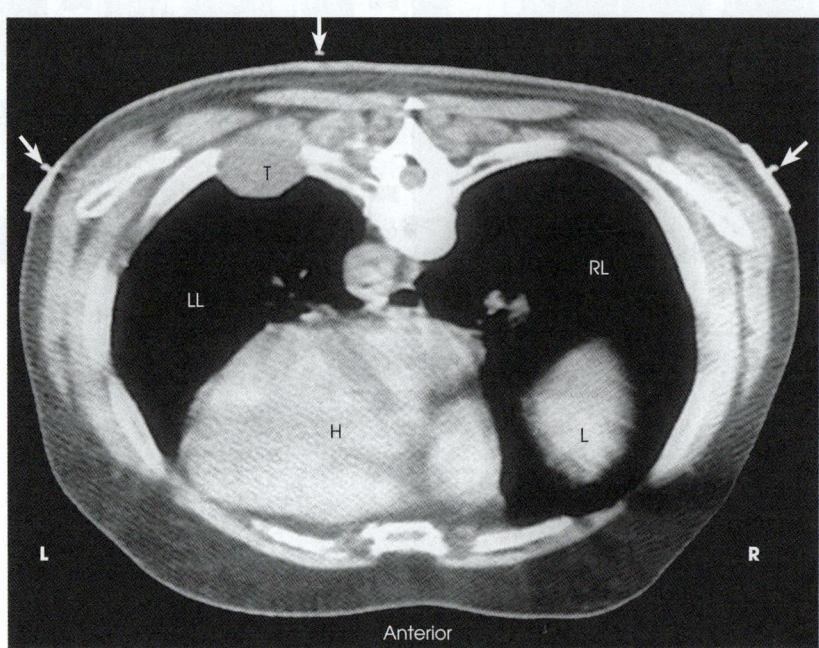

Fig. 25.43 Patient in prone position for radiation treatment planning. Radiopaque markers *(arrows)* show location of treatment field skin marks: tumor *(T)*, heart *(H)*, liver *(L)*, right lung *(RL)*, and left lung *(LL)*.

scanner housings; in other configurations, the scanner appears to be a single unit. Current PET/CT scanners are typically third-generation scanners and incorporate the latest in detector technology. PET/CT scanners are typically housed in the nuclear medicine department instead of the CT department. The CT scanner is used for attenuation correction and anatomic correlation for functional PET scans. In addition, many patients require a more detailed diagnostic CT examination. This requirement has forced nuclear medicine technologists to obtain additional education and certification in CT to perform the diagnostic CT exams. Refer to Chapter 29 for more details. Fig. 25.44 shows sagittal reconstructed CT spine images and the corresponding PET images with a PET/CT fusion image.

SPECT/CT IMAGING

Single photon emission computed tomography (SPECT) is a conventional nuclear imaging technique that is used to determine tissue function. In SPECT, the patient is given a radiopharmaceutical and is imaged with a gamma camera. An image is captured every 3 degrees (120 projections) until a full rotation around the patient is complete. SPECT is 100 times less sensitive than PET and is mainly useful in cardiac studies. Refer to the nuclear medicine chapter (Chapter 29) for more details.

QUALITY CONTROL

The goal of any quality assurance program in CT is to ensure that the system is producing the best possible image quality with the minimum amount of radiation to the patient. A CT system is a complex combination of sensitive and expensive equipment that requires systematic monitoring for performance and image quality. Most CT systems require daily, weekly, or biweekly quality assurance (QA) testing to ensure proper operation. In addition to QA testing, CT systems require preventive maintenance, which can be performed quarterly unless the manufacturer's service engineer or a private company recommends more frequent maintenance.

Increasingly, the technologist is assigned the responsibility of performing and documenting routine QA tests. Many technologists routinely perform daily test scans on a water phantom to measure the consistency of the CT numbers and to record the standard deviation. As data is recorded over time, the CT scanner's current operating condition and its performance over longer time periods can be evaluated. Many units are also capable of *air calibrations*, which do not require the water phantom and can be performed between patients for unit self-calibration.

A CT phantom is typically multisectioned and is constructed from plastic cylinders, with each section filled with test objects designed to measure the performance of specific parameters. Some phantoms are designed to allow numerous parameters to be evaluated with a single scan. The recommended quality assurance tests for evaluating routine performance include contrast scale and the mean CT number of water, high-contrast resolution, low-contrast resolution, laser light accuracy, noise, uniformity, slice thickness, and patient dose.

Radiation Dose

Calculating the radiation dose patients receive during CT examinations presents a unique set of circumstances. Typically, radiation received during radiologic examinations comes from a fixed source with delivery to the patient in one or two planes (e.g., anteroposterior [AP] and lateral projections). These exposure parameters typically produce a much higher entrance skin dose than the exit skin dose, which creates a large dose gradient across the patient. In contrast, CT exposures (helical/spiral) originate from a continuous source that rotates 360 degrees around the patient. This results in a radially symmetric radiation dose gradient within the patient.

Some equipment manufacturers have created an application to decrease the amount of radiation dose to patients in CT. This application can reduce the patient dose by 15% through the use of a pre-patent filtering technique and reduce the patient dose up to 25% with an ultrafast ceramic detector, as well as by using dose modulation. Utilizing these three items to decrease patient dose is described as automatic tube current modulation. Other developments are new hardware to reduce patient dose, including off-focal radiation suppression devices, beam shaping filters, z-axis efficiency with increased collimation, and improved data acquisition systems. Fig. 25.45 demonstrates the

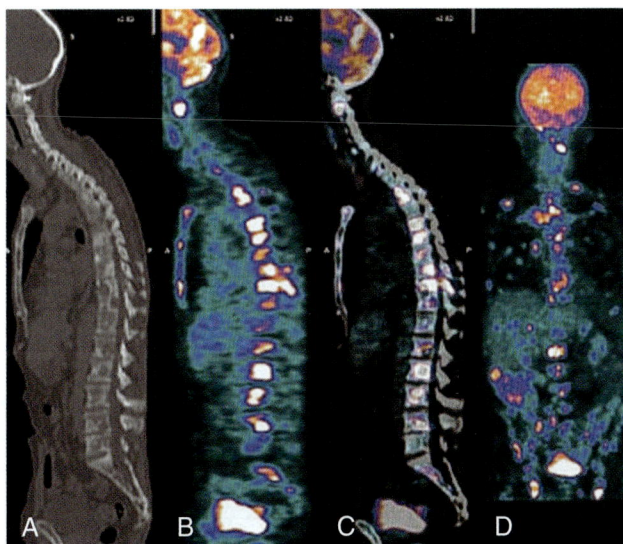

Fig. 25.44 (**A**) Sagittal reformatted CT scan. (**B**) Sagittal PET. (**C**) PET/CT fusion image. (**D**) Coronal PET.

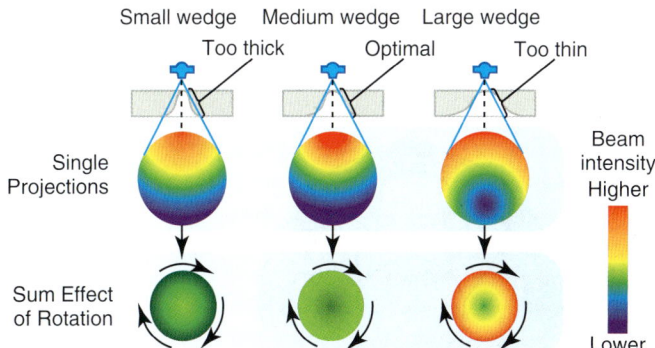

Fig. 25.45 Diagram represents selectable bowtie filters that reduce patient dose and improve image quality. These are referred to as SmartShape wedges on the Philips Brilliance iCT scanner. Note how correct wedge selection affects patient dose. Wedges are typically small (infants 0–18 months), medium (cardiac), and large (adult head and body). Wedge selection is built into scan protocols.

(Courtesy Philips Medical Systems.)

SmartShape wedge from Philips Medical Systems, which is an example of a beam-shaping filter. Note the dose reduction shown on the center image when the appropriate filter is applied. Z-axis efficiency reduces dose effects related to "overscanning," which occurs in helical or spiral scanning systems. CT data acquisition systems utilize higher efficiency detector material to minimize electronic noise. Software development has allowed dose optimization without degrading the image quality, which improves spatial resolution and low contrast detectability. For the pediatric population, dedicated protocols have been developed and should be included in a CT purchase.

Measurements of CT dose are typically performed using a circular CT dosimetry phantom that is made of polymethyl methacrylate (PMMA) with implanted thermoluminescent dosimeters (TLDs). The TLDs are positioned 1 cm below the surface around the periphery of the phantom and at the center (isocenter). The typical phantom sizes are 32 cm for body calculations and 16 cm for head calculations. For a single axial scan location (one full rotation of the tube, no table movement), the typical dose for the body phantom is 20 mGy at the periphery and 10 mGy at the isocenter. The typical dose for the head phantom is higher, at 40 mGy at the periphery and 40 mGy at the isocenter. See Fig. 25.46 for the body and Fig. 25.47 for the head. Patient dose is dependent on the size of the patient (e.g., the dose differs depending on whether the scan is for the head or body and whether the patient is a child or an adult).

Another component of dose to the patient is distribution of absorbed dose along the length of the patient from one single scan (full rotation at one table location). The radiation dose profile (Fig. 25.48) is not limited just to the slice location; the "tails" of the dose profile contribute to the absorbed dose outside of the primary beam. The size of the contribution to dose from the adjacent sections is directly related to the spacing of the slices, the width, and shape of the radiation profile.

The first method used to describe dose as a result of multiple scan locations is the *multiple scan average dose* (MSAD). MSAD is described as average dose resulting from scans over an interval length on the patient. Next is the *computed tomography dose index* (CTDI), which is calculated by using a normalized beam width and a standard of 14 contiguous axial slices. This method required a dose profile to be measured with TLDs or film, neither of which was convenient. To overcome the measurement limitations, another dose index, the $CTDI_{100}$, was developed. This dose index allowed profile calculations along the full length (100 mm) of a pencil ionization chamber and did not require nominal section widths. $CTDI_W$ was created to provide a weighted average of the center ($CTDI_{center}$) and peripheral ($CTDI_{periphery}$) measurements. The final descriptor is $CTDI_{vol}$, which accounts for the spiral/helical CT imaging that is used for specific protocols. The most common dose reporting method on present scanners used today is *dose-length product* (DLP). DLP is the total amount of exposure for a scan. DLP can be calculated by multiplying the length of the scan (cm) and the $CTDI_{vol}$. When reporting DLP, it is expressed as mGy/cm.

The most recent patient dose measurement to be published is size-specific dose estimate (SSDE). Just as the name says, the dose measurement is based on the size of the patient, and it takes into account pediatric-sized patients, whereas DLP and $CTDI_{vol}$ do not take into consideration pediatric patients. (See the AAPM Report 204 for further details.) Patient dose is part of the permanent record for each examination. Manufacturers display dose parameters in various ways. Fig. 25.49 is an example of how Philips Medical Systems displays dose information (note parameters within the blue box just above the "go" button). To assist in preventing excessive exposure to patients, the American Association of Physicists in Medicine (AAPM) published a position statement on "Notifications Levels Statement" with preestablished *notification values* for individual scans using $CTDI_{vol}$ (mGy). Notification values (NV) are predetermined and set up within the exam protocol; the technologist is notified when any scan series within the complete exam protocol exceeds the preset value. The alert value (AV) notifies the technologist when the cumulative dose index value exceeds the preset value. The dose checking systems will track and report all instances when established diagnostic reference levels (DRLs) have been exceeded.

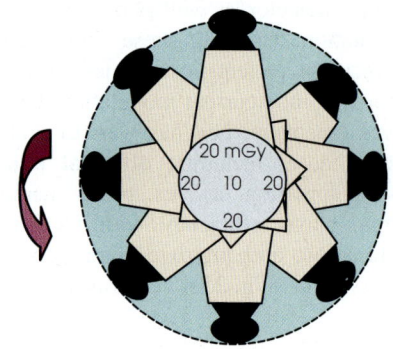

Fig. 25.46 CT dose profile for body.

(Data from McNitt-Gray MF: AAPM/RSNA physics tutorial for residents: topics in CT. Radiation dose in CT. *RadioGraphics* 22:1541, 2002.)

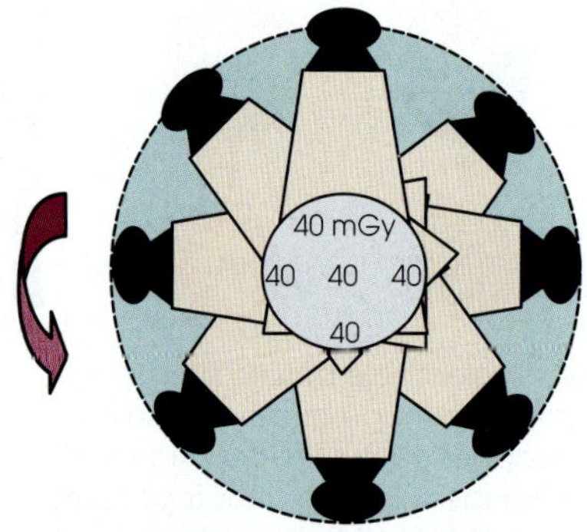

Fig. 25.47 CT dose profile for head.

(Data from McNitt-Gray MF: AAPM/RSNA physics tutorial for residents: topics in CT. Radiation dose in CT. *RadioGraphics* 22:1541, 2002.)

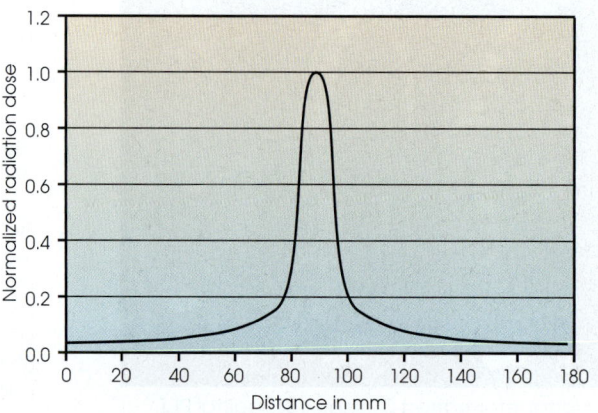

Fig. 25.48 Single-slice CT dose profile.

ESTIMATING EFFECTIVE DOSE

Effective dose takes into account where the radiation dose is being absorbed (e.g., which tissue or organ has absorbed the radiation). The International Commission on Radiological Protection (ICRP) sets the weighting factors for each radiosensitive organ (available at www.ICRP.org). Effective dose is measured in sieverts (Sv) or rems (100 rem = 1 Sv). The effective dose is determined by multiplying the DLP by a region-specific conversion factor. The conversion factors are 0.017 mSv/mGy per cm for chest imaging, 0.019 mSv/mGy per cm for pelvis imaging, and 0.0023 mSv/mGy per cm for head imaging. The conversion factor for head scans is considerably less because fewer radiosensitive organs are irradiated. (The DLP for a given chest examination is 375 mGy; the resulting estimated effective dose is 375 multiplied by 0.017, which equals 6.4 mSv.)

Factors That Affect Dose

The factors that directly influence the radiation dose to the patient are beam energy (kVp), tube current (mA), rotation or exposure time (seconds), section or slice thickness (beam collimation), object thickness and attenuation (size of the patient, pediatric vs. adult), pitch or section spacing (table distance traveled in one 360-degree rotation), dose reduction techniques (mA modulation), patient centering, distance from the tube to isocenter, amount of detectors, and z-scanning, as well as iterative and deep learning reconstruction. Improper patient centering can result in an increase in surface dose. A 3-cm centering mistake can increase the surface dose (breasts) by 18%. A 6-cm mistake can increase surface dose by up to 41%.

Each vendor has optimized the ability to use automatic exposure control (AEC) in CT, developing a product for automatic tube current modulation (ATCM), and calculating or using patient attenuation measurements in one or more planes. Fig. 25.50 shows a technique of mA modulation that uses an AP and lateral scout image to calculate patient thickness, which results in automatic mA adjustments during the scan (see *red line*). New "selectable" filters (Fig. 25.51) allow different filter applications based on body section or patient age or size. These filters can reduce dose by nearly 30% when using 120 kVp and 45% when using 80 kVp. Equipment manufacturers include an automated dose-optimized selection of the tube voltage, as in some instances a lower kVp may provide better images with a lower dose.

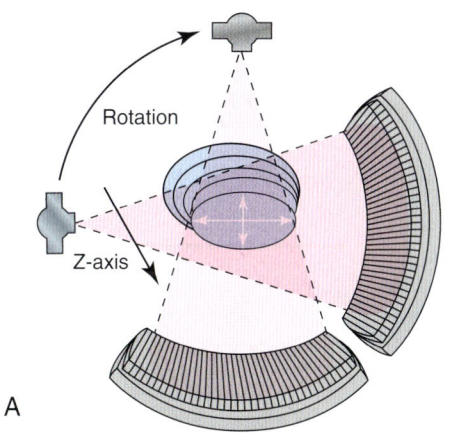

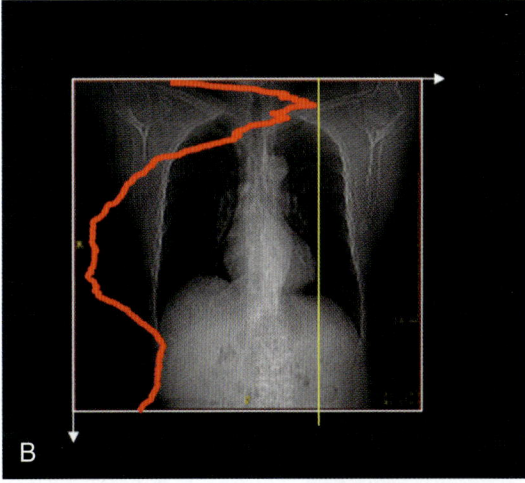

Fig. 25.49 Dose amounts must be reported for every series and protocol performed. Each manufacturer displays information differently. Note CTDI and DLP displayed inside the *blue box*.

(Courtesy Philips Medical Systems.)

Fig. 25.50 (**A**) AP and lateral scout images performed for mA modulation calculations. Note thickness difference A/P versus R/L. (**B**) Philips DoseRight automated tube current selection (ACS). *Red line* shows z-axis dose modulation. Note technique increase in shoulder and abdomen region and technique decrease in lung region.

(Courtesy Philips Medical Systems.)

Beam collimation (slice thickness) varies in single-detector scanners and multidetector scanners. Beam collimation for single-detector systems has minimal effect on dose; however, this is not the case for multidetector scanners. These scanners have multiple ways to scan and reconstruct images. A multidetector scanner can perform axial scans of 4 × 1.25 mm (5-mm beam width, 1.25-mm slice reconstruction), 4 × 2.5 mm (10-mm beam width, 2.25-mm slice reconstruction), and 4 × 5 mm (20-mm beam width, 5-mm slice reconstruction). The manufacturer designs and programs the scanning parameters that technologists select for examinations (Table 25.4). Advancement of technology allows patients to receive lower radiation dose based on software that adjusts the technical factors. Table 25.5 shows technical factors that lower the dose while producing quality images.

As mentioned earlier, patient size must be considered carefully when creating scan parameters. A small adult or pediatric patient absorbs less of the entrance radiation than a larger patient. This results in an exit radiation dose of higher intensity.

TABLE 25.4
Multidetector doses

Collimation (mm)	Total beam width (mm)	$CTDI_W$ head phantom (mGy)	$CTDI_W$ body phantom (mGy)
4 × 1.25	5	63	34
2 × 2.5	5	63	34
1 × 5	5	63	34
4 × 2.5	10	47	25
2 × 5	10	47	25
4 × 5	10	47	21

TABLE 25.5
Low-dose protocols (Philips Brilliance iCT)

Examination type	Scan mode	kVp	mAs	CTDIvol (mGy)
Adult abdomen and pelvis	Helical	120	160	11.4
Adult chest	Helical	140	20	2
Pediatric head	Helical	120	200	16.3

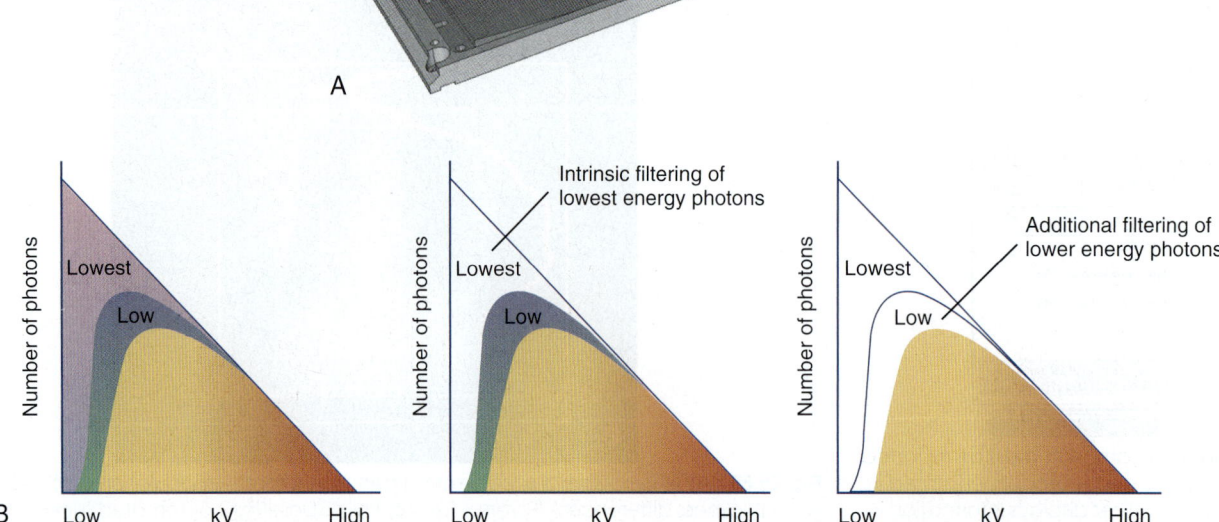

Fig. 25.51 (**A**) IntelliBeam adjustable filter that controls beam hardness (quality). Filters are used in conjunction with wedges to reduce patient dose. (**B**) Graph showing decrease in dose owing to elimination of low-energy photons *(far right diagram)*.

(Courtesy Philips Medical Systems.)

Radiation Dose Reduction and Safety

The following are best practice guidelines to follow to ensure lowest dose and patient safety within CT departments:

- Develop a comprehensive dose-reduction strategy (The Joint Commission gap analysis).
- Establish an exam request review process to eliminate unnecessary radiation—special consideration to multiphase exams.
- Utilize specific exam protocols with consideration given for reason of study, patient history, and as low as reasonably achievable (ALARA) principles.
- Institute specific exam protocol guidelines to ensure consistency across all sites.
- Appoint someone to audit and update exam protocols as needed.

Artificial Intelligence in Computed Tomography

Artificial intelligence has been at the forefront of all research. There are two types of subsets of artificial intelligence: machine learning and deep learning. Fig. 25.52 explains that machine learning (ML) is taught to perform a certain task and deep learning is created by numerous layers that resemble a human brain. The layers of deep learning are a unique type of artificial neural networks (ANN).

DEEP LEARNING RECONSTRUCTION (DLR)

Deep learning reconstruction (DLR), also known as deep learning image reconstruction (DLIR), is to ensure that the image quality and performance of dose, as well as the speed of the image reconstruction processes, are improved. Currently, GE has a DLR algorithm called TrueFidelity, and Canon's algorithm is referred to as Advanced Intelligent Clear-IR Engine (AiCE). With DLR/DLIR, studies have shown a decrease in image noise with a high-contrast resolution. This means that image quality has increased, creating better images and decreasing patient dose.

Advancements

With advancements in technology such as iterative reconstruction and deep learning algorithms, CT technologists have an increased responsibility to understand contrast dynamics and the spiral scan parameters of pitch, collimation, scan timing, and table speed.

Advancements in dose reduction, improvement in spatial resolution, and temporal resolution will continue. Manufacturers are working hard to improve ALARA practices and to meet or exceed the standards published by Image Gently, The Alliance for Radiation Safety in Pediatric Imaging (www.imagegently.org), and Image Wisely: Radiation Safety in Adult Medical Imaging (www.imagewisely.org).

Progress in computer power and design has provided workstations that can generate three-dimensional models, rotate the models along any axis, and display the models with varying parameters (Figs. 25.53 and 25.54). Digital subtraction CT, multimodality image superimposition, and translucent shading of soft tissue structures are some advanced applications. Advancements in virtual colonoscopy (Fig. 25.55), virtual bronchoscopy (Fig. 25.56), virtual cholangiopancreatography, and virtual labyrinthoscopy (inner ear) continue to evolve. As higher-quality images increase the accuracy of diagnosis and treatment, patient care will improve. Because of the superb diagnostic information and cost-effectiveness that CT provides, this imaging modality will continue to be a highly respected diagnostic tool.

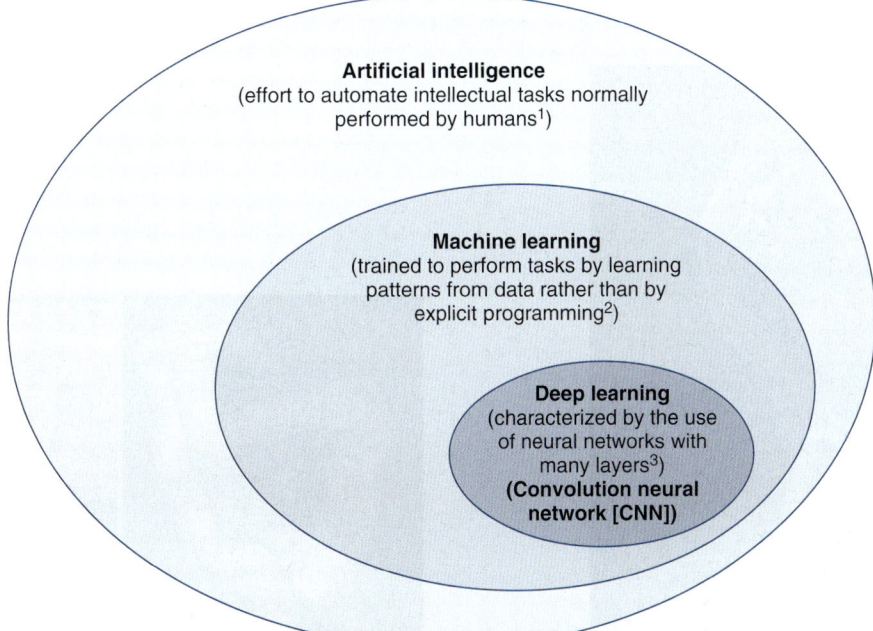

Fig. 25.52 Two subsets of artificial intelligence (AI) are machine learning (ML) and deep learning (DL) (which is a subset of ML).

(From Seeram E: *Computed tomography: physical principles, patient care, clinical applications, and quality control*, ed 5. St Louis, 2022, Elsevier. Definitions courtesy Chollet F. *Deep learning with Python.* Shelter Island, NY, 2018, Manning Publications[1]; Erickson BJ, Korfiatis P, Akkus Z, et al. Machine learning for medical imaging. *Radiographics,* 2017;37(2):505-515[2]; and Chartrand G, Cheng PM, Vorontsov E, et al. Deep learning: a primer for radiologists. *Radiographics,* 2017;37(7):2113-2131[3].)

New Technologies

With technology changing daily, health care engineers and scientists ensure that they stay on top of the new and advanced technologies. Siemens Healthineers has done just that with their new Photon-Counting CT machine. This CT machine is different from any other CT machine because instead of the x-ray photons being converted to light then an electrical signal, photon-counting allows the x-ray photon to go straight to an electrical signal. The technology will allow for a decrease in patient dose and an increase in contrast to noise ratio, along with higher spatial resolution.

Many patients are unable to come to the radiology department because they are not stable; however, the patient may have experienced a change in responsiveness, which could be indication for a CT scan. Fig. 25.57 shows a portable CT machine, which is strictly used for imaging a head on patients who may be in the ICU or the emergency room and unable to go to the radiology department. This machine allows for an increase in workflow efficiency, as well as for fast treatment decisions and a decrease in patient transportation.

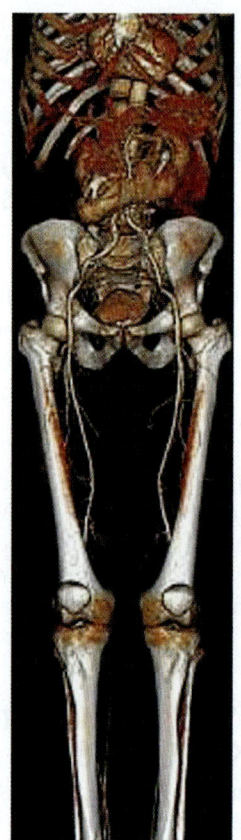

Fig. 25.53 Full-body three-dimensional reconstruction from 64-row CT scanner.

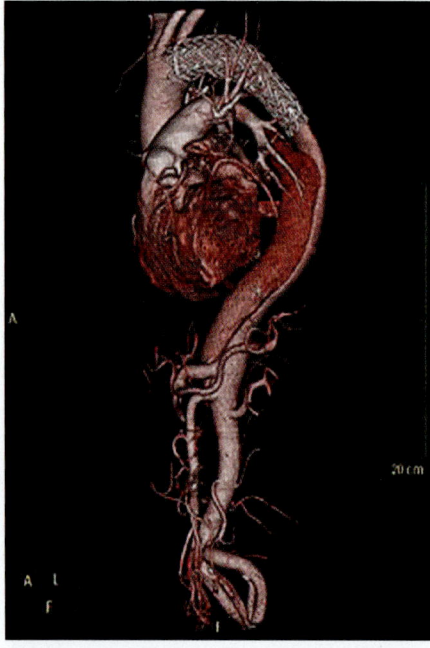

Fig. 25.54 Aortic arch stent shown on 500-mm three-dimensional reconstruction.

(Courtesy Philips Medical Systems.)

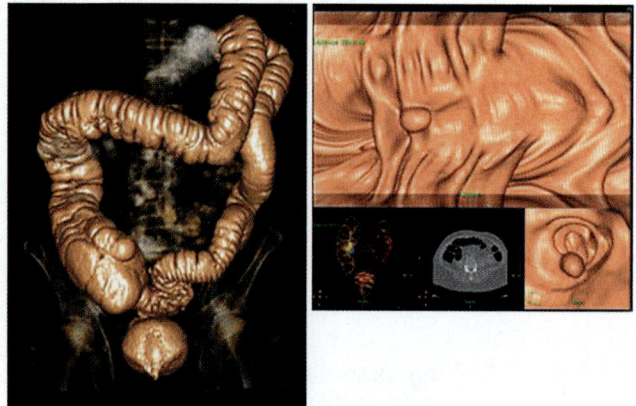

Fig. 25.55 CT colonography.

(Courtesy Philips Medical Systems.)

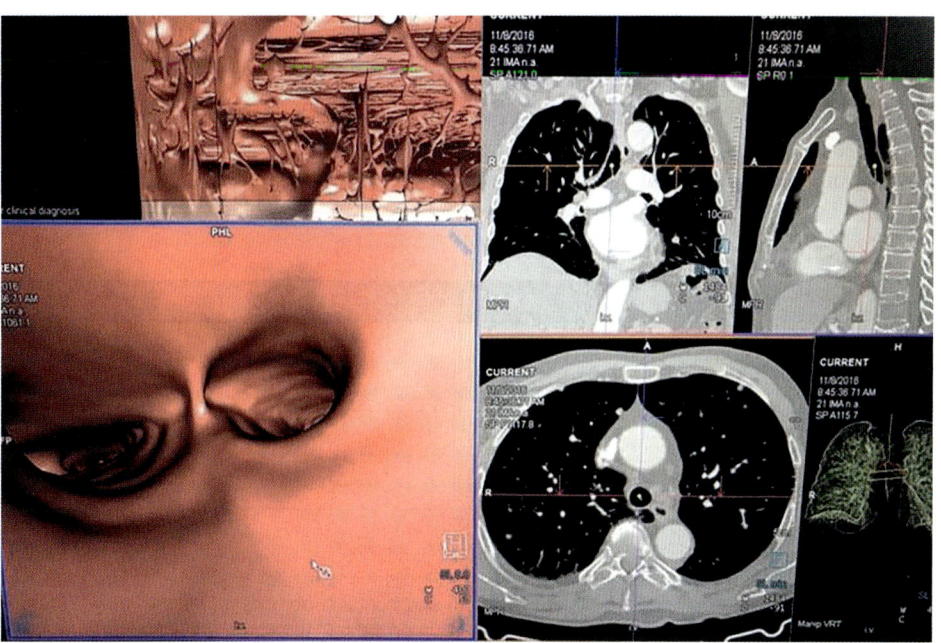

Fig. 25.56 Virtual CT bronchoscopy at the level of carina.

(From Patel ACH, Gulati P, Chidambaranathan N, et al., Eds. *Comprehensive textbook of clinical radiology. Volume I: Principles of clinical radiology, multisystem diseases & head and neck.* New Delhi, 2023, Elsevier India.)

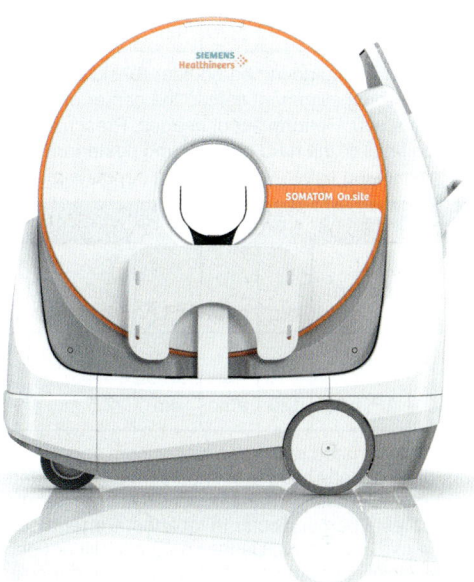

Fig. 25.57 Portable CT machine from Siemens Healthineers.

(Courtesy SOMATOM® On.site from Siemens Healthineers.)

Basic Computed Tomography Examination Protocols

It is impossible to list exact examination protocols due to the numerous scanner types, parameters, tube rotation speeds, and detector types that are used in CT imaging. Technical factors are directly related to the detector configuration that is used: number of detector rows and fixed array versus adaptive array. Many scans are performed using auto tube current modulation as opposed to fixed mA. The protocols listed below are basic CT scan values in close approximation for the various examinations using an adaptive array, 64-row scanner.

BASIC HEAD

Anatomic scan range	Scan type	Localizer scans	kVp	mAs	DFOV	Scan slice thickness	Recon slice thickness	Gantry tilt	Recon kernel	IV contrast	Oral contrast
Skull base through vertex of head	Axial sequential	AP, LAT	120	250 auto	~23 cm	5 mm	2.5 mm	Match skull base	Standard	Typically no*	No

Place patient in supine position with head in head holder. Ensure that patient is not rotated or tilted. Elevate table to bring coronal alignment light to the center of the skull. Landmark per equipment requirements (table movement for scout images). Perform scout images. Prescribe scan locations from skull base to vertex of head. Angle gantry to match skull base (occipital bone) (foramen magnum) and frontal bone (roof of orbits). Patient's chin should be tucked down toward the chest as much as possible; this avoids the lens of the eye from direct radiation. *If IV contrast ordered, 100 mL @ 1.0 mL/s. Delay 5 mins.

SINUSES

Anatomic scan range	Scan type	Localizer scans	kVp	mAs	DFOV	Scan slice thickness	Recon slice thickness	Gantry tilt	Recon kernel	IV contrast	Oral contrast
Starting above the frontal sinus and ending just below the hard palate	Helical	AP, LAT	120	200 auto	~16-18 cm	2.5 mm	0.625 mm	Usually none	Standard	No	No

Place patient in supine position with head in head holder (basic head positioning). Ensure that patient is not rotated or tilted. Elevate table to bring coronal alignment light to the center of the skull. Landmark per equipment requirements (table movement for scout images). Perform scout images. Prescribe scan locations to include entire frontal sinus to the maxillary sinus (or at the level of the hard palate), and posteriorly to include the sphenoid sinus. Volume scans can be performed with either positioning option with MPRs in opposite planes.

SOFT TISSUE NECK

Anatomic scan range	Scan type	Localizer scans	kVp	mAs	DFOV	Scan slice thickness	Recon slice thickness	Gantry tilt	Recon kernel	IV contrast	Oral contrast
At the level of the mid orbits to mid aortic arch	Helical	AP, LAT	120	150 auto	~20-24 cm	2.5 mm	1.25 mm	Usually none	Medium average	Yes*	No

Place patient supine on table with head resting on radiolucent sponge. Ensure that patient's head and neck are within table scan range. Ensure that patient's head and shoulders are not rotated or tilted. Elevate table to bring coronal alignment light to the center of the neck. Landmark per equipment requirements (table movement for scout images). Tip chin up to bring plane of teeth perpendicular to tabletop. Perform scout images. Prescribe scan locations at the level of the mid orbits to the mid aortic arch. Usually no gantry tilt needed; however, scans should be perpendicular to midcoronal plane. *Scans typically performed with IV contrast and a split bolus of first injection – 50 mL @ 2 min delay; second injection – 75 mL and start scan 25 seconds after the start of the second injection.

CERVICAL SPINE

Anatomic scan range	Scan type	Localizer scans	kVp	mAs	DFOV	Scan slice thickness	Recon slice thickness	Gantry tilt	Recon kernel	IV contrast	Oral contrast
Just above the base of the skull to below T2	Helical	AP, LAT	120	250 auto	~14 cm	3 mm	1.5 mm	Usually none	Sharp bone	No	No

Place patient supine on table with head resting on radiolucent sponge. Ensure that patient's head and neck are within table scan range. Ensure that patient's head and shoulders are not rotated or tilted. Elevate table to bring coronal alignment light to the center of the neck. Landmark per equipment requirements (table movement for scout images). Perform scout images. Prescribe scan locations from skull base/occipital condyles to below T2. Usually no gantry angle when scanning the entire C-spine. If individual vertebral bodies are of interest, gantry can be angled to match vertebral bodies/disc spaces. Volume scans performed with MPRs in sagittal and coronal planes.

ROUTINE CHEST

Anatomic scan range	Scan type	Localizer scans	kVp	mAs	DFOV	Scan slice thickness	Recon slice thickness	Gantry tilt	Recon kernel	IV contrast	Oral contrast
Above lung apices to below adrenal glands	Helical	AP, LAT	120	100 auto	~38 mm to include thorax margin	5 mm	2.5 mm	None	Standard	Yes*	No

Place 20-gauge needle in antecubital space, and ensure patency. Place patient in supine position with head on pillow, cushion under patient's knees for comfort. Ensure that patient is not rotated or tilted. Elevate table to bring coronal alignment light to the center of the chest. Landmark per equipment requirements (table movement for scout images). Bring patient's arms above their head and support with sponges/pillows for comfort and to protect IV site. Perform scout images. Prescribe scan locations from above lung apices to below adrenal glands. Define DFOV to include lateral margins of chest and use lateral scout to center DFOV to include anterior and posterior margins of the chest. Scans typically performed with IV contrast and a scan delay of 35 seconds. *80 mL @ 3.0 mL/s followed by 50 mL saline flush, 35-second delay.

ROUTINE ABDOMEN/PELVIS

Anatomic scan range	Scan type	Localizer scans	kVp	mAs	DFOV	Scan slice thickness	Recon slice thickness	Gantry tilt	Recon kernel	IV contrast	Oral contrast
Above hemidiaphragms to below the pubic symphysis	Helical	AP, LAT	120	200 auto	~38 mm to include the body margin	5 mm	2.5 mm	None	Standard	Yes*	Yes 24 hr/1 hr

Exams typically performed with oral contrast; give contrast 24 hours and 1 hour before exam or timing as requested by radiologist. Place 20-gauge needle in antecubital space, and ensure patency. Place patient in supine position with head on pillow, cushion under patient's knees for comfort. Ensure that patient is not rotated or tilted. Elevate table to bring coronal alignment light to the center of the abdomen/pelvis. Landmark per equipment requirements (table movement for scout images). Bring patient's arms above their head and support with sponges/pillows for comfort and to protect IV site. Perform scout images. Prescribe scan locations from above hemidiaphragms to below the pubic symphysis. Define DFOV to include lateral margins of abdomen and use lateral scout to center DFOV to include anterior and posterior margins of the abdomen. *Scans typically performed with IV contrast and a scan delay of 70 seconds. 125 mL @ 3.0 mL/s followed by 50 mL of saline flush.

Basic Computed Tomography Examination Protocols

EXTREMITY - KNEE

	Anatomic scan range	Scan type	Localizer scans	kVp	mAs	DFOV	Scan slice thickness	Recon slice thickness	Gantry tilt	Recon kernel	IV contrast	Oral contrast
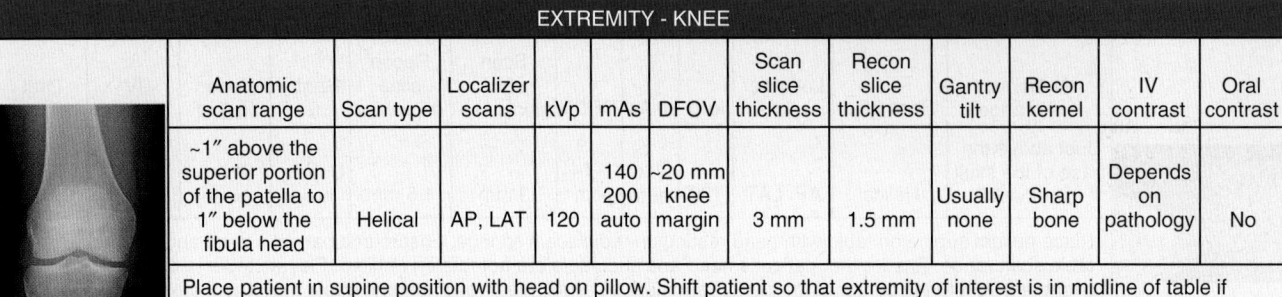	~1" above the superior portion of the patella to 1" below the fibula head	Helical	AP, LAT	140 120	200 auto	~20 mm knee margin	3 mm	1.5 mm	Usually none	Sharp bone	Depends on pathology	No

Place patient in supine position with head on pillow. Shift patient so that extremity of interest is in midline of table if possible. Extend leg of interest if possible. Ensure that patient is not rotated or tilted. Elevate table to bring coronal alignment light to the center of the knee. Landmark per equipment requirements (table movement for scout images). Flex the unaffected knee to bring leg and foot away from scan plane through affected knee if possible. Perform scout images. Prescribe scan locations from approximately 1" above the superior portion of the patella to 1" below the fibula head or to the area of interest. Define DFOV to include lateral margins of soft tissues and use lateral scout to center DFOV to include anterior and posterior margins of the knee. Volume scans performed followed by MPRs.

PEDIATRIC IMAGING

The following four points should be considered for pediatric imaging: (1) "Child size" the radiation dose, (2) scan only when necessary, (3) scan only indicated areas, (4) multiphase scanning is usually not indicated. Most protocols are adjusted based on patient weight as opposed to patient age, with 55 kg being the top of the scale for pediatric adjustments. Note: kVp and mAs values listed are typical low/high ranges for imaging based on patient weight.

PEDIATRIC PROTOCOLS

Anatomic region	Pediatric considerations	Scan type	Localizer scans	kVp	mAs	DFOV	Scan slice thickness	Recon slice thickness	Gantry tilt	Recon kernel	IV contrast	Oral contrast
Head	Avoid eyes with scan plane	Helical	AP, LAT	80 120	100 200 auto	16-25 cm	5 mm	2.5 mm	Match skull base	Standard	No	No
Soft tissue neck	Typically same coverage as adults	Helical	AP, LAT	80 120	20 80 auto	~20 cm	3 mm	1.5 mm	Usually none	Standard	Typically yes	No
C-spine	Typically entire C-spine, avoid eyes	Helical	AP, LAT	80 120	40 100 auto	10-14 cm	3 mm	1.5 mm	Usually none	Sharp bone	No	No
Chest	Restrict to area of interest, typically single phase for peds	Helical	AP, LAT	80 120	20 70 auto	Edge of anatomy to include lateral borders of the soft tissue	3 mm	1.5 mm	Usually none	Standard	Yes	No
Abdomen/ pelvis	Restrict to area of interest, typically single phase for peds	Helical	AP, LAT	80 120	40 100 auto	Edge of anatomy to include lateral borders of the soft tissue	5 mm 3 mm	2.5 mm 1.5 mm	Usually none	Standard	Yes	Yes
Extremities	Typically same coverage as adults	Helical	AP, LAT	80 120	50 150 auto	Edge of anatomy to include lateral borders of the soft tissue	3 mm	1.5 mm	Usually none	Sharp bone	Depends on pathology	No

Best Practices in Computed Tomography

Computed tomography technologists have a dual responsibility to understand not only the principles of CT but also the specific capabilities of their machines and the universal standards of workflow. The connections the CT technologist makes while selecting scan protocols and parameters are directly related to the image quality, safety, and radiation dose delivered to the patient. CT technologists are on the front lines of imaging with robust, highly specialized technical systems that support the patient's needs, ranging from trauma scans to lifesaving CT-guided procedures to low-dose, highly sensitive pediatric imaging. This section is a compilation of some useful advice from experienced CT technologists regarding best practices and universal guidelines for the practicing CT technologist.

1. *Workflow:* The CT technologist must know and understand the capabilities of their CT scanner system inside and out. With careful preparation and practice, the CT technologist must be ready to stop or pause the scanner and the injector at any moment. All of the preparation in the world will never account for each individual patient's experience while having a CT with IV contrast. If the CT technologist understands the ins and outs of their scanner and knows the general principles of CT and departmental CT protocols, as well as the basics of blood flow, the technologist will be able to think quickly and achieve the requested phase of contrast and blood flow even in unprecedented situations.

2. *Pathology:* The CT technologist is the final reviewer of the CT exam order. This includes understanding medical terminology that describes not only the patient's signs and symptoms, but also the pathology on which the provider is focusing for the patient's illness. It is imperative that the technologist, as the administrator of oral and IV contrast, understand and follow the radiologist protocol; this includes recognizing high thresholds for renal function lab values such as GFR (glomerular filtration rate) and creatinine. In addition, the technologist needs to be sure that the patient has no allergies or contraindications to IV or oral contrast administration. This knowledge and final review allow for high image quality, as the technologist will select the CT scanner protocol and IV contrast protocol based on the patient's pathology, weight, and phase of blood flow to be achieved.

3. *Positioning:* There is a perception that positioning in CT does not matter, as the reconstruction options and the tools to create them are endless; however, accurate positioning, minimization of motion, and clear breathing instructions do affect image quality. Equally important is to reduce the patient's cumulative radiation dose. As mentioned in the text, as little as a 3-cm centering mistake can cost the patient as much as an 18% increase in surface dose. Extremity positioning is equally vital, especially when performing CT imaging for preoperative planning protocols and vascular imaging on a traumatic extremity.

4. *CT department scanner protocols and scope of practice:* The CT technologist has a responsibility to know and understand departmental CT scanner protocols. The technologist is responsible for submitting the right CT exam on the right patient at the prescribed contrast timing, with prescribed speed, rotation time, and pitch. The scope of practice for a CT technologist can vary from state to state and from institution to institution. It is imperative that the technologist follow the ASRT Professional Practice Standards for Medical Imaging and Radiation Therapy and its advisory opinions.

5. *Pediatrics:* CT technologists must select the appropriate pediatric-designed protocol for the pediatric patient's imaging. In general, pediatric protocols should be designed with remarkably lower radiation dose thresholds than adult CT protocols. The same would correlate to any CT IV contrast injection and oral contrast protocols.

6. *Anticipation and attention to detail:* Anticipating the needs of the patient and recognizing any need for delayed imaging based on real-time pathology benefit the patient and the radiologist. Many times, the radiologist is in a separate workspace away from the CT scanner. Therefore, it is in the best interest of both the patient and the radiologist if the technologist notices pathology that would benefit from additional imaging. The technologist can reach out swiftly to the radiologist for a rapid prescription for additional images. Or the technologist may recognize pathology, such as an abscess, head bleed, or appendicitis, that needs urgent care. In these circumstances, the technologist can immediately reach out to the radiologist for prompt intervention. This practice can result in expedited care.

7. *Professionalism and adherence to practice standards:* It is inherent to a CT technologist to follow the code of ethics of the American Registry of Radiologic Technologists (ARRT). The ARRT has provided a foundation for assessment, knowledge, and skills that is expressed through a technologist's decision-making process. The focus for the CT technologist should always be to create high-quality CT imaging studies and to care for the patient as safely as possible at the lowest dose.

Definition of Terms

air calibration: Scan of air in gantry; based on a known value of –1000 for air, the scanner calibrates itself according to this density value relative to actual density value measured.

algorithm: Mathematic formula designed for computers to carry out complex calculations required for image reconstruction; designed for enhancement of soft tissue, bone, and edge resolution. Also referred to as *kernel*.

anisotropic spatial resolution: Spatial resolution of a voxel in which all three axes of the volume element are not equal. Slice thickness is not equal to pixel size.

aperture: Opening of the gantry through which the patient passes during the scan.

archiving: Storage of CT images on a long-term storage device, such as cassette tape, magnetic tape, CD/DVR, optical disk, or USB.

artifact: Distortion or an error in image that is unrelated to the subject being studied.

attenuation: Coefficient CT number assigned to measured remnant radiation intensity after attenuation by tissue density.

axial: Describes plane of an image as presented by CT scan; same as *transverse*.

bolus: Preset amount of radiopaque contrast medium injected rapidly per

IV administration to visualize high-flow vascular structures, usually in conjunction with dynamic scan; most often injected using a pressure injector.

channel: In multidetector CT, multiple rows of detectors (channels) are arranged along the longitudinal (z) axis of the patient. Each detector row (channel) consists of numerous elements.

computed tomography (CT): X-ray tube and detector assembly rotating 360 degrees around a specified area of the body; also called CAT (computed axial tomography) scan.

computed tomography dose index (CTDI): Radiation dose descriptor calculated with normalized beam widths for 14 contiguous sections or slices.

computed tomography dose index$_{100}$ (CTDI$_{100}$): Radiation dose descriptor calculated with the full length of a 100-mm pencil ionization chamber. Measures larger scan distances than CTDI, but only one location is calculated.

computed tomography dose index$_{vol}$ (CTDI$_{vol}$): Radiation dose descriptor that takes into account the parameters that are related to a specific imaging protocol. Considers helical pitch or axial scan spacing in its calculation. More accurate measure of dose per protocol.

computed tomography dose index (CTDI$_w$): Radiation dose descriptor that provides a weighted average of the center and peripheral contributions to dose within the scan plane. More accurate than CTDI$_{100}$, owing to calculations from more than one location.

CT angiography: Use of volumetric CT scanning with spiral technique to acquire image data that are reconstructed into three-dimensional CT angiograms.

CT number: Arbitrary number assigned by computer to indicate relative density of a given tissue; CT number varies proportionately with tissue density; high CT numbers indicate dense tissue, and low CT numbers indicate less dense tissue. All CT numbers are based on the density of water, which is assigned a CT number of 0. Also referred to as a *Hounsfield unit*.

contrast resolution: Ability to differentiate between small variations in density within the image.

curved planar reformations: Post-processing technique applied to stacks of axial image data that can be reconstructed into irregular or oblique planes.

data acquisition system (DAS): Part of detector assembly that converts analog signals to digital signals that can be used by the CT computer.

detector: Electronic component used for radiation detection; made of either high-density photo reactive crystals or pressurized stable gases.

detector array: a collection of detectors spaced closely together in a CT scan system. It senses the x-ray radiation.

detector assembly: Electronic component of CT scanner that measures remnant radiation exiting the patient, converting the radiation to an analog signal proportionate to the radiation intensity measured.

direct coronal: Describes position used to obtain images in coronal plane; used for head scans to provide images at right angles to axial images; patient is positioned prone for direct coronal images and supine for reverse coronal images.

dose length product (DLP): Commonly reported dose descriptor on CT scanners. Calculated by multiplying the CTDI$_{vol}$ by the length of the scan (cm). DLP = CTDI$_{vol}$ × scan length.

dynamic scanning: Process by which raw data are obtained by continuous scanning; images are not reconstructed but are saved for later reconstruction; most often used for visualization of high-flow vascular structures; can be used to scan an uncooperative patient rapidly.

extravasation: Leakage of IV contrast media into the surrounding soft tissues.

field of view (FOV): Area of anatomy displayed on the monitor; can be adjusted to include entire body section or a specific part of the patient anatomy being scanned.

gantry: Part of CT scanner that houses x-ray tube, cooling system, detector assembly, and DAS; often referred to by patients as the "doughnut."

gas-ionization detectors: Convert x-ray energy directly to electrical energy.

generation: Description of significant levels of technologic development of CT scanners; specifically related to tube/detector movement.

grayscale image: Analog image whereby each pixel in the image corresponds to a particular shade of gray.

helical CT: Data acquisition method that combines continuous gantry rotation with continuous table movement to form a helical path of scan data; also called *spiral CT*.

high-resolution scans: Use of scanning parameters that enhance contrast resolution of an image, such as thin slices, high matrices, high-spatial frequency algorithms, and small-display FOV.

host computer: Primary link between system operator and other components of imaging system.

Hounsfield unit (HU): Number used to describe average density of tissue; term is used interchangeably with *CT number*; named in honor of Hounsfield, who is generally given credit for development of the first clinically viable CT scanner.

image misregistration: Image distortion caused by combination of table indexing and respiration; table moves in specified increments, but patient movement during respiration may cause anatomy to be scanned more than once or not at all.

index: Table movement; also referred to as *table increments*.

isotropic spatial resolution: Spatial resolution of a voxel in which all three axes of the volume element are equal. Slice thickness is equal to pixel size.

mapping: Assignment of appropriate gray level to each pixel in an image.

matrix: Mathematical formula for calculation made up of individual cells for number assignment; CT matrix stores a CT number relative to the tissue density at that location; each cell or "address" stores one CT number for image reconstruction.

maximum intensity projection (MIP): Reconstruction of brightest pixels from stack of image data into a three-dimensional image.

multiplanar reconstruction (MPR): Post-processing technique applied to stacks of axial image data that can be reconstructed into other orientations or imaging planes.

multiple scan average dose (MSAD): Dose descriptor that calculates average dose resulting from a series of scans over an interval length of scans.

noise: Random variation of CT numbers around some mean value within a uniform object; noise produces a grainy appearance in the image.

partial volume averaging: Calculated linear attenuation coefficient for a pixel that is a weighted average of all densities in the pixel; the assigned CT number and ultimately the pixel appearance are affected by the average of the different densities measured within that pixel.

pixel (picture element): One individual cell surface within an image matrix used for image display.

post-processing techniques: Specialized reconstruction techniques that are applied to CT images to display the anatomic structures from different perspectives.

primary data: CT number assigned to the matrix by the computer; the information required to reconstruct an image.

protocol: Instructions for CT examination specifying slice thickness, table increments, contrast administration, scan diameter, and any other requirements specified by the radiologist.

quantum noise: Any noise in the image that is a result of random variation in the number of x-ray photons detected.

real time: Ability to process or reconstruct incoming data in milliseconds.

reconstruction: Process of creating a digital image from raw data.

region of interest (ROI): Measurement of CT numbers within a specified area for evaluation of average tissue density.

rendering: Process of changing the shading of a three-dimensional image; commonly used to increase depth perception of an image.

retrieval: Reconstruction of images stored on long-term device; can be done for extra film copies or when films are lost.

scan: Actual rotation of x-ray tube around the patient; used as a generic reference to one slice or an entire examination.

scan diameter: Also referred to as the zoom or focal plane of a CT scan; predetermined by the radiographer to include the anatomic area of interest; determines FOV.

scan duration: Amount of time used to scan an entire volume during a single spiral scan.

scan time: X-ray exposure time in seconds.

scintillation detectors: Convert x-ray energy into light, then light into electrical energy by a photodetector.

segmentation: Method of cropping or editing target objects from image data.

shaded surface display (SSD): Process used to generate three-dimensional images that show the surface of a three-dimensional object.

shading: Post-processing technique used in three-dimensional reconstructions to separate tissues of interest by applying a threshold value to isolate the structure of interest.

slice: One scan through a selected body part; also referred to as a *cut*; slice thickness can vary from 0.35 mm to 1 cm, depending on the examination.

slip ring: Low-voltage electrical contacts within the gantry designed to allow continuous rotation of an x-ray tube without the use of cables connecting internal and external components.

spatial resolution: Ability to identify visibly anatomic structures and small objects of high contrast.

spiral CT: Scanning method that combines a continuous gantry rotation with a continuous table movement to form a spiral path of scan data; also called *helical CT*.

streak artifact: Artifact created by high-density objects that result in an arc of straight lines projecting across the FOV from a common point.

system noise: Inherent property of a CT scanner; the difference between the measured CT number of a given tissue and the known value for that tissue; most often evaluated through the use of water phantom scans.

table increments: Specific amount of table travel between scans; can be varied to move at any specified increment; most protocols specify from 1 mm to 20 cm, depending on type of examination; also referred to as *indexing*.

table speed: Longitudinal distance traveled by the table during one revolution of the x-ray tube.

temporal resolution: Ability of CT system to freeze motions of the scanned object; the shortest amount of time needed to acquire a complete dataset.

threshold value: CT number used in defining the corresponding anatomy that comprises a three-dimensional object; any pixels within a three-dimensional volume having the threshold value (CT number) or higher would be selected for the three-dimensional model.

voxel (volume element): Individual pixel with the associated volume of tissue based on the slice thickness.

window: Arbitrary numbers used for image display based on various shades of gray; *window width* controls the overall gray level and affects image contrast; *window level* (center) controls subtle gray images within a certain width range and ultimately affects the brightness and overall density of an image.

Selected bibliography

AAPM Task Group 204. " Size-Specific Dose Estimates (SSDE) in Pediatric and Adult Body CT Examinations". 2011.

Bushong SC. *Radiologic Science for Technologists: Physics, Biology, and Protection*. 12th ed. St Louis: Elsevier; 2022.

Griffey RT, Sodickson A. Cumulative radiation exposure and cancer risk estimates in emergency department patients undergoing repeat or multiple CT. *AJR Am J Roentgenol*. 2009;192(4):887–892.

Haaga JR, Boll DT, et al., eds. *CT and MRI of the Whole Body, vols I and II*. 6th ed. St Louis: Elsevier; 2017.

Image Gently. *The Alliance for Radiation Safety in Pediatric Imaging Standards*. Available at: www.imagegently.org.

Image Wisely. *Radiation Safety in Adult Medical Imaging*. Available at: imagewisely.org.

Joemai RMS, Zweers D, Obermann WR, et al. Assessment of patient and occupational dose in established and new applications of MDCT fluoroscopy. *AJR Am J Roentgenol*. 2009;192(4):881–886.

Patel ACH, Gulati P, Chidambaranathan N, et al. *Comprehensive Textbook of Clinical Radiology. Volume I: Principles of Clinical Radiology, Multisystem Diseases & Head and Neck*. New Delhi: Elsevier India; 2023.

Seeram E. *Computed Tomography: Physical Principles, Patient Care, Clinical Applications, and Quality Control*. 5th ed. St Louis: Elsevier; 2023.

Zagoria RJ, Dyer R, Brady B. *Genitourinary Imaging: The Requisites*. 3rd ed. Philadelphia: Elsevier; 2016.

26
MAGNETIC RESONANCE IMAGING

ELIZABETH NELSON

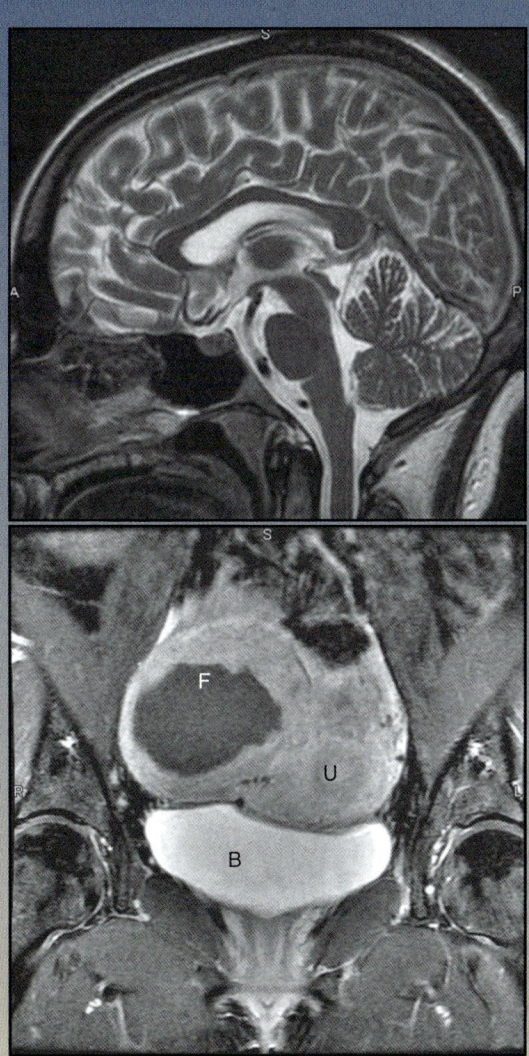

OUTLINE

Principles of Magnetic Resonance Imaging, 270
Comparison of Magnetic Resonance Imaging and Conventional Radiography, 270
Historical Development, 270
Physical Principles, 271
Equipment, 273
Safety of Magnetic Resonance Imaging, 283
Infection Control, 286
Examination Protocols, 287
Clinical Applications, 293
Advanced Clinical Applications, 303
Best Practices, 306
Conclusion, 306
Definition of Terms, 306

Principles of Magnetic Resonance Imaging

Magnetic resonance[a] imaging (MRI) is a noninvasive technique that produces computer-generated cross-sectional images similar to those of computed tomography (CT) (see Chapter 25). Ionizing radiation is not utilized to generate *magnetic resonance (MR)* images. MR images are created through the interactions of magnetic fields and radio frequency energy with biologic tissues.

An interesting historical note: MRI was originally called *nuclear magnetic resonance* (NMR) imaging, with the word *nuclear* indicating that the nonradioactive atomic nucleus played an important role in the technique. This term was dropped because of public apprehension about nuclear energy and nuclear weapons—neither of which is associated with MRI in any way.

---

[a]Almost all italicized words on the succeeding pages are defined at the end of this chapter.

Comparison of Magnetic Resonance Imaging and Conventional Radiography

Despite being the mainstay of medical imaging for more than a century, conventional radiography has two significant weaknesses.

On a radiograph, all body structures exposed to the x-ray beam are superimposed into one flat or two-dimensional (2D) image. This makes it extremely difficult to separate individual organs or anatomic structures from one another. In many instances, multiple projections must be acquired to visualize these important structures. Cross-sectional imaging techniques, such as MRI, can create three-dimensional (3D) images with little or no superimposition of structures.

Contrast, or the ability to discriminate between two slightly different tissue densities, is necessary for imaging soft tissue structures. Because conventional radiography depends on differences in x-ray *attenuation* within the object and the sensitivity of the recording medium, it is difficult for radiographs to detect small differences in contrast. Typically, conventional radiographs can distinguish only tissues with large differences in attenuation of the x-ray beam (e.g., air, fat, bone, and metal). Soft tissue structures such as the liver and kidneys cannot be separated by differences in x-ray attenuation alone. For these structures, differences are magnified using contrast agents. MRI can distinguish very small differences in contrast among tissues by manipulating biologic tissue with magnetic fields and radio waves.

Historical Development

In the mid-1940s, Felix Bloch, working at Stanford University, and Edward Purcell, working at Harvard University, discovered the principles of NMR. Their work led to the use of nuclear magnetic spectroscopy for the analysis of complex molecular structures and dynamic chemical processes. This technology is still in use today for the nondestructive testing of chemical compounds. In 1952, Bloch and Purcell were jointly awarded the Nobel Prize in Physics for their development of new methods for making precise nuclear magnetic measurements.

In 1969, Raymond Damadian proposed the first MRI body scanner. He discovered that the relaxation times (discussed later in this chapter) of tumors differed from the relaxation times of normal tissue. This finding suggested that if images of the body could be obtained by producing maps of relaxation rates, it would be possible to differentiate normal from abnormal tissues. In 1973, Paul Lauterbur published the first cross-sectional images of objects obtained with MRI techniques. These first images were crude, and only large objects could be distinguished. Sir Peter Mansfield demonstrated how the signals could be rapidly analyzed mathematically, which made it possible to develop useful imaging techniques. Since those discoveries, MRI technology has advanced rapidly. Very small structures are commonly imaged quickly and with increased resolution and contrast. In 2003, the Nobel Prize in Physiology or Medicine was jointly awarded to Lauterbur and Mansfield for their discoveries in MRI.

Physical Principles

SIGNAL PRODUCTION

The structure of an atom is often compared with the structure of the solar system, with the sun representing the central atomic *nucleus* and the planets representing the orbiting electrons. MRI uses the properties of the nucleus to generate the signal containing information that is used to construct the image. Clinical MRI scanners "image" hydrogen because it is the most abundant element in the body and is the strongest nuclear magnet on a per-nucleus basis.

Elements with odd atomic numbers, such as hydrogen, are called *MR-active nuclei* and have magnetic properties causing them to act like tiny bar magnets (Fig. 26.1). Ordinarily, in the absence of a strong magnetic field, these protons point in random directions, as shown in Fig. 26.2, creating no net magnetization. At this point, they are not useful for imaging. However, if the body is placed within a strong uniform magnetic field, the protons will attempt to align themselves in one of two orientations: with the main magnetic field (parallel) or against the main magnetic field (antiparallel). At equilibrium, a slight majority of hydrogen protons will align with (parallel to) the main magnetic field (also called the *longitudinal plane*), resulting in a slight net magnetization of the imaging volume.

The protons do not line up precisely with the external magnetic field, but at an angle, causing them to rotate around the magnetic field in a manner similar to the wobbling of a spinning top. This wobbling motion, depicted in Fig. 26.3, is called *precession* and occurs at a specific *frequency* (rate) for a given atom's nucleus in a magnetic field of a specific strength. These precessing protons can absorb energy only if that energy matches the frequency at which they are wobbling. In MRI, the energy to excite the protons comes from *radio frequency* (RF) energy, typically found in the FM band of the electromagnetic spectrum. The absorption of energy by the precessing protons is referred to as *resonance*. This resonant or precessional frequency, called the Larmor frequency, varies depending on the field strength of the MRI scanner. For example, in a 1 tesla (T) scanner, the Larmor frequency is 42.58 megahertz (MHz), but in a 3T scanner, the precessional frequency is 127.74 MHz.

When an *RF pulse* is applied at the Larmor frequency, the protons absorb the energy and begin to resonate, resulting in a reorientation of the net tissue magnetization into a plane perpendicular to the main magnetic field. This is known as the *transverse plane*. The protons in the transverse plane are also precessing at the same resonant frequency. Faraday's law of induction states that a moving magnetic field induces an electrical current in a wire; therefore, the precessing protons (a moving magnet) in the tissues create an electrical current, the MRI *signal*, in the receiving coil or *antenna*.

The MRI signal is picked up by this sensitive antenna or coil, amplified, and processed by a computer to produce a sectional image of the body, which is viewed on a computer monitor. Since the information is in a digital format, it can be post-processed for additional diagnostic information.

Many other odd-numbered nuclei in the body can be used in MRI. Nuclei from elements such as phosphorus and sodium provide useful and different diagnostic information, particularly in efforts to understand the metabolism of normal and abnormal tissues. Metabolic changes may prove to be more sensitive and specific in detecting abnormalities than the more physical and structural changes recognized by hydrogen MRI. Nonhydrogen nuclei may also be used for combined imaging and *spectroscopy*, in which small volumes of tissue may be analyzed for chemical content.

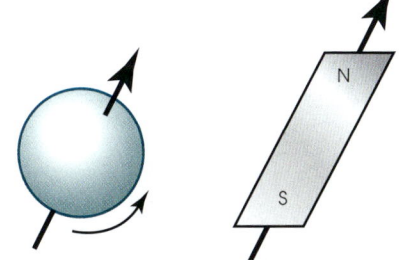

Fig. 26.1 A proton with magnetic properties can be compared to a tiny bar magnet. Curved arrow indicates that a proton spins on its own axis; this motion is different from that of precession.

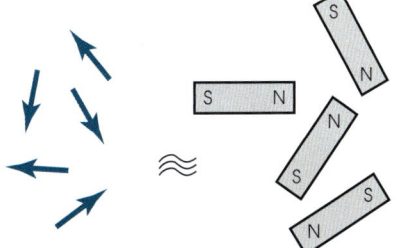

Fig. 26.2 In the absence of a strong magnetic field, the protons *(arrows)* point in random directions and cannot be used for imaging.

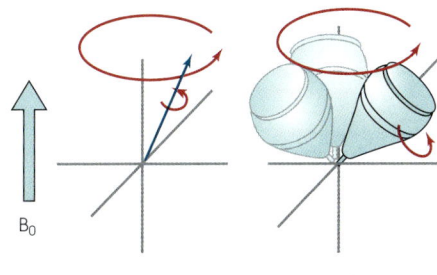

Fig. 26.3 Precession. The protons *(arrow)* and the toy top spin on their own axes. Both also rotate *(curved arrows)* around the direction of an external force in a wobbling motion called *precession*. Precessing protons can absorb energy through resonance. B_0 represents the external magnetic field acting on the nucleus. The toy top precesses under the influence of gravity.

SIGNIFICANCE OF THE SIGNAL

As mentioned earlier, conventional radiographic techniques, including CT, produce images based on a single property of tissue: x-ray attenuation or density. MR images are more complex because they contain information about a variety of tissue properties—proton density, relaxation rates, and flow phenomena. These properties contribute to the overall strength of the MRI signal. Computer processing converts signal strength to shades of gray on the image. Strong signals are represented by white in the image, and weak signals are represented by black.

One determinant of signal strength is the number of precessing protons in a given volume of tissue. Signal strength that depends on the concentration of protons is termed *proton density*. Most soft tissues, including fat, have a similar number of protons per unit of volume; therefore, the use of proton density characteristics alone separates these tissues poorly. Other tissues have few hydrogen nuclei per unit of volume; examples include the cortex of bone and air in the lungs. These tissues have a weak signal as a result of low proton density and can be easily distinguished from other tissues.

MRI signal intensity also depends on the relaxation times of the nuclei. *Relaxation* is the release of energy by the excited protons. Excited nuclei relax through two processes. The process of nuclei releasing their excess energy to the general environment or lattice (the arrangement of atoms in a substance) is called *spin-lattice relaxation*. The rate of this relaxation process is measured in milliseconds and is labeled as *T1*. *Spin-spin relaxation* is the release of energy by excited nuclei through interaction among themselves. The rate of this process is also measured in milliseconds but is labeled as *T2*.

Relaxation (T1 and T2) occurs at different rates in different tissues. The environment of a hydrogen nucleus in the spleen differs from that of one in the liver; therefore, their relaxation rates differ, and the MRI signals created by these nuclei differ. The different relaxation rates in the liver and spleen result in different signal intensities and appearances on the image, enabling the viewer to discriminate between the two organs. Similarly, many types of tissue, such as fat and muscle, can be distinguished based on the relaxation rates of their nuclei. The most important factor in tissue discrimination is the *relaxation time*.

The signals produced by MRI techniques contain a combination of proton density, T1, and T2 information. It is possible to obtain images "weighted" toward any one of these three parameters by manipulating nuclei with specific *pulse sequences*. In most imaging sequences, a short T1 (fast spin-lattice relaxation rate) produces a high signal on T1-weighted images. Conversely, a long T2 (slow spin-spin relaxation rate) generates a high signal on T2-weighted images.

The final property that influences image appearance is flow. For complex physical reasons, moving substances usually have weak MRI signals. With some specialized pulse sequences, the reverse may be true; see the discussion of magnetic resonance angiography (MRA) later in the chapter. With standard pulse sequences, flowing blood in vessels produces a low signal. It is easily distinguished from surrounding stationary tissues without the need for the contrast agents required by regular radiographic techniques. Stagnant blood, such as an acute blood clot, typically has a high signal due to its short T1 and long T2 relaxation times. Specific pulse sequences may facilitate the assessment of vessel patency or the determination of the rate of blood flow through vessels (Fig. 26.4).

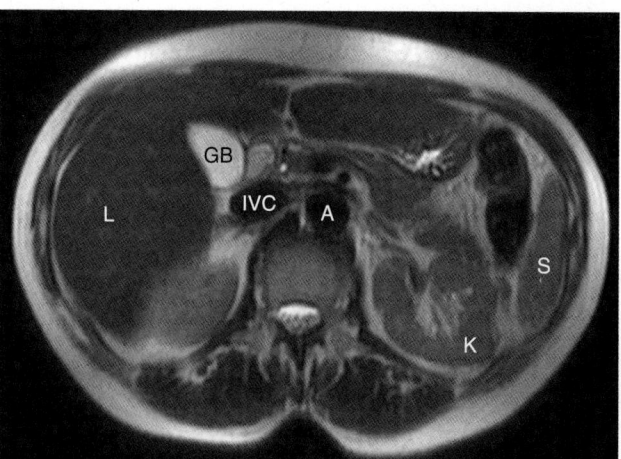

Fig. 26.4 T2-weighted image of an abdomen showing the flow void produced by flowing blood. *A,* Aorta; *GB,* gallbladder; *IVC,* inferior vena cava; *K,* kidney; *L,* liver; *S,* spleen.

Equipment

MRI requires a patient area (magnet room), an equipment room, and an operator's console. A separate diagnostic workstation is optional.

CONSOLE

The operator's console is used to control the imaging process (Fig. 26.5). At the console, the operator can interact with the system's computers and electronics to manipulate all necessary examination parameters. Images are viewed on a computer monitor to ensure that the examination is of diagnostic quality. Here, images can be manipulated, and hard copies of the exam produced if necessary. An independent workstation may be used to perform additional image manipulation or postprocessing when required.

EQUIPMENT ROOM

The equipment room houses all the electronics and computers necessary to complete the imaging process. The RF cabinet controls transmission of the radio wave pulse sequences. The gradient cabinet controls the time-varying magnetic fields necessary to localize the MRI signal. The array processors and computers receive and process the large amount of *raw data* received from the patient and construct the images the operator sees on the operator's console.

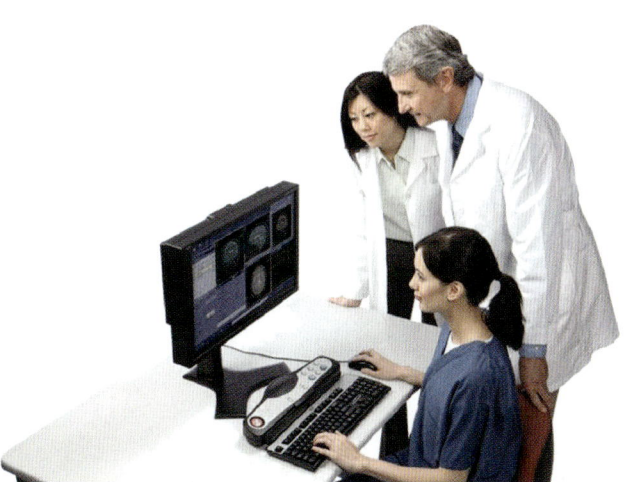

Fig. 26.5 Operator's console. This device controls the imaging process and allows visualization of images.

(Courtesy GE Healthcare.)

MAGNET ROOM

The magnet is the major component of the MRI system in the scanning room. It must be large enough to surround the patient and any antennas (coils) that are required for radio wave transmission and reception. Antennas are typically wound in the shape of a positioning device for a particular body part. These are commonly referred to as *coils*, or *RF antennas*. As the patient lies on the table, coils are placed either on, under, or around the part to be imaged. Once positioned, the patient is advanced into the center of the magnet (isocenter) (Fig. 26.6).

Various magnet types may be used to provide the strong uniform magnetic field required for imaging, as follows:

- *Resistive magnets* are simple but large electromagnets consisting of coils of wire. A magnetic field is produced by passing an electrical current through the wire coils. The greater the current, the higher the field strength. However, the electrical resistance of the wire coils produces heat, which limits the maximum strength of the magnetic field.
- *Superconductive (cryogenic) magnets* are also electromagnets. Their wire loops are cooled to very low temperatures with liquid helium to reduce electrical resistance. This permits higher magnetic field strengths than those produced by resistive magnets.
- *Permanent magnets* have a constant field that does not require additional electricity or cooling. Early permanent magnets were extremely heavy, even compared with the massive superconductive and resistive units. Because of their weight, these magnets were difficult to place for clinical use. The magnetic fields of permanent magnets do not extend as far away from the magnet *(fringe field)* as do the magnetic fields of other types of magnets. Fringe fields are a problem because of their effect on nearby electronic equipment.

Prior to the development of actively shielded magnets, installing an MRI system in the hospital was a challenge due to large magnetic fringe fields. Advances in magnet technology and the use of *passive* and *active shielding* have made the siting of MRI units less challenging. The fringe fields of both resistive and superconducting magnets can now be "pulled in" or reduced to lessen the interference with nearby electronic and computer equipment. This shielding also reduces the effect of metal objects such as elevators or automobiles moving near the magnetic fringe field.

Stray radio waves present another challenge in the placement of MRI units. The radio waves used in MRI may be of the same frequency as the radio waves used for other nearby radio applications. Stray radio waves can be picked up by the MRI antenna coils and interfere with normal image production. MRI facilities require specially constructed rooms, called *Faraday cages*, to shield the receiving antennas from outside radio interference.

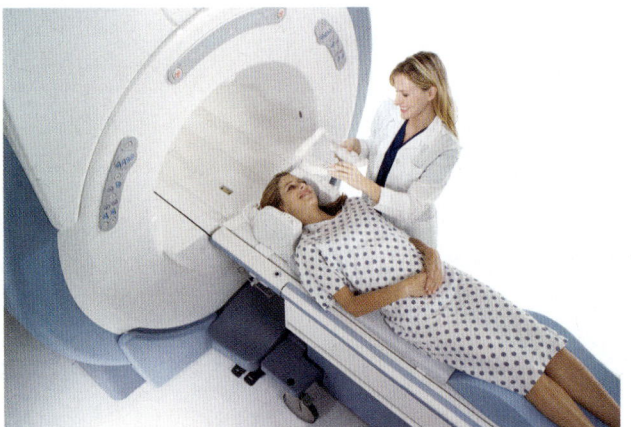

Fig. 26.6 Patient prepared for MRI.

(Courtesy GE Healthcare.)

TYPES OF MRI SCANNERS

Various MRI systems operate at different magnetic field strengths. Magnetic field strength is measured in *tesla* (T) or *gauss* *(G)*. There are a variety of MRI scanners that can be utilized for MR imaging, such as closed, open, extremity, point-of-care scanners, and scanners in hybrid MRI environments.

Closed scanners

Closed scanners have a cylindrical design that surrounds the patient. The side walls of the scanner are closed (Fig. 26.7). The main magnetic field, B_0, is oriented along the horizontal or z-axis. These scanners range from 0.55T to 7T in field strength. Traditionally, the bore aperture of closed units was 60 cm (23.6 inches). Patients often experience *claustrophobia* due to the confined dimensions of these scanners (Fig. 26.8). Claustrophobia can be a significant impediment to MRI in up to 20% of patients. Patient education is perhaps most important in preventing this problem, but medication, appropriate lighting, music, aromatherapy, air movement, and mirrors or prisms that enable a patient to look out of the scanner may be helpful. Claustrophobic patients may also find comfort in having a friend or family member present in the room during the scan. In addition, body habitus may prevent some patients from entering the magnet.

Wide-bore scanners can mitigate these challenges. These scanners can have a bore aperture of 70 cm (27.6 inches), 74 cm (29.1 inches) with an oval shape, or 80 cm (31.5 inches). The extra space reduces anxiety and accommodates patients of greater body habitus. Wide-bore scanners range in field strength from 0.55T to 3T.

Clinical 7T and research-oriented 11T MRI systems have been introduced. The advantages of these ultra-high field systems are significantly increased signal-to-noise ratio (SNR) and resolution. While ultra-high field systems provide high image quality, open scanners also produce quality images.

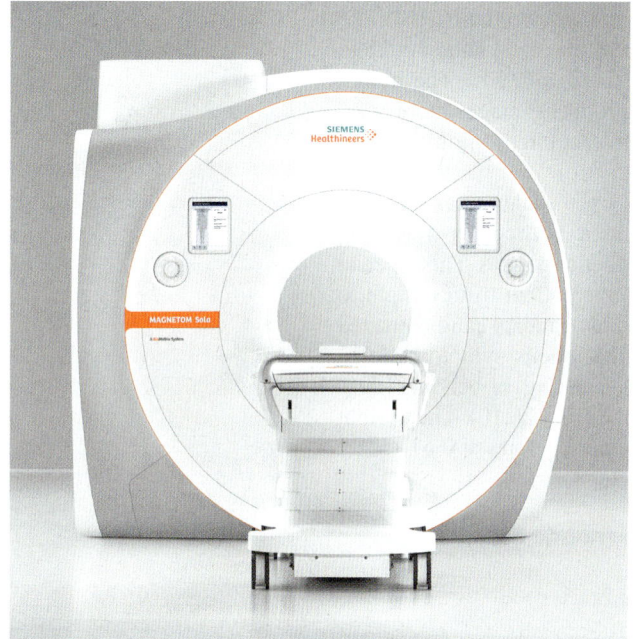

Fig. 26.7 Closed MRI scanner: 1.5T MAGNETOM Sola by Siemens Healthineers.

(Courtesy Siemens Healthineers.)

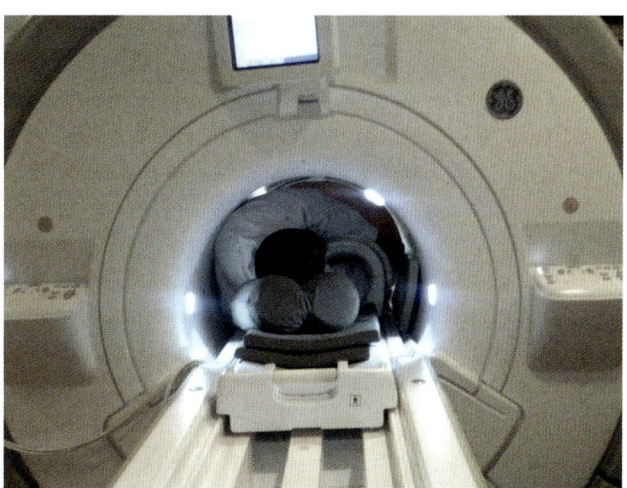

Fig. 26.8 Patient inside a superconducting 1.5T magnet. Some patients cannot be scanned because of claustrophobia.

(Courtesy GE Healthcare.)

Open scanners

Open scanners have a patient table placed between a top and bottom magnet, and the sides are completely open (Fig. 26.9). The open design alleviates anxiety and provides greater patient access during intraoperative or interventional procedures. The main magnetic field, B_0, is oriented along the vertical axis. Low-field open magnets range in field strength from 0.2T to 0.35T.[1] Mid-field open magnets range in field strength from 0.6T to 0.7T.[1] High-field open magnets range in field strength from 1.0T to 1.2T.[1] The higher field strength produces images more comparable to those acquired on closed 1.5T systems.

The upright open scanner has a motorized bed oriented between two vertical opposing magnetic poles.[2] This special bed can rotate the patient from upright to recumbent.[2] Thus, patients can be imaged in a position that elicits symptoms (e.g., supine, seated, standing, or bending [flexion, extension])[2] (Fig. 26.10). The upright open MRI scanner operates at 0.6T.[3]

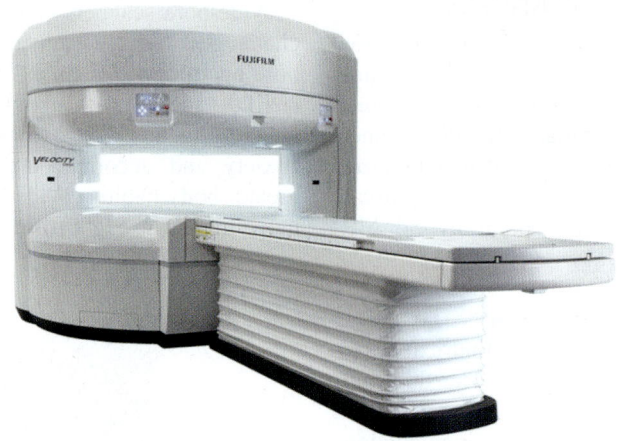

Fig. 26.9 Open MRI scanner: Fujifilm 1.2T Oasis Velocity.

(Courtesy Fujifilm.)

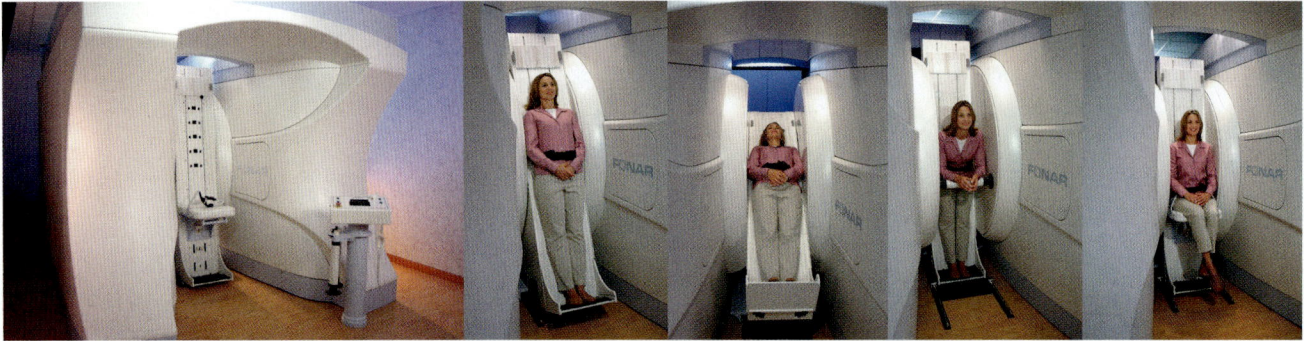

Fig. 26.10 UPRIGHT® Multi-Position™ MRI (aka STAND-UP® MRI).

(Courtesy FONAR Corporation.)

Similarly, the weight-bearing MRI scanner has a bed optimized to support standing oriented between two magnets. The weight-bearing MRI scanner operates at 0.25T.[4] The magnet and the patient can be rotated from 0 to 90 degrees, which allows patients to be scanned in the supine and weight-bearing positions[4] (Fig. 26.11). The appearance of pathology often changes when the patient moves from the supine to the weight-bearing position (Fig. 26.12).[4] Therefore, acquiring images in both the supine and weight-bearing positions can provide greater insight into the cause of a patient's symptoms.

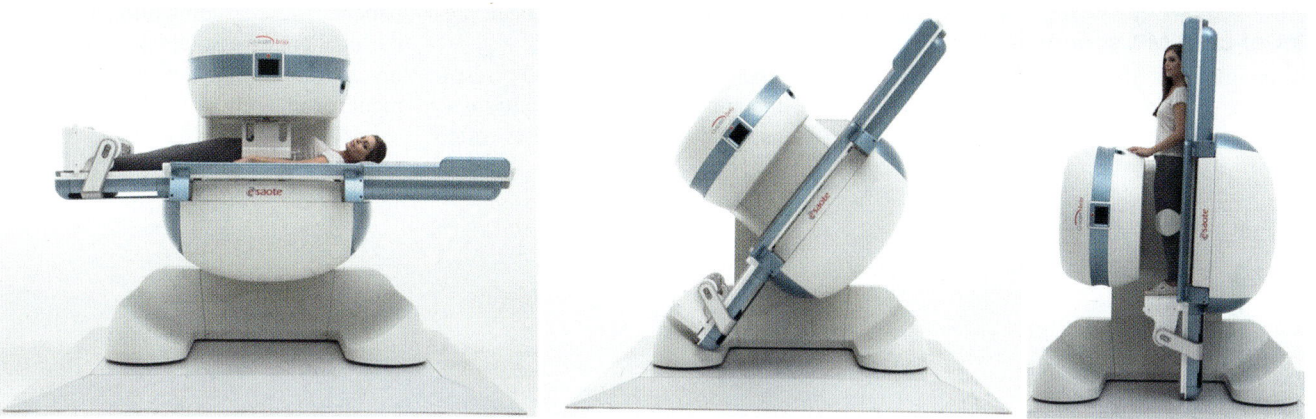

Fig. 26.11 Weight-bearing MRI scanner: 0.25T G-scan Brio Weight-Bearing MRI by Esaote.

(Courtesy Esaote.)

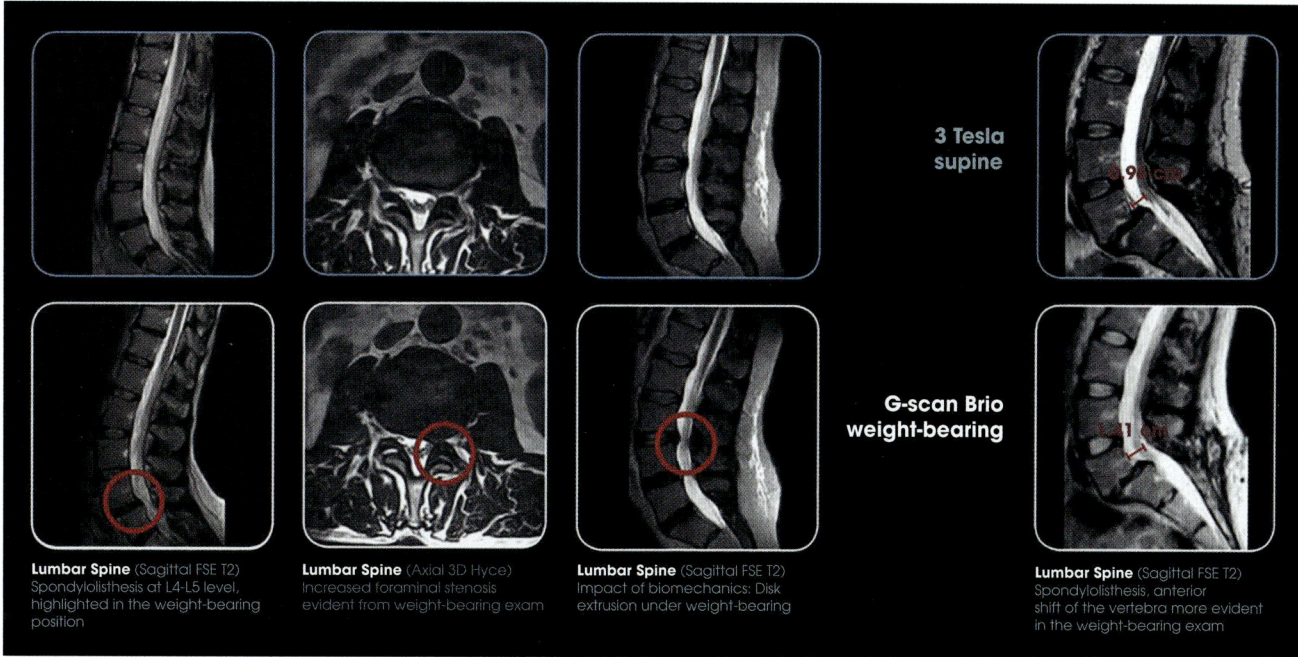

Fig. 26.12 Standing vs. supine positioning. Images reveal what supine MRI misses.

(Courtesy Esaote.)

Extremity magnets

Extremity magnets permit imaging in an open environment and are often utilized in orthopedic offices (Fig. 26.13). Extremity scanners range in field strength from 0.25T to 0.31T.[5] These systems can image the hands, wrists, elbows, knees, feet, and ankles. They allow the patient to recline comfortably during imaging. These units are lightweight, take up less space than conventional MRI scanners, and produce quality images (Fig. 26.14).

Point-of-care MRI scanners

MR imaging of the brain is essential for the development of treatment plans in emergency departments, adult and pediatric intensive care units, and the neonatal intensive care unit (NICU). Traditionally, critical patients were transported to the radiology department for MR imaging.

Transport from the inpatient unit to the MRI department presents several challenges. The imaging department may not have immediate scanner availability at the time of an emergent MRI request. Upon arrival in the radiology department, the patient may have to wait briefly in a holding area until the scan room has been prepared for their exam.

Additional staff such as nurses, respiratory therapists, nurse practitioners, physicians, and anesthesiologists often accompany high acuity patients to the MRI suite. These team members are responsible for monitoring vital signs, patient temperature, and administering sedation to the patient during imaging.

While some patients are stable enough to be transported to the MRI suite, others are too critical to leave the unit. Imaging is often delayed until the patient's condition stabilizes. Technological advancements have led to the development of point-of-care MRI systems that bring MRI to the patient. These systems mitigate several of the challenges associated with transporting a critical patient to the MRI department for imaging.

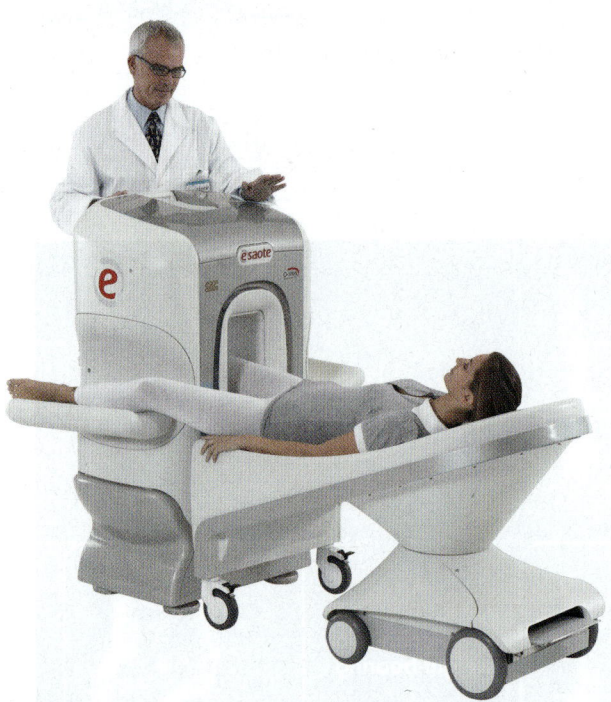

Fig. 26.13 Extremity MRI scanner: 0.31T O-scan Premium Extremity MRI scanner.

(Courtesy Esaote.)

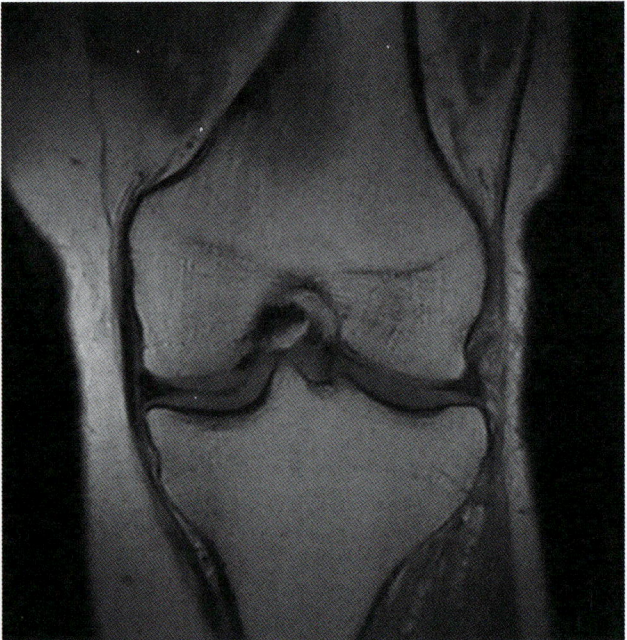

Fig. 26.14 Coronal T1-weighted image of the knee obtained with an O-scan Dedicated Extremity MRI scanner.

(Courtesy Esaote.)

Portable MR imaging system

The portable MR imaging system is designed for brain imaging in patients of all ages (Fig. 26.15).[6] The system has a permanent magnet and operates at 0.064T.[6] It has an open layout, which can alleviate anxiety and accommodate respiratory equipment. The acoustic noise generated is lower than that of conventional MRI systems, thereby reducing anxiety and the need for sedation.[7] The unit assures safety with a 5-gauss guard and requires no external shielding.[6] Thus, health care personnel and family members can remain in the room with the patient during imaging. In addition, medical equipment in the vicinity of the portable unit can remain nearby. The patient can remain in their hospital bed during imaging since the system requires only that the patient's head be positioned within the scanner. To initiate a scan, the portable unit is plugged into a standard electrical outlet and is ready to scan in minutes.[6] Imaging is directed from a tablet interface.[6] Currently, the following imaging sequences can be obtained: T1, T2, fluid-attenuated inversion recovery (FLAIR), and diffusion-weighted imaging (DWI) with an apparent diffusion coefficient (ADC) map.[6] These sequences can be acquired in the axial, sagittal, or coronal planes.[6] However, DWI can only be acquired in the axial plane.[6] Clinicians have found the portable imaging system to be useful in the assessment and follow-up evaluation of numerous neurologic conditions.

Neonatal point-of-care MRI system

The neonatal point-of-care MRI unit is designed specifically for installation and use in the NICU (Fig. 26.16).[8] It has a 1.0T permanent magnet, a horizontal B_0 field, and no external magnetic field.[8] This magnet has quiet imaging, which can reduce the need for sedation.[8] The patient bed is temperature controlled to support the needs of premature infants and has portals that allow for easy routing of tubing and monitoring equipment.[8] Currently, the system images only the brain. It accommodates infants weighing 1 kg to 4.5 kg (2.20 pounds to 9.92 pounds) with a maximum head circumference of 38 cm (14.9 inches).[8] The following pulse sequences can be obtained: 2D and 3D gradient echo, spin echo, fast spin echo, DWI with ADC maps, susceptibility-weighted imaging (SWI), and 2D and 3D MRA.[8] The following image contrasts can be obtained: T1 and T2.[8] Infants can undergo imaging in the NICU, resulting in quicker access to imaging, a reduced need for sedation, and less time out of the unit. This technology has been implemented in several institutions and found to be beneficial to patients and staff.

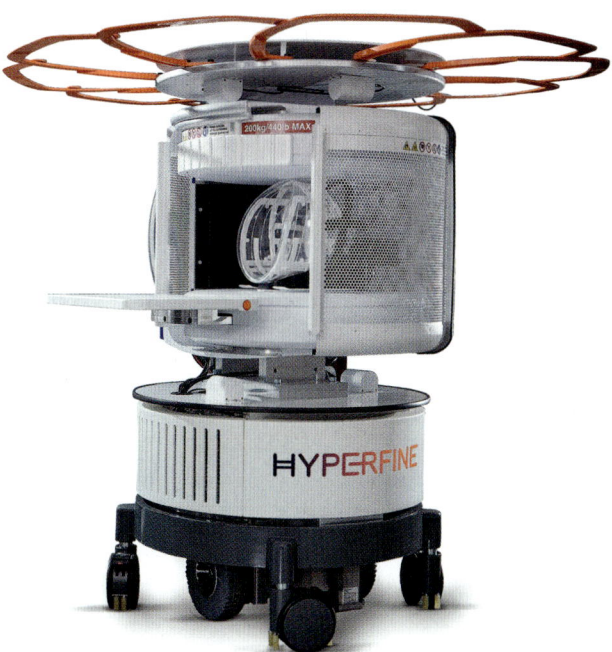

Fig. 26.15 The Hyperfine, Inc. *Swoop*® Portable MR Imaging® System.

(Courtesy Hyperfine, Inc.)

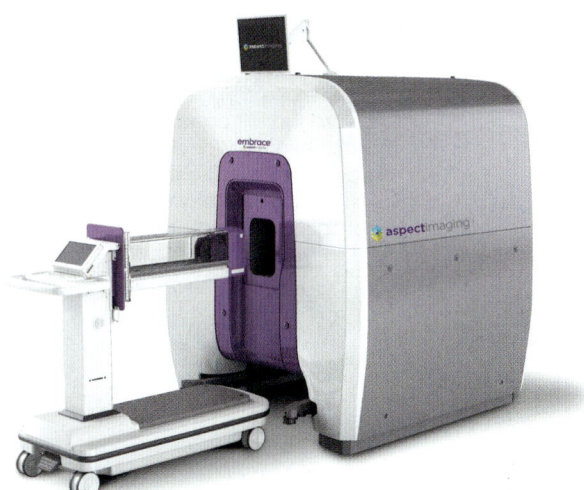

Fig. 26.16 Aspect Imaging Embrace® Neonatal Point-of-Care MRI System.

(Courtesy Aspect Imaging.)

Hybrid-MRI environments

MRI has been implemented in other areas outside of the radiology department, such as operating rooms, interventional suites, nuclear medicine, and radiation therapy. These hybrid MRI environments present special safety considerations, as all team members must be well versed in MR safety.

Intraoperative and interventional MRI

Intraoperative and interventional MRI units can have an open or closed design. Open systems allow greater access to the patient during procedures, as the sides of the unit are open. High-field open scanners are often utilized for intraoperative and interventional procedures. Closed units provide high image quality, but staff have limited access to the patient. Closed units utilized for intraoperative and interventional MRI procedures have a 70 cm (27.6 inch) bore aperture and range in field strength from 1.5T to 3T.

Intraoperative MRI suites are designed to provide efficient transfer of the patient between the operating theatre and the MRI unit (Fig. 26.17). Intraoperative MRI is often utilized during neurosurgical procedures.[9] Intraoperative MRI provides the surgeon with detailed images of the brain that guide the procedure.[9] The use of intraoperative MRI results in increased precision and better outcomes.[9]

Since the introduction of interventional MRI, techniques and clinical applications have significantly advanced.[10] Some clinical applications include localization of soft tissue diseases with poor soft tissue contrast, sclerotherapy of venous malformations, biopsy, and image-guided thermal ablation and cryoablation.[11] Interventional MRI procedures may be performed in various body regions.

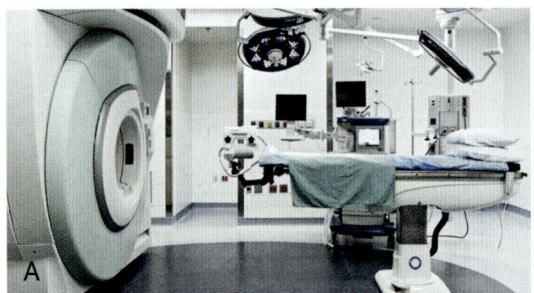
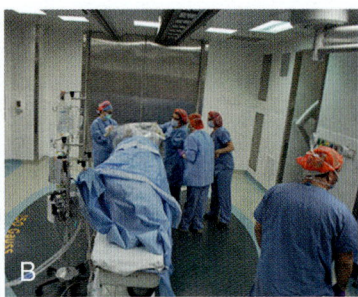
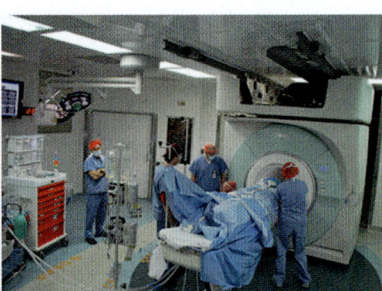

Fig. 26.17 (A) Massachusetts General Hospital neurosurgical operating room. IMRIS (Deerfield Imaging, Minnetonka, MN) magnet on left moving on ceiling-mounted rails toward the MR conditional operating table. (B) Patient is intubated and under general anesthesia on MR conditional operating table. Photo on left shows the operating room team preparing the patient before opening the magnet room doors. On right, the team is ensuring safe entry of the patient into the 70-cm bore IMRIS magnet in advance of obtaining intraoperative MR images.

(From Jones PS, Swearingen B: Intraoperative MRI for pituitary adenomas. *Neurosurg Clin N Am*, 2019;39(4):413–420.)

PET-MRI

A positron emission tomography (PET) scan is an imaging exam that can reveal the metabolic or biochemical function of tissues and organs.[12] The PET scan uses a radioactive drug called a tracer to show both typical and atypical metabolic activity.[12] PET images are combined with CT images via PET-CT scanners. Scanners capable of combining PET and MR images have been developed. PET-MR scanners resemble closed MRI systems but can acquire PET and MR images simultaneously (Fig. 26.18). Currently, these units have a 60 cm (23.6 inch) bore aperture and a field strength of 3T. Oncologists rely on PET-MR scans for cancer detection and staging, treatment planning, and to assess the response to treatment.[13] PET-MR scans can also be utilized in the study of neurologic diseases.[13]

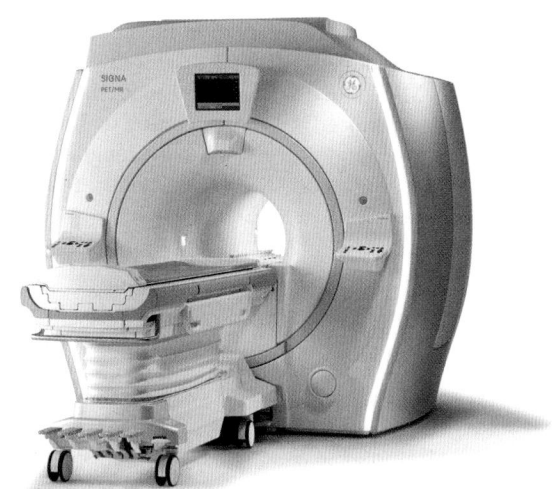

Fig. 26.18 SIGNA™ PET/MR.

(Courtesy GE Healthcare.)

MR-guided radiation therapy

MRI has been used in radiation treatment planning for many years. MR-guided radiation therapy has been introduced. The magnetic resonance linear accelerator (MR-Linac) combines MR imaging and radiation therapy into one unit. The MR-Linac resembles a closed MRI scanner. One MR-Linac has a field strength of 1.5T, a bore aperture of 70 cm (27.6 inches), and a short bore length[14] (Fig. 26.19). Daily MRI scans confirm the position, size, and shape of the area to be treated (Fig. 26.20). MR imaging during a treatment session monitors anatomic motion, which aids in precisely treating the target.

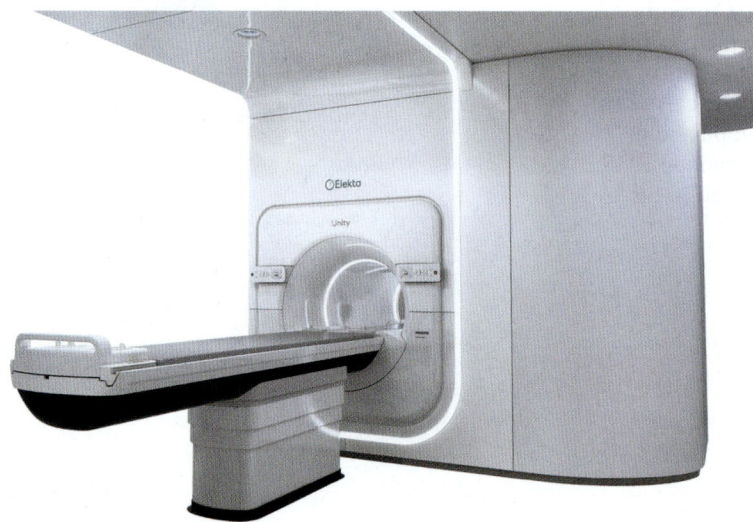

Fig. 26.19 Magnetic Resonance Linear Accelerator (MR-Linac): Elekta Unity MR-Linac.

(Courtesy of Elekta. https://www.elekta.com/company/newsroom/image-bank/.)

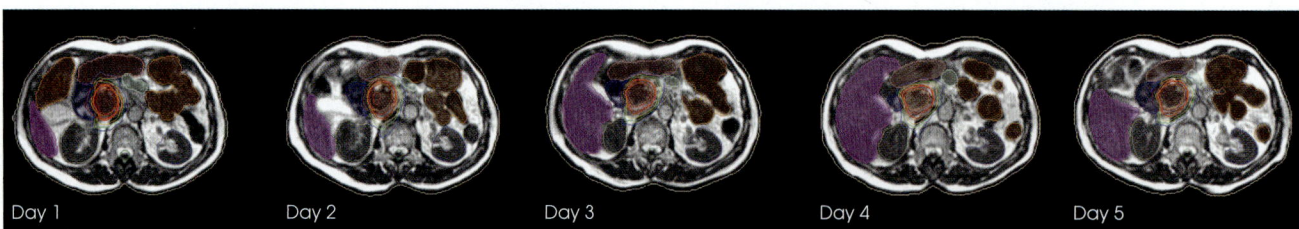

Fig. 26.20 Treatment-planning MR images over the course of 5 days. Images demonstrate changes in the position, shape, and size of the tumor and surrounding healthy tissue between treatments.

(Courtesy ViewRay Systems, Inc.)

Safety of Magnetic Resonance Imaging

MRI is generally considered safe, as it does not utilize ionizing radiation to generate images. However, the MRI environment can be a dangerous environment if safety guidelines are not followed.

ZONES

There are four designated zones within MRI facilities to promote safety (Fig. 26.21). *Zone I* is the area farthest from the magnet room and is freely accessible to the general public.

Zone II is an interface between the publicly accessible Zone I and the strictly controlled Zones III and IV.[15] Patients are under the supervision of MR personnel in Zone II. Zone II may include the reception area, screening area, and dressing rooms. Screening takes place in Zone II. Anyone entering the MRI environment (e.g., patients, visitors, and personnel) should be screened to ensure that they do not carry metallic objects into the magnet room or have medical devices within their bodies that could be adversely affected by exposure to strong magnetic fields.

A *ferromagnetic detection system* (FMDS) supplements the screening process. An FMDS detects ferrous objects that one may be carrying prior to entry into the exam room (Fig. 26.22). While an FMDS can detect ferrous objects, the system should not replace a thorough written and verbal screening.

Zone III is adjacent to the magnet room and poses a physical risk to unscreened patients or personnel, as the fringe field may extend into Zone III at some sites. Individuals must be properly screened prior to entering this restricted area. Access to Zone III is limited to employees who have completed proper training. Zone III houses the operator's console.

Zone IV houses the MRI scanner and poses the greatest risk to patients and personnel. Access to this area is highly restricted to prevent accidents, injuries, or death. No individual is allowed in Zone IV without being screened and supervised by level 2 MR personnel.

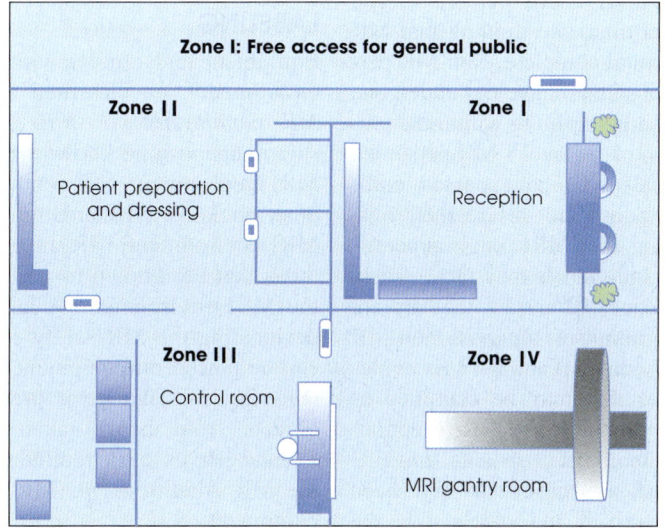

Fig. 26.21 Floor plan demonstrating the MRI environment divided into four zones to promote safety.

(From Sutton D, Aggarwal B: *Textbook of radiology and imaging,* ed 8, St Louis: Elsevier, 2022.)

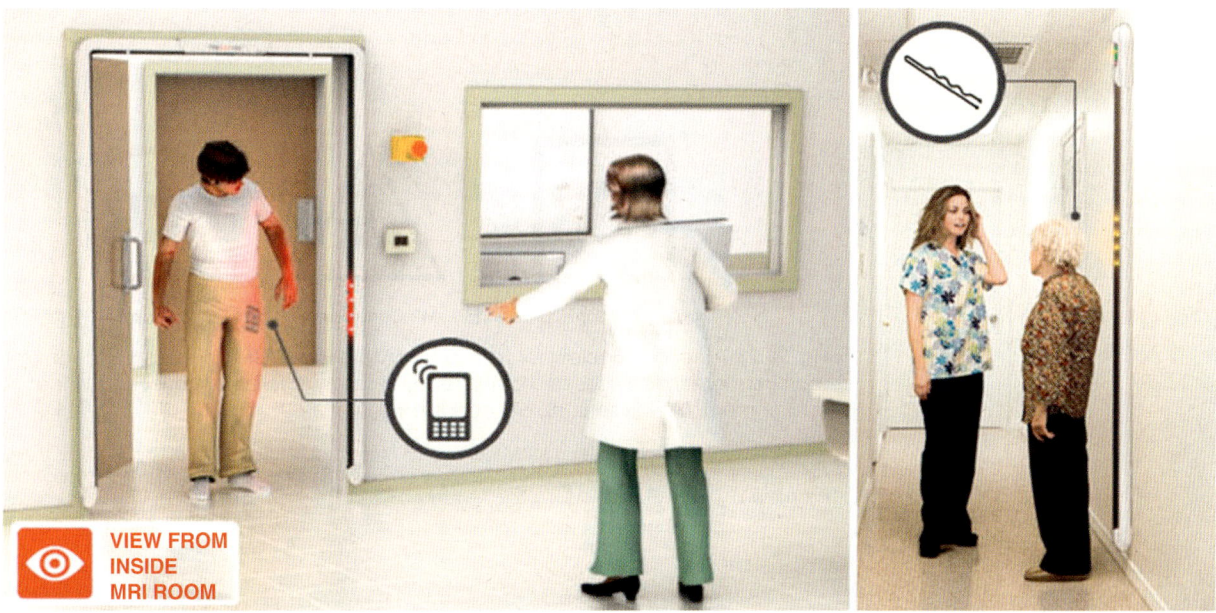

Fig. 26.22 Ferromagnetic detection systems serve as an additional safeguard to prevent ferrous objects from entering the magnet room. *Left,* FerrAlert® ferromagnetic entryway detection system by Kopp Development Inc. *Right,* FerrAlert® ferromagnetic prescreening detection system by Kopp Development Inc.

(Courtesy Kopp Development, Inc.)

PERSONNEL

Each MRI department should designate an *MR medical director (MRMD)*. This individual (physician) is well versed in MR safety and establishes MR safety policies and procedures for the site. The MRMD makes the final decision regarding scanning patients with implants or devices. This role is typically filled by a radiologist in the clinical setting. The MRMD is responsible for classifying personnel as *non-MR personnel*, *level 1 MR personnel*, and *level 2 MR personnel*. The MRMD determines the training that MR personnel should complete. Non-MR personnel are those who have not undergone formal MR safety training within the previous 12 months.[15] Level 1 MR personnel are individuals who have passed minimal safety training to ensure their own safety within the MRI environment.[15] While these individuals may move freely throughout Zones III and IV, they are not permitted to admit or supervise non-MR personnel in Zones III and IV.[15] Examples of employees that may be classified as level 1 MR personnel are MR receptionists and technologist assistants. Level 2 MR personnel are those who have been extensively trained and educated in the broader aspects of MR safety.[15] Examples of employees who may be classified as level 2 MR personnel are MRI technologists, radiologists, and radiology nurses. In hybrid-MRI environments, there may be additional staff members who complete level 2 training to ensure safety in these unique environments. The *MR safety officer (MRSO)* oversees MR safety practices within a facility.[15] A technologist typically serves in this role. The *MR safety expert (MRSE)* is an individual who serves as a resource to the MRMD and MRSO on MR safety issues. This role is typically filled by a physicist.

LABELING

Equipment and objects within the MRI environment are classified as *MR safe*, *MR conditional*, or *MR unsafe*. MR safe items pose no known hazards in the MRI environment. MR conditional items pose no known hazards in a specified MRI environment. MR unsafe items are those that are known to pose hazards in the MRI environment. A label (sticker) designating the MR safety classification can be placed on equipment and objects (Fig. 26.23). This helps prevent unsafe objects from being taken into Zone IV and serves as a reminder to follow the MR conditions for MR conditional equipment.

Medical devices implanted within patients are also classified as MR safe, MR conditional, or MR unsafe. The imaging team must verify the MR safety classification of medical devices prior to an MRI examination. Patients often have a device identification card that designates this classification. In the absence of a card, the imaging team can review operative records or consult the device manufacturer's implant registry to aid in identifying the device. Once the imaging team has confirmed the type of medical device implanted within the patient, the team can request information regarding the MR safety classification from the manufacturer. This information contains specific guidelines (MR conditions) for scanning a patient with an implanted device. MR conditions describe the limits for the static and time-varying magnetic fields (gradients, radio frequency) for an implanted device.

Some implanted devices such as MR conditional pacemakers and neurostimulators, require the device to be placed into a special mode prior to an MRI examination (MRI mode). Some devices can be placed into MRI mode by the patient, and others require that a representative from the manufacturer activate MRI mode. In these cases, collaboration with device representatives and other health care providers, such as the nursing staff, is necessary to select an optimal date and time for the MRI examination.

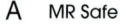

A MR Safe   B MR Conditional   C MR Unsafe

Fig. 26.23 American Society for Testing and Materials (ASTM) International icons for marking medical devices and other items for safety in the magnetic resonance environment. (**A**) MR safe. (**B**) MR conditional. (**C**) MR Unsafe.

(Reprinted with permission from ASTM F2503-23e1 Standard Practice for Marking Medical Devices and Other Items for Safety in the Magnetic Resonance Environment, copyright ASTM International, www.astm.org.)

BIOLOGIC EFFECTS

Opinions differ about the safety of the varying magnetic and RF fields to which the patient is directly exposed. Many studies in which experimental animal and cell culture systems were exposed to these fields over long periods have reported no adverse effects, whereas others have reported changes in cell cultures and embryos. RF energy is deposited in the patient during imaging and is dissipated as heat. The resulting changes seem to be lower than the levels considered clinically significant, even in areas of the body with poor heat dissipation, such as the lens of the eye. The significance of direct short-term exposure (i.e., exposure of a patient) and long-term exposure (i.e., exposure of an employee who works with MRI) is unclear. No clear association of MRI with adverse effects in humans has been proven, but research is continuing.

There are several temporary effects associated with the static and time-varying magnetic fields. Exposure to the static magnetic field can result in changes on electrocardiogram (ECG) tracings while a patient is within the magnet. ECG changes are the result of the movement of blood (conductive fluid) across a magnetic field, which induces a voltage.[16] The induced voltage distorts the ECG signal, which is observed as an elevation of the T-wave on ECG tracings.[17] (Fig. 26.24). This is referred to as the *magnetohydrodynamic effect*.[17] ECG tracings return to normal once the patient exits the magnetic field.

Exposure to the static magnetic field has been associated with vertigo, nausea, and nystagmus (uncontrollable movement of the eyes).[18] These sensations occur more frequently at higher field strengths. Personnel can reduce the occurrence of these effects by avoiding rapid movements within the static magnetic field.

Patients may visualize flashes of light (*magnetophosphenes*) as a result of the retina being stimulated by magnetic field–induced currents.[19]

The exposure to the time-varying magnetic field (gradients) may generate *peripheral nerve stimulation (PNS)*. PNS occurs due to the excitation of nerves from the electrical voltage potentials induced by rapidly changing magnetic gradients.[20] Patients experiencing PNS may feel tingling or tapping sensations during the MRI examination.[20] These sensations may be uncomfortable, but are not harmful to the patient.

HAZARDS

Forces associated with the static magnetic field are *translational force (missile effect), rotational force (torque), and Lenz forces*. Translational force (missile effect) refers to the ability of the fringe field to attract ferromagnetic objects and rapidly draw them into isocenter.[21] Rotational force (torque) refers to the long axis of ferrous objects becoming aligned with the orientation of the main magnetic field (B_0).[21] Lenz forces are characterized by the generation of opposing magnetic fields. Faraday's law indicates that a changing magnetic field will induce a voltage and subsequent current in an electrical conductor.[15] According to Lenz's law, the induced current will generate a magnetic field that opposes the main magnetic field (B_0).[15] Patients implanted with a device that is nonferrous, but electrically conductive, may experience sensations (e.g., tugging, pulling) associated with Lenz forces.[15] These sensations can be reduced by advancing the table to and from isocenter at a slower rate.

Hazards related to the static magnetic field have been well documented. Objects containing ferromagnetic metals (e.g., iron, nickel, cobalt) may be attracted to the magnet with sufficient force to injure patients or personnel who may be interposed between them. Scissors, oxygen tanks, and patient stretchers are among the many items that have been drawn into the magnetic fields at MRI sites. Metallic implants within patients or personnel may become displaced or dislodged and cause injury if they are in delicate locations. Examples include intracranial aneurysm clips, auditory implants, and metallic foreign bodies in the eye. Surgical clips, metal hardware, and artificial joints typically do not pose problems. Electromechanical implants such as non-MR conditional pacemakers or internal cardiac defibrillators can malfunction when they are exposed to strong magnetic fields or RF energy. Patients who have such implants should not be allowed near the magnet.

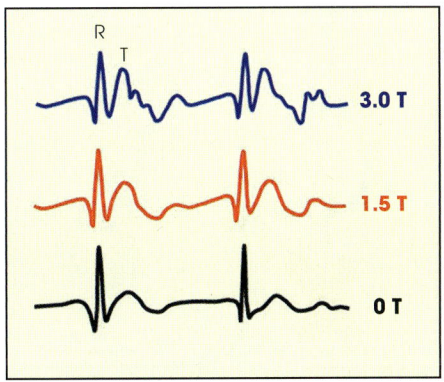

Fig. 26.24 When a patient is placed within the magnetic field, ECG tracings demonstrate an elevation of the T-wave (magnetohydrodynamic effect). The observed changes on ECG tracings increase as field strength increases.

(Courtesy of Allen D. Elster, MRIQuestions.com.)

Fortunately, manufacturers continue to develop MR safe and MR conditional implants, allowing these patients to be scanned safely under specific conditions.

The time-varying magnetic fields (gradients) in an MRI unit act on the machine itself, causing knocking or banging sounds. These noises can be loud enough to produce temporary or permanent hearing damage. Anyone in the magnet room during scanning must use earplugs or some other sound damping device to prevent auditory complications.

The time-varying magnetic fields (radio frequency) can produce thermal complications. Patients can receive burns from wires, such as ECG leads, and other monitoring devices that may touch their skin during MRI examinations. These injuries have included burns caused by currents induced in the wires or by heating of these wires. Such burns can be prevented by using MR safe or MR conditional ECG leads and monitoring devices. Burns can also be prevented by checking wires for frayed insulation, ensuring that no wire loops are within the magnetic field, and placing additional insulation between the patient and any wires exiting the scanner. Additional insulation should also be placed between the patient and the bore wall to prevent proximity burns. Furthermore, padding should be placed between points of skin-to-skin contact to prevent burns (Fig. 26.25). Many types of clothing are now manufactured with invisible metallic microfibers that can cause burns if they are within the volume of transmitted RF. Therefore, patients should remove street clothing and change into apparel provided by the facility.

PREGNANCY

MRI technologists and other health care providers are permitted to work in the MRI environment throughout all stages of pregnancy.[15] Staff may continue their daily duties in Zones III and IV; however, it is recommended that pregnant women not be present in Zone IV during scanning.[15] MRI examinations can be performed on pregnant patients, as MRI exposure has not been shown to have any adverse effects on a developing fetus.[15,22] The decision to proceed with an MRI examination on a pregnant patient is based on the medical benefits weighed against unknown potential risks.[15,22]

QUENCH

In superconductive magnet systems, rapid venting (*quench*) of the supercooled liquid gas (helium) from the magnet into the surrounding room space is a rare, but possible hazard. As the helium fills the magnet room, it replaces the oxygen, which can lead to unconsciousness or asphyxiation. Oxygen monitoring devices in the magnet or cryogen storage room can signal personnel when the oxygen concentration becomes too low. Personnel may then evacuate the area and activate ventilation systems to exchange the escaped gas for fresh air.

Infection Control

Because of the inherent dangers that exist within the MRI suite (e.g., projectiles, torque), developing and maintaining a strict infection-control protocol can be a challenge. Although it may be expected that all technologists will practice standard precautions, some may not realize that the cleanliness of the magnet room is typically their responsibility. In many institutions, housekeeping is not allowed in the magnet room. It is important for technologists to be aware of the infection-control policies of their institution. Research has shown that various pathogens, including methicillin-resistant *Staphylococcus aureus* (MRSA), will grow within the bore of the magnet. Therefore, technologists must be diligent in their practice of infection control.

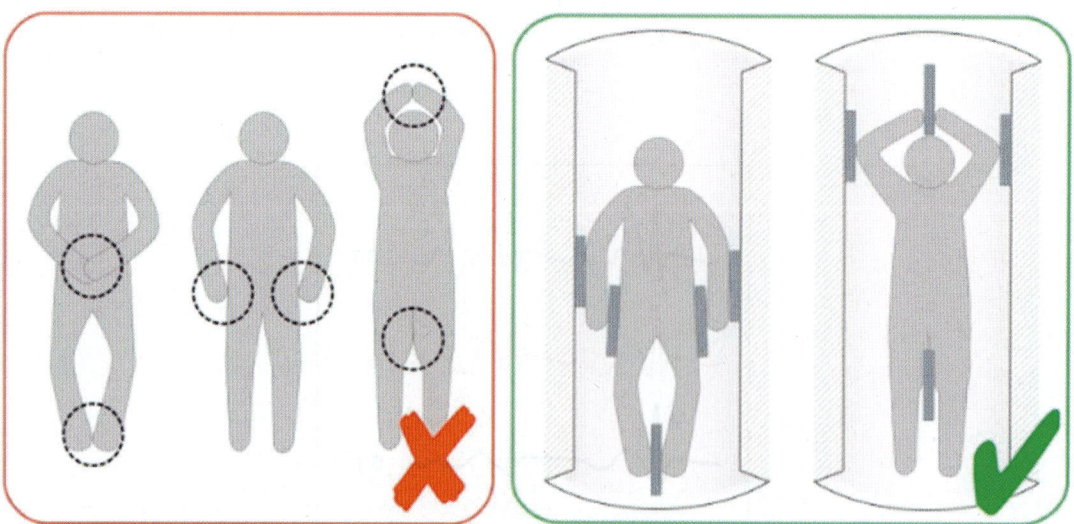

Fig. 26.25 Padding should be placed between points of skin-to-skin contact to prevent burns.

(Courtesy Siemens Healthineers.)

Examination Protocols

IMAGING PARAMETERS

The availability of many adjustable parameters, such as repetition time (TR), echo time (TE), acquisition plane, slice thickness, and imaging matrix make MRI a complex imaging technique. Knowledge of the patient's clinical condition or disease is also important in choosing the proper technique or exam protocol.

The operator may choose to obtain MR images in any orthogonal (i.e., sagittal, coronal, axial) or oblique plane. These are independently and directly acquired images with equal resolution in any plane (Fig. 26.26). 3D imaging is utilized when numerous thin *slices* or multiple imaging planes are desired. In this technique, data are collected simultaneously from a 3D block of tissue rather than from a series of slices. Special data collection techniques and subsequent computer analysis allow the technologist greater flexibility for post-processing (Fig. 26.27).

Slice thickness is an important parameter in the production of MRI signal and the visualization of pathology. More signal is available from a thicker slice than a thinner slice. Therefore, thicker slices may provide images that are less grainy (more signal to noise) but contain lower resolution, potentially hiding small pathologic lesions. Slice thickness is adjusted by the technologist based on the type of lesion under investigation.

Imaging matrix (the size of the pixel or voxel) affects not only MRI signal but also image resolution and scan time. A fine matrix has small pixels and voxels. It allows small lesions to be seen but contains less signal to noise and takes longer to acquire. A coarse matrix has large pixels and voxels. It contains more signal but can potentially hide small lesions. It is a balancing act for the technologist to adjust the matrix based on the part being imaged and the patient's condition.

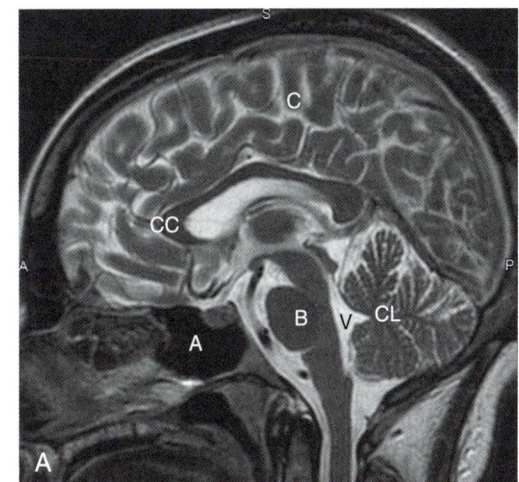
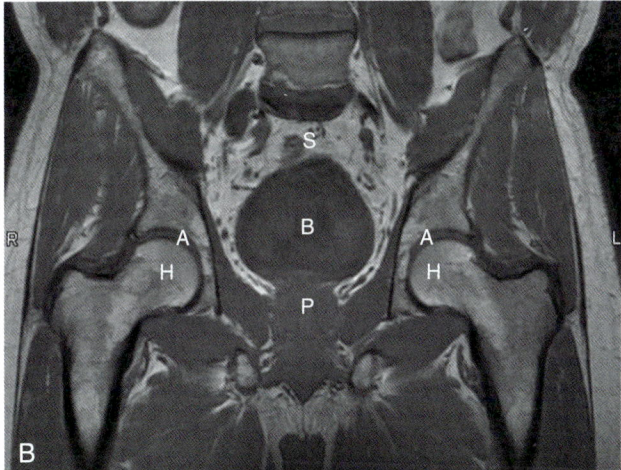

Fig. 26.26 Two images (different patients) from a 3T superconductive MRI scanner, showing excellent resolution of images. (**A**) This image shows remarkable anatomic detail in a midsagittal image of the head. *A*, Air in sinuses; *B*, brain stem; *C*, cerebrum; *CC*, corpus callosum; *CL*, cerebellum; *V*, ventricle. (**B**) This coronal image of the pelvis shows anatomic relationships of the prostate (*P*), which is enlarged and elevating the bladder (*B*). Hips (*H*) and acetabula (*A*) are also shown. A loop of the sigmoid (*S*) colon is on top of the bladder. This degree of resolution in coronal or sagittal images would be difficult to obtain by reformatting a series of transverse CT slices.

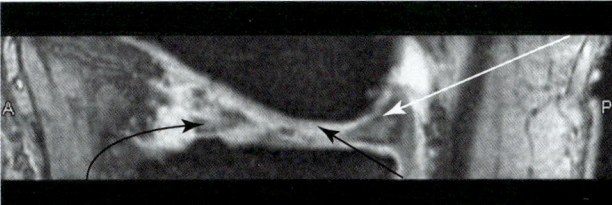

Fig. 26.27 Single slice from 3D acquisition of the knee on a 3T MRI unit. Data from an entire volume within the imaging coil are obtained concurrently. The data may be reconstructed into thin slices in any plane, such as the sagittal image shown here. This imaging sequence shows hyaline cartilage *(black arrow)* as a rim of fairly high signal intensity overlying the bone. Meniscal fibrocartilage *(white arrow)* has low signal intensity. High signal intensity from joint fluid in a tear *(curved arrow)* within the anterior horn of the meniscus is visualized.

ARTIFICIAL INTELLIGENCE

The addition of artificial intelligence to MRI software benefits patients and imaging teams. In MRI, there is a balance between SNR, resolution, and scan time.[23] Each is equally important, but optimizing one results in a tradeoff in the other two.[23] The development of deep learning algorithms has changed the paradigm in MRI. Technologists must no longer choose between SNR, resolution, and scan time.[23] This technology can differentiate between *noise* and true signal, but only uses true signal to reconstruct the image.[23] The application of deep learning algorithms produces images that have a higher SNR and resolution, fewer *artifacts*, and a significantly reduced scan time (Fig. 26.28). Shorter scan times make MRI exams more tolerable for patients. Imaging departments can provide quicker access to imaging, as they are able to scan more patients per day. Radiologists, referring physicians, and patients benefit from the improved image quality provided by this technology.

MRI examinations begin with a three-plane localizer. The resulting images are utilized to manually prescribe slices for subsequent sequences. When artificial intelligence is applied, a three-plane localizer is acquired and the system automatically identifies anatomic landmarks utilized for slice prescription.[24–26] These landmarks are used by the system to automatically prescribe slices for subsequent sequences.[24–26] This technology provides consistent slice prescription between initial and follow-up exams, which assists radiologists in comparing exams over time.[24–26]

PULSE SEQUENCES

A *pulse sequence* is a combination of gradients and RF pulses chosen to favor a particular tissue (contrast) as quickly as possible (speed) while minimizing artifacts and maximizing the SNR. Depending on the choice of pulse sequence and imaging parameters, the resulting images may be more strongly weighted toward proton density, T1, or T2 information. Depending on the relative emphasis given to these factors, normal anatomy (Fig. 26.29) or a pathologic lesion (Fig. 26.30) may be more easily recognized. It is not unusual for a lesion to stand out dramatically when one pulse sequence is used yet be nearly isointense (same signal intensity as surrounding normal tissue) with a different pulse sequence.

Pulse sequences are classed depending on the timing of the gradient and RF pulses. Although the discussion of pulse sequences is beyond the scope of this chapter, they can be divided into two major categories. *Spin echo* sequences yield true T1, T2, or proton density–weighted images and are the standard pulse sequences used for all routine imaging. Classic spin echo sequences tend to have long scan times, so researchers have developed fast or turbo spin echo, which can dramatically shorten the scan time. Another type of spin echo pulse sequence is inversion recovery. *Inversion recovery* is a sequence that can minimize or null the signal intensity of a particular tissue. The most common are short tau inversion recovery (STIR), which nulls fat signal, and FLAIR, which nulls signal from cerebrospinal fluid (CSF) in brain imaging. *Gradient echo* sequences are used where the scan time must be short, as in breath-hold abdominal scans. They generate T1 and T2 star (T2*)-weighted images. They are also used for imaging flowing blood (see the discussion of MRA later in this chapter) or pooling blood from hemorrhage or trauma (susceptibility-weighting). Researchers continue to develop new pulse sequences for specific applications.

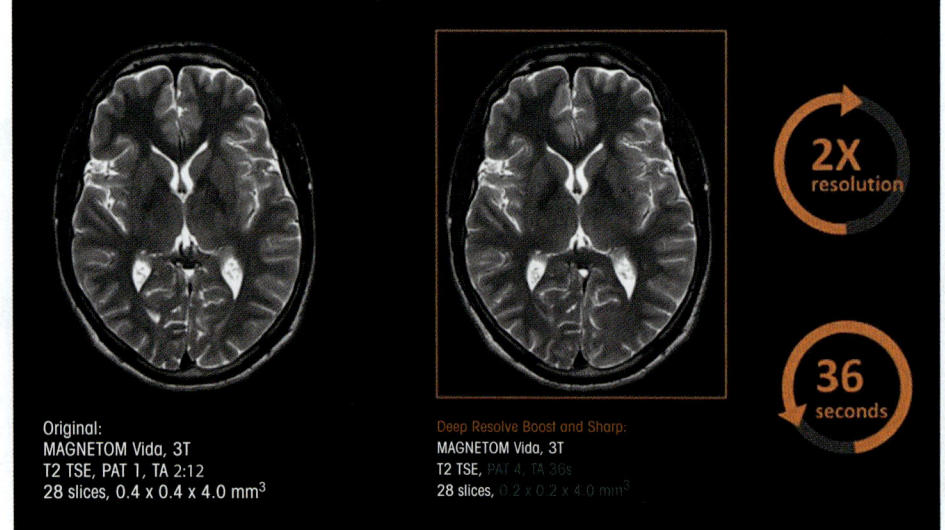

Fig. 26.28 Two axial T2-weighted images of the brain compare conventional image reconstruction (*left*) to image reconstruction using artificial intelligence (*right*). The use of artificial intelligence produces images with a high SNR and resolution, fewer artifacts, and a short scan time.

(Courtesy Siemens Healthineers.)

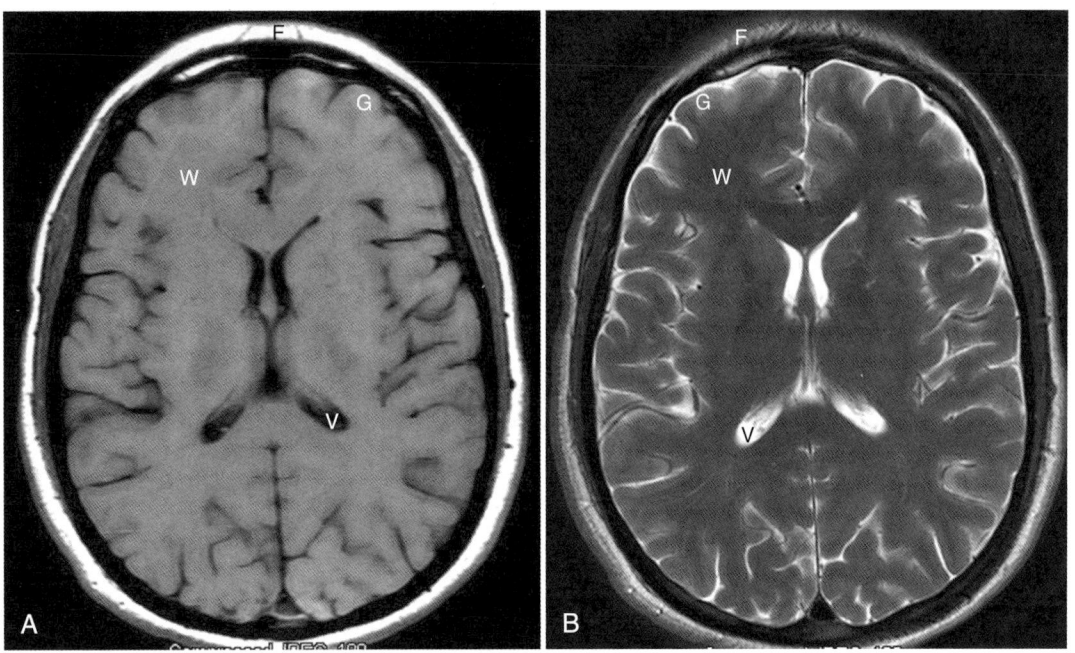

Fig. 26.29 Axial 3T images through a normal brain. (**A**) T1-weighted image shows relatively low differentiation of gray matter *(G)* and white matter *(W)* within the brain. (**B**) Heavily T2-weighted image shows improved differentiation between gray and white matter. Cerebrospinal fluid within the ventricles *(V)* also changes in appearance with a change in pulse sequence (low signal on T1-weighted image); fat *(F)* normally shows high signal intensity, whereas on the T2-weighted image, the signal intensity of fat is less than that of cerebrospinal fluid.

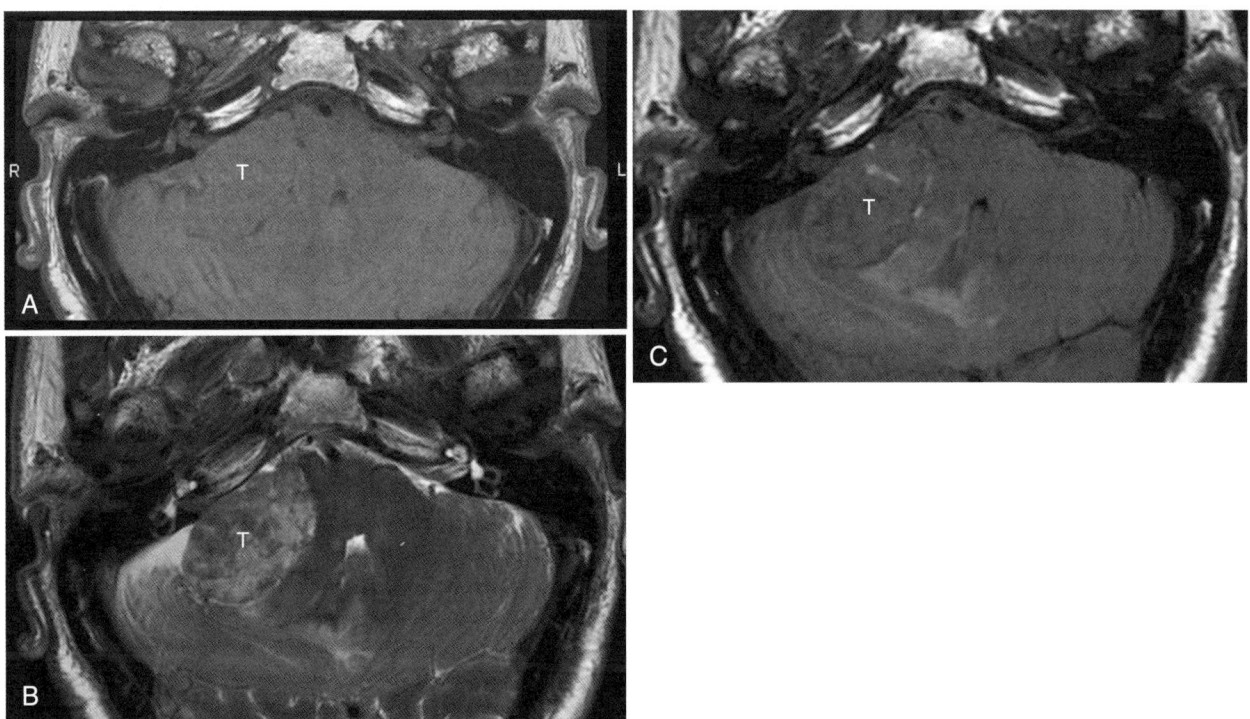

Fig. 26.30 Axial magnetic resonance imaging showing the use of different pulse sequences and their effect on the visualization of the cerebellopontine angle tumor. (**A**) T1-weighted image shows that limited contrast exists between the tumor *(T)* and normal brain. (**B**) The lesion becomes dramatically more obvious using the pulse sequence of the T2-weighted image. (**C**) The lesion is still visible on a FLAIR pulse sequence, but not as well as in the T2-weighted image. Choice of pulse sequence is critical. These images also show how the lack of bone artifact makes MRI superior to CT for imaging of posterior fossa lesions.

POSITIONING

Patient positioning for MRI is usually straightforward. Generally, the patient lies supine on a table that is subsequently advanced into the magnet. As previously discussed, it is important to ensure that the patient has no contraindications to MRI, such as an unsafe cardiac pacemaker or intracranial aneurysm clips. Claustrophobia may be a problem for some patients, as previously noted, because the imaging area is tunnel-shaped in most MRI system configurations (see Fig. 26.8).

COILS

Receiving *coils* are used for transmitting the RF pulse and/or receiving the MRI signal (as described earlier in the section on signal production). Some coils can both transmit and receive (transmit/receive coils), whereas others may only receive the signal (receive-only coils).

The body part to be examined determines the placement and shape of the surface or receiving coil that is used for imaging (Fig. 26.31). Most coils are round or oval, and the body part to be examined is inserted into the coil's open center. Some coils, rather than encircling the body part, are placed directly on the patient over the area of interest. Another form of receiving coil is the endocavity coil, which is designed to fit within a body cavity such as the rectum. This enables a receiving coil to be placed closer to an internal organ that may be distant from surface coils applied to the exterior body, as when imaging the prostate or uterus. Endocavity coils may also be used to image the wall of the cavity itself (Fig. 26.32).

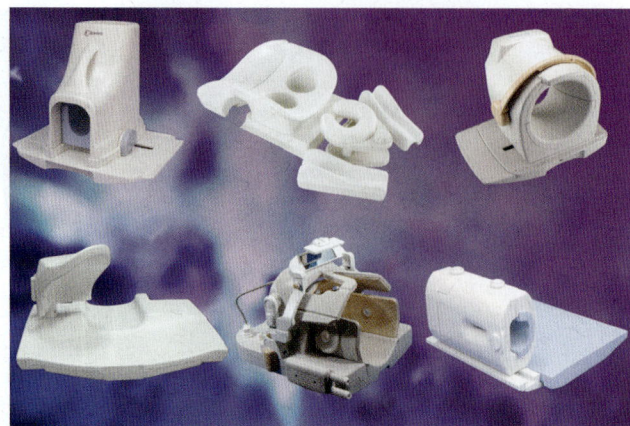

Fig. 26.31 Examples of coils used for magnetic resonance imaging. *Upper row, left to right,* Foot/ankle coil, breast coil, and knee coil. *Lower row, left to right,* Shoulder coil, functional head coil, and wrist coil.

(Courtesy Invivo Corporation.)

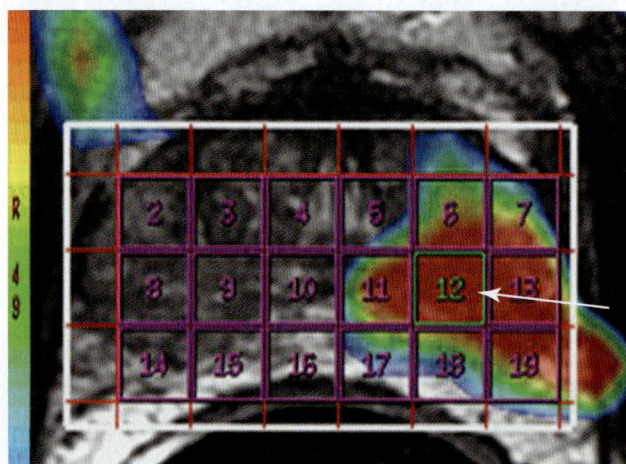

Fig. 26.32 Axial image of prostate obtained with an endorectal coil. The increased resolution allowed by the endorectal coil makes it possible to perform magnetic resonance spectroscopy *(PROSE)*. The spectroscopy map shows an elevated citrate level *(arrow),* consistent with tumor.

(Courtesy GE Healthcare.)

PATIENT MONITORING

Although most MRI sites are constructed so that the operator can see the patient during imaging, visibility is often limited, leaving the patient relatively isolated within the scan room (see Fig. 26.8). At most sites, intercoms are used for verbal communication with the patient, and all units have "call buttons" with which the patient may summon assistance. These devices may be insufficient, however, to monitor the health status of a sedated, anesthetized, or unresponsive patient. MR safe and MR conditional devices are available to monitor multiple physiologic parameters such as heart rate, respiratory rate, blood pressure, and oxygen concentration in the blood. The technologist should also monitor the patient visually and verbally during the exam.

CONTRAST MEDIA

Contrast agents widen the signal differences (contrast to noise) in MR images between various normal and abnormal structures. Gadolinium is a rare-earth metal with *paramagnetic* qualities and is commonly used as a contrast agent in MRI. In its pure or unchelated form, gadolinium is a toxic substance. Gadolinium is combined with a chelate to reduce its toxicity, thereby rendering it safe for routine clinical use. Pharmacologically, the intravenous (IV) administration of a gadolinium-based contrast agent acts similarly to an iodinated IV agent. It is distributed through the vascular system, and its major route of excretion is the urine. Gadolinium-based contrast agents (GBCAs) respect the blood-brain barrier (i.e., they do not leak out from the blood vessels into the brain substance unless the barrier has been damaged by a pathologic process).

GBCAs can be used in the evaluation of any body part, including the central nervous system and the musculoskeletal system. The most important clinical action of GBCAs is the shortening of the T1 relaxation time. In T1-weighted images, this provides a high-signal, high-contrast focus in areas where gadolinium has accumulated. As seen in Fig. 26.33, gadolinium-based contrast has leaked through the broken blood-brain barrier into the brain substance. In contrast-enhanced T1-weighted images, brain tumors or metastases are better distinguished from their surrounding edema than in routine T2-weighted images. GBCAs improve the visualization of small tumors or tumors with a signal intensity similar to that of a normal brain, such as meningiomas. Rapid IV injections of GBCAs are routinely used in dynamic imaging studies of body organs such as the liver and kidneys, similar to techniques using iodinated agents in CT. Contrast-enhanced MRA is routinely performed to image the blood vessels of the neck (carotid) and body.

In general, GBCAs are nonspecific; however, organ-specific agents have been developed, primarily for imaging the liver. Continued research facilitates the development of novel contrast agents to improve the specificity of MR imaging.

GBCAs are well tolerated, typically have fewer side effects than iodine-based contrast agents, and are not nephrotoxic. Nevertheless, patients with severe kidney disease and reduced renal function are susceptible to developing a life-threatening condition known as nephrogenic systemic fibrosis (NSF).

Gadolinium has been discovered in the brain and body tissues of patients who have received repeated doses of GBCAs. Retained gadolinium has been identified in patients with normal and abnormal renal function. The significance of gadolinium retention is still being studied. GBCAs should be used only when clinically necessary.

GBCAs are not typically administered to pregnant patients, as they cross the placenta.[22,27] However, GBCAs can be administered when there is the potential for a significant clinical benefit.[22,27] GBCAs can be administered to patients who are breastfeeding despite excretion into breast milk. Studies indicate that it is safe to continue breastfeeding following contrast-enhanced MRI examinations, as infants absorb only a small percentage of the ingested gadolinium.[27] However, breast milk can be expressed and discarded for a period of 12 to 24 hours after receiving the GBCA if mothers have concerns about infant safety.[27]

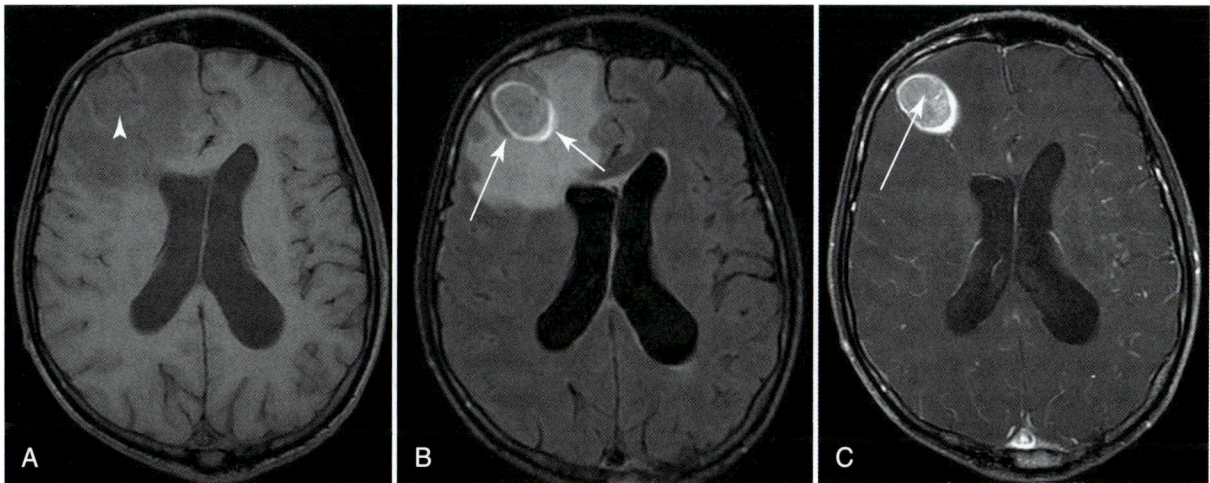

Fig. 26.33 Use of IV gadolinium-based contrast for lesion enhancement in axial images of the brain. **(A)** T1-weighted sequence. A single brain lesion *(arrowhead)* is seen as a focal area of low signal intensity in a large area of edema. The borders of the lesion are difficult to delineate. **(B)** FLAIR image. Areas of high signal *(arrows)* represent tumor and surrounding edema. **(C)** T1-weighted image obtained using similar parameters after IV administration of gadolinium-based contrast. Lesion borders and size *(arrow)* are much more conspicuous.

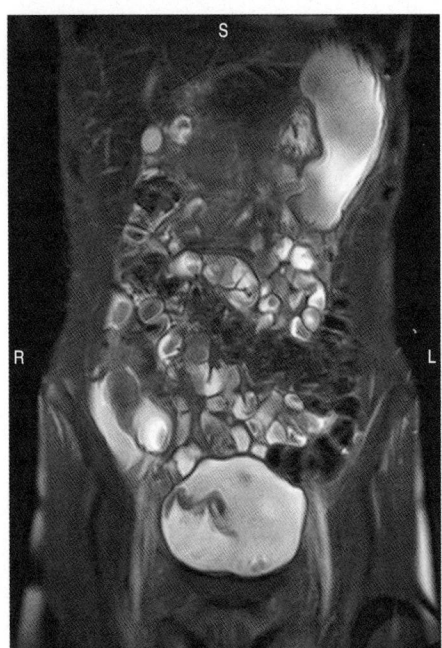

Fig. 26.34 Magnetic resonance enterography. An oral contrast agent provides distention of the small bowel, which promotes the evaluation of inflammatory bowel disease.

Oral contrast agents can be used in conjunction with GBCAs. Oral contrast agents are typically utilized for imaging of the small bowel. An oral contrast agent provides distention of the small bowel, which promotes the evaluation of inflammatory bowel disease (Fig. 26.34).

GATING

In imaging of the chest and abdomen, heart and breathing motion can degrade image quality. Even fast pulse sequences have difficulty freezing this type of motion. Respiratory and/or cardiac *gating* or triggering can be utilized to improve image quality. Cardiac gating and respiratory gating obtain data throughout the entire cardiac or respiratory cycle. With either cycle, the system records the points at which the data are acquired and then reconstructs that data motion-free. Cardiac or respiratory triggering uses a specific point in the cardiac or respiratory cycle to trigger the acquisition of data. Each method has its advantages and disadvantages, but the result of both methods is motion-free images (Fig. 26.35).

OTHER CONSIDERATIONS

When MRI was first introduced, long imaging times were required to produce diagnostic images. With advances in computer technology and pulse sequence developments, images can now be acquired more quickly, reducing the time the patient is in the scanner. These fast sequences can accentuate the bright signal of fluid, allowing for myelographic effects in spine imaging or arthrographic effects in joint imaging. New pulse sequences have been developed for specialized applications, such as the ability to perform dynamic scans and free-breathing abdominal imaging.

Quality assurance is important in complex technology such as MRI. Calibration of the unit is generally performed by service personnel. Routine scanning of phantoms by the technologist can be useful for detecting any problems that may develop.

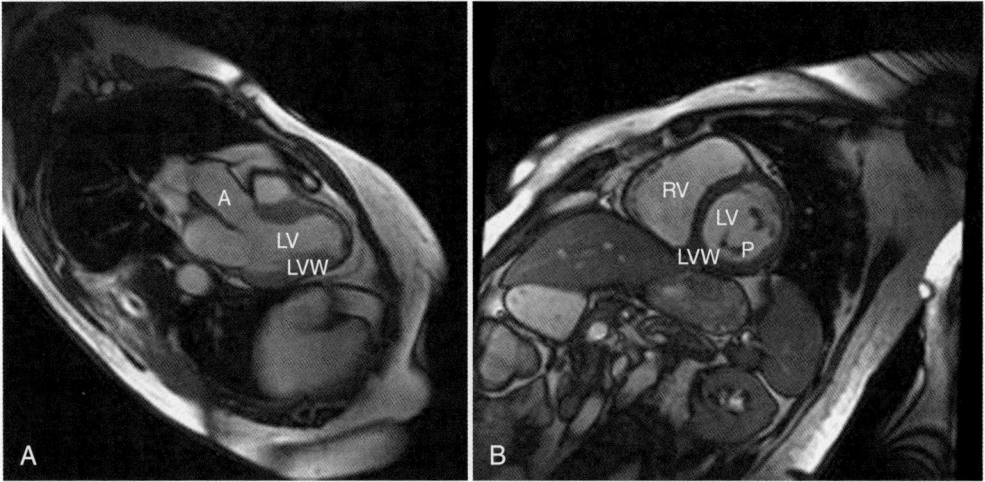

Fig. 26.35 Electrocardiogram-gated images of the heart. **(A)** Left ventricular outflow tract. **(B)** Short-axis images. *A*, Aorta; *LV*, left ventricle; *LVW*, left ventricular wall; *P*, papillary muscles; *RV*, right ventricle.

Clinical Applications
CENTRAL NERVOUS SYSTEM

MRI is the modality of choice for imaging of the central nervous system. It is routinely used in almost all examinations of the brain, except for acute trauma. MRI is superior in the brain because of its inherent ability to differentiate the natural contrast among tissues such as gray and white matter (see Fig. 26.29). This ability allows MRI to be more sensitive than CT in detecting changes in white matter disease, such as multiple sclerosis. The development of specialized pulse sequences, such as FLAIR, helps visualize lesions in the periventricular area that were previously difficult to detect. MRI is also superior at imaging the posterior fossa (cerebellum and brain stem) because cortical bone does not produce any signal in MRI. This area is often obscured on CT because of beam-hardening *artifact*. Almost all brain lesions—such as primary and metastatic tumors, pituitary tumors, acoustic neuromas (tumors of the eighth cranial nerve), and meningiomas—are better seen on MRI. The use of IV gadolinium-based contrast has allowed better differentiation and increased sensitivity in detecting these lesions (Fig. 26.36). Cerebral infarction is identified sooner using DWI compared with CT. DWI also gives MRI the ability to determine the age of lesions or differentiate acute from chronic ischemic changes.

MRI is also routinely used to image the spinal canal and its contents. The ability of MRI to image directly in the sagittal plane allows for the screening of a large area in a single examination. T2-weighted pulse sequences permit the separation of CSF and the spinal cord, as in myelography, without the use of a contrast agent (Fig. 26.37). Because of its inherent ability to differentiate slight changes in soft tissue contrast, MRI is exquisitely sensitive to cystic changes associated with tumors within the spinal cord. The visualization of bone marrow is useful in the detection and diagnosis of metastatic disease, pathologic and nonpathologic vertebral fractures, and discitis (infection). MRI is also commonly used in the imaging of disc disease. The posterior longitudinal ligament can be visualized in the sagittal plane. The sagittal and axial planes can show the severity of disc herniation (Fig. 26.38). The use of IV gadolinium-based contrast aids in differentiating between recurrent disc herniation and postoperative scar tissue, a crucial clinical distinction.

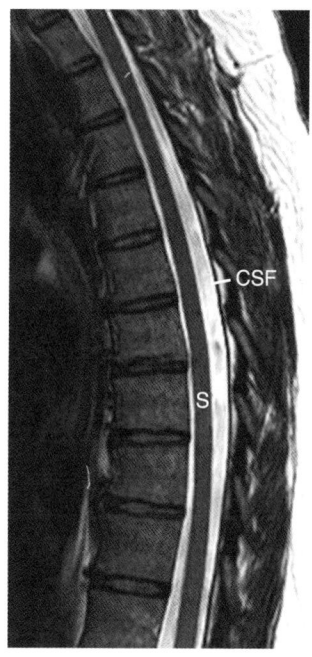

Fig. 26.37 Sagittal T2-weighted magnetic resonance imaging through the thoracic spine. High signal from cerebrospinal fluid *(CSF)* outlines the normal spinal cord *(S)*, giving a myelogram-like effect without the use of contrast agents.

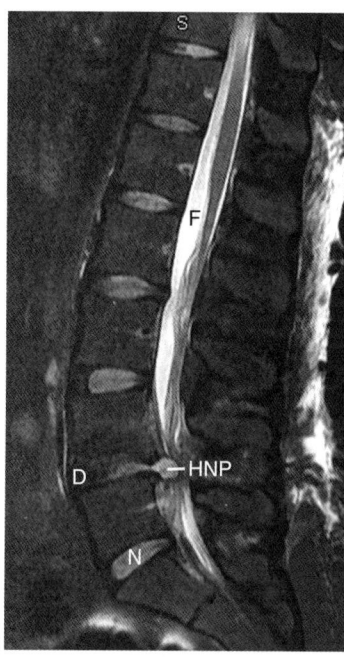

Fig. 26.38 Sagittal T2-weighted fat-suppressed image of the lumbar spine. The spinal canal is filled with high-signal-intensity cerebrospinal fluid *(F)*, except for low-signal-intensity linear nerve roots running within the spinal canal. Normal vertebral discs have a high-signal-intensity nucleus pulposus *(N)*. Desiccated discs *(D)* show low signal intensity. At L4-5, note the herniated nucleus pulposus *(HNP)* protruding into the spinal canal and compressing the nerve roots.

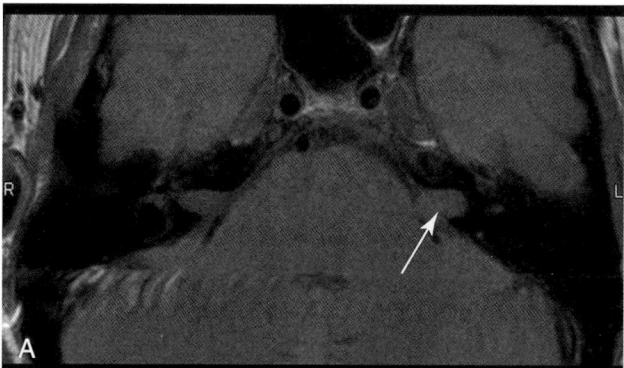 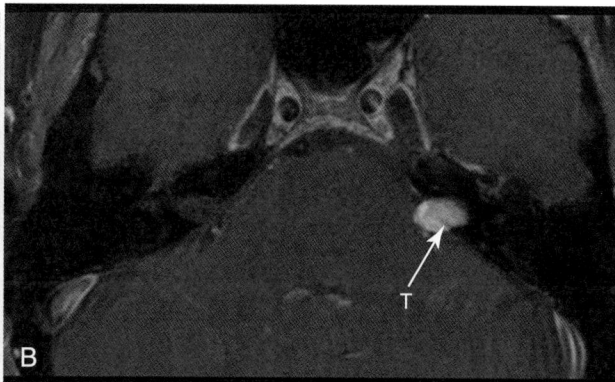

Fig. 26.36 Axial magnetic resonance imaging of the brain in a patient with an acoustic nerve tumor arising from the complex of the seventh and eighth cranial nerves. **(A)** Precontrast T1-weighted image shows an inhomogeneous area of abnormality *(arrows)*, with mass effect expanding the area of the nerve complex. **(B)** Image obtained at the same level after contrast enhancement. Active tumor *(T)* shows high signal intensity.

CHEST

Ultrafast pulse sequences and software algorithms have made it possible to obtain motion-free images of the chest and heart. Cardiac gating (imaging only during a certain part of the cardiac cycle), respiratory gating or triggering, breath-hold scans, and ultrafast imaging sequences have enabled MRI to excel at cardiac imaging. MRI can show anatomy and produce functional data (e.g., ejection fractions, chamber volume) similar to nuclear medicine and echocardiography. Studies of congenital heart disease, imaging of masses, and heart muscle viability are now routine (Fig. 26.39). MRI may also be used to image the chest wall, thoracic outlet, and brachial plexus region.

Breast MRI, once used only sparingly, has become an essential part of breast imaging. It is routinely used to screen high-risk patients preoperatively, to define the extent of disease, and to screen the contralateral breast for additional disease (Fig. 26.40). Patients also undergo breast MRI to monitor the response to adjuvant therapies, such as chemotherapy or radiation. In addition, breast MRI is the method of choice for imaging ruptured breast implants.

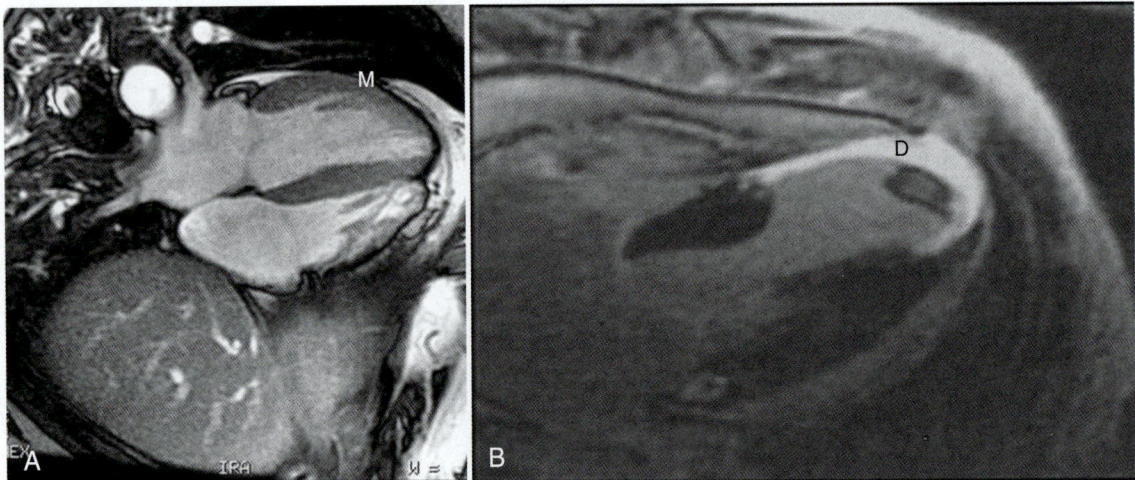

Fig. 26.39 Cardiac MRI: four-chamber view from two different patients. **(A)** Steady-state free precession (SSFP) image showing normal myocardium in the wall of the left ventricle *(M)* before the administration of contrast. **(B)** Delayed-enhancement image (inversion recovery) showing bright signal in the wall of the left ventricle, representing infarcted or dead myocardium *(D)*.

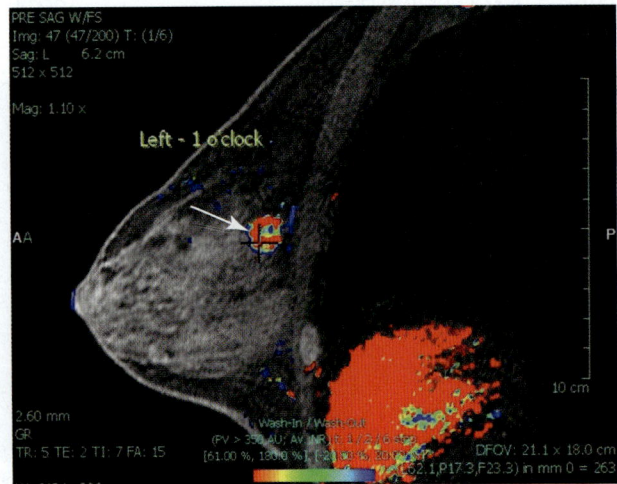

Fig. 26.40 MRI of the breast is post-processed and showing contrast wash-in and wash-out. The patient is a 68-year-old woman with an enhancing mass in the left breast at the 1 o'clock position *(arrow)*.

ABDOMEN

Abdominal imaging is also affected by respiratory motion. The use of ultrafast scanning techniques and the ability to acquire 2D and 3D volumes in a breath-hold scan have made MRI extremely useful in the evaluation of abdominal pathology. Free breathing and motion correction pulse sequences permit imaging of patients with a limited breath-hold capacity. MRI is not typically used as a primary diagnostic tool; however, it can further evaluate questionable results from other modalities such as CT and ultrasound. One exception is liver imaging, in which MRI may be more sensitive in detecting primary and metastatic tumors. The use of liver-specific IV contrast agents improves the detection and characterization of liver lesions. MRI can predict the histologic diagnosis of certain abnormalities such as hepatic hemangiomas, which have a distinctive appearance (Fig. 26.41). Moreover, the use of in-phase and out-of-phase images can distinguish between benign and malignant adrenal tumors. The use of heavily T2-weighted images can identify abnormalities within the gallbladder, biliary duct, and the pancreatic duct (Fig. 26.42).

Quantitative imaging techniques complement the standard MR imaging exam. These techniques gauge the severity of disease, guide the development of treatment plans, and monitor the response to treatment.

Magnetic resonance elastography combines MR imaging with low-frequency vibrations to create a visual map (elastogram) that shows the stiffness of body tissues.[28] Currently, MR elastography is used to detect stiffening of the liver caused by fibrosis and inflammation in chronic liver disease[28] (Fig. 26.43).

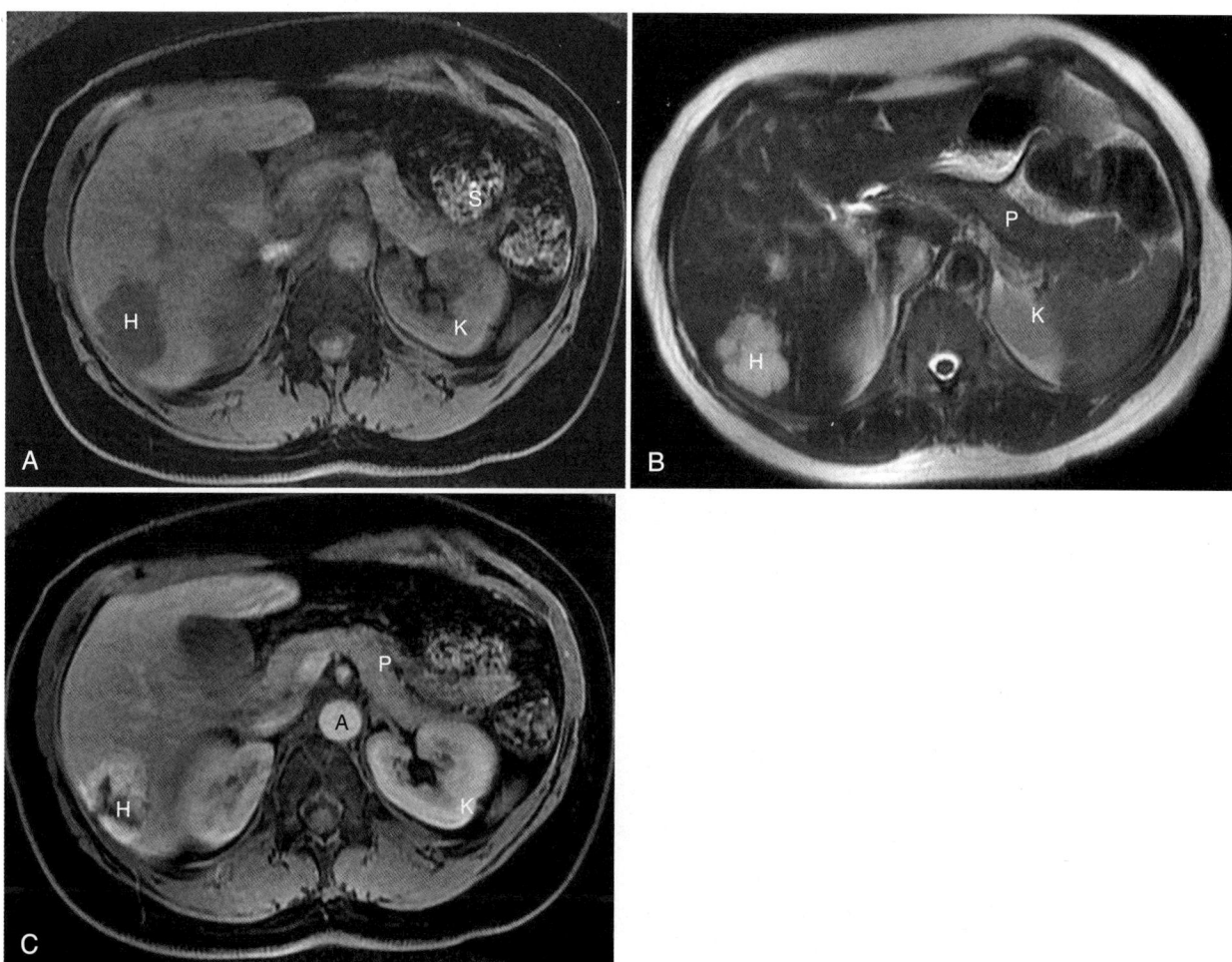

Fig. 26.41 Multiple images through the liver of a patient with hemangioma (H). (**A**) Axial T1-weighted fat-suppressed image before contrast administration. (**B**) Axial T2-weighted image. (**C**) Axial T1-weighted fat-suppressed image postcontrast. This image shows the classic fill-in of contrast material from the periphery of the lesion toward the center. MRI also shows the other abdominal organs and their relationship quite well: kidneys (K), pancreas (P), stomach (S), and aorta (A).

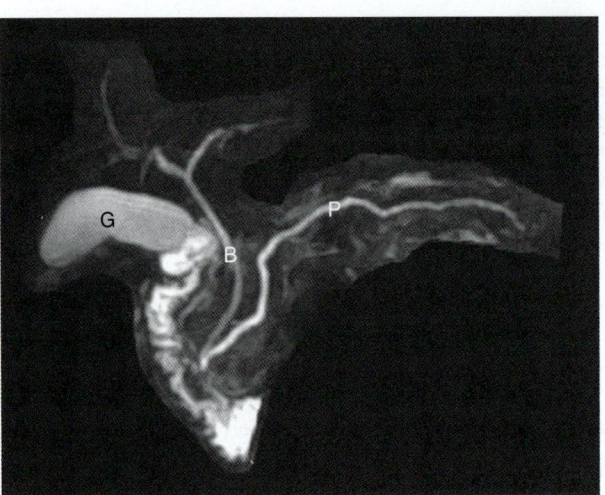

Fig. 26.42 Magnetic resonance cholangiopancreatography (MRCP). Heavily T2-weighted images specially designed to image the gallbladder (G) and the biliary (B) and pancreatic ducts (P).

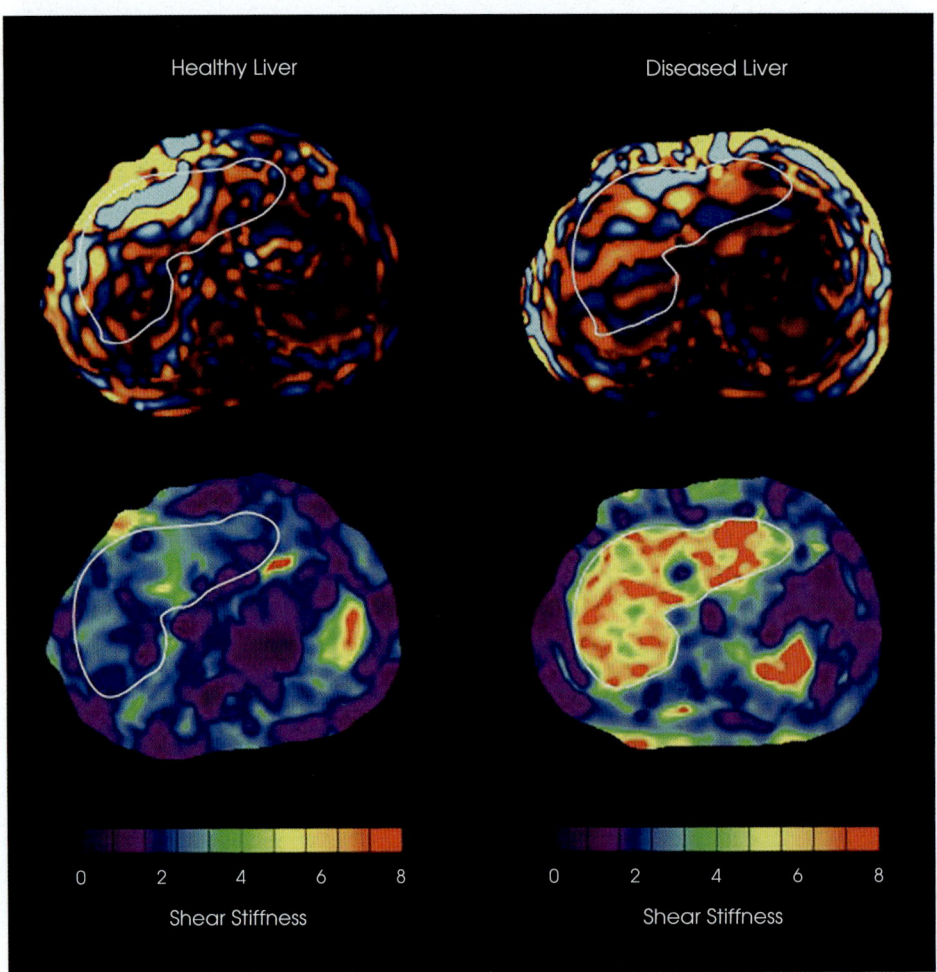

Fig. 26.43 Magnetic resonance elastography. Elastograms comparing a healthy liver and a diseased liver.

(Courtesy GE Healthcare.)

Sequences that measure the amount of fat and iron present in the liver have been introduced (Fig. 26.44). The prevalence of hepatic steatosis or fatty liver disease has increased.[29] The liver is one of the main iron storage organs and the first to show iron overload.[30] Determining the presence and severity of hepatic steatosis and iron overload is essential to prevent complications.

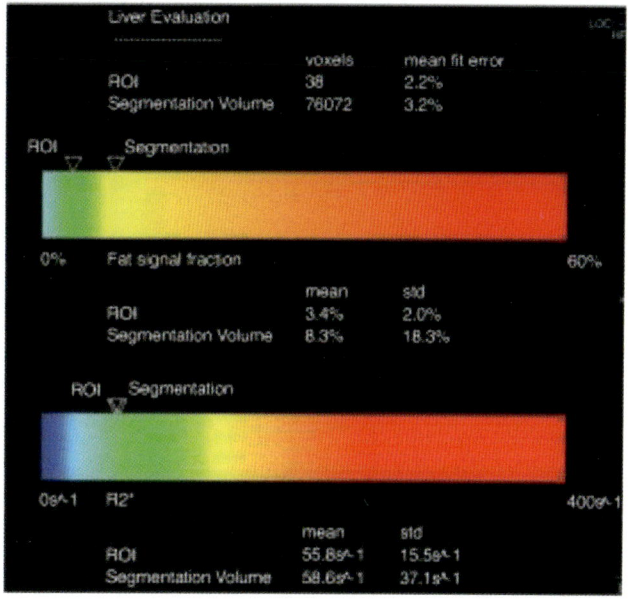

Fig. 26.44 Proton density fat fraction (PDFF) and R2 star (R2*) values show the hepatic fat signal fraction of 3.4%, suggestive of normal parenchyma (<5% is normal). Also, note normal R2* values are suggestive of an absence of hepatic parenchymal iron deposition.

(From Sutton D, Aggarwal B: *Textbook of radiology and imaging*, ed 8, St Louis: Elsevier, 2022.)

PELVIS

Respiratory motion has little effect on the structures of the pelvis. Therefore, these structures can be better visualized than structures in the upper abdomen. The ability of MRI to image in the coronal and sagittal planes is helpful in examining the curved surfaces in the pelvis. Bladder tumors are shown well, including tumors at the dome and base of the bladder, which can be difficult to evaluate in the transverse dimension. In the prostate (see Fig. 26.32), MRI is useful in detecting a neoplasm and its spread. In the female pelvis, MRI can be used to image benign and malignant conditions (Fig. 26.45). In addition, MRI can be used during pregnancy to evaluate fetal and placental abnormalities.

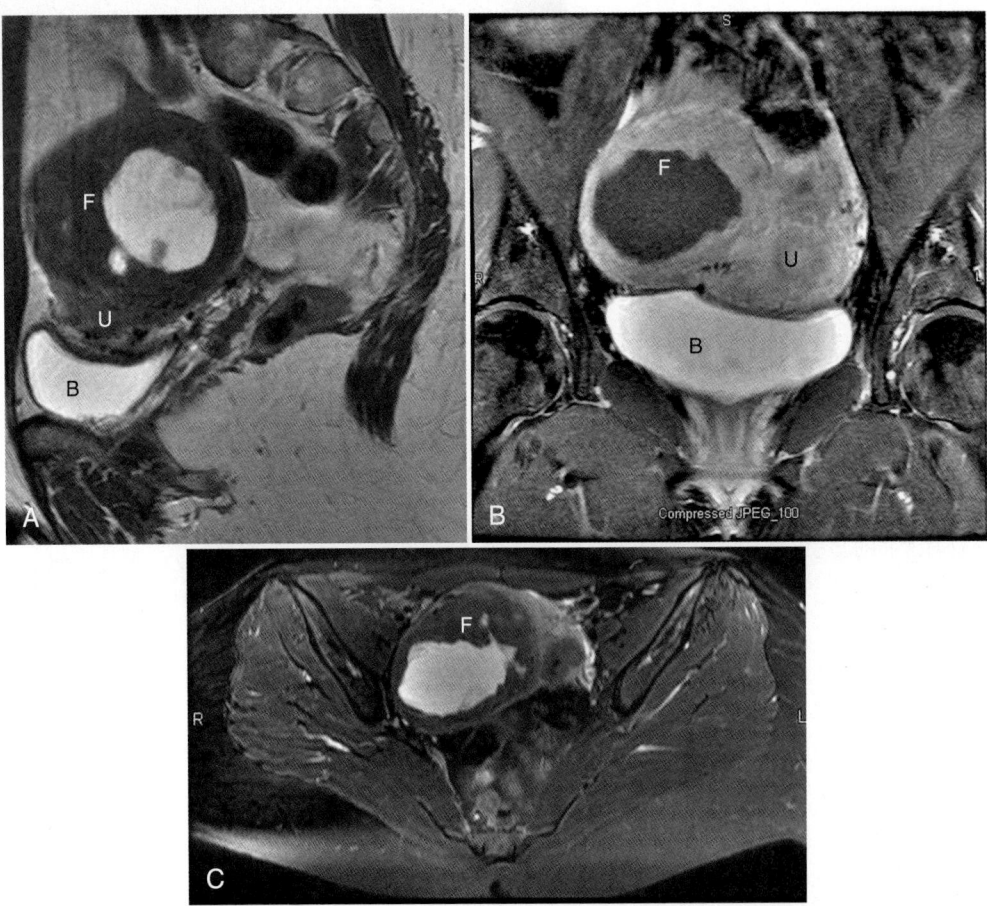

Fig. 26.45 Multiple images through a female pelvis. (**A**) Sagittal T2-weighted image. (**B**) Coronal T1-weighted fat-suppressed image after the administration of contrast. (**C**) Axial T2-weighted fat-suppressed image. All images show the different components of a uterine fibroid *(F)*. The relationship between the uterus *(U)* and bladder *(B)* is shown well using multiple imaging planes.

MUSCULOSKELETAL SYSTEM

The ability to image in multiple planes with excellent soft tissue contrast, as well as the ability to image bone marrow, has rapidly expanded the role of MRI in musculoskeletal imaging. The lack of bone artifact in MRI permits excellent visualization of the bone marrow (Fig. 26.46) and facilitates more effective diagnosis of pathologic conditions such as stress fractures and avascular necrosis (Fig. 26.47). Local staging of soft tissue and bone tumors is best accomplished with MRI (Fig. 26.48).

MRI has become the imaging modality of choice for small and large joints. It has replaced radiographic arthrography in all joints. MR arthrography is now routinely performed. The ability to assess damage to ligaments, tendons, and menisci, as well as to quantify the loss of cartilage, is very helpful in treating osteoarthritis of the knee and other joints (see Fig. 26.27). Quantitative imaging also monitors the degree of tissue healing following orthopedic surgical procedures[31] (Fig. 26.49)

Follow-up MR imaging can be limited by magnetic susceptibility artifact after surgery during which orthopedic hardware is implanted. Pulse sequences that significantly reduce the severity of the artifact have been developed (Fig. 26.50). Thus, technologists can acquire images of higher quality when orthopedic hardware is present.

A pulse sequence with a zero TE has been introduced.[32] This sequence evaluates tissues that have extremely short T2 relaxation times.[32] In conventional pulse sequences, the signal for these tissues has decayed before the time of signal detection.[32] The zero TE images have a CT-like appearance and provide 3D rendering capabilities (Fig. 26.51). This sequence can evaluate bone morphology, calcifications, ossification, and fractures.[32]

Similarly, a pulse sequence with an ultrashort TE has been introduced.[33] This sequence is gradient echo based and evaluates tissues with extremely short T2* relaxation times. In conventional gradient echo sequences, the signal for these tissues has decayed before the time of signal detection. This sequence also produces images with a CT-like appearance.[33]

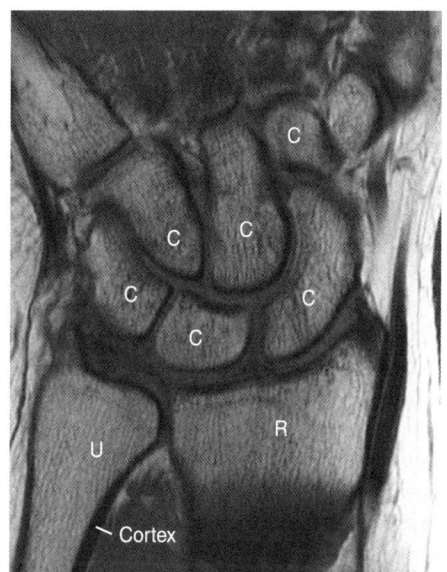

Fig. 26.46 Coronal T1-weighted image of the wrist acquired using a surface coil to improve the visualization of superficial structures. Marrow within the carpal bones *(C)*, radius *(R)*, and ulna *(U)* has high signal as a result of its fat content. A thin black line of low-signal cortex surrounds the marrow cavity of each bone, and trabecular bone can be seen as low-signal detail interspersed within marrow.

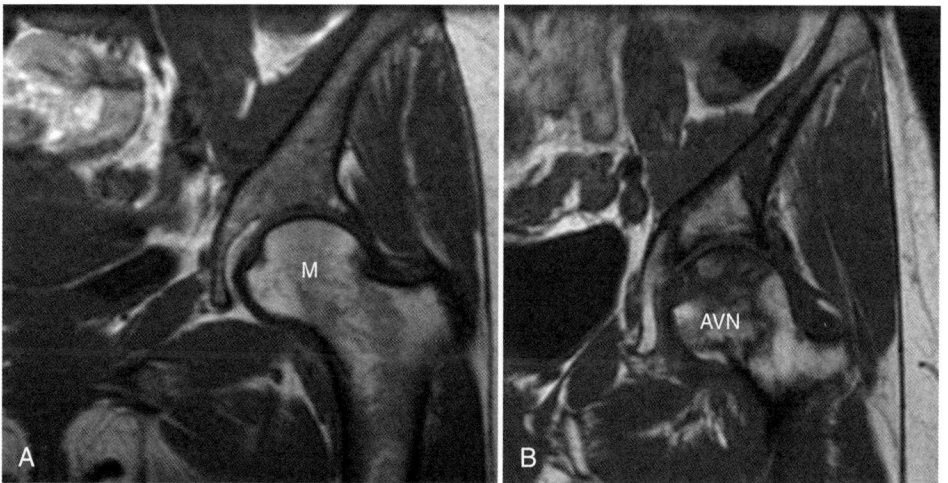

Fig. 26.47 Two coronal T1-weighted images of the left hip from different patients. **(A)** Normal bone marrow signal *(M)*. **(B)** Abnormal bone marrow signal consistent with avascular necrosis *(AVN)*.

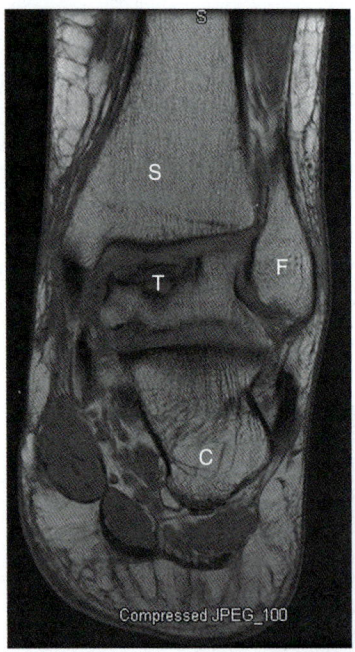

Fig. 26.48 Coronal T1-weighted image of the ankle. Bone marrow shows high signal intensity because of fat. Osteochondral defect seen in the dome of the talus (*T*) shows low signal intensity. *C,* Calcaneus; *F,* fibula; *S,* tibia.

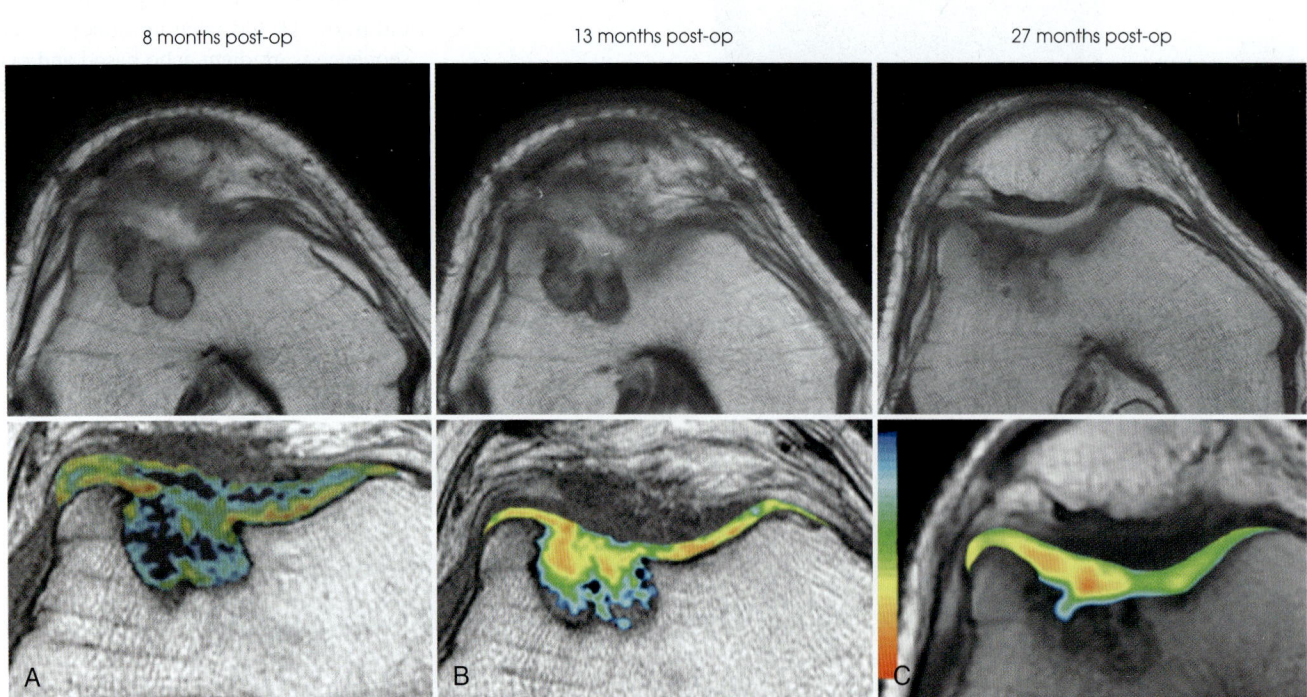

Fig. 26.49 Axial T2 mapping sequence of the knee. Late teen with biphasic scaffold plugs into the trochlea. The T2 maps demonstrate progressive organization of repaired tissue. (**A**) 8 months post-op. (**B**) 13 months post-op. (**C**) 27 months post-op.

(Courtesy GE Healthcare.)

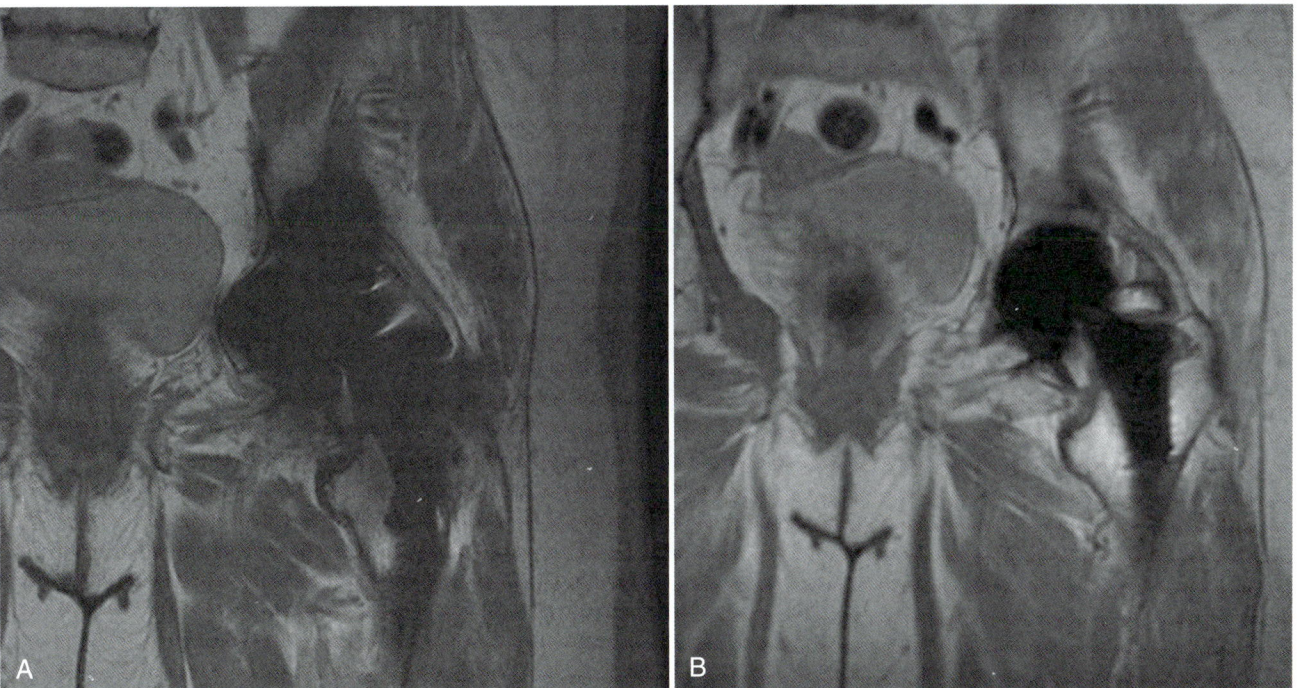

Fig. 26.50 Orthopedic hardware can degrade image quality. (**A**) Fast spin echo coronal T1-weighted image demonstrating magnetic susceptibility artifact from a hip prosthesis. (**B**) Coronal T1-weighted metal suppression image demonstrating the reduction in the magnetic susceptibility artifact from a hip prosthesis.

(Courtesy GE Healthcare.)

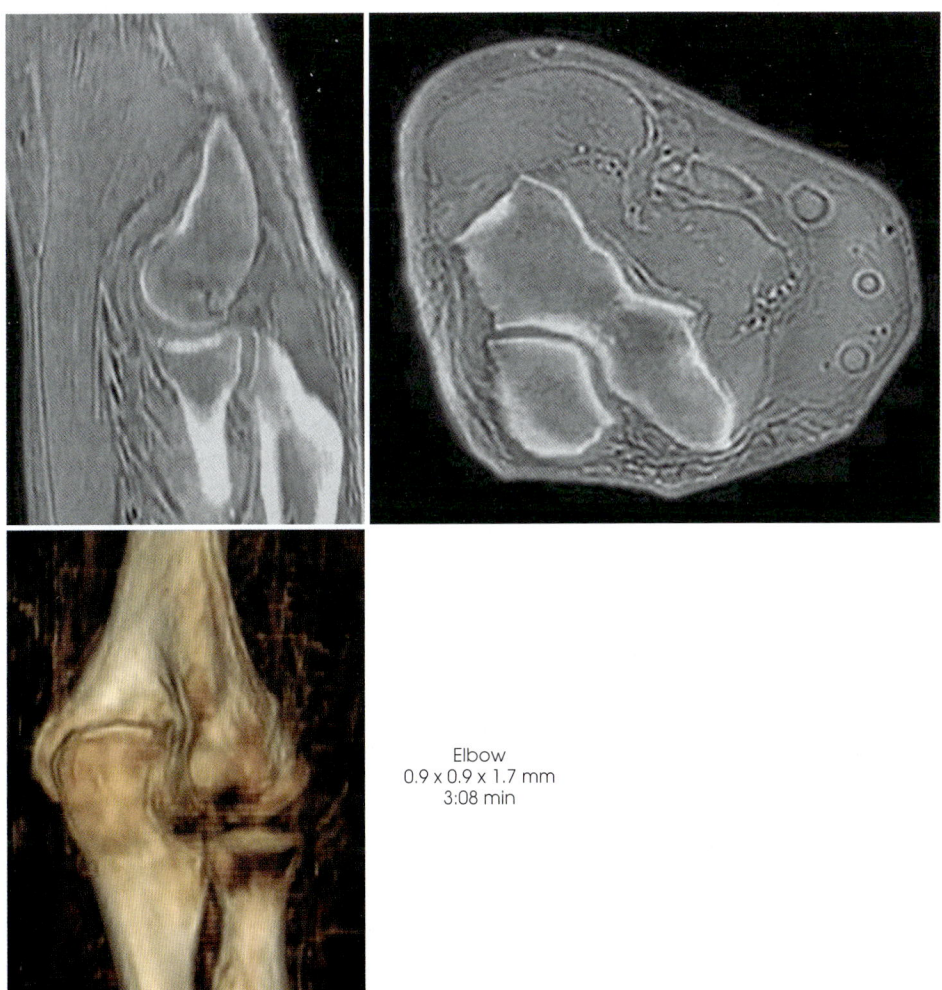

Elbow
0.9 x 0.9 x 1.7 mm
3:08 min

Fig. 26.51 Zero TE images of the elbow have a CT-like appearance and provide 3D rendering capabilities.

(Courtesy GE Healthcare.)

VESSELS

MRA is the imaging of vascular structures. Two techniques used to obtain images of flowing blood are time-of-flight (TOF) and phase-contrast (PC) imaging. With either of these techniques, MRAs can be obtained in 2D or 3D volumes. In TOF imaging, a special pulse sequence is used to suppress the MRI signal from the anatomic area surrounding the vessels of interest. Consequently, signal is given only by material that is outside the area of study when the signal-suppressing pulse occurs. Incoming blood appears bright, whereas stationary tissue is suppressed (Fig. 26.52). PC imaging takes advantage of the shifts in phase, or orientation, experienced by moving spins. Special pulse sequences enhance these effects in flowing blood, producing a bright signal in vessels when the unchanging signal from stationary tissue is subtracted. PC imaging is used when data about the velocity and direction of blood flow are needed.

TOF imaging can be used with the injection of IV gadolinium-based contrast material. Gadolinium shortens the T1 relaxation time of blood, which increases its signal intensity. This allows a decrease in imaging time (breath-hold sequences) and 3D volume imaging in the long axis of the vessel. Imaging of the carotid (Fig. 26.53), thoracic, abdominal, and pelvic arteries (Fig. 26.54) is possible in this way. With the use of a moving table, the aorta can be imaged from the heart to the feet. This is routinely performed to screen for lesions in the peripheral vasculature. Vascular imaging can be used to look for dissections, aneurysms, arteriovenous malformations, plaque, stenosis, and occlusions.

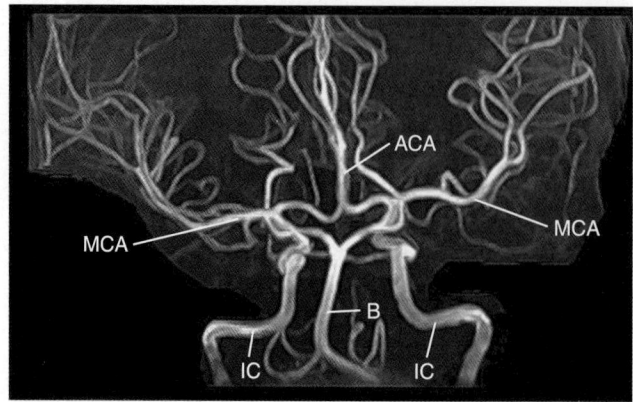

Fig. 26.52 MRA shows intracranial arterial vessels in the AP view. *ACA,* Anterior cerebral arteries; *B,* basilar artery; *IC,* internal carotids; *MCA,* middle cerebral artery. In the center is the circle of Willis.

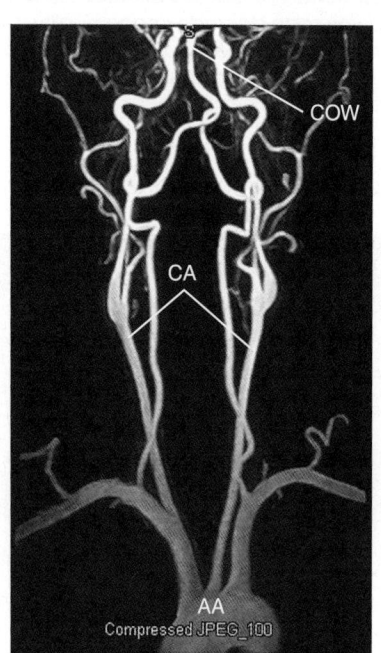

Fig. 26.53 Contrast-enhanced MRA shows carotid arteries *(CA)* from the aortic arch *(AA)* to the circle of Willis *(COW)*.

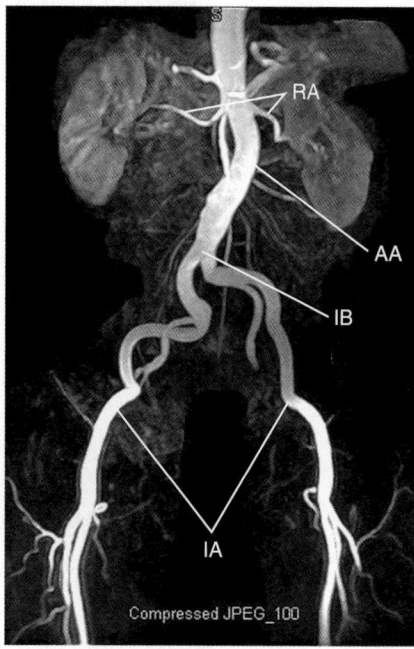

Fig. 26.54 Contrast-enhanced MRA of the abdominal aorta *(AA)* shows the renal arteries *(RA),* iliac bifurcation *(IB),* and iliac arteries *(IA)*.

Advanced Clinical Applications

DIFFUSION AND PERFUSION

The sensitivity of MRI to motion can be a handicap or a potential source of information. Motion artifacts interfere with upper abdominal images, yet flow-sensitive pulse sequences can image flowing blood in blood vessels.

Specialized techniques have been developed that can image the *diffusion* and *perfusion* of molecules within matter. Molecules of water experience diffusion or random motion. This random motion can be affected by cellular membranes and structures, which in turn affects the rate of such diffusion. These microscopic motions can be detected by specialized MRI pulse sequences that can image their rate and direction. Diffusion and perfusion motion differ among tissue types. Diffusion patterns of gray matter in the brain differ from the diffusion patterns in more directionally oriented fiber tracts of white matter. This concept is currently used in diffusion tensor imaging.

Diffusion and perfusion imaging are most often used in the brain to visualize ischemic changes, such as stroke. Recovery from acute stroke can be predicted by viewing the mismatch between the diffusion and perfusion images. Diffusion and perfusion imaging can produce clinically significant images that may help us understand white matter degenerative diseases (e.g., multiple sclerosis, ischemia, infarction) (Fig. 26.55), develop possible therapies to return blood flow to underperfused brain tissue, and characterize brain tumors. Similar applications for the rest of the body have been developed, allowing diffusion and perfusion imaging to be used in imaging of the abdominal and pelvic organs, as well as the spine.

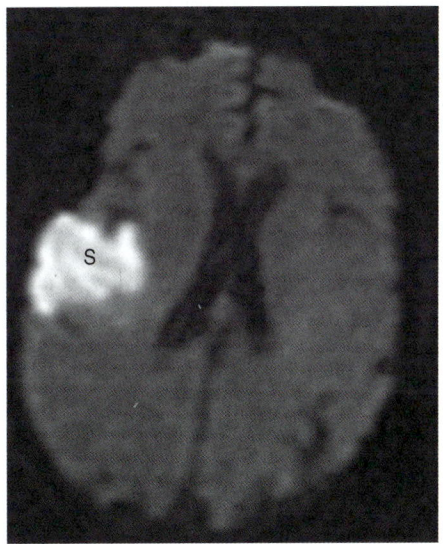

Fig. 26.55 Diffusion-weighted image shows acute ischemic infarct (stroke) *(S)* in the territory of the right middle cerebral artery. Lack of diffusion in this area turns it bright on this heavily T2-weighted image.

SPECTROSCOPY

In routine MRI, the purpose is to produce detailed pictures of the anatomy being imaged. This is accomplished by spatially localizing the MRI signal in a volume of tissue. In magnetic resonance spectroscopy (MRS), the result is a graph, or spectrum, of the chemical composition of the volume of tissue being "imaged." This graph denotes not only the chemical compounds present, but also the quantity of each compound, and the ratios between the compounds. In pathologic conditions in which the imaging characteristics are similar or difficult to interpret, MRS can add vital information, leading to a more accurate interpretation.

MRS is most commonly used in the brain. It can be helpful in diagnosing metabolic conditions, tumor recurrence versus necrosis, and pathologic processes (Fig. 26.56). The use of MRS is becoming more widespread in breast and prostate imaging to differentiate between normal and abnormal tissue. It has also been used to study normal physiologic changes such as those seen in muscle contraction (Fig. 26.57).

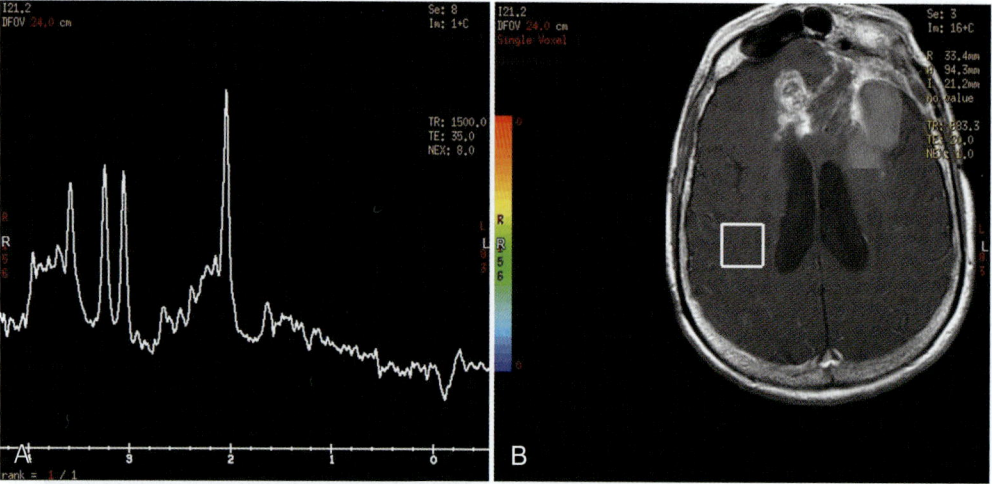

Fig. 26.56 Routine spectroscopy in a patient with a primary brain tumor. Voxel shows normal brain spectra in an area unaffected by the brain tumor.

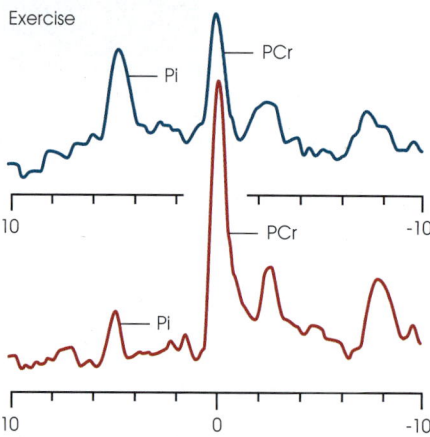

Fig. 26.57 Spectra from human muscle before *(red line)* and during *(blue line)* exercise. Thin horizontal lines represent separate baselines for each spectrum. Each peak represents a different chemical species, and the area under the peak down to the baseline indicates the amount of substance present. The inorganic phosphate *(Pi)* peak increases with exercise as energy-rich phosphocreatine *(PCr)* is used to provide energy for muscle contraction.

FUNCTIONAL MAGNETIC RESONANCE IMAGING

Functional MRI (fMRI) records active areas of the brain during certain activities or after the introduction of stimuli, such as visual or auditory stimuli. Blood oxygen level–dependent (BOLD) imaging uses the differences in the magnetic properties of oxygenated and deoxygenated blood to visualize active areas of the brain. The human body is composed of approximately 50% oxygenated and 50% deoxygenated blood. Oxygenated blood displays diamagnetic properties; that is, it does not affect molecules in the surrounding area. Deoxygenated blood is a paramagnetic substance, which increases T2* decay and decreases the availability of signals in the area immediately surrounding it (magnetic susceptibility artifact). Because of this increase in magnetic susceptibility artifact, it is possible for MRI to measure the difference between oxygenated and deoxygenated blood. As blood flow increases to areas of activation, the MRI scanner distinguishes the subtle differences in signal and registers the area of brain activity.

Currently, fMRI is used in many areas of research to increase our understanding of human brain anatomy and function. Studies involving the visual cortex, memory, Alzheimer's disease, schizophrenia, and many other topics have been performed through fMRI. fMRI may prove useful in areas of lie detection and mind reading. It holds promise for the future of MRI, not only as a diagnostic tool, but also as a predictor of future behaviors and disease processes.

WHOLE-BODY MRI

Whole-body MRI (WB-MRI) has been an emerging technique over the past several years. WB-MRI is now commonly used to determine the extent of malignant bone disease and the response to treatment.[34] WB-MRI is recommended in both international and national imaging guidelines for several types of cancer and the assessment of cancer-associated conditions and syndromes.[35] WB-MRI acquires images of the entire body in a single imaging session. Today's scanners permit imaging from the head to the feet using multichannel coils and multistation imaging. Images are acquired in stations and post-processed to form a single image (Fig. 26.58). A variety of imaging contrasts and sequences may be obtained, including T1 with or without *fat suppression*, T2 with or without fat suppression, STIR, and DWI.[34,35]

MR NEUROGRAPHY

MR neurography is used to evaluate peripheral nerve disorders that are the result of trauma, tumors, inflammation, radiation damage, compression, or entrapment.[36,37] It is also used to locate and grade nerve injuries.[36] Imaging can be performed anytime following an injury, whereas electrodiagnostic testing requires a waiting period for abnormalities to become apparent. MR neurography images gauge the severity of disease, facilitate the development of treatment plans, and monitor the response to treatment. This technique can image peripheral nerves in any body region, but is commonly utilized in the evaluation of the brachial plexus, lumbosacral plexus, thoracic outlet, and sciatic nerves.[37]

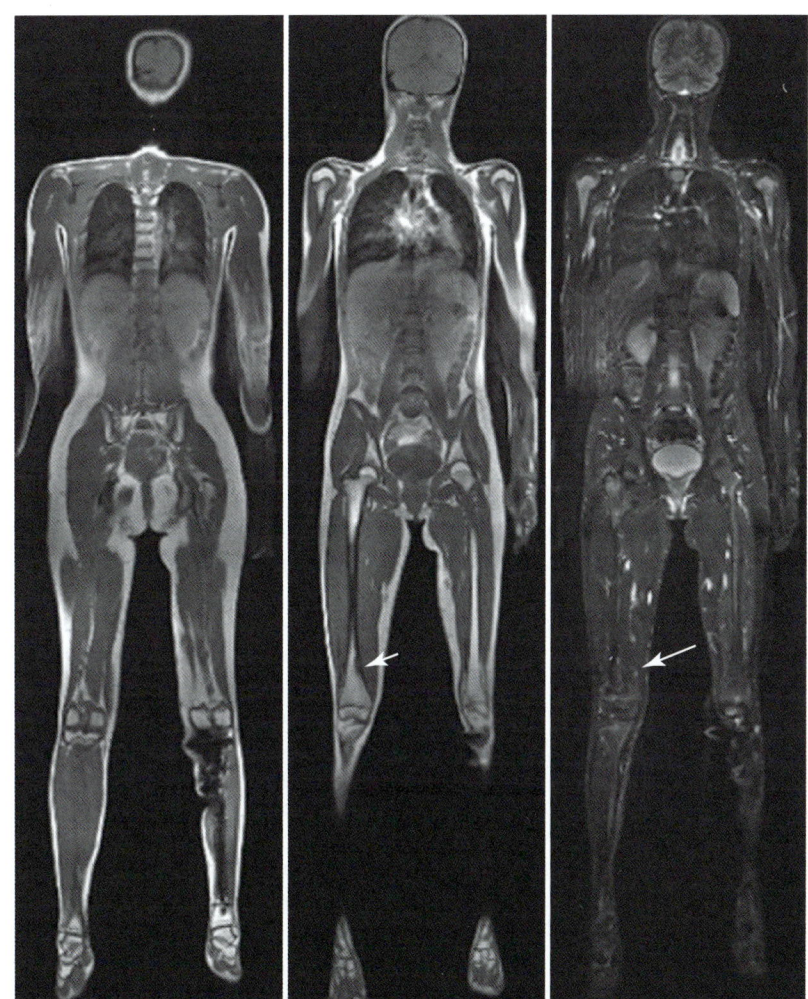

Fig. 26.58 WB-MRI. Images are acquired in stations and post-processed to create a single image.

(From Farina A, Gasperini C, Aparisi Gomez MP, et al. The role of FDG-PET and whole-body MRI in high grade bone sarcomas with particular focus on osteosarcoma. *Semin Nucl Med*, 2022;52(5):635–646.)

Best Practices

The production of high-quality diagnostic MR images requires the technologist to master a myriad of imaging parameters and options while at the same time paying strict attention to patient and staff safety. The following best practices will serve as a guide for the MRI technologist.

SAFETY

The MRI environment is a dangerous and potentially lethal environment. The primary responsibility of the MRI technologist is the safety of all individuals within this magnetic environment.

The technologist must have sufficient knowledge and understanding to perform the following responsibilities:
- Serve as a gatekeeper to the magnet room (Zone IV) to ensure the safety of patients, visitors, and staff.
- Screen all equipment, staff, patients, and visitors to prevent any unsafe objects/devices from entering the magnet room (Zone IV).
- Prescreen patients for the presence of implanted devices that require further investigation and/or coordination with device representatives.
- Use a ferromagnetic detection system (FMDS) to supplement the written and verbal screening process.
- Label equipment (e.g., wheelchairs, stretchers, oxygen tanks) as MR safe, MR conditional, or MR unsafe.
- Change patients into MRI-appropriate attire for exams (i.e., no street clothes).
- Use appropriate padding between the patient and the bore wall, between areas of skin-to-skin contact, and between cables/wires and the patient to prevent burns.
- Provide patients, visitors, and staff who remain within the magnet room during scanning with appropriate hearing protection.
- Clean equipment after each patient to prevent the transmission of pathogens.
- Implement a time-out during which the imaging team verifies the following: correct patient, exam, laterality, protocol, proper screening, and contrast dose.

APPROPRIATE PATIENT SETUP/EXAM PROTOCOL

Choosing the appropriate coil, patient position, and exam protocol requires a unique knowledge base. The technologist must be an integral part of this equation by modeling the following behaviors:
- Thinking outside the box for patient positioning and coil usage. Patients are not always able to tolerate the standard positioning or coil used for a procedure.
- Collaborating with radiologists on what sequences are most important for various exams.
- Utilizing time reduction techniques, such as parallel imaging.
- Making use of motion reduction techniques to improve image quality.
- Utilizing pulse sequences that acquire multiple contrasts (e.g., in-phase, out-of-phase, fat, water) in a single scan to reduce the duration of the exam.
- Incorporating the use of artificial intelligence to decrease scan time, improve image quality, reduce variability among technologists, and increase consistency across follow-up exams.
- Understanding the need and use of contrast media.

PATIENT MANAGEMENT

MRI's unique environment presents challenges that require the technologist to have above-average patient care and communication skills. The technologist may demonstrate this expertise by carrying out the following tasks:
- Explaining the procedure to the patient on their level (e.g., adult vs. child).
- Paying attention to nonverbal cues that signify claustrophobia, pain, or discomfort. The technologist can then make modifications to the patient position or imaging technique to ensure a successful exam.
- Communicating with the patient throughout the exam. This reduces anxiety, gives the patient a sense of how much time remains, and lets the patient know that they are not alone.
- Using distraction techniques such as lighting, music, prism glasses, airflow, and aromatherapy to combat claustrophobia. Medication and an accompanying friend or family member may also be helpful.

Conclusion

Since its development in the 1970s, MRI has evolved into an advanced, widely used tool that is necessary for the diagnosis, staging, and treatment of disease. Today, MRI is the imaging modality of choice for studying the central nervous and musculoskeletal systems. The role of MRI in breast, cardiac, and body imaging continues to expand. Quantitative techniques, MR spectroscopy, fMRI, WB-MRI, and MR neurography will enhance its usefulness.

MRI's ability to utilize multiple biological parameters in its image acquisition, the development of new pulse sequences and more sensitive hardware, and the use of organ-specific contrast agents will keep MRI at the forefront of the imaging world.

Definition of Terms

active shielding: A set of superconducting coils positioned outside the primary coils, but still inside the cryostat. An electric current moves in the opposite direction of the primary current. This produces a magnetic field that counteracts the primary magnetic field, which results in a reduced magnetic fringe field.

antenna: Device for transmitting or receiving radio waves.

artifact(s): Spurious finding in or distortion of an image.

attenuation: Reduction in energy or amount of a beam of radiation when it passes through tissue or other substances.

claustrophobia: The fear of being in a small or confined place and being unable to escape.

coil: Single or multiple loops of wire (or another electrical conductor such as tubing) designed to produce a magnetic field from current flowing through the wire or to detect a changing magnetic field by voltage induced in the wire.

contrast: Degree of difference between two substances in some parameter, with the parameter varying depending on the technique used (e.g., attenuation in radiographic techniques or signal strength in MRI).

cryogenic: Relating to extremely low temperature (see *superconductive magnet*).

diffusion: Spontaneous random motion of molecules in a medium; a natural and continuous process.

fat suppression: An imaging technique that reduces the signal intensity of fat tissue. On fat-suppressed images, the fat tissue is made to be of a lower, darker signal intensity than the surrounding structures.

ferromagnetic detection system (FMDS): System that identifies ferrous objects that one is carrying on their person prior to entry into the magnet room.

frequency: Number of times that a process repeats itself in a given period (e.g., the frequency of a radio wave is the number of complete waves per second).

fringe field: Portion of the magnetic field that extends away from the confines of the magnet; it cannot be used for imaging but can affect nearby equipment or personnel.

gating: Organizing data so that the information used to construct the image comes from the same point in the cycle of a repeating motion, such as a heartbeat. The moving object is "frozen" at that phase of its motion, thus reducing image blurring.

gauss (G): Unit of magnetic field strength (see *tesla*).

gradient echo: A pulse sequence that uses a gradient instead of a 180-degree RF refocusing pulse to generate T1 and T2*-weighted images.

inversion recovery: Standard pulse sequence available on most MRI scanners; the name indicates that the direction of longitudinal magnetization is reversed (inverted) before relaxation (recovery) occurs.

Lenz forces: Forces characterized by opposing magnetic fields. Faraday's law indicates that a changing magnetic field will induce a voltage and subsequent current in an electrical conductor.[15] According to Lenz's law, the induced voltage will generate a magnetic field that opposes the main magnetic field.[15]

level 1 MR personnel: Individuals who have passed minimal safety training to ensure their own safety within the MRI environment.

level 2 MR personnel: Individuals who have been extensively trained and educated in the broader aspects of MR safety.

longitudinal plane: This plane corresponds to the direction of the main magnetic field in superconducting magnets and is the location of protons awaiting excitation.

magnetohydrodynamic effect: Effect that results in the elevation of the T-wave on ECG tracings while a patient is within the magnetic field. ECG changes are the result of the movement of blood (conductive fluid) across a magnetic field, which induces a voltage.[16] The induced voltage distorts the ECG signal, which is observed as an elevation of the T-wave on ECG tracings.[17]

magnetophosphenes: Flashes of light visualized while in the magnetic field. These are thought to be the result of the retina being stimulated by magnetic field–induced currents.[19]

magnetic resonance (MR): Process by which certain nuclei, when placed in a magnetic field, can absorb and release energy. This technique can be used for chemical analysis or to produce cross-sectional images of body parts. Computer analysis of the radio wave data is required.

MR conditional: An item that has been demonstrated to pose no known hazards in a specified MRI environment with specified conditions of use.

MR medical director (MRMD): An individual (physician) who is well versed in MR safety, establishes MR safety policies and procedures, defines personnel classifications and necessary training, and determines whether patients with implants and devices can be scanned.[15]

MR safe: An item that poses no known hazards in any MRI environment.

MR safety expert (MRSE): An individual who serves as an MR safety resource to the MR medical director and MR safety officer.[15]

MR safety officer (MRSO): An individual who oversees MR safety practices within a facility.[15]

MR unsafe: An item that is known to pose hazards in the MRI environment.

noise: Random contributions to the total signal that arise from stray external radio waves, imperfect electronic apparatus, or other interference. Noise cannot be eliminated but can be minimized; it tends to degrade the image by interfering with accurate measurement of the true MRI signal, similar to the difficulty in maintaining a clear conversation in a noisy room.

non-MR personnel: Individuals who have not completed formal MR safety training within the past 12 months.

nuclear magnetic resonance (NMR): Another name for magnetic resonance; this term is not commonly used.

nucleus: The central portion of an atom, composed of protons and neutrons.

paramagnetic: Referring to materials that alter the magnetic field of nearby nuclei. Paramagnetic substances are not directly imaged by MRI, but instead change the signal intensity of the tissue where they localize, acting as MRI contrast agents. Paramagnetic agents shorten the T1 and T2 relaxation times of the tissues they affect—actions that tend to have opposing effects on signal intensity. An increase in signal intensity is observed on T1-weighted images and a decrease in signal intensity is observed on T2-weighted images.

passive shielding: The placement of ferromagnetic material in the walls of the examination room or around the magnet to reduce the fringe field. Passive shielding is heavy and expensive. It is not typically used in modern MRI suites.

perfusion: Flow of blood through the vessels of an organ or anatomic structure; usually refers to blood flow in the small vessels (e.g., capillary perfusion).

peripheral nerve stimulation (PNS): A tingling or tapping sensation experienced by some patients due to the time-varying (gradient) magnetic field.

permanent magnet: An object that produces a magnetic field without requiring an external supply of electricity.

precession: Rotation of an object around the direction of a force acting on that object. This should not be confused with the axis of rotation of the object itself (e.g., a spinning top rotates on its own axis, but it may also precess [wobble] around the direction of the force of gravity that is acting on it).

proton density: Measure of proton (i.e., hydrogen, because its nucleus is a single proton) concentration (number of nuclei per given volume); one of the major determinants of MRI signal strength in hydrogen imaging.

pulse: *See radio frequency (RF) pulse.*

pulse sequence(s): A coordinated series of gradient activations and RF transmissions designed to excite nuclei in such a way that their energy release has varying contributions from proton density, T1, or T2 processes.

quench: In superconductive magnet systems, the rapid venting of the supercooled liquid gas (helium) from the magnet.

radio frequency (RF) pulse: A short burst of radio waves. If the radio waves are of the appropriate frequency, they can give energy to nuclei that are within a magnetic field by the process of resonance. The length of the pulse determines the amount of energy given to the nuclei.

raw data: Information obtained by radio reception of the MRI signal as stored by a computer. Specific computer manipulation of these data is required to construct an image from them.

relaxation time: Measure of the rate at which nuclei, after stimulation, release their absorbed energy.

resistive magnet: Simple electromagnet in which electricity passing through coils of wire produces a magnetic field; can be turned on and off.

resonance: Process of energy absorption by an object that is tuned to absorb energy of a specific frequency only. All other frequencies do not affect the object (e.g., if one tuning fork is struck in a room full of tuning forks, only the forks tuned to that identical frequency would vibrate [resonate]).

rotational force (torque): Refers to the long axis of ferrous objects becoming aligned with the orientation of the main magnetic field (B_0).

signal: In MRI, induction of current into a receiver coil by precessing magnetization.

slice(s): Cross-sectional image(s); can also refer to the thin section(s) of the body from which data are acquired to produce the image(s).

spectroscopy: An imaging technique that produces a spectrum instead of an MR image. The values for the various chemicals of the spectrum aid in determining the presence of a disease process.

spin echo: Standard MRI pulse sequence that can provide T1-weighted, T2-weighted, or proton density–weighted images. The name indicates that a declining MRI signal is refocused to gain strength (similar to an echo) before it is recorded as raw data.

spin-lattice relaxation: Release of energy by excited nuclei to their general environment; one of the major determinants of MRI signal strength. T1 is a rate constant measuring spin-lattice relaxation. Also called T1 relaxation.

spin-spin relaxation: Release of energy by excited nuclei as a result of interaction among themselves; one of the major determinants of MRI signal strength. T2 is a rate constant measuring spin-spin relaxation. Also called T2 relaxation.

superconductive magnet: Electromagnet in which the coils of wire are cooled to an extremely low temperature so that resistance to the conduction of electricity is nearly eliminated (superconductive).

T1: Spin-lattice relaxation.

T2: Spin-spin relaxation.

tesla (T): Unit of magnetic field strength; 1T equals 10,000 gauss or 10 kilogauss (other units of magnetic field strength). The earth's magnetic field approximates 0.5 gauss.

translational force (missile effect): The ability of the fringe field to attract ferromagnetic objects and rapidly draw them into isocenter with considerable force.

transverse plane: The plane perpendicular to the longitudinal plane where the MRI signal can be measured.

Zone I: The area that is farthest from the magnet room and is freely accessible to the general public.

Zone II: An interface between the publicly accessible Zone I and the strictly controlled Zones III and IV.

Zone III: An area that is adjacent to the magnet room and poses a physical risk to unscreened patients or personnel.

Zone IV: The area that houses the MRI scanner and poses the greatest risk to patients and personnel.

References

1. Washington Open MRI. *Misunderstanding field strength*. n.d. Available at: https://washingtonopenmri.com/misunderstanding-field-strength/. (Accessed November 4, 2023).
2. Fonar Corporation. *The upright MRI*. n.d. Available at: https://www.fonar.com/upright-mri.html. (Accessed November 4, 2023).
3. Fonar Corporation. *Upright MRI specifications*. n.d. Available at: https://www.fonar.com/specifications.html. (Accessed November 4, 2023).
4. Esaote. *The tilting MRI: The key to confidence (G-scan Brio)*. n.d. Available at: https://www.esaote.com/dedicated-mri/mri-systems/p/g-scan-brio/. (Accessed November 4, 2023).
5. Elster AD. *Brands of scanners*. n.d. Questions and Answers in MRI [website]. Available at: https://mriquestions.com/brands-of-scanners.html. (Accessed November 4, 2023).
6. Hyperfine. *Meet Swoop portable MR imaging system*. n.d. Available at: https://20597499.fs1.hubspotusercontent-na1.net/hubfs/20597499/Brochures%20and%20White%20Papers/Swoop%20System%20Brochure.pdf. (Accessed November 4, 2023).
7. Hyperfine. Swoop portable MR imaging system: Frequently asked questions; 2023. Available at: https://hyperfine.io/swoop/frequently-asked-questions; 2023. (Accessed November 4, 2023).
8. Aspect Imaging Ltd. *Embrace point of care imaging technology*. n.d. Available at: https://embracemri.com/technology-2/. (Accessed November 4, 2023).
9. OHSU Doernbecher Children's Hospital. *Intraoperative MRI (iMRI)*. n.d. Available at: https://www.ohsu.edu/doernbecher/intraoperative-mri-imri. (Accessed November 4, 2023).
10. Reiser MF, Hricak H, Knauth M. *Interventional Magnetic Resonance Imaging*. Berlin: Springer; 2012.
11. Thompson SM, Gorny KR, Koepsel EMK, et al. Body interventional MRI for diagnostic and interventional radiologists: Current practice and future prospects. *Radiographics*. 2021;41(6):1785–1801.
12. Mayo Clinic. *Positron Emission Tomography Scan*; 2023. Available at: https://mayoclinic.org/tests-procedures/pet-scan/about/pac-20385078. (Accessed November 4, 2023).
13. Siemens Healthineers. *Biograph mMR: Simultaneous MR and PET imaging*. n.d. Available at: https://www.siemens-healthineers.com/en-us/magnetic-resonance-imaging/mr-pet-scanner/biograph-mmr. (Accessed November 4, 2023).
14. Elekta Group. Elekta Unity. Two worlds, one future; 2020. Available at: https://www.elekta.com/products/radiation-therapy/unity/assets/Elekta-Unity-Brochure.pdf. (Accessed November 4, 2023).
15. American College of Radiology (ACR) Committee on MR Safety. *ACR manual on MR safety*. Reston, VA: American College of Radiology; 2020. Available at https://www.acr.org/-/media/ACR/Files/Radiology-Safety/MR-Safety/Manual-on-MR-Safety.pdf. (Accessed November 4, 2023).
16. McRobbie DW, Moore EA, Graves MJ. *MRI from Picture to Proton*. 3rd ed. Cambridge University; 2017.
17. Elster AD. *B_0 effect on EKG*. n.d. Questions and Answers in MRI [website]. Available at: https://mriquestions.com/magnet-changes-ekg.html. (Accessed November 4, 2023).
18. Shellock FG, Crues JV. *MRI Bioeffects, Safety, and Patient Management*. Playa Del Rey, CA: Biomedical Research Publishing Group; 2014.
19. Elster AD. *Magnetophosphenes*. n.d. Questions and Answers in MRI [website]. Available at: https://mriquestions.com/flickering-lights.html. (Accessed November 4, 2023).
20. Elster AD. *Stimulation by gradients*. n.d. Questions and Answers in MRI [website]. Available at: https://mriquestions.com/nerve-stimulation.html. (Accessed November 4, 2023).
21. Elster AD. *Forces on metal objects*. n.d. Questions and Answers in MRI [website].

21. Available at: https://mriquestions.com/forces-on-metal.html. (Accessed November 4, 2023).
22. American College of Obstetricians and Gynecologists' Committee on Obstetric Practice. Committee Opinion No. 723: Guidelines for diagnostic imaging during pregnancy and lactation. *Obstet Gynecol*. 2017;130(4):e210–e216. Available at: https://www.acog.org/clinical/clinical-guidance/committee-opinion/articles/2017/10/guidelines-for-diagnostic-imaging-during-pregnancy-and-lactation. (Accessed November 4, 2023).
23. GE Healthcare. *AIR™ Recon DL* [video]; 2020. Available at: https://www.youtube.com/watch?v=t0wl0ulSIWE. (Accessed November 4, 2023).
24. GE Healthcare. *AIR X™. Prescribing precision MRI slices*; 2023. Available at: https://www.gehealthcare.com/products/magnetic-resonance-imaging/mr-workflow-solutions/air-x-mri-slices. (Accessed November 4, 2023).
25. Siemens Healthineers. *AutoAlign*. n.d. Available at https://www.siemens-healthineers.com/en-us/magnetic-resonance-imaging/options-and-upgrades/clinical-applications/autoalign. (Accessed November 4, 2023).
26. Philips. *SmartExam brain*. n.d. Available at: https://www.usa.philips.com/healthcare/product/HCNMRB514/smartexam-brain-mr-clinical-application. (Accessed November 4, 2023).
27. American College of Radiology (ACR) Committee on Drugs and Contrast Media. *ACR Manual on Contrast Media*. Reston: VA: American College of Radiology; 2023. Available at: https://www.acr.org/-/media/ACR/Files/Clinical-Resources/Contrast_Media.pdf. (Accessed November 4, 2023).
28. Mayo Clinic. *Magnetic Resonance Elastography*; 2022. Available at: https://www.mayoclinic.org/tests-procedures/magnetic-resonance-elastography/about/pac-20385177. (Accessed November 4, 2023).
29. Starekova J, Hernando D, Pickhardt PJ, et al. Quantification of liver fat content with CT and MRI: state of the art. *Radiology*. 2021;301(2):250–262.
30. Labranche R, Gilbert G, Cerny M, et al. Liver iron quantification with MR imaging: a primer for radiologists. *Radiographics*. 2018;38(2):392–412.
31. GE Healthcare. *Orthoworks: Characterizing cartilage before and after surgery*. n.d. Available at: https://www.gehealthcare.com/-/jssmedia/files/g/2020/08/21/glb_mr_signaworks_orthoworks_characterizing-cartilage.pdf?rev=-1. (Accessed November 4, 2023).
32. GE Healthcare. *oZTEo for MR Bone Imaging*; 2022. Available at: https://www.gehealthcare.com/-/jssmedia/gehc/us/files/products/magnetic-resonance-imaging/mr-applications/ozteo/sell-sheet-ozteo-jb19307xx.pdf?rev=-1. (Accessed November 4, 2023).
33. Ultra short TE multi-echo (UTE multi-echo). *Canon Medical Systems [website]*. 2022. Available at https://global.medical.canon/products/magnetic-resonance/good-to-know#ultrashort. (Accessed November 8, 2023).
34. Winfield JM, Blackledge MD, Tunariu N, et al. Whole-body MRI: a practical guide for imaging patients with malignant bone disease. *Clin Radiol*. 2021;76(10):715–727.
35. Petralia G, Padhani AR, Pricolo P, et al. Whole-body magnetic resonance imaging (WB-MRI) in oncology: recommendations and key uses. *Radiol Med*. 2019;124(3):218–233.
36. Siemens Healthineers. *MR neurography*. n.d. Available at: https://www.magnetomworld.siemens-healthineers.com/clinical-corner/protocols/neurology-neurography/neurography. (Accessed November 4, 2023).
37. University of California San Francisco Department of Radiology & Biomedical Imaging. *MR neurography/MR imaging of peripheral nerves (PNI)*. n.d. Available at: https://radiology.ucsf.edu/patient-care/services/mr-neurography. (Accessed November 4, 2023).

Selected bibliography

American College of Radiology (ACR) Committee on MR Safety. *ACR Manual on MR Safety*. Reston: VA: American College of Radiology; 2020. Available at: https://www.acr.org/-/media/ACR/Files/Radiology-Safety/MR-Safety/Manual-on-MR-Safety.pdf. (Accessed November 4, 2023).

Bloch F. Nuclear induction. *Physiol Rev*. 1946;70:460.

Burghart G, Finn CA. *Handbook of MRI Scanning*. St Louis: Elsevier; 2010.

Bushong SC, Clarke G. *MRI Physical and Biological Principles*. 4th ed. St Louis: Elsevier; 2015.

Damadian R. Tumor detection by nuclear magnetic resonance. *Science*. 1971;171(3976):1151–1153.

Kelley LL, Petersen CM. *Sectional Anatomy for Imaging Professionals*. 3rd ed. St Louis: Elsevier; 2013.

Purcell EM, Torrey HC, Pound RV. Resonance absorption by nuclear magnetic moments in a solid. *Physiol Rev*. 1946;69:37.

Shellock FG. *Magnetic Resonance Procedures: Health Effects and Safety*. Boca Raton, FL: CRC Press; 2001.

Shellock FG. *Reference Manual for Magnetic Resonance Safety, Implants, and Devices: 2018*. Playa Del Rey, CA: Biomedical Research Publishing Group; 2018.

Shellock FG, Crues JV. *MRI Bioeffects, Safety, and Patient Management*. Playa Del Rey, CA: Biomedical Research Publishing Group; 2014.

Westbrook C, Kaut Roth C, Talbot J. *MRI in Practice*. 4th ed. Oxford: Wiley-Blackwell; 2011.

27

VASCULAR, CARDIAC, AND INTERVENTIONAL RADIOGRAPHY

JESSICA COOPER; RICHARD RYAN WALL

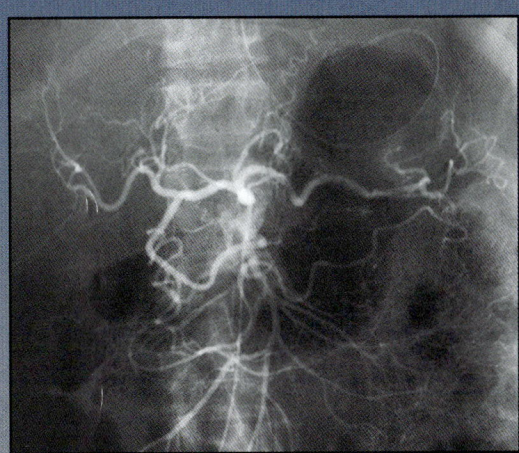

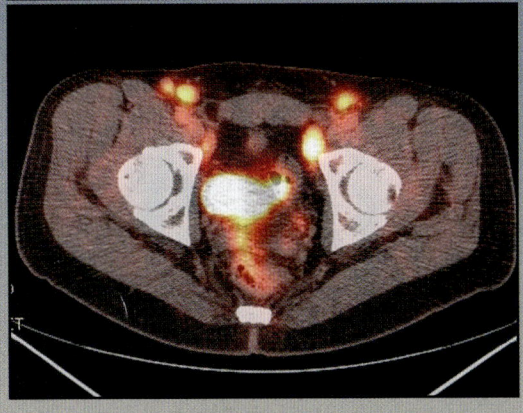

OUTLINE

Historical Development, 312
ANATOMY, 314
Circulatory System, 314
Blood-Vascular System, 315
Lymphatic System, 318
ANGIOGRAPHY, 320
Definitions and Indications, 320
Angiography Team, 321
Preparation of Angiographic Procedure Room, 321
Radiation Protection, 322
Contrast Media, 322
Injection Techniques, 323
Angiographic Imaging Techniques, 323
Angiographic Imaging Equipment, 324
Angiographic Procedures, 326
ANGIOGRAPHY PROCEDURES, 334
Aortography, 334
Peripheral Angiography, 340
CEREBRAL ANGIOGRAPHY, 342
Cerebral Anatomy, 342
Technique, 345
Aortic Arch Angiogram, 348
Extracranial Carotid and Vertebral Arteriography, 348
Intracranial Anterior Circulation, 349
Posterior Circulation, 351
Venography, 353

INTERVENTIONAL RADIOLOGY, 356
Percutaneous Transluminal Angioplasty and Stenting, 356
Abdominal Aortic Aneurysm Endografts, 358
Transcatheter Embolization, 360
Vena Cava Filter Placement, 364
Transjugular Intrahepatic Portosystemic Shunt, 368
Pharmacologic Thrombolysis and Mechanical Thrombectomy, 369
Other Procedures, 370
Nonvascular Interventional Procedures, 370
Vascular and Interventional Radiology: Present and Future, 371
CARDIOVASCULAR INTERVENTIONAL RADIOGRAPHY, 372
Cardiac Catheterization, 372
Diagnostic Cardiac Procedures, 379
Interventional Cardiac Procedures, 386
Congenital Defects, 396
Electrophysiology (EP), 396
Interventional Cardiology: Present and Future, 401
Best Practices in Vascular, Cardiac, and Interventional Radiology, 402
Definition of Terms, 402

Historical Development

In January 1896, just 10 weeks after the announcement of Roentgen's discovery of x-rays, Haschek and Lindenthal announced that they had produced a radiograph showing the blood vessels of an amputated hand using a thick emulsion of chalk, known as Teichmann's mixture, as a contrast medium. This work heralded the beginning of angiography. However, the advancement of angiography was hindered by the lack of suitable contrast media and low-risk techniques to deliver the media to the desired location. By the 1920s, researchers were using sodium iodide as a contrast medium to produce lower limb angiography studies. The contrast medium was either injected through a needle that punctured the vessel or through a ureteral catheter that passed into the body through a surgically exposed peripheral vessel.

The first human cardiac catheterization was reported in 1929 by Forssman, a 25-year-old surgical resident who passed a catheter, via an arm vein, into his own heart and then walked to the radiology department, where a chest radiograph was produced to document his medical achievement. Catheterization of the heart soon became a valuable tool used primarily for diagnostic purposes. Through the 1940s, the basic catheterization study remained relatively uncomplicated and easy for physicians to perform; however, the risk to the patient was significant.

In 1952, shortly after the development of a flexible thin-walled catheter, Seldinger announced a *percutaneous*[a] method of catheter introduction. The Seldinger technique eliminated the surgical risk, which exposed the vessel and tissues. This technique is described in detail later in this chapter. Selective coronary *angiography* was first reported by Sones in 1959, when he inadvertently injected contrast media into the right coronary artery of a patient who was undergoing routine aortography. In 1962, Ricketts and Abrams described a percutaneous method for selective coronary angiography. This method was further perfected in the late 1960s with the introduction of preshaped catheters designed to engage the ostium of the right and left coronary arteries.

Innovations in guidewire and catheter technology continued alongside increased research into intraluminal treatments or endovascular interventions. It has been said that the "Fathers of Interventional Radiology and Cardiology" were Charles Dotter and Andreas Grüntzig, respectively. Dotter performed the first successful dilation of a superficial femoral artery in 1964 using coaxial catheters. In the November 1964 edition of *Circulation*, percutaneous transluminal angioplasty (PTA) was described by Dotter with coauthor Dr. Melvin Judkins. In 1966, Dotter

---
[a]Almost all italicized words on the succeeding pages are defined at the end of this chapter.

fabricated a reinforced balloon dilating catheter, but it was not used on patients. Dr. Werner Portsman (Berlin, Germany) introduced "*Korsett Balloon Kather*," an 8-Fr outer Teflon catheter with four longitudinal slits in 1973. A latex balloon catheter was inflated inside the longitudinal slits. In September 1977, Dr. Andreas Grüntzig successfully used a balloon PTA to treat a left anterior descending coronary artery stenosis. Grüntzig and Hopff introduced the double-lumen, balloon-tipped catheter. One lumen allows the passage of a guidewire and fluids through the catheter. The other lumen communicates with a balloon at the distal end of the catheter. When inflated, the balloon expands to a size much larger than the catheter. Double-lumen balloon catheters for angioplasty are available in sizes ranging from 3 to 9 Fr, with attached balloons varying in length and expanding to diameters of 2 to 20 mm or more. Transluminal angioplasty can be performed in virtually any vessel that can be reached percutaneously with a catheter. In 1978, Molnar and Stockum described the use of balloon angioplasty for dilation of strictures within the biliary system. Balloon angioplasty is also conducted in venous structures, ureters, and the gastrointestinal tract.

Expandable metallic stents were developed in the 1980s. Andrew Cragg, Charles Dotter, Cesare Gianturco, Dierk Maas, Julio Palmaz, and Hans Wallsten were the first stent pioneers. These stents were composed primarily of a stainless steel alloy or of nitinol (an alloy of nickel and titanium with a thermal memory) and were self-expandable or balloon expandable. Three stents available for use in 1985 were the Gianturco Z, Palmaz, and Wallstent. Dotter continued the advancement of cardiovascular procedures by first using Streptokinase for selective pharmacologic *thrombolysis*. In the 1980s, Urokinase was used for this widely performed procedure. In the 1990s and early 2000s, developments in thrombolysis were due to the advancement of fibrinolytic agents *(recombinant tissue plasminogen activators)*.

Therapeutic vascular occlusion procedures began in 1931 with an open surgical *embolization* of a carotid cavernous fistula. Dr. Shoji Ishimore used Gelfoam pieces through a polyethylene tube into an exposed carotid artery. It was not until the 1980s and 1990s, however, that *transcatheter embolization* became popular with the advancement of embolization agents, such as gelatin sponges (Gelfoam), polyvinyl alcohol (Ivalon), liquid and rapidly solidifying polymers including cyanoacrylate glue, coils, and detachable balloons.

Early angiograms consisted of single radiographs or the visualization of vessels by fluoroscopy. Because the advantage of *serial imaging* within angiography was recognized, cassette changers, roll film changers, cut film changers, cine, and serial spot-filming/digital devices were developed. Until the early 1990s, most angiograms recorded flowing contrast media in a series of images that required rapid film changers or *cinefluorography* devices; however, presently, digital subtraction angiography (DSA) systems are used almost exclusively.

The resolution possible with early digital equipment was a drawback to the use of digital imaging in angiography. Larger matrix size, the obvious solution to this problem, allowed for acceptable resolution but also created another problem: how to acquire and store large volumes of digital information. In the late 1970s and early 1980s, the high-speed parallel transfer disk was introduced to solve the acquisition and short-term storage problem. This new disk acquired and stored an entire coronary angiogram and made real-time digital playback during the procedure possible. Permanent storage of the digital images remained a problem, however. Floppy disk and computer tape storage were inadequate solutions because they required significant time and supplies. Long-term storage of large amounts of digital images has benefited from advances in computer technology, which provide high-speed, large-capacity methods of storage capable of acquiring large amounts of data (terabytes) with very high resolution.

Current imaging equipment has increased image quality while reducing patient dose and can produce images up to a rate of 30 frames per second. DSA imaging and faster data processing provide the interventionalist with a variety of tools for image manipulation, analysis, and measurement that are almost immediately available, dramatically reducing patient procedure time and allowing for diagnostic and interventional procedures to occur simultaneously.

Over the last 50 years, there have been tremendous advances in radiologic and cardiovascular medicine and technology. Radiographic imaging and recording equipment, physiologic monitoring equipment, and cardiovascular pharmaceuticals and supplies became increasingly reliable. The use of computers in cardiovascular interventional laboratories has facilitated the development of this rapidly growing subspecialty of the cardiovascular medical and surgical sciences. These advances and trends have enabled angiography to evolve from a simple diagnostic investigation to its current state as a sophisticated diagnostic study and interventional procedure.

ANATOMY

Circulatory System

The *circulatory system* has two complex systems of intimately associated vessels. Through these vessels, fluid is transported throughout the body in a continuous, unidirectional flow. The major portion of the circulatory system transports blood and is called the *blood-vascular system* (Fig. 27.1). The minor portion, called the *lymphatic system*, collects fluid from the tissue spaces. This fluid is filtered throughout the lymphatic system, which conveys it back to the blood-vascular system. The fluid conveyed by the lymphatic system is called *lymph*. Together, the blood-vascular and lymphatic systems carry oxygen and nutritive material to the tissues. They also collect and transport carbon dioxide (CO_2) and other waste products of metabolism from the tissues to the organs of excretion: the skin, lungs, liver, and kidneys.

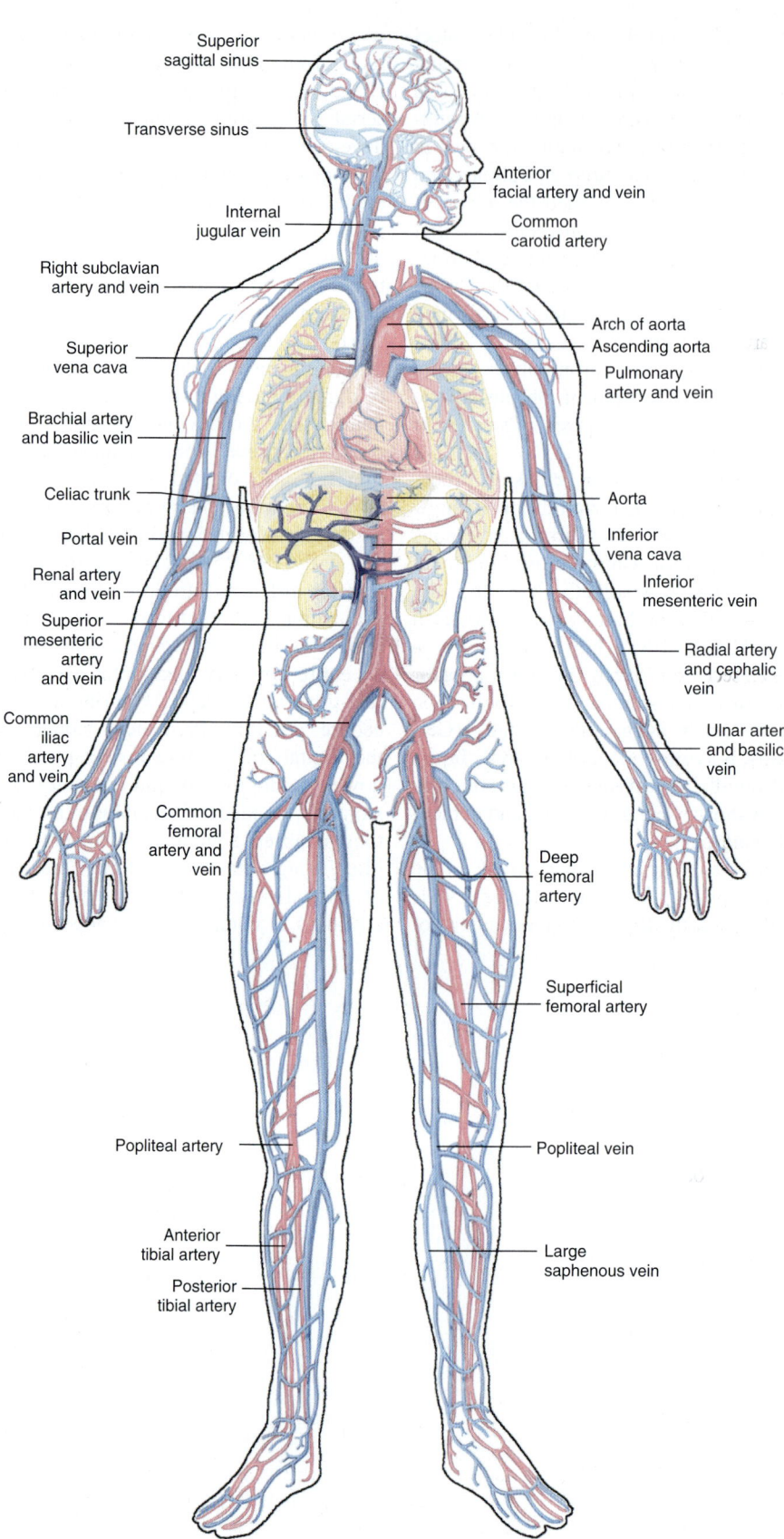

Fig. 27.1 Major arteries and veins: *red*, arterial; *blue*, venous; *purple*, portal.

Blood-Vascular System

The blood-vascular system consists of the *heart*, *arteries*, *capillaries*, and *veins*. The *heart* serves as a pumping mechanism to keep the blood in constant circulation throughout the vast system of blood vessels. *Arteries* convey the blood *away* from the heart. *Veins* convey the blood *back* toward the heart.

Two circuits of blood vessels branch out of the heart (Fig. 27.2). The first circuit is the arterial circuit or the *systemic circulation*, which carries oxygenated blood to the organs and tissues. Every organ has its own vascular circuit that arises from the trunk artery and leads back to the trunk vein for return to the heart. The systemic arteries branch out, treelike, from the aorta to all parts of the body. The arteries are usually named according to their location. The systemic veins usually lie parallel to their respective arteries and are given the same names.

The second circuit is the *pulmonary circulation*, which takes blood to the lungs for CO_2 exchange and for the reoxygenation of the blood, which is carried back to the arterial systemic circulation. The pulmonary trunk arises from the right ventricle of the heart, passes superiorly and posteriorly for a distance of about 5 cm (2 inches), and then divides into two branches, the right and left pulmonary arteries. These vessels enter the root of the respective lung and, following the course of the bronchi, divide and subdivide to form a dense network of capillaries surrounding the alveoli of the lungs. Through the thin walls of the capillaries, the blood discharges CO_2 and absorbs oxygen from the air contained in the alveoli. The oxygenated blood passes onward through the pulmonary veins for return to the heart. In pulmonary circulation, the deoxygenated blood is transported by the pulmonary arteries, and the oxygenated blood is transported by the pulmonary veins.

Two main trunk vessels arise from the heart. The first is the aorta for systemic circulation: the arteries progressively diminish in size as they divide and subdivide along their course, finally ending in minute branches called *arterioles*. The arterioles divide to form the capillary vessels, and the branching process is then reversed: the *capillaries* unite to form *venules*, the beginning branches of the veins, which unite and reunite to form larger and larger vessels as they approach the heart. These venous structures empty into the right atrium, then into the right ventricle, and then into the second main trunk that arises from the heart—the pulmonary trunk, or the pulmonary circulation. The process of oxygen exchange is carried out in small venous structures and then in larger and larger pulmonary veins. The pulmonary veins join to form four large veins (two from each lung), which empty into the left atrium, then into the left ventricle, and then into the aorta, which starts the circulation again throughout the body.

The pathway of venous drainage from the abdominal viscera to the liver is called the *portal system*. In contrast to the systemic and pulmonary circuits, which begin and end at the heart, the portal system begins in the capillaries of the abdominal viscera and ends in the capillaries and sinusoids of the liver. The blood is filtered and then exits the liver via the hepatic venous system, which empties into the *inferior vena cava (IVC)* just proximal to the right atrium.

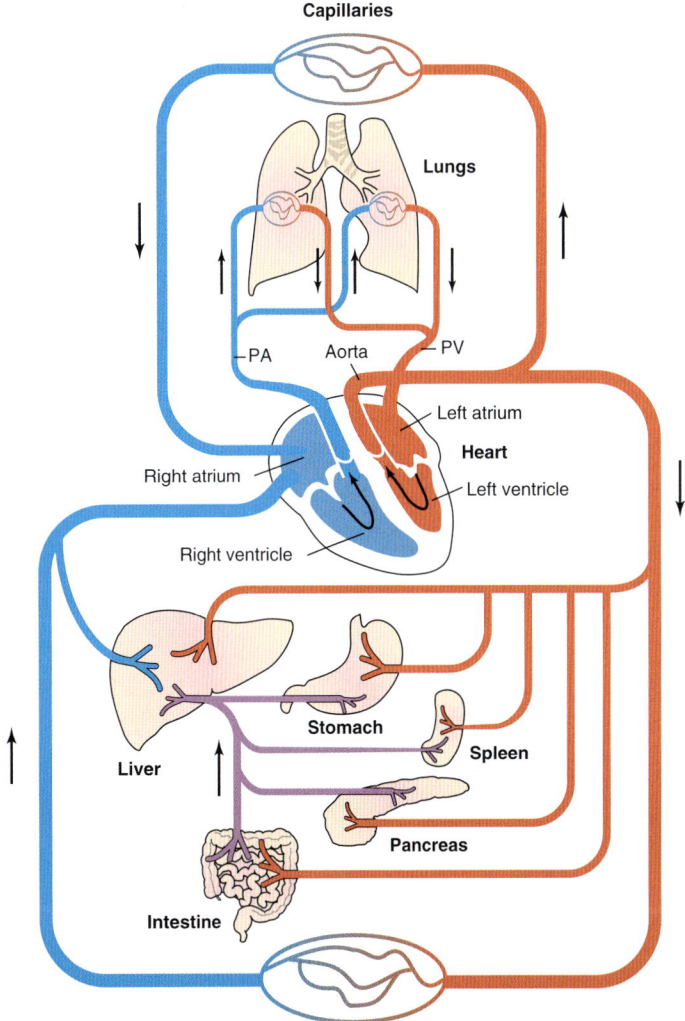

Fig. 27.2 Pulmonary, systemic, and portal circulation: oxygenated *(red)*, deoxygenated *(blue)*, and nutrient-rich *(purple)* blood.

The systemic veins are arranged in a superficial set and in a deep set with which the superficial veins communicate; both sets converge at a common trunk vein. The systemic veins end in two large vessels opening into the heart: the *superior vena cava (SVC)* leads from the portion of the body above the diaphragm, and the IVC leads from below the level of the diaphragm.

The capillaries connect the arterioles and venules to form networks that pervade most organs and all other tissues supplied with blood. The capillary vessels have exceedingly thin walls through which the essential functions of the blood-vascular system take place: the blood constituents are filtered out, and the waste products of cell activity are absorbed. The exchange takes place through the medium of tissue fluid, which is derived from the blood plasma and is drained off by the lymphatic system for return to the blood-vascular system. The tissue fluid undergoes modification in the lymphatic system. As soon as this tissue fluid enters the lymphatic capillaries, it is called *lymph*.

The *heart* is the central organ of the blood-vascular system and functions solely as a pump to keep the blood in circulation. It is shaped like a cone and measures approximately 12 cm (4.75 inches) in length, 9 cm (3.5 inches) in width, and 6 cm (2.5 inches) in depth. The heart is situated obliquely in the central mediastinum, primarily to the left of the midsagittal plane. The base of the heart is directed superiorly, posteriorly, and to the right. The apex of the heart rests on the diaphragm against the anterior chest wall and is directed anteriorly, inferiorly, and to the left.

The muscular wall of the heart is called the *myocardium*. Because of the force required to drive blood through the extensive systemic vessels, the myocardium is about three times as thick on the left side (the arterial side) as on the right (the venous side). The membrane that lines the interior of the heart is called the *endocardium*. The heart is enclosed in the double-walled *pericardial sac*. The exterior wall of this sac is fibrous. The thin, closely adherent membrane that covers the heart is referred to as the *epicardium* or, because it also serves as the serous inner wall of the pericardial sac, the *visceral pericardium*. The narrow, fluid-containing space between the two walls of the sac is called the *pericardial cavity*.

The heart is divided by septa into right and left halves, with each half subdivided by a constriction into two cavities or chambers. The two upper chambers are called *atria*. Each *atrium* consists of a principal cavity and a lesser cavity called the *auricle*. The two lower chambers of the heart are called *ventricles*. The opening between the right atrium and right ventricle is controlled by the right atrioventricular (tricuspid) valve, and the opening between the left atrium and left ventricle is controlled by the left atrioventricular (mitral or bicuspid) valve.

The atria and ventricles separately contract (*systole*) in pumping blood and relax or dilate (*diastole*) in receiving blood. The atria precede the ventricles in contraction; while the atria are in systole, the ventricles are in diastole. One phase of contraction (referred to as the heartbeat) and one phase of dilation are called the *cardiac cycle*. In the average adult, one cardiac cycle lasts 0.8 seconds. The heart rate, or number of pulsations per minute, varies with size, age, and gender. Heart rate is faster in small persons, young individuals, and females. The heart rate is also increased with exercise, food, and emotional disturbances.

The atria function as receiving chambers. The superior and IVC empty into the right atrium (Fig. 27.3); the two right and left pulmonary veins empty into the left atrium. The ventricles function as distributing chambers. The right side of the heart handles the venous, or deoxygenated, blood, and the left side handles the arterial, or oxygenated, blood. The left ventricle pumps oxygenated blood through the aortic valve into the aorta and the systemic circulation. The three major portions of the aorta are the ascending aorta, the aortic arch, and the descending aorta. The right ventricle pumps deoxygenated blood through the pulmonary valve into the pulmonary trunk and the pulmonary circulation.

Blood is supplied to the myocardium by the right and left coronary arteries. These vessels arise in the aortic sinus immediately superior to the aortic valve (Fig. 27.4). Most of the cardiac veins drain into the coronary sinus on the posterior aspect of the heart, and this sinus drains into the right atrium (Fig. 27.5).

The ascending aorta arises from the superior portion of the left ventricle and passes superiorly and to the right for a short distance. It then arches posteriorly and to the left and descends along the left side of the vertebral column to the level of L4, where it divides into the right and left common iliac arteries. The common iliac arteries pass to the level of the lumbosacral junction and divide into the internal iliac, or hypogastric, artery and the external iliac artery. The internal iliac artery passes into the pelvis. The external iliac artery passes to a point about midway between the anterior superior iliac spine and pubic symphysis and then enters the upper thigh to become the common femoral artery.

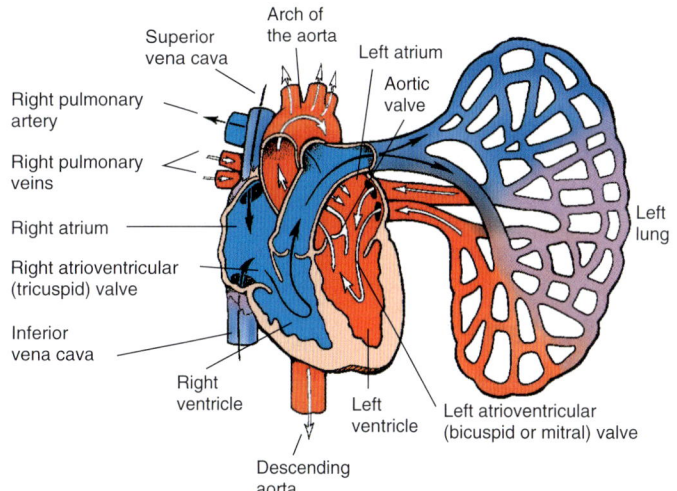

Fig. 27.3 Heart and great vessels: deoxygenated blood flow *(black arrows)*; oxygenated blood flow *(white arrows)*.

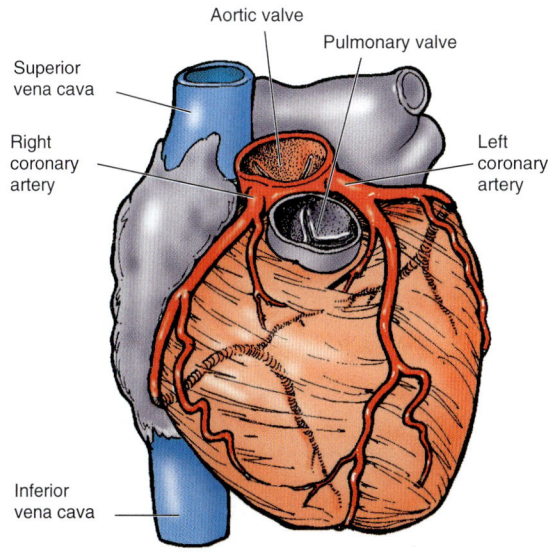

Fig. 27.4 Anterior view of coronary arteries.

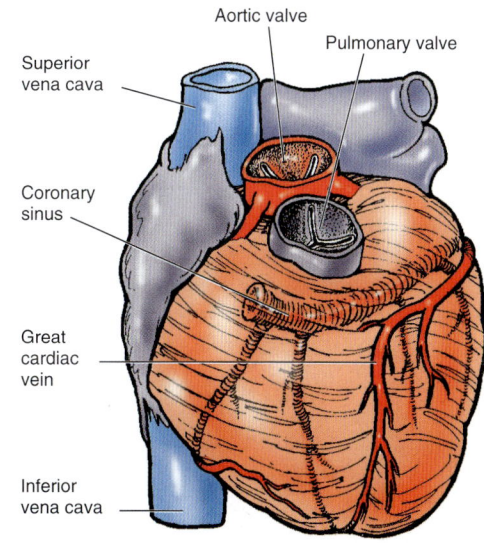

Fig. 27.5 Anterior view of coronary veins.

The velocity of blood circulation varies with the rate and intensity of the heartbeat. Velocity also varies in the different portions of the circulatory system based on distance from the heart. The speed of blood flow is highest in the large arteries arising at or near the heart because these vessels receive the full force of each wave of blood pumped out of the heart. The arterial walls expand with the pressure from each wave. The walls then rhythmically recoil, gradually diminishing the pressure of the advancing wave from point to point, until the flow of blood is normally reduced to a steady, nonpulsating stream through the capillaries and veins. The beat, or contraction and expansion of an artery, may be felt with the fingers at several points and is called the *pulse*.

Complete circulation of the blood through the systemic and pulmonary circuits, from a given point and back again, requires about 23 seconds and an average of 27 heartbeats. In certain contrast examinations of the cardiovascular system, tests are conducted to determine the circulation time from the point of contrast media injection to the site of interest.

Lymphatic System

The lymphatic system consists of an elaborate arrangement of closed vessels that collect fluid from the tissue spaces and transport it to the blood-vascular system. Almost all lymphatic vessels are arranged in two sets: (1) a superficial set that lies immediately under the skin and accompanies the superficial veins and (2) a deep set that accompanies the deep blood vessels and with which the superficial lymphatics communicate (Fig. 27.6). The lymphatic system lacks a pumping mechanism, such as the heart of the blood-vascular system. The lymphatic vessels are richly supplied with valves to prevent backflow, and the movement of the lymph through the system is believed to be maintained primarily by extrinsic pressure from the surrounding organs and muscles.

The lymphatic system begins in complex networks of thin-walled, absorbent capillaries situated in the various organs and tissues. The capillaries unite to form larger vessels, which form networks and unite to become still larger vessels as they approach the terminal collecting trunks. The terminal trunks communicate with the blood-vascular system.

The lymphatic vessels are small in caliber and have delicate, transparent walls. Along their course, the collecting vessels pass through one or more nodular structures called *lymph nodes*. The nodes occur singly but are usually arranged in chains or groups of 2 to 20. The nodes vary from the size of a pinhead to the size of an almond or larger. They may be spherical, oval, or kidney shaped. Large groupings of lymph nodes are typically found in the neck, armpits, and groin. Each node has a hilum through which arteries and veins enter, and *efferent lymph vessels* emerge. *Afferent lymph vessels* do not enter at the hilum, but rather enter the node opposite the hilum and break into wide capillaries that surround the lymph follicles and form a canal known as the *peripheral* or *marginal lymph sinus*. This network of capillaries continues into the medullary portion of the node, where absorption and interchange of tissue fluids and cells occur. The capillaries then converge into several efferent lymph vessels that leave the node at the hilum. In addition to the lymphatic capillaries, blood vessels, and supporting structures, each lymph node contains masses, or follicles, of lymphocytes that are arranged around its circumference.

Lymphocytes are added to the lymph inside the lymph nodes. It is thought that most of the lymph is absorbed by the venous system from these nodes, and only a small portion of the lymph is passed on through the conducting vessels to the terminal trunks.

The main terminal trunk of the lymphatic system is called the *thoracic duct*. The lower, dilated portion of the duct is known as the *cisterna chyli*. The thoracic duct receives lymphatic drainage from all parts of the body below the diaphragm and from the left half of the body above the diaphragm. The thoracic duct extends from the level of L2 to the base of the neck, where it ends by opening into the venous system at the junction of the left subclavian and internal jugular veins.

Three terminal collecting trunks—the right jugular, the subclavian, and the bronchomediastinal trunks—receive the lymphatic drainage from the right half of the body above the diaphragm. These vessels open into the right subclavian vein separately or occasionally after uniting to form a common trunk called the *right lymphatic duct*.

Lymphography is seldom performed in current practice because of the superior imaging capabilities of magnetic resonance imaging (MRI), computed tomography (CT), and positron emission tomography (PET) (Fig. 27.7). A more detailed description of lymphography is provided in previous editions of this text.

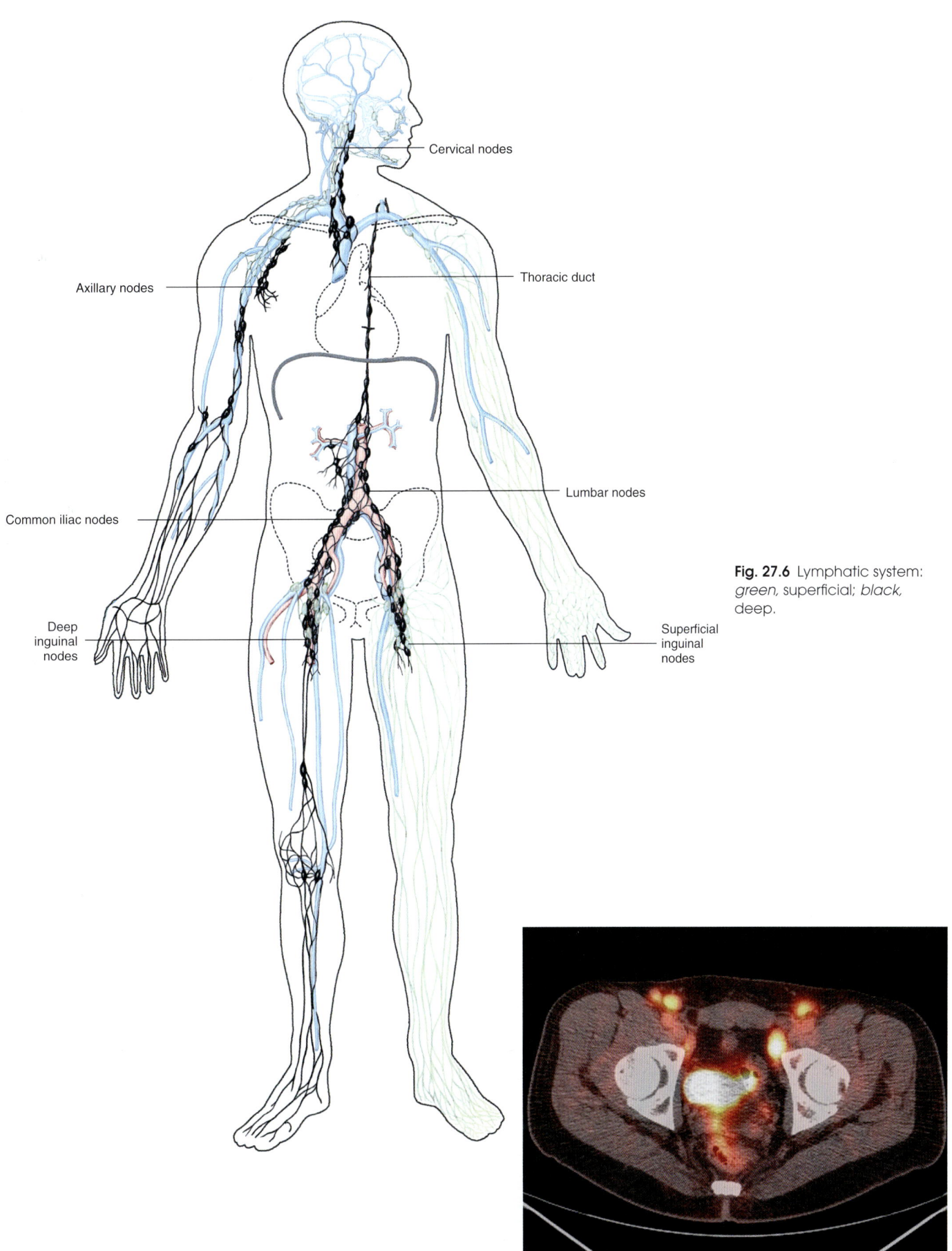

Fig. 27.6 Lymphatic system: *green,* superficial; *black,* deep.

Fig. 27.7 Axial PET/CT of lymph nodes with lymphoma.

Lymphatic System

ANGIOGRAPHY

Definitions and Indications

Angiography is a general term that describes the radiologic examination of vascular structures within the body after the introduction of a contrast media or gas. This procedure is primarily used to identify the anatomy or pathologic process of blood vessels. Angiography procedures include *arteriography* and *venography*. Examinations are more precisely named for the specific blood vessel opacified and the method of injection (e.g., renal arteriography).

Blood vessels are not normally visible on conventional radiography because no natural contrast exists between them and other soft tissues of the body. These vessels must be filled with a radiopaque contrast media to delineate them for radiography. Today computerized tomography angiography (CTA) and magnetic resonance angiography (MRA) are commonly performed *noninvasive* diagnostic angiographic studies. These imaging studies are discussed in subsequent chapters. This chapter will discuss *minimally invasive* angiography, in which radiographic images of vessels are taken as iodinated contrast is injected via catheters placed percutaneously into the vessels. Most angiographic procedures are performed to investigate anatomic variances, such as vascular disease, tumor, or injury; however, some evaluate the motion or function of an organ, such as the heart. Minimally invasive angiographic procedures can be purely diagnostic or, as is most commonly the case, a combination of both diagnostic and interventional (therapeutic) procedures. Many vascular pathologies are amenable to some type of percutaneous vascular intervention or treatment immediately after a diagnosis is confirmed with angiography.

Chronic cramping leg pain after physical exertion, a condition known as *claudication*, may prompt a physician to order an arteriogram of the lower limbs to determine whether atherosclerosis is diminishing the blood supply to the leg muscles. A *stenosis* or *occlusion* is commonly caused by *atherosclerosis* and is an indication for an interventional procedure such as percutaneous transluminal angioplasty. Cerebral angiography is performed to detect and verify the existence and exact position of an intracranial vascular lesion such as an *aneurysm*. An aneurysm can be treated with interventional procedures such as coil embolization.

Angiographic procedures of the heart are usually performed by interventional cardiologists rather than radiologists; however, there are many shared techniques and similarities between vascular interventional radiology and cardiac catheterization and interventional cardiology.

Angiography Team

The angiography team primarily consists of the physician (interventional radiologist, interventional cardiologist, or interventional neuroradiologist), one or more radiologic technologists, and one or more registered nurses. Other specialists, such as an anesthetist or respiratory technologist, may be necessary, depending on the patient's condition. Over the years, angiography rooms have developed from relatively simple diagnostic imaging rooms to large interventional suites comparable to operating rooms (ORs) with multiple imaging capabilities. These suites can accommodate a high volume of high-risk, high-acuity patients and require a large number of multimodality personnel to perform effective procedures.

The radiologic technologist is a key member of the angiography team and must receive dedicated education in either vascular interventional or cardiac interventional radiography. The technologist prepares the angiographic room, assists the physician with angiographic imaging, ensures that necessary supplies are readily available, and is often a scrub assistant to the physician. The technologist is also actively involved in patient education, patient positioning, preparing angiographic and medical equipment, maintaining a sterile field during procedures, and ensuring that radiation protection and safety measures are followed. The primary role of the nurse is to manage the overall patient care, including sedating and monitoring the patient and documenting the procedure. In some cardiac catheterization facilities, technologists with additional training and certification may also administer procedural medications, monitor the patient, and record patient *hemodynamic data*. Clear communication regarding the roles and responsibilities of staff during a procedure is essential.

Preparation of Angiographic Procedure Room

The angiography suite and every item in it should be scrupulously clean. The room should be fully prepared, with every item needed or likely to be needed on hand before the patient is admitted. Cleanliness and advance preparation are important in procedures that must be carried out under aseptic conditions. The technologist should observe the following guidelines in preparing the room:

- Ensure that patient information is entered correctly on acquisition equipment.
- Check the angiographic equipment and all working parts of the equipment, and adjust the controls for the procedure being performed.
- Ensure that all patient safety equipment is available, including emergency equipment.
- Ensure that all appropriate sterile supplies for the procedure are available as needed.

A comprehensive angiography suite contains a considerable amount of equipment other than angiographic imaging equipment (Fig. 27.8). Patient monitoring systems are necessary to record patient electrocardiogram (ECG) data, blood pressure readings, and pulse oximetry pre-, peri-, and immediately postprocedure. Emergency equipment must be readily available, including resuscitation equipment (e.g., a defibrillator for the heart) and anesthesia apparatus. Other imaging equipment, such as ultrasound, may be required for certain procedures or situations. Interventional devices often require accessory equipment to function. It is important for the technologist to understand when and how each piece of equipment is used and operated in a safe manner.

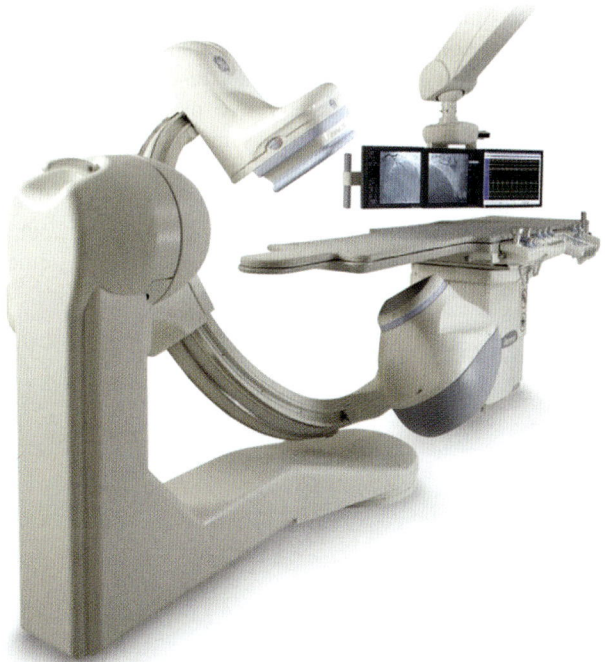

Fig. 27.8 Modern single-plane digital angiography suite.

(Courtesy GE Medical.)

Radiation Protection

Radiation protection during angiography is extremely important for patients and staff. Angiography procedures, especially interventional procedures, can include extended periods of fluoroscopy and multiple imaging sequences. The technologist is expected to know how to effectively use the imaging equipment to produce quality images while limiting the radiation dose.

There are many radiation safety features inherent in angiography equipment, such as shielding, collimators, low-dose parameters for imaging, low pulse rates for fluoroscopy, and last image hold on monitors designed to limit the radiation dose. Keeping the IR as close to the patient as possible reduces radiation scatter, and keeping the tube as far from the patient as possible reduces skin dose. All staff must wear lead protective clothing during fluoroscopy studies and maintain as much distance as possible from the tube during exposures. Lead-equivalent shielding should be utilized as much as possible to reduce the radiation dose to staff; when possible, staff should leave the examination room when imaging sequences are performed. Angiography suites are designed to allow observation of the patient at all times and provide adequate protection to the physician and staff. These goals are usually accomplished with leaded glass observation windows between the examination room and control room.

Contrast Media

Opaque contrast media containing organic iodine solutions are most commonly used in angiographic studies. Iodine absorbs x-ray energy, resulting in radiopaque images of iodinated filled structures. The iodine in the contrast media is incorporated into water-soluble molecules formed as triiodinated benzene rings, meaning there are three iodine atoms on each particle in solution (a 3:1 ratio).

Although usually tolerated, the injection of iodinated contrast media may cause undesirable consequences. The contrast medium is subsequently filtered out of the bloodstream by the kidneys. It causes physiologic cardiovascular side effects, including peripheral vasodilation, hypotension, and renal toxicity. It may also produce nausea and an uncomfortable burning sensation. Most significantly, the injection of iodinated contrast media may invoke allergic reactions. These reactions may be moderate (e.g., hives, slight difficulty in breathing) and require minimal treatment, or they may be severe and require immediate medical intervention. Severe reactions are characterized by a state of shock in which the patient exhibits shallow breathing and a high pulse rate and may lose consciousness. The administration of contrast media is one of the significant risks in angiography.

There are two major classes of triiodinated contrast: ionic and nonionic. Ionic contrast agents have high solubility, low viscosity, and high osmolar properties. Nonionic contrast agents have high viscosity and low osmolar properties. Nonionic contrast media cause fewer physiologic cardiovascular side effects, less intense sensations, and fewer allergic reactions.

Another type of contrast medium is a dimer, in which the two benzene rings are bonded together as the anion. Ionic contrast media with a dimer result in six iodine atoms for every two particles in solution, which yields the same 3:1 ratio as nonionic contrast media. The ionic dimer has advantages over the ionic monomeric molecule, primarily by reducing osmolality, but it lacks some of the properties of the nonionic molecule. Nonionic contrast media can also be found as a dimer, which yields a ratio of 6:1 because it does not dissociate into two particles, producing an osmolality similar to blood.

All forms of iodinated contrast media are available in various iodine concentrations. The agents of higher concentration are more opaque. Typically, 30% iodine concentrations (300 mg/mL) are used for cerebral and limb arteriography, whereas 35% concentrations (350 mg/mL) are used for visceral angiography. Peripheral venography may be performed with 30% or lower concentrations. Ionic agents of higher concentration and nonionic agents are more viscous and produce greater resistance in the catheter during injection.

Patients with a predisposition to allergic reaction may be pretreated with a regimen of antihistamines and steroids to help prevent anaphylactic reactions to contrast media. Patients who have a history of severe reaction to iodinated contrast media or with compromised renal function may undergo procedures in which CO_2 is used as a contrast agent. CO_2 is less radiopaque than blood and appears as a negative or void in angiographic imaging. CO_2 is approved for use only below the diaphragm because the possibility of emboli is too great near the brain. CO_2 imaging is possible only in the DSA environment because it requires a narrow contrast window and the ability to stack or combine multiple images to provide a single image free of bubbles or fragmented vascular opacification. Specific kVp values should be employed to display the CO_2 optimally in contrast to the rest of the body. Faster imaging rates are also required, usually 10 frames per second, because the CO_2 dissipates quickly within the blood.

Injection Techniques

Angiography primarily involves placing the catheter within a vessel and injecting a contrast media so that the vessel and its major branches are opacified. In a selective injection, the catheter tip is positioned into the orifice of a specific artery so that only that specific vessel is opacified. This technique has the advantage of more densely opacifying the vessel and limiting the superimposition of other vessels.

A contrast medium may be injected by hand with a syringe, but ideally, it should be injected with an automatic injector. The major advantage of automatic injectors is that a specific quantity of contrast media can be injected during a predetermined period. Another advantage to automatic injectors is the ability to operate these remotely from a shielded control room. This reduces radiation exposure to physician and staff while still allowing visualization of images and patient. Automatic injectors have controls to set the injection rate, injection volume, and maximum pressure. Another useful feature, the linear rate rise, sets a time interval during which the injector gradually achieves the set injection rate. This rate rise may prevent a catheter from being dislodged from its target vessel by reducing sudden catheter motion during contrast injection.

Because the opacifying contrast media are carried away from the area of interest by blood flow, the injection and demonstration of opacified vessels usually occur simultaneously. The injector is often electronically connected to the rapid serial radiographic imaging equipment to coordinate the timing between the injector and the onset of imaging.

Angiographic Imaging Techniques

Under fluoroscopic guidance, the intravascular catheter is positioned within the target vessel and a suitable imaging position and field of view are selected. At this point, an image that does not have a large dynamic range should be established; no part of the image should be significantly brighter than the rest of the image. This image can be accomplished by proper positioning, but it often requires the use of compensating filters. Most imaging systems have built-in compensating filters. If compensating filters are not properly placed, image quality is reduced significantly. Automatic controls in the system adjust the exposure factors so that the brightest part of the image is at that level. An unusually bright spot satisfies the automatic controls and causes the rest of the image to lie at significantly reduced levels, where the camera performance is worse. Proper positioning and technique are essential for high-quality imaging.

As the imaging sequence begins, an image that will be used as a subtraction mask (without contrast media) is acquired, digitized, and stored in the digital memory. Images are produced when the x-ray tube is energized, and x-ray exposures are taken in rapid sequence at 65 to 95 kVp and between 5 and 1000 mAs. The dose for each exposure may be the same as that used for a single conventional radiograph. As there is potential for high patient dose in angiography, it is important to utilize all methods available to decrease patient dose while maintaining optimal imaging quality. Images can be acquired at variable rates, from 1 image every 2 to 3 seconds up to 30 images per second.

The *acquisition rate* or imaging rate can also be varied during an imaging sequence or run. Most commonly, images are acquired at a faster rate during the passage of contrast media through the arteries, or atrial phase, and then at a reduced rate in the venous phase, during which the blood flow is much slower. This procedure minimizes the radiation exposure to the patient but provides a sufficient number of images to show the clinical information. Each of these digitized images is electronically *subtracted* from the mask, and the subtraction image is amplified (contrast enhanced) and displayed in real time so that the subtraction images appear essentially instantaneously during the imaging procedure. The images are simultaneously stored on a *digital imaging system*.

Some DSA equipment allows the table or the image receptor, such as a flat panel detector system, to be moved during acquisition. The movement is permitted to "follow" the flow of contrast media as it passes through the arteries. Sometimes called the "bolus chase" or "DSA stepping" method, this technique is particularly useful for evaluating the arteries in the pelvis and lower limb. Previously, several separate imaging sequences would be performed with the image receptor positioned in a different location for each sequence, requiring an injection of contrast media for each sequence. The bolus chase method requires only one injection of contrast media, and the imaging sequence follows (or "chases") the contrast media as it flows down the limb. The imaging sequence may be preceded or followed by a duplicate sequence without contrast media injection to enable subtraction. Occasionally, this method may need to be repeated because the contrast media in one leg may flow faster than in the other.

Misregistration, a major problem in DSA, occurs when the mask and the images displaying the vessels filled with contrast media do not exactly coincide. Misregistration is sometimes caused by voluntary movements of the patient, but it is also caused by involuntary movements, such as bowel peristalsis or heart contractions. Preparing the patient by describing the sensations associated with injection of contrast media and the importance of holding still can help eliminate voluntary movements. It is also important to have the patient suspend respiration during the imaging sequence.

During the imaging procedure, the subtraction images appear on the display monitor (Fig. 27.9).

Often a preliminary diagnosis can be made at this point. Some *post-processing* is performed after each exposure sequence to improve visualization of the anatomy of interest or to correct misregistration. The processed images are available on the computer monitor for review by the radiologist. As more advanced imaging software becomes available, more involved post-processing, including quantitative analysis, can be performed before the end of the procedure, allowing for accurate periprocedural diagnosis and treatment planning.

In most institutions, DSA images are stored in a *picture archive and communication system (PACS)*. These digital images can be transmitted via a computer network throughout the hospital or to remote locations for consultation with an expert or referring physician.

Angiographic Imaging Equipment

Rapid serial imaging used in angiography requires x-ray tubes to have high heat load ratings and multiple focal-spot sizes. Large focal-spot sizes of 0.8 to 1.2 mm are most capable of withstanding a high heat load and are used for abdominal and thoracic angiography. Small focal-spot sizes of 0.4 to 0.6 mm provide more detailed imaging and are used for cerebral and peripheral angiography. Magnification studies require focal spot sizes of 0.1 to 0.3 mm. X-ray tubes may have to be specialized to satisfy these extreme demands. Rapid serial imaging also necessitates radiographic generators with high-power output. Because short exposure times are needed to compensate for all patient motion, the generators must be capable of producing high-milliampere output. Imaging systems may be used either singly or in combination at right angles to obtain simultaneous frontal and lateral images of the vascular system under investigation with one injection of contrast media. This arrangement of units is called a *biplane imaging system* (Fig. 27.10). These biplane imaging systems are considered optimal for carotid, cerebral, and pediatric angiographic procedures.

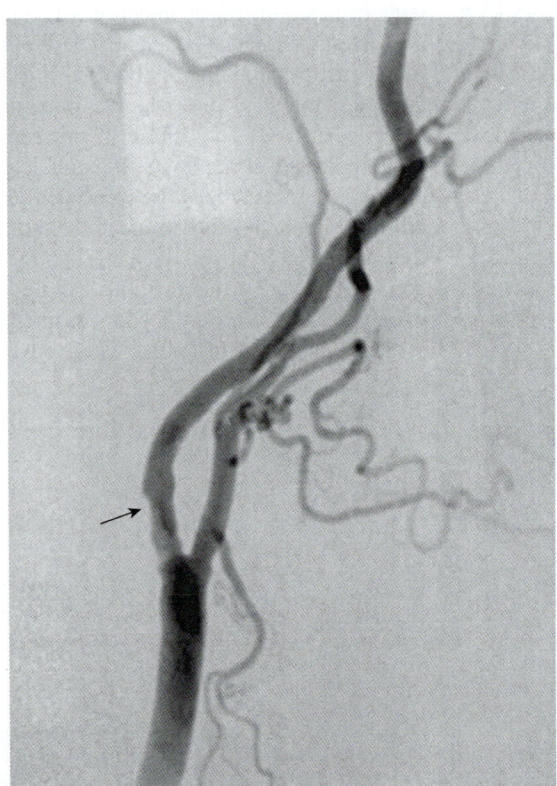

Fig. 27.9 DSA image of common carotid artery showing stenosis *(arrow)* of internal carotid artery.

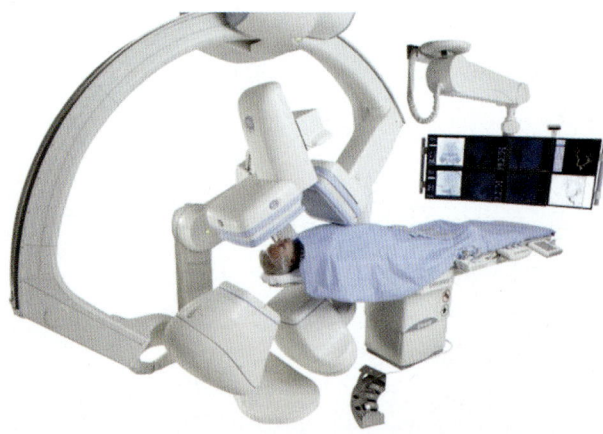

Fig. 27.10 Modern biplane digital angiography suite.

(Courtesy GE Medical.)

MAGNIFICATION

Magnification occurs intentionally and unintentionally in angiographic imaging sequences. Different magnification levels can be utilized by employing different focusing filters inside the image receptor. Varying the distance of the image receptor can increase this type of magnification. Intentional use of magnification can result in a significant increase in resolution of fine-vessel recorded detail. Fractional focal-spot tubes of 0.3 mm or less are necessary for direct radiographic magnification techniques. The selection of a fractional focal spot necessitates the use of low milliamperage. Short exposure time (1 to 200 ms) is necessary because of the size and load capacity of the smaller focal spot.

The formula for manual magnification is as follows:

$$M = \frac{SID}{SOD} \text{ or } \frac{SID}{SID - OID}$$

The SID is the *source-to-image receptor distance*, the SOD is the *source-to-object distance*, and the OID is the *object-to-image receptor distance*. For a 2:1 magnification study using an SID of 102 cm (40 inches), the focal spot and the image receptor are positioned 50 cm (20 inches) from the area of interest. A 3:1 magnification study using a 102-cm (40-inch) SID is accomplished by placing the focal spot 33 cm (13 inches) from the area of interest and the image receptor 68 cm (27 inches) from the area of interest.

Unintentional magnification occurs when the area of interest cannot be placed in direct contact with the image receptor. The magnification that occurs as a result of these circumstances is frequently 20% to 25%. A 25% magnification occurs when a vessel within the body is 20 cm (8 inches) from the image receptor—OID of 20 cm (8 inches)—and the SID is 102 cm (40 inches).

Angiographic images do not represent vessels at their actual size, and this must be considered when direct measurements are made from angiographic images. Increasing SID while maintaining OID can reduce unintentional magnification. When any measurement is necessary, the DSA post-processing quantitative analysis programs require the radiologist to calibrate the system by measuring an object in the imaging field of known value. Some systems calibrate by using the known position of the table, the image receptor, and x-ray tube and the tube angulation.

THREE-DIMENSIONAL INTRAARTERIAL ANGIOGRAPHY

To acquire a three-dimensional model of a vascular structure, a C-arm is rotated around the region of interest (ROI) at speeds up to 60 degrees per second. The C-arm makes a preliminary sweep while mask images are acquired. Images are acquired at 7.5 to 30 frames per second. The C-arm returns to its initial position, and a second sweep is initiated. Just before the second sweep, a contrast medium is injected to opacify the vascular anatomy. The second sweep matches mask images from the first sweep, producing a rotational subtracted DSA sequence. The DSA sequence is sent to a three-dimensional rendering computer where a three-dimensional model is constructed. This model provides an image that can be manipulated and analyzed. It has proved to be a valuable tool for interventional approaches and for evaluation before surgery. Various methods of vessel analysis are available with three-dimensional models. Aneurysm volume calculation, interior wall analysis, bone fusion, and device display all are possible (Figs. 27.11 and 27.12).

Angiographic Procedures

Angiographic imaging systems place the image receptor above the tabletop and the x-ray tube below. Generally, for angiographic procedures, patients lie supine, with the central ray located below, entering the posterior of the patient first, then exiting the anterior of the patient on its course to the image receptor. The position of the central ray technically results in PA projections; however, commonly used projections and tube angulations in angiography are described as AP projections. For example, a 45-degree left anterior oblique (LAO) is obtained by rotating the image receptor 45 degrees toward the patient's left; a 30-degree cranial projection is obtained by rotating the image receptor 30 degrees toward the patient's head. Fluoroscopy is often used to determine the final position and angulation of the central ray required to achieve the desired image.

PATIENT CARE

Before the angiographic procedure, it is necessary to explain the procedural process, risks, benefits, and alternative options to the patient and/or their family. Written informed consent is obtained to document that the patient gives their permission to proceed with the procedure. Informed consent is a legal document required for most angiographic procedures. Potential risks or complications of minimally invasive angiography include vasovagal reaction; stroke; heart attack; death; infection; bleeding at the puncture site; nerve, blood vessel, or tissue damage; and allergic reaction to the contrast media. Bleeding at the puncture site is usually easily controlled with pressure on the site. Blood vessel and tissue damage may require a surgical procedure. A vasovagal reaction is characterized by sweating and nausea caused by a decrease in blood pressure. The patient's legs should be elevated, and intravenous (IV) fluids may be administered to help restore blood pressure. Moderate allergic reactions to iodinated contrast media, such as hives and congestion, are usually controlled with medications and may not require treatment. Severe allergic reactions may result in shock, which is characterized by shallow breathing, high pulse rate, and possibly loss of consciousness. Angiography is performed only if the benefits of the examination outweigh the risks.

Patients are usually restricted to clear liquid intake and routine medications before undergoing angiography. Adequate hydration from liquid intake may minimize kidney damage caused by iodinated contrast media. Solid food intake is restricted to reduce the risk of aspiration related to vomiting.

Contraindications to angiography are determined by physicians and include previous severe allergic reaction to iodinated contrast media, severely impaired renal function, impaired blood clotting factors, pregnancy, and inability to undergo a surgical procedure or general anesthesia.

Risks of general anesthesia are greater than the risks associated with most angiographic procedures; therefore, conscious sedation is given, when applicable, to minimize patient discomfort and reduce anxiety.

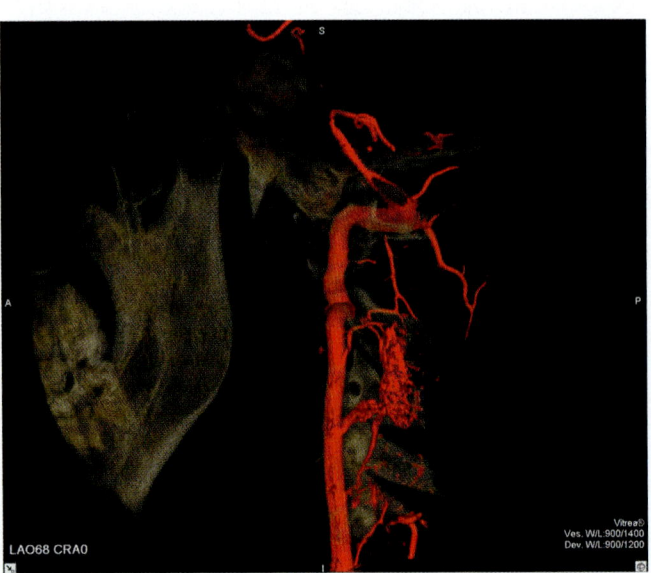

Fig. 27.11 Three-dimensional angiography provides for reconstruction of the skeletal vessels and the anatomy.

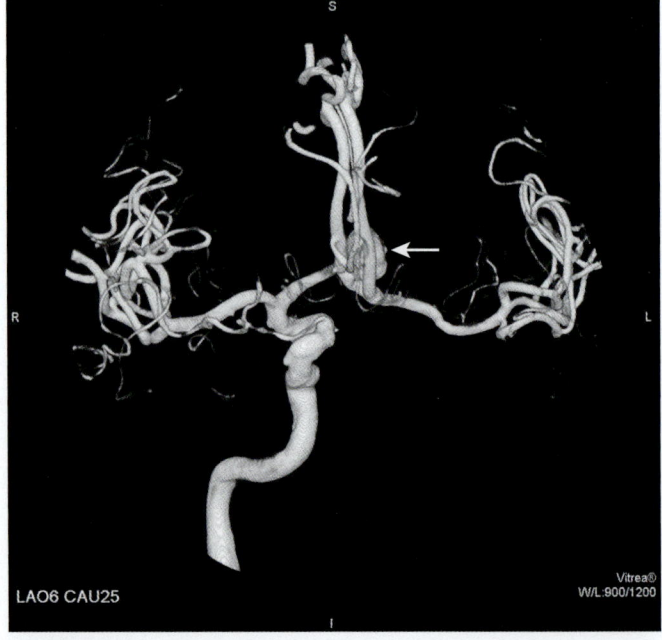

Fig. 27.12 Three-dimensional reconstruction of left internal carotid artery. Note the anterior communicating artery aneurysm *(arrow)*.

PREPROCEDURE

A preprocedure checklist is a useful tool to maximize patient safety during the procedure. A checklist may include the following:
- The planned procedure
- Indications for the procedure
- Patient history and physical examination (H&P) to include medications, allergies, previous surgeries, sedation risks, possible pregnancy
- Laboratory blood work (within appropriate date parameters): CBC, renal profile, PT/INR
- Verification of informed consent
- The preferred vascular access site
- Expected discharge arrangements

Prior to the procedure, the patient's vital signs (i.e., ECG, blood pressure monitoring, *pulse oximetry*) are recorded. The agreed-on site for vascular access is visually assessed and, for arteriography, arterial pulses distal to the arterial access site are assessed. The strength of distal pulses is documented prior to the procedure and will be assessed again postprocedure. Numerous sites can be used for vascular access and catheter introduction. The specific sites vary according to procedure, the age and body habitus of the patient, the preference of the physician, and vascular disease. The most frequent sites used for arteriography are the femoral and radial arteries. For venography and venous interventions, the brachial, axillary, subclavian, jugular, femoral, or popliteal veins may be chosen.

Periprocedure

Infection complications from percutaneous vascular access are rare; however, best practices in sterile technique are essential. The chosen vascular access site is exposed, shaved when necessary, and cleaned with an antimicrobial solution. Chlorhexidine-based skin preparations are most commonly used. The scrub assistant or the physician will drape and adhere sterile coverings around the exposed vascular access site, ensuring an adequate sterile field will be maintained throughout the procedure. The following considerations are taken when preparing the skin site and surrounding sterile field: providing adequate space to safely prepare, handle, and store opened sterile supplies during the procedure, such as access needles, guidewires, catheters, and sterile solutions; having the ability to move angiographic equipment into multiple angles around the patient without disrupting the sterile field; having the ability to incorporate additional imaging or interventional equipment into the sterile field; and knowing the location of patient monitoring devices, cables, and IV and fluid lines that are covered by sterile drapes.

Time-out

Immediately before vascular access is obtained, a time-out procedure is performed. This is a universal protocol in which all procedural team members stop what they are doing and collectively verify that the patient in the room is the correct patient for the correct procedure on the correct body part.

VASCULAR ACCESS AND CATHETERIZATION

Historically, the common femoral artery was the most commonly used arterial access site for angiography because it was associated with the fewest risks. The radial artery is quickly becoming the preferred access site, especially during cardiac catheterization, as the radial artery is superficial and more accessible than the femoral artery, which allows for more control of bleeding. Accessing the radial artery also results in a more comfortable postcatheterization recovery for the patient.

Catheterization for filling vessels with contrast media is preferred to needle injection of the media. The advantages of catheterization are as follows:
- The risk of *extravasation* is reduced.
- Most body parts can be reached for selective injection.
- The patient can be positioned as needed.
- The catheter can be safely left in the body while radiographs are being examined.

In 1952, shortly after the development of a flexible thin-walled catheter, Seldinger[1] announced a percutaneous method of catheter introduction. Seldinger described the method as puncture of both walls of the vessel (the anterior and posterior walls). The steps of the Seldinger technique are described in Fig. 27.13. The modified Seldinger technique allows for puncture of the anterior wall only and has become the preferred method. With this percutaneous technique, the arteriotomy or venotomy is no larger than the external diameter of the catheter, or vascular sheath used, minimizing bleeding. Patients can usually resume normal activity within 24 hours after the examination. Most outpatient angiographic studies can be performed in the morning, allowing the patient to be discharged later that same day. The risk of infection is less than in surgical procedures because the vessel and tissues are not exposed.

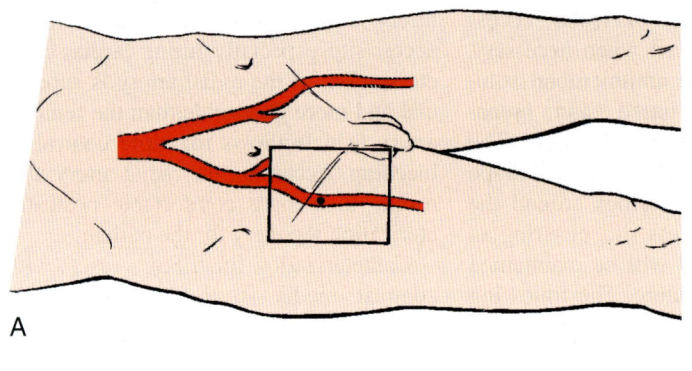

Fig. 27.13 Seldinger technique. (**A**) The ideal puncture occurs in the femoral artery just below the inguinal ligament. (**B**) Beveled compound needle containing an inner cannula that pierces through the artery. (**C**) Needle is withdrawn slowly until there is blood flow. (Modified Seldinger would puncture only here, on the anterior wall.) (**D**) The needle's inner cannula is removed, and a flexible guidewire is inserted. (**E**) Needle is removed; pressure fixes the wire and reduces hemorrhage. (**F**) Catheter is slipped over the wire and into the artery. (**G**) Guidewire is removed, leaving the catheter in the artery.

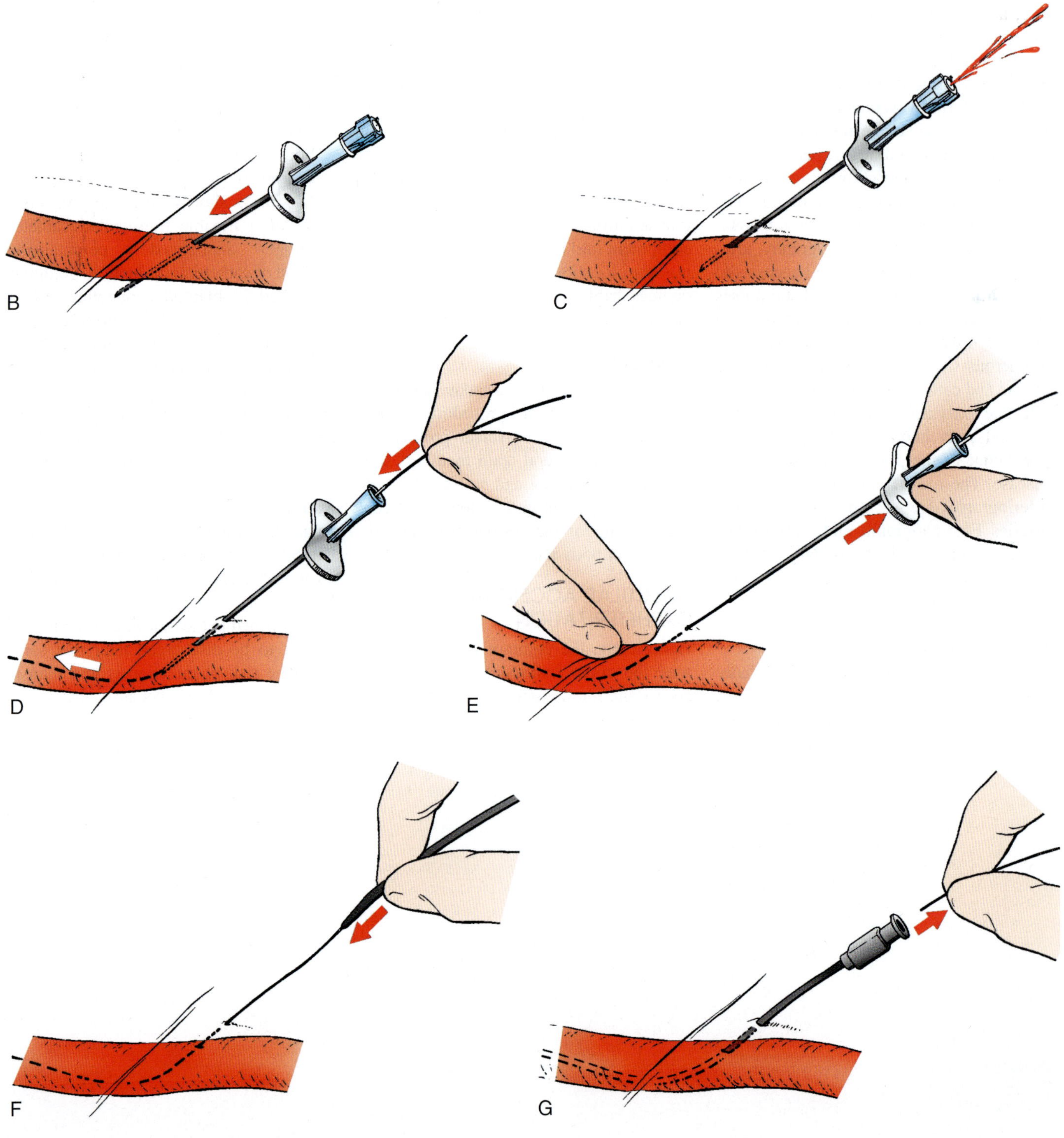

After the needle is introduced into the appropriate vessel, a guidewire is threaded through the needle and into the vascular system. The needle is removed over the guidewire and a catheter is then threaded onto and over the guidewire. Under fluoroscopic guidance, the guidewire and catheter are maneuvered to the desired location inside the patient by pushing, pulling, and turning the end of the catheter outside the patient. The guidewire helps to stabilize, manipulate, and guide the catheter while reducing any damage to the lumen of the vessel. When the wire is removed from the catheter, the catheter is aspirated to ensure blood return and then infused, or flushed, with sterile solution, most commonly heparinized saline, to help prevent clot formation. If multiple catheter exchanges are expected, a vascular sheath may be used. Assisting the physician in the catheterization process is often the responsibility of the technologist.

Vascular needles

Numerous vascular access needles are available for percutaneous procedures. Needle size is based on the external diameter of the needle and is assigned a gauge size. To allow for appropriate guidewire matching, the internal diameter of the needle must be known. Vascular access needles come in different types, sizes, and lengths. The most commonly used access needle for adult angiographic or cardiovascular procedures is an 18-gauge needle that is 7 cm (2.75 inches) long. This particular needle is compatible with a 0.035-inch guidewire, which is the most frequently used guidewire in cardiovascular procedures. Appropriate needle size is predicated on the type or size of guidewire needed, the size of the patient, and the vessel to be accessed. To decrease the chances of vascular complications, the smallest-gauge needle that meets the above-mentioned criteria is used for vascular access. Access needles for pediatric patients come in smaller gauge sizes with shorter lengths (Fig. 27.14).

Guidewires

Guidewires are used in angiography and other special procedures as a platform over which the catheter is advanced. To decrease the possibility of complications, the guidewire should be advanced into the vasculature ahead of the catheter. After the guidewire is positioned in the area of interest, the position of the guidewire is fixed, and the catheter is advanced until it meets the tip of the guidewire. Similar to needles, guidewires come in various sizes, shapes, and lengths, and care must be taken to match the proper guidewire to the selected access needle and catheter. The diameter of the guidewire is measured in inches. Common diameters are between 0.010 inches and 0.038 inches. Guidewire lengths typically range from 40 cm to 300 cm.

Most guidewires are constructed of stainless steel, with a core or mandrel encased circumferentially within a tightly wound spiral outer core of spring wire. The mandrel gives the guidewire its stiffness and body. The length of the mandrel within the wire determines the flexibility of the wire. The shorter the mandrel, the more flexible the wire and the more likely it is to traverse tortuous anatomy. A safety ribbon is built into the tip of the guidewire to prevent wire dislodgment in case the wire fractures. Many stainless steel guidewires are coated with polytef (Teflon) to provide lubricity and to decrease the friction between the catheter and wire. Similarly, the Teflon coating is thought to help decrease the thrombogenicity of the guidewire.

Plastic alloy guidewires consist of a hydrophilic plastic polymer coating. These wires provide a smooth outer coating with a pliable tip and exhibit a high degree of torque or maneuverability (Fig. 27.15).

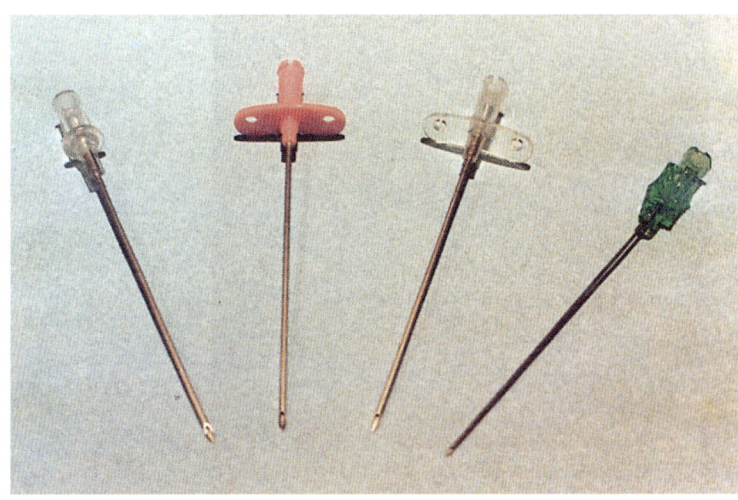

Fig. 27.14 Various needles used during catheterization.

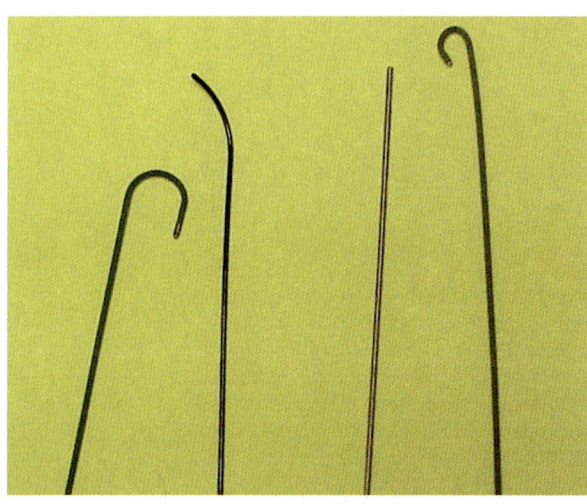

Fig. 27.15 A guidewire allows the user a high degree of torque and maneuverability. Various lengths and shaped tips are available.

Micropuncture access sets

Micropuncture access sets allow vascular access using a smaller-gauge needle, typically 21-gauge that accepts a 0.018-inch guidewire. Once the 0.018 guidewire is in the vessel, a coaxial short access catheter with a removable inner dilator is advanced over the 0.018 guidewire. The wire and inner dilator are removed, leaving the access catheter in the vessel. The access catheter has a lumen that will accept a 0.038 guidewire (Fig. 27.16).

Angiographic catheters

Angiographic catheters are manufactured in various forms, each with a particular advantage in size, shape, maneuverability or torque, and maximum injection rate (Fig. 27.17). Sizes of catheters are categorized by diameter and length. Catheter diameter is measured in French (Fr) sizes, with 1 Fr being equivalent to 0.33 mm or 0.013 inches. Common angiographic catheters range in size from 3 Fr (0.039 inch) to 8 Fr (0.105 inch). For diagnostic catheters, French sizes refer to the outer diameter of the catheter. Not all catheters of the same French size have the same inner diameter or lumen size. The lumen size is usually printed on the catheter packaging. It is important to know the lumen size of a catheter to ensure the correct fit for guidewires, microcatheters, and interventional devices. Commonly used catheters vary in length from 40 cm to 100 cm, although specialized microcatheters can be as long as 150 cm.

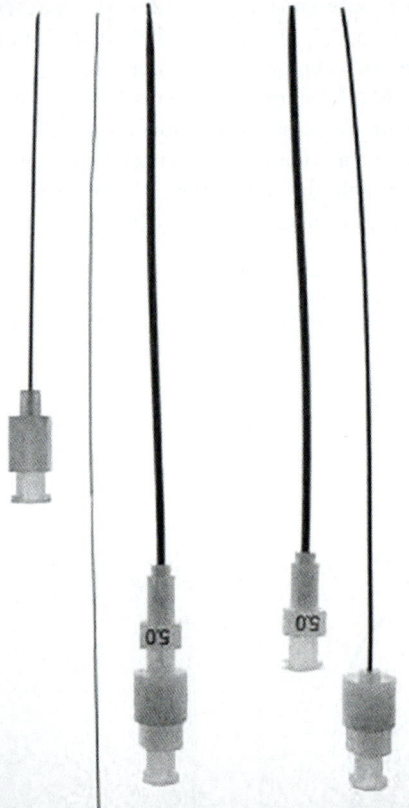

Fig. 27.16 Micropuncture access set. From left: 21-gauge needle; 0.018 guidewire; 5-Fr coaxial short access catheter with 3-Fr removable inner dilator; 5-Fr access catheter with 3-Fr inner dilator removed (accepts 0.038 guidewire; 3-French inner dilator).

(From Kaufman JA: Fundamentals of angiography. In Kaufman JA, Lee MJ, editors: *Vascular and interventional radiology: the requisites*, 2nd ed, 2014, Elsevier.)

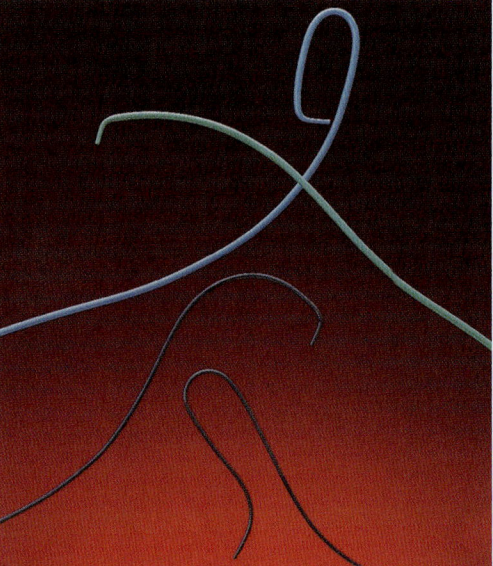

Fig. 27.17 Selected catheter shapes used for angiography.

(Courtesy Cook, Inc., Bloomington, IN.)

Catheters are made of pliable plastic to straighten for insertion over the guidewire. The catheters normally resume their original shape after the guidewire is withdrawn. Some catheters have multiple side holes to facilitate high-volume and high-pressure injection rates of contrast media, which are optimal for angiographic imaging in large vascular structures, such as in the aorta. These are commonly known as "flush" catheters. An example of a flush catheter is a pigtail catheter, which has a tightly curled catheter tip with multiple side holes and allows a large bolus of contrast media to be injected very quickly and safely. Maximum injection pressure rates and flow rates are listed on catheter packaging to prevent catheter damage and possible harm to the patient during automatic pressure injections. Selective catheters have only an end hole, allowing contrast media to be injected in one direction only. These "end-hole" catheters are available in many predetermined designs or shapes that help physicians maneuver the catheter tip into the origin of a particular vessel for selective contrast media injections.

Microcatheters and microguidewires are often used for distal, or superselective, catheterization. These microcatheter systems are usually threaded through a diagnostic catheter, or a specialized guiding catheter, coaxially for additional support during superselective procedures (Fig. 27.18).

Introducer sheaths

Introducer sheaths are frequently used in angiographic procedures when multiple catheter exchanges are expected or to assist with vascular closure at the end of the procedure. When the sheath has been placed, controlled access of the vasculature is ensured while reducing vessel trauma by limiting numerous catheter passages through the vessel wall.

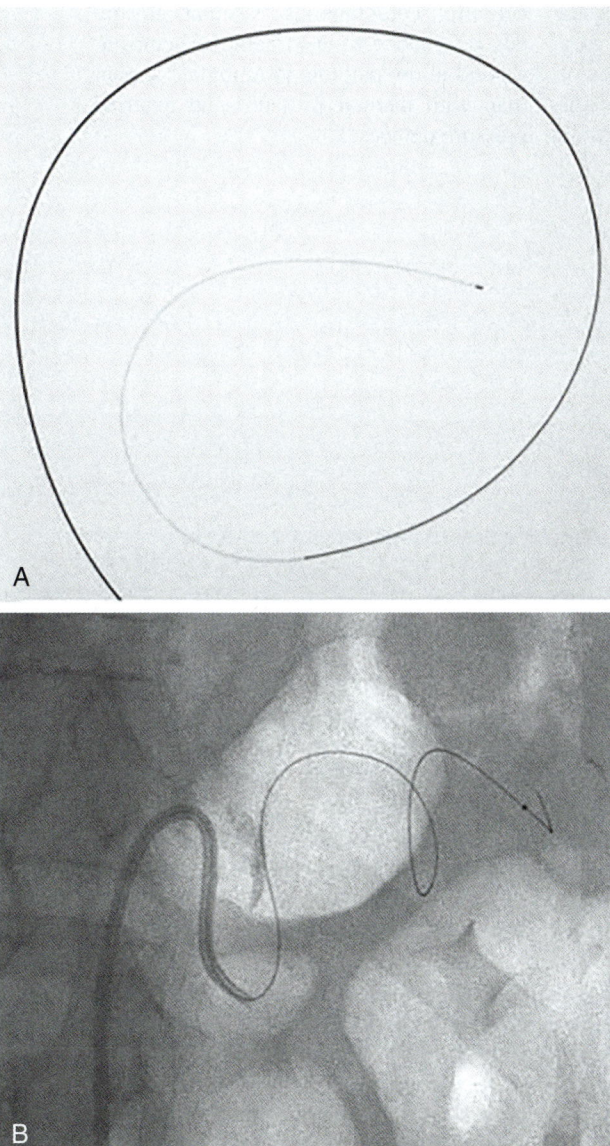

Fig. 27.18 (**A**) Typical microcatheter that tapers from 3-Fr to 2.3-Fr with radiopaque marker at tip. (**B**) Microcatheter is advanced over a 0.016-inch guidewire into distal splenic artery through a larger diagnostic selective catheter.

(From Kaufman JA: Fundamentals of angiography. In Kaufman JA, Lee MJ, editors: *Vascular and interventional radiology: the requisites,* 2nd ed, 2014, Elsevier.)

Introducer sheaths are short catheters consisting of a slotted, rubberized back-bleed valve and a sidearm extension port. The back-bleed valve prevents the loss of blood volume during catheter exchanges or guidewire manipulations. The sidearm extension port may be used to infuse medications, monitor blood pressure, or inject contrast media to visualize the vessel or adjacent vessels.

Similar to angiographic catheters, introducer sheaths come in various French sizes and lengths. Unlike catheters, however, introducer sheaths are identified according to the French size catheter they can accommodate, e.g., a 5-Fr introducer sheath will accept a 5-Fr catheter. To accomplish this, the outer diameter of an introducer sheath is 1.5 to 2 Fr sizes larger than the catheter it can accept; hence a 5-Fr introducer has an outer diameter of nearly 7 Fr. Typically, introducer sheaths range in length from 10 to 90 cm (4 to 35 inches) (Fig. 27.19).

POSTPROCEDURE

When the examination is complete, the catheter and sheath are removed. Pressure is applied to the site until complete hemostasis is achieved, while maintaining adequate blood flow through the vessel. Pressure can be applied manually by staff, by external pressure devices, or with percutaneous vascular closure devices. These percutaneous devices, considered internal closure devices, were designed for closing arteriotomies in the femoral artery after using sheath sizes between 4 and 8 Fr (Fig. 27.20). These devices work either by placing a collagen plug, a thrombin-collagen slurry, or a sealant gel between the artery and the skin, or by closing the arteriotomy with suture or a small surgical clip. Percutaneous vascular closure devices reduce time to achieve hemostasis and allow patients to ambulate sooner than with manual pressure and external pressure devices.

After procedures using common femoral arterial access, the patient remains supine and is placed on complete bed rest for 2 to 6 hours to decrease the chances for the development of bleeding or *hematoma* at the access site. Manual pressure and external pressure devices are used to obtain hemostasis for radial arteriotomies. Postprocedure recovery from radial arterial access is considered more comfortable for patients; only the affected arm is immobilized, allowing the patient to sit upright immediately postprocedure and often allowing them to ambulate sooner than with femoral arterial access. Obtaining hemostasis after venous access is achieved with manual pressure at the site.

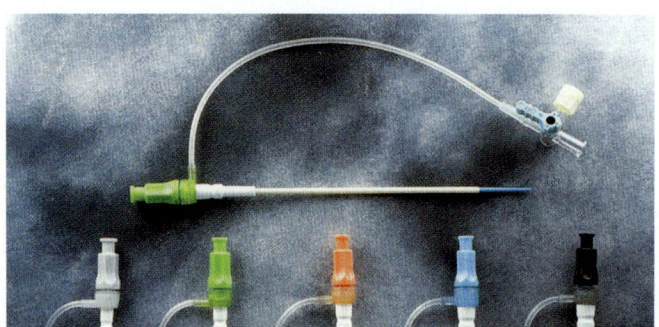

Fig. 27.19 Various types of introducer sheaths used during catheterization.

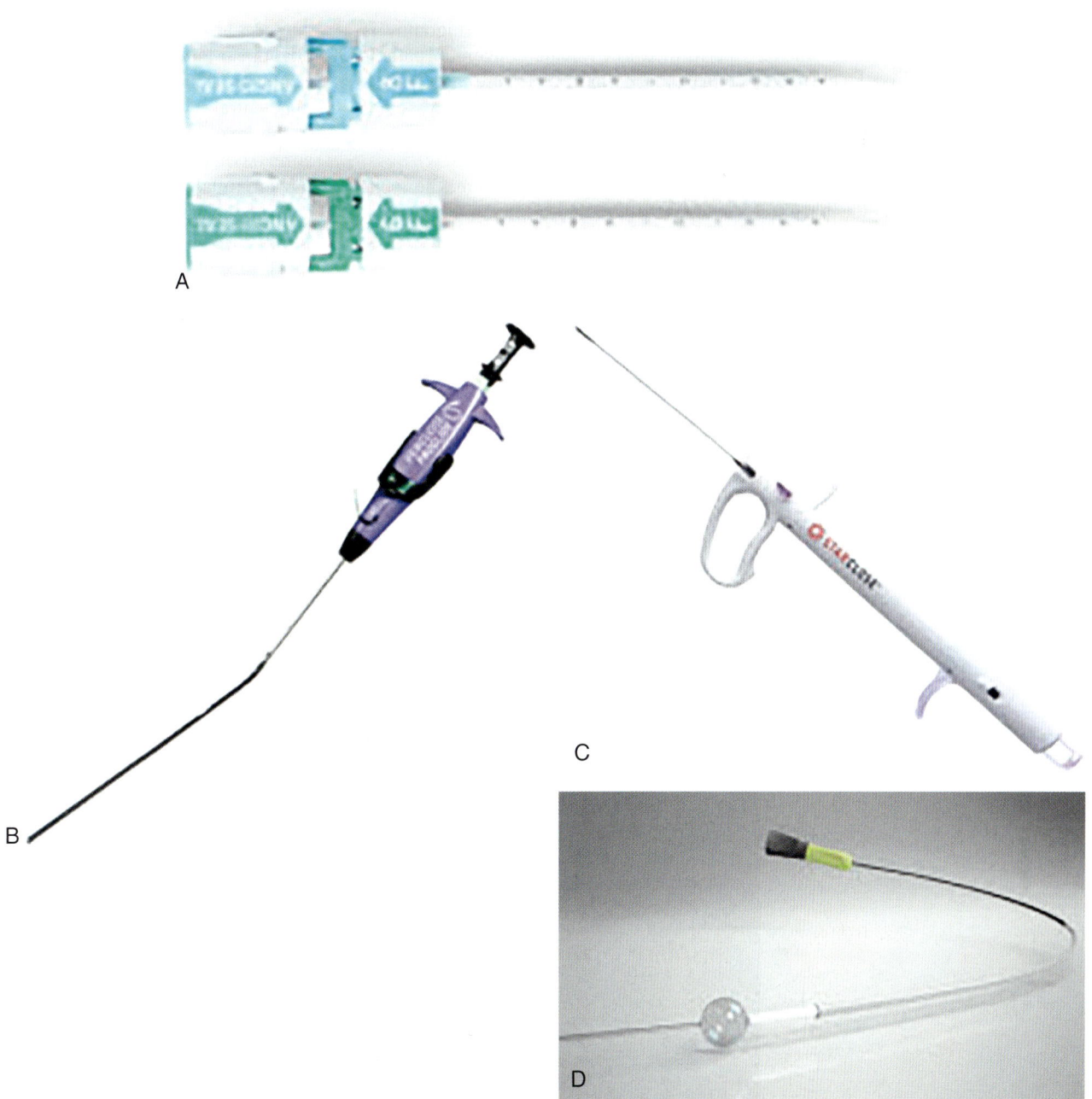

Fig. 27.20 Vascular closure devices. (**A**) Angio-Seal; (**B**) Perclose; (**C**) StarClose; (**D**) Mynx.

(A, Courtesy St. Jude Medical, Inc., St. Paul, MN; B and C, courtesy Abbott Vascular, Redwood City, CA; D, courtesy AccessClosure, Inc., Santa Clara, CA.)

ANGIOGRAPHY PROCEDURES

Aortography

Visualization of the aorta is achieved by placing a multihole, or flush, catheter into the aorta at the desired level, using the modified Seldinger technique. *Aortography* is usually performed with the patient in the supine position for simultaneous frontal and lateral imaging, with the central ray perpendicular to the imaging system.

THORACIC AORTOGRAPHY

Catheter-directed thoracic aortography is performed to evaluate congenital pathology, to accurately measure and assess aortic anatomy prior to endovascular intervention, and to assess postinterventional or postsurgical conditions.

When performing this exam, the technologist will do the following:

- For best results, increase lateral SID so that magnification is reduced.
- Consider a 45-degree LAO projection (or a 45-degree right posterior oblique [RPO]), which often produces an adequate study of the aorta.
- For lateral projections, move the patient's arms superiorly so that they do not appear in the field of view.
- For all projections, direct the perpendicular central ray to the center of the chest at the level of T7. The entire thoracic aorta should be visualized, including the proximal brachiocephalic, carotid, and subclavian vessels.
- Contrast media injection rates range from 15 to 25 mL/s for a total volume of 30 to 50 mL.
- Make the exposure at the end of suspended inspiration (Fig. 27.21).

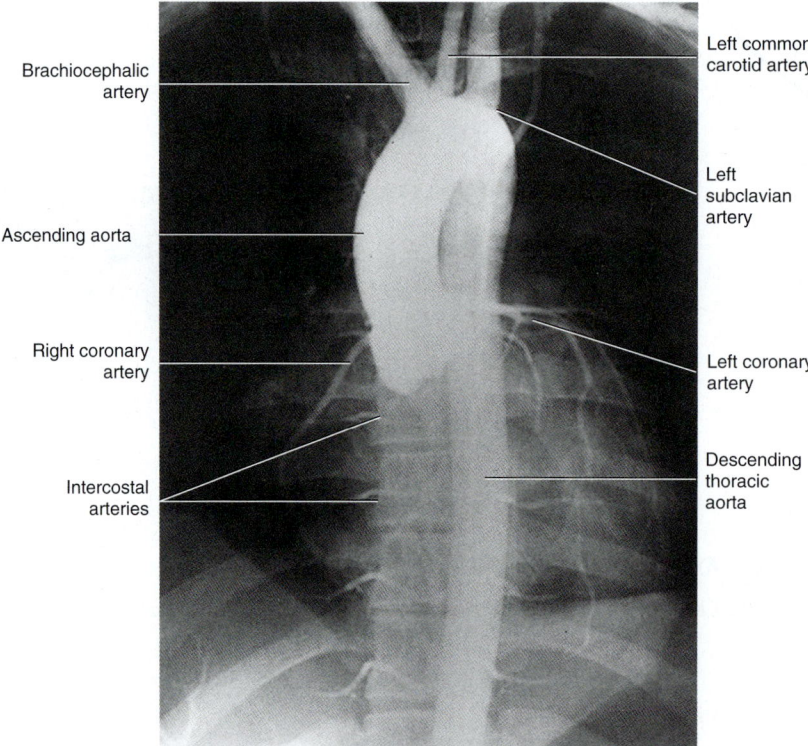

Fig. 27.21 AP thoracic aorta that also shows right and left coronary arteries.

ABDOMINAL AORTOGRAPHY

Abdominal aortography may be performed to accurately measure and assess aortic anatomy and pathology immediately prior to endovascular intervention. It may also be performed to assess postinterventional and postsurgical conditions.

- Direct the perpendicular central ray at the level of L2 so that the aorta is visualized from the diaphragm to the aortic bifurcation.
- The AP projection shows best the renal artery origins, the aortic bifurcation, and the course and general condition of all abdominal visceral branches.
- The lateral projection best shows the origins of the celiac and superior mesenteric arteries because these vessels arise from the anterior abdominal aorta.
- For the lateral projection, move the patient's arms superiorly so that the arms are out of the image field.
- Usually, collimate the field in the anterior aspect of the lateral projection. Filters may be necessary to reduce the image contrast in the field of view. Superficial bowel gas in the anterior aspect and the lumbar spine in the posterior aspect are both present in the field of view.
- Contrast media injection rates range from 15 to 20 mL/s for a total volume of 25 to 40 mL.
- Make the exposure at the end of suspended expiration (Figs. 27.22 and 27.23).

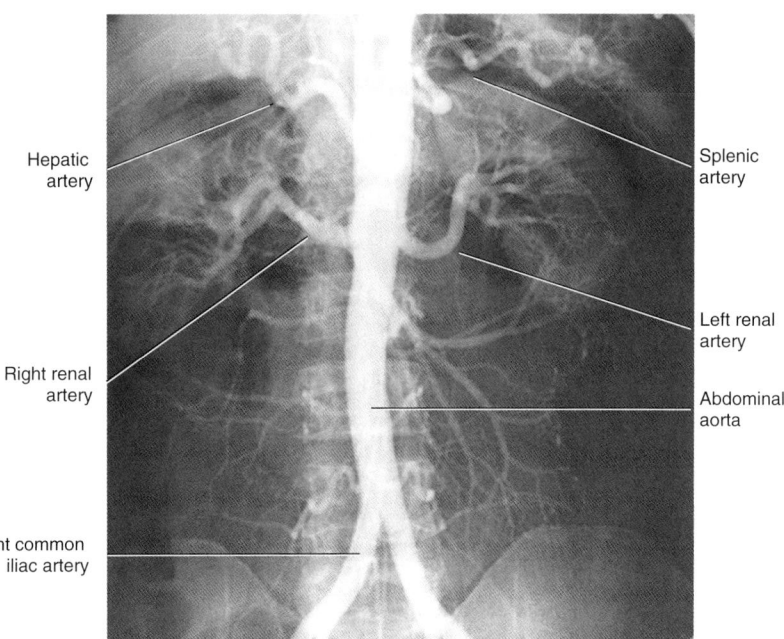

Fig. 27.22 AP abdominal aorta.

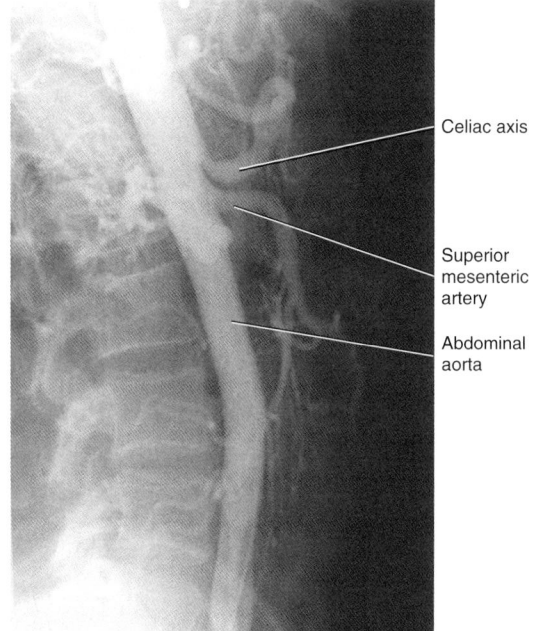

Fig. 27.23 Lateral abdominal aorta.

VISCERAL ARTERIOGRAPHY

Abdominal visceral arteriographic studies (Fig. 27.24) are usually performed to visualize tumor vascularity; to accurately identify the extent of atherosclerotic disease, thrombosis, or occlusion; and to locate the site of bleeding. An appropriately shaped catheter is introduced and advanced into the orifice of the desired artery.

- Position the patient in the supine position.
- Direct the central ray perpendicular to the image receptor.
- If necessary, use oblique projections to improve visualization or avoid superimposition of vessels.
- For all abdominal visceral studies, obtain angiograms during suspended expiration.

Selective abdominal visceral arteriograms are described in the following sections.

Celiac arteriogram

The celiac artery normally arises from the aorta at the level of T12 and carries blood to the stomach and proximal duodenum, liver, spleen, and pancreas.

- For the angiographic examination, center the patient to the image receptor.
- Direct the central ray to L1 (Fig. 27.25).
- Contrast media injection rates range from 5 to 10 mL/s for a total volume of 20 to 35 mL.
- To visualize the portal venous system, it is necessary to extend the imaging sequence.

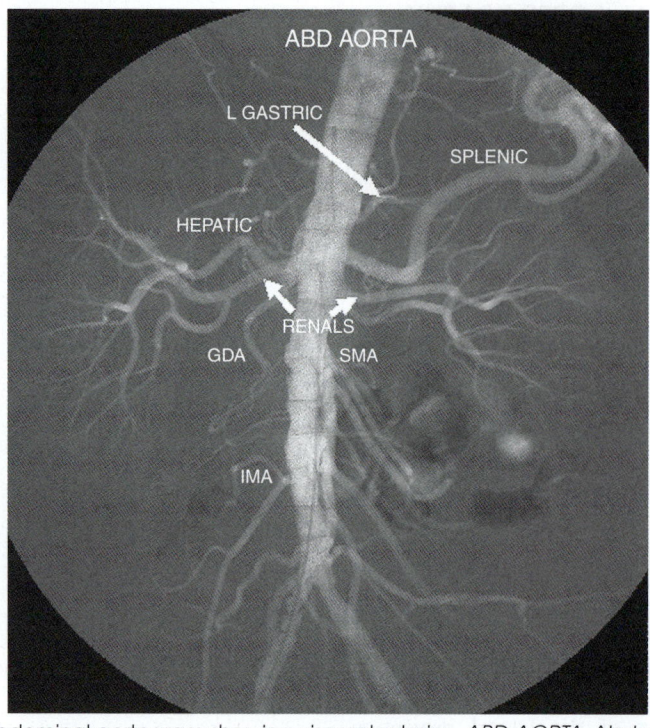

Fig. 27.24 Abdominal aortogram showing visceral arteries. *ABD AORTA,* Abdominal aorta; *GDA,* gastroduodenal artery; *IMA,* inferior mesenteric artery; *SMA,* superior mesenteric artery.

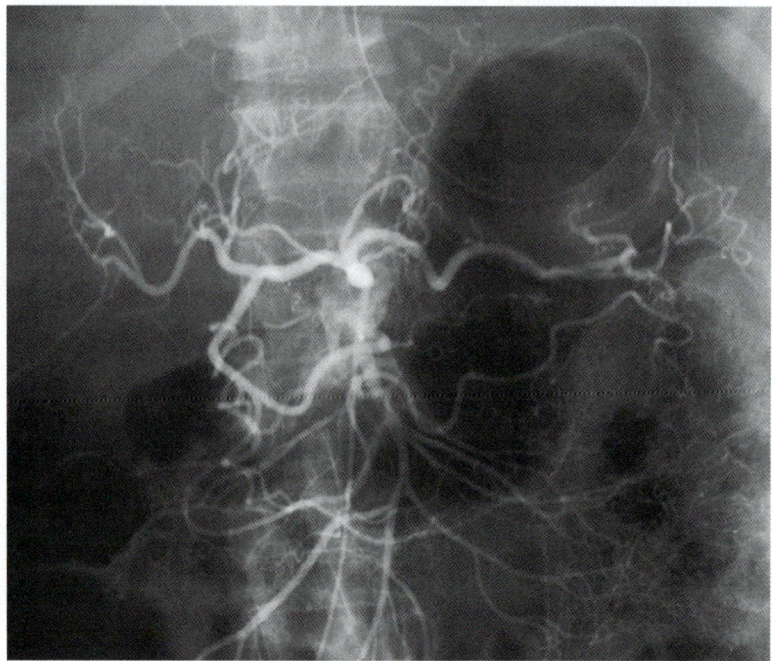

Fig. 27.25 Superselective celiac artery injection.

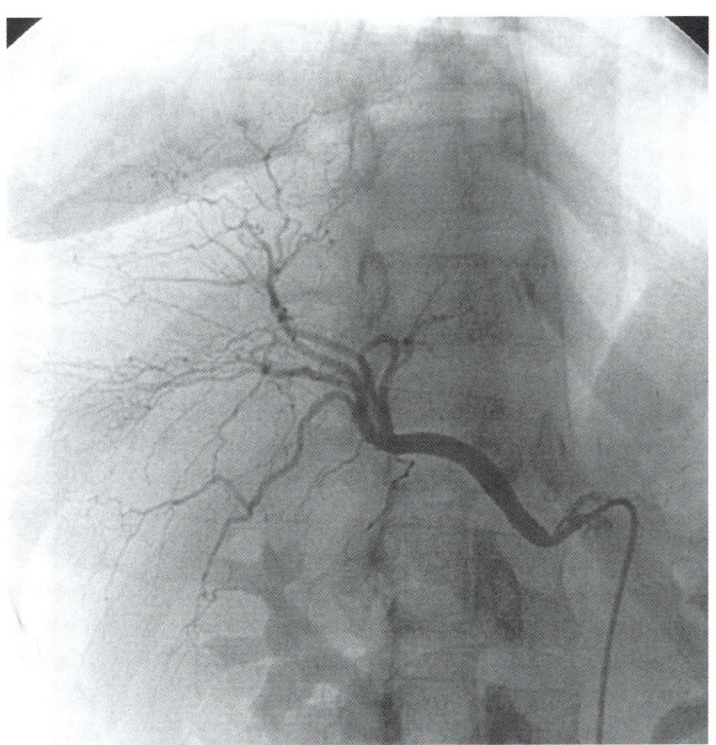

Fig. 27.26 Superselective hepatic artery injection.

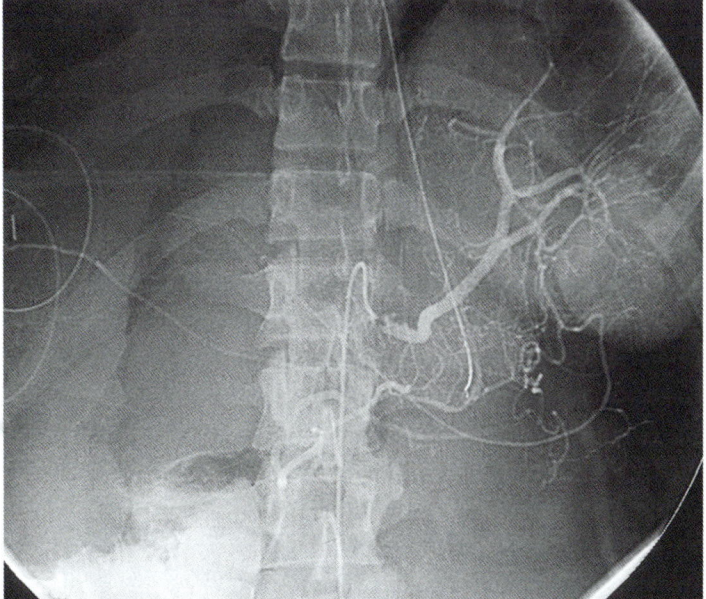

Fig. 27.27 Superselective splenic artery injection.

Hepatic arteriogram

The common hepatic artery branches from the right side of the celiac artery and supplies circulation to the liver, stomach and proximal duodenum, and pancreas.

- Position the patient so that the upper and right margins of the liver are at the respective margins of the image receptor (Fig. 27.26).
- Contrast media injection rates range from 5 to 10 mL/s for a total volume of 10 to 30 mL.

Splenic arteriogram

The splenic artery branches from the left side of the celiac artery and supplies blood to the spleen and pancreas.

- Position the patient to place the left and upper margins of the spleen at the respective margins of the image receptor (Fig. 27.27).
- Injection of the splenic artery can show the portal venous system on the late venous images.
- To show the portal vein, center the patient to the image receptor.
- Contrast media injection rates range from 5 to 10 mL/s for a total volume of 10 to 30 mL.

Superior mesenteric arteriogram

The superior mesenteric artery (SMA) supplies blood to the small intestine and the ascending and transverse colon. It arises at about the level of L1 and descends to L5–S1.

- To visualize the SMA, center the patient to the midline of the image receptor.
- Direct the central ray to the level of L3 (Fig. 27.28).
- It may be necessary to inject a number of times with overlapping fields of view to visualize the entire area supplied by the SMA.
- Contrast media injection rates range from 5 to 10 mL/s for a total volume of 10 to 35 mL.
- When attempting to visualize bleeding sites, extend the exposure duration to 60 seconds or as requested by the radiologist.

Inferior mesenteric arteriogram

The inferior mesenteric artery (IMA) supplies blood to the splenic flexure, descending colon, and rectosigmoid area. It arises from the left side of the aorta at about the level of L3 and descends into the pelvis.

- To visualize the IMA best, use a 15-degree right anterior oblique (RAO) or left posterior oblique (LPO) projection that places the descending colon and rectum at the left and inferior margins of the image (Fig. 27.29).
- It may be necessary to inject a number of times with overlapping fields of view to visualize the entire area supplied by the IMA.
- Contrast media injection rates range from 3 to 5 mL/s for a total volume of 9 to 15 mL.

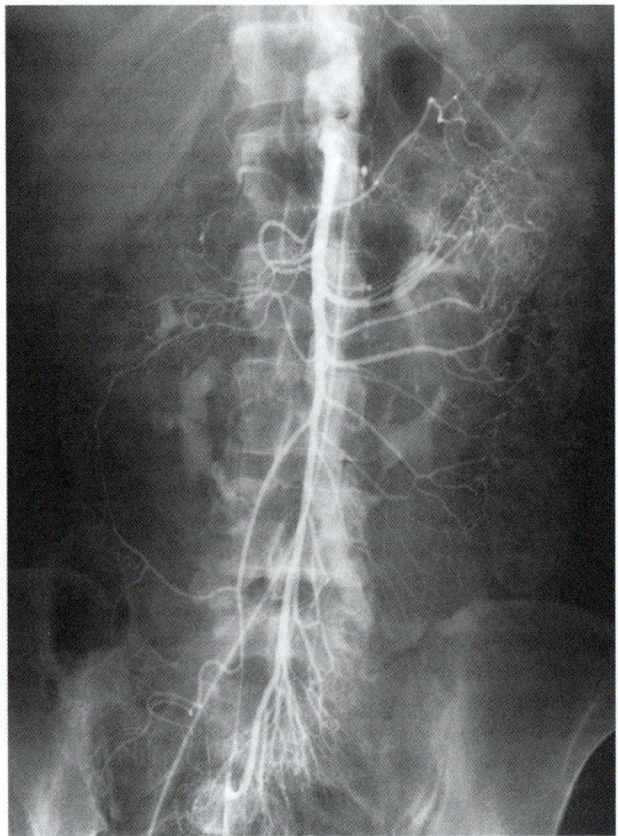

Fig. 27.28 Selective SMA injection.

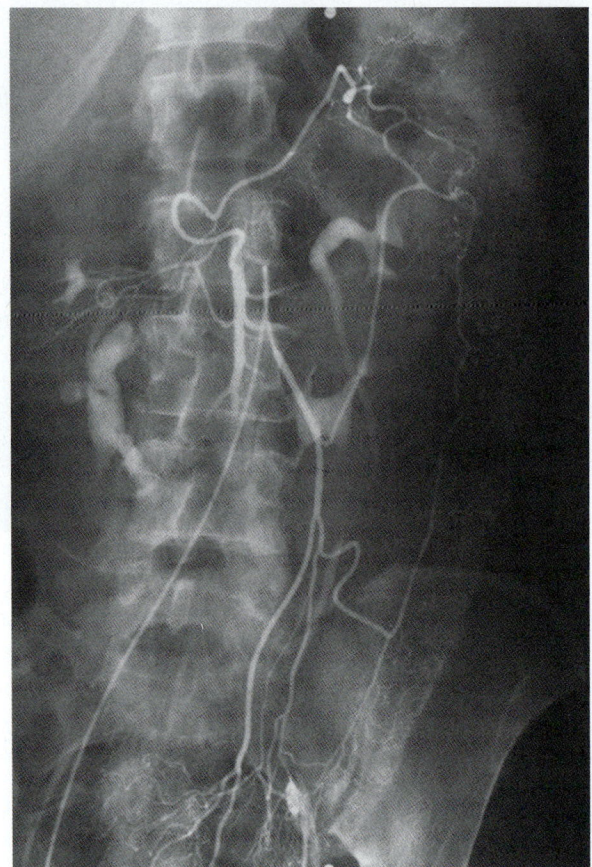

Fig. 27.29 Selective IMA injection.

Renal arteriogram

The renal arteries arise from the right and left side of the aorta between L1 and L2 and supply blood to the respective kidney.

- A renal flush aortogram may be accomplished by injecting 10 to 20 mL/s for a total volume of 20 to 40 mL of contrast media through a catheter with multiple side holes positioned in the aorta at the level of the renal arteries.
- For a right renal arteriogram, position the patient so that the central ray enters at the level of L2 midway between the center of the spine and the patient's right side.
- For a selective left renal arteriogram, position the patient so that the central ray enters at the level of L1 midway between the center of the spine and the patient's left side (Fig. 27.30).

A representative selective renal injection is 5 mL/s for a 10-mL total volume.

Other arteriograms

Other arteries branching from the aorta may be selectively studied to show anatomy and possible pathology. The positioning for these procedures depends on the area to be studied and the surrounding structures; these procedures may include spinal, bronchial, phrenic, adrenal, or lumbar arteriograms.

PULMONARY ARTERIOGRAPHY

Pulmonary arteriography is most commonly performed prior to interventional procedures such as thrombolysis, thrombectomy, embolization, balloon angioplasty, and stent placement. Unlike other arteriograms, pulmonary arteriography is performed using venous access, most commonly the internal jugular, subclavian, or femoral vein. Under fluoroscopic control, a catheter is directed through the vena cava and right side of the heart and into the pulmonary arteries. Depending on the location of pathology, catheter placement is either within the main pulmonary arteries or selective for more localized imaging (Fig. 27.31).

- Position the patient in the supine position.
- Image in both AP and oblique views.
- Multiple views may be required to cover apex and base of lung.
- Contrast media injection rates range from 10 to 20 mL/s for a total volume of 20 to 40 mL.
- Make exposures at end of suspending inspiration.

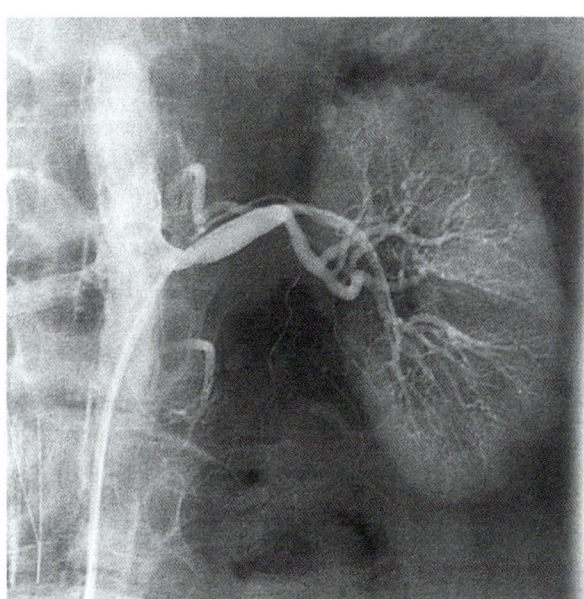

Fig. 27.30 Selective left renal artery injection in early arterial phase.

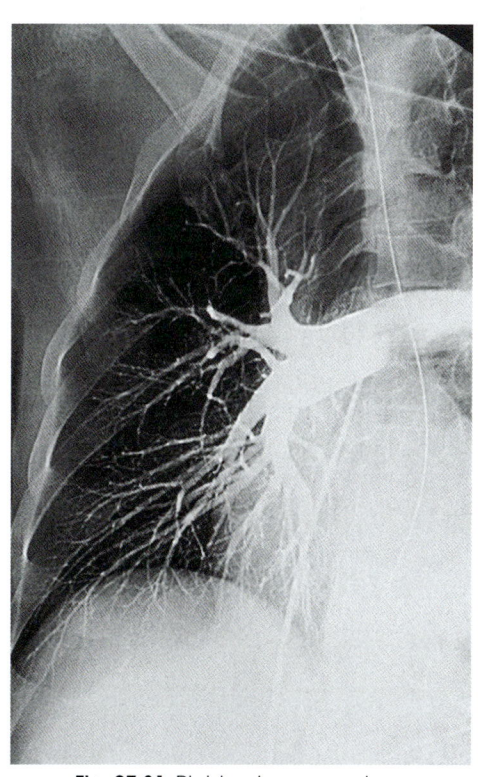

Fig. 27.31 Right pulmonary artery.

Peripheral Angiography
LOWER LIMB ARTERIOGRAMS

Aortofemoral arteriography is usually performed to accurately assess vascular pathology prior to intervention. The catheter tip is positioned superior to the aortic bifurcation so that bilateral arteriograms are obtained simultaneously. When only one leg is to be examined, the catheter tip is placed below the bifurcation, or the contrast media is injected through a catheter or sheath placed in the femoral artery on the side of interest.

- For a bilateral examination, place the patient in the supine position for single-plane AP projections and center the patient to the midline of the image receptor. Images include the area from the renal arteries to the ankles (Fig. 27.32).
- Internally rotate the legs 30 degrees.
- Subtracted or unsubtracted bolus chase selections can be used to follow the contrast media down the legs, or alternately, a number of stationary DSA imaging sequences can be performed to cover the area of interest.
- Make exposures of the opacified lower abdominal aorta and aortic bifurcation with the patient in suspended expiration.
- Examinations of a specific area of the leg, such as the popliteal fossa or foot, are occasionally performed.
- AP or lateral projections, or both, may be obtained with the patient centered to the designated area.
- Contrast media injection rates range from 5 to 10 mL/s for a total of 40 to 60 mL for bolus chase, or from 5 to 10 mL/s for a total of 10 to 30 mL for stationary DSA sequences.

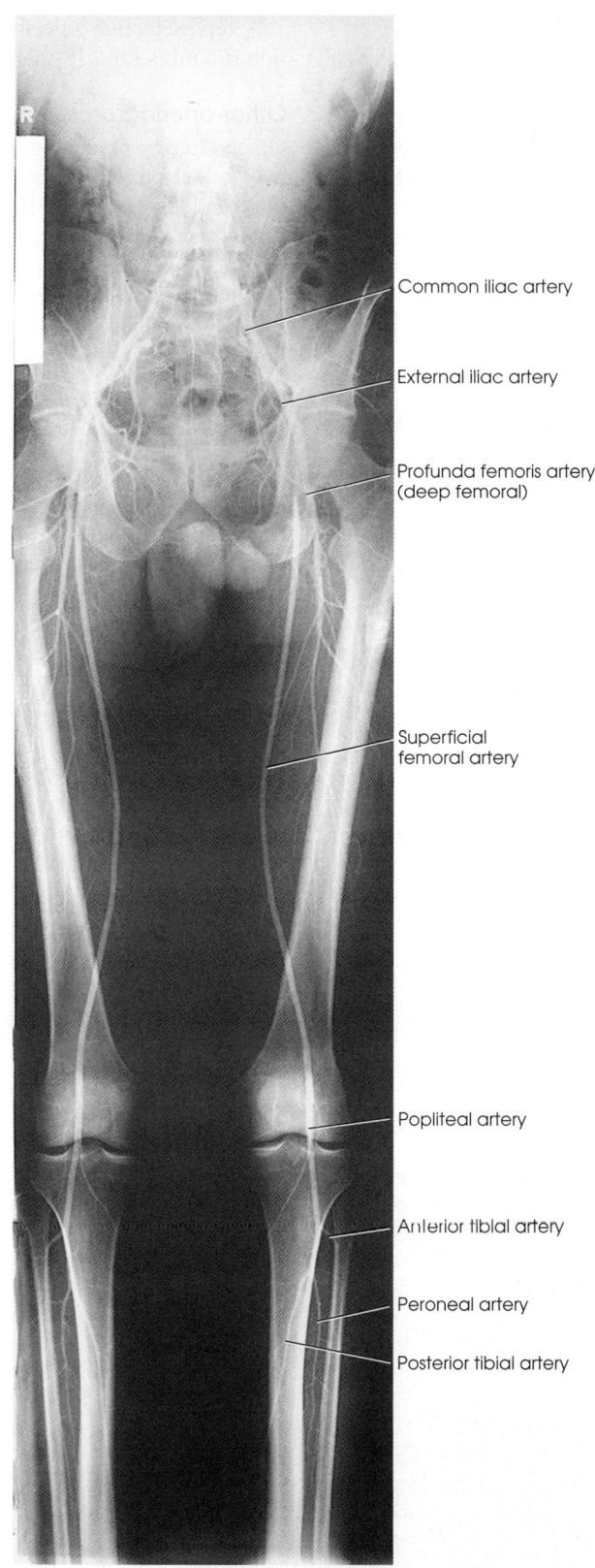

Fig. 27.32 Normal abdominal aortogram and bilateral femoral arteriogram in late arterial phase.

UPPER LIMB ARTERIOGRAMS

Upper limb arteriography is most often performed to evaluate traumatic injury, atherosclerotic disease, or other vascular lesions. Arteriograms are obtained by introducing a catheter, most often at a femoral artery site, for selective injection into the subclavian or axillary artery. The contrast media may also be injected at a more distal site through a catheter. The area to be radiographed may be a hand or another selected part of the arm or the entire upper extremity and thorax. When pathology is suspected in the brachiocephalic arteries, an arch aortogram is performed.

- The recommended projection is a true AP projection with the arm extended and the hand supinated. Hand arteriograms may be obtained in the supine or prone arm position (Figs. 27.33 and 27.34).
- The injection varies from 3 to 4 mL/s through a catheter positioned distally to 10 mL/s through a proximally positioned catheter.

Images are obtained by using a bolus chase technique or by performing serial runs over each segment of the extremity.

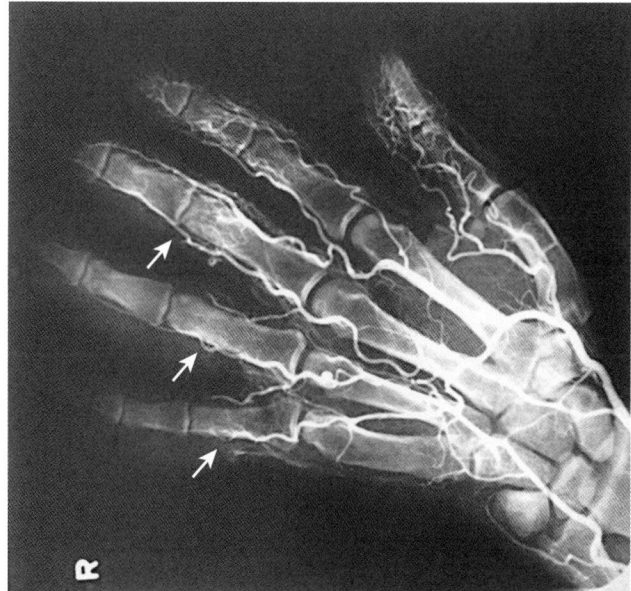

Fig. 27.33 Right hand arteriogram (2:1 magnification) showing severe arterial occlusive disease *(arrows)* affecting digits after cold temperature injury.

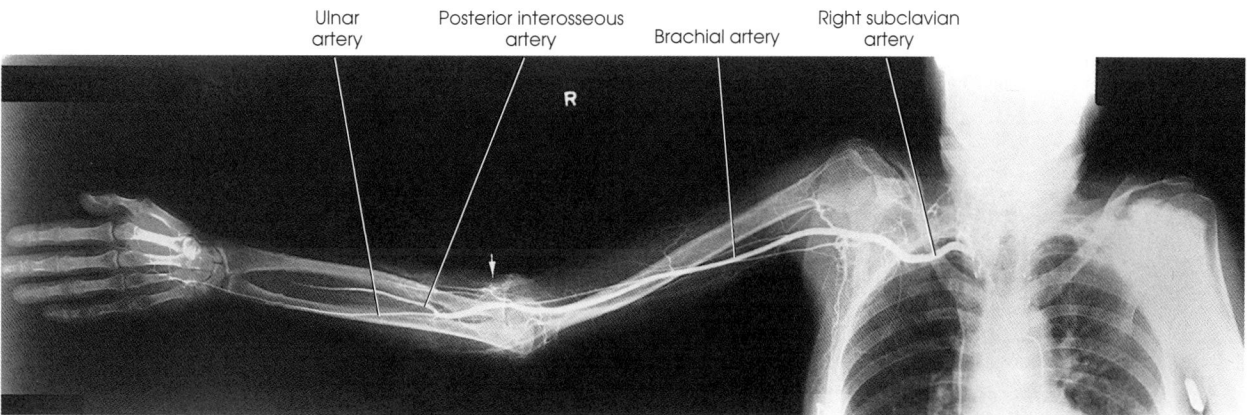

Fig. 27.34 Right subclavian artery injection showing iatrogenic occlusion of radial artery *(arrow)*.

CEREBRAL ANGIOGRAPHY

Cerebral Anatomy

Cerebral angiography demonstrates the blood vessels of the brain. The procedure was introduced by Egas Moniz[2] in 1927. It is performed to investigate intracranial vascular lesions such as aneurysms, arteriovenous malformations (AVMs), tumors, atherosclerotic or stenotic lesions, and acute thrombus (blood clot).

The brain is supplied by four trunk vessels or great vessels (Fig. 27.35): the right and left common carotid arteries, which supply the anterior circulation, and the right and left vertebral arteries, which supply the posterior circulation. These paired arteries branch from the arch of the aorta and ascend through the neck.

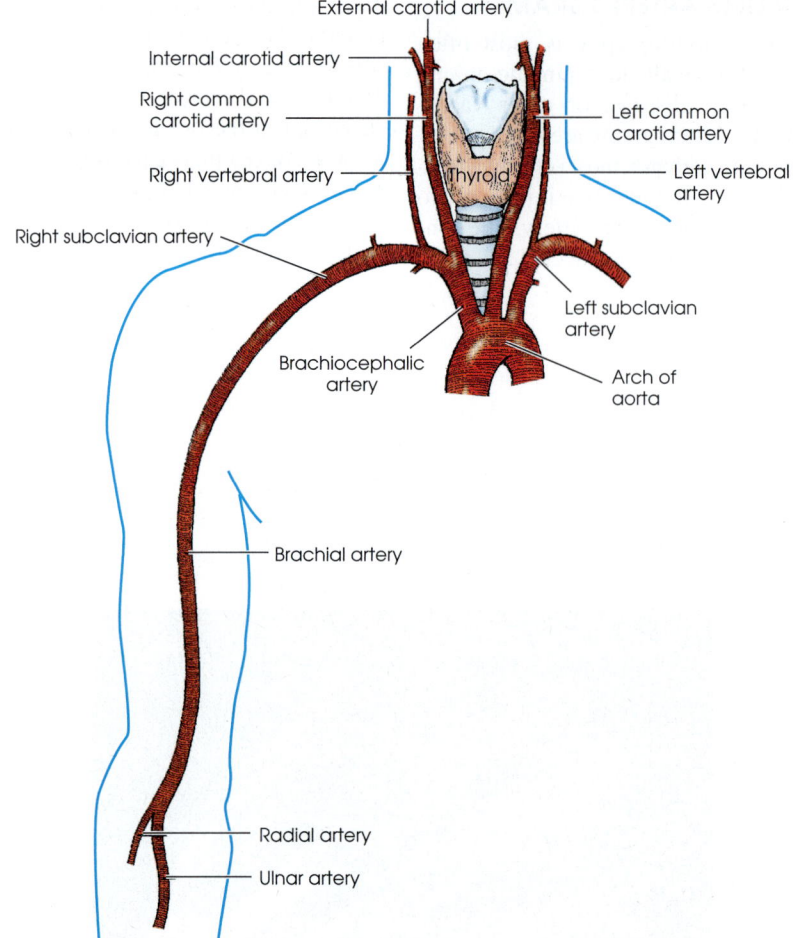

Fig. 27.35 Major arteries of upper chest, neck, and arm.

The first branch of the aortic arch is the *innominate artery* or the *brachiocephalic artery*. It bifurcates into the right common carotid artery (CCA) and the right subclavian artery. The second branch of the aortic arch is the left CCA, followed by the left subclavian artery. Each of the vessels originates directly from the aortic arch. Both vertebral arteries most commonly take their origins from the subclavian arteries. Although this branching pattern is common in most patients, there can be some *anomalous* origins of these great vessels. Each CCA passes superiorly and laterally alongside the trachea and larynx to the level of C4 and then divides into internal and external carotid arteries (ECAs). The ECA contributes blood supply to the extracranial and extra-axial circulation. There can be some collateral circulation into the internal carotid circulation in some situations. The internal carotid artery (ICA) enters the cranium through the carotid foramen of the temporal bone and bifurcates into the anterior and middle cerebral arteries (Fig. 27.36). These vessels branch and rebranch to supply the anterior circulation of the respective hemisphere of the brain.

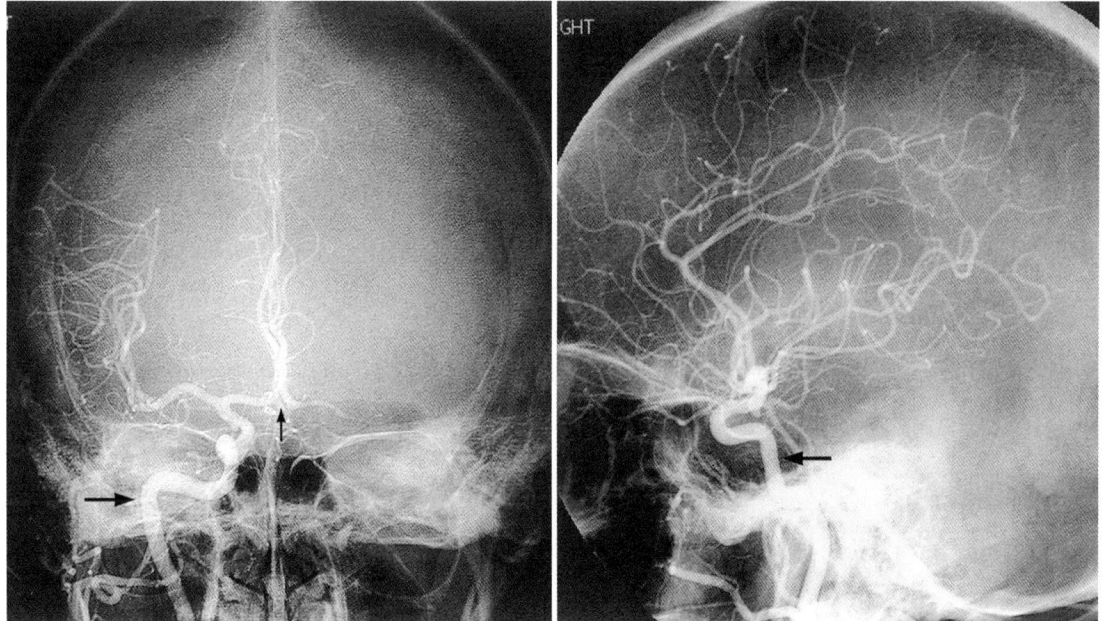

Fig. 27.36 Right common carotid artery injection showing right internal carotid artery *(arrows)* and anterior cerebral blood circulation, including reflux across anterior communicating artery *(small arrow)*.

The vertebral arteries ascend through the cervical transverse foramina and pass medially to enter the cranium through the foramen magnum. The vertebral arteries unite to form the basilar artery, which, after a short superior course along the posterior surface of the dorsum sellae, bifurcates into the right and left posterior cerebral arteries. The blood supply to the posterior fossa (cerebellum) originates from the vertebral and basilar arteries (Fig. 27.37).

The anterior and posterior cerebral arteries are connected by communicating arteries at the level of the midbrain to form the *circle of Willis*. The anterior communicating artery forms an anastomosis between the anterior cerebral arteries, which communicate between the right and left hemispheres. The right and left posterior communicating arteries each form an anastomosis between the ICA and the posterior cerebral artery, connecting the anterior and posterior circulation. Illustrations that detail intracerebral circulation are provided in Figs. 27.38 and 27.39.

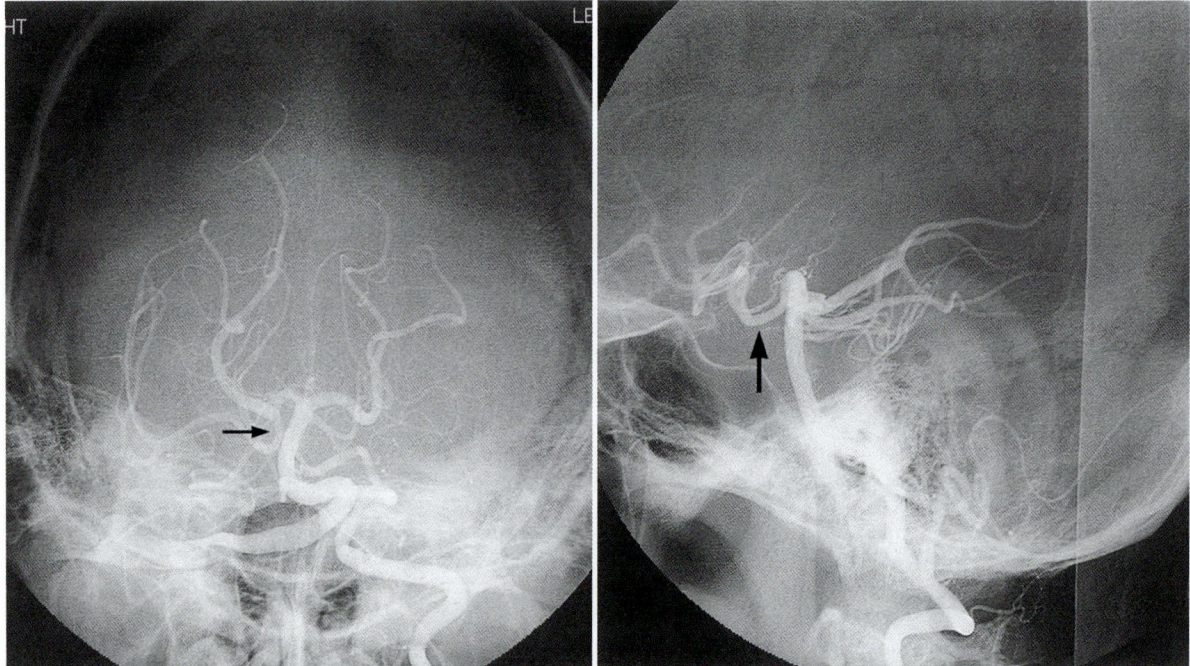

Fig. 27.37 Left vertebral artery injection showing posterior cerebral blood circulation, including reflux into posterior communicating artery *(arrows)*.

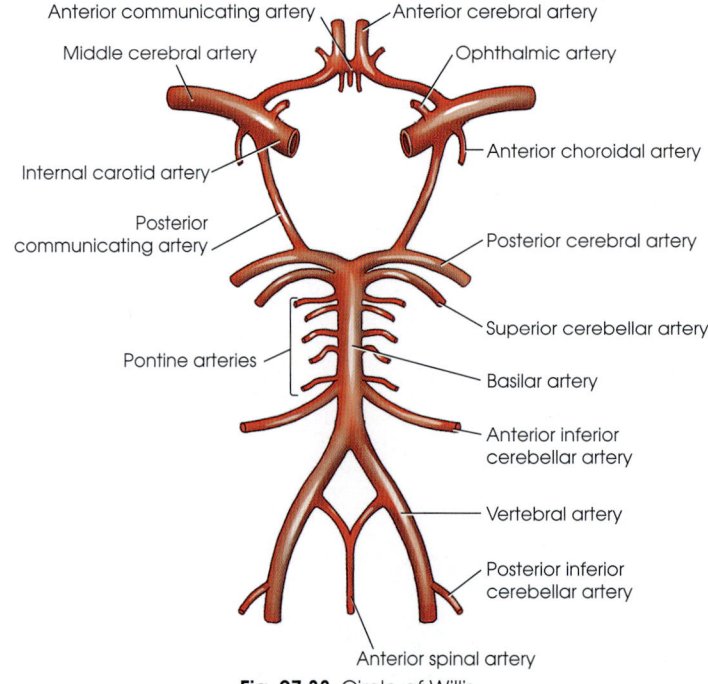

Fig. 27.38 Circle of Willis.

Technique

Catheter-directed cerebral angiography should be performed only in facilities equipped to produce studies of high technical quality with minimal risk to the patient. Rapid-sequence biplane imaging with DSA electronically coupled with an automatic injector is employed almost universally in cerebral angiography. Collimating to the area of the head and neck is essential for improving image quality in a nonmagnified study.

Cerebral angiography is performed either by using a femoral arterial approach or a radial arterial approach. Selective catheterization techniques allow the internal and external carotid circulation to be studied separately, which is particularly useful in delineating the blood supply of cerebral tumors and vascular malformations.

The final position of the catheter depends on the information sought from the angiographic study. When atherosclerotic disease of the extracranial carotid, subclavian, and vertebral arteries is being evaluated, injection of the aortic arch with imaging of the extracranial portion of these vessels is an appropriate way to begin.

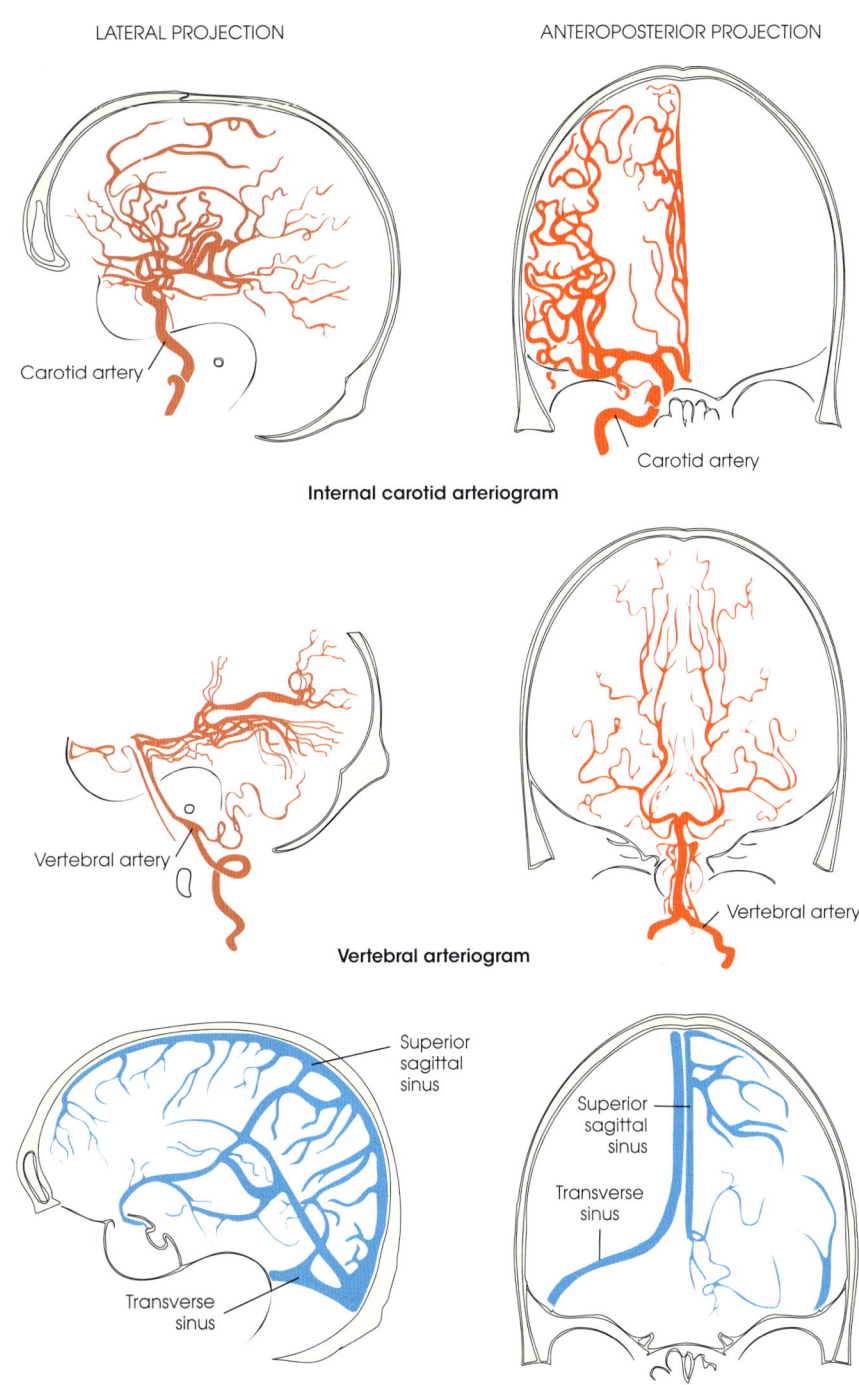

Fig. 27.39 Diagram of intracranial circulation: arterial and venous phase.

(From Bean BC: A chart of the intracerebral circulation, ed 2. *Med Radiogr Photogr* 34:25, 1958; courtesy Dr. Berton C. Bean and Eastman Kodak Co.)

CIRCULATION TIME AND IMAGING PROGRAM

Egas Moniz[3] stated that the transit time of the cerebral circulation is only 3 seconds for the blood to circulate from the ICA to the jugular vein, with the circulation time being slightly prolonged by the injected contrast solution. Greitz,[4] who measured the cerebral circulation time as "the time between the points of maximum concentration (of contrast media) in the carotid siphon and in the parietal veins," found a normal mean value of 4.13 seconds. Certain pathologic conditions significantly alter the cerebral circulation time. AVMs shorten the transit time; vascular occlusions or arterial vasospasm may cause a considerable delay.

A standard angiographic program should include at least one image taken before the arrival of contrast media to serve as a subtraction mask and then rapid-sequence images at 2 to 4 images per second in the AP and lateral projections during the arterial phase (first 1½ to 2½ seconds) of the arteriogram (Fig. 27.40). After the arterial phase, imaging may be slowed to one image per second for the capillary, or parenchymal, phase (Fig. 27.41) and maintained at one image per second or every other second for the venous phase (Fig. 27.42) of the angiogram. The entire program should cover 7 to 10 seconds, depending on the preference of the angiographer. The imaging program can be tailored to optimally demonstrate the suspected pathologic condition.

Injections at rates of 5 to 9 mL/s for 1 to 2 seconds are most often employed in the cerebral vessels, with variations dependent on vessel size and the patient's circulatory status.

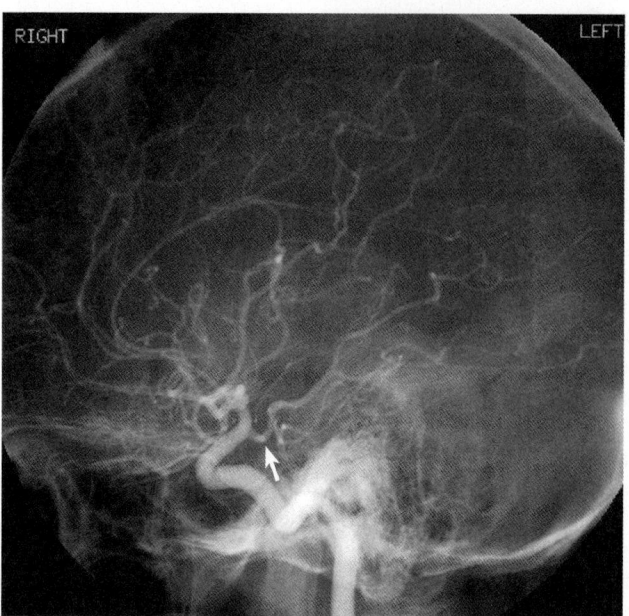

Fig. 27.40 Right internal carotid injection, lateral projection, shows arterial phase of circulation. Note posterior communicating artery *(arrow)*.

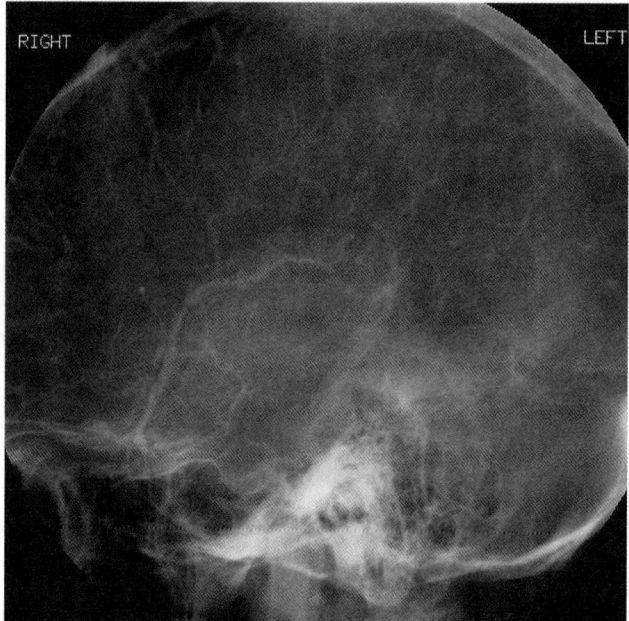

Fig. 27.41 Right internal carotid injection, lateral projection, shows capillary phase of carotid circulation.

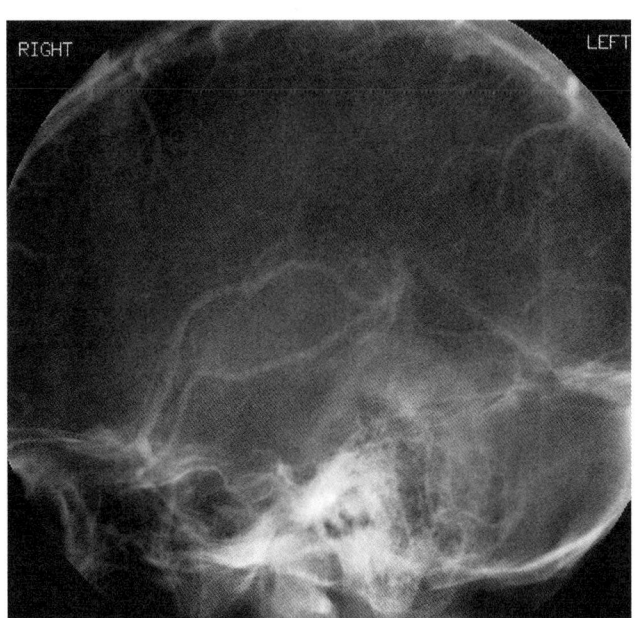

Fig. 27.42 Right internal carotid injection, lateral projection, shows venous phase of circulation.

POSITION OF HEAD

The centering and angulation of the central ray required to show the anterior circulation differ from those required to show the posterior circulation. The same head position is used for the basic AP and lateral projections of both regions.

- Adjust the patient's head so that it lies symmetrically in the headholder; the midsagittal plane is perpendicular to the horizontal plane.
- Place the infraorbitomeatal line (IOML) perpendicular to the horizontal plane.
- Angle the central ray for caudally inclined AP and AP oblique projections.

This chapter discusses the most frequently employed images and reasonably standard specifications for obtaining them.

The number of radiographs required for satisfactory delineation of a lesion depends on the nature and location of the lesion. Oblique projections or variations in central ray angulation are used to separate the vessels that overlap in the basic positions and to evaluate any existing abnormality.

Aortic Arch Angiogram

An aortic arch angiogram is most commonly obtained to visualize atherosclerotic or occlusive disease of the extracranial or common carotid, vertebral, and subclavian arteries. A catheter with multiple side holes is positioned in the ascending thoracic aorta so that the subsequent injection fills all of the vessels simultaneously.

SIMULTANEOUS BIPLANE OBLIQUE PROJECTIONS

For best results, simultaneous biplane oblique projections are produced so that superimposition of vessels is minimized (Fig. 27.43).

- Place the image receptor in a 35-degree LAO position. This position opens the aortic arch and clearly demonstrates the origins of the brachiocephalic, left common carotid, and left subclavian arteries.
- Raise the patient's chin to superimpose the inferior margin of the mandible onto the occiput so that as much of the neck as possible is exposed in the frontal image.
- Move the patient's shoulders inferiorly so that they are removed as much as possible from the lateral image.
- Position the lateral image receptor in a 35- to 45-degree RAO position to better demonstrate the bifurcation of the brachiocephalic and the origin of the left vertebral artery.
- The image receptor is positioned to include the inferior border of the aortic arch at the bottom of the imaging field.

Extracranial Carotid and Vertebral Arteriography

The most common vascular pathology in the extracranial carotid and vertebral arteries is atherosclerotic disease resulting in stenosis or occlusion. The majority of these stenoses are located at the bifurcation of the CCA or proximal ICA. Risk of stroke in patients with a high-grade stenosis, equal to or greater than 70%, is very high. Angiography of the extracranial carotid and vertebral arteries is often performed to verify the degree of occlusive disease demonstrated on prior noninvasive imaging and to plan appropriate endovascular or surgical intervention. Selective injections are performed at the origin of the right CCA, left CCA, and the vertebral arteries.

Selective catheter angiography of the ECA is performed to demonstrate vascular anatomy and pathology of extracranial branches supplying the neck, face, and scalp.

COMMON CAROTID ARTERIOGRAPHY

- Adjust the patient's head so that the head lies symmetrically in the headholder.
- Raise the patient's chin to superimpose the inferior margin of the mandible onto the occiput so that as much of the neck as possible is exposed in the frontal image.
- Move the patient's shoulders inferiorly so that the shoulders are removed as much as possible from the lateral image.
- The CCA is usually visualized with three projections: AP, 45-degree oblique, and lateral.
- A representative injection rate is 5 mL/s for a total of 10 mL.
- It is important for the patient to hold respirations and prevent any movement, including swallowing, during exposures to minimize misregistration of DSA images.

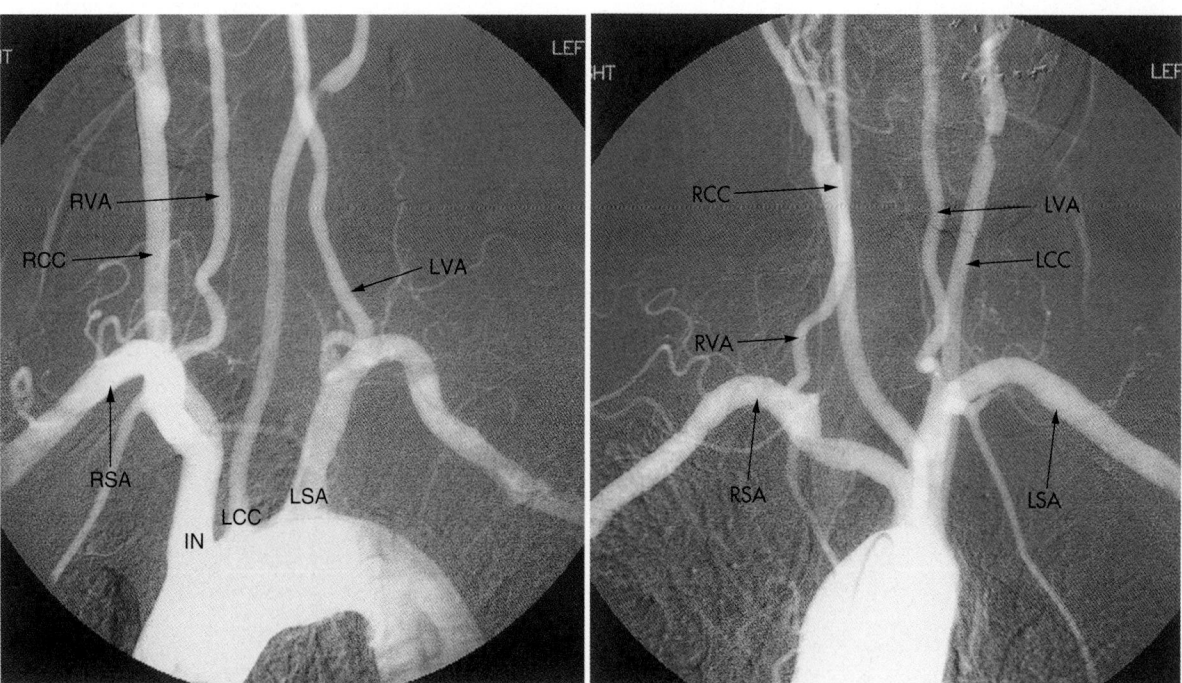

Fig. 27.43 Digital subtracted images of thoracic aortogram showing the origins of the great vessels. *IN,* Innominate; *LCC,* left common carotid; *LSA,* left subclavian artery; *LVA,* left vertebral artery; *RCC,* right common carotid; *RSA,* right subclavian artery; *RVA,* right vertebral artery.

VERTEBRAL ARTERIOGRAPHY

- The patient's position is the same as in common carotid arteriography.
- The extracranial vertebral artery is visualized in the AP and lateral projections.
- Position the central ray more posterior in the lateral plane to include the posterior aspect of the spine.
- A representative injection rate is 5 mL/s for a total of 8 mL.

EXTERNAL CAROTID ARTERIOGRAPHY

- The patient's position is the same as in common carotid arteriography.
- The ECA is routinely visualized in the AP and lateral projections.
- Increase the field of view to include the mandible and the soft tissue of the skull.
- Position the central ray more anterior in the lateral plane to include the facial structures.
- Close collimation and additional filters may be necessary to reduce image contrast and prevent image burnout.
- A representative injection rate is 3 mL/s for a total of 6 mL.
- If possible, warn the patient of heat sensation from the contrast media in facial tissue.

Intracranial Anterior Circulation

LATERAL PROJECTION

- Adjust the patient's head so that the skull lies symmetrically; the midsagittal plane is perpendicular to the horizontal plane.
- Place the IOML perpendicular to the horizontal plane.
- Perform lateral projections of the anterior, or carotid, circulation with the central ray directed horizontally to a point slightly cranial to the auricle and midway between the forehead and the occiput. This centering allows for patient variation (Figs. 27.44 to 27.46).
- A representative injection rate for a selected ICA is 6 mL/s for a total of 8 mL.

NOTE: See Fig. 27.39 for assistance in identifying the cerebral vessels in the image.

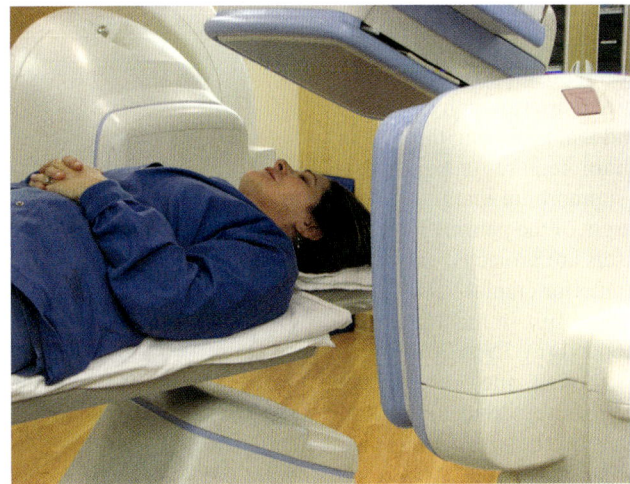

Fig. 27.44 Cerebral angiogram: lateral projection as part of a biplane setup.

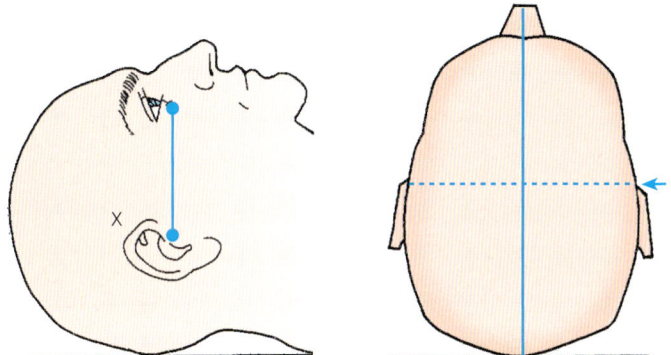

Fig. 27.45 Lateral projection.

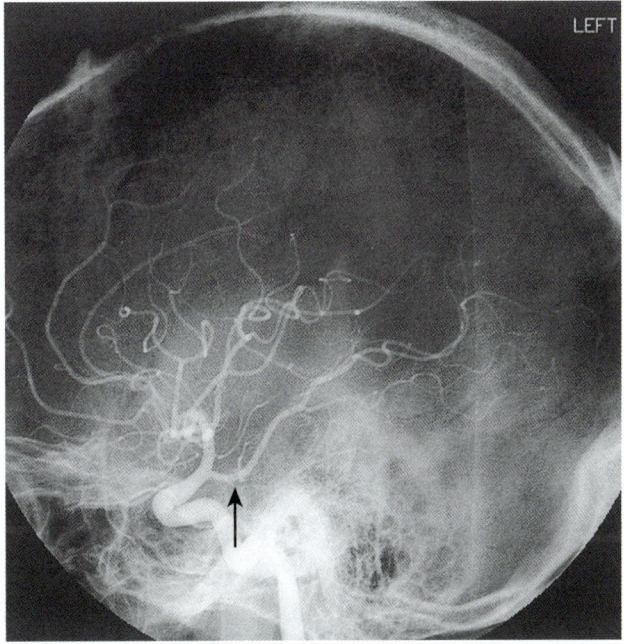

Fig. 27.46 Left internal carotid artery injection. Cerebral angiogram: lateral projection showing anterior circulation. Note posterior communicating artery *(arrow)*.

AP AXIAL PROJECTION (SUPRAORBITAL)

The patient's head position is the same as in common carotid arteriography.

- Keep in mind that achieving the goal in this angiogram requires superimposition of the supraorbital margins on the superior margin of the petrous ridges so that the vessels are projected above the floor of the anterior cranial fossa.
- To obtain this result in most patients, direct the central ray 15 to 20 degrees caudally, directing the central ray through the frontal bone and EAM to the center of the image receptor (Figs. 27.47 to 27.49).

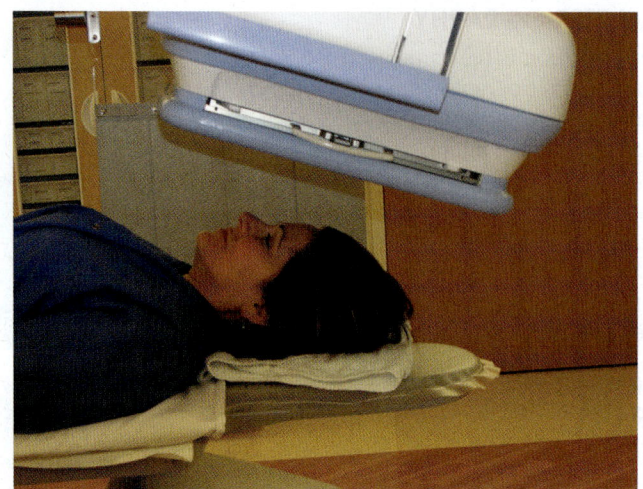

Fig. 27.47 Carotid angiogram: PA axial (supraorbital) projection.

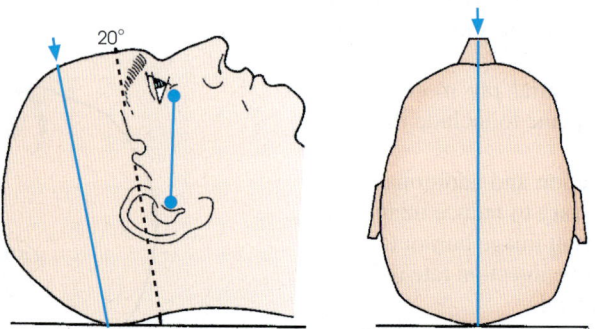

Fig. 27.48 AP axial (supraorbital).

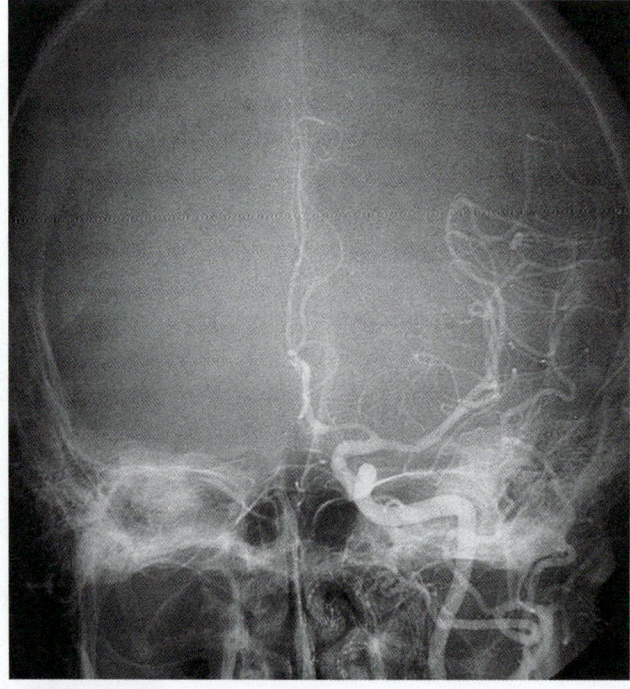

Fig. 27.49 Left common carotid artery injection showing AP axial (supraorbital) projection. Arterial phase of circulation.

AP AXIAL OBLIQUE PROJECTION (TRANSORBITAL)

The oblique transorbital projection shows the internal carotid bifurcation and the anterior communicating and middle cerebral arteries within the orbital shadow.
- From the position for the basic AP projection, rotate the patient's head approximately 30 degrees away from the injected side, or angle the central ray 30 degrees toward the injected side.
- Angle the central ray 20 degrees cephalad, and center it to the midorbit of the injected side (Figs. 27.50 and 27.51).

Posterior Circulation
LATERAL PROJECTION
- Adjust the patient's head so that the skull lies symmetrically; the midsagittal plane is perpendicular to the horizontal plane.
- Place the IOML perpendicular to the horizontal plane.
- Perform lateral projections of the posterior, or vertebral, circulation with the central ray directed horizontally to the mastoid process at a point about 1 cm superior to and 2 cm posterior to the EAM.
- Restrict the exposure field to the middle and posterior fossae for lateral studies of the posterior circulation (Figs. 27.52 and 27.53). Inclusion of the entire skull is neither necessary nor, from the standpoint of optimal technique, desirable.

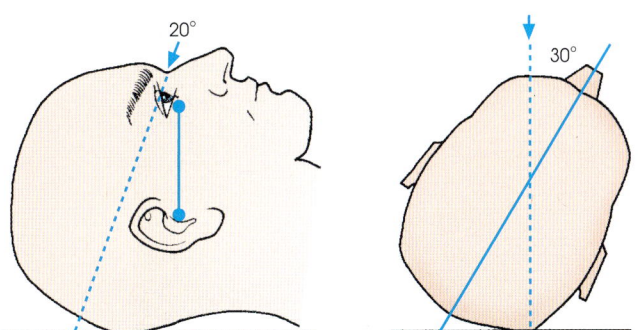

Fig. 27.50 AP axial oblique (transorbital) projection.

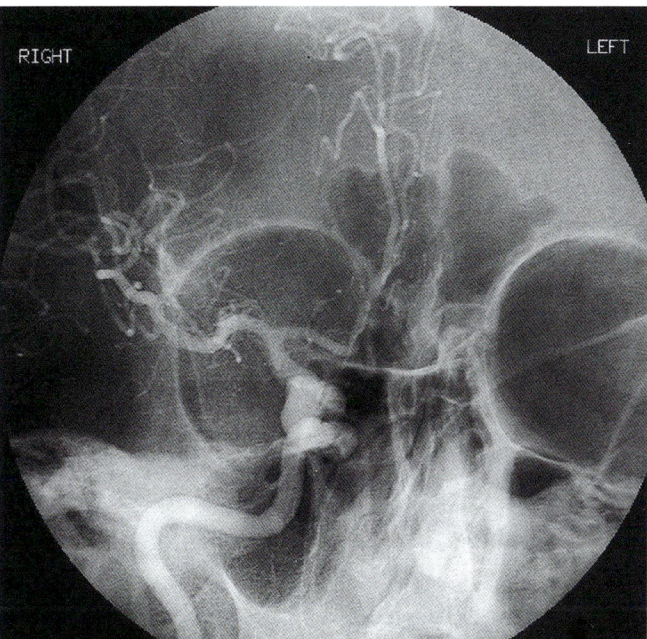

Fig. 27.51 Right internal carotid artery injection showing AP axial oblique (transorbital) projection.

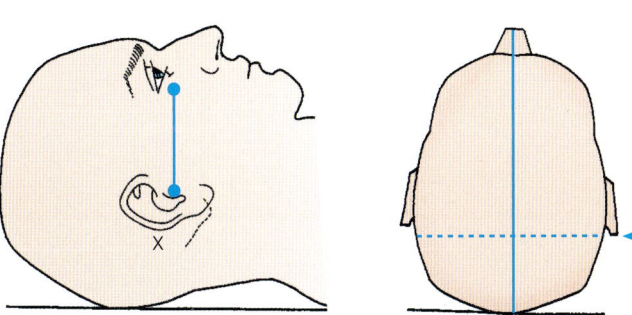

Fig. 27.52 Lateral projection for posterior circulation.

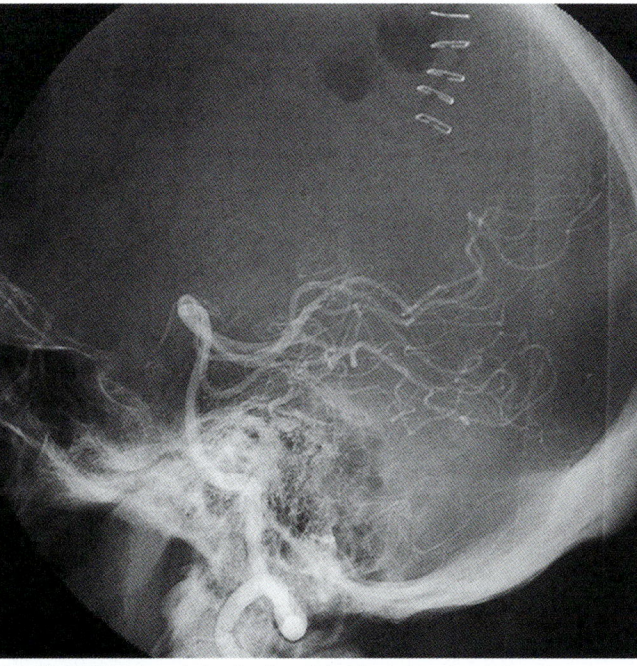

Fig. 27.53 Right vertebral artery injection showing lateral projection of vertebrobasilar system.

- A representative injection rate is 5 mL/s for a total of 8 mL.

AP AXIAL PROJECTION

- Adjust the patient's head so that the skull lies symmetrically; the midsagittal plane is perpendicular to the horizontal plane.
- Place the IOML perpendicular to the horizontal plane.
- Direct the central ray to the region approximately 4 cm (1.5 inches) superior to the glabella at an angle of 30 to 35 degrees caudad. The central ray exits at the level of the EAM. For this projection, the supraorbital margins are positioned approximately 2 cm (0.75 inch) below the superior margins of the petrous ridges (Figs. 27.54 and 27.55).

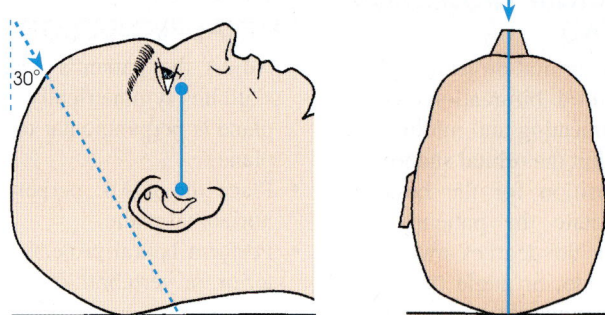

Fig. 27.54 AP axial projection for posterior circulation.

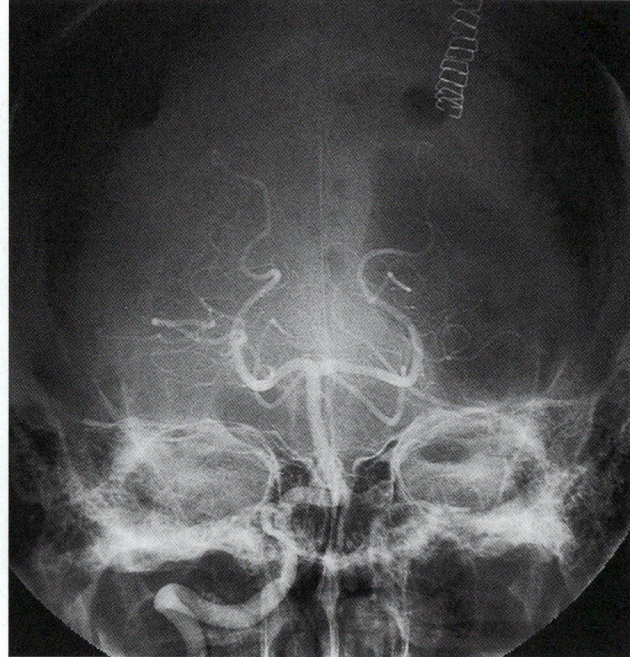

Fig. 27.55 Right vertebral artery injection showing AP axial projection of vertebrobasilar system.

Venography

Venography

Venous blood in veins flows proximally toward the heart. Injection into a central venous structure may not opacify the peripheral veins that *anastomose* to it. The position of peripheral veins can be indirectly documented, however, by the filling defect from unopacified blood in the opacified central vein. This phenomenon is often used to locate the position of renal veins on an IVC venogram.

UPPER LIMB VENOGRAMS

Upper limb venography is most often performed to look for thrombosis or occlusions. The contrast medium is injected through a needle, IV line, or catheter into a superficial vein at the elbow or wrist. Radiographs should cover the vasculature from the wrist or elbow to the SVC (Fig. 27.56). Contrast media injections are usually performed by hand rather than automatic injection. Injection rates and imaging rates will vary, depending on suspected pathology and site of injection.

LOWER LIMB VENOGRAMS

Lower limb venography is performed to accurately visualize thrombosis of the deep veins of the leg prior to intervention. Ultrasound of the legs is the first-line diagnostic tool to diagnose deep vein thrombosis. CT or MRI venography can also be performed for noninvasive diagnostic imaging. In cases in which interventional procedures are expected to be performed, lower limb venography can also be obtained with contrast media injected through a sheath or catheter placed directly into the popliteal vein with the patient prone (Fig. 27.57).

SUPERIOR VENACAVOGRAM

Venography of the SVC is performed primarily to rule out the existence of thrombus or the occlusion of the SVC. Superior opacification of the SVC results from injection through a catheter positioned in the axillary, subclavian, or jugular veins. Radiographs should include the opacified subclavian vein, brachiocephalic vein, SVC, and right atrium (Fig. 27.58).

INFERIOR VENACAVOGRAM

Venography of the IVC is performed primarily to identify the location of the renal veins for placement of an IVC filter. The contrast media are injected through a catheter with multiple side holes and inserted through the femoral vein and positioned in the common iliac vein or the inferior aspect of the IVC (Fig. 27.59).

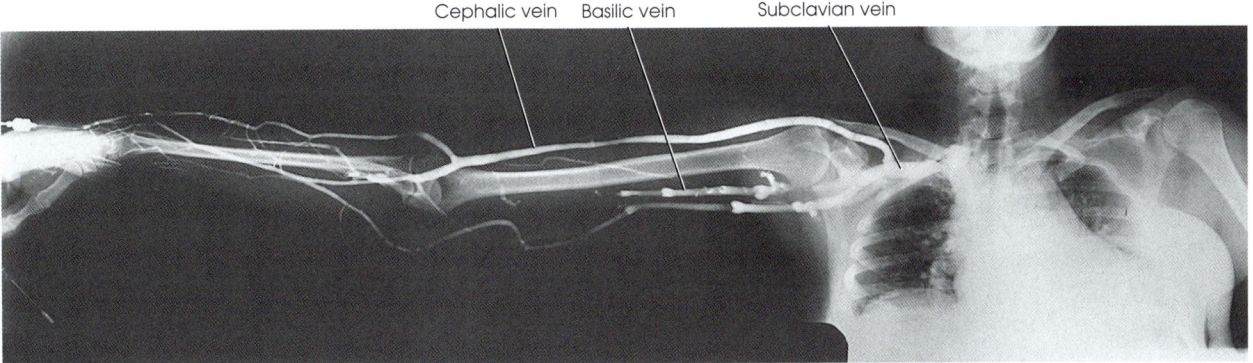

Fig. 27.56 Normal right upper limb venogram.

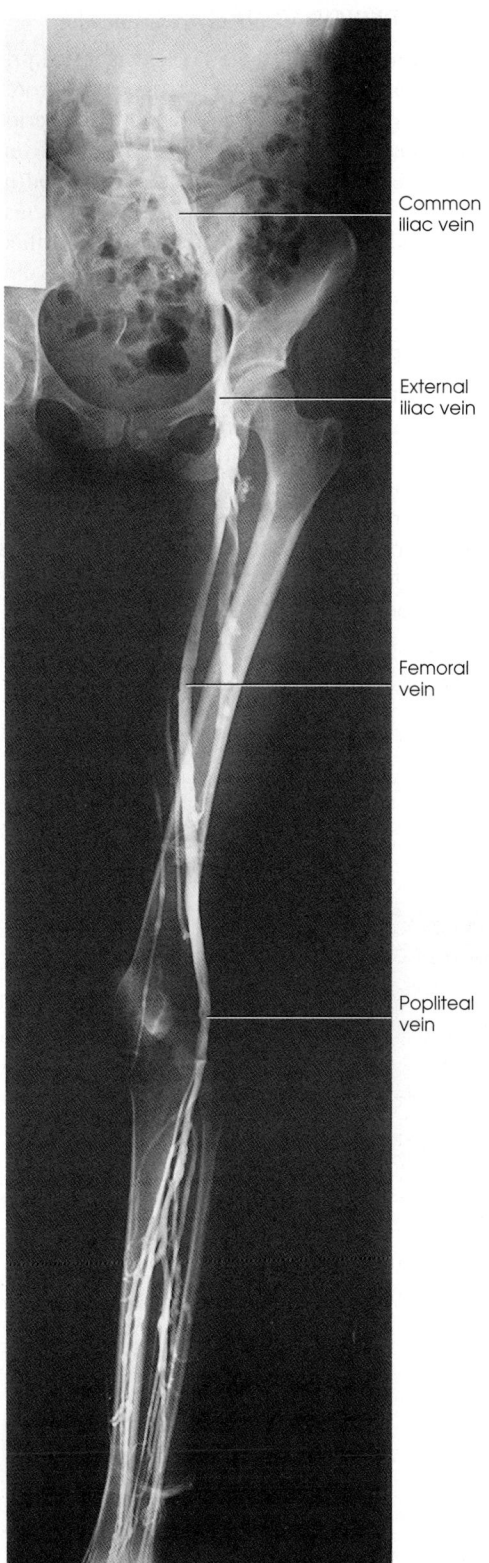

Fig. 27.57 Normal left lower limb venogram.

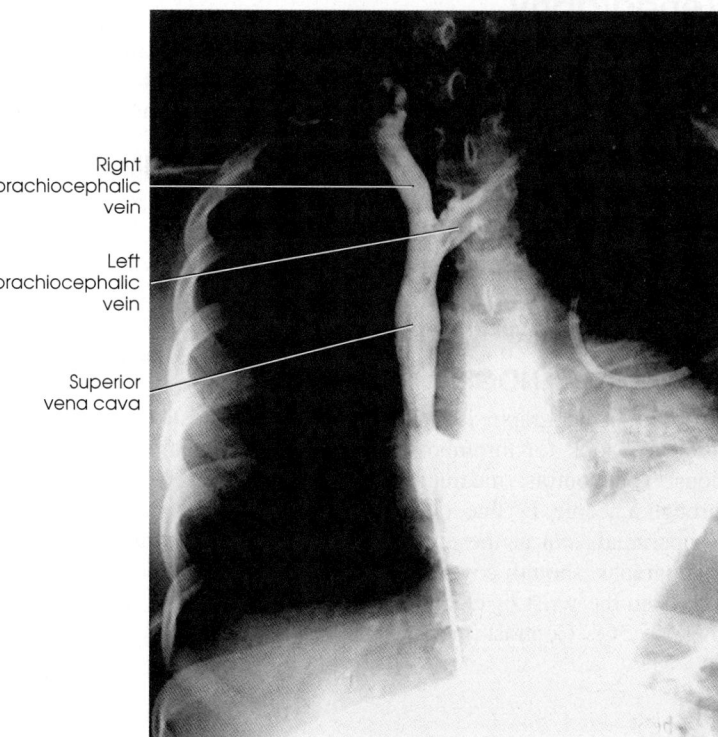

Fig. 27.58 AP superior vena cava.

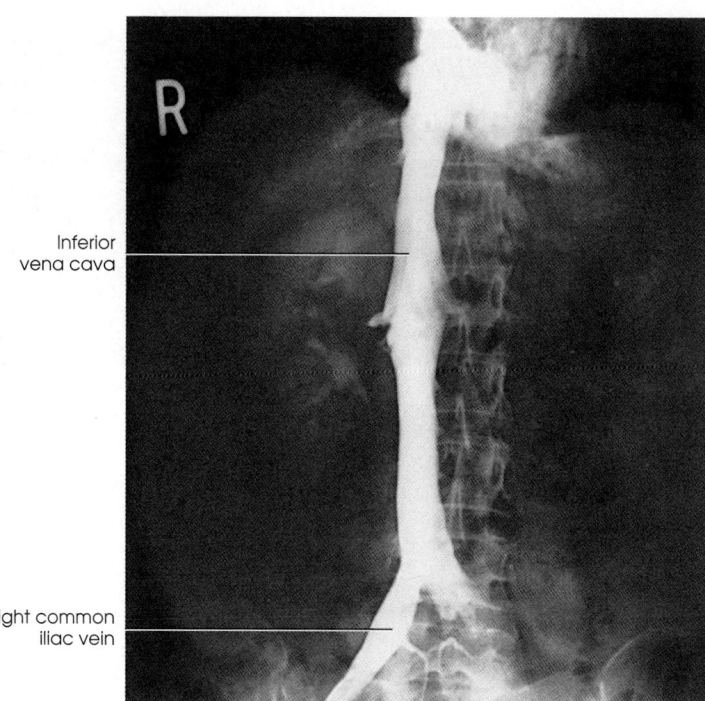

Fig. 27.59 AP inferior vena cava.

VISCERAL VENOGRAPHY

The visceral veins are often visualized by extending the imaging program of the corresponding visceral arterial injection. The veins that drain the small bowel are normally visualized by extending the imaging program of a superior mesenteric arteriogram. Portal venography (Fig. 27.60) can be performed by injecting the portal vein directly from a percutaneous approach, but it is usually accomplished by late-phase imaging of a splenic artery injection or SMA injection.

HEPATIC VENOGRAM

Hepatic venography is usually performed to rule out stenosis or thrombosis of the hepatic veins. These veins can also be catheterized to obtain pressure measurements from the interior of the liver. The hepatic veins carry blood from the liver to the IVC. (The portal vein carries nutrient-rich blood from the viscera to the liver.) The hepatic veins are most easily catheterized from a jugular vein or an upper limb vein approach, but a femoral vein approach may also be used.

- Place the patient in the supine position for AP or PA projections that include the liver tissue and the extreme upper IVC (Fig. 27.61).
- Make exposures at the end of suspended expiration.

RENAL VENOGRAM

Renal venography is usually performed to rule out thrombosis of the renal vein. The renal vein is also catheterized for blood sampling, usually to measure the production of renin, an enzyme produced by the kidney when it lacks adequate blood supply. The renal vein is most easily catheterized from a femoral vein approach.

- Place the patient in the supine position for a single-plane AP or PA projection.
- Center the selected kidney to the image receptor, and collimate the field to include the kidney and area of the IVC (Fig. 27.62).
- Make exposures at the end of suspended expiration.

Over the years the role of minimally invasive angiography as a primary diagnostic tool has diminished as noninvasive diagnostic imaging techniques have evolved. The majority of angiography procedures today are vascular interventional procedures; however, conventional angiographic methods, such as vascular access, guidewire and catheter manipulations, and precise imaging, will always be the foundation for vascular interventional procedures.

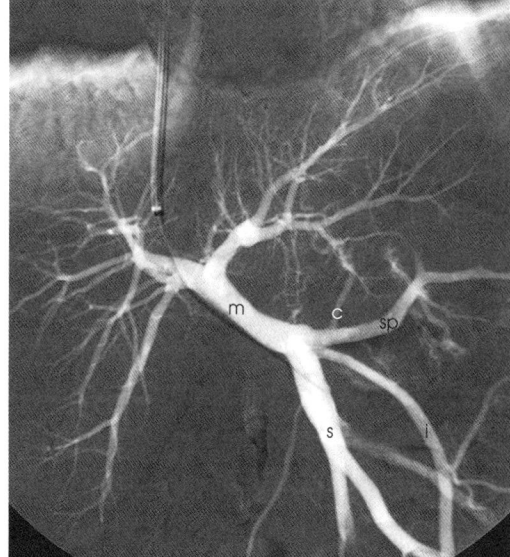

Fig. 27.60 Portal venogram. *c*, Coronary varices; *i*, inferior mesenteric vein; *m*, main portal vein; *s*, superior mesenteric vein; *sp*, splenic vein.

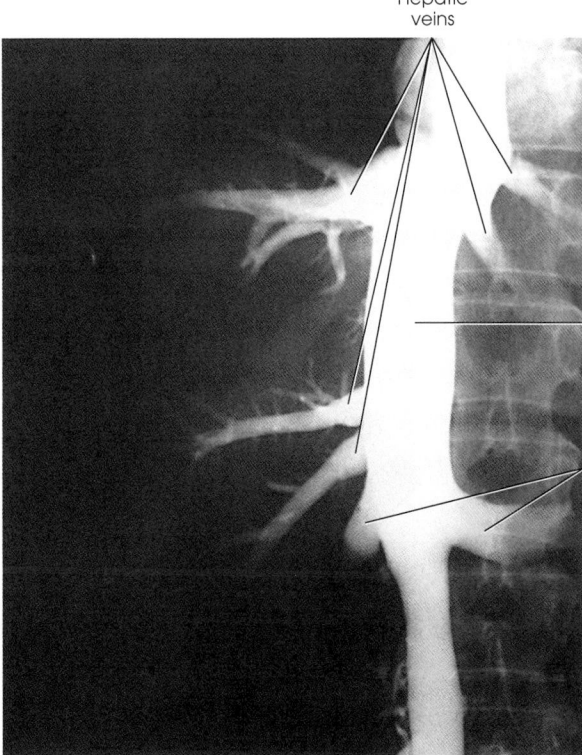

Fig. 27.61 Hepatic vein visualization from reflux from inferior vena cava injection. (Note reflux into bilateral renal veins.)

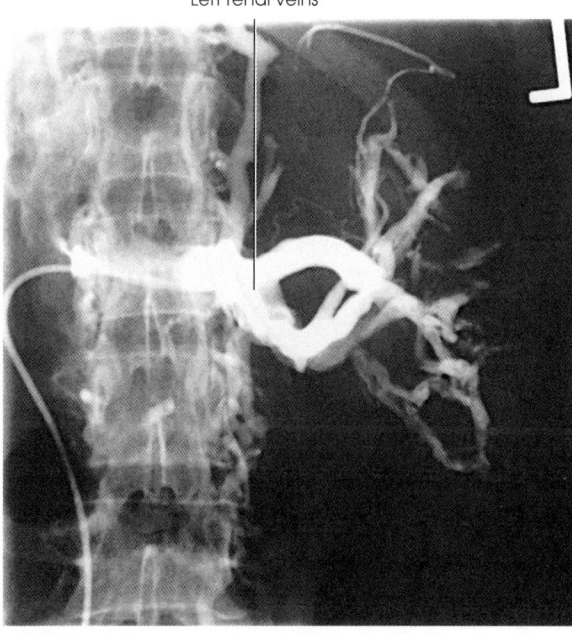

Fig. 27.62 Selective left renal venogram. AP projection.

INTERVENTIONAL RADIOLOGY

Interventional radiology has a therapeutic rather than diagnostic purpose in that it intervenes in, or interferes with, the course of a disease process or other medical condition. Interventional radiologic procedures reduce hospital stays in many patients and help some patients avoid surgery, with consequent reductions in medical costs. Since the conception of this form of radiology in the early 1960s, its realm has become so vast and sophisticated that publishers of periodicals struggle to keep abreast of this rapidly advancing specialty.

Every interventional radiologic procedure must include two integral processes. The first is the interventional or medical side of the procedure, in which a highly skilled interventionalist uses wires, catheters, and special medical devices (e.g., occluding coils, stents) to improve the patient's status or condition. The second process involves the use of fluoroscopy and radiography to guide and document the progress of the steps taken during the first process. A radiologic technologist must receive special education in either vascular interventional or cardiac interventional radiography. This skilled technologist has an important role in assisting the physician in interventional procedures.

The more frequently performed interventional procedures are described in this section. Specific cardiac interventions are described later in the chapter. Resources containing more detailed information are cited in the selected bibliography at the end of the chapter.

Percutaneous Transluminal Angioplasty and Stenting

PTA is a therapeutic radiologic procedure designed to dilate or reopen stenotic or occluded areas within a vessel using a catheter introduced by the Seldinger technique. In 1964, Dotter and Judkins[5] first described PTA using a coaxial catheter method. First, a guidewire is passed through the narrowed area of a vessel. A smaller catheter is then passed over the guidewire through the stenosis to begin the dilation process. Finally, a larger catheter is passed over the smaller catheter to cause further dilation. This method is referred to as the "Dotter method." Although this method can achieve dilation of stenosis, it has the significant disadvantage of creating an arteriotomy as large as the dilating catheters, and it is seldom used as a first-line therapy.

In 1974, Grüntzig and Hopff[6] introduced the double-lumen, balloon-tipped catheter. One lumen allows the passage of a guidewire and fluids through the catheter. The other lumen communicates with a balloon at the distal end of the catheter. When inflated, the balloon expands to a size much larger than the catheter. Double-lumen angioplasty balloon catheters are available in sizes ranging from 3 to 9 Fr, with attached balloons varying in length and expanding to diameters of 2 to 20 mm or more (Fig. 27.63).

Fig. 27.64 illustrates the process of *balloon angioplasty*. The stenosis is initially identified on a previously obtained angiogram. The balloon diameter used for a procedure is often the measured diameter of the normal artery adjacent to the stenosis. The angioplasty procedure is often performed at the same time and through the same catheterization site as the initial diagnostic examination.

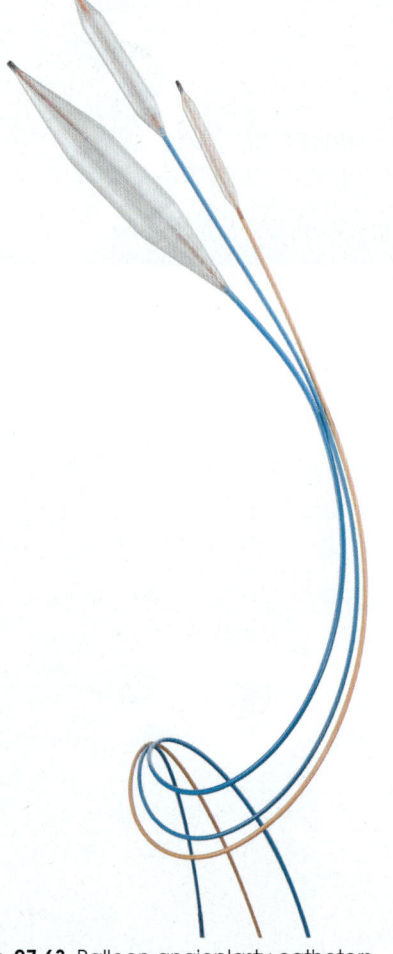

Fig. 27.63 Balloon angioplasty catheters with varied diameters and lengths.

(2014 C. R. Bard, Inc. Used with permission. Bard is a registered trademark of C. R. Bard, Inc.)

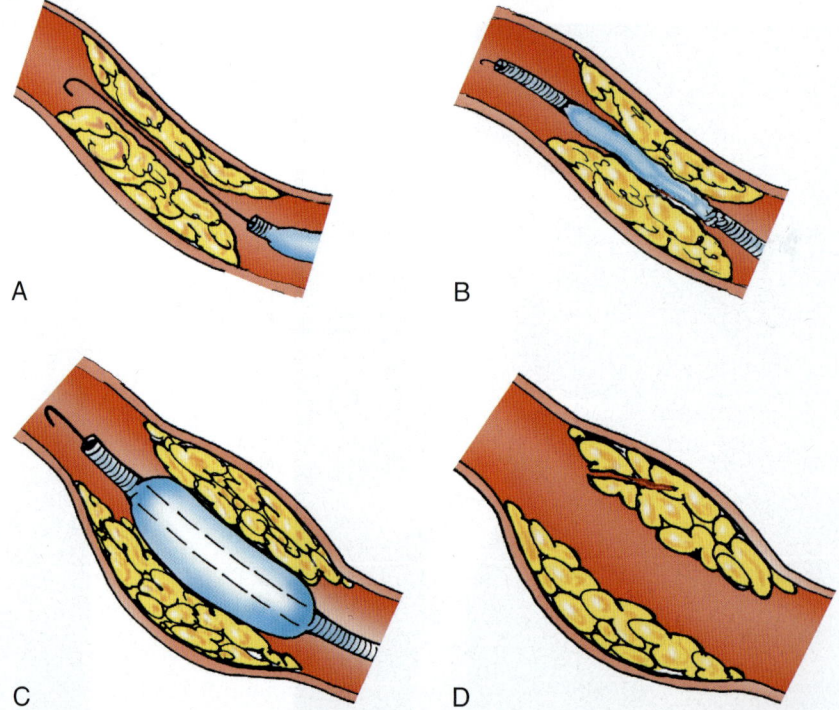

Fig. 27.64 Balloon angioplasty of atherosclerotic stenosis. **(A)** Guidewire advanced through stenosis. **(B)** Balloon across stenosis. **(C)** Balloon inflated. **(D)** Postangioplasty stenotic area.

After the guidewire is positioned across the stenosis, the angiographic catheter is removed over the wire. The angioplasty balloon catheter is introduced and directed through the stenosis over the guidewire. The balloon is usually inflated with a diluted contrast media mixture for 15 to 45 seconds, depending on the degree of stenosis and the vessel being treated. The balloon is deflated and repositioned or withdrawn from the lesion. Contrast media can be injected through the angioplasty catheter for a repeat angiogram to determine whether the procedure was successful. The success of the angioplasty procedure may also be determined by comparing transcatheter blood pressure measurements from a location distal and a location proximal to the lesion site. Nearly equal pressures indicate a reopened stenosis.

Transluminal angioplasty can be performed in virtually any vessel that can be reached percutaneously with a catheter (Figs. 27.65 and 27.66). In 1978, Molnar and Stockum[7] described the use of balloon angioplasty for dilation of strictures within the biliary system. Balloon angioplasty is

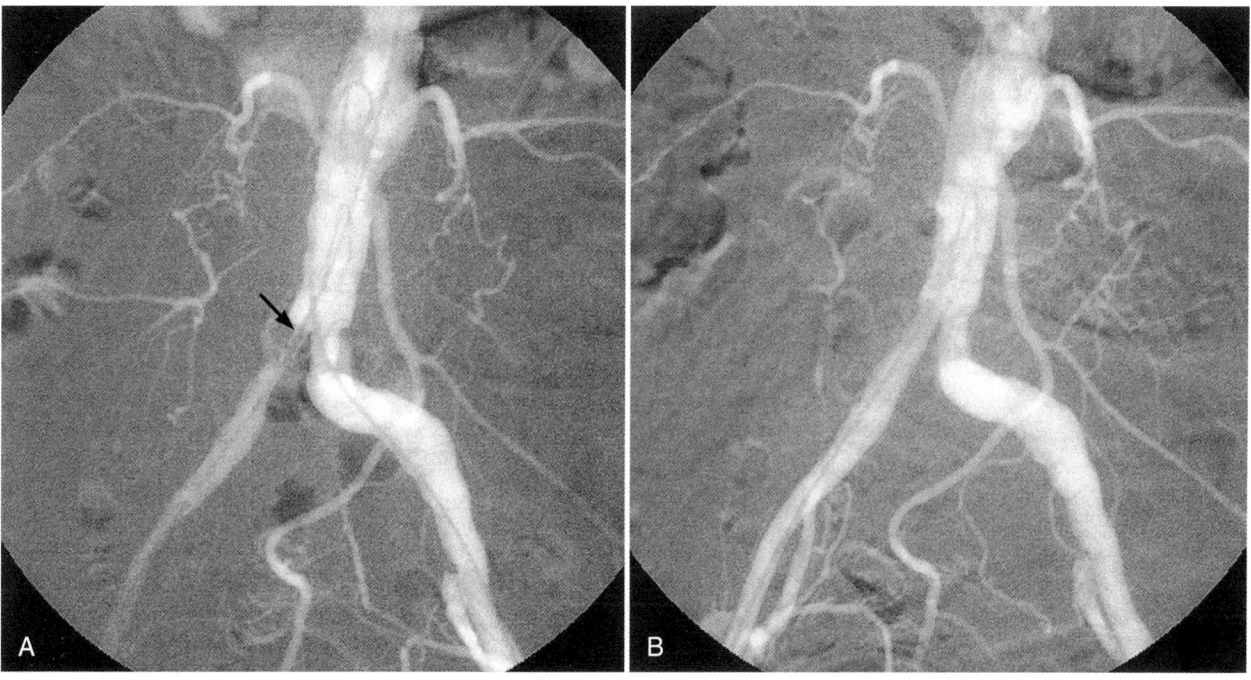

Fig. 27.65 Digital subtracted images of the abdominal aortogram and bilateral iliac arteries. **(A)** High-grade stenosis of right common iliac artery *(arrow).* **(B)** Abdominal aortogram and bilateral iliac arteries, postangioplasty, showing widely patent iliac system.

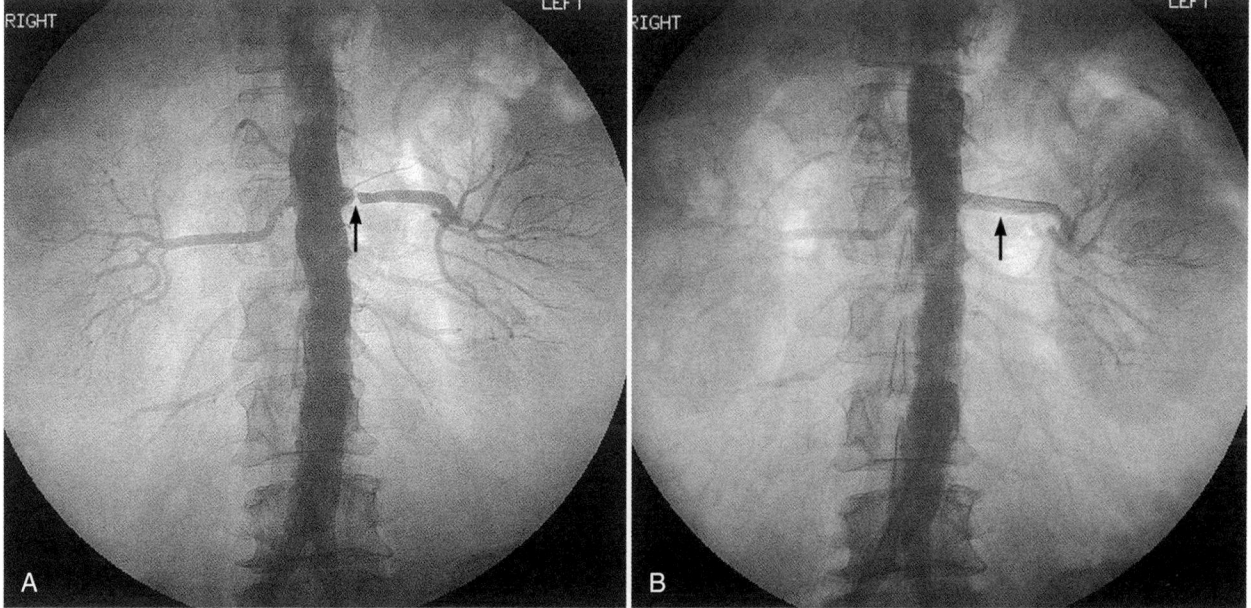

Fig. 27.66 Abdominal aortogram before and after angioplasty of the left renal artery. **(A)** High-grade stenosis of left renal artery *(arrow).* **(B)** Postangioplasty and stent placement within left renal artery *(arrow).*

also conducted in venous structures, ureters, and the gastrointestinal tract.

Balloon angioplasty has been used successfully to manage various diseases that cause arterial narrowing. The most common form of arterial stenosis treated by transluminal angioplasty is caused by atherosclerosis. Dotter and Judkins[5] speculated that this atheromatous material was soft and inelastic and could be compressed against the artery wall. Later research showed, however, that the plaque does not compress. If plaque surrounds the inner diameter of the artery, the plaque cracks at its thinnest portion as the arterial lumen is expanded. Continued expansion cracks the inner layer of the arterial wall, the *intima*, then stretches and tears the middle layer, the *media*, and finally stretches the outer layer, the *adventitia*. The arterial lumen is increased by permanently enlarging the artery's outer diameter. Restenosis, when it occurs, is usually caused by deposits of new plaque rather than arterial wall collapse. Angioplasty involving the arteries of the heart, *percutaneous transluminal coronary angioplasty* (*PTCA*), is generally performed in the cardiac catheterization laboratory. PTCA is discussed later in this chapter.

Another percutaneous treatment of vessel stenoses is the placement of vascular stents. A vascular *stent* is composed of a metal material, stainless steel, or nitinol that can be covered or uncovered with a surgical graft material. The stent is introduced through a catheter system and positioned across a stenosis. When deployed, the stent applies *radial force* to the stenosis to keep the narrowed area spread apart. These devices remain in the vessel permanently (Figs. 27.67 and 27.68).

The success of PTA and/or stent placement in the management of atherosclerosis has made it a significant alternative to surgical procedures in the treatment of this disease. PTA is not indicated in all cases, however. Long segments of occlusion may be best treated by surgery. PTA has a lower risk than surgery but is not totally risk-free. Generally, patients must be able to tolerate the surgical procedure that may be required to repair vessel damage that can be caused by PTA. Unsuccessful transluminal angioplasty and stent procedures rarely prevent or complicate necessary subsequent surgery. In selected cases, the procedure is effective and almost painless and can be repeated as often as necessary, with no apparent increase in risk to the patient. The recovery time is often no longer than the time required to stabilize the arteriotomy site, usually a matter of hours, and general anesthesia is normally not required.

Abdominal Aortic Aneurysm Endografts

An interventional therapy started in the late 1990s treats abdominal aortic aneurysms (AAAs) with a transcatheter approach and stenting. AAAs historically have been treated with an open repair of the aneurysm by a vascular surgeon. This approach has risks associated with abdominal surgery and a long hospital stay for recovery of the incision. The stent graft or endograft is a metal stent covered in synthetic graft material that comes in pieces or one intact device, depending on the manufacturer (Fig. 27.69). A cutdown approach to bilateral femoral arteries is done, and sheaths and delivery catheters are advanced to deliver the device. A large amount of planning is done before a

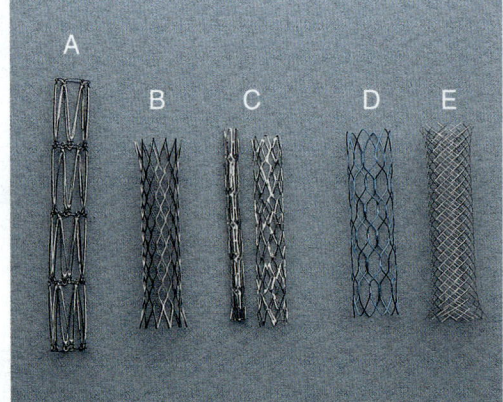

Fig. 27.67 Intravascular stents. (**A**) Gianturco-Rosch biliary Z-stent. (**B**) Memotherm. (**C**) Palmaz; unexpanded and expanded. (**D**) Symphony. (**E**) Wallstent.

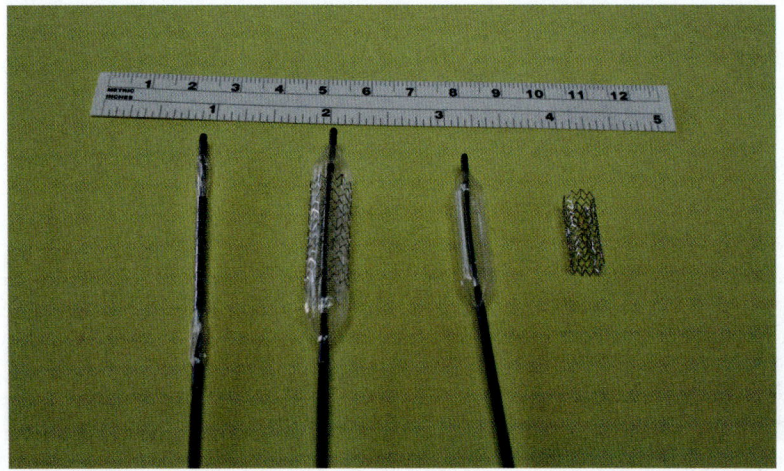

Fig. 27.68 Stent and balloon for angioplasty shown collapsed and inflated.

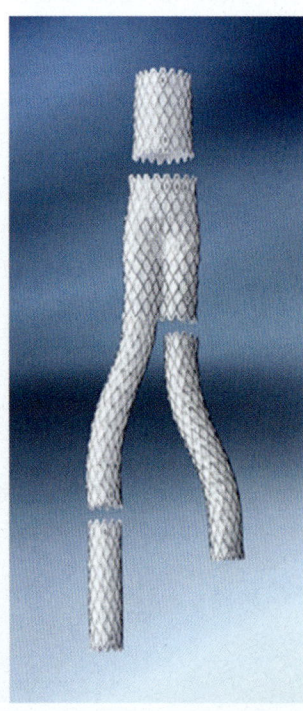

Fig. 27.69 Stent graft or endograft used to repair aneurysm in the aorta and iliac region.

patient can undergo this approach to treating AAA. Patients preferably should have an AAA that is infrarenal or occurring below the renal arteries. The endograft would occlude any arteries originating from the portion of the aorta being treated. Some newer AAA endograft devices are designed to treat aneurysms that extend to involve the renal artery and even mesenteric artery origins. These fenestrated endografts are usually custom made for each individual patient (Fig. 27.70).

Preliminary abdominal and iliac arteriograms may be obtained using a calibrated catheter that the interventionalist or vascular surgeon can use for measuring (Fig. 27.71). CT is the preferred imaging

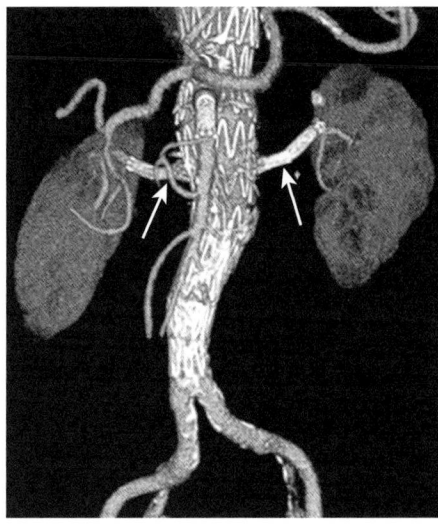

Fig. 27.70 Fenestrated, or branched, endograft. Volume rendering of a computed tomographic angiography showing a fenestrated endograph (Zenith, Cook, Bloomington, IL). There are extensions into both renal arteries *(arrows)*, the superior mesenteric artery, and celiac artery.

(From Kaufman JA: Abdominal aorta and pelvic arteries. In Kaufman JA, Lee MJ, editors: *Vascular and interventional radiology: the requisites*, 2nd ed, 2014, Elsevier. Courtesy Roy Greenberg, MD, Cleveland, OH.)

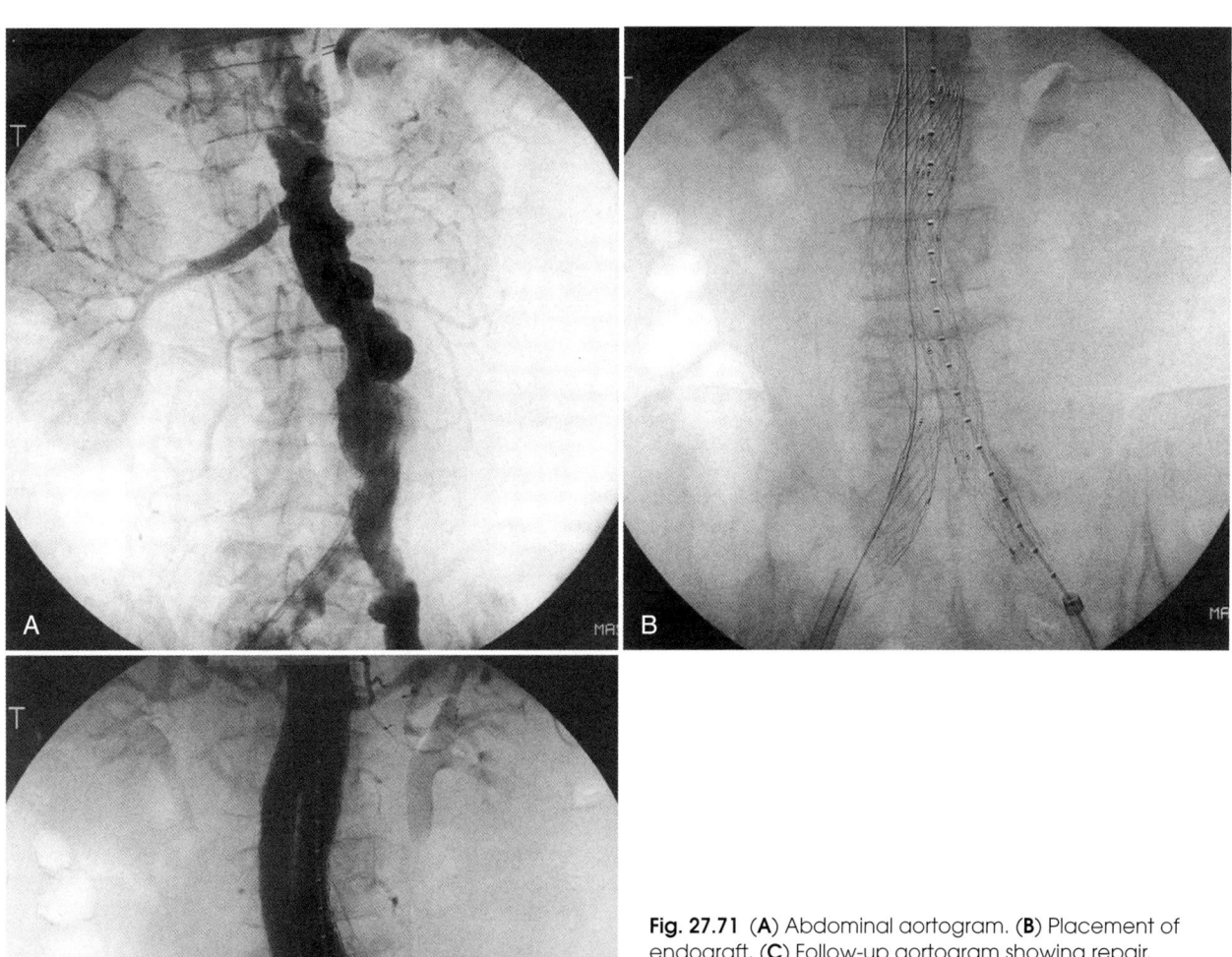

Fig. 27.71 (**A**) Abdominal aortogram. (**B**) Placement of endograft. (**C**) Follow-up aortogram showing repair.

modality and is used as the primary source for measurements. This procedure is usually performed in a hybrid angiography suite with OR capabilities to reduce the need to move the patient should complications arise requiring open surgery. Alternatively, they are performed in the OR using a portable C-arm with DSA capability.

Transcatheter Embolization

Transcatheter embolization was first described by Brooks[8,9] in 1930. He described vessel occlusion for closure of arteriovenous fistula. Transcatheter embolization involves the therapeutic introduction of various substances to occlude or drastically reduce blood flow within a vessel (Box 27.1). The three main purposes for embolization are (1) to stop active bleeding sites, (2) to control blood flow to diseased or malformed vessels (e.g., tumors or AVMs), and (3) to stop or reduce blood flow to a particular area of the body before surgery.

The patient's condition and the situation must be considered when choosing an embolic agent. The interventionalist usually identifies the appropriate agent to be used. Embolic agents must be administered with care to ensure that they flow to the predetermined vessel or target without embolizing nontarget vessels. Embolization can be a permanent treatment; the effects on the lesion are irreversible. Many embolic agents are available (Box 27.2), and the choice of agent depends on whether the occlusion is to be temporary or permanent (Table 27.1).

Temporary agents such as Gelfoam or Avitene may be used as a means to reduce the pressure head of blood to a specific site. These temporary agents reduce flow into a bleeding site so that hemostasis may be achieved. Temporary agents can also be used to prevent inadvertent embolization of normal vessels.[b]

---

[b]Gelfoam is the trademark for a sterile, absorbable, water-insoluble, gelatin-based sponge.

BOX 27.1
Lesions amenable to embolization

Aneurysm
Pseudoaneurysm
Hemorrhage
Neoplasms
   Malignant
   Benign
Arteriovenous malformations
Arteriovenous fistula
Infertility (varicocele)
Impotence owing to venous leakage
Redistribution of blood flow

BOX 27.2
Embolic agents

Particulate agents
Polyvinyl alcohol
Embosphere
Avitene
Gelfoam

Metal coils
Gianturco coils
Detachable coils
   Platinum
   Coated

Vascular occluder plug
Liquid agents (occluding, sclerosing)
   Ethanol
   Thrombin
   Hypertonic glucose
   Sodium tetradecyl sulfate
   Ethibloc
   EVAL
   Onyx
Detachable balloons
   Latex—Debrun
   Silicone—Hieshima
Liquid adhesives
   N-butyl 2-cyanoacrylate
Autologous material

TABLE 27.1
Particulate agent sizes

Agent	Size
Gelfoam powder	40–60 μ
Gelfoam sponges	Pledgets-torpedoes
Avitene	100–150 μ
Polyvinyl alcohol	100–1200 μ
Embosphere	100–1200 μ

Vasoconstricting drugs can be used to reduce blood flow temporarily. Vasoconstrictors such as vasopressin (Pitressin) drastically constrict vessels, resulting in hemostasis.

When permanent occlusion is desired, as in trauma to the pelvis that causes hemorrhage or when vascular tumors are supplied by large vessels, stainless steel coils may be used. This coil (Fig. 27.72), which functions to produce thrombogenesis, is simply a looped segment of guidewire with Dacron fibers attached to it. The coil is initially straight and is easily introduced into a catheter that has been placed into the desired vessel. This coil is then deployed by being pushed out of the catheter tip with a guidewire. The coil assumes its looping shape immediately as it enters the bloodstream. It is important that the catheter tip be specifically placed in the vessel so that the coil springs precisely into the desired area. Numerous coils can be placed as needed to occlude the vessel. Detachable coils are mounted on a wire and are deployed either manually or with an electrical current to allow for more precise placement. If the placement is not correct, the coil can be removed without being deployed. Newer generations of coils promise more effective embolization by using various coatings on the outside of the coil. One such coil uses a coating that initiates a foreign body/scarring response. Another type of coil is coated with an expansile gel that swells in the presence of

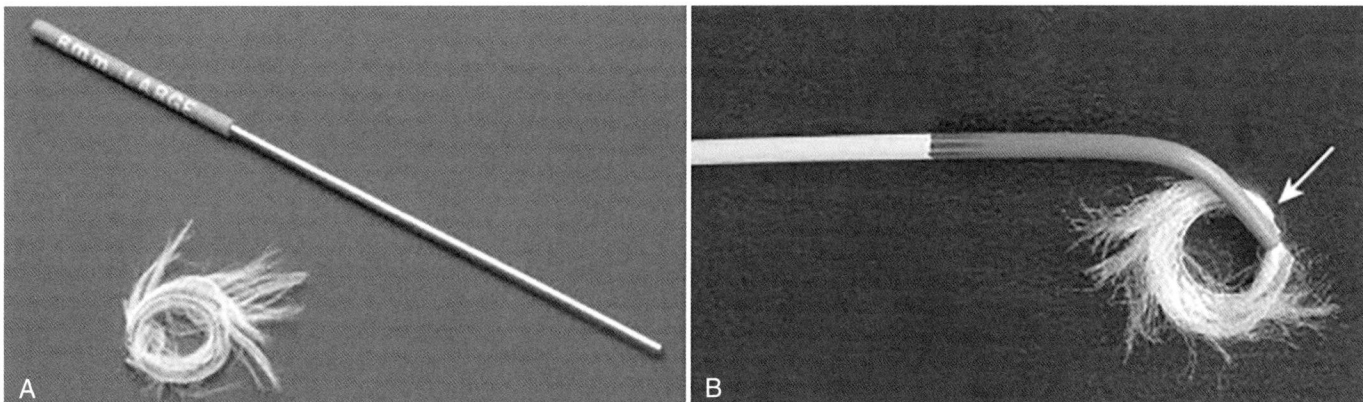

Fig. 27.72 Embolization coils. (**A**) Coils are packaged preloaded in tubes. Shown is a Gianturco stainless steel coil with polyester fibers. (**B**) The coil is delivered through a catheter *(arrow)*. The coil can be pushed with a guidewire, or injected.

(A, Courtesy Cook Group, Bloomington, IN. From Kaufman JA: Vascular interventions. In Kaufman JA, Lee MJ, editors: *Vascular and interventional radiology: the requisites*, 2nd ed, 2014, Elsevier.)

blood, occluding the vessel (Fig. 27.73). Another permanent occlusion device is a vascular plug, which is deployed by manually unscrewing the device from the delivery wire when in the desired position within the vessel. The vascular plug is used for large-vessel occlusion.

Fig. 27.74 shows a hypervascular uterine fibroid that was causing significant symptoms. Embolization of this uterine fibroid was successfully accomplished with total occlusion of the lesion. Embolization combined with arterial catheter directed infusion of chemotherapy drugs is known as *chemoembolization*. This is most commonly performed for treatment of primary and metastatic hepatic lesions. In recent years embolic spheres or *microspheres* have been designed to absorb therapeutic agents, such as chemotherapy drugs, to ensure a more controlled and sustained release of the drug.[10]

Radioembolization is also used to treat hepatic lesions. This procedure uses radioactive microspheres to both cut off blood supply to the tumor and to destroy tumor tissue by emitting powerful, but short, penetrating beta radiation. Radioembolism procedures may be completed using multiple modalities. Some treatments require intraprocedural 3D reconstruction spins. This allows for precise placement of the radioactive microspheres. In procedures such as ^{90}Y hepatic malignancy treatments, preprocedural anatomy mapping is required for the determination of tumor vascularity, embolization of nontarget extrahepatic vessels, and injection of a ^{99m}Tc-MAA radioisotope. Following the interventional procedure, the patient is taken to nuclear medicine to determine the radioisotope uptake in the lungs and surrounding tissues of the malignancy. If uptake levels are determined to be safe, the patient will return to the interventional suite about 2 weeks after the mapping procedure. Hepatic arteriography is performed to place microcatheters into the tumor vasculature and inject the ^{90}Y microspheres. The patient is taken to nuclear medicine after this procedure also. Radiotherapy is delivered for 10 to 14 days following the procedure.

Transcatheter embolization is also used in the cerebral vasculature of the brain. Vascular lesions, such as aneurysms, AVMs, and tumors, can be managed using multiple embolic agents, PVA, or tissue adhesive. Microcatheters (2 or 3 Fr) are passed through a larger catheter, a coaxial system that is positioned in the cerebral vessels. The smaller catheter is manipulated into the appropriate cerebral vessel, and if possible, into the aneurysm itself. The embolic materials are delivered through the microcatheter until the appropriate embolization is achieved (Fig. 27.75).

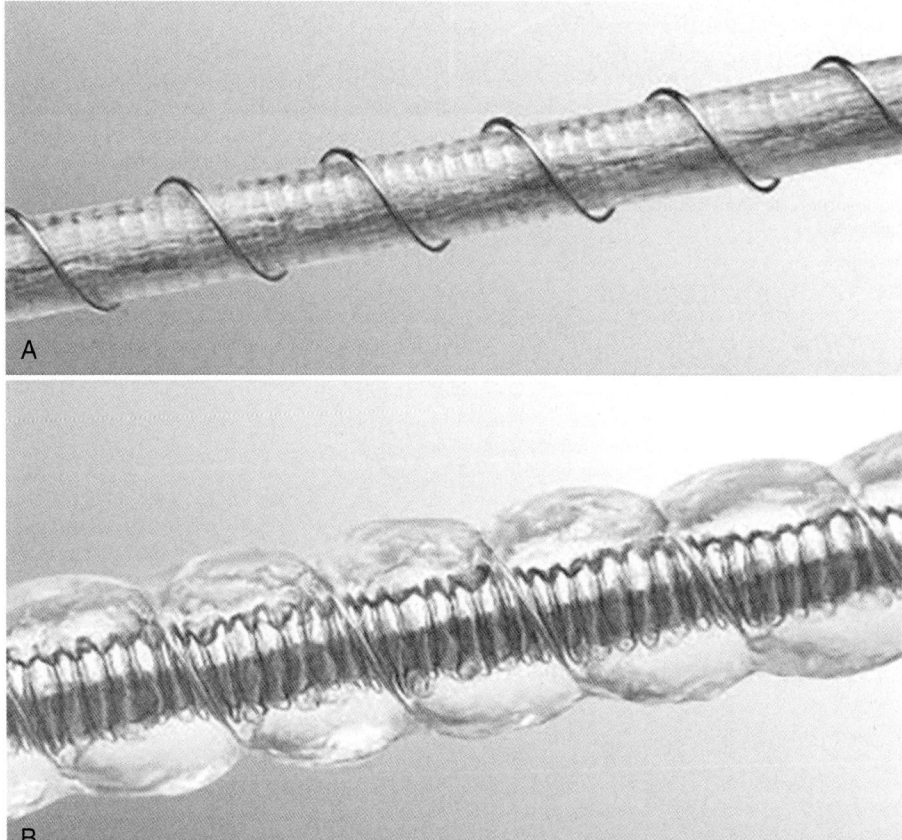

Fig. 27.73 Coil coated with a hydrogel that swells when in contact with blood. (**A**) Coil as packaged. (**B**) Coil after hydration. The process requires approximately 20 minutes in the blood to complete.

(Courtesy MicroVention Inc., Tustin, CA. From Kaufman JA: Vascular interventions. In Kaufman JA, Lee MJ, editors: *Vascular and interventional radiology: the requisites*, 2nd ed, 2014, Elsevier.)

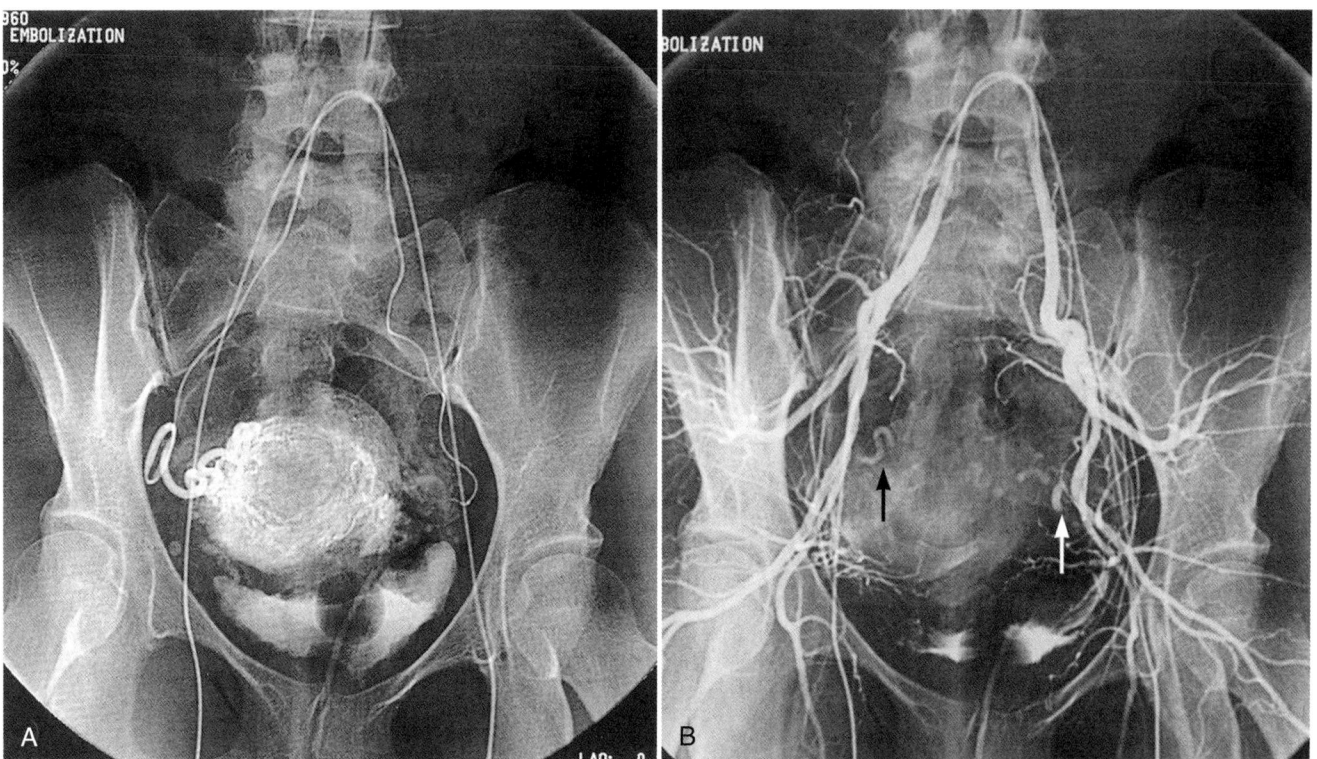

Fig. 27.74 Hypervascular uterine fibroid. (**A**) Bilateral uterine artery injections using coaxial microcatheters, showing hypervascular uterine fibroid. (**B**) Bilateral iliac artery injections, postembolization, showing total occlusion of both uterine arteries *(arrows)*.

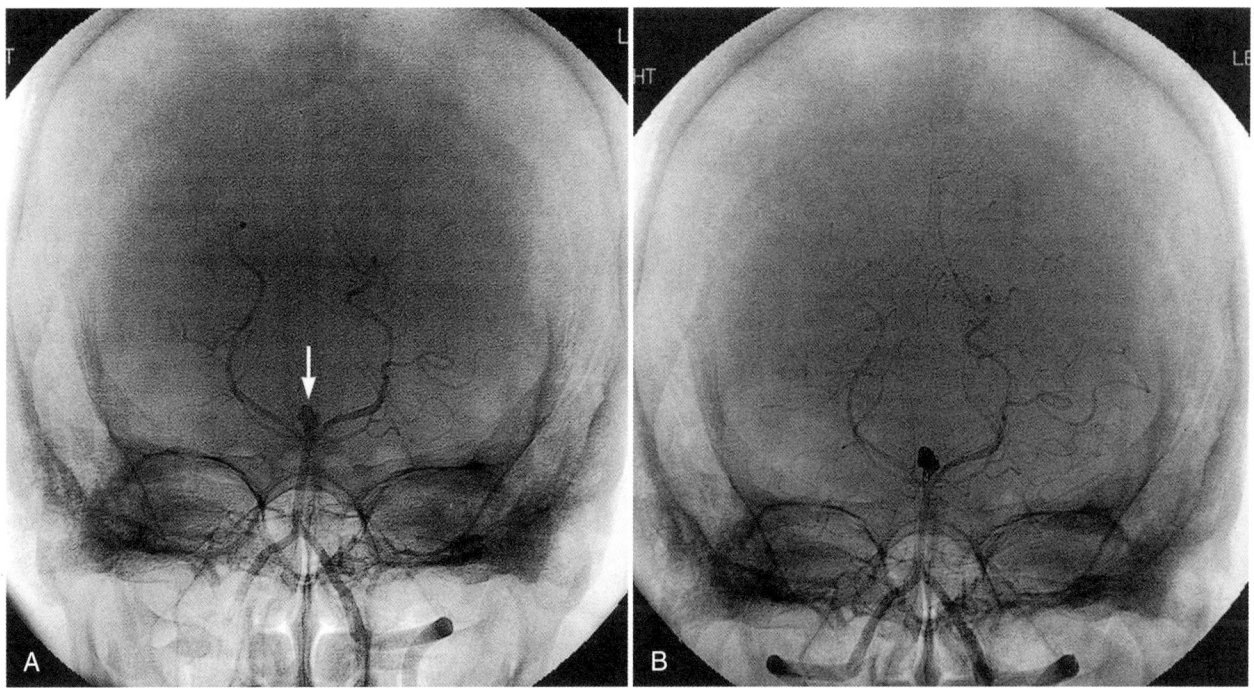

Fig. 27.75 Left vertebral artery injection. (**A**) Basilar tip aneurysm *(arrow)*. (**B**) Left vertebral artery injection postembolization with the use of Guglielmi detachable coils (GDCs).

Vena Cava Filter Placement

Vena cava filters are designed to trap venous emboli from migrating to the pulmonary arteries, causing a pulmonary embolus (PE). Most commonly, filters are placed in the IVC, although filters can also be placed in the SVC when necessary. A PE is a blood clot that forms as a thrombus and usually develops in the deep veins of the leg. When such a thrombus becomes dislodged and migrates, it is called an *embolus*. An embolus originating in the leg may migrate through the IVC and right side of the heart and finally lodge in the pulmonary arteries. A filter can be percutaneously placed in the IVC to trap such an embolus.

Lower limb vein thrombosis is not an indication for IVC filter placement. Normally, blood-thinning medications are administered to treat deep vein thrombosis. When anticoagulant therapy is contraindicated due to an increased risk for hemorrhage, filter placement may be indicated. Filter placement itself has associated risks, including thrombosis of the vein through which the filter is introduced and thrombosis of the vena cava. These risks normally are not life threatening. IVC filter placement is not a treatment for deep vein thrombosis of the leg but a therapy intended to reduce the chance of pulmonary embolism.

The idea of interrupting the pathway of an embolus is not a new one. Surgical interruption of the common femoral vein was first described in 1784, and surgical interruption of the IVC was described in 1868. These procedures and the partial surgical interruption procedures that evolved from them had a high rate of complications, not only owing to the surgical process but also owing to inadequate venous drainage from the lower limbs. Catheterization technology led to the development of detachable balloons for occluding the IVC, but that procedure also resulted in complications because of inadequate venous flow from the lower limbs.

The first true filter designed to trap emboli while maintaining vena cava patency was introduced in 1967 by Mobin-Uddin. It consisted of six metal struts joined at one end to form a conical shape that was covered by a perforated plastic canopy. Because of this filter's striking resemblance to an open umbrella, vena cava filters of all types for many years were referred to as "umbrella filters."

Today IVC filters are available in various shapes. All of these filters are initially compacted inside an introducer catheter delivery system and assume their functional shape as they are released (Fig. 27.76). The introducers are passed through sheaths ranging in size from 6 to 15 Fr.

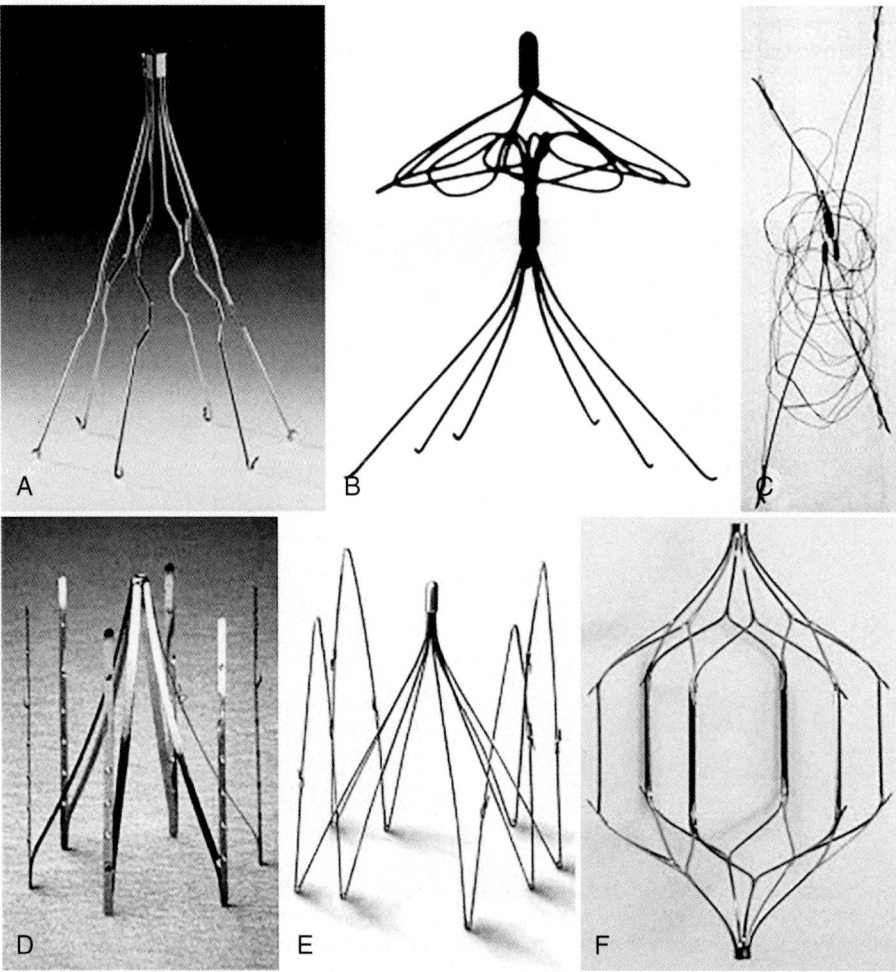

Fig. 27.76 Examples of permanent inferior vena cava (IVC) filters. **(A)** Greenfield (Boston Scientific); **(B)** Simon Nitinol (Bard); **(C)** Bird's Nest (Cook); **(D)** Vena Tech (B. Braun Medical); **(E)** Vena Tech LP (B. Braun Medical); **(F)** TrapEase (Cordis Corporation). Optional IVC filters.

Continued

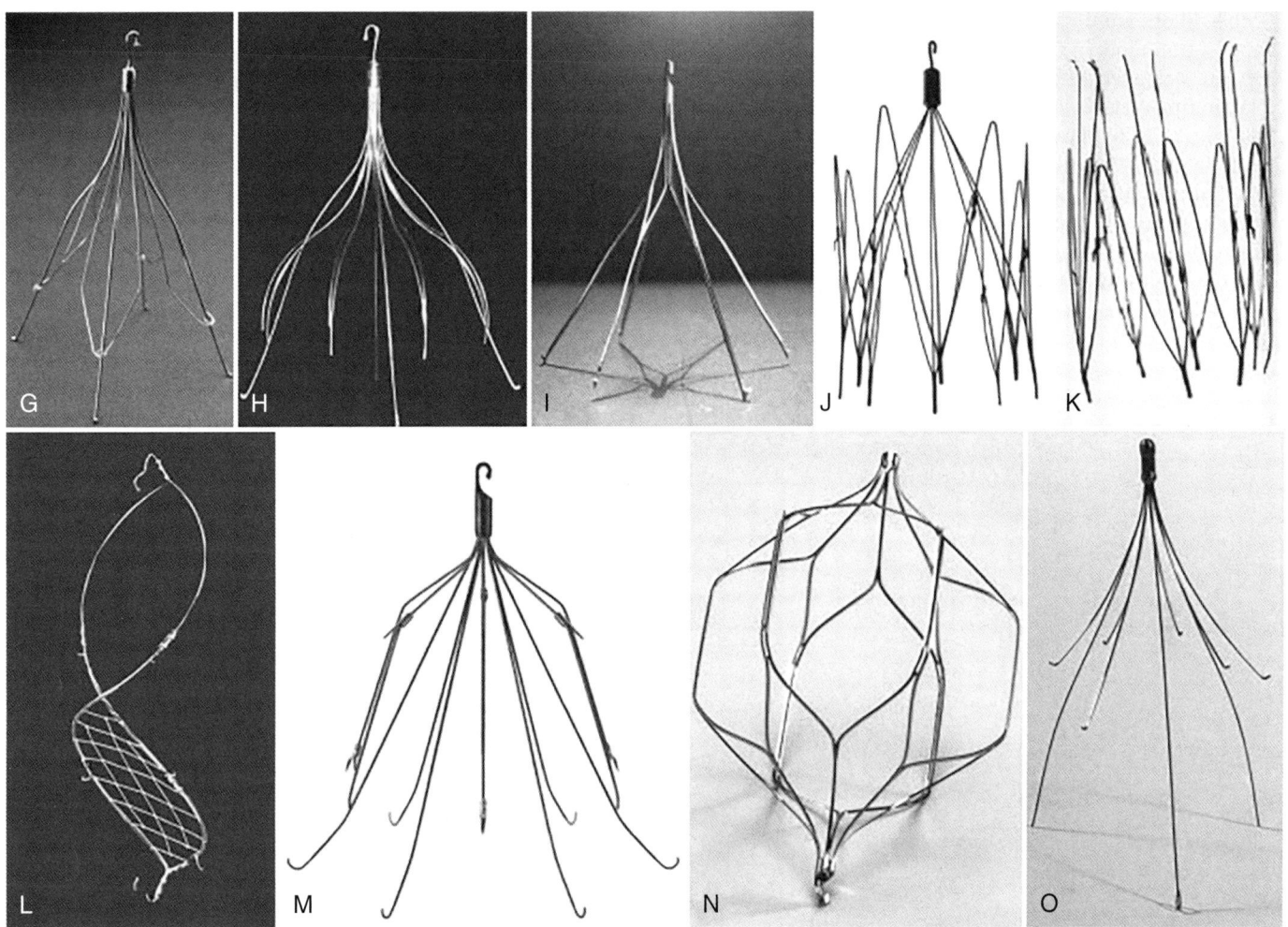

Fig. 27.76, cont'd (**G**) Gunther Tulip (Cook); (**H**) Celect (Cook); (**I**) Option (Argon Medical); (**J**) Convertible filter in closed position (B. Braun Medical); (**K**) Convertible filter with cap removed (B. Braun Medical); (**L**) Crux filter (Crux BioMedical); (**M**) Meridian (Bard); (**N**) OPTEASE (Cordis); (**O**) ALN (ALN Implants).

(From Kaufman JA: Inferior vena cava and tributaries. In Kaufman JA, Lee MJ, editors: *Vascular and interventional radiology: the requisites*, 2nd ed, 2014, Elsevier.)

Most filters are designed as a conical shape to trap clots in the central lumen. They are designed to be placed in vena cava ranging up to 20 to 30 mm in diameter. Fig. 27.76 shows the currently available IVC filters. Several newer filters are designed to be retrievable within a specified time frame. These are known as optional filters, as physicians have the option to remove the filter or leave the filter in permanently, depending on the risks and benefits to the patient. These retrievable filters have hooks, either at the top or bottom, that allow them to be grasped by a catheter snare device and removed percutaneously (Fig. 27.77).

Regardless of whether the filter is permanent or temporary, the purpose is to prevent new onset of PE by trapping venous emboli. These filters do not treat preexisting clots.

The filters are percutaneously inserted through a femoral, jugular, or antecubital vein, usually for placement in the IVC just inferior to the renal veins. Placement inferior to the renal veins is important to prevent renal vein thrombosis, which can occur if the vena cava is occluded superior to the level of the renal veins by a

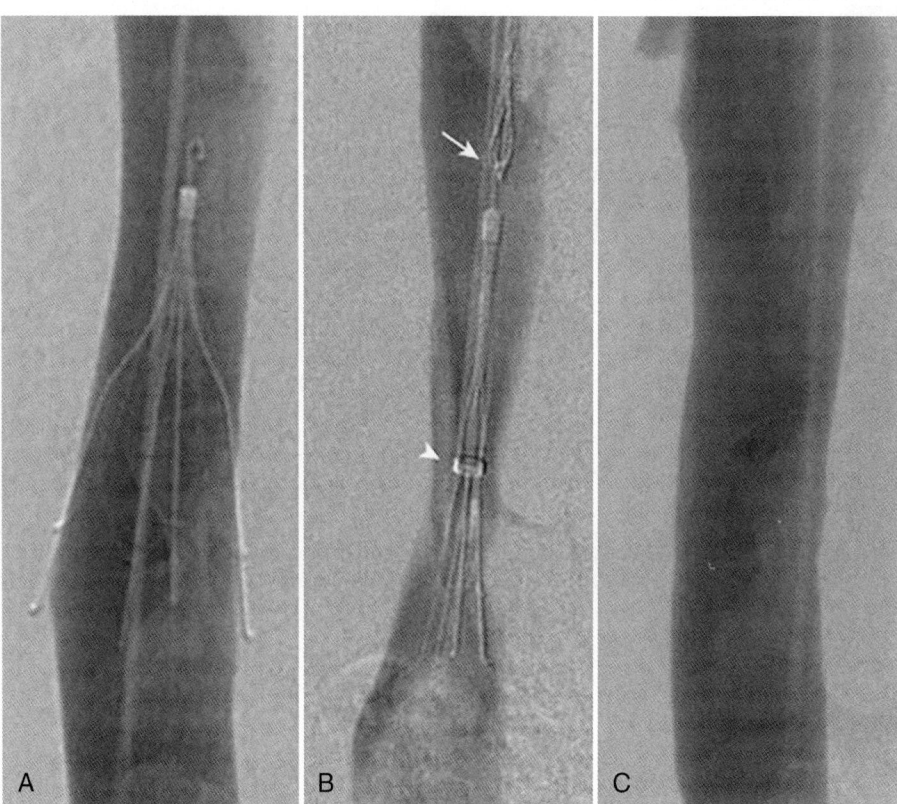

Fig. 27.77 The process of filter retrieval. (**A**) Initial cavogram confirming patency of the filter and inferior vena cava (IVC) (Gunther Tulip, Cook Medical). (**B**) The filter has been snared *(arrow)* and the sheath *(arrowhead)* advanced over the filter to constrain it. The sheath is advanced over the feet of the filter for safe removal. (**C**) Completion cavogram after filter removal showing a normal IVC.

(From Kaufman JA: Inferior vena cava and tributaries. In Kaufman JA, Lee MJ, editors: *Vascular and interventional radiology: the requisites*, 2nd ed, 2014, Elsevier.)

large thrombus in a filter. An inferior vena cavogram is performed using the modified Seldinger technique. The inferior vena cavogram defines the anatomy, including the level of the renal veins, determines the diameter of the vena cava, and rules out the presence of a thrombus (Fig. 27.78). The diameter of the vena cava may influence the choice of filter as each filter has a maximum diameter. If the patient's IVC diameter is larger than the filter's maximum diameter, there is an increased risk of filter migration toward the patient's heart, which could result in serious complications.

Filter insertion from the jugular or antecubital approach may be indicated if a thrombus is present in the iliac veins and/or in the IVC. The filter insertion site is dilated to accommodate the filter introducer. The filter remains sheathed until it reaches the desired level and is released from its introducer by the interventionalist. The introducing system is then removed, and external compression is applied to the venotomy site until hemostasis is achieved. A postplacement image is obtained to document the location of the filter (Fig. 27.79).

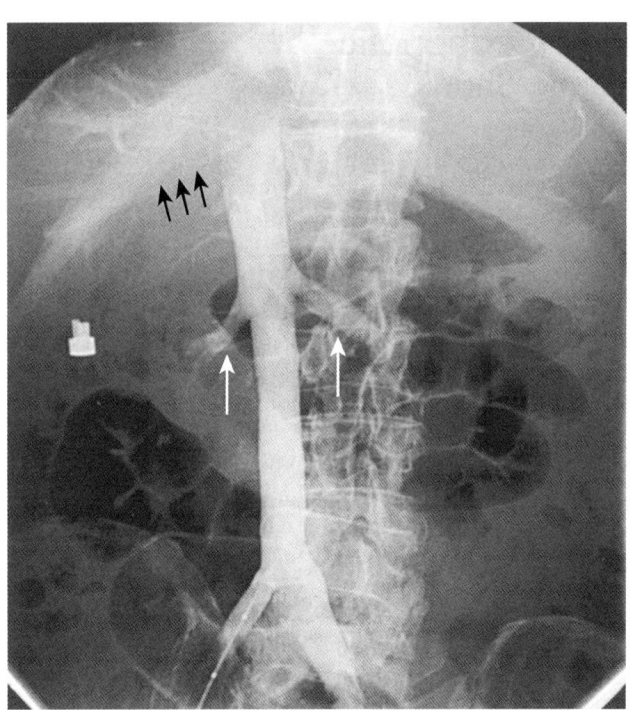

Fig. 27.78 Inferior vena cavogram. Note reflux into renal veins *(white arrows)* and hepatic veins *(black arrows)*.

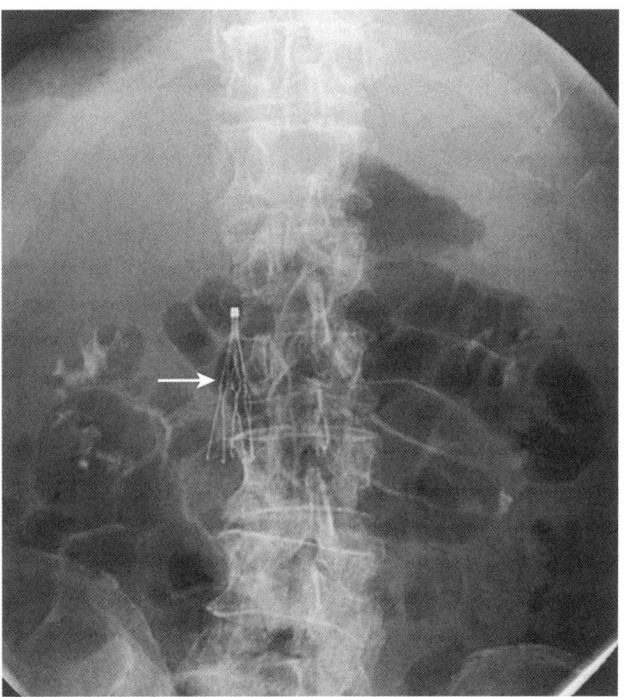

Fig. 27.79 Postplacement image showing Greenfield filter in place *(arrow)*.

Transjugular Intrahepatic Portosystemic Shunt

The *portal circulation* consists of blood from the digestive organs, which drains into the liver. The portal system consists of the splenic vein, the superior mesenteric vein, and the inferior mesenteric vein. The blood passes through the liver tissue and is returned to the IVC via the hepatic veins. Disease processes can increase the resistance of blood flow through the liver, elevating the blood pressure of the portal circulation—a condition known as *portal hypertension*. It may cause the blood to flow through collateral veins. Venous *varices* are the result and can be life threatening if they bleed. The creation of a portosystemic shunt can decrease portal hypertension and the associated variceal bleeding by allowing the portal venous circulation to bypass its normal course through the liver. The percutaneous intervention for creating an artificial low-pressure pathway between the portal and hepatic veins is called a *transjugular intrahepatic portosystemic shunt (TIPS)*.

Prior to a TIPS procedure, ultrasonography is used to confirm patency of the portal venous system. Hepatic venography and portography are performed during a TIPS procedure to delineate anatomy. Transcatheter blood pressure measurements are often used to confirm the existence of a pressure gradient between the portal and hepatic veins.

The most common approach for a TIPS procedure is from a right internal jugular venous puncture site to the middle or right hepatic vein. A hepatic venogram may be obtained using contrast material or CO_2 or both. CO_2 typically allows for better visualization of the portal vein during wedged hepatic venography. A special long needle is passed into the hepatic vein and advanced through the liver tissue into the portal vein. The needle is exchanged for an angioplasty balloon catheter, and the tract through the liver tissue is dilated. An angiographic catheter may be passed through the tract and advanced into the splenic vein for a splenoportal venogram. An intravascular stent is positioned across the tract to maintain its patency (Figs. 27.80 and 27.81). The tract and stent may be enlarged further with an angioplasty balloon catheter until the desired reduction in pressure gradient between the portal and hepatic veins is achieved. If large gastric or splenic varices persist after the shunt creation, embolization of these varices using coils, sclerosants, or glue may be performed. Once the shunt is created, portal pressures are reduced, and flow through the varices is diverted, the sheath is removed from the internal jugular vein, and external pressure is applied until hemostasis at the venotomy occurs.

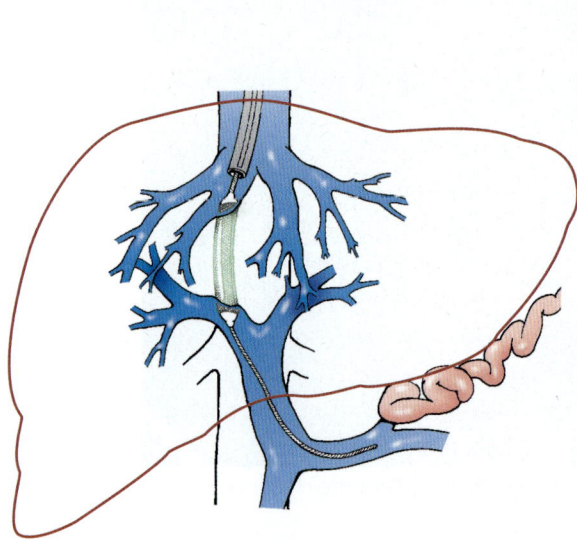

Fig. 27.80 Intravascular stent placement in a TIPS procedure.

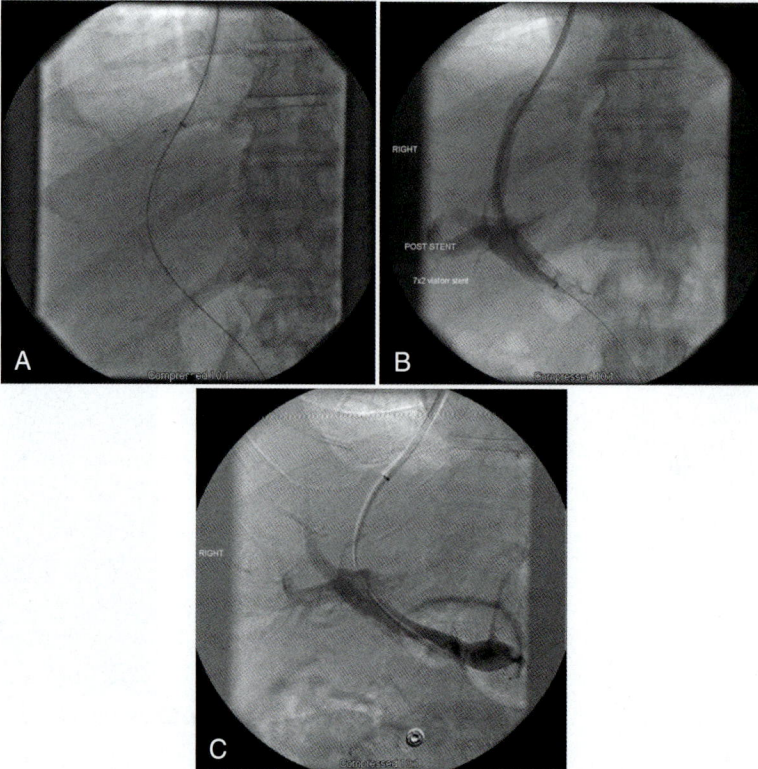

Fig. 27.81 TIPS procedure. (**A**) Stent placement. (**B**) Stent with contrast. (**C**) Initial contrast agent injection.

Pharmacologic Thrombolysis and Mechanical Thrombectomy

When an angiogram shows a thrombus (blood clot) within a vessel, interventional catheters and devices can be used to remove the thrombus and restore blood flow in both arterial and venous systems. These methods are effective in restoring arterial blood flow quickly in acute emergent situations such as large vessel ischemic stroke, limb-threatening ischemia, large PE, and acute myocardial infarction (MI), discussed later in this chapter. Pharmacologic thrombolysis uses blood clot–dissolving medications that are infused through an angiographic catheter positioned against the thrombus. Special infusion catheters with side holes are manipulated directly into the clot. Periodic repeat *angiograms* evaluate the progress of *lysis* (dissolution). The catheter may have to be advanced under fluoroscopic control to keep it against or in the clot as lysis progresses.

Mechanical thrombectomy uses catheters and/or devices to physically remove the clot. Mechanisms for physical thrombus removal include aspiration, extraction, maceration, and fragmentation. Fig. 27.82 demonstrates mechanical thrombectomy in the cerebral arteries using specialized aspiration catheters and a stent retriever device to restore blood flow to brain tissue. The most recent advancements in mechanical thrombectomy include treatments for pulmonary embolisms and deep vein thrombosis. These devices eliminate the need for thrombolytics and ICU stays. The aspiration and extraction devices can remove large acute and chronic clot burdens in one procedure. Figure 27.83 demonstrates the Inari Medical FlowTriever aspiration of a saddle pulmonary embolism. This device uses a controlled-vacuum syringe system and mesh discs to safely remove clots and minimize blood loss.

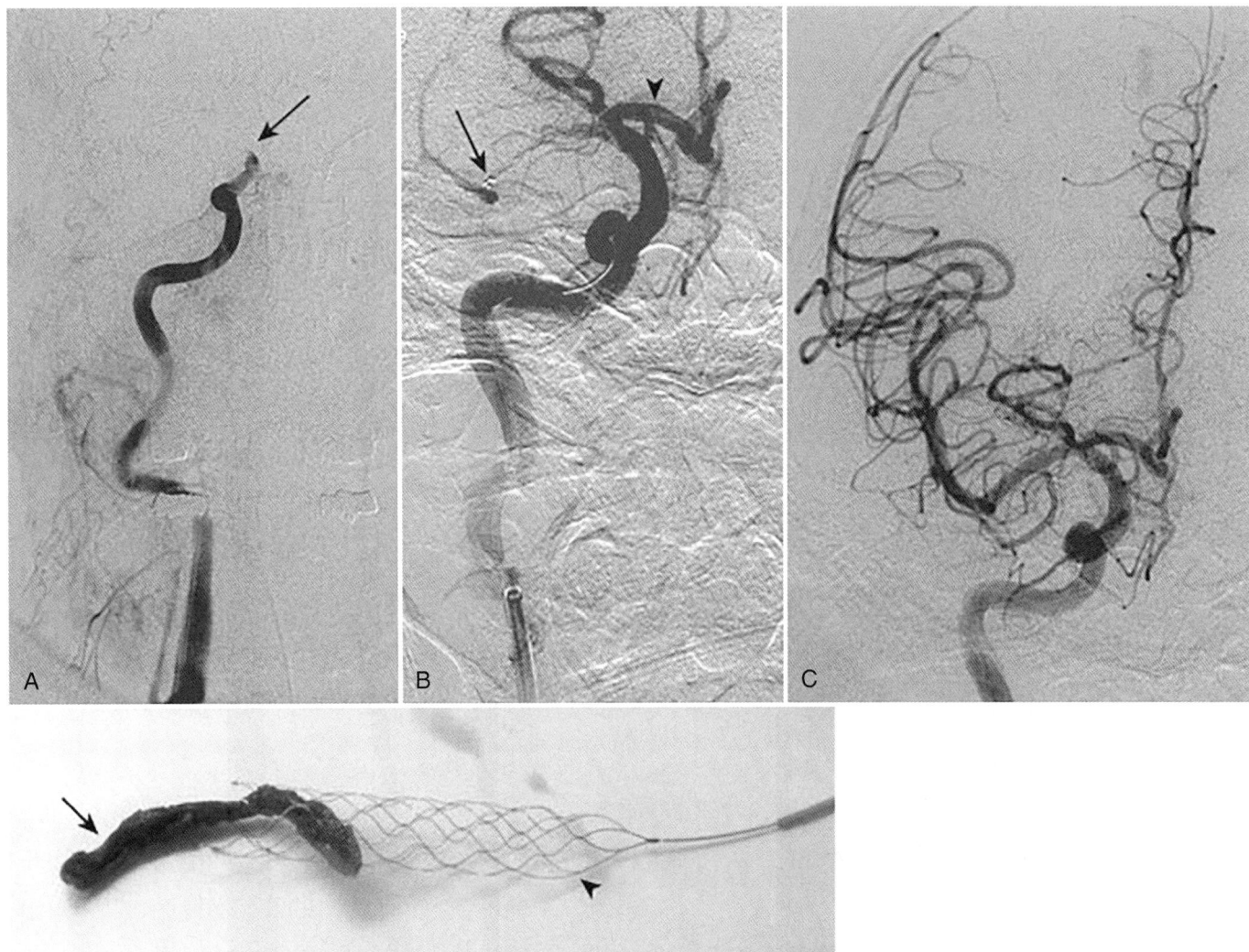

Fig. 27.82 Stroke intervention with a thrombus retrieval device (the Solitaire retrievable stent, Medtronic, Minneapolis, MN). **(A)** Carotid arteriogram showing abrupt occlusion in right internal carotid artery *(arrow)*. **(B)** Arteriogram after first pass with stent retriever showing right anterior cerebral artery is now open *(arrowhead)*. **(C)** Completion arteriogram showing reperfusion in the right anterior and middle cerebral arteries. **(D)** The thrombus *(arrow)* removed, trapped in the stent retriever *(arrowhead)*.

(From Kaufman JA, Nesbit GM: Carotid and vertebral arteries. In Kaufman JA, Lee MJ, editors: *Vascular and interventional radiology: the requisites*, 2nd ed, 2014, Elsevier.)

Other Procedures

The insertion of vascular access catheters, such as central lines, hemodialysis catheters, tunneled catheters for long-term use, and implantable vascular access devices, such as port-a-caths used for chemotherapy infusion, are often performed in interventional radiology.

Interventional devices can be used to remove foreign bodies, such as catheter fragments or broken guidewires, percutaneously from the vasculature. Various snares can be used for this purpose. A snare catheter introduced using the Seldinger technique is manipulated under fluoroscopic control to grasp the foreign body. The snare and foreign body are then withdrawn as a unit.

Nonvascular Interventional Procedures

In addition to vascular interventional procedures, there are many nonvascular interventional procedures that are performed in interventional radiology. Technologists are expected to have comprehensive knowledge of anatomy and pathophysiology of the gastrointestinal, biliary, and urinary systems, and to demonstrate an understanding of interventional procedures such as needle biopsy, percutaneous drainage, and stent placement. Common nonvascular interventional procedures include but are not limited to:

- Percutaneous nephrostomy catheter placement: to externally drain urine from the pelvis of the kidney.
- Percutaneous ureteral stent placement: to provide an internal pathway for urine to flow from the kidney to the bladder, through an obstructed or damaged ureter.
- Percutaneous gastrostomy and gastrojejunostomy: to place direct gastrointestinal (GI) feeding tubes and/or drainage tubes into the most appropriate section of the GI tract.
- Percutaneous biliary drainage and/or stent placement: to relieve biliary obstruction, to divert bile in the presence of a bile leak, or to externally drain infected bile.
- Vertebroplasty/kyphoplasty: treatment for vertebral compression fractures using a bone cement and potentially balloons or devices to restore vertebrae height.

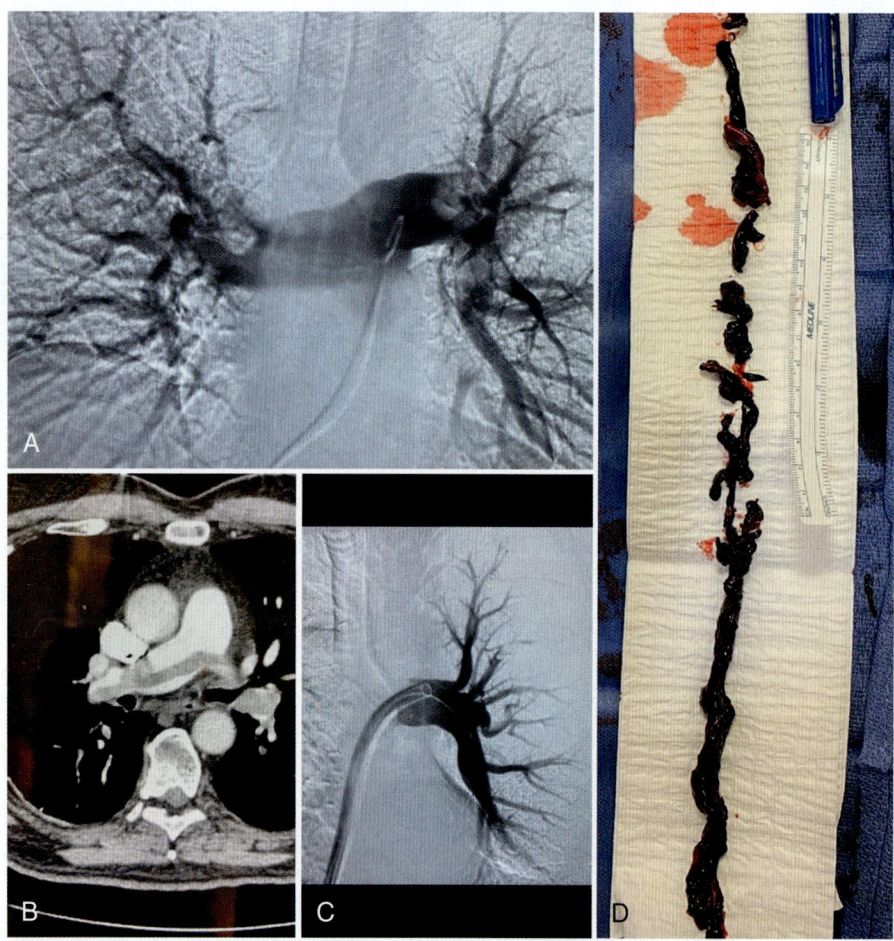

Fig. 27.83 Pulmonary embolism intervention with an aspiration device (Inari Medical FlowTriever). **(A)** Angiogram demonstrating insufficient contrast filling the pulmonary arteries. **(B)** Axial CT image. The white demonstrates the pulmonary artery filled with contrast, while the dark linear void is the embolus. **(C)** Angiogram shows the contrast-filled left pulmonary arteries postembolectomy. **(D)** Emboli removed using the FlowTriever.

(Courtesy of NEA Baptist Hospital in Jonesboro, AR.)

Vascular and Interventional Radiology: Present and Future

As previously mentioned, the field of interventional radiology is continually and rapidly evolving.

New catheters, guidewires, and medical devices are constantly being introduced with the ultimate aim of improving patient outcomes by performing less invasive procedures. More complex diseases and more critically ill patients are being treated with interventional procedures, a change that has led to incorporating dedicated angiography equipment into the OR, or ensuring that the angiography suite is OR compatible, allowing for dedicated anesthesia support and the potential to quickly convert percutaneous procedures to open surgical procedures. These suites are often considered *hybrid suites*. In these suites, interventionalists will often work alongside vascular, cardiothoracic, and neurosurgeons in complicated procedures that use both percutaneous and open surgical techniques. These procedures are highly technical, and a team approach is crucial.[11] The cardiovascular and interventional technologist plays an active role in this multidisciplinary interventional team (Fig. 27.84).

The imaging capabilities of angiographic equipment have also evolved dramatically. Increased image resolution at lower radiation dose is a primary goal within angiography, and manufacturers are continually developing ways to meet this goal.

Other imaging advancements include incorporating cross-sectional and 3D imaging into the angiography suite. Most angiographic equipment manufacturers now offer the capability to perform cone beam CT acquisitions using the C-arm. These CT acquisitions allow for high-quality 3D imaging and advanced image processing without the need for additional imaging equipment. Some larger facilities have integrated CT and even MRI scanners into the angiography suite to assist with image guidance for procedures.

Advances in medical imaging software and applications have allowed for multimodality fusion imaging. This allows images from other modalities to be projected onto and incorporated into the live fluoroscopic image so that the image moves in conjunction with the fluoroscopy image to assist with catheter placement during interventional procedures.

Currently, research is being conducted into the use of robotics in interventional radiology and cardiovascular interventions. Robotic angiographic instruments have been designed to manipulate needles, guidewires, and medical devices, such as balloon angioplasty catheters. It is thought that the use of these robotics could drastically reduce radiation exposure to the interventionalist, allow for easier and safer navigation of tortuous vasculature, and allow for MRI-guided interventions to be faster and more accurate.

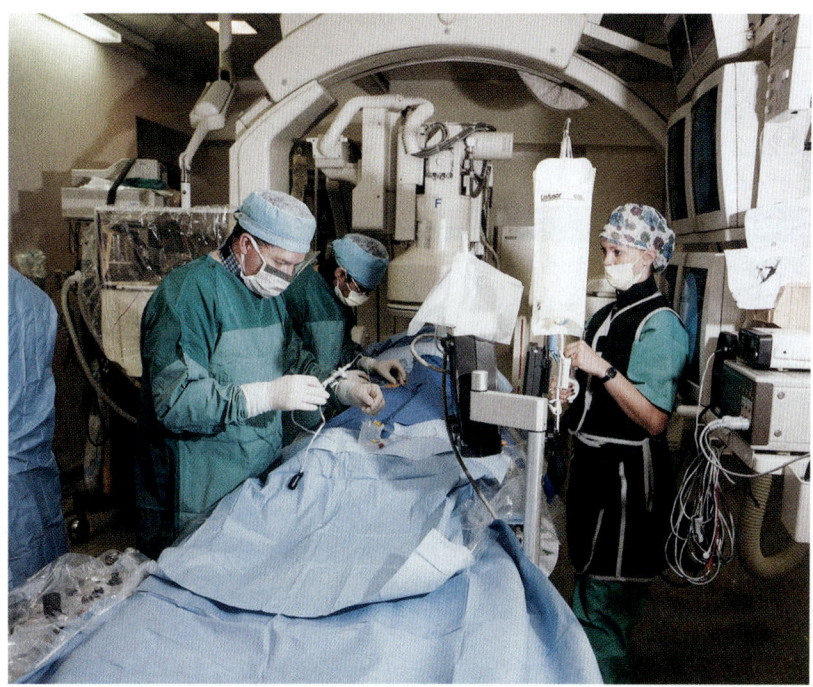

Fig. 27.84 The technologist plays an active role on the interventional team by assisting the interventionalist *(left)* or by circulating within the angiography suite *(right)*.

CARDIOVASCULAR INTERVENTIONAL RADIOGRAPHY

Cardiovascular interventional radiography is a branch of cardiology that covers diagnostic and interventional procedures that utilize radiographic imaging of the heart. These procedures include cardiac catheterization, structural heart interventions, and electrophysiology procedures. The most common of these procedures is the cardiac catheterization.

Cardiac Catheterization

Cardiac catheterization is a comprehensive term used to describe a minimally invasive percutaneous procedure involving the introduction of specialized catheters into the heart and surrounding vasculature for diagnostic evaluation and possible intervention associated with cardiovascular-related disorders in children and adults. Cardiac catheterization is classified as either a diagnostic or an interventional procedure. The primary purpose of diagnostic procedures is to collect data necessary to evaluate the patient's condition. Cardiac interventional procedures involve the application of therapeutic measures through catheter-based systems or other mechanical means to treat disorders of the vascular and conduction systems within the heart.

GENERAL INDICATIONS

Cardiac catheterization is performed to identify the anatomic and physiologic condition of the heart. The data gathered during catheterization provides the physician with information to develop management strategies for patients who have cardiovascular disorders. *Coronary angiography* is performed to accurately visualize coronary anatomy and pathology. The anatomic information gained from this procedure may include the presence and extent of obstructive coronary artery disease, thrombus formation, coronary artery collateral flow, coronary anomalies, aneurysms, and spasms. Coronary artery size can also be determined. Often the goal of coronary angiography is to evaluate and plan the most appropriate coronary interventional procedure (e.g., PTCA, intracoronary stent, or atherectomy).

Coronary artery disease is the most common disorder necessitating catheterization of the adult heart. This disease is caused primarily by the accumulation of fatty intracoronary *atheromatous* plaque, which leads to *stenosis* and *occlusion* of the coronary arteries. Coronary artery disease is symptomatically characterized by chest pain (angina pectoris) or a heart attack (MI). Treatment of coronary artery disease includes medical, surgical, and catheter-directed interventions.

Diagnostic cardiac catheterization of an adult patient with coronary artery disease is conducted to assess the appropriateness and feasibility of various therapeutic options. Cardiac catheterization provides *hemodynamic* and *angiographic* data to document the presence and severity of the disease. In selected circumstances, postoperative catheterization is performed to assess the results of surgery.

Diagnostic studies of the adult heart also aid in evaluating a patient who has confusing or obscure symptoms (e.g., chest pain of undetermined cause). These studies are also used to assess diseases of the heart not requiring surgical intervention, such as certain cardiomyopathies.

In children, diagnostic heart catheterization is employed to evaluate congenital and valvular disease, disorders of the cardiac conduction system, and selected cardiomyopathies. Interventional techniques are also performed in children, primarily to alleviate symptoms associated with certain congenital heart defects.

The indications for cardiac catheterization are established by a special task force comprised of the American College of Cardiology and the American Heart Association (ACC/AHA). The indications are summarized in Table 27.2. Commonly performed procedures based on diagnosis are also presented. The ACC/AHA[11] has

TABLE 27.2

Indications for cardiac catheterization

Indications	Procedures
1. Suspected or known coronary artery disease	
a. New-onset angina	LV, COR
b. Unstable angina	LV, COR
c. Evaluation before a major surgical procedure	LV, COR
d. Silent ischemia	LV, COR, ERGO
e. Positive ETT	LV, COR, ERGO
f. Atypical chest pain or coronary artery spasm	LV, COR, ERGO
2. Myocardial infarction	
a. Unstable angina postinfarction	LV, COR
b. Failed thrombolysis	LV, COR, RH
c. Shock	LV, COR, RH
d. Mechanical complications (ventricular septal defect)	LV, COR, RH (rupture of wall or papillary muscle)
3. Sudden cardiovascular death	LV, COR, R + L
4. Valvular heart disease	LV, COR, R + L, AO
5. Congenital heart disease (before anticipated corrective surgery)	LV, COR, R + L, AO
6. Aortic dissection	AO, COR
7. Pericardial constriction or tamponade	LV, COR, R + L
8. Cardiomyopathy	LV, COR, R + L, BX
9. Initial and follow-up assessment for heart transplant	LV, COR, R + L, BX

AO, Aortography; *BX*, endomyocardial biopsy; *COR*, coronary angiography; *ERGO*, ergonovine provocation of coronary spasm; *ETT*, exercise tolerance test; *LV*, left ventriculography; *R + L*, right and left heart hemodynamics; *RH*, right heart oxygen saturations and hemodynamics (e.g., placement of Swan-Ganz catheter).
From Kern MJ: *The cardiac catheterization handbook,* 4th ed, 2003, Mosby.

classified the indications and appropriateness for coronary angiography by placing the previously discussed disease categories into three classifications, as follows:

- Class 1: Conditions for which there is general agreement that coronary angiography is justified
- Class 2: Conditions for which coronary angiography is frequently performed, but for which a divergence of opinion exists with respect to its justification in terms of value and appropriateness
- Class 3: Conditions for which coronary angiography ordinarily is not justified

Other procedures that may be performed concurrently with coronary angiography are listed in Table 27.3. Some of these procedures are discussed later in the text.

TABLE 27.3
Procedures that may accompany coronary angiography

Procedures	Comment
1. Central venous access (femoral, internal jugular, subclavian)	Used as IV access for emergency medications or fluids, temporary pacemaker (pacemaker not mandatory for coronary angiography)
2. Hemodynamic assessment	
a. Left heart pressures (aorta, left ventricle)	Routine for all studies
b. Right and left heart combined pressures	Not routine for coronary artery disease; mandatory for valvular heart disease; routine for CHF, right ventricular dysfunction, pericardial diseases, cardiomyopathy, intracardiac shunts, congenital abnormalities
3. Left ventricular angiography	Routine for all studies; may be excluded with high-risk patients, left main coronary or aortic stenosis, severe CHF
4. Internal mammary selective angiography	Not routine unless used as coronary bypass conduit
5. Pharmacologic studies	
a. Ergonovine	Routine for coronary vasospasm
b. IC/IV/sublingual nitroglycerin	Optionally routine for all studies
6. Aortography	Routine for aortic insufficiency, aortic dissection, aortic aneurysm, with or without aortic stenosis; routine to locate bypass grafts not visualized by selective angiography
7. Digital subtraction angiography	Not routine for coronary angiography; excellent for peripheral vascular disease
8. Cardiac pacing and electrophysiologic studies	Arrhythmia evaluation
9. Interventional and special techniques	Intracoronary flow-pressure for lesion assessment Coronary angioplasty (PTCA) Myocardial biopsy Transseptal or direct left ventricular puncture Balloon catheter valvuloplasty Conduction tract catheter ablation
10. Arterial closure devices	Available for patients with conditions prone to puncture site bleeding

CHF, Congestive heart failure; *PTCA,* percutaneous transluminal coronary angioplasty.
From Kern MJ: *The cardiac catheterization handbook,* 4th ed, 2003, Mosby.

CONTRAINDICATIONS, COMPLICATIONS, AND ASSOCIATED RISKS

While cardiac catheterization has inherent risk factors, most physicians agree that the only absolute contraindications to this procedure are the refusal of the procedure by a mentally competent person and the lack of adequate equipment or catheterization facilities.

There are few contraindications for cardiac catheterization when the appropriateness of the procedure is based on the benefit-risk ratio. Relative contraindications according to the guidelines of the ACC/AHA[11] include the following:

- Active gastrointestinal bleeding, anemia
- Anticoagulation, or known bleeding disorder
- Electrolyte imbalance
- Infection and fever
- Medication intoxication (digitalis, phenothiazine)
- Pregnancy
- Recent stroke
- Renal failure
- Uncontrolled congestive heart failure
- Uncooperative patient

Some of these conditions may be temporary, or they may be treated and reversed before cardiac catheterization is attempted.

As with any invasive procedure, complications can be expected during cardiac catheterization. The Society for Cardiac Angiography and Interventions (SCAI) reviewed catheterizations in more than 300,000 patients from three different time periods and found that the major complication rate for the entire group was less than 2%. As the severity of the patient's disease increases, however, so do the risks associated with the procedure.

The risks of cardiac catheterization vary according to the type of procedure and the status of the patient undergoing the procedure. Significantly influencing the outcome of the procedure is the stability of the patient's condition before the procedure. Patients presenting with left main coronary stenosis are at a significantly higher risk of complications from coronary angiography than patients who have no left main coronary stenosis. The SCAI database identified the main predictors of major complications after cardiac catheterization and determined that the following increased the risk of complications:[12]

- Moribund patient (patient with poor response to life-threatening condition)
- Cardiogenic shock
- Acute MI (within 24 hours)
- Renal insufficiency
- Cardiomyopathy

The expected benefits of cardiac catheterization must be weighed against the associated risks when determining whether to perform the procedure.

SUPPLIES AND EQUIPMENT

Cardiovascular equipment consists of a wide variety of supplies and equipment used to perform the procedure. In addition to the equipment mentioned previously for vascular angiographic procedures, there are variations in catheter design to accommodate the coronary arteries. Because of the complexity and vast number of different types of procedures performed in a cardiac catheterization laboratory, only a few of the most used items are discussed.

Sheaths

Sheaths are an essential supply used in almost every cardiac cath case. A sheath is a short, hollow plastic tube with a one-way valve and a side port (Fig. 27.85). Once vascular access is obtained, a sheath is inserted over a guidewire to maintain access without blood loss. The valve on the sheath allows for the introduction of other equipment such as catheters, guidewires, balloons, or stents without significant blood loss.

Guidewires

Guidewires are critical to a safe vascular procedure. A guidewire is a thin, flexible piece of metal that has either a curved or floppy tip. Guidewires are inserted to help guide catheters and other equipment through the vasculature without damaging the walls of the vessels. Guidewires come in a multitude of sizes, tip shapes, lengths, and stiffness.

Catheters

The catheters used for left heart cardiac catheterization are similar to the angiographic catheters previously described except that cardiac catheters are specifically shaped for the cardiac vasculature (Fig. 27.86). Left heart catheterization involves accessing the arterial system to locate the coronary arteries and left side of the heart. Right heart catheterization involves accessing the venous system to locate the right side of the heart and the pulmonary arteries. Specialized catheters are used for right heart catheterization procedures. In contrast to angiographic catheters, the main purpose of which is to serve as a conduit for contrast media, right heart catheters are typically flow-directed catheters that use an inflated balloon on the tip of the catheter to ease passage through the various chambers of the heart. Various types of flow-directed catheters are capable of performing more tasks than the standard angiographic catheter. Depending on the type of procedure to be performed, the cardiologist determines which catheter(s) to use.

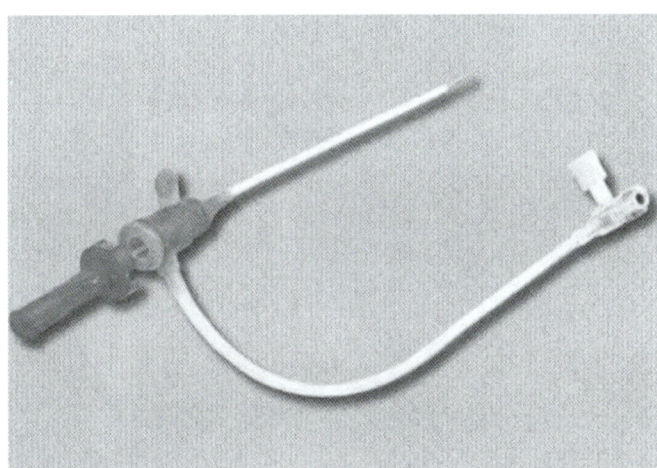

Fig. 27.85 Arterial introducer sheath.

(From Peate I, Macleod J: *Pudner's nursing the surgical patient*, 4th ed, 2021, Elsevier.)

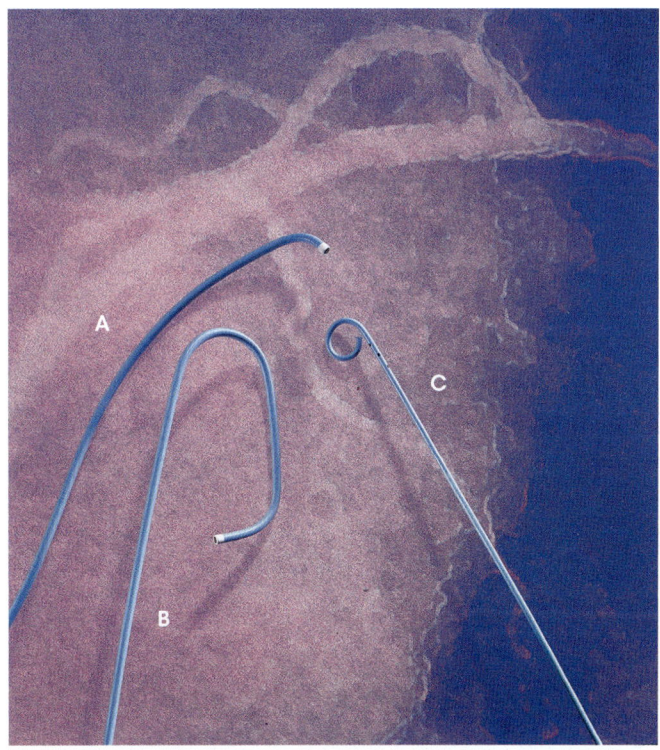

Fig. 27.86 Catheters used during cardiac catheterization. (**A**) Judkins right. (**B**) Judkins left. (**C**) Pigtail.

(Courtesy Cordis Corp., Miami, FL.)

Catheters placed in a patient's vasculature can function as a fluid-filled column for hemodynamic data or as a conduit for contrast media, thrombolytic agents, or mechanical devices. Blood samples can be drawn directly from selected cardiac chambers for the purpose of *oximetry* or other laboratory analysis. To perform these and other tasks, three or four valves (*stopcocks*) are combined to form a *manifold*, which is attached to the proximal end of the catheter (Fig. 27.87). Using a manifold allows such functions as drawing blood samples, administering medications, and recording blood pressure without disconnecting from the catheter.

Balloons

The main method of coronary intervention is balloon angioplasty. An angioplasty balloon is a long, thin catheter with a small balloon mounted on the tip. This catheter is directed into the blocked artery, and the balloon is inflated to open the blockage. These balloons come in multiple diameters and lengths. There are also two main types of balloons: compliant and noncompliant. The compliance of a balloon refers to how the balloon will inflate when a portion of it is compressed.

Stents

Stent placement is the final goal of angioplasty in most cases. A stent is flexible metal mesh in the shape of a tube. Stents come collapsed and mounted on a balloon catheter. Once in position, the balloon is inflated, and the stent is deployed. The stent holds the vessel open and pushes the plaque against the wall. Stents come in a variety of diameters and lengths as well. There are two main types of stents commonly used: bare metal and drug-eluting stents (DES). A DES is a stent coated in a specific drug that will prevent any tissue regrowth through the stent after placement. A bare metal stent does not have any drug coating.

Contrast media

Injection of contrast media is essential for angiographic visualization of the cardiac anatomy. Several iodinated radiographic contrast media are approved for intravascular, intracardiac, and intracoronary use in adults and children. Transient (temporary) ECG changes during and immediately after the injection of contrast media are common.

Pressure injector

A pressure injector is a tool used to administer radiographic contrast media (Fig. 27.88) during cardiac catheterization. The pressure injector is used to inject a large amount (25 to 50 mL) of contrast material into the ventricles (the main pumping chambers of the heart), the aortic root, or the pulmonary vessels. Because the coronary arteries are of small caliber and of low flow rate, administration of contrast media into these structures generally does not require a high-pressure injector. Instead, most physicians opt for manual injection using an angiographic control syringe and manifold system. However, newer pressure injectors have settings that allow for low pressure, controlled injections into the coronary arteries. This allows the cardiologist a great amount of consistency of the amount and force with which the contrast is injected into the arteries. This enhanced control allows for improved imaging and more accurate contrast counting.

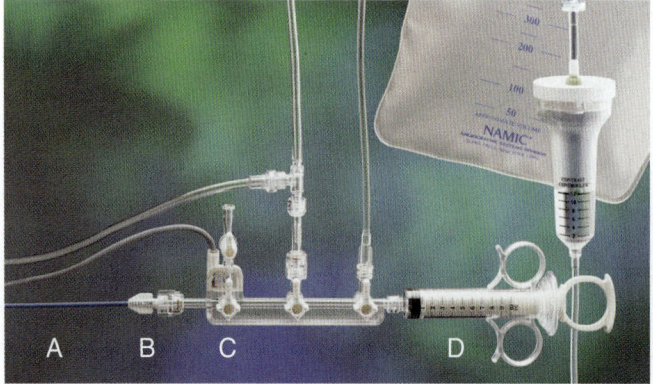

Fig. 27.87 Disposable three-valve Compensator Morse manifold, with a Selector catheter (**A**), rotating adapter (**B**), pressure transducer (**C**), and angiographic control syringe (**D**).

(Courtesy SCHNEIDER/NAMIC, Glens Falls, NY.)

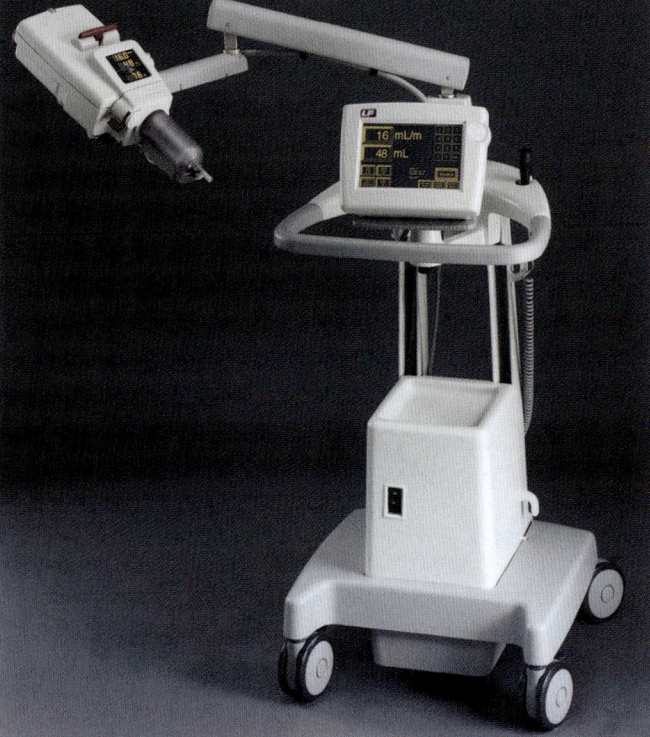

Fig. 27.88 The Angiomat (ILLUMENA) high-pressure injector for radiographic contrast media.

(Courtesy Liebel-Flarsheim, a product of Mallinckrodt, Inc., Cincinnati, OH.)

Equipment

The imaging equipment found in the cardiac catheterization laboratory is essentially the same as the equipment found in the vascular angiography suite. The catheterization laboratory requires a system capable of producing fluoroscopic images with the greatest amount of recorded detail available. Maximum resolution from the optical system is crucial because of the small size of the cardiac anatomy, which must be imaged while in motion. The imaging used for cardiac studies is typically 15 to 30 frames per second, compared with 2 to 6 frames per second used for peripheral imaging. The motion of the heart beating requires this increased frame rate to visualize these small arteries properly. The imaging equipment necessary to produce high-resolution imaging is described in the earlier section on DSA procedures.

Physiologic equipment

The physiologic monitor is essential to cardiac catheterization procedures. It is used to monitor and record vital patient functions, including electrical activity (ECG)[c] within the heart and blood pressure (hemodynamic) within the various intracardiac chambers (Fig. 27.89). The patient's ECG and hemodynamic pressures are continuously displayed throughout the various types of procedures. Selective samplings of ECG and hemodynamic pressures are recorded for permanent documentation.

For the collection of hemodynamic data during catheterization, the physiologic recorder (receiving information in electrical form) must be connected to the catheter (carrying information as physical fluid pressure). Devices called *pressure transducers* are interfaced between the manifold and the physiologic recorder to convert fluid (blood) pressure into an electrical signal.

For a standard cardiac catheterization procedure, four channels of the physiologic recorder are usually prepared: Two for ECG recordings and two for pressure recordings. A physiologic recorder can have as many as 32 channels.

Other equipment

Because of the nature of the patient's condition, the inherent risks of cardiac catheterization, and the types of procedures performed, each catheterization room should have the following equipment available:

- A fully equipped emergency cart. The cart typically contains emergency medications, cardiopulmonary resuscitation equipment, intubation equipment, and other related supplies (Fig. 27.90).
- Oxygen and suction.
- Whole-blood oximeters, used to determine the oxygen saturation of the blood samples obtained during adult and pediatric catheterizations (Fig. 27.91).
- Defibrillator, used to treat life-threatening arrhythmias. Ideally the defibrillator would also have the ability to pace externally. Some laboratories have two defibrillators available in case one fails.
- Temporary pacemaker to treat potential asystole or symptomatic bradycardia.
- Pulse oximeter to monitor and assess level of oxygenation noninvasively during sedation.
- Noninvasive blood pressure monitoring capabilities.

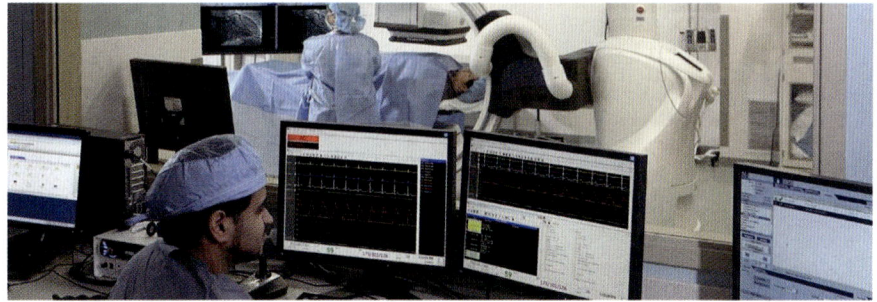

Fig. 27.89 Computer-based physiologic monitor used to monitor patient ECG and hemodynamic pressures during cardiac catheterization.

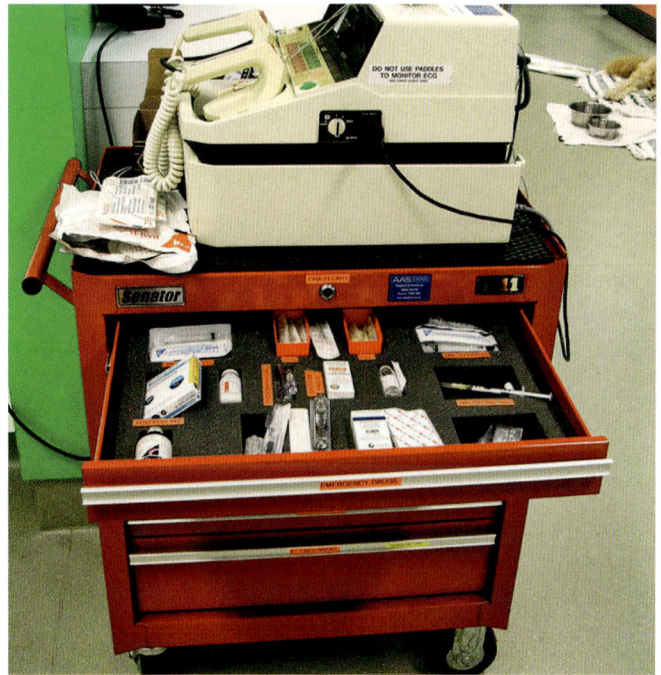

Fig. 27.90 Standard emergency resuscitation cart and defibrillator unit.

- Equipment to perform cardiac output studies.
- Intraaortic balloon pump, used to increase myocardial perfusion and cardiac output during interventional procedures.
- An activated clotting time (ACT) machine, used to monitor blood coagulation while using high-dose heparin or other anticoagulants during procedures.

In addition to the basic coronary angiogram and left and right heart studies, many effective tools are available to diagnose and treat coronary artery disease (Table 27.4).

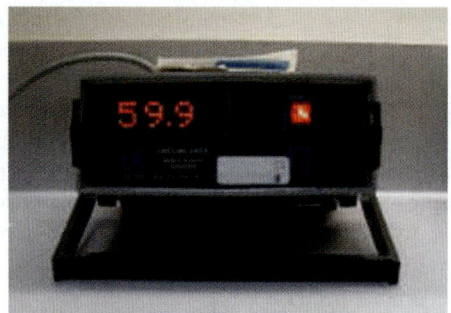

Fig. 27.91 Oximeter used to measure oxygen saturation in blood.

TABLE 27.4
Tools for diagnosis and treatment of coronary artery disease

Equipment	Use	Diagnostic or therapeutic
Pressure wire	Measures blood flow across lesion to determine severity of stenosis	Diagnostic
IVUS	Internal vessel visualization of stenosis, plaque, stent position	Diagnostic
OCT (optical coherence tomography)	Laser light to image the inside of the vessel wall	Diagnostic
Rotablator	Rotational atherectomy of intraluminal plaque or calcium	Therapeutic
Rheolytic thrombectomy	High-velocity saline spray for thrombectomy	Therapeutic
The Crosser	Study device to chronic total occlusions	Therapeutic

IVUS, Intravascular ultrasound; *OCT*, optical coherence tomography.

PRECATHETERIZATION CARE

Before the catheterization is performed, the procedure is explained, and informed consent is obtained. A preprocedure checklist is used to ensure that all the necessary patient medical history, physical examinations, noninvasive imaging, and laboratory blood tests have been performed and reviewed prior to the procedure.

Various medications are frequently administered for sedation and control of nausea. Typically, patients are not allowed anything to eat or drink for 4 to 6 hours before the procedure. During all catheterizations, a protocol (or detailed record) of every aspect of the procedure is maintained.

CATHETER INTRODUCTION

The most frequent sites used for cardiac catheterization are the femoral and radial area. The brachial, axillary, jugular (neck), and subclavian (chest) areas may also be chosen.

For catheterization of the artery or vein, the percutaneous approach is employed (see the modified Seldinger technique, which is described and illustrated in Fig. 27.13). On rare occasions, if the percutaneous approach cannot be used, a cutdown technique is employed. This technique requires that a small incision be made in the skin to allow for direct visualization of the artery or vein that the physician wants to catheterize. The skin is aseptically prepared, infiltrated with local anesthetic, and the vessel or vessels are bluntly dissected and exposed. After an opening is created in the desired vessel (arteriotomy or venotomy), the catheter is introduced and advanced toward the heart.

POSTCATHETERIZATION CARE

When the catheterization procedure is completed, all catheters are removed. If a cutdown approach was used, the arteriotomy or venotomy is repaired as appropriate. If a percutaneous approach was used, multiple techniques can be employed to obtain hemostasis. Manual pressure may be placed on the puncture site until bleeding is controlled. For femoral arteriotomies internal closure devices may be used. These devices are deployed under the skin against the artery wall and include a collagen seal, suture-mediated devices, or a metal clip. For radial arteriotomies, an external pressure device is often used that allows gradual reduction of pressure at the site after a prescribed time, usually over 1 to 2 hours. For venotomies, manual pressure for 5 to 10 minutes is usually sufficient to obtain hemostasis. Once hemostasis is achieved, these wound sites are cleaned and dressed to minimize the risk of infection.

The puncture site must be observed for hemorrhage or hematoma, and the status of the distal pulse is recorded on the protocol record before the patient leaves the catheterization laboratory. Vital signs should be monitored regularly after the catheterization. The ingestion of fluids should be encouraged, and pain medication may be indicated.

Cardiac catheterization is often performed on an outpatient or same-day treatment basis. The patient is monitored for 4 to 8 hours in a recovery area and then allowed to go home. Instructions for home care recovery procedures are usually given to the patient or a family member before the patient leaves the recovery area. At this time, any prescriptions the physician recommends for long-term use will be discussed with the patient and their family members.

Diagnostic Cardiac Procedures

LEFT HEART CATHETERIZATION (LHC)

Catheterization of the left side of the heart is performed to evaluate heart function, to measure hemodynamic pressures in the aorta and left ventricle, and to access the right and left coronary arteries. The catheter may be introduced through the radial, brachial, or femoral artery and advanced over a guidewire to the ascending aorta. When in the ascending aorta, the guidewire is removed, and the catheter is aspirated and flushed to prevent migration of any air bubbles.

A normal aortic valve prevents backward flow of contrast media into the left ventricle during injection, whereas an insufficient valve does not (Fig. 27.92). Left ventriculography provides information about valvular competence, interventricular septal integrity, and the efficiency of the pumping action of the left ventricle (ejection fraction) (Fig. 27.93). Mitral regurgitation is another example of valvular incompetence, and angiographically, it is seen as the backward flow of contrast media from the left ventricle into the left atrium or pulmonary veins (Fig. 27.94).

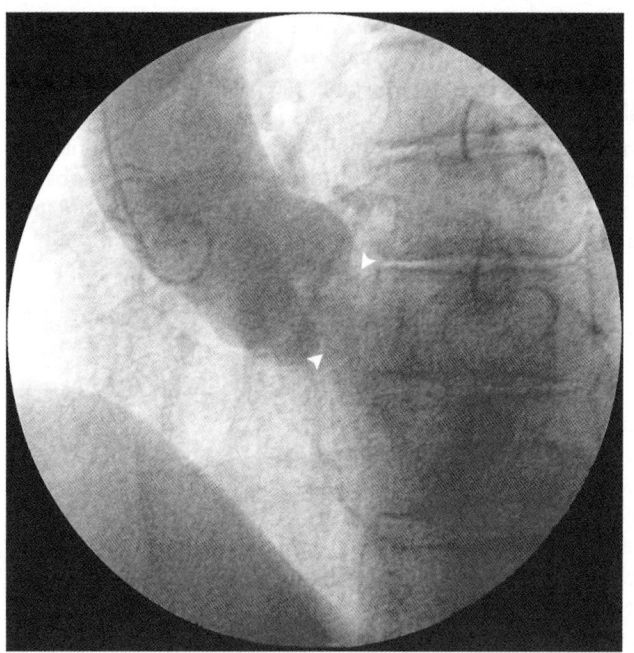

Fig. 27.92 Aortic root injection showing aortic insufficiency with contrast agent flowing back into left ventricle *(arrowheads)*.

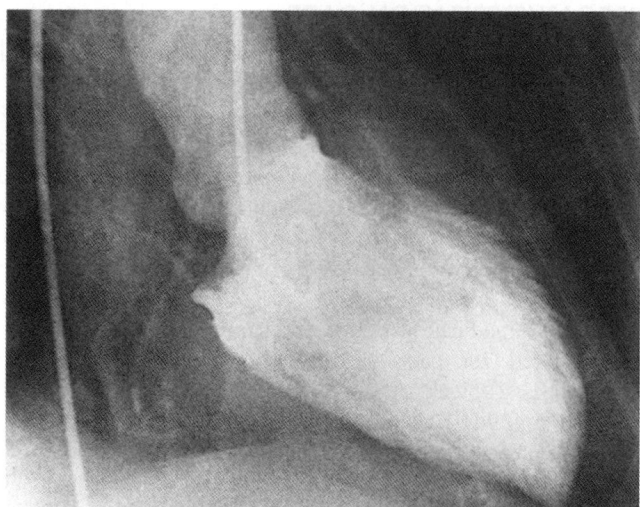

Fig. 27.93 Normal left ventriculogram during diastole.

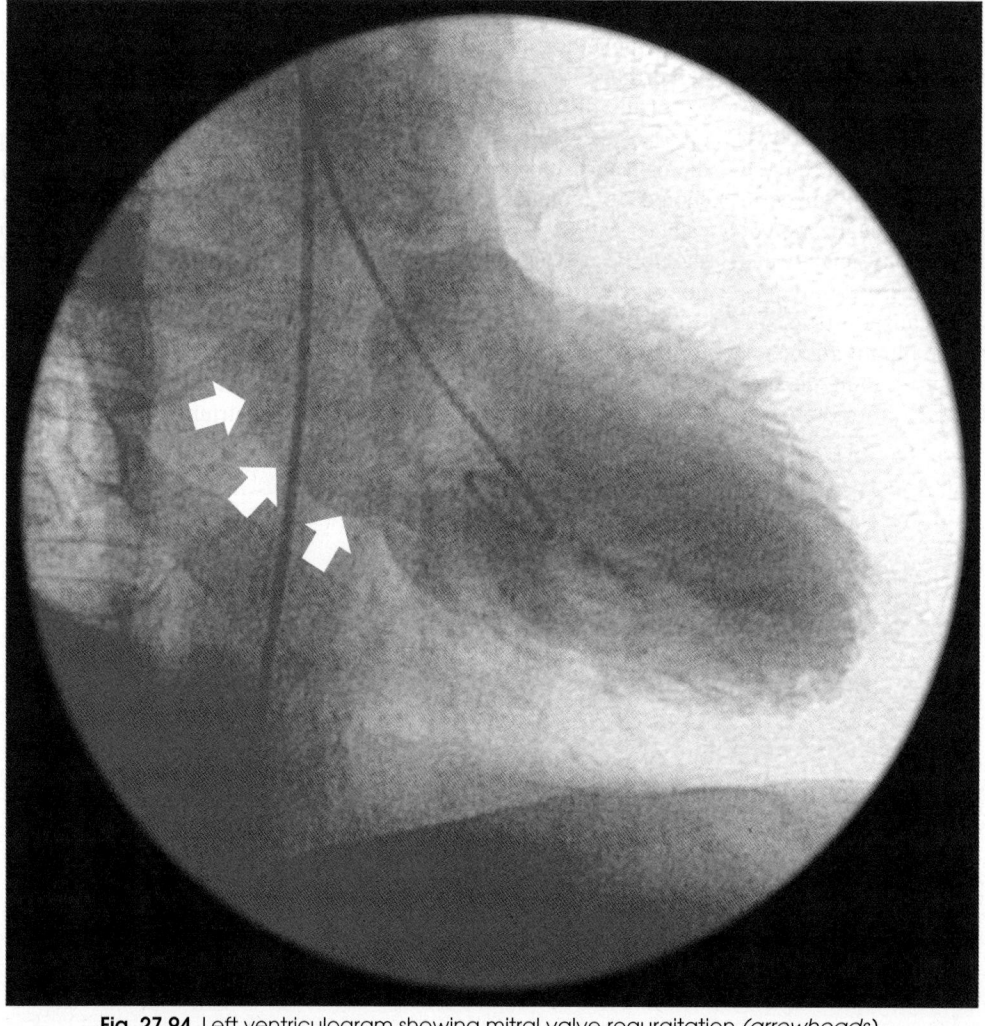

Fig. 27.94 Left ventriculogram showing mitral valve regurgitation *(arrowheads)*.

Computer *planimetry* software calculates how well the ventricle functions (Fig. 27.95). The presence of aortic valve stenosis is determined as the blood pressure measurements are repeated while the catheter is withdrawn across the aortic valve. Normal flow of blood through the aortic valve allows the systolic pressure in the left ventricle to match the systolic pressure in the aorta. When the systolic blood pressure in the left ventricle is greater than the systolic blood pressure in the aorta, aortic stenosis is present.

SELECTIVE CORONARY ANGIOGRAPHY

Selective angiography of the right coronary artery and left coronary artery is performed, with different projections used for each coronary artery to prevent superimposition with overlapping structures. Coronary angiography allows the extent of intracoronary stenosis to be evaluated (Figs. 27.96 to 27.101).

Because of the complexity of the anatomy involved, the variations in patient body habitus, and the presence of anomalies, a comprehensive guide for angiographic projections is difficult to establish. Projections commonly used during coronary angiography are listed in Table 27.5. The cardiologist determines the projections that best show the artery of interest. Coronary arteriograms are obtained in nearly all catheterizations of the left side of the heart.

RIGHT HEART CATHETERIZATION (RHC)

The right heart catheterization (RHC) is another commonly performed procedure. During right heart catheterization, venous access is established in the femoral, antecubital fossa, internal jugular, or subclavian vein. Then a catheter called a Swan-Ganz (Fig. 27.102) is inserted and advanced to the vena cava, into the right atrium, across the tricuspid valve, to the right ventricle, and through the pulmonary valve to the pulmonary artery, until it is wedged distally in the pulmonary artery. Pressure measurements and oximetry are performed in each of the heart chambers as the catheter is advanced. The pressure measurements are used to determine the presence of disorders such as valvular heart disease, congestive heart failure, pulmonary hypertension, and certain cardiomyopathies. The oximetry data are used to determine the presence of an intracardiac shunt, as well as obtaining measurements for a Fick calculation of the cardiac output. Finally, the catheter is positioned in

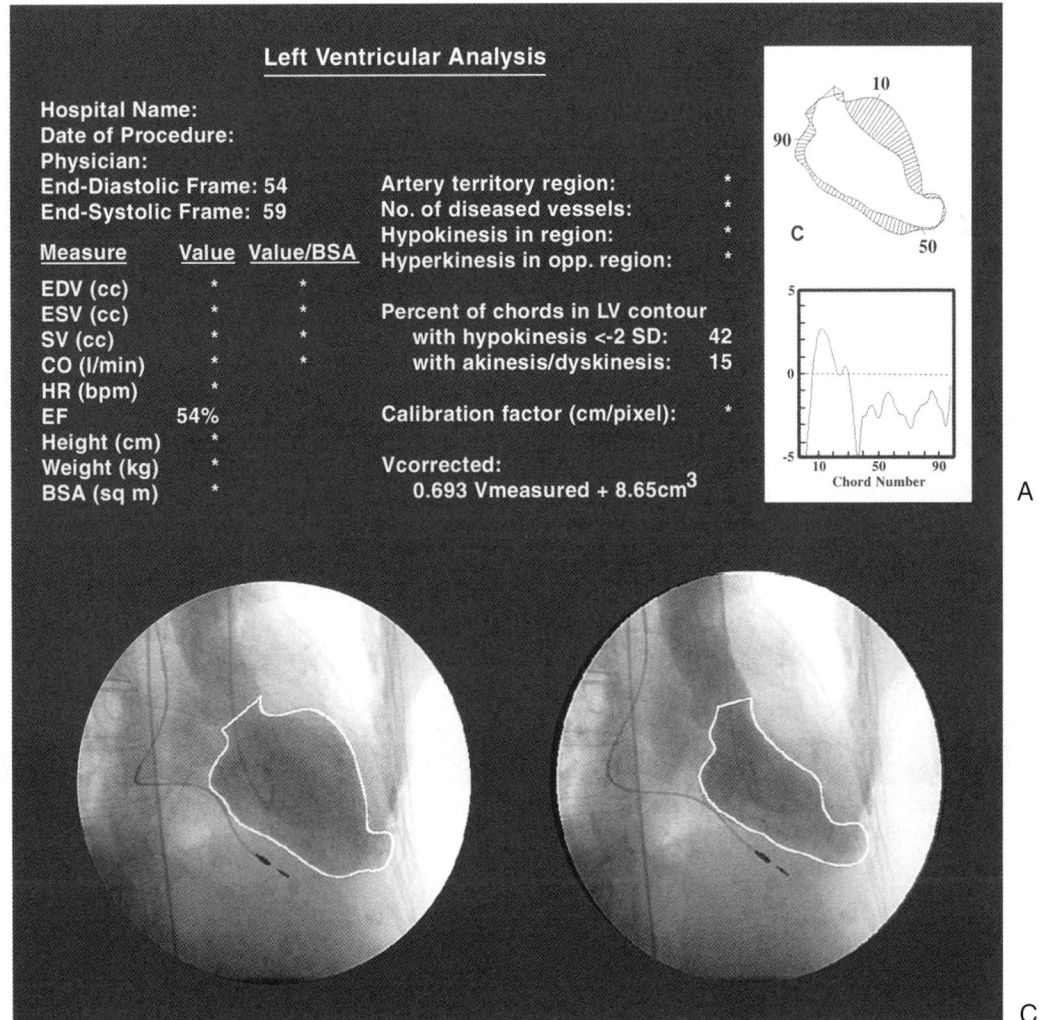

Fig. 27.95 Computerized planimetry for evaluation of left ventricular ejection fraction. **(A)** Digital representation of when the diastolic and systolic phases of contraction are superimposed. **(B)** Diastolic phase of contraction of the heart. **(C)** Systolic phase of contraction of the heart.

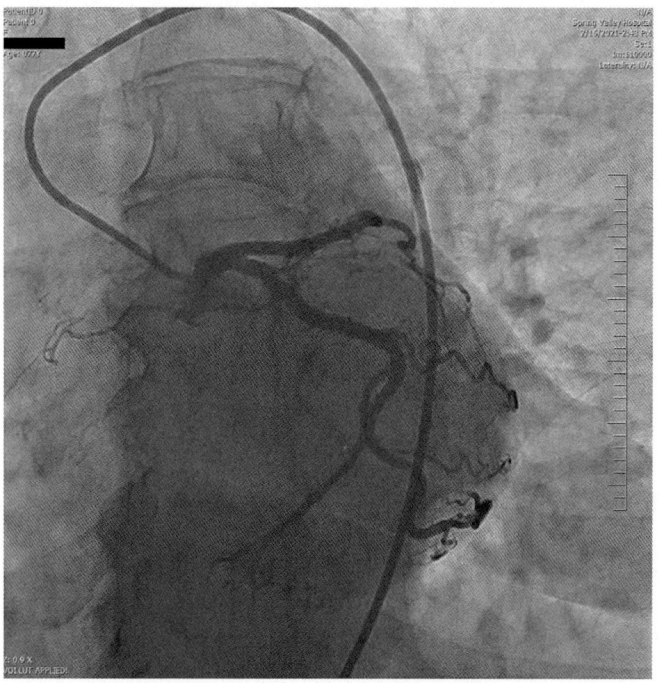

Fig. 27.96 Normal left anterior descending (LAD) and circumflex coronary arteries in the LAO caudal view.

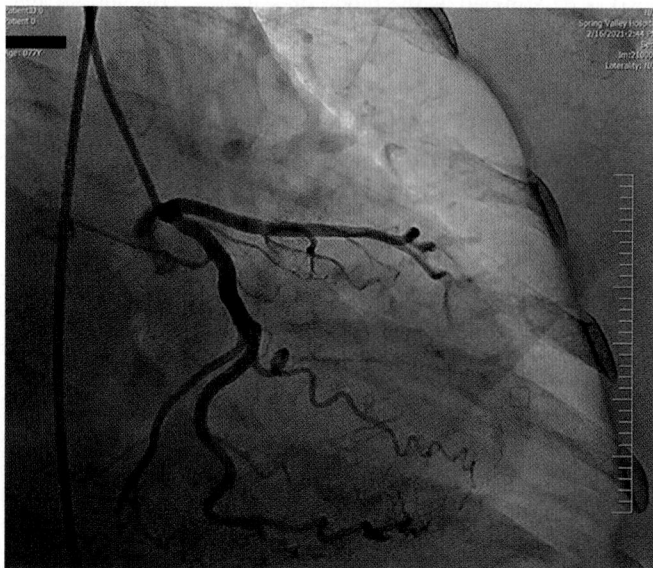

Fig. 27.98 Normal left anterior descending (LAD) and circumflex coronary arteries in the RAO caudal view.

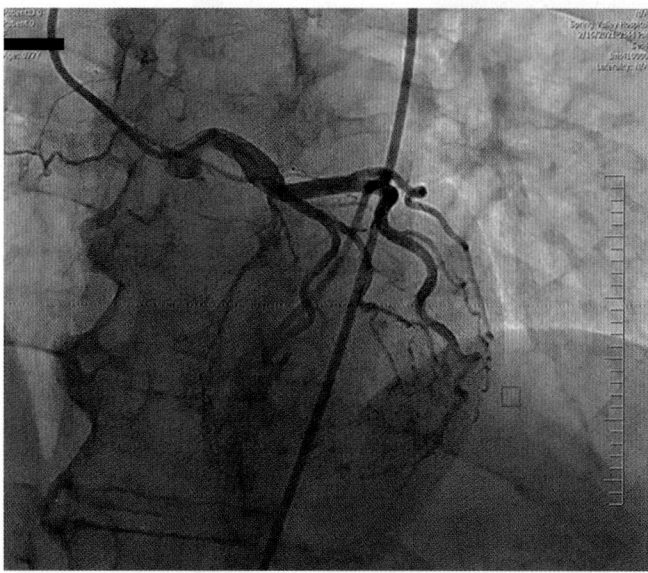

Fig. 27.97 Normal left anterior descending (LAD) and circumflex coronary arteries in the LAO cranial view.

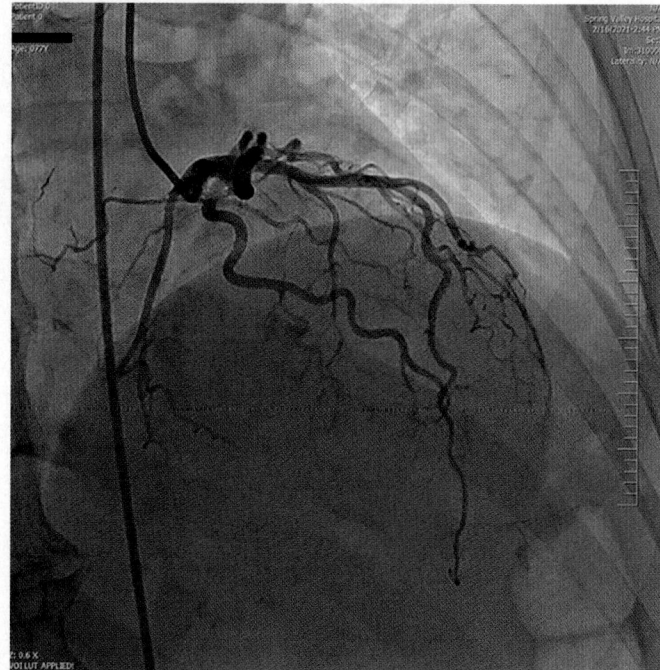

Fig. 27.99 Normal left anterior descending (LAD) and circumflex coronary arteries in the RAO cranial view.

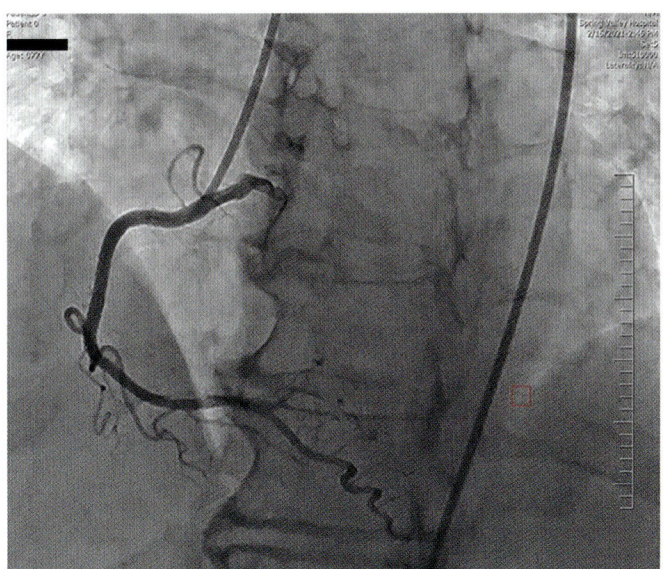

Fig. 27.100 Normal right coronary artery in the LAO view.

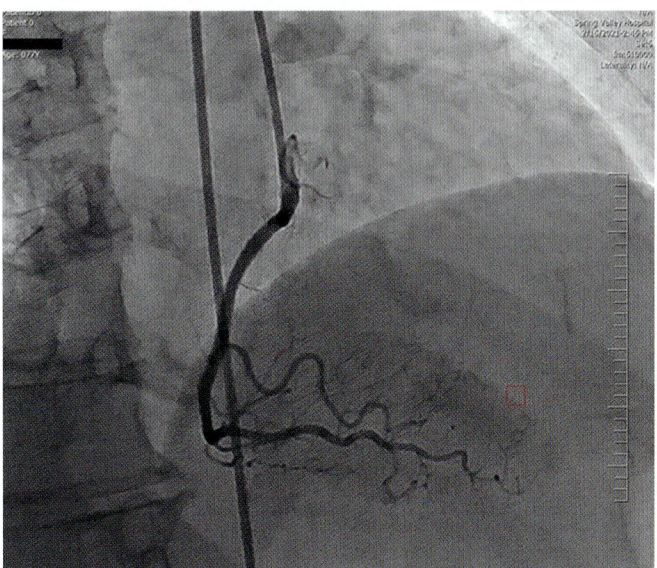

Fig. 27.101 Normal right coronary artery in the RAO view.

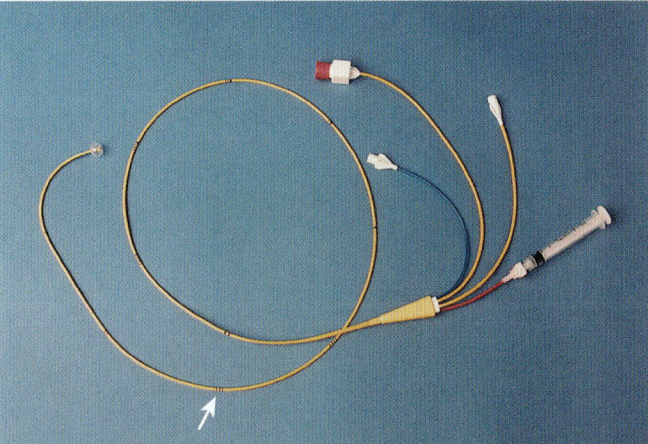

Fig. 27.102 Typical Swan-Ganz catheter.

(From Mann DL, Zipes DP, Libby P, et al., Eds: *Braunwald's heart disease: a textbook of cardiovascular medicine,* 10th ed, Elsevier, 2015.)

the proximal pulmonary artery and injections of saline are performed. This is called thermodilution cardiac output. A thermostat built into the catheter measures the temperature of the blood. The rapid injection of saline causes the temperature to drop and then return to normal as the blood is pumped through the PA. These measurements create a wave on a graph. The computer then calculates the cardiac output based on this graph.

Assessment of valvular disease such as aortic or mitral valve stenosis requires measurement of the valve area. While there are several equations for valve area, they all require pressure measurements on both sides of the valve. For example, to measure aortic valve area simultaneous measurements of the left ventricular and aortic pressures are needed, as well as the cardiac output. The mitral valve area requires measurements of the left ventricle and left atrium or pulmonary capillary wedge pressure. These valve area measurements are critical to planning for structural heart interventions such as transcatheter aortic valve replacement (TAVR). Exercise hemodynamics are often required in the evaluation of valvular heart disease when symptoms of fatigue and dyspnea are present. In such cases, simultaneous catheterization and pressure measurements of the right and left heart are performed at rest and during peak exercise. Exercise may be achieved by the patient pedaling a stationary bicycle ergometer that is placed on top of the examination table, by using an arm ergometer, or by lifting weights. Alternatively, exercise, or stress on the heart, can be induced pharmacologically (with medication), with the use of temporary pacing wires, or with a rapid bolus infusion of fluids.

TABLE 27.5

Common angiographic angles for specific coronary arteries

Coronary artery	Vessel segment	Projections
Left coronary artery	Left main	PA or RAO 5–15 degrees
	Left anterior descending	LAO 30–40 degrees, cranial 20–40 degrees
		RAO 5–15 degrees, cranial 15–45 degrees
		RAO 20–40 degrees, caudal 15–30 degrees
		RAO 30–50 degrees
		Lateral
	Circumflex	RAO 20–40 degrees, caudal 15–30 degrees
		LAO 40–55 degrees, caudal 15–30 degrees
		LAO 40–60 degrees
Right coronary artery	Middle right	LAO 20–40 degrees
		RAO 20–40 degrees
	Posterior descending	LAO 5–30 degrees, cranial 15–30 degrees

ENDOMYOCARDIAL BIOPSY

Endomyocardial biopsy is performed to provide a tissue sample for direct pathologic evaluation of cardiac muscle. This is especially common when looking for signs of possible rejection in patients with a history of heart transplant. A special biopsy catheter with a bioptome tip (Fig. 27.103) is advanced under fluoroscopic control from either the jugular or the femoral vein to the right ventricle (Fig. 27.104). After the bioptome is advanced into the ventricle, the jaws of the device are opened, and the catheter is advanced to the ventricular septum. After the bioptome is in contact with the septum, its jaws are closed, and a gentle tugging motion is applied to retrieve the tissue sample. Several biopsy specimens are acquired in this manner. The specimens are immediately fixed in either glutaraldehyde or buffered formalin before being sent for pathologic evaluation. Endomyocardial biopsy is frequently used to monitor cardiac transplantation patients for early signs of tissue rejection and to differentiate between various types of cardiomyopathies.

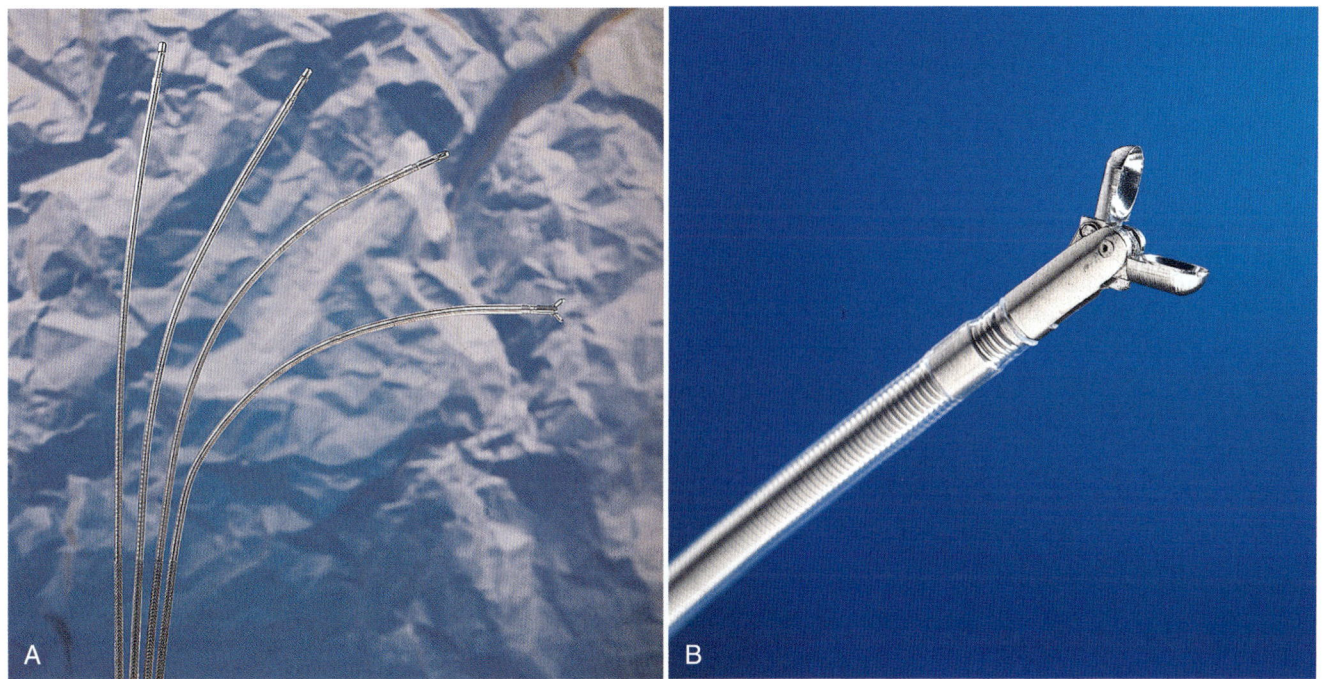

Fig. 27.103 (**A**) Standard biopsy catheters. (**B**) Bioptome catheter tip used for myocardial biopsy. The jaws on the tip close and take a "bite" from the inside of the heart muscle.

(Courtesy Cordis Corp., Miami, FL.)

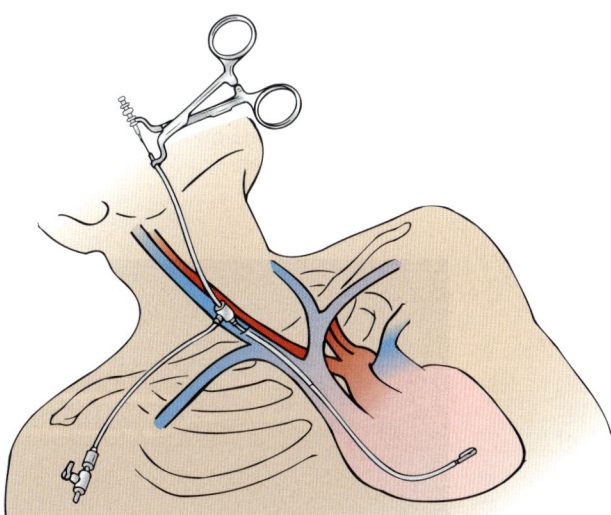

Fig. 27.104 Bioptome tip in the right ventricular apex points toward the ventricular septum.

Interventional Cardiac Procedures

Because of the risks associated with mechanical interventions of the vascular system, openheart surgical facilities must be immediately available. Coronary occlusion is a major complication requiring emergency surgery in patients undergoing catheter-based mechanical interventions.

Interventional pharmacologic procedures in adults consist of the therapeutic administration of medications that may be given before the patient reaches the cardiac catheterization laboratory. A thrombolytic agent can be used in the early hours of an acute MI in an effort to modify its course. Estimates indicate that thrombotic coronary artery occlusion is present in 75% to 85% of patients with acute MI. If reperfusion of the ischemic myocardium is effective, scarring is reduced. Reperfusion in the early stages of MI offers greater potential for heart muscle salvage. ST segment elevation MI is determined from a 12-lead ECG performed in the field or in the emergency department. These patients are the most critical and typically have a complete or almost complete blockage of a coronary artery. Rapid reperfusion to the heart muscle must be performed to minimize damage.

PERCUTANEOUS CORONARY INTERVENTION (PCI)

Interventional cardiac catheterization techniques requiring special-purpose catheters have expanded significantly since the late 1970s. PTCA is a technique that employs balloon dilation of a coronary artery stenosis to increase blood flow to the heart muscle. Grüntzig performed the first successful PTCA in 1977.

During PTCA, a specially designed guiding catheter is placed into the orifice of the stenotic coronary artery (Fig. 27.105). A steerable guidewire is inserted through the guide catheter and advanced across the stenotic area; it serves as a support platform so that balloons and stents can be advanced across the stenosis. Once a PTCA balloon has been inserted, controlled and precise inflations of the balloon are used to fracture and compress the fatty deposits against the muscular wall of the artery. This compression, in conjunction with the stretching of the external vessel diameter, is necessary for successful angioplasty. The balloon is deflated to allow rapid reperfusion of blood to the heart muscle. The inflation procedure, followed by arteriography, may be repeated several times until a satisfactory degree of patency is observed (Fig. 27.106). The limiting factor of PTCA is restenosis, which occurs in approximately 30% to 50% of patients who undergo the procedure. Restenosis of the coronary artery after revascularization is the major factor in failed long-term outcomes. Due to this high restenosis rate, balloon-expandable coronary stent placement, rather than PTCA alone, is now commonly performed.

There are several different stent designs (Fig. 27.107). Drug-coated or drug-eluting stents (DES) were designed to reduce or inhibit restenosis that occurs after a revascularization procedure. Drugs are chemically bound or coated on a stent. The drug is released in small amounts over time to inhibit restenosis. The various drugs reduce restenosis by limiting the proliferation of smooth muscle cells or reducing the rate at which this occurs. However, drug-eluting stents are more prone to the development of a blood clot in the stent. This necessitates that all patients who undergo stent placement with DES be placed on a dual anti-platelet drug regimen for at least 1 year. Later generations of DES have reduced the recommended amount of time in the drug regimen.

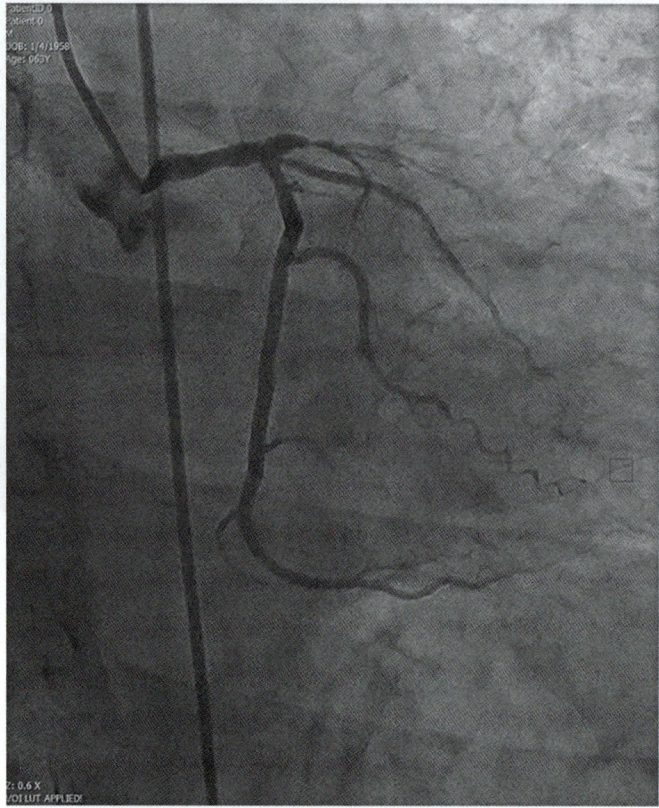

Fig. 27.105 Occluded LAD coronary artery before PTCA. Complete occlusion with no blood flow distal to the lesion.

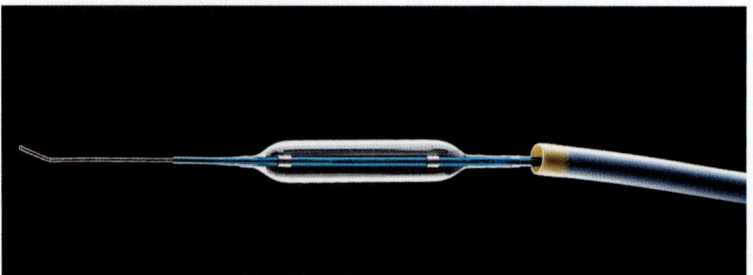

Fig. 27.106 Standard coronary angioplasty balloon. Shown fully inflated.

(Courtesy Cordis Corp., Miami, FL.)

Bare metal stents are used as an alternative to DES. Factors such as patient age, ability to maintain dual anti-platelet therapy, and extent of the disease are some of the determining factors. The procedure is the same as that for DES placement and is performed in the same manner. For optimal stent deployment, the stent is centered across the entire length of the stenosis. Deployment of the stent is achieved with the inflation and deflation of the angioplasty balloon. After the stent is deployed, the angioplasty balloon is removed, and a high-pressure balloon is advanced within the stent. Inflation of the high-pressure balloon is performed to embed the metallic struts of the stent in the walls of the artery (Fig. 27.108). Restenosis rates are lower in patients receiving intracoronary stents than in patients who undergo conventional angioplasty. Major concerns following stent placement are dissections at the proximal and distal ends of the stent and incomplete apposition of the stent against the vessel wall.

ADVANCED PCI TECHNIQUES
Cutting balloon

A cutting balloon is a special type of angioplasty balloon that has a set of blades mounted to the outside of the balloon. When the balloon is inflated, the blades will cut into plaque in the artery, causing what is called positive remodeling and weakening the structure of the plaque itself. This allows for better stent expansion and apposition. Cutting balloons also increase the risk of causing a dissection, or tear, in the intima of the vessel. A similar type of balloon was developed to reduce this type of complication, called a scoring balloon. Instead of blades, scoring balloons have squared off metal wires wrapped around the balloon. When inflated, the metal will dig into the plaque like a cutting balloon. Both types of balloons are commonly used in PCI.

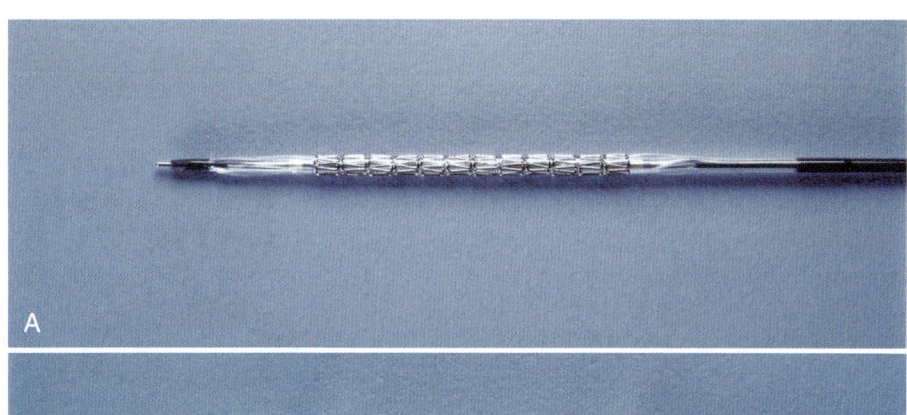
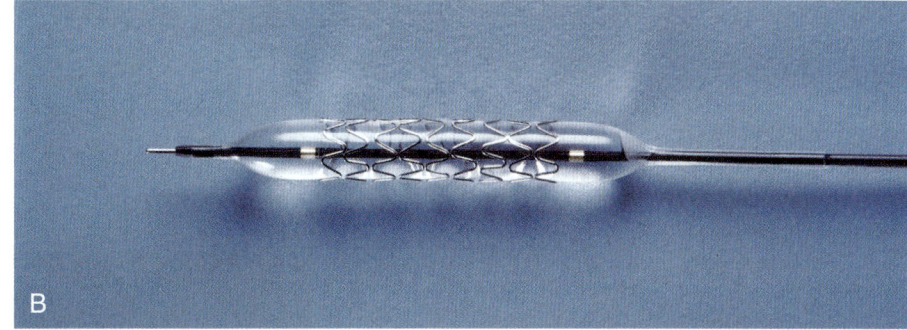

Fig. 27.107 Coronary artery stent balloon system. Shown (**A**) mounted on the balloon and (**B**) fully expanded.

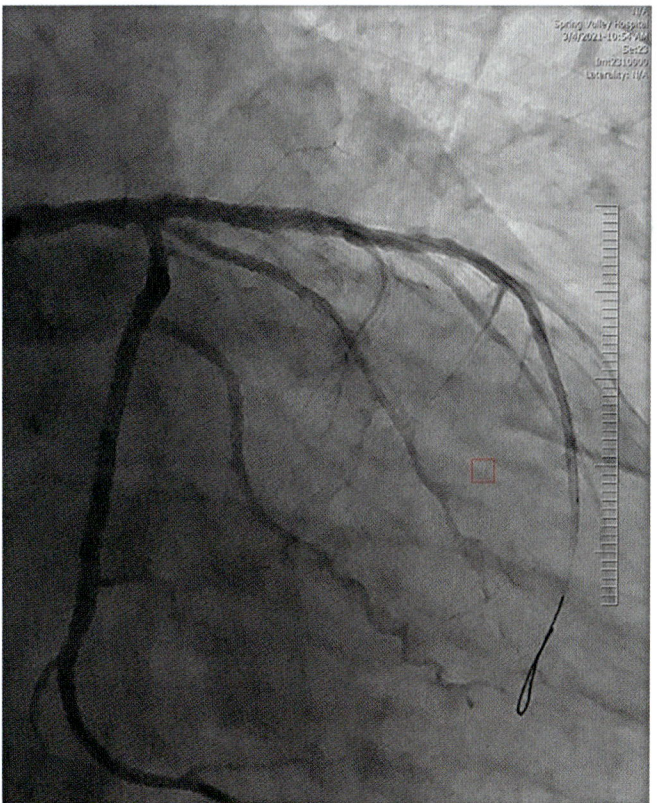

Fig. 27.108 Coronary arteriogram after PTCA in the same patient as in Fig. 27.106.

Intravascular lithotripsy

Recent developments in the treatment of calcified lesions led to the development of intravascular lithotripsy balloons. These balloons contain multiple small filaments that create tiny explosions inside the balloon while inflated. These explosions create shock waves that transmit energy through the fluid medium in the balloon and into the calcium in the vessel walls, fracturing it. Once the calcium in the vessel wall is fractured, it becomes more flexible, allowing for adequate balloon and stent expansion.

Rotational atherectomy

Rotational atherectomy devices can be used in the treatment of coronary artery disease. These devices have been indicated for use in the treatment of atherosclerotic coronary artery disease. Commonly referred to as percutaneous transluminal coronary rotational atherectomy (PTCRA), this procedure is used in conjunction with PTCA or stenting. Rotational atherectomy devices are used to "grind" down severely calcified coronary lesions. The tip of the catheter (1.25 to 2.5 mm in diameter) resembles a football and is embedded with microscopic diamond particles, which rotate on a special type of guidewire between 160,000 and 200,000 rpm (Figs. 27.109 and 27.110).

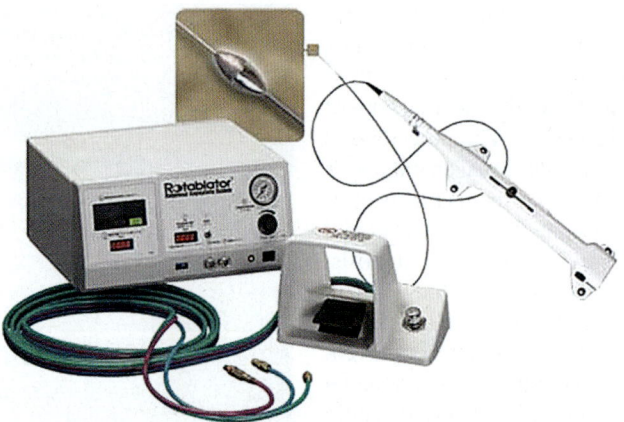

Fig. 27.109 Rotablator rotational atherectomy catheter with advancer unit. Insert shows football-shaped burr.

(Courtesy Boston Scientific.)

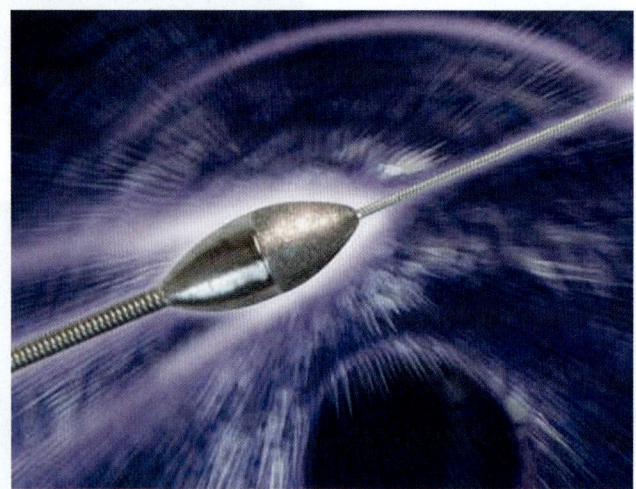

Fig. 27.110 Atherectomy catheter burr.

(Courtesy Boston Scientific.)

Prior to rotational atherectomy, the cardiologist should consider the need for a temporary pacemaker in case of a rapid decrease in heart rate during atherectomy passes. Standard angioplasty guide catheter positioning techniques are used to position a guidewire distal to the targeted lesion. A rotational atherectomy burr size is selected and advanced over the special guidewire just proximal to the lesion. A special solution is mixed and used to help lubricate the system, as well as to keep the artery from spasming. This solution includes the lubricant, normal saline, and usually small amounts of the drugs nitroglycerin and verapamil, which relax the smooth muscle of the arteries and dilate the capillary bed. At this point, the burr is activated, and the plaque and calcium are pulverized and reduced to the size of a blood cell (Fig. 27.111). The pulverized material is removed by the reticuloendothelial system. After an adequate amount of plaque is cleared, standard PTCA or stenting techniques are employed to maintain artery patency. PTCRA has proven to be beneficial in the treatment of highly calcified lesions and in-stent restenosis compared with PTCA alone (Fig. 27.112).

ADVANCED IMAGING TECHNIQUES

Although coronary angiography remains the gold standard for the diagnosis of coronary artery disease, advanced imaging techniques such as intravascular ultrasound (IVUS), optical coherence tomography (OCT), fractional flow reserve (FFR), and instant wave-free ratio (IFR) offer further diagnostic and interventional information that cannot be appreciated by angiography alone.

Intravascular ultrasound (IVUS)

IVUS utilizes a catheter-mounted ultrasound array that can be inserted directly into the vasculature, allowing for a full 360-degree circumference visualization of the vessel wall, providing information regarding vascular pathology and longitudinal and volumetric measurements This information better facilitates the guidance of catheter-based interventions. The intervention-associated potential of IVUS is the ability to optimize the type and size of device being used and to determine proper apposition of the stent after deployment against the artery wall.

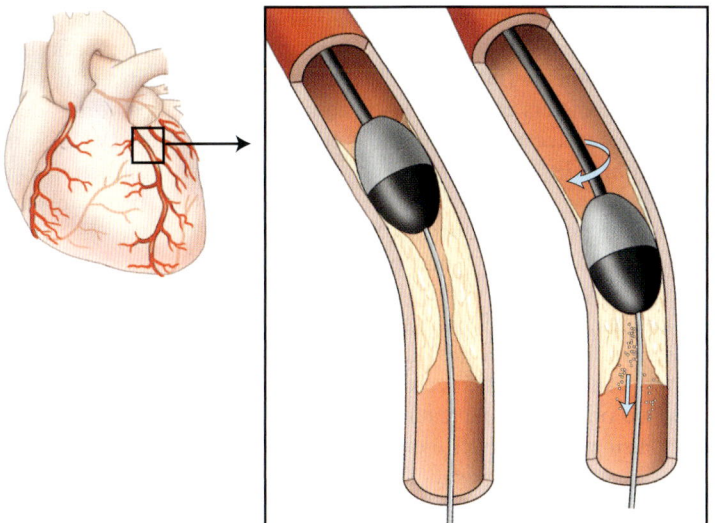

Fig. 27.111 Rotational atherectomy burr being advanced into a coronary artery lesion.

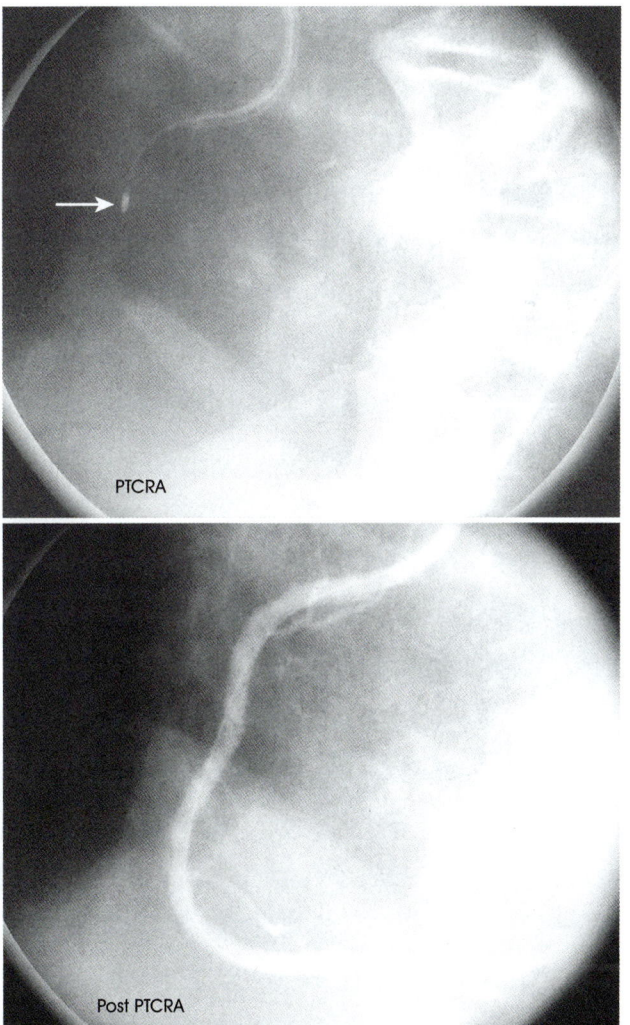

Fig. 27.112 PTCRA. *Arrow* points to burr of catheter. After PTCRA, a widely patent right coronary artery is shown.

Components consist of the ultrasound unit, recording device, transducer, pullback device, and catheter (Fig. 27.113). The intravascular catheters employ 20- to 40-MHz silicon piezoelectric crystals and range in size from 5 Fr on the proximal end of the catheter to 2.9 Fr at the distal end. During the procedure, the IVUS catheter is advanced over the guidewire that was previously placed within the artery being imaged. The IVUS catheter is advanced distal to the targeted lesion, at which time the transducer and recording device are turned on. Slowly, the catheter is withdrawn, using the pullback device to maintain a consistent withdrawal of the catheter and to help ascertain the length of the targeted lesion. Documentation of IVUS catheter position can be obtained with angiography. The images are stored on the hard drive of the IVUS system and can be retrieved for the cardiologist to review, take measurements, and print (Figs. 27.114 and 27.115).

At present, IVUS remains an integral part of coronary interventions being performed. With advances in stent designs, brachytherapy, local drug delivery, and future technologies, IVUS will remain a vital source for information in improving the outcomes of percutaneous coronary interventions. The clinical use of IVUS imaging and other improved computerized image enhancements should allow for more precise data collection and more tailored methods of determining the interventional method to use in treating coronary artery disease.

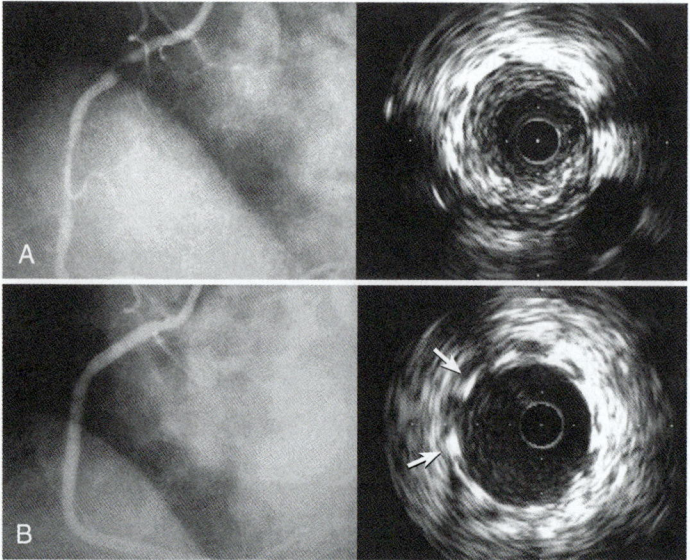

Fig. 27.114 IVUS images shown on the right correlated with angiography images on the left. **A** demonstrates a significant narrowing of the coronary artery angiographically and is correlated with the plaque burden shown in the IVUS image. *Arrows* in **B** show the echogenicity of the stent struts during IVUS.

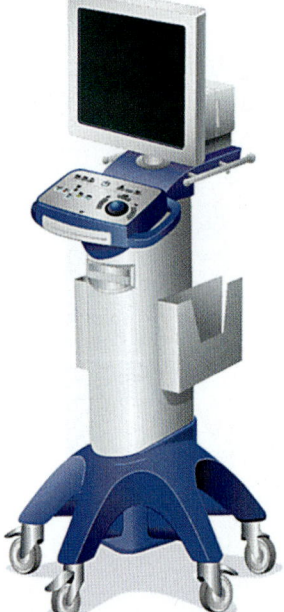

Fig. 27.113 IVUS unit. Shown here are the keyboard and monitor.

(Courtesy Volcano.)

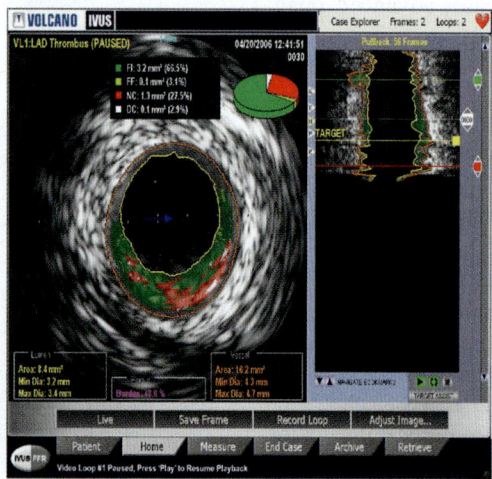

Fig. 27.115 IVUS artery images.

Optical coherence tomography (OCT)

A newer diagnostic tool available to visualize intravascular structures is optical coherence tomography (OCT). OCT is similar to IVUS in that it is an imaging device mounted on a catheter that is inserted directly into a blood vessel. However, OCT uses infrared laser light, as opposed to ultrasound waves, to identify plaque rupture, stent apposition, dissection, and vessel size. The OCT catheter is positioned in the artery and calibrated. Then a bolus of contrast is injected into the artery. The contrast displaces the opaque blood, briefly replacing it with contrast, which allows the light waves to pass through and image the vessel. This process creates extremely high-resolution images with improved visualization of calcified plaques. The only limitation to using OCT imaging is if the patient has significantly impaired renal function and contrast use should be minimized (Fig. 27.116).

Fractional flow reserve (FFR)/instant wave-free ratio (IFR)

FFR is a diagnostic tool used to determine whether a lesion is significantly impairing blood flow in a coronary artery. The FFR device consists of a tiny pressure sensor mounted on a guidewire. The wire is inserted through a guide catheter into the coronary arteries. The FFR wire is advanced past the lesion in question. A vasodilator such as adenosine is then administered. This dilates the coronary arteries, mimicking the heart being under stress. The arterial line pressure wave is then compared to the FFR pressure wave. The ratio between the arterial pressure and the FFR wire pressure is then used to determine whether the lesion is significantly reducing blood flow.

IFR is a diagnostic tool almost the same as FFR with one exception. IFR does not require the use of vasodilators to calculate the ratio. In fact, IRF and FFR are simply different measurements using the same pressure wire and the same computer system.

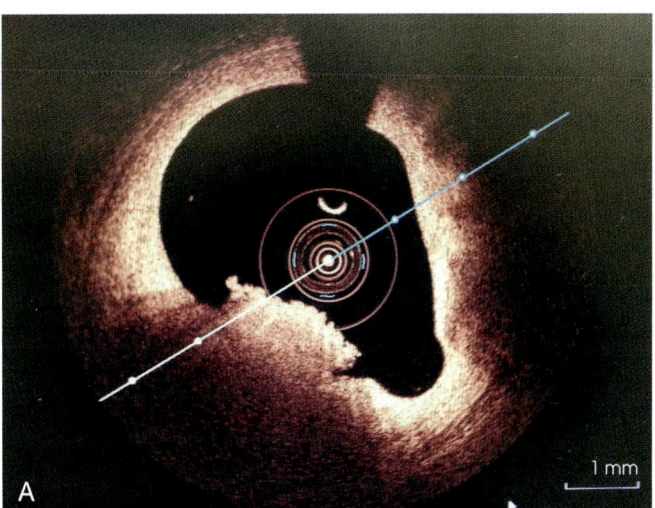
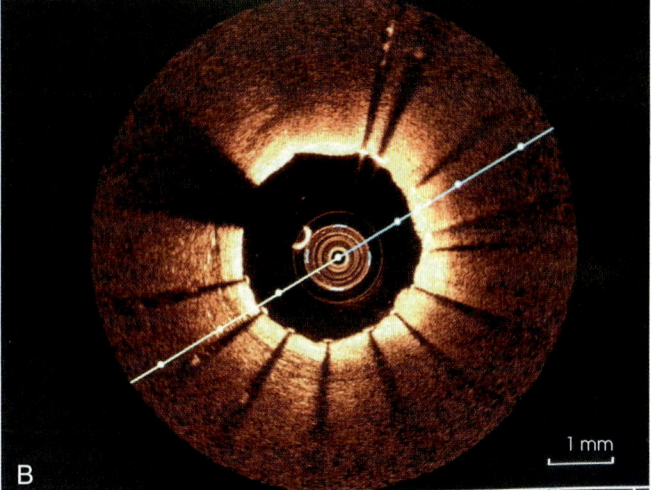

Fig. 27.116 (**A**) OCT demonstrating plaque burden inside a coronary artery. (**B**) OCT of coronary artery post stent deployment.

CARDIOVASCULAR SUPPORT PROCEDURES

Temporary transvenous pacemaker (TTVP)

The placement of a temporary transvenous pacemaker (TTVP) is a common cardiovascular support procedure employed for the treatment of certain arrhythmias, such as bradycardia and third-degree or complete heart block. A temp pacer catheter is inserted through the venous system and directed into the right ventricle. It is then connected to a pacing box that delivers a set amount of milliamperes (mA) at a set rate (BMP) (Fig. 27.117). The pacer is tested by pacing faster than the underlying heart rate until pacer capture is established. Then the mA is slowly turned down until capture is lost. The mA just before capture is lost is called the threshold, or the lowest energy level that still paces the heart muscle. Once position is verified the catheter is secured in place. TTVPs are also used in some structural heart procedures to rapidly pace the heart to temporarily reduce cardiac output, allowing for more precise positioning of a valvuloplasty balloon or valve replacement.

Intraaortic balloon pump (IABP)

An intraaortic balloon pump (IABP) is a cardiac support device used to treat cardiogenic shock by increasing perfusion of the coronary arteries. The IABP device consists of a large balloon mounted on a catheter and the pump itself. The balloon size ranges from 30 cc to 50 cc, depending on the patient's height. The balloon is inserted through the femoral artery and is positioned in the descending aorta with the distal end above the renal arteries. Once in position, the balloon is primed with helium gas. A sensor in the balloon tip measures the aortic blood pressure and provides a timing trigger so that the balloon is inflated during systole, or when the heart contracts, and deflated when the heart relaxes into diastole. This technique is called counter pulsation. This timing forces more blood into the coronary arteries, thereby increasing coronary perfusion and reducing stress on the heart. IMBPs are commonly used in patients post MI who have undergone PCI and may still be in cardiogenic shock. In these cases, the balloon pump may be left in for a few hours to a few days. In some cases, IABPs are used preemptively in complex PCI cases in which the patient is at high risk.

Percutaneous left ventricular support device

A percutaneous left ventricular support device is a catheter-mounted pump that is inserted via the arterial system into the left ventricle (Fig. 27.118). The pump works by drawing in blood through the end of the catheter that is in the LV and pumping it out a port on the catheter positioned in the aortic root. This action augments the heart's own cardiac output, increasing circulation to the coronary arteries (as well as to the rest of the body), and allows for deceased cardiac workload. This type of device is used in severe cases of cardiogenic shock or preemptively in complex PCI cases in which the patient is at high risk. These devices should not be confused with left ventricular assist devices (LVAD), which are surgically implanted into the heart and are meant for long-term use. LV support devices are meant for short-term use, a couple of weeks at the maximum.

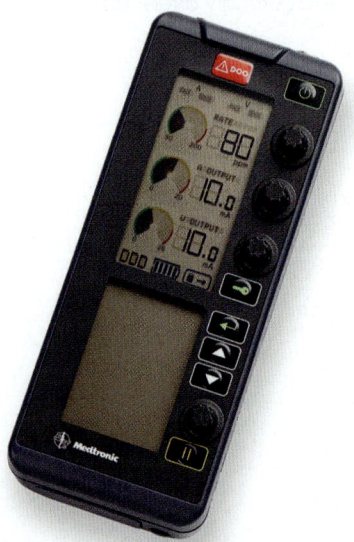

Fig. 27.117 Temporary external, dual-chamber demand pacemaker.

(© 2024 Medtronic. All rights reserved. Used with permission of Medtronic.)

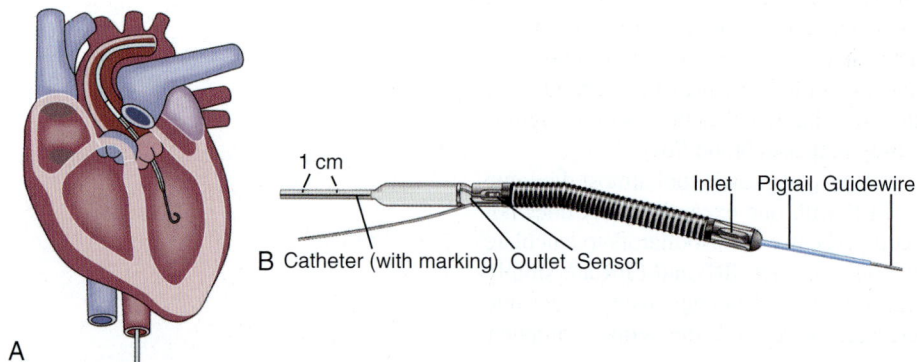

Fig. 27.118 (**A**) A left ventricular support device shown in proper position in the left ventricle. (**B**) The pump itself shown in more detail.

(A, courtesy of AbioMed; B, from Libby P, Bonow RO, Mann DL, et al.: *Braunwald's heart disease: a textbook of cardiovascular medicine*, 12th ed, 2022, Elsevier.)

STRUCTURAL HEART PROCEDURES
Balloon aortic valvuloplasty (BAV)/ balloon mitral valvuloplasty (BMV)

Many procedures previously performed by open surgery, such as cardiac valve replacements, are now being performed percutaneously in the catheterization laboratory or in a hybrid angiography/OR suite. Percutaneous valve stenosis treatment, known as valvuloplasty, has been performed for many years. Balloon aortic valvuloplasty (BAV) is often a first-line treatment for aortic stenosis prior to a transcatheter aortic valve replacement (TAVR). In fact, BAV is often performed during the TAVR procedure as well, to prep the native valve prior to replacement. A BAV procedure requires the placement of a temporary pacemaker to rapid-pace the heart during the balloon inflation. The procedure is performed through an arterial access in the common femoral artery. A series of catheters and guidewires is used to cross the aortic valve. Once across, the valvuloplasty balloon is inserted and directed over a guidewire across the aortic valve. Rapid pacing is initiated, usually at 180 bpm. This drastically reduces the cardiac output, thereby reducing the movement of the balloon. The balloon is briefly inflated, then deflated, and rapid pacing is terminated. Results can be verified by comparing the gradient across the valve pre- and post-BAV.

For mitral valve stenosis, balloon valvuloplasty is considered the initial mechanical treatment. The mitral valve is accessed by passing a needle from the right atrium across the septum into the left atrium (transseptal access). A specially designed balloon catheter, called an Inoue balloon, is then passed into the left atrium and manipulated to cross the mitral valve. The mitral valve is then carefully dilated, in multiple stages, under continual transmitral pressure gradient and echocardiographic monitoring.

Percutaneous mitral valve repair

The percutaneous mitral valve repair is much less invasive than the standard surgical mitral valve repair for the treatment of severe mitral regurgitation. The clip pinches together the two leaflets of the mitral valve, reducing the overall valve area and the amount of backflow into the left atrium. The procedure utilizes both fluoroscopy and transesophageal echocardiogram (TEE) for visualization of the mitral valve morphology and function, as well as the placement of the clip. Venous access is obtained in the right femoral vein and a catheter is advanced into the right atrium. A septal puncture is then performed, allowing for access into the left atrium. The clip delivery system is inserted and passed through the septal puncture and directed through the mitral valve leaflets. The clip is then opened and slightly withdrawn until it grasps both leaflets of the mitral valve. Once positioning is verified, it is deployed. Once deployed, the clip position is confirmed with TEE, and any residual mitral regurgitation is assessed. Finally, the delivery system is removed, and the septal puncture site is visualized to determine whether a septal occlusion device is necessary. Upon completion the venous access site is closed.

Transcatheter aortic valve replacement (TAVR)

Transcatheter aortic valve replacement, or TAVR, is a procedure used to percutaneously replace the aortic valve, as opposed to open-heart surgery. TAVR has become much more common, with many facilities building structural heart programs. The procedure is multidisciplinary, with cardiologists and cardiothoracic surgeons working together, as well as the cardiac cath lab and open-heart surgery teams. The TAVR procedure workup requires using multiple imaging modalities, including cardiac catheterization, transesophageal echocardiogram (TEE), and computed tomography, to accurately assess valvular anatomy and function. The procedure itself is usually performed in the cardiothoracic OR or in a hybrid angiography/OR suite to quickly convert the percutaneous procedure to an open-heart surgery if required.

The TAVR procedure involves the insertion of multiple catheters, under fluoroscopy guidance, to visualize the aortic valve. A temporary pacemaker is also placed at this point. Once all these catheters are in position, the new valve is prepared and inserted on its delivery system. TAVR valves can be either self-expanding or balloon expandable, depending on the manufacturer. Once the TAVR valve is positioned across the aortic valve, the heart is rapidly paced to reduce movement of the delivery system, and the valve is deployed (Fig. 27.119). Afterward the valve position and function are verified with fluoroscopy and either transthoracic or transesophageal echocardiography. Once the procedure is complete, the percutaneous access sites are closed and the patient is sent to recovery.

Patent foramen ovale closure (PFO)

A patent foramen ovale, or PFO, is a connection between the right and left atria. This connection is present when a person is still in utero but closes quickly after birth. In some cases, the connection doesn't fully close and there is still a patent connection between the atria. This connection increases a person's risk for embolic stroke. When a PFO is found in an adult, it is often the best course to close the connection to prevent further risk. In a PFO closure procedure a catheter and wire are inserted through the femoral vein and directed across the PFO into the left atrium. This is done under fluoroscopy guidance with either TEE or intracardiac echocardiography (ICE) imaging. Once the guidewire is in position, a septal occlusion device is inserted and deployed across the septum, covering the PFO in both chambers. The position is verified by echocardiography and the venous access site is closed.

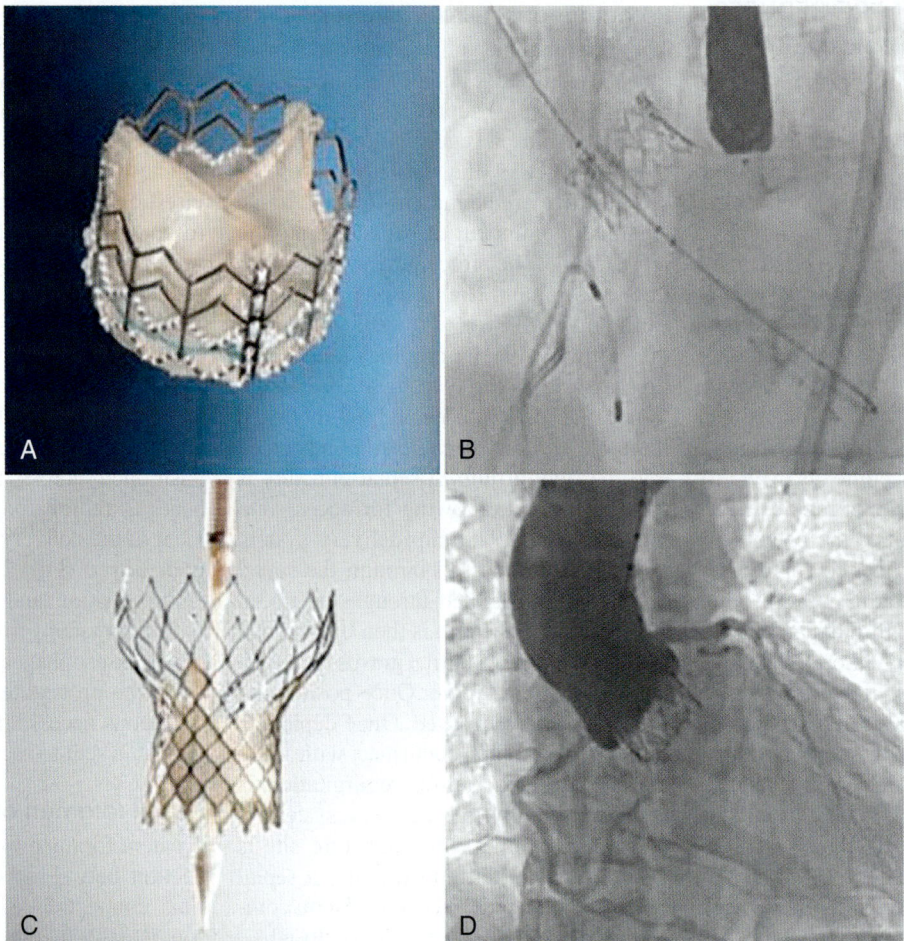

Fig. 27.119 Percutaneous aortic valves deployed during TAVR procedures. (**A**) The Edwards Sapien valve. (**B**) Fluoroscopic image of the Sapien valve deployed. (**C**) The CoreValve by Medtronic. (**D**) Aortogram image showing a deployed CoreValve.

(From Steinberg DH, Staubach S, Franke J, et al.: Defining structural heart disease in the adult patient: current scope, inherent challenges and future directions. *Eur Heart J Suppl* 12(E):E2–E9, 2010.)

Left atrial appendage occlusion device

Conditions such as atrial fibrillation, or A-fib, cause slow-moving blood in the atria, which in turn can lead to blood clots. Blood clots in the left atria tend to form in the left atrial appendage. Placement of a left atrial appendage occlusion device can reduce the risk of stroke and pulmonary embolism secondary to a clot from the left atrial appendage. The procedure is performed through femoral venous access. A catheter and wire are inserted and directed into the right atria. Then, under fluoroscopic and echocardiographic guidance a device is inserted to puncture the atrial septum to allow for access to the left atrium. Once in the left atrium, the atrial appendage is visualized via echo and the occlusion device is directed into position and deployed (Fig. 27.120). Placement is confirmed with echocardiography and the venous access site is closed.

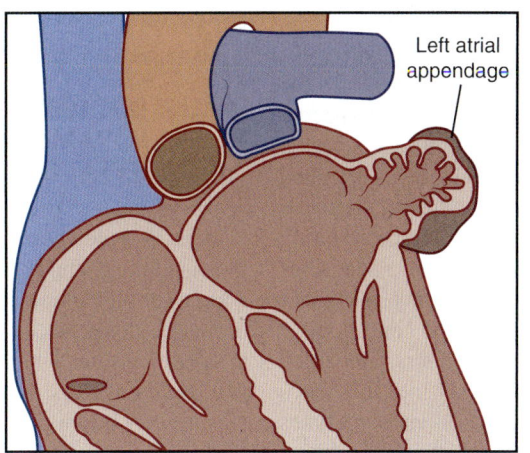

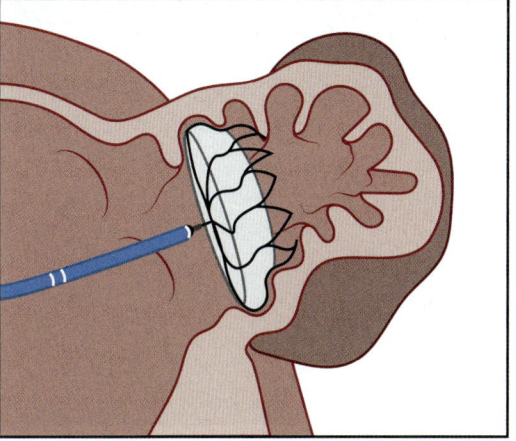

Fig. 27.120 (**A**) Left atrial appendage. (**B**) Left atrial appendage occlusion device. (**C**) Watchman closure device placed.

(From Stromberg HK: *Medical-surgical nursing: concepts and practice,* 5th ed, 2023, Elsevier.)

Congenital Defects

A primary indication for diagnostic catheterization studies in children is the evaluation and documentation of specific anatomy, hemodynamic data, and selected aspects of cardiac function associated with congenital heart defects. Methods and techniques used for catheterization of the heart vary depending on age, heart size, type and extent of defect, and other coincident pathophysiologic conditions.

Pediatric cardiac catheters are often introduced percutaneously into the femoral vein and, in older children, sometimes into the femoral artery. In very young patients, it may be possible to pass a catheter from the right atrium to the left atrium (allowing access to the left side of the heart) through either a patent foramen ovale (PFO) or a preexisting atrial septal defect. If the atrial septum is intact, temporary access to the left atrium may be obtained using a transseptal catheter system (Fig. 27.121). With the transseptal catheter system, a long introducer and needle are used to puncture the right atrial septum of the heart to gain access to the left atrium if access cannot be attained as previously described.

PATENT DUCTUS ARTERIOSUS, PATENT FORAMEN OVALE, AND ATRIAL SEPTAL DEFECT CLOSURE

A patent ductus arteriosus is sometimes evident in a newborn. In utero, the pulmonary artery shunts blood flow into the aorta through the ductus arteriosus, which normally closes after birth. Patent ductus arteriosus occurs when this channel fails to close spontaneously. In some instances, closure can be induced with medication. If this measure is unsuccessful and the residual shunt is deemed significant, surgical closure (ligation) of the vessel is appropriate.

For some patients, occlusion of a patent ductus arteriosus can be accomplished in the catheterization laboratory. A catheter containing an occlusion device, similar to an umbrella, is advanced to the ductus. After the position of the lesion is confirmed by angiography, the occluder is released. Subsequent clotting and fibrous infiltration permanently stop the flow and subsequent mixing of blood. Specific transcatheter closure devices are available to close a PFO, an opening between the right and left atria, and other atrial septal defects. A PFO can be the cause of stroke in an adult patient. Occluder devices have shown positive results in treatment of the PFO.

BALLOON SEPTOSTOMY

Balloon septostomy may be used to enlarge a PFO or preexisting *atrial septal defect*. Enlargement of the opening enhances the mixing of right and left atrial blood, thereby improving the level of systemic arterial oxygenation. Transposition of the great arteries is a condition for which atrial septostomy is performed.

Balloon septostomy requires a catheter similar to the type used in PTCA. The balloon is passed through the atrial septal opening into the left atrium, inflated with contrast media, and snapped back through the septal orifice. This maneuver causes the septum to tear. Often the technique must be repeated until the septal opening is sufficiently enlarged to allow the desired level of blood mixing as documented by oximetry, intracardiac pressures, and angiography.

Electrophysiology (EP)

Electrophysiology involves the analysis, diagnosis, and treatment of conditions affecting the electrical conduction systems of the heart. This includes the diagnostic EP procedure, ablations, pacemaker/defibrillator implants, and loop recorder implants. EP procedures are usually performed in a dedicated EP room, although implant procedures can be performed in any cath lab room. EP procedures require specialized equipment for cardiac mapping and RF or cryoablations.

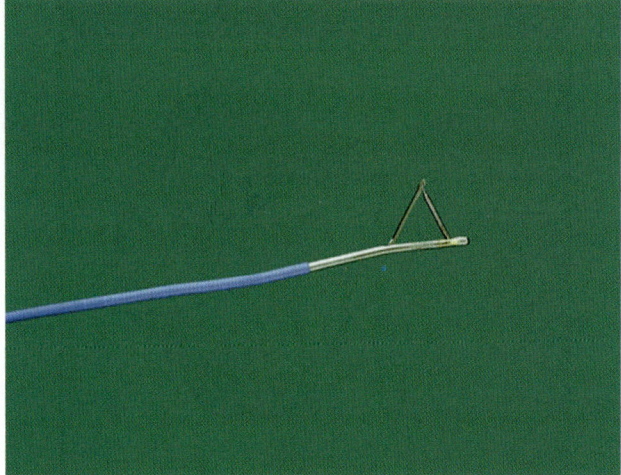

Fig. 27.121 Blade on catheter tip used to incise septal walls in pediatric interventional procedures.

DIAGNOSTIC PROCEDURES

The electrophysiology (EP) study involves the collection of sophisticated data to facilitate detailed mapping of the electrical conduction system within the heart. The procedure involves the placement of numerous multipolar electrode catheters in specific areas of the heart (Fig. 27.122). These placements include the high right atrium (HRA), the bundle of His, the coronary sinus (CS), and the apex of the right ventricle (RV). EP studies are used to analyze the conduction system, induce arrhythmias, evaluate existing arrhythmias, and determine the effects of therapeutic measures in treating arrhythmias.

Electrode catheters are introduced into the femoral vein, internal jugular vein, or subclavian vein. Because several catheters are used, multiple access sites are needed. It is common to have three introducer sheaths placed within the same vein. The catheters consist of several insulated wires, each of which is attached to an electrode on the catheter tip that serves as an interface with the intracardiac surface. The arrangements of the electrodes on the catheter allow its dual function of recording the electrical signals of the heart (intracardiac electrograms) and pacing the heart. The pacemaker function has a variety of purposes. First, it allows the physician to accurately measure the time it takes for an impulse to travel through the conduction system. Second, it allows for assessment of the health of the conduction system based on the responses of the tissue to various pacing maneuvers. Finally, it allows for the induction of premature electrical impulses to determine possible arrhythmias. After the precise defect is characterized, an appropriate course of therapy can be undertaken. Cardiac ablations, pacemakers, and internal cardiac defibrillators are the most common treatments for arrhythmias. In some cases, surgical intervention is required.

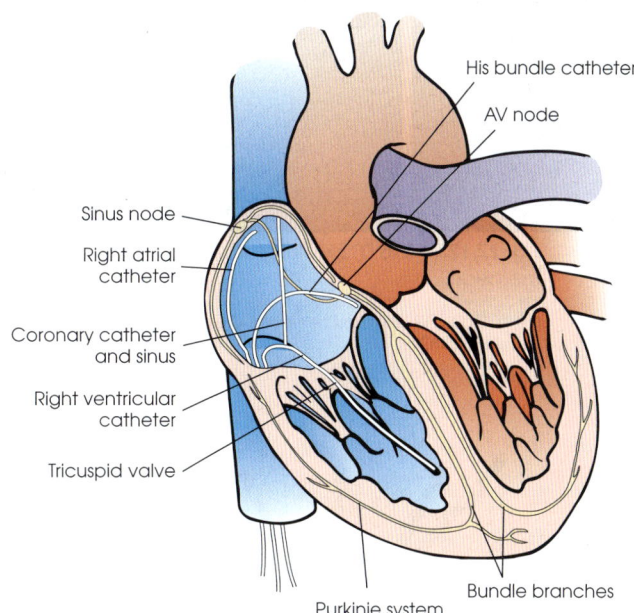

Fig. 27.122 Catheter positions for routine electrophysiologic study. Multipolar catheters are positioned in the high right atrium near the sinus node, in the area of the atrioventricular apex, and in the coronary sinus.

Electrophysiology mapping

A significant part of electrophysiology is to map the structures of the heart and the conduction system in the areas of interest. This process is threefold. First, the cardiologist will map areas of the conduction system by visualizing the electrical signals, called electrograms, as the EP catheters are moved around the heart (Fig. 27.123). This allows them to identify critical structures such as the AV node and the bundle of His. This process can also be used to track arrhythmias that occur periodically. By using computer-matching technology, the physician can find a specific area that is generating an arrhythmia and reproduce it. Second, in some cases, an intracardiac echo (ICE) catheter is inserted. This catheter takes ultrasound pictures from the inside of the heart. These images can be used to begin to create a 3D computer model of certain structures of the heart. Finally, dedicated mapping catheters are inserted to further generate and refine the 3D map, as well as to record other data (Fig. 27.124). These 3D maps can then be overlaid with a color spectrum representing voltage of signal from the tissues or the timing of the tissue activation. The allows the physician to have a map of areas that may need treatment. This map correlated with analysis of the electrograms allows for targeted treatment.

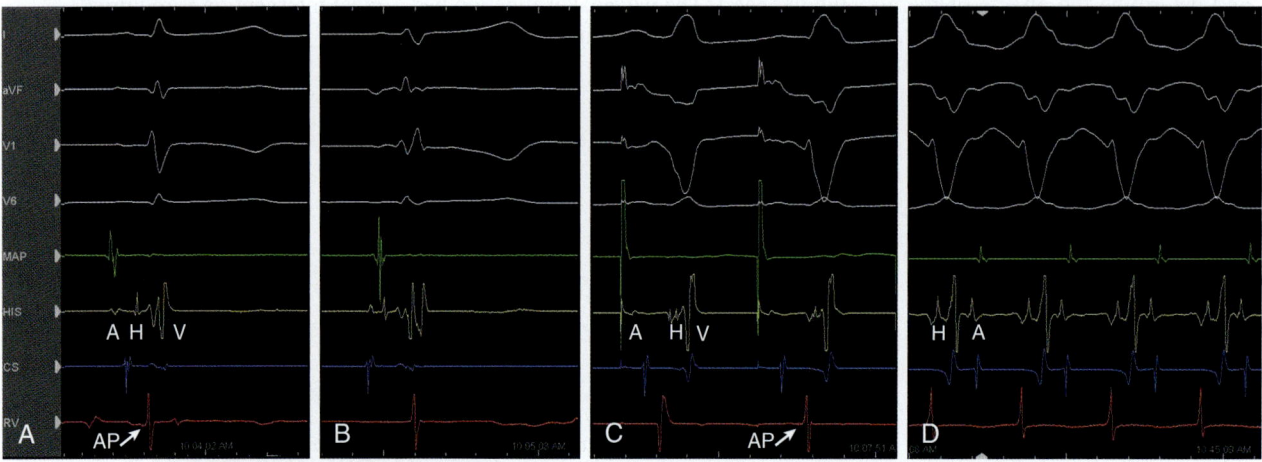

Fig. 27.123 (**A to D**) Electrograms from electrophysiology catheters at different positions in the heart.

(From Zipes DP, Jalife J, Stevenson WG: *Cardiac electrophysiology: from cell to bedside,* 7th ed, Elsevier, 2018.)

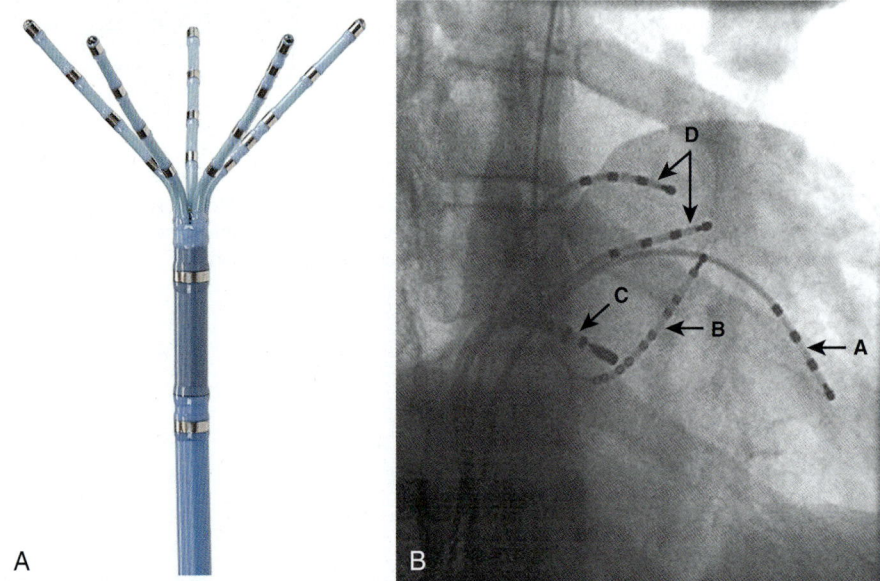

Fig. 27.124 (**A**) An electrophysiology mapping catheter. Note the multiple arms with multiple electrodes on each. (**B**) Fluoroscopic image with catheters shown are: right ventricular (a), coronary sinus (b), bundle of His (c), and atrial (d).

(A, Courtesy Biosense Webster, Inc., Irvine, CA, USA. B, from Hampton J, Adam D: *The ECG made practical,* 7th ed, 2019, Elsevier.)

INTERVENTIONAL CONDUCTION PROCEDURES

Radiofrequency (RF) ablation

A common interventional procedure to treat disorders of the conduction system is radiofrequency (RF) ablation. Several different arrhythmias previously treated with ICD implantation or drug therapy can now be treated with RF ablation. The procedure is normally performed at the time of the diagnostic EP study if an underlying mechanism or arrhythmogenic focus is identified.

RF ablation is achieved by delivering a low-voltage, high-frequency alternating current directly to the endocardial tissue through a specially designed ablation catheter. The current desiccates the underlying abnormal myocardial conduction tissue and creates a small, discrete burn lesion. Localized RF lesions create areas of tissue necrosis and scar, subsequently destroying or isolating the arrhythmogenic focus. Several RF lesions may be necessary to eliminate the abnormal conduction. RF ablation is commonly used in the treatment of atrial flutter and atrial fibrillation.

In the case of atrial flutter, the abnormal conduction crosses around the right atria in a circular pattern. The placement of a "flutter line" or ablation of the tissue of the tricuspid isthmus, the area between the tricuspid valve and the IVC, blocks the circular pattern of conduction, breaking the arrhythmia. Follow-up electrophysiologic testing is performed to document the resolution of the arrhythmia. Results are verified by pacing an EP cath placed in the coronary sinus and observing the cycle length, or the amount of time it takes for the impulse to travel across the atrium of each beat. A normal cycle length is around 800 to 1000 milliseconds while the cycle length in atrial flutter is usually around 150 to 200 milliseconds.

The combination of permanent pacemaker placement with subsequent RF ablation of the atrioventricular (AV) node is becoming the preferred treatment for chronic atrial fibrillation with rapid ventricular responses. The atrioventricular junction is destroyed intentionally; consequently, the rapid, irregular electrical impulses from the atrium are not conducted into the ventricle. A pacemaker is implanted, and a more consistent, regular heart rate is achieved.

Cryoablation

Cryoablation is an alternative procedure to RF ablation, often used in EP labs. Cryoablation utilizes balloon catheters that produce extreme cold temperatures to create lesions or scars in specific areas of the heart to block the conduction of arrhythmias. It is often used in the treatment of atrial fibrillation (A-fib). In most cases of A-fib, abnormal conduction of signals from the pulmonary veins causes a disruption of signals in the atria, leading to atrial fibrillation. In cryoablation the ablation balloon catheter is directed into the ostium of each pulmonary vein and inflated and cooled to around minus 60 degrees (Fig. 27.125). This scars the tissue around the opening of the vein, preventing electrical signals from conducting into the atria. Once the cryoablation is complete, results can be verified by inserting an EP catheter into the pulmonary vein and pacing it. If a signal conducts into the atria, the ablation process needs to be repeated.

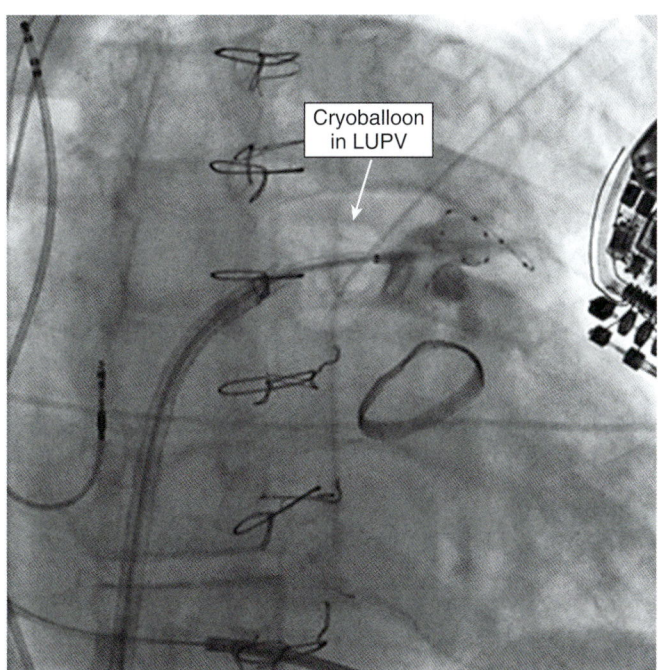

Fig. 27.125 The fluoroscopic image shows the inflated cryoballoon at the antrum of the left upper pulmonary vein. A small puff of contrast into the vein confirms good balloon positioning.

(From Gatzoulis MA, Webb GD, Daubeney PEF: *Diagnosis and management of adult congenital heart disease*, 3rd ed, 2018, Elsevier.)

Electrophysiology device implants

Permanent implantation of an antiarrhythmic device is another interventional procedure performed in cardiac catheterization laboratories. Antiarrhythmic devices include pacemakers for patients with bradyarrhythmia or disease of the electrical conduction system of the heart and implantable cardioverter defibrillators (ICDs) for patients with lethal ventricular tachyarrhythmias originating from the bottom of the heart (Fig. 27.126).

Permanent pacemaker (PPM)

Placement of a PPM is a common procedure in the cath lab and EP lab. It is usually performed under local anesthesia with conscious sedation. The left upper chest is the most common implant site. The left subclavian vein is accessed, and a special type of sheath that can peel apart is inserted. The pacemaker leads (electrically insulated wires with distal electrodes) are inserted through these sheaths. Pacemakers can have a single RV lead, RV and RA leads, or RV, RA, and coronary sinus (CS) leads. The number of leads is determined by the implanting physician based on the patient's condition. For example, a patient with persistent atrial fibrillation (A-fib) will have no need of a lead to pace the RA. In another example, patients with a wide QRS on their ECG will need a CS lead to pace the LV and synchronize with the RV. The leads are manipulated so that their tips are in direct contact with the right ventricular or right atrial endocardium, or both. The leads are tested for stimulation and sensing properties to ascertain proper functioning before they are attached to the pulse generator. If the lead is in good position, it is secured by screwing the tip directly into the myocardium. At this point the peel away sheath is removed, and the process is repeated for subsequent leads. After testing is completed, the proximal end of the lead is attached to a battery (pacemaker or ICD) and implanted in a subcutaneous or subpectoral pocket created in the thorax. The incision is then closed, and the device is checked and programmed. Current pacemakers have a longevity of 5 to 10 years, and ICDs have a longevity of 6 to 8 years.

Newer pacemaker technologies allow the elimination of pacemaker leads, although at present they are only available as an alternative to single-lead pacemakers. A small pacemaker device is delivered through a catheter and embedded directly into the right ventricle. This leadless pacemaker is intended for patients with atrial fibrillation or other dangerous arrhythmias, such as bradycardia-tachycardia syndrome.

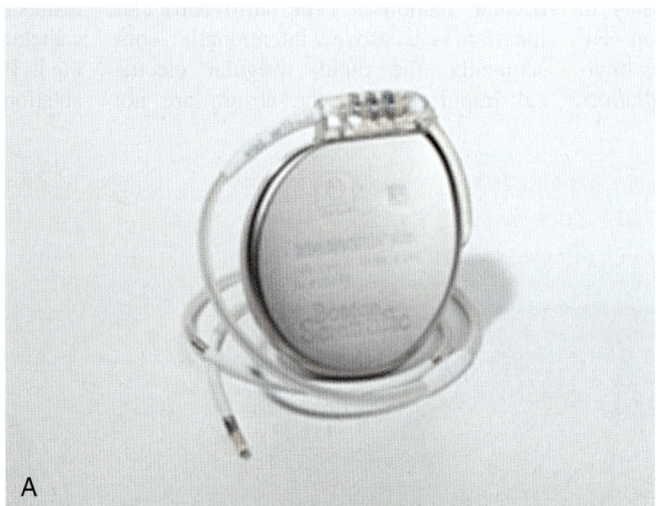

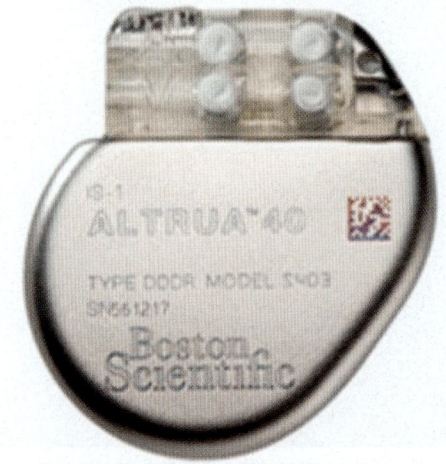

Fig. 27.126 (**A**) Single-chamber ICD. (**B**) Dual-chamber pacemaker.

(Used with permission of Boston Scientific Corporation. Boston Scientific Corporation 2013 or its affiliates. All rights reserved.)

Implanted cardioverter defibrillator (ICD)

The implantation of an ICD follows the same process as that of a PPM (Fig. 27.127). However, ICD implantation requires conscious sedation or general anesthesia, depending on the type of testing required at the time of implantation. During the procedure defibrillation threshold testing may be performed to determine the amount of energy required to defibrillate a patient from ventricular tachycardia or fibrillation. This process is done under general anesthesia and involves inducing an arrhythmia and allowing the ICD to recognize it, charge, and deliver the energy needed to defibrillate the patient. A backup external defibrillator is always connected to the patient and is charged and ready if the ICD fails to defibrillate the patient.

Loop recorder

A loop recorder is a small implantable device smaller than a stick of gum that is implanted under the skin of the chest close to the heart to record information about the electrical signals of the heart. It is usually implanted in patients with a history of losing consciousness for unknown reasons or in those who experience intermittent heart palpitations. The device can record the patient's heart rhythms when signaled by an external trigger or even a smart phone application. If a patient begins to feel palpations or starts to lose consciousness, then the patient, or someone else, can trigger the system to record. The information is downloaded directly to the cardiologist's office via the patient's home wireless network. The device is meant to be temporary and can be both implanted and removed in the physician's office setting under local anesthesia.

Interventional Cardiology: Present and Future

Existing and new interventional procedures will continue to provide patients with viable, relatively low-risk, financially reasonable alternatives to open-heart surgery. The area of transcatheter guidance in structural heart interventions, such as valve replacement, is continuing to grow rapidly. New guidelines have opened the TAVR procedure to moderate- and low-risk patients. New generations of TAVR valves have seen reductions in the need for post-op pacemaker placement, as well as improved patient outcomes. Research is being conducted on transcatheter replacement of the mitral valve as well. These procedures, while minimally invasive for the patient, are technically complex and require multimodality imaging, both in planning for and performing the procedure. Advances in 3D/4D transesophageal echocardiography (TEE) and cardiac CTA have assisted in procedure planning. The ability to use cardiac *fusion imaging* software in the angiographic suite has greatly improved visualization during the procedure. Cardiac fusion imaging software overlays both CTA and TEE images onto the live fluoroscopy image. The images can also be incorporated into the live fluoroscopy image so that the image moves in conjunction with the fluoroscopy image to assist with catheter and device manipulation.

One recent development has seen the widespread adoption of leadless pacemakers in certain cases. A leadless pacemaker is a device about the size of a pen cap that is implanted directly into the patient's right ventricle. This device eliminates the need for leads and a surgical incision in the chest for the generator. Once in position the device senses the underlying heart rhythm and paces the heart as needed. The latest iteration currently under development can even sense the rhythm of the atria based on the sound of the valve opening and closing.

Research is currently being conducted on advances in IVUS imaging as well. A new IVUS imaging algorithm will soon hopefully be able to directly measure the IFR of a vessel during an IVUS pullback. This would eliminate the need for extra supplies and provide cardiologists with crucial data during IVUS imaging.

As the practice of interventional cardiology evolves to include more complex and therefore longer procedures, innovative technology is being explored to reduce radiation exposure to both patients and staff, and to make the cardiac catheterization laboratory more ergonomically friendly. The use of remote-controlled robotics in percutaneous coronary intervention is thought to be a way to reduce some of the occupational hazards to interventional radiologists. Research is currently being conducted to evaluate patient safety and the technical and clinical performance of these robotic systems in manipulating needles, guidewires, catheters, and stents. Despite changes in cardiovascular technology and medical techniques, cardiac catheterization laboratories continue to provide the essential patient care services necessary for the diagnosis and treatment of a vast number of cardiovascular-related diseases.

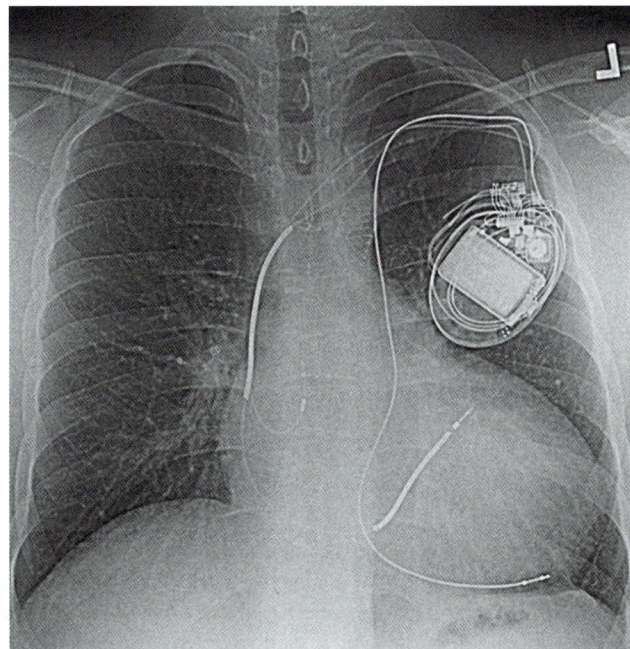

Fig. 27.127 A chest x-ray showing a dual-lead ICD.

(From Gatzoulis MA, Webb GD, Daubeney PEF: *Diagnosis and management of adult congenital heart disease*, 3rd ed, 2018, Elsevier.)

Best Practices in Vascular, Cardiac, and Interventional Radiology

Vascular and cardiac interventional technologists have a fundamental role in vascular and cardiac angiographic procedures. The technologist prepares the angiographic room, assists the physician with angiographic imaging, ensures that necessary supplies are readily available, and is often a scrub assistant to the physician. The technologist is actively involved in patient education, patient positioning, preparing angiographic and medical equipment, maintaining a sterile field during procedures, and ensuring that radiation protection and safety measures are followed. Cardiac interventional technologists also receive additional training for monitoring and documenting hemodynamic data during cardiac procedures. Often technologists perform these tasks under emergent and stressful conditions, when time is a critical factor in improving patient outcomes. The following best practices provide some guidelines for the vascular and cardiac interventional technologists.

1. *Effective communication and teamwork:* In critical medical situations, such as during angiographic and interventional procedures, it is vital to communicate effectively with fellow team members. Technologists should practice the following: verify pertinent information and ensure that expectations are aligned, ask for clarification where necessary, ask for assistance where necessary, be prepared to assist when possible, and prioritize patient safety measures.
2. *Preparation:* When preparing the room for the procedure, technologists should verify the expected procedure, the expected supplies to be used, and the patient's condition with the physician. Preparing the room as much as possible before the patient arrives in the procedural room will allow for effective use of procedural time.
3. *Attention to departmental protocol and scope of practice:* The technologist should know the department's protocols and practice them within their own competence and abilities.
4. *Universal protocol:* All angiographic team members are responsible for ensuring that the three steps of the universal protocol are adhered to (where applicable) prior to any invasive procedure. These steps include the pre-procedural verification checklist, site marking, and the "time-out" procedure.
5. *Informed consent and documentation:* All angiographic team members are responsible for ensuring that informed consent is given prior to invasive procedures. Technologists must be knowledgeable of facility policies regarding the informed consent process, including documentation and alternative decision-maker issues, as well as exceptional circumstances, such as ST-elevation myocardial infarction (STEMI).
6. *Infection control:* The interventional suite should be treated as an OR environment. Access should be limited to essential personnel only. Personnel must wear proper attire and be trained to follow strict aseptic practices. The procedure room, patient devices, and angiographic equipment must be cleaned thoroughly between cases. Surgical hand scrub should be performed immediately before putting on sterile gown and gloves. Maximum sterile barrier precautions should be utilized. All staff must ensure that the sterile field is maintained and not contaminated. Packaging for sterile supplies must be checked for expiration dates and signs of damage before opening.
7. *Radiation safety:* All angiographic procedures should be performed while keeping the radiation dose as low as reasonably achievable (ALARA). All personnel in the procedure room should wear personal radiation protective equipment, including lead aprons, radiation badges, thyroid shields, and leaded glasses for those nearest the radiation source. Technologists should be mindful of and remind visiting personnel, such as anesthesia or respiratory staff, the importance of time, intensity, distance, and shielding with fluoroscopy procedures.
8. *Certification training and continuing education:* Ideally, technologists should obtain Vascular Interventional (VI), Cardiac Interventional (CI), or Registered Cardiovascular Invasive Specialist (RCIS) certification and comply with continuing education requirements for these certifications. Additional training and education pertaining to angiographic equipment, imaging applications, patient monitoring devices, angiographic and interventional devices, and new procedures are essential to function effectively in the fields of interventional radiology and cardiovascular interventions. Documentation for technologists' competency should be reviewed and updated regularly to reflect additional training. Technologists should also be encouraged to join professional organizations, attend national meetings, and be actively involved in staying current in their field.

Definition of Terms

ablation: A surgical procedure used to remove or cause the destruction of function of a body tissue.

acquisition rate: The rate at which angiographic images are taken; measured in frames per second (f/s).

activated clotting time (ACT): A lab test used to determine the amount of time before a patient's blood begins to form clots. Commonly used during interventional procedures.

adventitia: The outermost layer of connective tissue that surrounds a blood vessel.

afferent lymph vessel: Vessel carrying lymph toward a lymph vessel.

anastomose: Join.

aneurysm: Sac formed by local enlargement of a weakened artery wall.

angina pectoris: Severe form of chest pain and constriction near the heart; usually caused by a decrease in the blood supply to cardiac tissue; most often associated with stenosis of a coronary artery as a result of atherosclerotic accumulations or spasm. Pain generally lasts for a few minutes and is more likely to occur after stress, exercise, or other activity resulting in increased heart rate.

angiography: Radiographic demonstration of blood vessels after the introduction of contrast media.

anomaly: Variation from the normal pattern.

aortic dissection: Tear in inner lining of the aortic wall that allows blood to enter and track along the muscular coat.

aortography: Radiographic examination of the aorta.

arrhythmia: Variation from normal heart rhythm.

arrhythmogenic: Producing an arrhythmia.
arteriography: Radiologic examination of arteries after injection of a radiopaque contrast medium.
arteriole: Very small arterial vessel.
arteriosclerotic: Indicative of a general pathologic condition characterized by thickening and hardening of arterial walls, leading to general loss of elasticity.
arteriotomy: Surgical opening of an artery.
arteriovenous malformation: Abnormal anastomosis or communication between an artery and a vein.
artery: Large blood vessel carrying blood away from the heart.
atherectomy: Excision of atherosclerotic plaque.
atheromatous: Characteristic of degenerative change in the inner lining of arteries caused by the deposition of fatty tissue and subsequent thickening of arterial walls that occurs in atherosclerosis.
atherosclerosis: Condition in which fibrous and fatty deposits on the luminal wall of an artery may cause obstruction of the vessel.
atrium: One of the two upper chambers of the heart.
balloon angioplasty: See *percutaneous transluminal angioplasty (PTA)*.
balloon aortic valvuloplasty (BAV): The inflating of a balloon across the aortic valve to treat aortic stenosis or to prep the valve for transcatheter aortic valve replacement (TAVR) placement.
balloon mitral valvuloplasty (BMV): The inflation of a balloon across the mitral valve to treat mitral stenosis.
bare metal stent: A type of stent without any drug coating.
bifurcation: Place where a structure divides into two branches.
biplane: Two x-ray exposure planes 90 degrees from one another, usually frontal and lateral.
blood vascular system: Vascular system comprising arteries, capillaries, and veins, which convey blood.
bradyarrhythmia: Irregular heart rhythm in conjunction with bradycardia.
bradycardia: Any heart rhythm with an average heart rate of less than 60 beats/min.
capillary: Tiny blood vessel through which blood and tissue cells exchange substances.
cardiac output: Amount of blood pumped from the heart per given unit of time; can be calculated by multiplying stroke volume (amount of blood in milliliters ejected from the left ventricle during each heartbeat) by heart rate (number of heartbeats per minute). A normal resting adult with a stroke volume of 70 mL and a heart rate of 72 beats/min has a cardiac output of approximately 5 L/min.
cardiomyopathies: Relatively serious group of heart diseases typically characterized by enlargement of the myocardial layer of the left ventricle and resulting in decreased cardiac output; hypertrophic cardiomyopathy is a condition often studied in the catheterization laboratory.
cinefluorography: Same as cineradiography; the production of a motion picture record of successive images on a fluoroscopic screen.
claudication: Cramping of the leg muscles after physical exertion because of chronically inadequate blood supply.
coagulopathy: Any disorder that affects the blood-clotting mechanism.
collateral: Secondary or accessory.
cryoablation: An ablation procedure utilizing extreme cold to scar myocardial tissue.
cutting balloon: A type of angioplasty balloon fitted with small blades to increase positive remodeling of coronary lesions.
diastole: Relaxed phase of the atria or ventricles of the heart during which blood enters the chambers; in the cardiac cycle at which the heart is not contracting (at rest).
drug-eluting stent (DES): A type of stent that has a drug coating designed to reduce tissue growth through the struts of the stent.
dyspnea:
Labored breathing.
efferent lymph vessel: Vessel carrying lymph away from a node.
ejection fraction: Measurements of ventricular contractility expressed as the percentage of blood pumped out of the left ventricle during contraction; can be estimated by evaluating the left ventriculogram; normal range is 57% to 73% (average 65%). A low ejection fraction indicates failure of the left ventricle to pump effectively.
electrophysiology (EP): A branch of cardiology that focuses on disease of the cardiac conduction system.
electrophysiology (EP) study: A procedure during which a patient's conduction system is evaluated.
embolization: The artificial or natural formation of an embolus.
embolus: Foreign material, often thrombus, that detaches and moves freely in the bloodstream.
endocardium: Interior lining of heart chambers.
epicardium: Exterior layer of heart wall.
ergometer: Device used to imitate the muscular, metabolic, and respiratory effects of exercise.
extravasation: Escape of fluid from a vessel into the surrounding tissue.
fractional flow reserve (FFR): A method of evaluating the degree to which coronary blood flow is affected by a lesion while the heart is under stress.
fibrillation: Involuntary, chaotic muscular contractions resulting from spontaneous activation of single muscle cells or muscle fibers.
Fick cardiac output: A method of estimating the cardiac output by comparing the oxygen saturations in the pulmonary arteries and the aorta.
French size: Measurement of catheter sizes; 1 French = 0.33 mm; abbreviated Fr.
guidewire: Tightly wound metallic wire over which angiographic catheters are placed.
hematoma: Collection of extravasated blood in an organ or a tissue space.
hemodynamics: Study of factors involved in circulation of blood. Hemodynamic data typically collected during heart catheterization are cardiac output and intracardiac pressures.
hemostasis: Stopping of blood flow in a hemorrhage.
iatrogenic: Caused by a therapeutic or diagnostic procedure.
implantable cardioverter defibrillator (ICD): An implanted device that monitors the patient's heart rhythm and can pace the heart as well as defibrillate a patient's heart automatically when it senses an arrythmia.
in-stent restenosis: Renarrowing of an artery inside a previously placed stent.
innominate or brachiocephalic artery: First major artery of the aortic arch supplying the cerebral circulation.
instant wave-free ratio (IFR): A method of evaluating the degree to which coronary blood flow is affected by a lesion without the need for the heart to be under stress. See *fractional flow reserve (FFR)*.
intervention: Therapeutic modality—mechanical or pharmacologic—used to modify the course of a disease process.

interventricular septal integrity: Continuity of the membranous partition that separates the right and left ventricles of the heart.

intima: Innermost endothelial layer of a blood vessel.

intraaortic balloon pump (IABP): A cardiovascular support device consisting of a large balloon placed in the aorta and inflated with helium in sync with the heartbeat to increase coronary perfusion.

intracoronary stent: Metallic device placed within a coronary artery across a region of stenosis.

intravascular lithotripsy (IVL): An advanced PCI technique that uses specially designed balloons to generate a shock wave inside a blood vessel to break up calcium deposits.

intravascular ultrasound (IVUS): An imaging method that utilizes sound waves to visualize the internal structures of blood vessels.

introducer sheath: Plastic tubing placed within the vasculature through which other catheters may be passed.

ischemic: Indicative of a local decrease of blood supply to myocardial tissue associated with temporary obstruction of a coronary vessel, typically as a result of thrombus (blood clot).

left atrial appendage occlusion device: A device designed to occlude the left atrial appendage to lower the risk of stroke in patients with slow blood flow in the atria.

lesion: Injury or other damaging change to an organ or tissue.

loop recorder: A small implantable device that records a patient's cardiac rhythm.

lymph: Body fluid circulated by the lymphatic vessels and filtered by the lymph nodes.

lymph vessels: See afferent and efferent lymph vessel.

lysis: Decomposition, destruction, or breakdown.

mandrel: Inner metallic core of a spiral wound guidewire.

meninges: Three membranes that envelop the brain and spinal cord.

minimally invasive: Minimizing surgical incisions to reduce trauma to the body.

misregistration: Occurs when the two images used to form a subtraction image are slightly displaced from one another.

modified Seldinger technique: A technique commonly used to access blood vessels.

myocardial infarction (MI): Acute ischemic episode resulting in myocardial damage and pain; commonly referred to as a heart attack.

myocardium: Muscular heart wall.

neointimal hyperplasia: Hyperproliferation of smooth muscle cells and extracellular matrix secondary to revascularization.

nephrotoxic: Chemically damaging to the kidney cells.

noninvasive imaging: Imaging that does not require the introduction of instruments into the body.

nonocclusive: Not completely closed or shut; allowing blood flow.

occlusion: Obstruction or closure of a vessel, such as a coronary vessel, as a result of foreign material, thrombus, or spasm.

optical coherence tomography (OCT): An intravascular image method that utilizes light to visualize vascular structures.

oximetry: Measurement of oxygen saturation in blood.

oxygen saturation: Amount of oxygen bound to hemoglobin in blood, expressed as a percentage.

patency: State of being open or unobstructed.

patent foramen ovale: Opening between the right atrium and left atrium that normally exists in fetal life to allow for the essential mixing of blood. The opening normally closes shortly after birth.

percutaneous: Introduced through the skin.

percutaneous left ventricular support device: A small pump that is inserted through the femoral or subclavian arteries and placed in the left ventricle to increase perfusion to the body.

percutaneous mitral valve repair: A percutaneous procedure designed to place a small clip on the mitral valve to treat severe mitral regurgitation.

percutaneous transluminal angioplasty (PTA): Surgical correction of a vessel from within the vessel using catheter technology.

percutaneous transluminal coronary angioplasty (PTCA): Manipulative interventional procedure involving the placement and inflation of a balloon catheter in the lumen of a stenosed coronary artery for the purpose of compressing and fracturing the diseased material, allowing subsequent increased distal blood flow to the myocardium.

percutaneous transluminal coronary rotational atherectomy (PTCRA): Manipulative interventional procedure to remove atherosclerotic plaque from within the coronary artery using a high-speed rotational burr.

percutaneously: Performed through the skin.

pericardium (pericardial sac): Fibrous sac that surrounds the heart.

permanent pacemaker (PPM): A device implanted that can detect a patient's heart rate and pace the heart as needed.

planimetry: Mechanical tracing to determine the volume of a structure.

pledget: Small piece of material used as a dressing or plug.

portal circulation (portal system): System of vessels carrying blood from the organs of digestion to the liver.

postprocessing: Image processing operations performed when reviewing an imaging sequence.

pressure transducer: See transducer.

pulmonary circulation: System of vessels carrying blood from the heart to the lungs and back to the heart.

pulse: Regular expansion and contraction of an artery that is produced by ejection of blood from the heart.

pulse oximetry: Measurement of oxygen saturation in the blood via an optic sensor placed on an extremity.

radial force: A force exerted from the center of a radius, used in endovascular stents.

radiofrequency (RF) ablation: An ablation procedure utilizing RF energy to scar myocardial tissue.

reperfusion: Reestablishment of blood flow to the heart muscle through a previously occluded artery.

restenosis: Narrowing or constriction of a vessel, orifice, or other type of passageway after interventional correction of primary condition.

rotational burr atherectomy: Ablation of atheroma through a percutaneous transcatheter approach using a high-speed rotational burr.

serial imaging: Acquisition of images in rapid succession.

stenosis: Narrowing or constriction of a vessel, an orifice, or another type of passageway.

stent: Wire mesh or plastic conduit placed to maintain flow.

systemic circulation: System of vessels carrying blood from the heart out to the body (except the lungs) and back to the heart.

systole: Contraction phase of the atria or ventricles of the heart during which blood is ejected from the chambers; point in the cardiac cycle at which the heart is contracting (at work).

tachyarrhythmia: Irregular heart rhythm in conjunction with tachycardia.

tachycardia: Any heart rhythm having an average heart rate in excess of 100 beats/min.

targeted lesion: Area of narrowing within an artery where a revascularization procedure is planned.

temporary transvenous pacemaker (TTVP): A small catheter inserted into the right ventricle in order to pace the heart temporarily.

thermodilution cardiac output: A method of measuring the cardiac output that utilizes a saline injection into the pulmonary artery measuring the temperature change across time.

thrombogenesis: Formation of a blood clot.

thrombolytic: Capable of causing the breakup of a thrombus.

thrombosis: Formation or existence of a blood clot.

thrombus: Blood clot obstructing a blood vessel or cavity of the heart.

transcatheter aortic valve replacement (TAVR): A procedure designed to percutaneously replace the aortic valve.

transducer: Device used to convert one form of energy into another. Transducers used in cardiac catheterization convert fluid (blood) pressure into an electrical signal displayed on a physiologic monitor.

transesophageal echocardiogram (TEE): A procedure in which echocardiographic images of the heart are taken using a special echo probe placed in the esophagus.

transposition of the great arteries: Congenital heart defect requiring interventional therapy. In this defect, the aorta arises from the right side of the heart, and the pulmonary artery arises from the left side of the heart.

valvular competence: Ability of the valve to prevent backward flow while not inhibiting forward flow.

varices: Irregularly swollen veins.

vasoconstriction: Temporary closure of a blood vessel using drug therapy.

vein: Vessel that carries blood from the capillaries to the heart.

venography: Radiologic study of veins after injection of radiopaque contrast media.

venotomy: Surgical opening of a vein.

ventricle: One of two larger pumping chambers of the heart.

venule: Any of the small blood vessels that collect blood from the capillaries and join to become veins.

References

1. Seldinger SI. Percutaneous selective angiography of the aorta: preliminary report. *Acta Radiol (Stockh)*. 1956;45:15.
2. Egas Moniz AC. L'encéphalographie artérielle, son importance dans la localisation des tumeurs cérébrales. *Rev Neurol*. 1927;2:72.
3. Egas Moniz AC. *L'angiographie Cérébrale*. Paris: Masson & Cie; 1934.
4. Greitz T. A radiologic study of the brain circulation by rapid serial angiography of the carotid artery. *Acta Radiol*. 1956;46(Suppl 140):1–123.
5. Dotter CT, Judkins MP. Transluminal treatment of arteriosclerotic obstruction: description of a new technique and preliminary report of its application. *Circulation*. 1964;30:654–670.
6. Grüntzig A, Hopff H. Perkutane rekanalisation chronischer arterieller verschlüsse mit einem neuen dilatationskatheter; modifikation der dotter-technik. *Deutsch Med Wochenschr*. 1974;99(49):2502–2511.
7. Molnar W, Stockum AE. Transhepatic dilatation of choledochoenterostomy strictures. *Radiology*. 1978;129(1):59–64.
8. Brooks B. The treatment of traumatic arteriovenous fistula. *South Med J*. 1930;23:100.
9. Brooks B. Discussion. In: Nolan L, Taylor AS, eds. Pulsating Exophthalmos. *Trans South Surg Assoc*. 1931;43:176.
10. Kaufman J, Lee M. *Vascular and Interventional Radiology: The Requisites*. 2nd ed. Philadelphia: Elsevier; 2014.
11. Scanlon PJ, Faxon DP, Audet AM, et al. ACC/AHA guidelines for coronary angiography: a report of the American College of Cardiology/American Heart Association Task Force on Practice Guidelines (Committee on Coronary Angiography). *J Am Coll Cardiol*. 1999;33(6):1756–1824.
12. Laskey W, Boyle J, Johnson LW. Multivariable model for prediction of risk of significant complication during diagnostic cardiac catheterization: the Registry Committee of the Society for Cardiac Angiography and Interventions. *Cathet Cardiovasc Diagn*. 1993;30(3):185–190.

Selected bibliography

Ahn SS, Concepcion B. Current status of atherectomy for peripheral arterial occlusive disease. *World J Surg*. 1996;20(6):635–643.

Burke TH, Shetty PC, Sanders WP. Cardiovascular and interventional technologists: their growing role in the interventional suite. *J Vasc Interv Radiol*. 1997;8(4):720.

Coldwell DM, Stokes KR, Yakes WF. Embolotherapy: agents, clinical applications, and techniques. *Radio-Graphics*. 1994;14(3):623–643.

Colombo A, Hall P, Nakamura S, et al. Intracoronary stenting without anticoagulation accomplished with intravascular ultrasound guidance. *Circulation*. 1995;91(6):1676–1688.

Danielkutty C, Weiss D, Kliger CA. *Cardiac fusion imaging provides benefits for transcatheter guidance in structural heart interventions*. Diagnostic and Interventional Cardiology (DAIC) [website]. 2018. https://www.dicardiology.com/content/cardiac-fusion-imaging-provides-benefits-transcatheter-guidance-structural-heart. (Accessed August 5, 2024.)

Dorffner R, Thurnher S, Polterauer P, et al. Treatment of abdominal aortic aneurysms with transfemoral placement of stent-grafts: complications and secondary radiologic intervention. *Radiology*. 1997;204(1):79–86.

Dyet JF. Endovascular stents in the arterial system—current status. *Clin Radiol*. 1997;52(2):83–108.

Eustace S, Buff B, Kruskal J, et al. Magnetic resonance angiography in transjugular intrahepatic portosystemic stenting: comparison with contrast hepatic and portal venography. *Eur J Radiol*. 1994;19(1):43–49.

Fillmore DJ, Miller FJ, Fox LF, et al. Transjugular intrahepatic portosystemic shunt: midterm clinical and angiographic follow-up. *J Vasc Interv Radiol*. 1996;7(2):255–261.

Kandarpa K. Technical determinants of success in catheter-directed thrombolysis for peripheral arterial occlusions. *J Vasc Interv Radiol*. 1995;6(6 pt 2 Suppl):55S–61S.

Kandarpa K, Machan L. *Handbook of Interventional Radiologic Procedures*. 4th ed. Lippincott Williams & Wilkins; 2011.

Kassamali RH, Ladak B. The role of robotics in interventional radiology. *Quant Imaging Med Surg*. 2015;5(3):340–343.

Kaufman J, Lee M. *Vascular and Interventional Radiology: The Requisites*. 2nd ed. Philadelphia: Elsevier; 2014.

Kern MJ, et al. *The Cardiac Catheterization Handbook*. 6th ed. Philadelphia: Elsevier; 2016.

Kerns SR, Hawkins IF Jr, Sabatelli FW. Current status of carbon dioxide angiography. *Radiol Clin North Am*. 1995;33(1):15–29.

Kirschner R, Orlowski T, Deyo K. Meeting OR standards in the interventional procedure room and cardiac catheterization laboratory. *J Radiol Nurs*. 2009;28(2):43.

Laine C, Venditti L, Localio R, et al. Combined cardiac catheterization for uncomplicated ischemic heart disease in a Medicare population. *Am J Med*. 1998;105(5):373–379.

Le Roux PD, Winn HR. Management of cerebral aneurysms. How can current management be improved? *Neurosurg Clin N Am*. 1998;9(3):421–433.

Naidu SS, Aronow HD, Box LC, et al. SCAI expert consensus statement: 2016 best practices in the cardiac catheterization laboratory: (endorsed by the Cardiological Society of India, and Sociedad Latino Americana de Cardiologia Intervencionista; Affirmation of value by the Canadian Association of Interventional Cardiology). *Catheter Cardiovasc Interv*. 2016;88(3):407–423.

Nelson PK. Kricheff II: Cerebral angiography. *Neuroimaging Clin N Am*. 1996;6:1.

Norris TG. Principles of cardiac catheterization. *Radiol Technol*. 2000;72(2):109–136.

Pieters PC, Miller WJ, DeMeo JH. Evaluation of the portal venous system: complementary roles of invasive and noninvasive imaging strategies. *Radiographics*. 1997;17(4):879–895.

Rees CR, Niblett RL, Lee SP, et al. Use of carbon dioxide as a contrast medium for transjugular intrahepatic portosystemic shunt procedures. *J Vasc Interv Radiol*. 1994;5(2):383–386.

Rogers CG Jr, Paolini RM, O'Leary JP. Intrahepatic vascular shunting for portal hypertension: early experience with the transjugular intrahepatic porto-systemic shunt. *Am Surg*. 1994;60(2):114–117.

Scanlon PJ, Faxon DP, Audet AM, et al. ACC/AHA guidelines for coronary angiography: a report of the American College of Cardiology/American Heart Association Task Force on Practice Guidelines (Committee on Coronary Angiography). *J Am Coll Cardiol*. 1999;33(6):1756–1824.

Seldinger SI. Percutaneous selective angiography of the aorta: preliminary report. *Acta Radiol (Stockh)*. 1956;45:15.

Snopek A. *Fundamentals of Special Radiographic Procedures*. 5th ed. Elsevier; 2006.

Viñuela F, Duckwiler G, Mawad M. Guglielmi detachable coil embolization of acute intracranial aneurysm: perioperative anatomical and clinical outcome in 403 patients. *J Neurosurg*. 1997;86(3):475–482.

Weisz G, Metzger DC, Caputo RP, et al. Safety and feasibility of robotic percutaneous coronary intervention: PRECISE (Percutaneous Robotically-Enhanced Coronary Intervention) Study. *J Am Coll Cardiol*. 2013;61(15):1596–1600.

28
DIAGNOSTIC MEDICAL SONOGRAPHY
SUSANNA L. OVEL

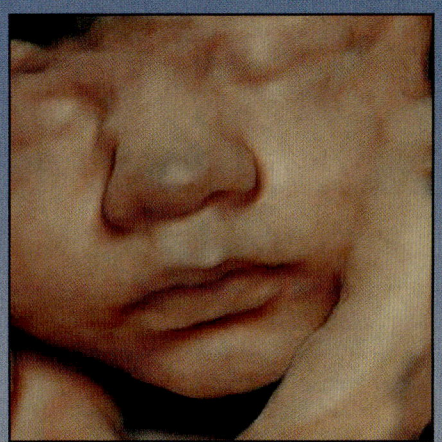

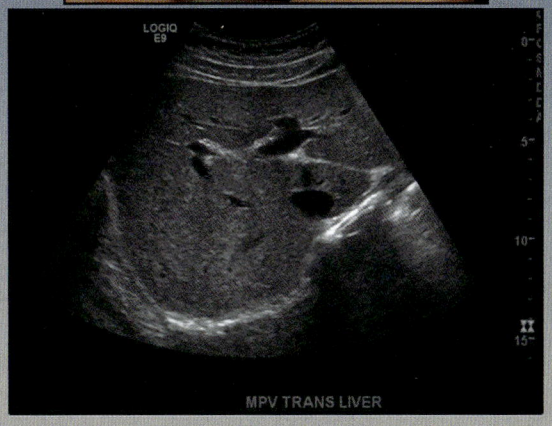

OUTLINE

Principles of Diagnostic Ultrasound, 408
Historical Development, 409
Physical Principles, 410
Anatomic Relationships and
 Landmarks, 411
Clinical Applications, 412
Cardiologic Applications, 430
Best Practices In General Sonography, 432
Conclusion, 432
Definition of Terms, 433

Principles of Diagnostic Ultrasound

Diagnostic medical sonography[a] is a general term used to encompass abdominal, breast, cardiac, gynecologic, obstetric, and vascular sonography. *Registered diagnostic medical sonographers* (RDMSs) specialize in abdominal sonography, obstetrics/gynecology imaging, breast sonography, musculoskeletal imaging, or pediatric sonography. *Registered diagnostic cardiac sonographers* (RDCSs) specialize in fetal, pediatric, or adult echocardiography. *Registered vascular technologists* (RVTs) specialize in abdominal vasculature imaging, as well as imaging of arteries and veins of the upper and lower extremities, imaging of extracranial arteries and veins, transcranial duplex sonography, and physiologic vascular testing in pediatric and adult patients. One overall physics examination, encompassing sonographic principles, hemodynamics, and instrumentation, is required for all these specialties.[a]

Diagnostic medical sonography employs high-frequency transducers ranging from 2 to 50 MHz. The transducer emits short pulses of ultrasound (pulse waves) into the human body. The transducer receives real-time reflections or frequency shifts from structures or vessels along the sound waves path, and they are displayed as a grayscale, color Doppler, spectral, or duplex image. Velocity of the red blood cells can be calculated using the Doppler equation. Pulse wave, continuous wave, and color Doppler techniques show blood flow direction, flow resistance and turbulence within the vessel, and regurgitation of the cardiac chamber.

Diagnostic medical sonography has evolved into a unique imaging tool. Sonography was previously thought to be a completely noninvasive technique. However, with the introduction of intracavity and intraluminal transducers, the collection of diagnostic data of the pelvic and cardiovascular regions has been shown to improve patient management and care.

CHARACTERISTICS OF DIAGNOSTIC MEDICAL SONOGRAPHERS

The diagnostic medical sonographer uses complicated equipment, independent judgment, and systematic problem-solving skills to acquire quality images and technical data for assistance in a patient's diagnosis, management, and care. Integrity and honesty are important qualities in all medical professionals. In sonography, these character traits are crucial because almost 90% of observed data are discarded. After each examination, the sonographer provides the reading physician with a technical report detailing the size and description of normal and abnormal anatomy and/or hemodynamics, along with possible differential diagnostic considerations when anomalies and abnormalities are visualized.

Similar to radiography, diagnostic medical sonography has national standardized protocols for each examination. The sonographer has the ability to expand on basic examination protocols when additional information is needed without fear of ionizing radiation. In-depth knowledge of pathophysiology, laboratory values, and other medical imaging modalities (i.e., computed tomography [CT] or magnetic resonance imaging [MRI]) are important parts of sonography education.

Physical requirements play an additional role in sonography. Sonographers must be able to aid in moving patients and medical equipment. Attention to the use of proper body mechanics is essential (Fig. 28.1). Repetitive usage injury or syndrome of the neck, shoulder, elbow, wrist, and back has been documented. The sonographer should be in good physical, emotional, and nutritional health, and should possess a dedication to continual learning. The career can be exciting and rewarding, as well as stressful, demanding, frustrating, and, occasionally, depressing.

---

[a] Almost all italicized words on the succeeding pages are defined at the end of this chapter.

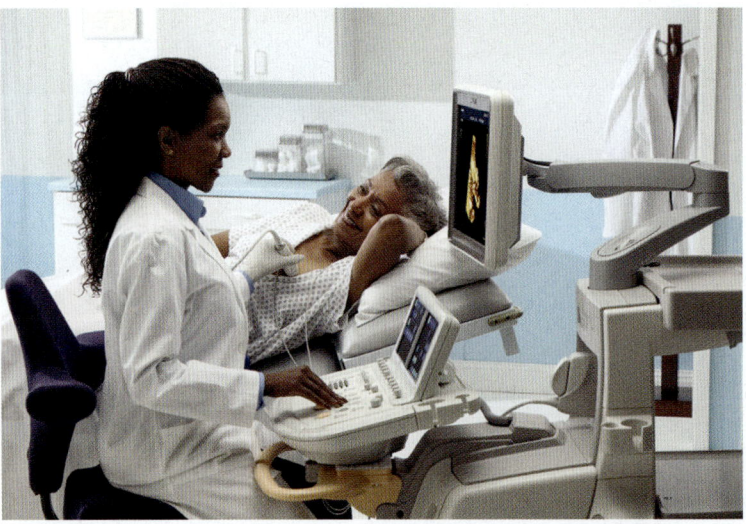

Fig. 28.1 Sonographer performing an ultrasound examination.

(Courtesy Philips Medical Systems.)

RESOURCE ORGANIZATIONS

Resource organizations devoted exclusively to ultrasound include the American Society of Echocardiography (ASE), the Society of Diagnostic Medical Sonography (SDMS), the American Institute of Ultrasound in Medicine (AIUM), the Society of Radiologists in Ultrasound (SRU), and the Society for Vascular Ultrasound (SVU). The International Foundation for Sonography Education and Research (IFSER) is a unique organization devoted to the educators of ultrasound.

Historical Development

Ultrasound began with the discovery of the piezoelectric effect in 1880 by Jacques and Pierre Curie. This discovery allowed for the future construction of transducers to generate and receive sound waves in water. In 1915, the first sonar-type device was developed by Paul Langevin to locate submarines. After World War II, research was conducted on medical applications of ultrasound. Between 1940 and 1962, various medical applications were researched and developed. In 1962, the first compound B-scanner was developed with the support of the US Public Health Services and the University of Colorado. Medical imaging using ultrasound was launched in 1963 with a handheld articulated arm compound B-mode (brightness mode) scanner. The original imaging was bi-stable (black and white only) until 1973, when grayscale imaging was developed by a group in Australia. By 1980, the digital scan converter, allowing 64 shades of gray in the ultrasound image, was developed. In the mid-1980s, ultrasound could be imaged in real time. Not only could sonographers image more reflected intensities, but they could also view live motion of the human anatomy.

Christian Andreas Doppler described the changes in the frequency of transmitted waves when relative motion occurred between the source of the wave and an observer. The first Doppler ultrasound device for medical use was created in the late 1950s in Japan. A prototype of a continuous wave Doppler soon followed, with the reported ability to assess blood flow using the Doppler frequency shift. In the mid-1960s, Dr. Eugene Strandness, at the University of Washington, began research on the use of Doppler ultrasound to detect vascular disease. The first pulsed Doppler technique was developed in 1974 by engineer Donald Baker. Color Doppler was established in 1983 in Japan. However, it was not until 1987 that color Doppler launched in the United States.

For the present-day general sonographer, it may be inconceivable that a diagnosis could be made using only bi-stable and static grayscale scanners to image human anatomy and the presence of abnormalities. The present-day vascular and cardiac sonographers would likely feel the same with the lack of color Doppler to aid in assessing vessel pathology and hemodynamics in vascular and cardiac imaging. Technological advances have benefited medical ultrasound with the use of high-frequency, multihertz, intracavity, and intraluminal transducers, together with three-dimensional, four-dimensional, and panoramic imaging. New technologies, such as elastography, fusion imaging, parallel processing, and contrast-enhanced ultrasound imaging, are allowing the diagnosis of pathology without the risks of ionizing radiation and invasive procedures. Most recently, a wireless transducer used with a smartphone, tablet, or laptop allows imaging in areas remote from the medical setting.

The ALARA principle (As Low As Reasonably Achievable) was developed to reduce biological effects in humans and the fetus. When used as a clinical imaging tool, diagnostic ultrasound has not been associated with any harmful biological effects and is generally accepted as a safe imaging modality.

Physical Principles

PROPERTIES OF SOUND WAVES

Sound waves are traveling variations of pressure, density, and particle motion. Matter must be present for sound to travel; it cannot travel through a vacuum. Sound carries energy, not matter, from one place to another. Vibrations from one molecule carry to the next molecule along the same axis. These oscillations continue until friction causes the vibrations to cease.

Ultrasound refers to sound waves beyond the audible range (>20 kHz). Diagnostic medical sonography can use frequencies of up to 50 MHz.

Acoustic impedance

Sound travels through tissues at different speeds, depending on the density and stiffness of the medium. The acoustic impedance of a medium determines how much of the wave transmits to the next medium (Fig. 28.2).

Velocity of sound

Propagation speed is the speed at which a sound wave travels through a medium. It is determined by the density and stiffness of a medium. In soft tissue, the propagation speed of sound is 1540 m/s. Bone shows a very high propagation speed (4080 m/s), whereas air shows the lowest propagation speed (330 m/s).

TRANSDUCER SELECTION

Diagnostic ultrasound transducers operate on the principle of piezoelectricity. The *piezoelectric effect* states that some materials produce a voltage when deformed by an applied pressure. Diagnostic ultrasound transducers convert electrical energy into acoustic energy during transmission, and acoustic energy into electrical energy for reception. Transducers routinely operate in a frequency range of 2 to 20 MHz for diagnostic applications. Transducers may be linear, convex, sector, or vector in construction (Fig. 28.3). Higher frequencies are used in intracavity and intraluminal transducers, as well as for visualizing the extremities or superficial structures. Lower frequencies are needed for deeper structures of the thoracic cavity, abdomen, and pelvis. Lower frequencies provide necessary penetration depth at the expense of *detail resolution*.

Pulse wave transducers transmit pulses of sound and receive returning echoes, producing a grayscale ultrasound image. A continuous wave transducer produces a continuous wave of sound and is composed of a separate transmit and receive element within a single transducer assembly. Continuous wave transducers do not produce an image.

VOLUME SCANNING AND THREE-DIMENSIONAL AND FOUR-DIMENSIONAL IMAGING

Volume scanning allows for quick "sweeps" of specific areas of the body or fetus. These sweeps give volume data that can be rendered even after the patient has left the ultrasound department. Three-dimensional imaging systems allow the sonographer to acquire volume data. The sonographer can reconstruct these data into a three-dimensional image on the ultrasound machine or at a workstation. With four-dimensional imaging, the ultrasound system can acquire and display three-dimensional images in real time.

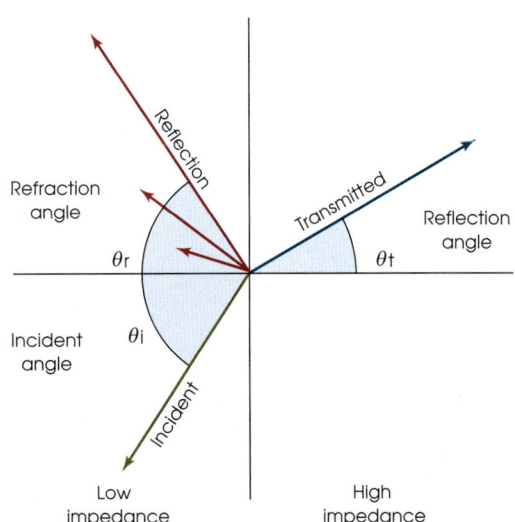

Fig. 28.2 Relationship among incident, reflected, and transmitted waves.

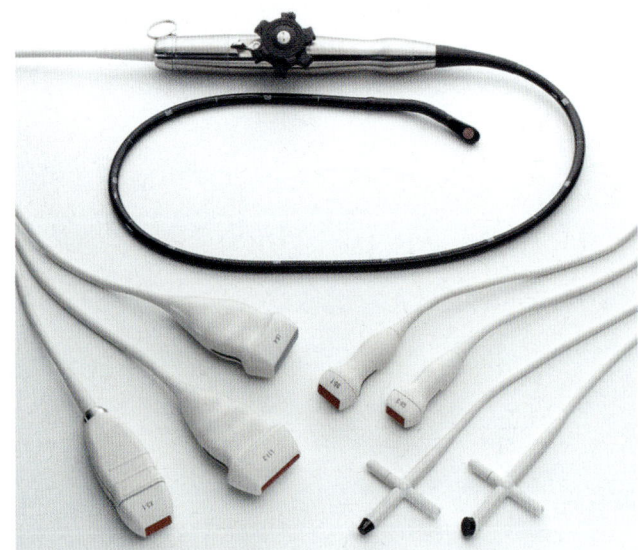

Fig. 28.3 Various ultrasound transducers.

(Courtesy Philips Medical Systems.)

Anatomic Relationships and Landmarks

The use of anatomic landmarks to define specific areas of the human body is an important part of the imaging and orientation skills of the sonographer. The middle hepatic vein is a sonographic landmark used to locate the division between the left and right hepatic lobes (Fig. 28.4A). The main lobar fissure is used to locate the gallbladder fossa (Fig. 28.4B). The ovaries are located medial and anterior to the iliac vessels (Fig. 28.4C). The use of anatomic landmarks is a routine part of many sonographic examinations.

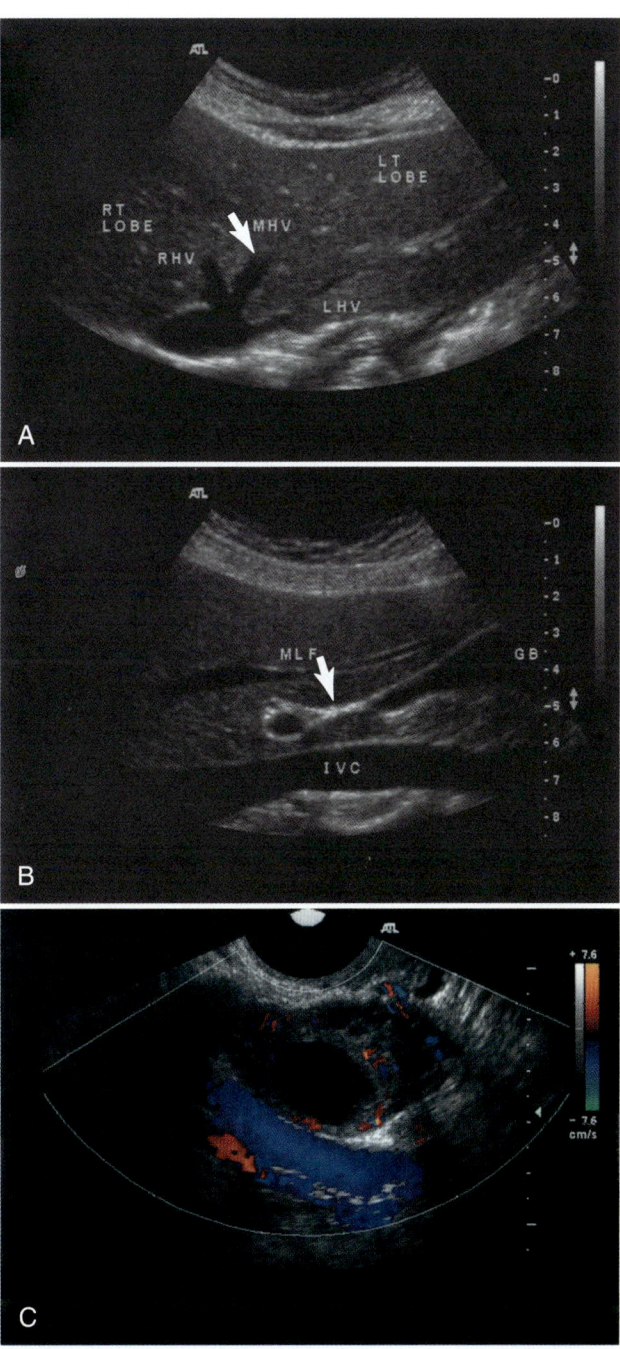

Fig. 28.4 (**A**) Transverse sonogram of liver showing middle hepatic vein (MHV) dividing left and right hepatic lobes. (**B**) Sagittal image of main lobar fissure (MLF) and its relationship to gallbladder (GB). (**C**) Sagittal color Doppler image of right ovary lying anterior and medial to iliac vessels. *IVC,* Inferior vena cava; *LHV,* left hepatic vein; *RHV,* right hepatic vein.

(B, Courtesy Paul Aks, BS, RDMS, RVT.)

Clinical Applications

CHARACTERISTICS OF THE SONOGRAPHIC IMAGE

The sonographer uses specific terms to characterize the sonographic image. If the echo pattern is similar throughout a structure or mass, it is termed *homogeneous* (Fig. 28.5A). If the echo pattern is dissimilar throughout a structure or mass, it is termed *heterogeneous* (Fig. 28.5B). Internal composition of a structure or mass is described using the terms *anechoic* (without internal echoes), *echogenic* (with internal echoes), and *complex* (containing anechoic and echogenic regions) (Fig. 28.6). The sonographer also uses descriptive terms to describe the borders of a mass. Are the borders calcified, smooth or irregular, thin or thick?

Imaging artifacts are an additional concern for the sonographer. Acoustic artifacts include reflections that are missing, not real, improperly positioned, or of improper brightness, number, shape, or size (Fig. 28.7). By understanding the physical principles of sound waves and the ultrasound system, the sonographer can better comprehend the real-time images.

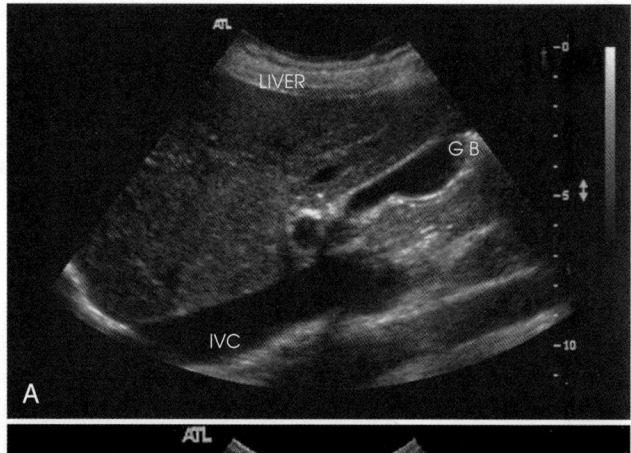

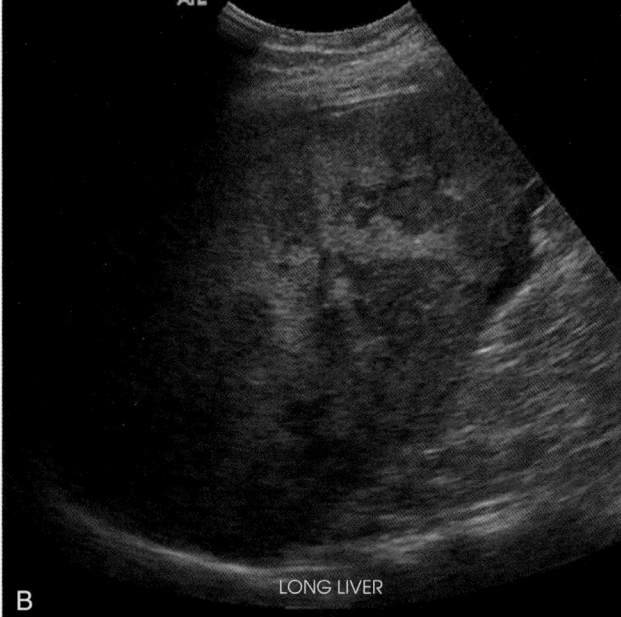

Fig. 28.5 (**A**) Sagittal sonogram of normal homogeneous liver. (**B**) Sagittal sonogram of heterogeneous liver parenchyma.

(B, Courtesy Susanna Ovel, RT, RDMS, RVT.)

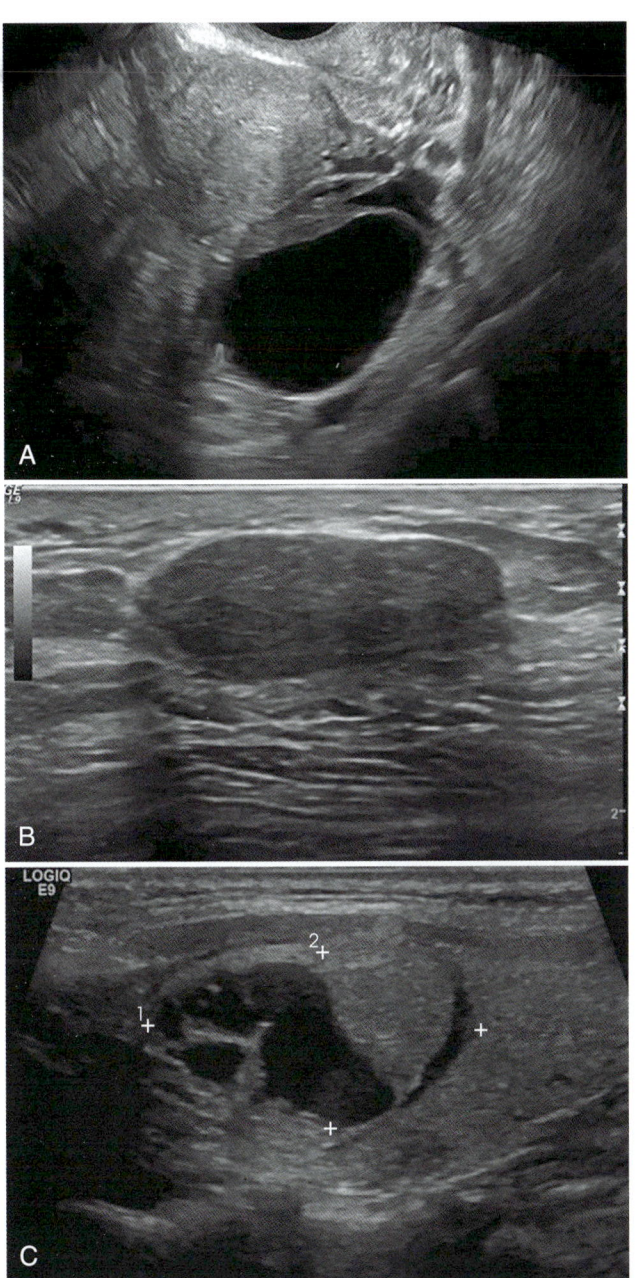

Fig. 28.6 (**A**) Endovaginal sonogram of anechoic ovarian cyst. (**B**) Echogenic superficial mass. (**C**) Transverse sonogram of complex thyroid mass.

(Courtesy Susanna Ovel, RT, RDMS, RVT.)

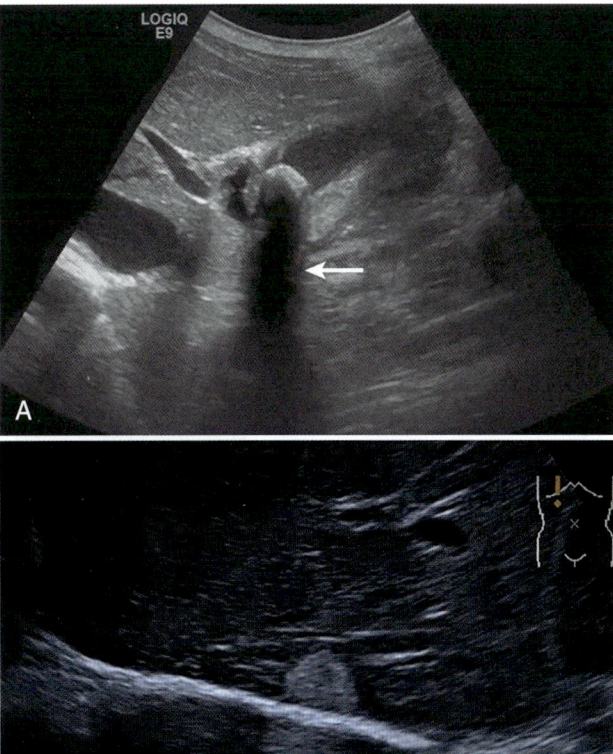

Fig. 28.7 (**A**) Gallstone demonstrating posterior acoustic shadowing *(arrow)*. (**B**) Mirror image of a hepatic hemangioma.

(A, Courtesy Susanna Ovel, RT, RDMS, RVT. B, Courtesy Ravi D Kadasne, MD.)

ABDOMEN AND RETROPERITONEUM

The abdominal ultrasound examination generally includes a survey of the liver, pancreas, gallbladder, spleen, great vessels, and kidneys in the sagittal and transverse planes (Figs. 28.8 and 28.9). Specific protocols are followed to image size, shape, and echogenicity of the organ *parenchyma* and anatomic relationships of the surrounding structures. Doppler flow patterns of the upper abdominal blood vessels may be included. Patients are examined in two different body positions (i.e., supine and decubitus). The use of two positions shows the mobility of gallstones and repositions interfering bowel gas. Air reflects most of the sound wave, making visualization of the abdominal and retroperitoneal structures difficult. Abdominal examinations are typically scheduled in the morning, with the patient fasting 6 to 8 hours before the sonogram.

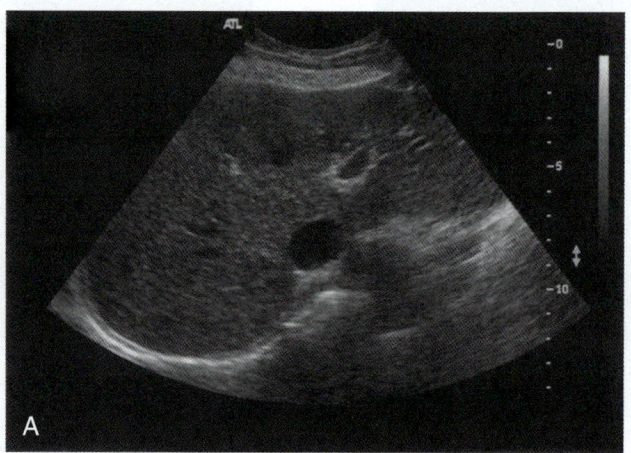

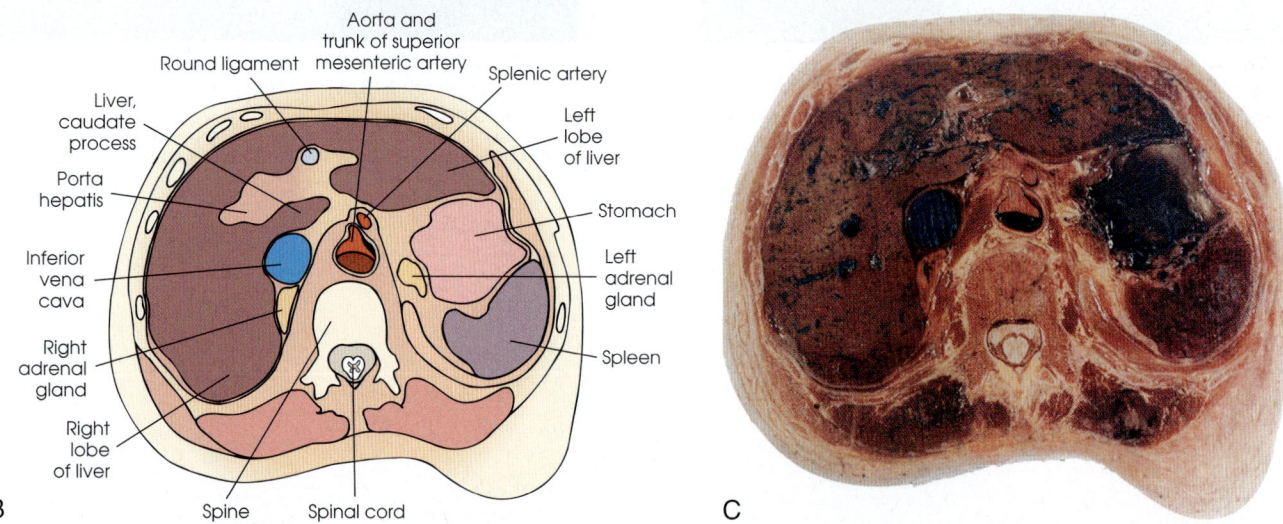

Fig. 28.8 (**A**) Transverse sonogram of right upper quadrant over right lobe of liver. (**B**) Line drawing of gross anatomic section. (**C**) Gross anatomic section at approximately same level as A.

The retroperitoneal ultrasound examination includes a survey of the great vessels, kidneys, and bladder in the sagittal and transverse planes before and after voiding. Specific protocols are followed to image the size, shape, cortical thickness, and echogenicity of the renal parenchyma. Anterior-posterior diameters of the inferior vena cava, aorta, and common iliac arteries are measured and documented. Doppler flow patterns of the great vessels and kidneys may be included. Retroperitoneum examinations can be scheduled in the morning or afternoon, with the patient drinking 8 to 16 oz of water 1 hour before the sonogram.

To produce an adequate survey of the abdominal and retroperitoneal cavities, the sonographer must fully understand the patient's clinical history. Although ultrasound cannot diagnose the specific pathology of a lesion or condition, a complete clinical picture may lead to more specific differential diagnostic considerations.

Liver and biliary tree

Sonographic examinations of the liver and biliary tree are generally requested in patients with right upper quadrant pain or elevations in liver function laboratory tests. The liver is assessed for size and echogenicity of the parenchyma. Under normal circumstances, the liver parenchyma appears moderately echogenic and homogeneous. Some types of liver pathologies shown on ultrasound include hepatic steatosis, cirrhosis, cavernous hemangioma, and hepatoma (Fig. 28.10). Doppler evaluation of the hepatic artery, hepatic veins, and portal veins is included with a patient history or suspicion of cirrhosis, portal hypertension, portal vein thrombosis, and Budd-Chiari syndrome.

The biliary tree includes the gallbladder, as well as the intrahepatic and

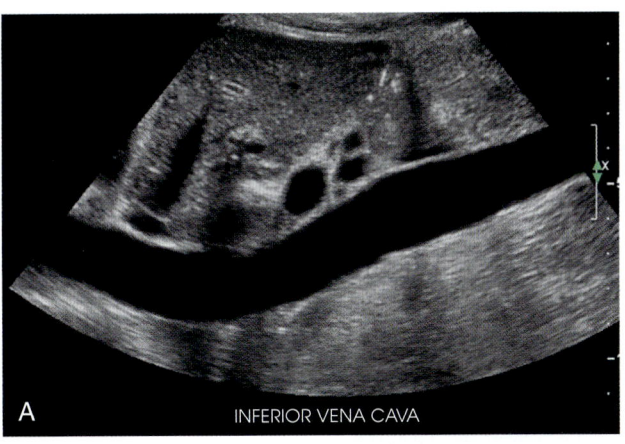

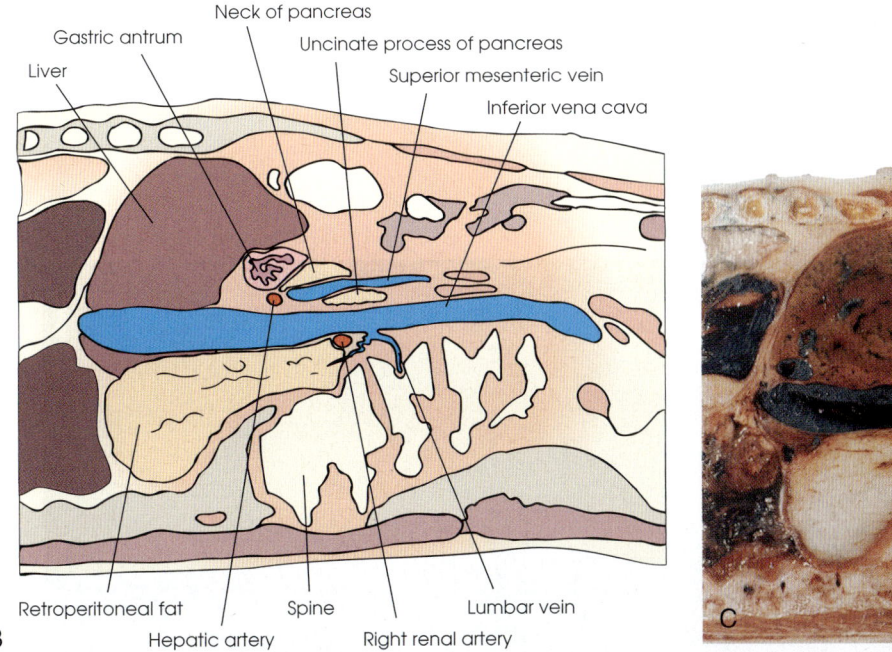

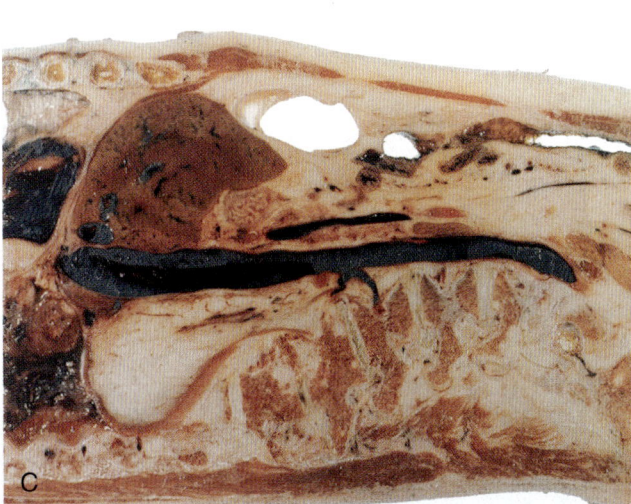

Fig. 28.9 (**A**) Sagittal sonogram of the liver and inferior vena cava. (**B**) Line drawing of gross anatomic section. (**C**) Gross anatomic section at approximately same level as A.

(A, Courtesy Susanna Ovel, RT, RDMS, RVT.)

extrahepatic bile ducts. The gallbladder is evaluated for size, wall thickness, and absence of internal echoes. Under normal circumstances, the gallbladder is a pear-shaped anechoic structure located in the gallbladder fossa on the posterior surface of the liver (Fig. 28.11). The intrahepatic biliary ducts converge near the *porta hepatis*, forming the common hepatic duct. The cystic duct joins the common hepatic duct to form the extrahepatic common bile duct. The biliary tree is evaluated for size and evidence of intraductal stones or masses. Some abnormalities of the biliary tree shown on ultrasound include intrahepatic and extrahepatic biliary obstruction, cholelithiasis, and cholecystitis (Fig. 28.12).

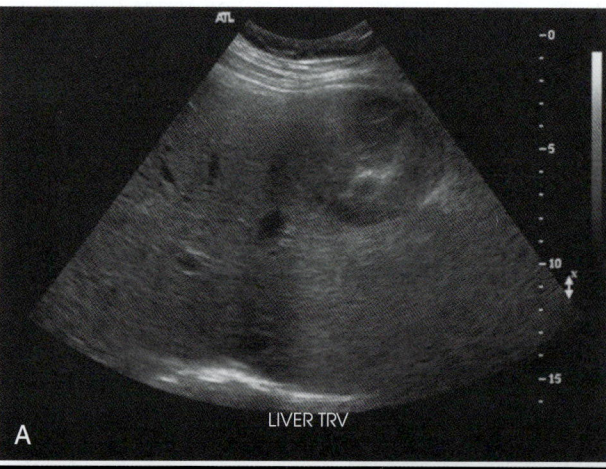

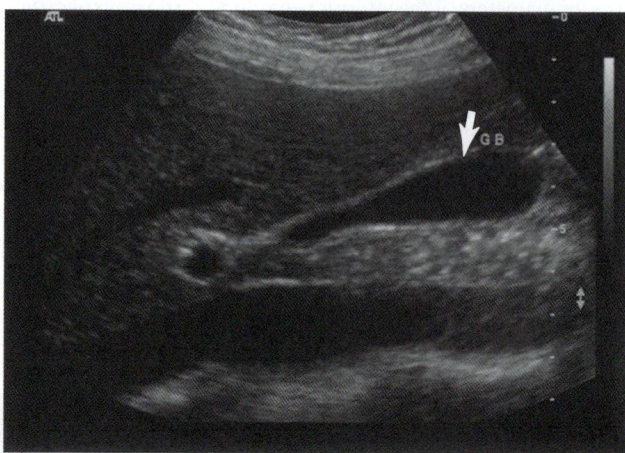

Fig. 28.11 Sagittal sonogram of normal gallbladder (*arrow*).

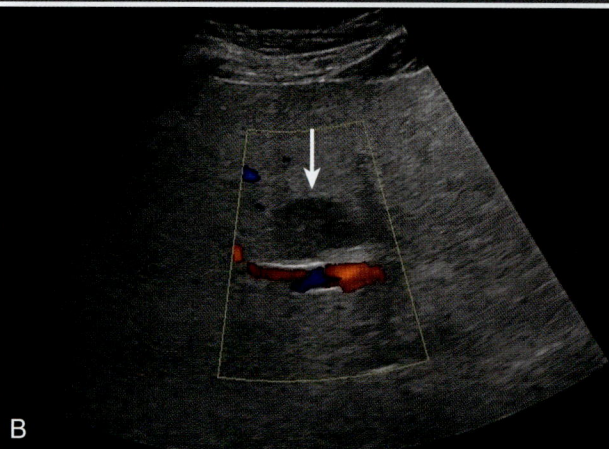

Fig. 28.10 (A) Transverse sonogram of liver shows a complex mass in the left lobe. (B) Sonogram of liver shows hepatic steatosis with small area of normal liver parenchyma anterior to porta hepatis (*arrow*).

(A, Courtesy Paul Aks, BS, RDMS, RVT. B, Courtesy Susanna Ovel, RT, RDMS, RVT.)

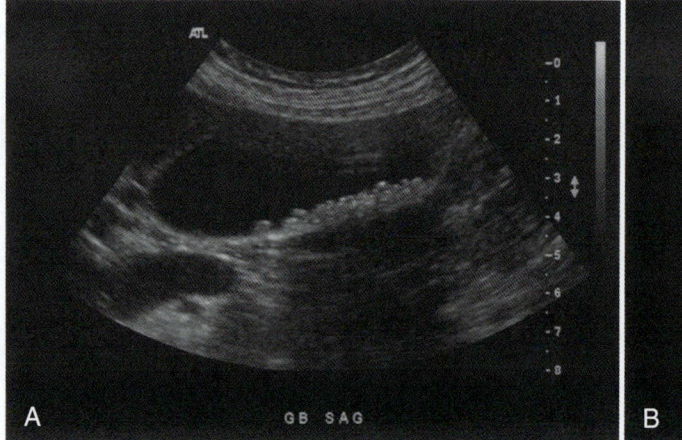
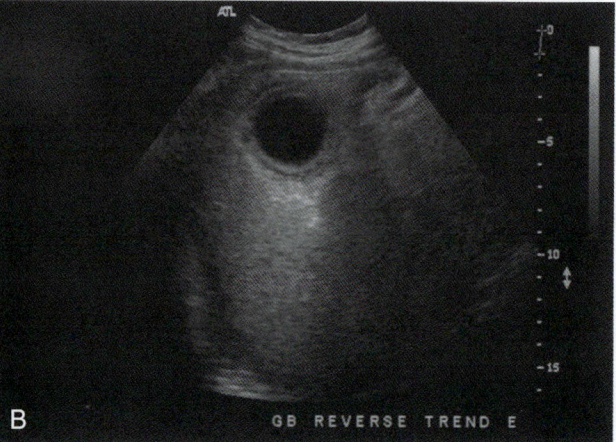

Fig. 28.12 (A) Sagittal sonogram of gallbladder showing multiple small gallstones with posterior acoustic shadowing. (B) Transverse sonogram of acute cholecystitis.

Pancreas

The pancreas is an elongated organ oriented in a transverse *oblique plane* in the epigastric and left hypochondriac regions of the retroperitoneal cavity. The head of the pancreas lies in the descending portion of the duodenum and is lateral to the superior mesenteric artery. The body is the largest portion, lying anterior to the superior mesenteric artery and splenic vein (Fig. 28.13). The tail is the most superior portion lying posterior to the antrum of the stomach and generally extends toward the splenic hilum. The echogenicity of the pancreas varies depending on the amount of fat but should appear homogeneous throughout the organ. Ultrasound examinations of the pancreas are requested in patients with a history of unexplained weight loss, epigastric pain, and elevation in pancreatic enzymes or liver function laboratory tests. The pancreas is evaluated for size and echogenicity of the parenchyma. The distal common bile duct is routinely measured in the posterior lateral portion of the head of the pancreas. Some abnormalities of the pancreas shown on ultrasound include inflammation, calcifications, abscess formation, and benign or malignant neoplasms (Fig. 28.14).

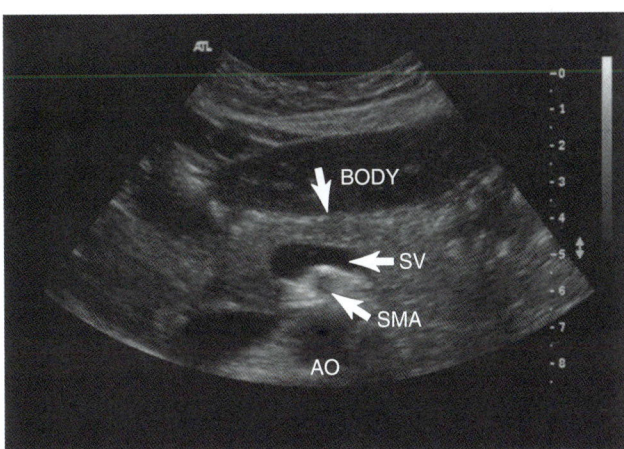

Fig. 28.13 Transverse sonogram of normal pancreas. The body of the pancreas lies anterior to splenic vein *(SV)*, superior mesenteric artery *(SMA)*, and aorta *(AO)*.

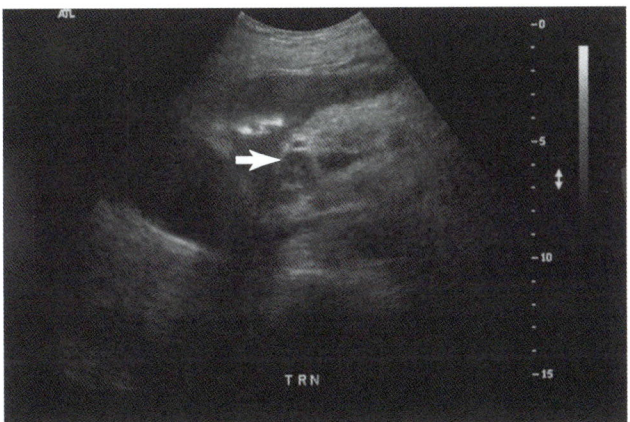

Fig. 28.14 Transverse sonogram shows hypoechoic mass in head of the pancreas *(arrow)*.

Spleen

The spleen is the predominant organ in the left upper quadrant, located inferior to the diaphragm and anterior to the left kidney. Ultrasound examinations of the spleen are requested in patients with a history of abdominal trauma, chronic liver disease, and leukocytosis. An increase in hepatic pressures from liver disease may cause an abnormal increase in the size of the spleen (Fig. 28.15). The normal spleen appears moderately echogenic, similar to the normal liver parenchyma. The spleen is evaluated for size and echogenicity of the parenchyma. Some abnormalities of the spleen shown on ultrasound include splenomegaly, splenic rupture, calcifications, or abscess formation. Doppler evaluation of the splenic artery and vein is included with a patient history or suspicion of portal hypertension.

Kidneys and bladder

The kidneys are bean-shaped structures lying in a *sagittal* oblique plane lateral to the psoas muscles in the retroperitoneal cavity (Fig. 28.16). Ultrasound examinations of the kidneys and bladder are requested in patients with a history of urinary tract infection, flank pain, hematuria, and an increase in creatinine levels. The normal adult renal cortex shows a moderate- to low-level echo pattern, *hypoechoic*, to the liver and spleen. The renal sinus is the most echogenic portion of the kidney and is considered *hyperechoic* to the surrounding structures. The kidneys are evaluated for contour, size, cortical thickness, dilation of calyces (hydronephrosis), and echogenicity of the renal parenchyma. Ultrasound guidance is used to localize the kidney during renal biopsy procedures and to evaluate for any postbiopsy complications.

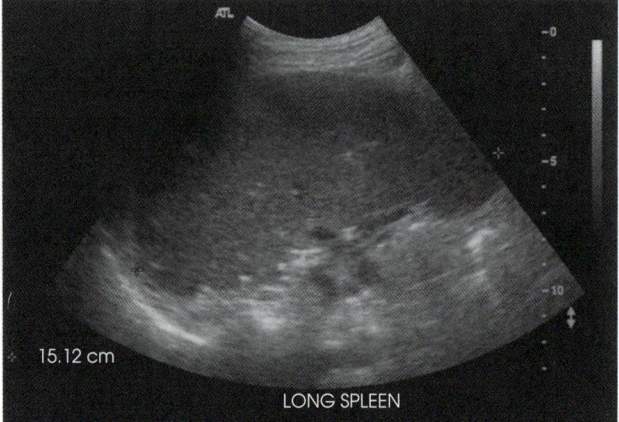

Fig. 28.15 Sagittal sonogram of enlarged spleen measuring greater than 15 cm in length (splenomegaly).

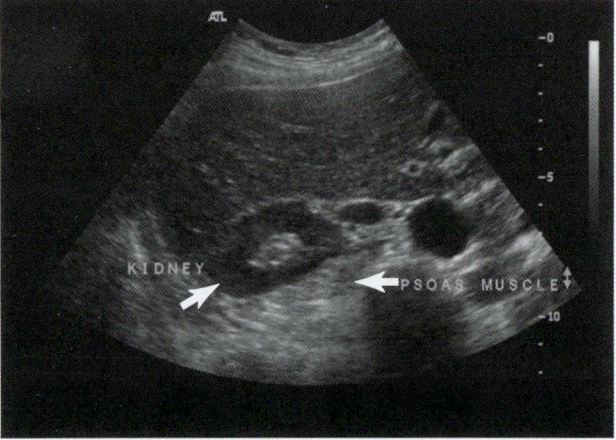

Fig. 28.16 Transverse sonogram of right kidney lying posterior to the liver and lateral to the psoas muscle.

Ultrasound is a useful imaging tool to monitor a renal transplant. The transplant is typically placed superficially in the right iliac fossa. Sonograms of the transplant include grayscale images to evaluate size, contour, echogenicity, and cortical thickness. The renal artery and vein are evaluated with Doppler, checking for intimal thickening, stenosis, and thrombosis.

A partially distended urinary bladder is evaluated for wall thickness, contour, and evidence of neoplasm. Postvoid imaging is included to evaluate the amount of residual urine and competence of the ureteral valves. Abnormalities of the kidneys and bladder shown on ultrasound include urinary obstruction, nephrolithiasis, abscess formation, cortical thinning, and benign and malignant neoplasms (Fig. 28.17).

MUSCULOSKELETAL STRUCTURES

The musculoskeletal system provides movement of the body parts and organs. Ultrasound examinations of the musculoskeletal structures are requested in patients with a history of trauma, palpable mass, and chronic pain. On ultrasound, normal muscles show a low to medium shade of gray echo pattern with hyperechoic striations throughout. Tendons appear homogeneous with hyperechoic linear bands. Some abnormalities of the musculoskeletal system shown on ultrasound include muscle or tendon tears, inflammation, hematoma, and edema (Fig. 28.18).

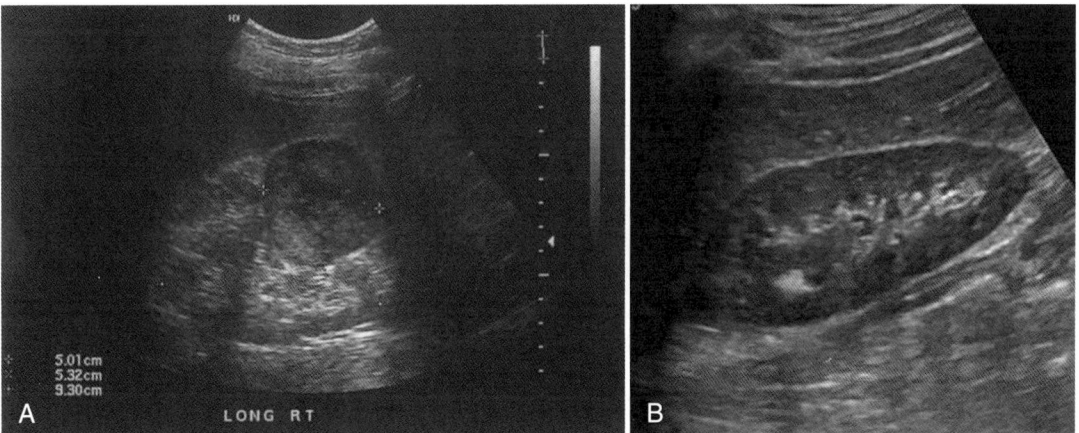

Fig. 28.17 (A) Sagittal sonogram shows hypoechoic mass in anterior right kidney. (B) Sagittal sonogram of right kidney shows hyperechoic kidney stone.

(Courtesy Susanna Ovel, RT, RDMS, RVT.)

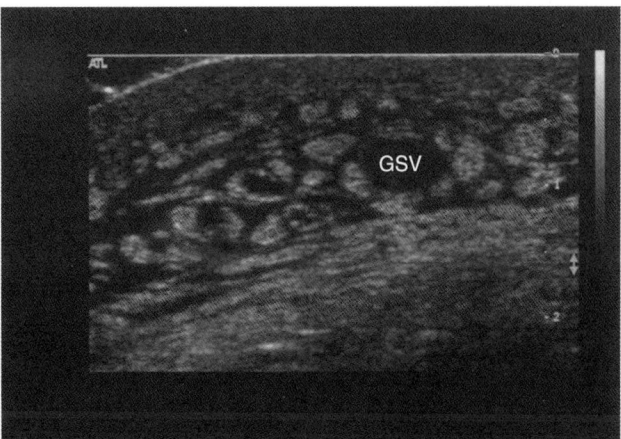

Fig. 28.18 Transverse sonogram of medial thigh shows tissue edema surrounding great saphenous vein (GSV).

SUPERFICIAL STRUCTURES

Superficial structures image well with ultrasound and include soft tissues, thyroid glands, breast, scrotum, penile, and the abdominal wall. The echogenicity of the thyroid glands and testes is similar, showing a moderately echogenic parenchymal pattern. Breast tissue varies depending on the amount of fat content. In sonography, all breast tissues are compared with the medium-level echo pattern of normal breast fat. Abdominal wall ultrasound examinations may be requested to rule out evidence of herniation or hematoma. Soft tissue ultrasound examinations are generally requested to evaluate a specific mass. Abnormalities of the superficial structures shown on ultrasound include inflammation, herniation, hematomas, vascular abnormalities, and benign and malignant neoplasms (Figs. 28.19 and 28.20).

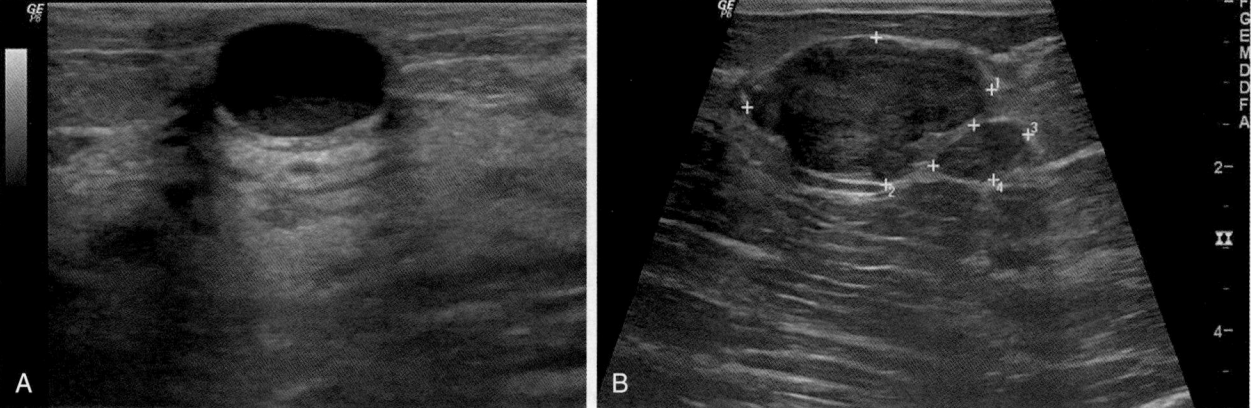

Fig. 28.19 (**A**) Breast cyst with debris is shown demonstrating well-defined borders, fluid-fluid level, and increased through transmission. (**B**) Fibroadenomas *(calipers)* demonstrate well-defined borders and may have some increased transmission; however, the internal echo pattern is solid and homogeneous. Benign lesions typically demonstrate a mass wider rather than tall.

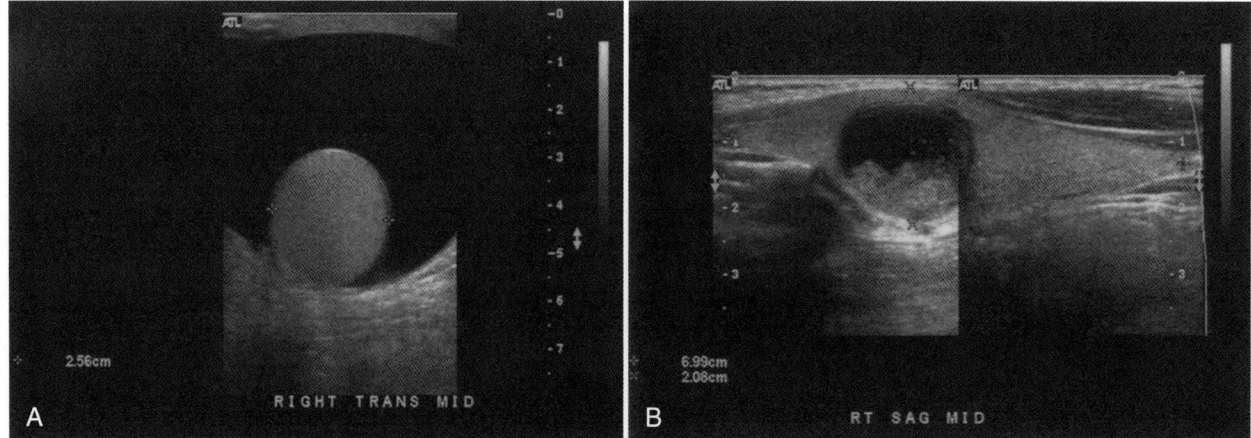

Fig. 28.20 (**A**) Transverse sonogram of right testis surrounded by anechoic fluid (hydrocele). (**B**) Sagittal image of complex thyroid mass.

(Courtesy Paul Aks, BS, RDMS, RVT.)

PEDIATRIC SONOGRAPHY

The goal of pediatric imaging is to perform a study with the lowest amount of radiation and the least amount of sedation. Ultrasound is becoming one of the most widely used imaging modalities, and it is frequently the initial imaging modality in infants and children. A specialty examination to include all general pediatric examinations was implemented in 2015 to replace the existing neonatal neurosonography specialty.

Normal sonographic appearance of anatomy in infants and children can differ from that of the adult patient. This new specialty examination covers the abdomen, pelvis, and small parts, along with pediatric-specific examinations. Examples of pediatric-specific examinations include the gastrointestinal tract for pyloric stenosis and intussusception (Fig. 28.21), infant spine for tethered cord, infant hips for developmental dysplasia of the hip (Fig. 28.22), and neonatal brain for hydrocephalus and intraventricular hemorrhage (Fig. 28.23).

Infants and children pose a challenge to the sonographer. A detailed understanding of the normal and abnormal sonographic appearances of pediatric anatomy is necessary to accurately assess and quickly image the pediatric patient.

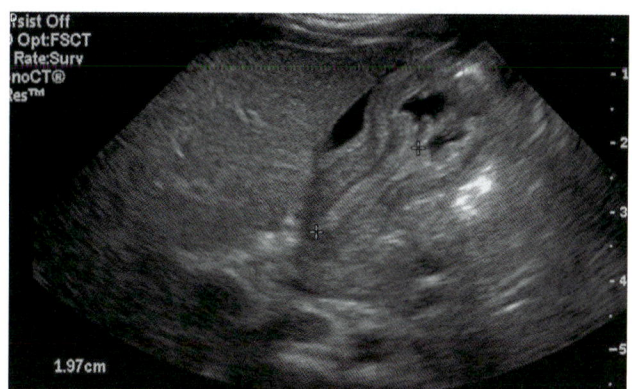

Fig. 28.21 Sagittal image of the pylorus in a case of pyloric stenosis.

(Courtesy Susanna Ovel, RT, RDMS, RVT.)

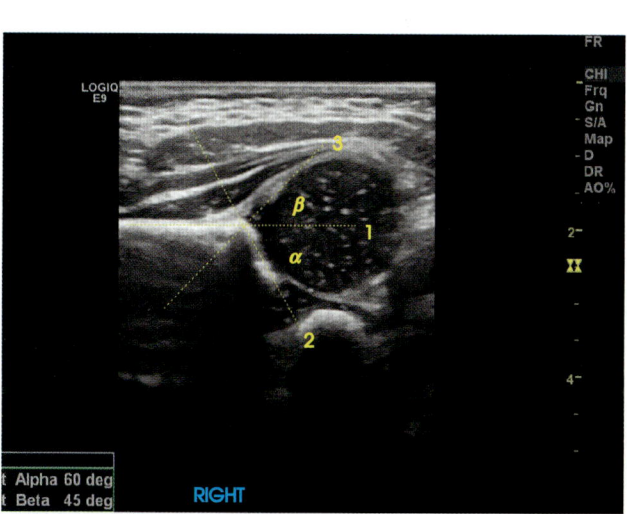

Fig. 28.22 Coronal image demonstrating the Graf angles in a normal infant hip.

(Courtesy Susanna Ovel, RT, RDMS, RVT.)

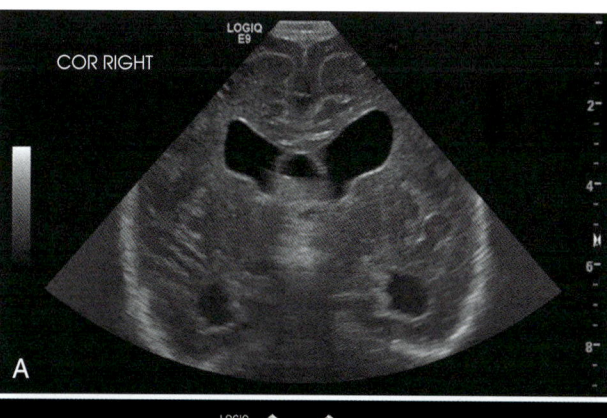

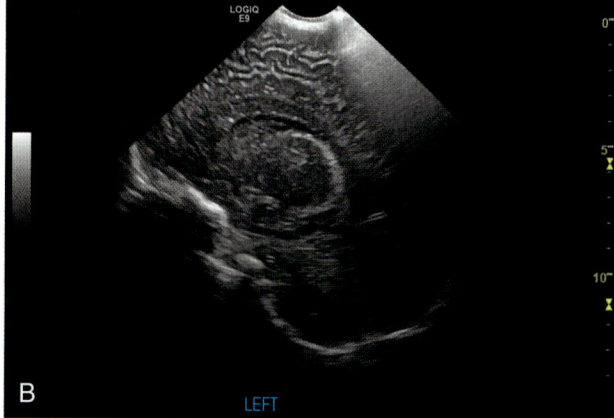

Fig. 28.23 **(A)** Coronal sonogram in a neonate showing bilateral ventriculomegaly of frontal horns. **(B)** Normal sagittal sonogram of left lateral ventricle.

(Courtesy Susanna Ovel, RT, RDMS, RVT.)

GYNECOLOGIC APPLICATIONS
Anatomic features of the pelvis

The pelvis is divided into the true and false pelvis by the *iliopectineal line*. The *false pelvis* contains loops of bowel and is bound by the abdominal wall, the ala of the iliac bones, and the base of the sacrum. The *true pelvis* contains the female reproductive organs, urinary bladder, distal ureters, and bowel (Fig. 28.24). It is bound by the symphysis pubis, sacrum, and coccyx. The pelvic floor is formed by ligaments and the levator ani, piriformis, and coccygeus muscles.

The *retrouterine pouch or pouch of Douglas* lies between the uterus and the rectum. Free fluid routinely accumulates in this area. All pelvic recesses should be imaged on all transabdominal and endovaginal sonograms.

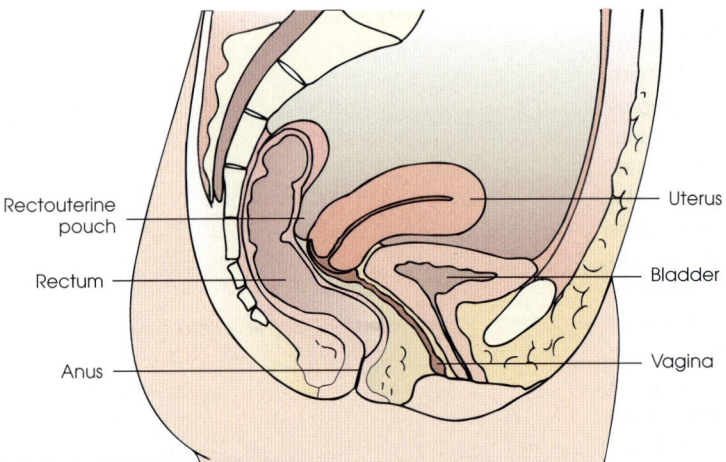

Fig. 28.24 Sagittal line drawing of female pelvis.

Sonography of the female pelvis

Sonography of the female pelvis is clinically useful in the premenarche, menarche, and postmenopausal periods. Pelvic ultrasound examinations are requested for assessment of a pelvic mass, pelvic pain, or abnormal uterine bleeding; infertility monitoring; and localization of an intrauterine device.

A complete transabdominal examination of the female pelvis includes evaluation and documentation of the distended urinary bladder, uterus, cervix, endometrial canal, vagina, ovaries, adnexal regions, pelvic recesses, and supporting pelvic musculature. The full bladder helps to reposition the intestines laterally into the false pelvis. The urinary bladder also serves as an *acoustic window* and anechoic landmark in transabdominal imaging. Transabdominal allows the sonographer to evaluate the entire pelvic area for pathology and peristalsis of the bowel (Fig. 28.25).

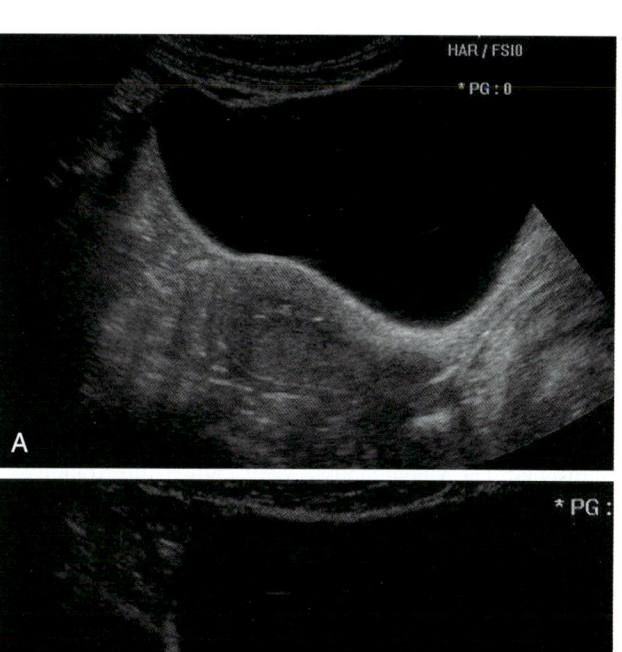
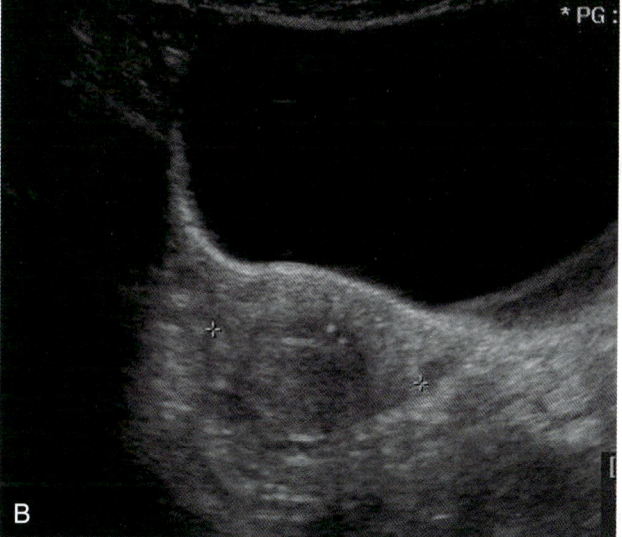

Fig. 28.25 (**A**) Transabdominal sagittal sonogram of uterus. (**B**) Transabdominal transverse sonogram of uterus.

Endovaginal transducers show excellent detail resolution of the uterine endometrium at the expense of penetration depth and acoustic windows (Fig. 28.26). Endovaginal sonography should be used in conjunction with a transabdominal pelvic examination. A high-frequency transducer is inserted into the vaginal canal to evaluate the uterus, endometrium, ovaries, adnexal regions, and pelvic recesses in the sagittal and coronal planes (Fig. 28.27).

The normal adult uterine myometrium appears homogeneous and moderately echogenic on ultrasound. The echogenicity and thickness of the normal endometrium vary with the menstrual cycle but should not exceed 14 mm in anteroposterior diameter. Normal ovaries appear moderately echogenic, with small functional cysts (follicles) of varying size and number. Monitoring the number and size of *follicular cysts* is a common practice in infertility treatment. Ultrasound is used to aid the gynecologist in determining when the ovum is ready for stimulation with high doses of human chorionic gonadotropin. Some abnormalities of the female pelvis shown on ultrasound include congenital malformation, leiomyoma, endometrial polyp, ovarian cyst, and tubal ovarian abscess (Fig. 28.28).

OBSTETRIC APPLICATIONS

Obstetric sonography is probably the most well-known ultrasound examination. An obstetric sonogram allows the obstetrician to view and monitor the developing *embryo* and *fetus*. Routine screening examinations are requested between 16 and 24 *gestational weeks* to measure *gestational age,* evaluate fetal anatomy, localize placental placement, assess amniotic fluid, and evaluate cervical competence. Evaluation of the fetus is relatively easy because the fetus occupies a fluid-filled *gestational sac,* an excellent acoustic window for ultrasound.

In the first trimester, endovaginal imaging is more likely to image an early gestational sac, yolk sac, amniotic cavity, and embryo (Figs. 28.29 and 28.30). The number of viable embryos is easily diagnosed with a first-trimester sonogram. The gestational sac may be visualized at 4.5 gestational weeks, and embryo cardiac activity can be identified at 5.5 gestational weeks with endovaginal sonography. By the ninth gestational week, the cerebral hemispheres and limb buds are evident. By the 12th gestational week, the fetus has a skeletal body.

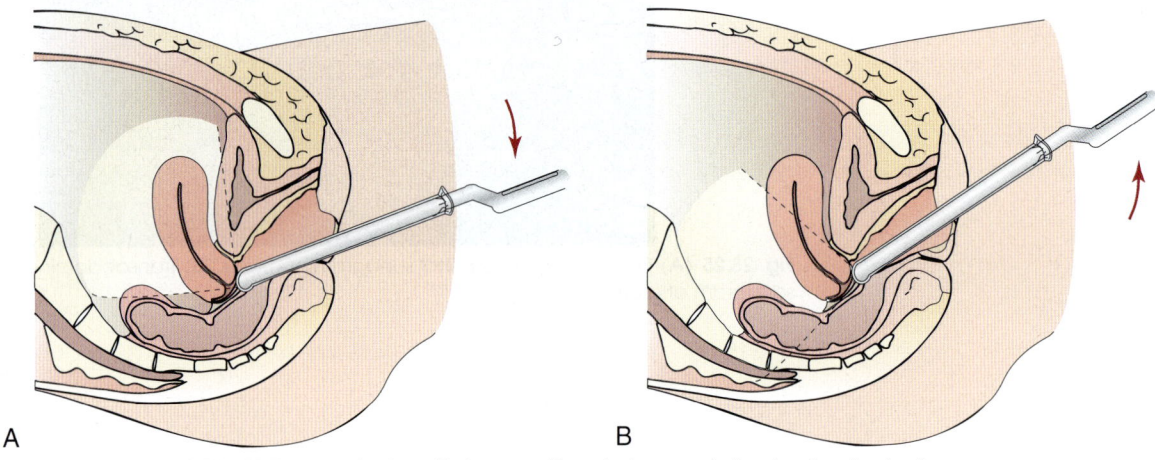

Fig. 28.26 (**A**) Transvaginal sagittal scan with anterior angulation to visualize better the fundus of normal anteflexed uterus. (**B**) Transvaginal sagittal scan with posterior angulation to visualize better cervix and rectouterine recess.

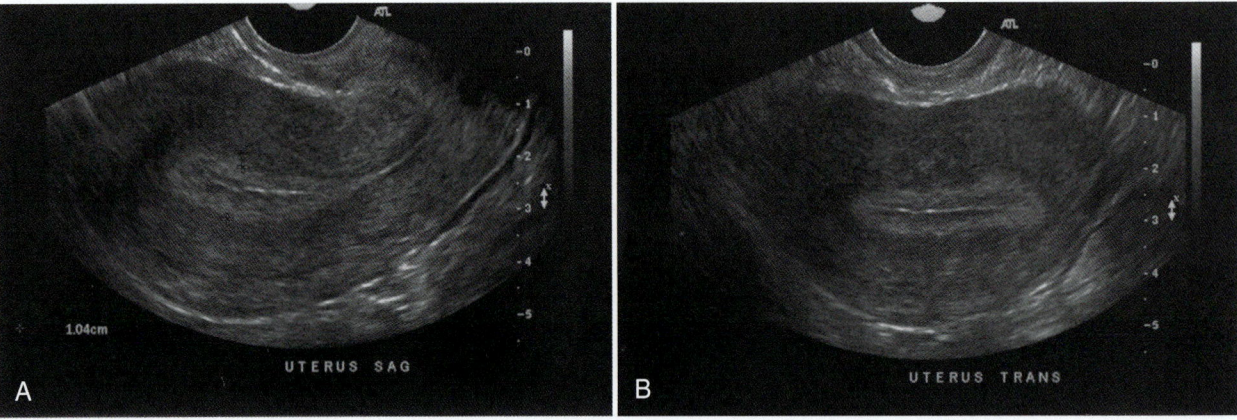

Fig. 28.27 (**A**) Endovaginal sagittal sonogram of uterus. (**B**) Coronal sonogram of uterus.

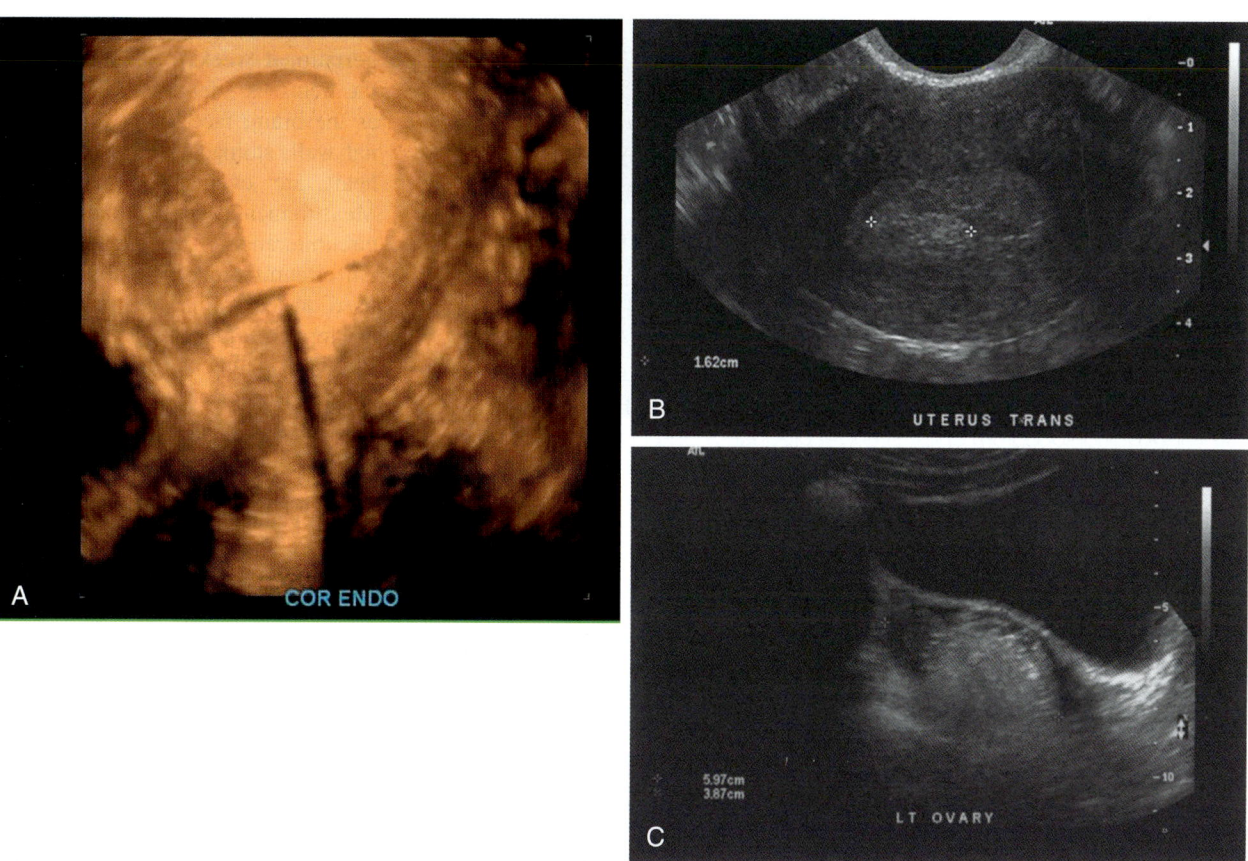

Fig. 28.28 (**A**) Volumetric coronal sonogram of uterine cervix showing improper location of an intrauterine device. (**B**) Coronal image of the endometrium showing a hyperechoic neoplasm *(calipers)*. (**C**) Sagittal image of complex left ovarian mass.

(A and C, Courtesy Paul Aks, BS, RDMS, RVT.)

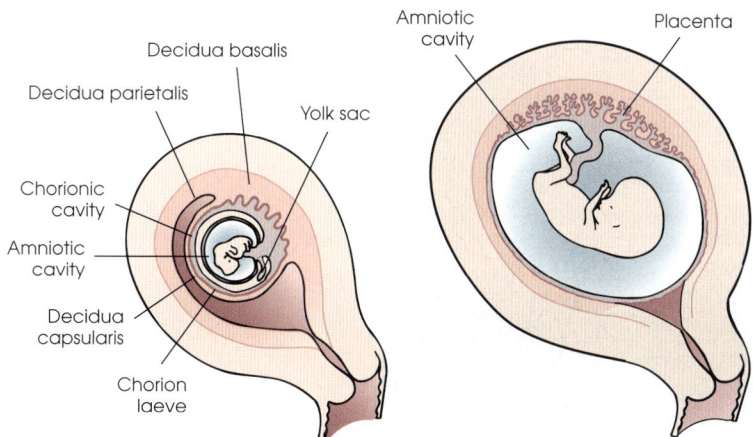

Fig. 28.29 First-trimester representations of developing embryo and yolk sac within amniotic and chorionic cavities of the uterus.

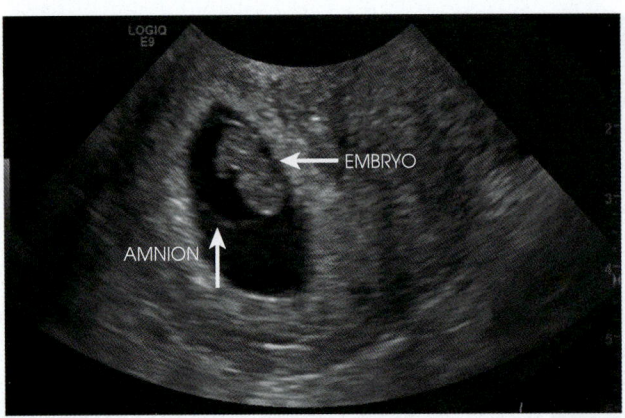

Fig. 28.30 Endovaginal sonogram of first-trimester pregnancy. The embryo and amnion are easily visualized within the fluid-filled gestational sac.

(Courtesy Susanna Ovel, RT, RDMS, RVT.)

During the second trimester (13–28 gestational weeks), detailed anatomy of the fetus is identified. Structures such as the brain, face, limbs, spine, abdominal wall, stomach, kidneys, bladder, and heart are evaluated and documented. Measurements of the biparietal diameter, circumference of the fetal head, abdominal circumference, and femur length are used to determine gestational age and are termed *biometric measurements* (Fig. 28.31). Documentation of the placenta, amniotic fluid, cervical length, and fetal position is also included.

In the third trimester (29–40 gestational weeks), the fetus grows an additional 10 cm (4 inches) in length and gains 2000 to 2800 g in weight (4–6 lb). Third-trimester ultrasound examinations are generally

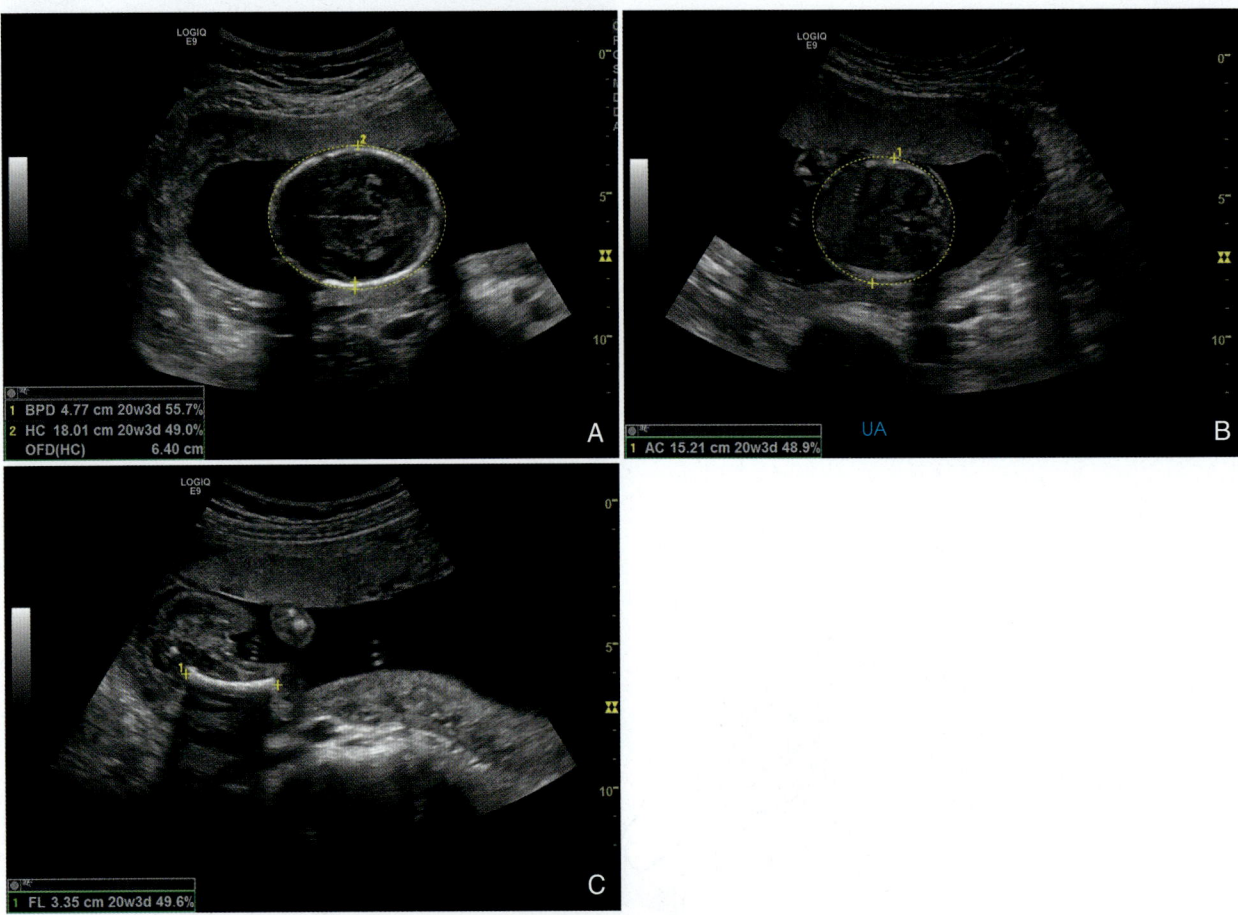

Fig. 28.31 (A) Biparietal diameter *(BPD)* is measured from outer to inner border of the cranium, perpendicular to falx cerebri in a plane that passes through the third ventricle and thalami. Fetal head circumference is measured from outer-to-outer border of the cranium in a plane that must include the cavum septi pellucidi (CSP) and tentorial hiatus. (B) Abdominal circumference is a cross-sectional measurement slightly superior to cord insertion at junction of left and right portal veins. (C) Femur length *(FL)* is measured parallel to femoral shaft at level of femoral head cartilage and distal femoral condyle.

(Courtesy Susanna Ovel, RT, RDMS, RVT.)

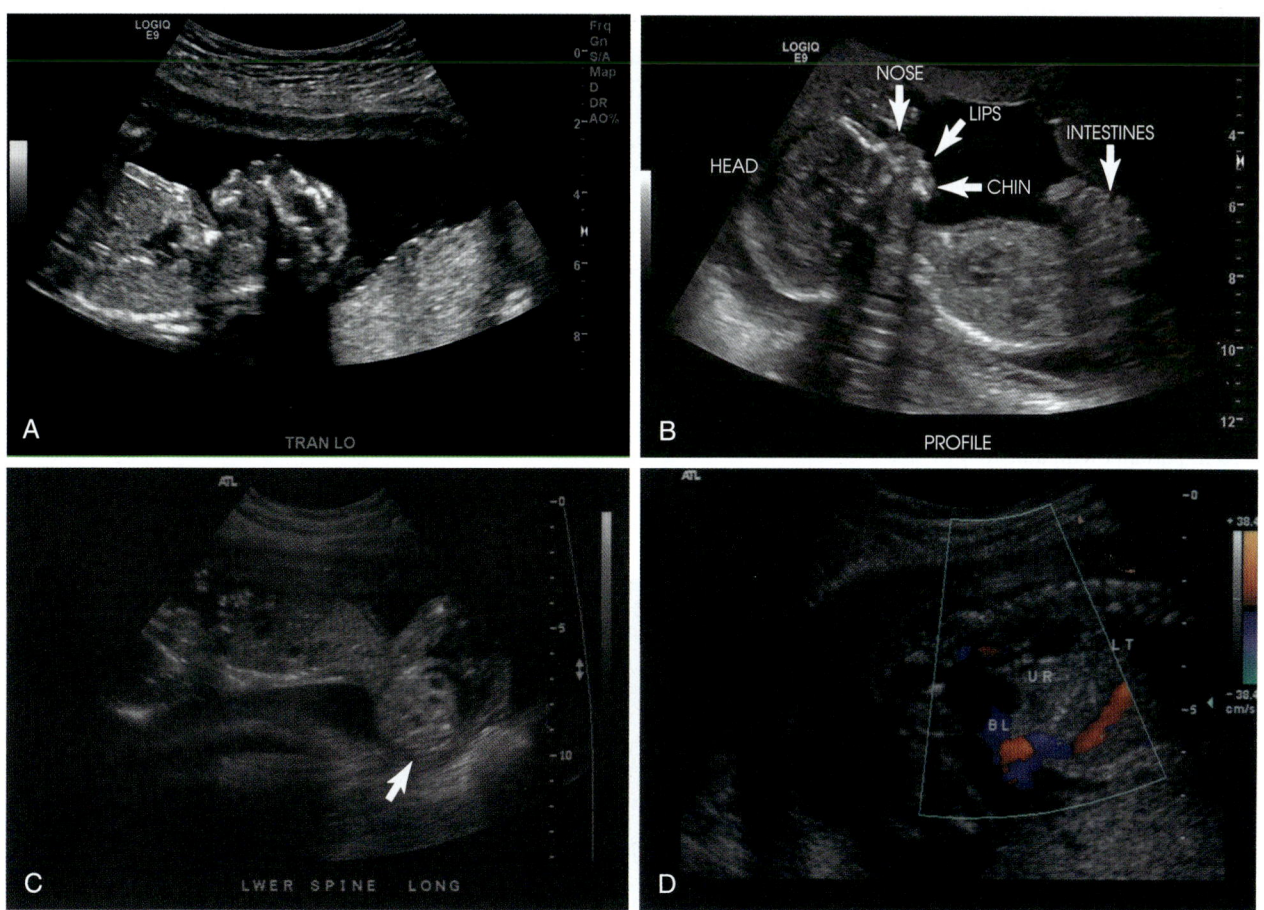

Fig. 28.32 (**A**) Early second-trimester sonogram of the fetal facial profile showing anencephaly. (**B**) Sagittal image of early second-trimester fetus showing gastroschisis. (**C**) Sagittal image of second-trimester fetus showing sacral teratoma *(arrow)*. (**D**) Sagittal image of left kidney showing hydronephrosis.

(A and B, Courtesy Susanna Ovel, RT, RDMS, RVT; C, courtesy B. Alex Stewart, RT, RDMS.)

requested to evaluate fetal growth and position, amniotic fluid volume, and placental placement.

Obstetric sonography is a safe imaging modality for evaluating normal and abnormal development of embryologic and fetal anatomy. A detailed ultrasound examination can assess complications of pregnancy, such as ectopic pregnancy, fetal demise, neural tube defects, nuchal cord, skeletal or limb anomalies, cardiac defects, gastrointestinal and genitourinary defects, and head anomalies (Fig. 28.32). Evaluation of the fetus using three-dimensional and four-dimensional imaging is not presently a routine part of obstetric screening examinations (Fig. 28.33).

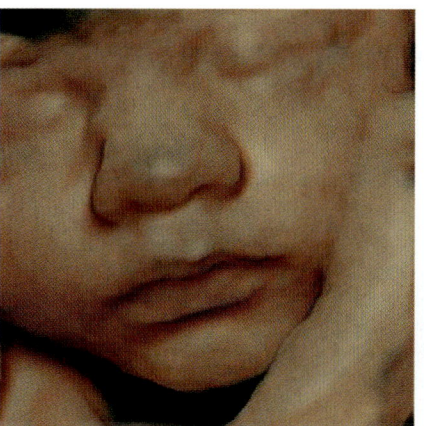

Fig. 28.33 Three-dimensional sonogram of second-trimester fetal face.

(Courtesy Jeanette Burlbaw, BS, RDMS, FSDMS, FAIUM.)

VASCULAR APPLICATIONS

Sonography applications for evaluating the hemodynamics and anatomy of vascular structures continue to increase. Color Doppler imaging and spectral analysis can evaluate blood flow characteristics of the vascular structures in the neck, upper and lower extremities, abdomen, and pelvis. RVTs have specialized education and training in arterial and venous anatomy, hemodynamics, arterial and venous abnormalities, and additional physiologic vascular testing (i.e., pulse volume recording).

Abdominal duplex examinations are requested in patients with a history or suspicion of portal hypertension, mesenteric ischemia, renal artery stenosis, and portal vein thrombosis. Spectral analysis of blood flow velocity and direction is evaluated and documented. Specific criteria are used to diagnose the degree of arterial narrowing shown on the spectral analysis.

The extracranial carotid arteries are evaluated using duplex sonography (Fig. 28.34). Arterial patency, blood flow velocity, resistance, direction, and evidence of turbulence are evaluated with color Doppler and spectral analysis. The highest flow velocities in the common carotid, internal carotid, external carotid, vertebral, and subclavian arteries are recorded. The velocity difference between the common and internal carotid arteries is used to diagnose the degree or percentage of stenosis (i.e., 50%) (Fig. 28.35).

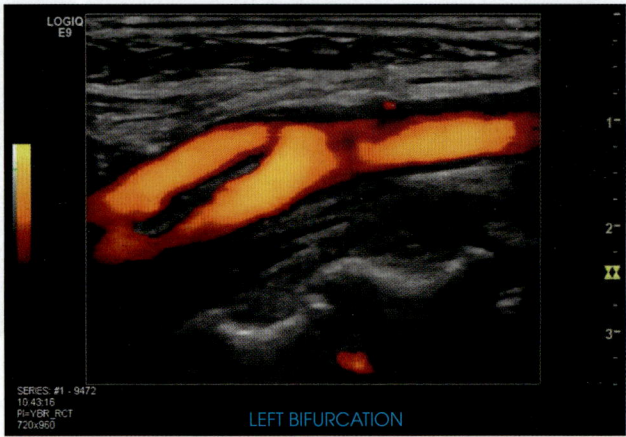

Fig. 28.34 Sagittal sonogram of carotid artery and bifurcation into internal and external carotid arteries.

(Courtesy Susanna Ovel, RT, RDMS, RVT.)

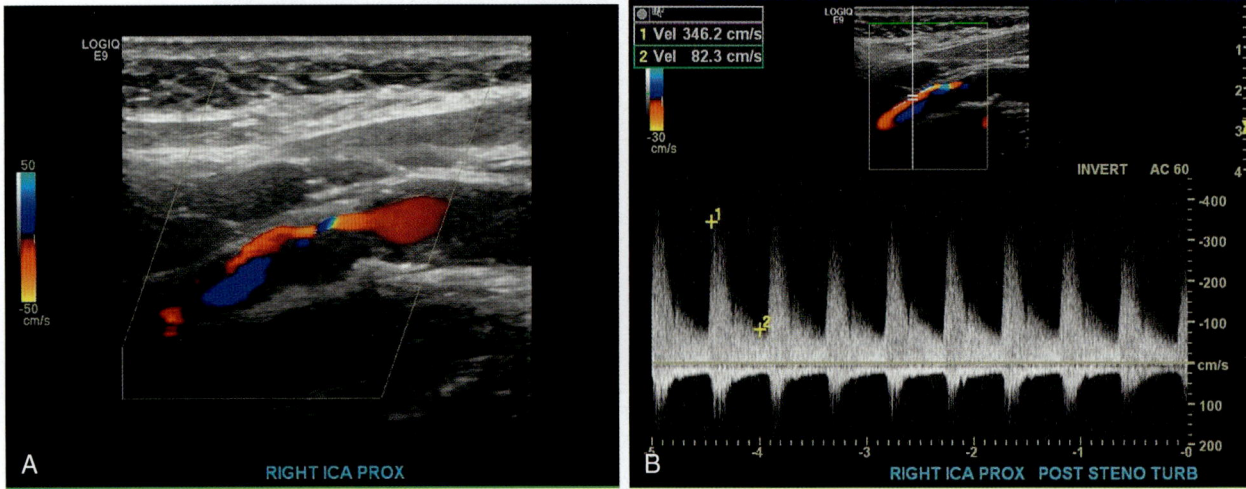

Fig. 28.35 (A) Sagittal image of carotid artery with high-grade stenosis in proximal internal carotid artery. (B) Color Doppler and spectral analysis show increases in flow velocity in stenotic internal carotid artery.

Duplex sonograms of the lower extremity arterial arteries are requested in patients with symptoms of claudication, rest pain, a decrease in palpable pedal pulse, and bypass graft surveillance. Patients with a clinical history of hypertension, cigarette smoking, and diabetes mellitus have an increased risk of developing peripheral arterial disease. Duplex examination of the lower extremities begins at the distal aorta. The common and external iliac arteries are examined for any inflow abnormalities. The common femoral, deep femoral, popliteal, anterior tibial, posterior tibial, and peroneal arteries are evaluated in grayscale with color Doppler and spectral analysis for patency, plaque formation, increases in flow velocity, and, when applicable, degree of stenosis. Upper extremity arterial duplex examinations are requested in patients with arm or hand pain, asymmetric blood pressures, and changes in skin pallor. Using duplex sonography, the subclavian, axillary, brachial, ulnar, and radial arteries are evaluated for patency, plaque formation, increase in flow velocities, and, when applicable, degree of stenosis.

Duplex sonographic examination of the lower extremity veins is an inexpensive imaging modality to evaluate for deep vein thrombosis and venous insufficiency. Acute or chronic leg pain, edema, changes in skin pigmentation, and varicose veins are indications for a lower extremity venous duplex sonogram.

When evaluating for deep vein thrombosis, the deep system is evaluated for patency and phasic flow. Incompetence of the venous valve is the most common cause of varicose vein development. When evaluating for venous insufficiency, the deep venous system is evaluated for patency and valve competency. The small and great saphenous veins are measured and evaluated for patency, valve competency, and association with varicosities. Visible perforator veins are also evaluated for patency and valve competency. The sonographer provides a technical report to the reading physician detailing the findings regarding evidence of lower extremity deep vein thrombosis, venous insufficiency, and possible source of varicosities (Fig. 28.36). Upper extremity venous examinations are requested in patients with indwelling catheters, arm or hand swelling, and arm pain. The internal jugular, subclavian, axillary, brachial, cephalic, and basilic veins are evaluated for patency and *phasic flow*.

Additional physiologic testing is used to evaluate peripheral arterial and venous flow. The ankle/brachial index (ABI), venous return time, and pulse volume recording are examples of nonimaging vascular testing.

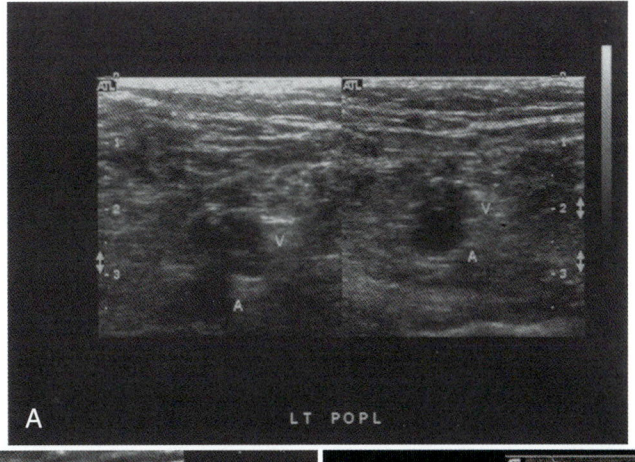

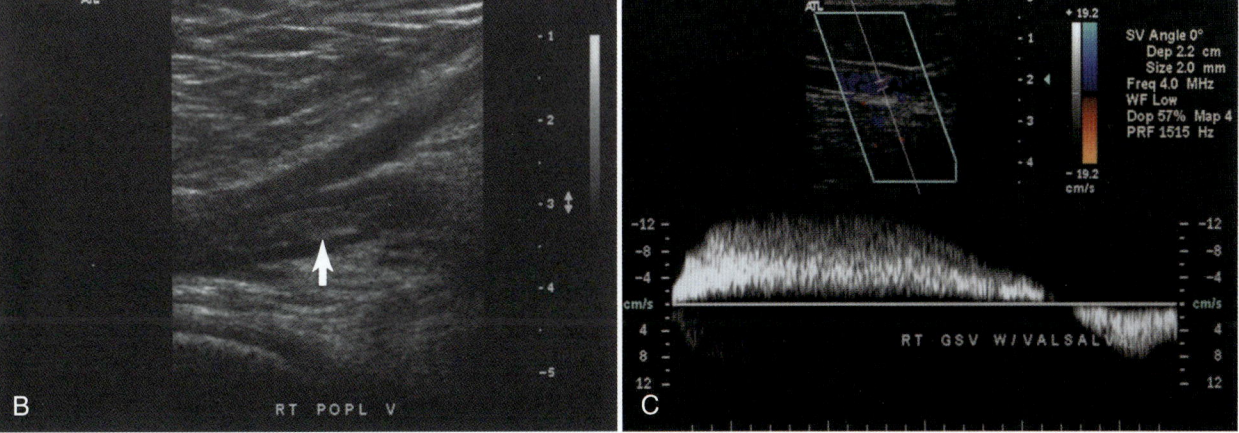

Fig. 28.36 (**A**) Transverse sonograms of popliteal artery and vein without compression *(left image)* and with compression *(right image)* showing a deep vein thrombosis. (**B**) Sagittal sonogram of popliteal vein showing echogenic thrombus *(arrow)*. (**C**) Spectral analysis of great saphenous vein shows venous reflux during Valsalva maneuver signifying venous incompetence at this level.

Cardiologic Applications

Real-time echocardiography of the fetal, neonatal, pediatric, and adult heart has proven to be a tremendous diagnostic aid for the cardiologist and internist. Multiple imaging windows are used to image cardiac anatomy in detail, including the four chambers of the heart, four heart valves (mitral, tricuspid, aortic, and pulmonic), interventricular and interatrial septa, muscular wall of the ventricles, papillary muscles, and chordae tendineae cordis. Difficult cases can be imaged using a transesophageal technique in which the transducer is passed from the mouth, through the esophagus, and then to the orifice of the stomach.

PROCEDURE FOR ECHOCARDIOGRAPHY

The echocardiographic examination begins with the patient in a left lateral decubitus position. This position allows the heart to move away from the sternum and fall closer to the chest wall, providing a better cardiac "window," or open area, for the sonographer to image. The transducer is placed in the third, fourth, or fifth intercostal space to the left of the sternum. The protocol for a complete echocardiographic examination includes images in the long axis, short axis, apical, and suprasternal windows (Fig. 28.37). Contrast agents improve visualization of viable myocardial tissue.

CARDIAC PATHOLOGY

Echocardiography is used to evaluate many cardiac conditions. Atherosclerosis or previous rheumatic fever may lead to scarring, calcification, and thickening of the valve leaflets. With these conditions, valve tissue destruction continues, causing stenosis and regurgitation of the leaflets and subsequent chamber enlargement.

The effects of subacute bacterial endocarditis can also be evaluated with echocardiography. With this infectious process, multiple small vegetations form on the endocardial surface of the valve leaflets, causing the leaflets to tear or thicken, with resultant severe regurgitation into subsequent cardiac chambers. The echocardiogram of a patient with congestive cardiomyopathy shows generalized four-chamber enlargement, valve regurgitation, and the threat of thrombus formation along the nonfunctioning ventricular wall. The pericardial sac surrounds the ventricles and right atrium, and may fill with fluid, impairing normal cardiac function.

Analysis of ventricular function and serial evaluation of patients after a myocardial infarction are accomplished with two-dimensional echocardiography and, in some cases, stress dobutamine echocardiography. Complications of myocardial infarction include rupture of the ventricular septum, development of a left ventricular aneurysm in the weakest area of the wall, and coagulation of thrombus in the akinetic or immobile apex of the left ventricle (Fig. 28.38).

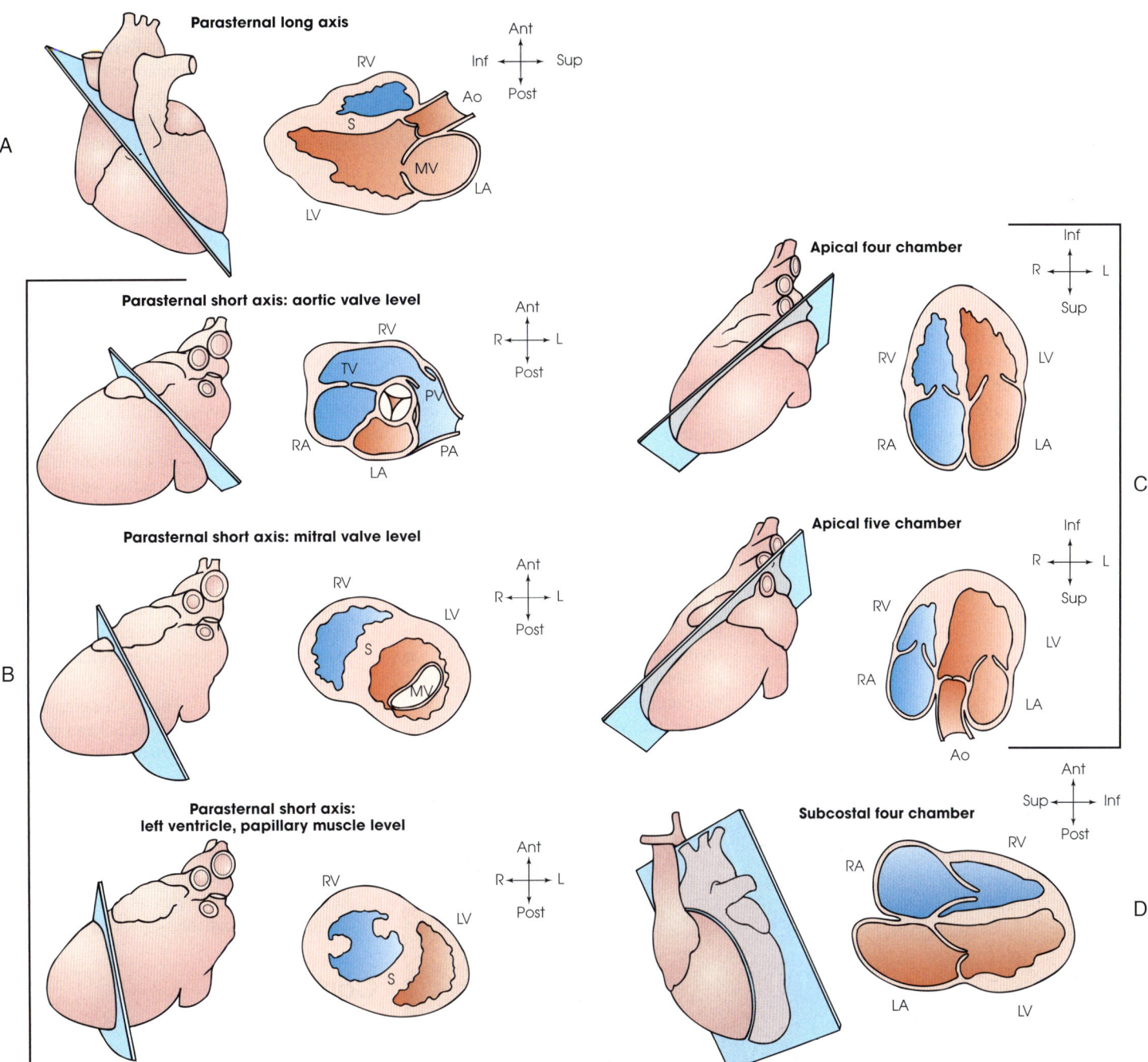

Fig. 28.37 (**A**) Parasternal long-axis drawing. (**B**) Parasternal short-axis drawings at various levels: aortic valve level; mitral valve level; and left ventricle, papillary muscle level. (**C**) Apical four-chamber image and apical five-chamber image. (**D**) Subcostal four-chamber image. *Ao,* Aorta; *LA,* left atrium; *LV,* left ventricle; *MV,* mitral valve; *PA,* pulmonary artery; *PV,* pulmonic valve; *RA,* right atrium; *RV,* right ventricle; *S,* septum; *TV,* tricuspid valve.

Congenital heart lesions

Echocardiography has been used to diagnose congenital lesions of the heart in fetuses, neonates, and young children. The cardiac sonographer is able to assess abnormalities of the four cardiac valves, determine the size of the cardiac chambers, assess the interatrial and interventricular septum for the presence of shunt flow, and identify the continuity of the aorta and pulmonary artery with the ventricular chambers to look for abnormal attachment relationships.

A premature infant has an improved chance of survival if the correct diagnosis is made early. If the neonate is cyanotic, congenital heart disease or respiratory failure may be rapidly diagnosed with echocardiography. Critical cyanotic disease in a premature infant may include hypoplastic left heart syndrome, transposition of the great vessels with pulmonary atresia, or severe tetralogy of Fallot.

Best Practices In General Sonography

The following best practices are guidelines for performing sonographic examinations. Ultrasound uses high-frequency sound waves instead of potentially harmful radiation. Real-time imaging and cine loop technology make it easier to accommodate patient movement. Cine loop technology saves the last several seconds of real-time imaging. The sonographer can scroll back and document the best image.

1. *Interaction with the patient:* When interacting with the patient, the sonographer's vocabulary, body language, and tone of voice should reflect a calming environment. Fear is the most likely cause of uncooperative behavior. Decreasing or eliminating the patient's unease is essential for sonography, especially in the pediatric patient.
2. *Speed:* Due to the possible short attention span of younger pediatric patients and pain or discomfort in the adult patient, the sonographer should document imaging protocols as quickly as possible. Most protocols require specific measurements, which should be made and recorded after completion of the exam.
3. *Accuracy:* Knowledge in normal anatomy, congenital anomalies, pathologies, and normal appearance of adult and pediatric anatomy is essential. Understanding sonography physics and instrumentation is crucial. Continuing education is essential to retain imaging accuracy.
4. *Positioning:* Maintaining a specific or steady position is not as crucial in sonographic imaging. Ingenuity is handy for adult and pediatric positioning. Understanding patient limitations and fears is crucial in achieving the best diagnostic images. Having a parent hug their child when scanning the kidneys may give the child a sense of security.
5. *Practice standard precautions:* The sonographer should practice standard precautions before, during, and after every ultrasound examination. Examination tables, pillow(s), the ultrasound machine, and transducers should be disinfected after every patient. Proper personal protective equipment (PPE) should be used with every examination.
6. *Professionalism:* The sonographer needs to possess ethical conduct and professionalism with all patients. Interacting with the pediatric patient is unique. Not only is the sonographer interacting with the patient, but they are also interacting with the patient's parents. The perception of the sonographer's professionalism by family members is relevant when interacting with all patients.

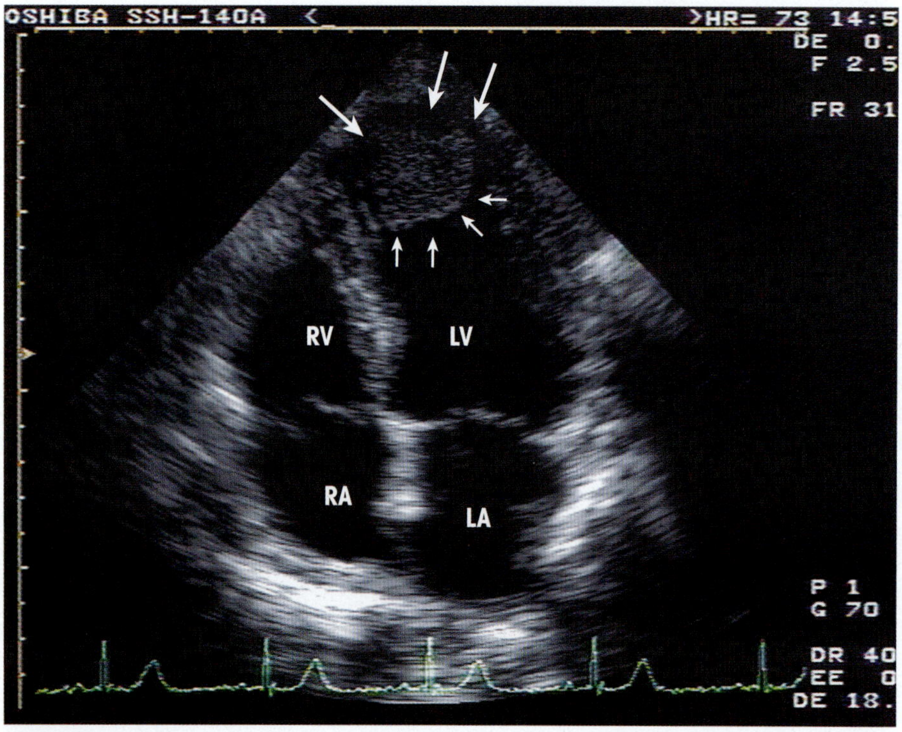

Conclusion

The contribution of diagnostic ultrasound to clinical medicine has been assisted by technologic advances in instrumentation and transducer design, an increased ability to process the returned echo information, and an improved methodology for three-dimensional reconstruction of images. The development of high-frequency *endovaginal*, *endorectal*, and *transesophageal transducers* with endoscopic imaging has aided the visualization of previously difficult areas. Improved computer capabilities and advances in teleradiography have enabled the sonographer to obtain more information and process multiple data points to obtain a comprehensive report from the ultrasound study. Color-flow Doppler has made it possible for the sonographer to distinguish the direction

Fig. 28.38 Apical four-chamber image with large apical thrombus. This thrombus (*arrows*), which is distinguished from an artifact because of its location in a region with abnormal wall motion, is attached to the apical endocardium, has well-defined borders, and moves in the same direction as the apex. *LA,* Left atrium; *LV,* left ventricle; *RA,* right atrium; *RV,* right ventricle.

and velocity of arterial and venous blood flow from vascular and other pathologic structures in the body. Doppler has allowed the sonographer to determine the exact area of obstruction or leakage present, and to precisely determine the degree of turbulence within a vessel or cardiac chamber.

Modifications in transducer design have improved resolution in superficial structures, muscles, and tendons. Advancements in equipment and transducer design have also improved the results of ultrasound examinations in neonates and children. Increased sensitivity allows the sonographer to define the texture of organs and glands with more detail and greater tissue differentiation. Improvements in resolution have aided the visualization of small cleft palate defects, abnormal development of fingers and toes, and small spinal defects. The ability to image the detail of the fetal heart has assisted in the early diagnosis of congenital heart defects.

Advanced research and development of computer analysis and tissue characterization of echo reflections should contribute further to the total diagnostic approach using ultrasound. Various abdominal contrast agents continue to be investigated to improve visualization of the stomach, the pancreas, and the small and large intestines. Cardiac contrast agents are already being used to improve the visualization of viable myocardial tissue within the heart. Saline and other contrast agents are being injected into the endometrial cavity to outline the lining of the endometrium for the purpose of distinguishing polyps and other lesions from the normal endometrium.

Ultrasound has rapidly emerged as a powerful, inexpensive, diagnostic imaging modality with various applications in patient management and care. Expected advancements include further developments in transducer design, image resolution, tissue characterization applications, color-flow sensitivity, and four-dimensional reconstruction of images.

Definition of Terms

acoustic window: Ability of sonography to visualize a particular area. The full urinary bladder is a good acoustic window to image the uterus and ovaries in a transabdominal sonogram. The intercostal margins may be a good acoustic window to image the liver parenchyma.

anechoic: Property of being free of echoes or without echoes.

ankle/brachial index (ABI): Ratio of ankle pressure to brachial pressure to provide a general guide to help determine the degree of disability of the lower extremity.

attenuation: Weakening of the sound wave as it propagates through a medium.

axial resolution: Ability to distinguish two structures along a path parallel to the sound beam.

biometric measurements: Fetal measurements to include biparietal diameter, head circumference, abdominal circumference, and femur length to assess fetal age and growth.

biparietal diameter (BPD): Largest dimension of the fetal head perpendicular to the midsagittal plane; measured by ultrasonic visualization and used to measure fetal development.

color-flow Doppler: Velocity in each direction is quantified by allocating a pixel to each area; each velocity frequency change is allocated a color.

complex: Containing anechoic and echogenic areas.

continuous wave ultrasound: Wave in which cycles repeat indefinitely; consists of a separate transmit and receive transducer housed within one assembly.

coronal image plane: Anatomic term used to describe a plane perpendicular to the sagittal and transverse planes of the body.

detail resolution: Includes axial and lateral resolution.

Doppler effect: Shift in frequency or wavelength, depending on the conditions of observation; caused by relative motions among sources, receivers, and medium.

Doppler ultrasound: Application of Doppler effect to ultrasound to detect movement of a reflecting boundary relative to the source, resulting in a change of the wavelength of the reflected wave.

duplex imaging: Combination of grayscale real-time imaging and color or spectral Doppler.

echogenic: Refers to a medium that contains echo-producing structures.

embryo: Term used for a developing zygote through the 10th week of gestation.

endometrium: Inner layer of the uterine canal.

endorectal transducer: High-frequency transducer that can be inserted into the rectum to visualize the bladder and prostate gland.

endovaginal transducer: High-frequency transducer (and decreased penetration) that can be inserted into the vagina to obtain high-resolution images of the pelvic structures.

false pelvis: Region above the pelvic brim.

fetus: Term used for the developing embryo from the 11th gestational week until birth.

follicular cyst: Functional or physiologic ovulatory cyst consisting of an ovum surrounded by a layer of cells.

frequency: Number of cycles per unit of time, usually expressed in hertz (Hz) or megahertz (MHz) (a million cycles per second).

gestational sac: Fluid-filled structure normally found in the uterus containing the pregnancy.

gestational weeks: Length of time calculated from the first day of the last menstrual period; also known as gestational age.

grayscale: Range of amplitudes (brightness) between white and black.

heterogeneous: Having a mixed composition.

homogeneous: Having a uniform composition.

hyperechoic: Increase in echogenicity when compared to another structure or normal expected echo pattern.

hypoechoic: Decrease in echogenicity when compared to another structure or normal expected echo pattern.

iliopectineal line: Bony ridge on the inner surface of the ileum and pubic bones that divides the true and false pelvis.

isoechoic: Having a texture nearly the same as that of the surrounding parenchyma.

lateral resolution: Ability to distinguish two structures lying perpendicular to the sound beam.

noninvasive technique: Procedure that does not require the skin to be broken or an organ or cavity to be entered (e.g., taking the pulse).

oblique plane: Slanting direction or any variation that is not starting at a right angle to any axis.

parenchyma: Functional tissue or cells of an organ or gland.

phasic flow: Normal venous respiratory variations.

piezoelectric effect: Conversion of pressure to electrical voltage or conversion of electrical voltage to mechanical pressure.

porta hepatis: Region in hepatic hilum containing common duct, proper hepatic artery, and main portal vein.

posterior acoustic enhancement: Increase in reflection amplitude from structures that lie behind a weakly attenuating structure (i.e., cyst).

posterior acoustic shadowing: Reduction in reflection amplitude from reflectors lying behind a strongly reflecting or attenuating structure.

pulse wave ultrasound: A transducer emits short pulses of ultrasound into the human body and receives reflections from the body before emitting another pulse of sound.

real-time imaging: Teleradiograph with rapid frame rate visualizing moving structures or scan planes continuously.

reflection: Redirection (return) of a portion of the sound beam back to the transducer.

refraction: Phenomenon of bending wave fronts as the acoustic energy propagates from the medium of one acoustic velocity to a second medium of differing acoustic velocity.

resolution: Measure of ability to display two closely spaced structures as discrete targets.

retrouterine pouch: Pelvic space located anterior to the rectum and posterior to the uterus; also known as pouch of Douglas.

sagittal: Plane that travels vertically from the top to the bottom of the body along the *y*-axis.

scattering: Diffusion or redirection of sound in several directions on encountering a particle suspension or rough surface.

sound wave: Longitudinal waves of mechanical energy propagated through a medium.

transducer: Device that converts energy from one form to another.

transverse: Plane that passes through the width of the body in a horizontal direction.

true pelvis: Region of the pelvis found below the pelvic brim.

ultrasound: Sound with a frequency greater than 20 kHz.

velocity of sound: Speed with direction of motion specified.

Selected bibliography

Curry RA, Prince M. *Sonography: Introduction to Normal Structure and Function*. 5th ed. Philadelphia: Elsevier; 2021.

Hagen-Ansert SL. *Textbook of Diagnostic Ultrasonography* (Vols I and II). 9th ed. St Louis: Elsevier; 2022.

Kremkau FW. *Diagnostic Ultrasound Principles and Instrumentation*. 10th ed. St Louis: Elsevier; 2021.

Norton ME, Scoutt LM, Feldstein VA. *Callen's Ultrasonography in Obstetrics and Gynecology*. 6th ed. Philadelphia: Elsevier; 2017.

Ovel S. *Sonography Exam Review: Physics, Abdomen, Obstetrics and Gynecology*. 3rd ed. St Louis: Elsevier; 2019.

Pellerito JS, Polak JE. *Introduction to Vascular Ultrasonography*. 7th ed. St Louis: Elsevier; 2020.

Rumack CM, Levine D. *Diagnostic Ultrasound*. 5th ed. St Louis: Elsevier; 2018.

29
NUCLEAR MEDICINE AND MOLECULAR IMAGING
RAYMOND J. JOHNSON

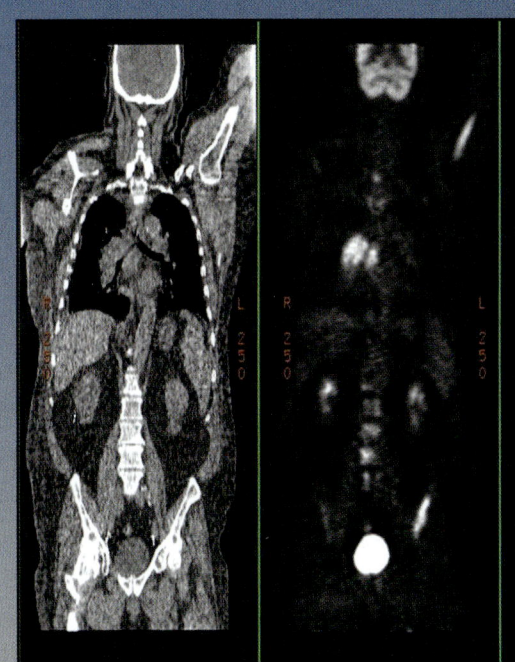

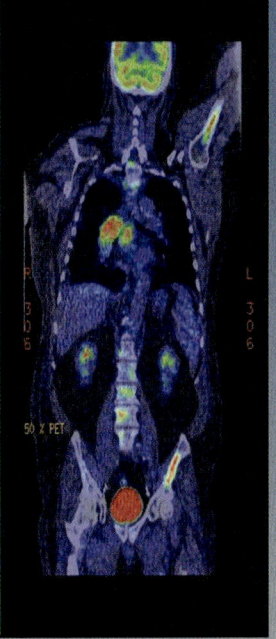

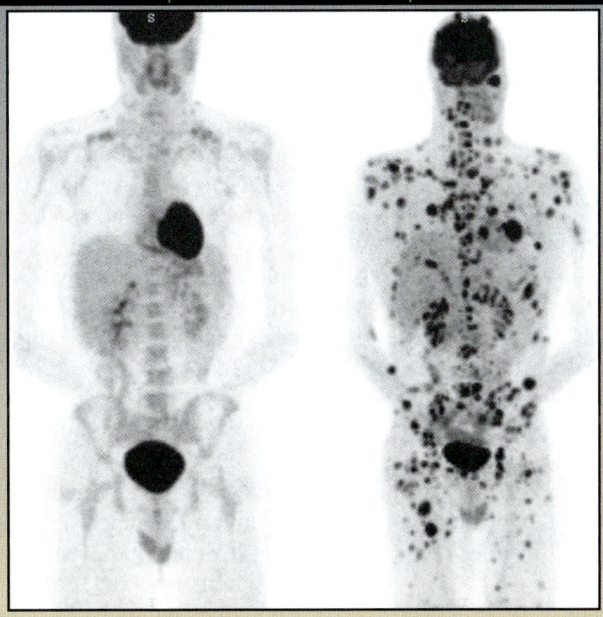

OUTLINE

Principles of Nuclear Medicine, 436
Historical Development, 436
Positron Emission Tomography, 436
Comparison With
  Other Modalities, 437
Physical Principles of Nuclear
  Medicine, 439
Radiopharmaceutical Dosing, 443
Radiation Safety in Nuclear
  Medicine, 444
Instrumentation in Nuclear
  Medicine, 445
Imaging Methods, 449
Clinical Nuclear Medicine, 453
Principles and Facilities in Positron
  Emission Tomography (PET), 460
Clinical PET, 472
Future of Nuclear Medicine, 475
Best Practices, 477
Conclusion, 477
Definition of Terms, 478

Principles of Nuclear Medicine

Nuclear medicine is an imaging modality that focuses on the use of radioactive materials called *radiopharmaceuticals*.[a] Radiopharmaceuticals are used for diagnosis, therapy, and medical research. In contrast to typical radiographic procedures that determine the presence of disease based on structural appearance, nuclear medicine explores the physiologic function of the body.

To begin a nuclear medicine procedure, the radiopharmaceutical, commonly referred to as a *radiotracer* or *tracer*, is introduced into the body through a multitude of ways. These include, but are not limited to, injection (intravenous, intradermal, intramuscular, or intrathecal), ingestion, or inhalation. Different radiotracers are used to study different regions of the body. Specific tracers are selected based on their ability to localize in specific organs and/or tissues. Radiotracers undergo radioactive decay to produce gamma-ray emissions. A special piece of equipment, known as a *gamma* or *scintillation camera,* is used to transform these emissions into images that provide information about the function and anatomy of the organ or system being studied. Physicians attempt to prescribe the lowest amount of radiotracer for each exam to reduce the radiation exposure to the patient without compromising image quality.

Nuclear medicine procedures are performed by a team of specially educated professionals: a nuclear medicine physician, a specialist with extensive education in the basic and clinical science of medicine who is licensed to use radioactive materials; a nuclear medicine technologist, who performs the tests and is educated in the theory and practice of nuclear medicine procedures; a medical physicist, who is experienced in the technology of nuclear medicine and the care of the equipment; and a radiopharmacist, who is qualified to prepare the necessary radiopharmaceuticals.

Historical Development

John Dalton is considered the father of the modern theory of atoms and molecules. In 1803, Dalton, an English schoolteacher, stated that all atoms of a given element are chemically identical, unchanged by chemical reaction, and combine in a ratio of simple numbers. Dalton measured atomic weights in reference to hydrogen, to which he assigned the value of 1 (the atomic number of this element).

The discovery of x-rays by Wilhelm Conrad Röntgen in 1895 was a great contribution to physics and the care of the sick. A few months later, another physicist, Antoine Henri Becquerel, discovered naturally occurring radioactive substances. In 1898, Marie Curie discovered two new elements in the uranium ore pitchblende. Curie named these trace elements polonium (after her homeland, Poland) and radium. Curie also coined the terms *radioactive* and *radioactivity*.

GENERAL NUCLEAR MEDICINE

In 1923, George de Hevesy, often called the "father of nuclear medicine," developed the tracer principle. He coined the term "radioindicator" and extended his studies from inorganic to organic chemistry. The first radioindicators were naturally occurring substances such as radium and radon. The invention of the *cyclotron* by Ernest Lawrence in 1931 made it possible for de Hevesy to expand his studies to a broader spectrum of biologic processes by using ^{32}P (phosphorus-32), ^{22}Na (sodium-22), and other cyclotron-produced (synthetic) radioactive tracers.

Radioactive elements then began to be produced in *nuclear reactors*. This method was developed by Enrico Fermi and colleagues in 1946. The nuclear reactor greatly extended the ability of the cyclotron to produce more radioactive tracers. A key development was the introduction of the *gamma camera* by Hal Anger in 1958. In the early 1960s, Edwards and Kuhl made the next advancement in nuclear medicine with the development of a crude single photon emission computed tomography (SPECT) camera known as the MARK IV. With this new technology, it was possible to create three-dimensional images of organ function instead of the two-dimensional images created previously. It was not until the early 1980s, when computers became fast enough to acquire and process all of the information successfully, that SPECT imaging could become a standard practice.

One of the first organs to be examined by nuclear medicine studies using *external radiation detectors* was the thyroid. In the 1940s, investigators found that the rate of incorporation of radioactive iodine by the thyroid gland was greatly increased in hyperthyroidism (the overproduction of thyroid hormones) and greatly decreased in hypothyroidism (the underproduction of thyroid hormones). Over the years, tracers and instruments were developed to allow almost every major organ of the body to be studied by application of the tracer principle. Subsequently, images were made of structures such as the liver, spleen, brain, and kidneys. Currently, the emphasis of nuclear medicine studies is more on function and pathology than anatomic structure.

Positron Emission Tomography

With the development of more suitable *scintillators,* such as sodium iodide (NaI), and more sophisticated nuclear counting electronics, positron coincidence localization became possible. In 1951, Wrenn demonstrated the use of positron-emitting radioisotopes for the localization of brain tumors. Gordon Brownell further developed instrumentation for similar studies. The next major advancement came in 1967, when Sir Godfrey Hounsfield demonstrated the clinical use of computed tomography (CT). The mathematics of positron emission tomography (PET) image *reconstruction* is similar to that used for CT reconstruction techniques. Instead of x-rays from a point source traversing the body and being detected by a single or multiple detector(s), as in CT, PET imaging uses two opposing detectors to count pairs of 511-keV photons simultaneously that originate from a single positron–electron annihilation event.

From 1967 to 1974, significant developments occurred in computer technology, scintillator materials, and *photomultiplier tube* (PMT) design. In 1975, the first closed-ring transverse positron emission tomograph was built for imaging by Michel M. Ter-Pogossian and Michael E. Phelps.

Developments now continue on two fronts that have accelerated the use of PET. First, scientists are approaching the theoretic limits (1–2 mm) of PET scanner resolution by employing smaller, more efficient scintillators and PMTs. Microprocessors tune and adjust the entire ring of *detectors* that surround the patient.

---

[a] Almost all italicized words on the succeeding pages are defined at the end of this chapter.

Each ring within the PET unit may contain 1000 detectors, and the entire unit may be composed of 30 to 60 rings. The second major area of development is in the design of new PET radiopharmaceuticals. Agents are being developed to measure blood flow, metabolism, protein synthesis, lipid content, receptor binding, and many other physiologic parameters and processes.

During the mid-1980s, PET was used predominantly as a research tool. However, by the early 1990s, clinical PET centers had been established, and PET was routinely used for diagnostic procedures on the brain, heart, and tumors. In the mid- to late 1990s, three-dimensional PET systems that eliminated the use of interdetector *septa* were developed. This allowed for the radiopharmaceutical dose to be reduced by approximately six- to tenfold. New image reconstruction methods have been developed to better characterize the distribution of annihilation photons from these three-dimensional systems.

HYBRID IMAGING: PET/CT, AND PET/MRI

Beginning in 2000, major nuclear medicine camera manufacturers developed combined PET and CT systems that can simultaneously acquire PET functional images and CT anatomic images. Both modalities are coregistered or exactly matched in size and position. The success of these camera systems led to the development of combined SPECT and CT systems, as well. Significant benefits have resulted in the diagnosis of metastatic disease due to the precise localization and function of the tumor site being routinely identified. In addition to anatomic registration, CT has allowed for improved attenuation correction (AC) in PET and SPECT. By accurately mapping the different densities in the body, more accurate reconstruction methods can be applied to raw PET and SPECT image data. This in turn reduces background noise and increases image sharpness. Rapid enhancements and developments continue to occur within this modality.

In addition to the hybrid fusion of PET and CT, the first PET/magnetic resonance imaging (MRI) system was approved by the U.S. Food and Drug Administration (FDA) for customer purchase in 2011. The integration of PET and MRI is not straightforward and challenges the technical design of both systems. PET/MRI merges the metabolic ability of PET imaging with the morphologic imaging of MRI (see Chapter 26) to generate diagnostic images for oncologic, cardiologic, and neurologic purposes.

Comparison With Other Modalities

Nuclear medicine is predominantly used to measure human cellular, organ, or system function. A parameter that characterizes a particular aspect of human physiology is determined from the measurement of the radioactivity emitted by a radiopharmaceutical in a given volume of tissue. In contrast, conventional radiography measures the structure, size, and position of organs or human anatomy by determining x-ray transmission through a given volume of tissue. X-ray attenuation by structures interposed between the x-ray source and the radiographic image receptor provides the contrast necessary to visualize an organ. CT creates cross-sectional images by computer reconstruction of multiple x-ray transmissions (see Chapter 25). The characteristics of radiologic imaging modalities are compared in Table 29.1.

TABLE 29.1
Comparison of imaging modalities

Modality information	PET	SPECT	MRI	CT
Measures	Physiology	Physiology	Anatomy (physiology)[a]	Anatomy
Resolution	3–5 mm	8–10 mm	0.5–1 mm	1–1.5 mm
Technique	Positron annihilation	Gamma emission	Nuclear magnetic resonance	Absorption of x-rays
Potential harm	Radiation exposure	Radiation exposure	None known	Radiation exposure
Use	Research and clinical	Clinical	Clinical (research)[a]	Clinical
No. of examinations per day	4–12	5–10	10–15	15–20

[a]Secondary function.

SPECT is a conventional nuclear imaging technique that is used to determine tissue function. Because SPECT employs collimators and lower energy photons, it is less sensitive (by 10^1–10^5) and less accurate than PET. Generally, PET resolution is better than SPECT resolution by a factor of 2 to 10. PET easily accounts for photon loss through attenuation by performing a *transmission scan*. This is difficult to achieve and not routinely done with SPECT imaging; however, newly designed SPECT instrumentation that couples a low-output x-ray CT to the gamma camera for the collection of attenuation information is now being used to correct for gamma attenuation. Software approaches are also being investigated that assign known *attenuation coefficients* for specific tissues to segmented regions of images for analytic AC of SPECT imaging data.

The differences between the various imaging modalities can be highlighted using a study of brain blood flow as an example. Without an intact circulatory system, an intravenously injected radiotracer cannot make its way into the brain for distribution throughout the brain's capillary network, ultimately diffusing into cells that are well perfused. For radiographic procedures, such as CT, structures within the brain may be intact, but there may be impaired or limited blood flow to and through major vessels within the brain. Under these circumstances, the CT scan may appear almost normal despite reduced blood flow to the brain. If the circulatory system at the level of the capillaries is not intact, a PET scan can be performed, but no perfusion information is obtained because the radioactive water used to measure blood flow is not transported through the capillaries and diffused into the brain cells.

Additional pitfalls involve the image-enhancing contrast agents and radiation dose to the patient. Contrast agents used in many radiographic studies may cause a toxic reaction (e.g., a warm uncomfortable feeling all over the body or even a severe allergic reaction). The x-ray dose to the patient in these radiographic studies is greater than the radiation dose in most nuclear imaging studies. An additional benefit is that the radiotracers used in PET studies are similar to the body's own biochemical constituents and are administered in very small amounts. This biochemical compatibility of the tracers within the body minimizes the risks to the patient because the tracers are not found to be toxic. At the same time, trace amounts minimize any alterations of the body's *homeostasis*.

An imaging technique that augments CT and PET is MRI (see Chapter 26). Images obtained with PET and MRI are shown in Fig. 29.1. MRI is used primarily to measure anatomy or morphology. In contrast to CT, which derives its greatest image contrast from varying tissue densities (bone from soft tissue), MRI better differentiates tissues by their proton content and the degree to which the protons are bound in lattice structures. The tightly bound protons of bone make it virtually transparent to MRI.

CT, MRI, and other anatomic imaging modalities provide complementary information to nuclear medicine imaging and PET. These imaging modalities benefit from *image coregistration* with CT and MRI by pinpointing physiologic function with precise anatomic locations. Greater emphasis is being placed on multimodality image coregistration between PET, CT, SPECT, and MRI for brain research and tumor localization throughout the body (Fig. 29.2). All new PET imaging systems are fused with a CT scanner for AC and anatomic positioning information. Many SPECT imaging systems incorporate CT technology for the same purposes.

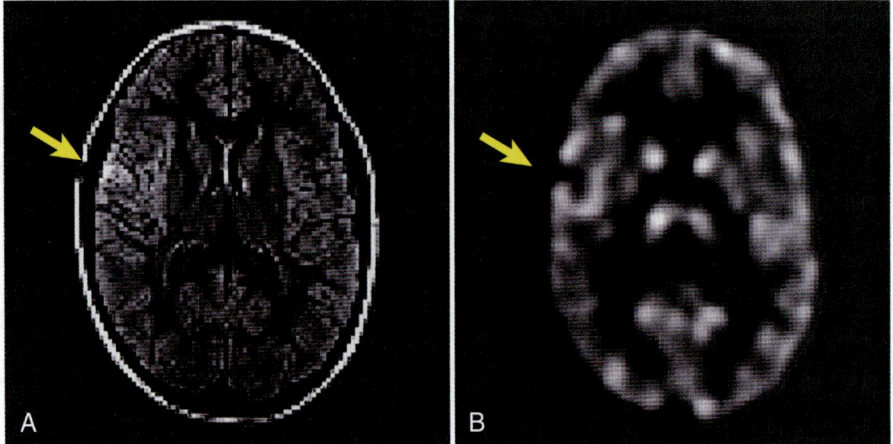

Fig. 29.1 Coregistered MRI and PET scans. *Arrows* indicate an abnormality on the anatomic image (**A**, MRI scan) and the functional image (**B**, PET scan). ^{18}F-FDG PET image depicts hypometabolic area of seizure focus *(arrow)* in a patient with a diagnosis of epilepsy.

Physical Principles of Nuclear Medicine

An understanding of radioactivity must precede an attempt to grasp the principles of nuclear medicine and how images are created using radioactive compounds. The term *radiation* is taken from the Latin word *radii*, which refers to the spokes of a wheel leading out from a central point. The term *radioactivity* is used to describe the radiation of energy in the form of high-speed *alpha* or *beta particles* or waves (gamma rays) from the nucleus of an atom.

BASIC NUCLEAR PHYSICS

The basic components of an atom include the nucleus (which is composed of varying numbers of protons and neutrons) and the orbiting electrons (which revolve around the nucleus in distinct energy levels). Protons have a positive electrical charge, electrons have a negative charge, and neutrons are electrically neutral. Protons and neutrons have masses nearly 2000 times the mass of the electron; thus the nucleus is responsible for most of the mass of an atom (~99%). The Bohr atomic model (Fig. 29.3) can describe this configuration. The total number of protons, neutrons, and electrons in an atom determines its chemical and physical characteristics, including stability.

The term *nuclide* is used to describe an atomic species with a particular arrangement of protons and neutrons within the nucleus. Elements with the same number of protons but a different number of neutrons are referred to as *isotopes*. Isotopes have the same chemical properties as one another because the total number of protons and electrons is the same. They differ simply in the total number of neutrons contained in the nucleus. The neutron-to-proton ratio in the nucleus determines the stability of the atom. At certain ratios, atoms may become unstable, and a process known as spontaneous *decay* can occur as the atom attempts to regain stability. Energy is released in various ways during this decay process, as it approaches its *ground state*.

Radionuclides decay by the emission of alpha, beta, and/or gamma radiation. For most radionuclides to reach their ground state, it usually requires multiple decay steps and various decay processes. This can include any array of, alpha, beta, positron, or *electron capture*, decay processes. These decay methods determine the types of particles or gamma rays given off as the radionuclide decays.

To explain this process better, investigators have created decay schemes to show the details of how a *parent* nuclide decays to its *daughter* and/or eventual ground state (Fig. 29.4A). A decay scheme is a simple illustration depicting how a radionuclide decays. Each radionuclide has its own unique decay scheme, similar to a fingerprint, which identifies the type(s) of decay, the energy associated with each process, the probability of a particular decay process occurring, and the rate of change to the ground state element (Fig. 29.4B).

Radioactive decay is considered a purely random and spontaneous process that can be mathematically defined by complex equations and represented by average decay rates. The term *half-life* is used to describe the time it takes for a quantity of a particular radionuclide to decay to one-half of its original activity or one-half of the original number of atoms through spontaneous disintegration. The rate of decay has an exponential function, which can be plotted on a linear scale (Fig. 29.4C). If plotted on a semilogarithmic scale, the decay rate would be represented as a straight line. Radionuclide half-lives can range anywhere from milliseconds to years. The half-lives of most radionuclides used in nuclear medicine range from several seconds to several days.

NUCLEAR PHARMACY (RADIOPHARMACY)

Naturally occurring radionuclides have very long half-lives (i.e., thousands of years). These natural radionuclides are unsuitable for nuclear medicine imaging because of limited availability and the high-absorbed dose a patient would receive. The radionuclides used in nuclear medicine (general and PET) are produced in nuclear reactors, generators, or *particle accelerators (cyclotrons)*. Radionuclides

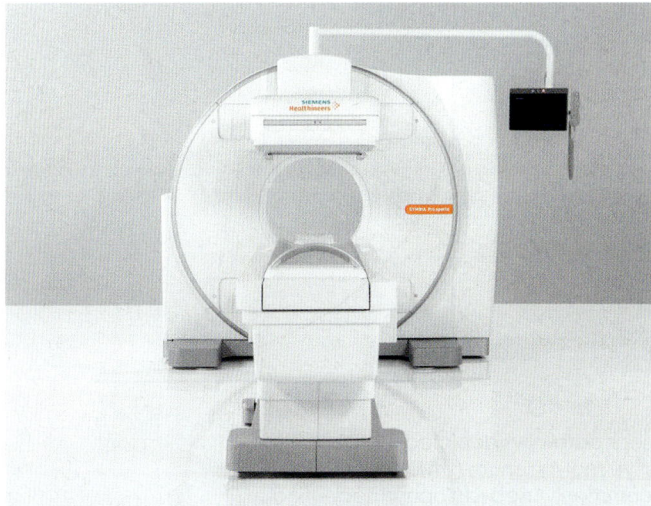

Fig. 29.2 SPECT/CT scanner unit, which combines two sets of images (SPECT and CT) into one hybrid image, providing interpreters with both anatomic and physiologic perspectives.

(Courtesy of Siemens Medical Solutions USA, Inc.)

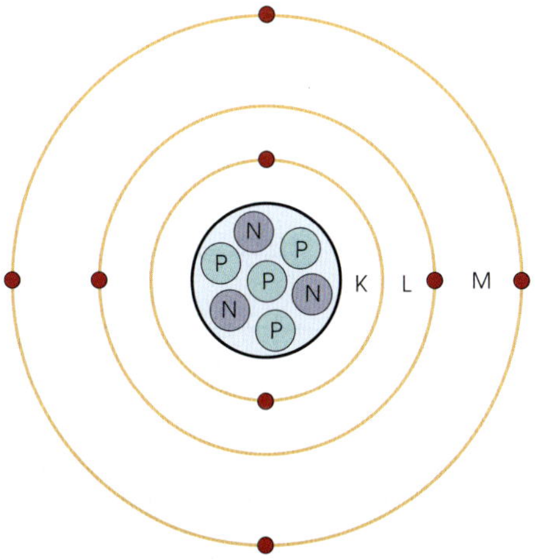

Fig. 29.3 Diagram of Bohr atom containing a single nucleus of protons (*P*) and neutrons (*N*) with surrounding orbital electrons of varying energy levels (e.g., *K, L, M*).

can be created in nuclear reactors either by inserting a target element into the reactor core where it is irradiated or by separating and collecting the *fission* byproducts. One of these byproducts is molybdenum-99 (^{99}Mo), which is used in the production of technetium-99m (^{99m}Tc) through a *generator system*. The radionuclides for nuclear medicine are also produced in particle accelerators or cyclotrons through nuclear reactions created between high-speed particles and specific targets. The number of protons in the target nucleus is changed when it is bombarded by the high-speed charged particles, and a new element or radionuclide is produced.

Radionuclides used for general nuclear medicine procedures include ^{99m}Tc, ^{123}I (iodine), ^{131}I (iodine), ^{111}In (indium), ^{201}Tl (thallium), and ^{67}Ga (gallium). When pharmaceuticals are compounded with these high atomic weight radionuclides, they often do not mimic the physiologic properties of naturally occurring substances found in the body. This is due to their size, mass, and different chemical properties. Compounds labeled with traditional nuclear medicine radionuclides are also found to be poor radioactive *analogs* for other natural substances. Imaging studies with these agents are qualitative and emphasize nonbiochemical properties.

Radionuclides used in PET include ^{11}C (carbon), ^{13}N (nitrogen), and ^{15}O (oxygen). The elements hydrogen, carbon, nitrogen, and oxygen are the predominant constituents of natural compounds found in the body. Different from common nuclear medicine radionuclides, these emit positrons, have low atomic weight, and can directly replace their stable isotopes in substrates, metabolites, drugs, and other biologically active compounds. This is also achieved without disrupting any bodily biochemical mechanisms and processes. For example, the most commonly used PET radionuclide, ^{18}F (fluorine), can replace hydrogen in many molecules,

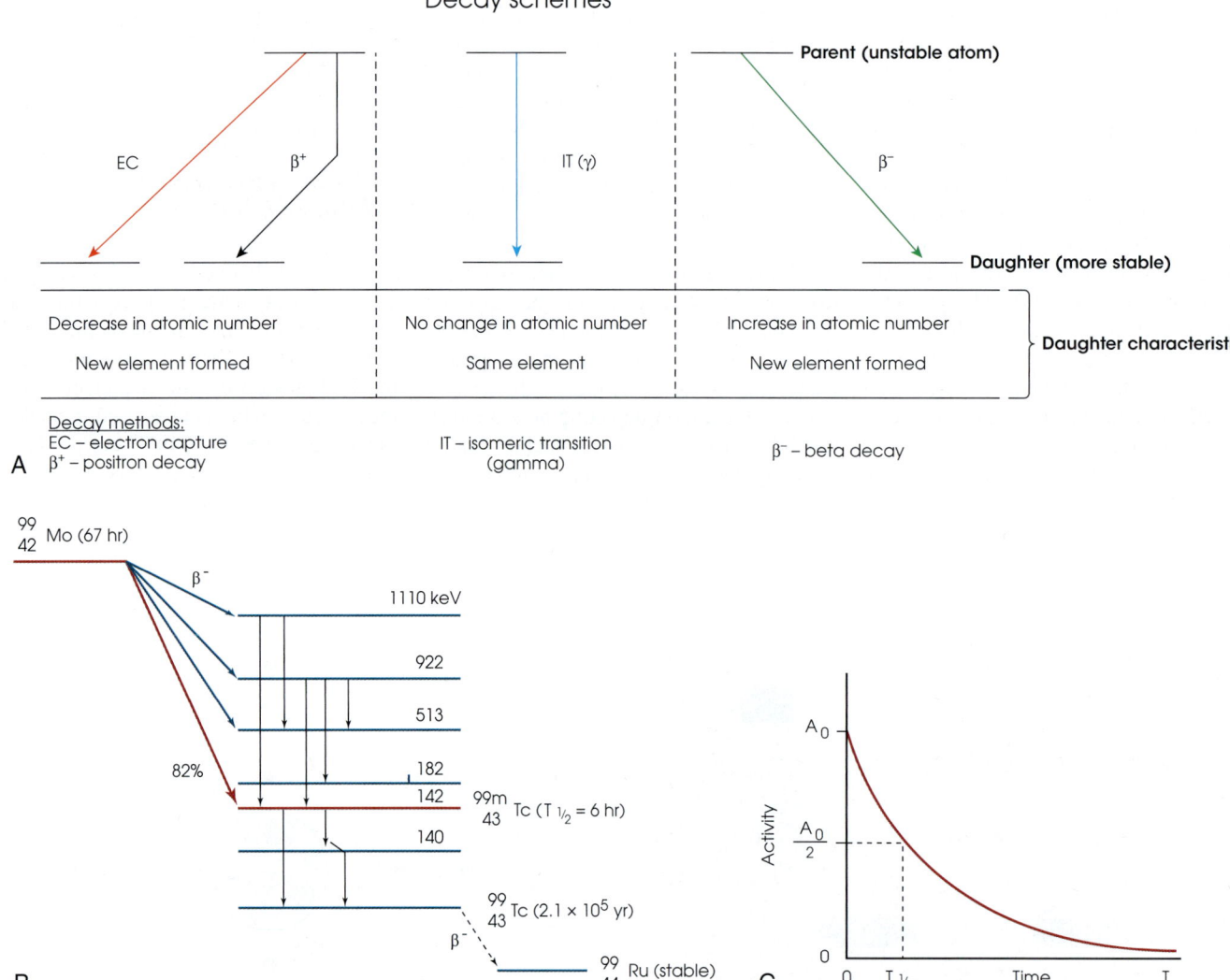

Fig. 29.4 (**A**) Four types of decay schemes with linear pathways depicted. (**B**) Decay scheme illustrating the method by which radioactive molybdenum (^{99}Mo) decays to radioactive technetium (^{99m}Tc), one of the most commonly used radiopharmaceuticals in nuclear medicine. (**C**) Graphic representation showing the rate of physical radioactive decay of a radionuclide. The *y (vertical)* axis represents the amount of radioactivity, and the *x (horizontal)* axis represents the time at which a specific amount of activity has decreased to one-half of its initial value. Every radionuclide has an associated half-life that is representative of its rate of decay.

providing an even greater assortment of biologic analogs.

The most commonly used radionuclide in nuclear medicine is ^{99m}Tc, which is produced in a generator system. This apparatus has the ability to make the desirable short-lived radionuclides (the *daughters*) readily available. These are formed by the decay of relatively longer-lived radionuclides (the *parents*). The generator system uses ^{99}Mo as the parent; ^{99}Mo has a half-life of 66.7 hours and decays (86% of the time) to a daughter product known as *metastable* ^{99m}Tc. Because ^{99m}Tc and ^{99}Mo are chemically different, they can easily be separated through an ion-exchange column. ^{99m}Tc exhibits nearly ideal characteristics for use in nuclear medicine examinations, including a relatively short physical half-life of 6.04 hours and a high-yield of low-energy gamma photons (98.6% at 140-keV) (see Fig. 29.4B).

A radiopharmaceutical generally has two components: a radionuclide and a *pharmaceutical*. The pharmaceutical is a biologically active compound chosen on the basis of its preferential localization or participation in the physiologic function of a given organ. A radionuclide is the radioactive material used to tag the pharmaceutical, which allows for the localization of the compound within the body (Fig. 29.5). After the radiopharmaceutical is administered, the target organ is localized by means of the physiologic pharmaceutical distribution, and the radiation emitted from it can be detected by imaging instruments or gamma cameras.

The following characteristics are desirable in an imaging radiopharmaceutical:
- Ease of production, low cost, and readily available
- Lowest possible radiation dose to the patient
- Primary photon energy between 100 and 400 keV
- Physical half-life greater than the time required to prepare the material, deliver it, and use it
- Effective half-life longer than the examination time
- Suitable chemical forms for rapid localization
- Different uptake in the structure to be detected than in the surrounding tissue
- Low toxicity in the chemical form administered to the patient
- Stability or near-stability

Because most radiopharmaceuticals are administered intravenously, they need to be sterile and *pyrogen-free*. They also need to undergo all of the quality control measures required of conventional drugs.

A commonly used radiopharmaceutical is ^{99m}Tc tagged to a macroaggregated albumin (MAA). After intravenous injection, this substance follows the pathway of blood flow to the lungs, where it is distributed throughout and trapped in the small pulmonary capillaries (Fig. 29.6). Blood

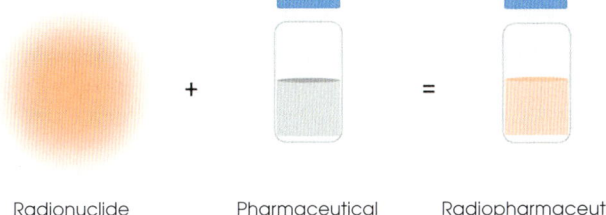

Fig. 29.5 A radionuclide is chosen based on the characteristics of its gamma emission and ability to tag to a specific pharmaceutical; the pharmaceutical is chosen based on its ability to localize to a specific organ or function. When combined, a radiopharmaceutical, or *tracer*, is formed.

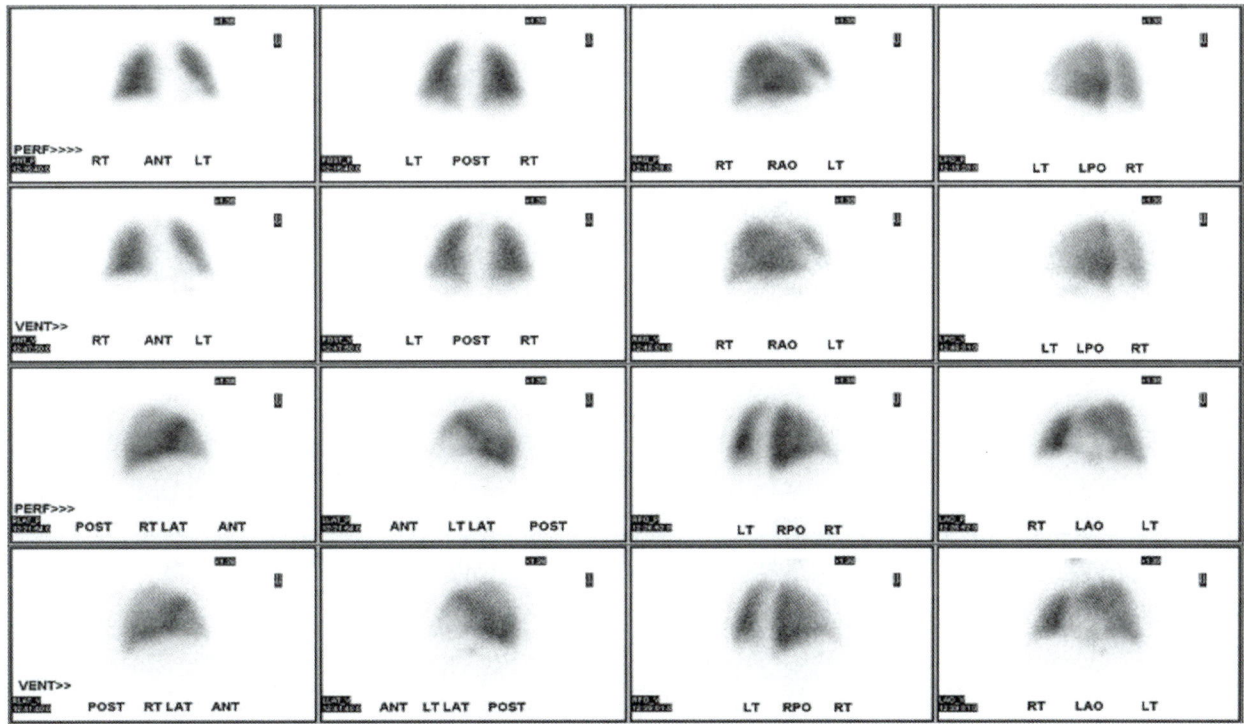

Fig. 29.6 Normal ventilation/perfusion lung scan using 40 mCi of ^{99m}Tc-diethylenetriamine pentaacetic acid (DTPA) (ventilation) and 5 mCi of ^{99m}Tc-macroaggregated albumin (MAA) (*perfusion*) on a large field-of-view gamma camera. Ventilation imaging is provided in the first and third rows. Perfusion imaging is displayed in the second and fourth rows. This provides the radiologist to identify discrepancies between ventilation and perfusion within each view.

clots along the pathway prevent this radiopharmaceutical from distributing in the area beyond the clot. As a result, the image shows a void or clear area, often described as *photopenia* or a *cold spot*. More than 30 different radiopharmaceuticals are used in nuclear medicine (Table 29.2).

Radioactivity is measured using either the *becquerel* (Bq), which corresponds to the decay rate, expressed as 1 disintegration per second (dps), or as the *curie* (Ci), which equals 3.73×10^{10} dps, relative to the number of decaying atoms in 1 g of radium.

TABLE 29.2
Radiopharmaceuticals used in nuclear medicine

Radionuclide	Symbol	Physical half-life	Chemical form	Diagnostic use
Carbon	^{11}C	20.4 min	Sodium acetate	Oncology and myocardial imaging
			Choline	Oncology imaging
Fluorine	^{18}F	110 min	Fluorodeoxyglucose	Oncology and myocardial hibernation
			Sodium fluoride	Bone imaging
Gallium	^{67}Ga	77 h	Gallium citrate	Inflammatory process and tumor imaging
Indium	^{111}In	67.4 h	DTPA	Cerebrospinal fluid imaging
			Ibritumomab tiuxetan	Localization of tumor
			OctreoScan (pentetreotide)	Neuroendocrine tumors
			Oxine	White blood cell/abscess imaging
Iodine	^{123}I	13.3 h	Sodium iodide	Thyroid function and imaging
	^{131}I	8 days	Sodium iodide	Thyroid function, imaging, and therapy
Nitrogen	^{13}N	10 min	Ammonia	Myocardial perfusion
Oxygen	^{15}O	2.03 min	Water (^{15}O)H$_2$O	Oncology and myocardial blood flow agent
			Gas	Cerebral blood flow imaging
Rubidium	^{82}Rb	75 s	Rubidium chloride	Cardiovascular imaging
Technetium	^{99m}Tc	6 h	Sodium pertechnetate	Imaging of brain, thyroid, scrotum, salivary glands, renal perfusion, and pericardial effusion; evaluation of left-to-right cardiac shunts
			Sulfur colloid	Imaging of liver and spleen and renal transplants, lymphoscintigraphy
			Macroaggregated albumin	Lung imaging
			Sestamibi	Cardiovascular imaging, myocardial perfusion
			DTPA	Brain and renal imaging
			DMSA	Renal imaging
			MAG3	Renal imaging
			Diphosphonate	Bone imaging
			Pyrophosphate	Bone and myocardial imaging
			Red blood cells	Cardiac function imaging
			HMPAO	Functional brain imaging and white blood cell/abscess imaging
			Neurolite (Bicisate)	Brain imaging
			Myoview (Tetrofosmin)	Myocardial perfusion
			Cardiolite (Sestamibi)	Myocardial perfusion
Thallium	^{201}Tl	73.5 h	Thallous chloride	Myocardial imaging
Xenon	^{133}Xe	5.3 days	Xenon gas	Lung ventilation imaging

DMSA, Dimercaptosuccinic acid; *DTPA*, diethylenetriamine pentaacetic acid; *HMPAO*, hexamethylpropyleneamine oxime; *MAG3*, mertiatide.

Radiopharmaceutical Dosing

Prescribed radiopharmaceutical doses vary, depending on the radionuclide used, the examination to be performed, the pathology involved, and the size (kg) and the age of the patient. A radiologist or authorized user will usually set an acceptable dose range to administer an adult patient based on the factors listed above. Pediatric patients only receive a fraction of the adult dose. Currently, there are several formulas used to calculate an appropriate pediatric dose (Fig. 29.7). All pediatric doses provided in this chapter reference the *North American Consensus Guidelines for Pediatric Administered Radiopharmaceutical Activities*.

Pediatric dose formulas:

A) North American Consensus Guidelines*:

  mCi / kg (with min and max)

B) European Association of Nuclear Medicine (EANM)**:

  Activity to be administered = baseline activity × multiplier

C) Body weight:

  mCi / kg (with min and max)

D) Body surface area (BSA):

$$\frac{\sqrt{Mass\ (kg) \times height\ (cm)}}{3600} = BSA$$

E) Clark's rule (assumes adult weight of 70 kg):

$$\frac{(Adult\ dose) \times (Child's\ weight\ in\ kg)}{70\ kg} = Activity\ to\ be\ administered$$

F) Webster's rule (age based):

$$\frac{(Adult\ dose) \times (Patient's\ age + 1)}{Age + 7} = Activity\ to\ be\ administered$$

G) Young's rule (age based):

$$\frac{(Adult\ dose) \times (Patient's\ age)}{Age + 12} = Activity\ to\ be\ administered$$

H) Fried's rule (age based):

$$\frac{(Adult\ dose) \times (Patient's\ age\ in\ months)}{150} = Activity\ to\ be\ administered$$

*The North American Consensus Guidelines has created a weight-based table (mCi/kg) identifying pediatric doses based on the isotope, radiopharmaceutical (RP), and exam.

**The EANM created a dosing reference card. Depending on the isotope and RP, a *Class* (A, B, or C) and *Baseline Activity* are assigned. Using the card, the patient's weight is referenced against the class, providing a *multiplier*. This is then multiplied by the Baseline Activity to identify the prescribed dose.

Fig. 29.7 Pediatric dose formulas.

Radiation Safety in Nuclear Medicine

The radiation protection requirements in nuclear medicine differ from the general radiation safety measures used for diagnostic radiography. The radionuclides employed in nuclear medicine are in liquid, solid, or gaseous form. Because of the nature of radioactive decay, these radionuclides continuously emit radiation (in contrast to diagnostic x-rays, which can be turned on and off mechanically). Thus, special radiation safety precautions are required.

Technologists and nuclear pharmacists are required to wear appropriate radiation monitoring (dosimetry) devices, such as radiation badges and thermoluminescent dosimetry (TLD) rings, to monitor radiation exposure to the body and hands. The *ALARA* (as low as reasonably achievable) principle/program applies to all nuclear medicine personnel at all times.

Generally, the quantities of radioactive tracers used in nuclear medicine present no significant hazard. Nonetheless, care must be taken to reduce unnecessary exposure. The high concentrations or activities of the radionuclides used in a nuclear pharmacy necessitate the establishment of a designated preparation area. These elected rooms are called *hot labs* and usually contain isolated ventilation, protective lead, or leaded glass shielding for vials and syringes, absorbent materials, and gloves. The handling and administration of diagnostic doses to patients warrants the use of gloves and a lead or tungsten syringe shield, which is especially effective for reduction of exposure to the technologist's hands and fingers (Fig. 29.8).

Any spilled radioactive material continues to emit radiation and must be cleaned up and contained immediately. Because radioactive material that contacts the skin can be absorbed and may not be easily washed off, it is very important to wear appropriate personal protective equipment (e.g., lab coat and gloves) when handling radiopharmaceuticals.

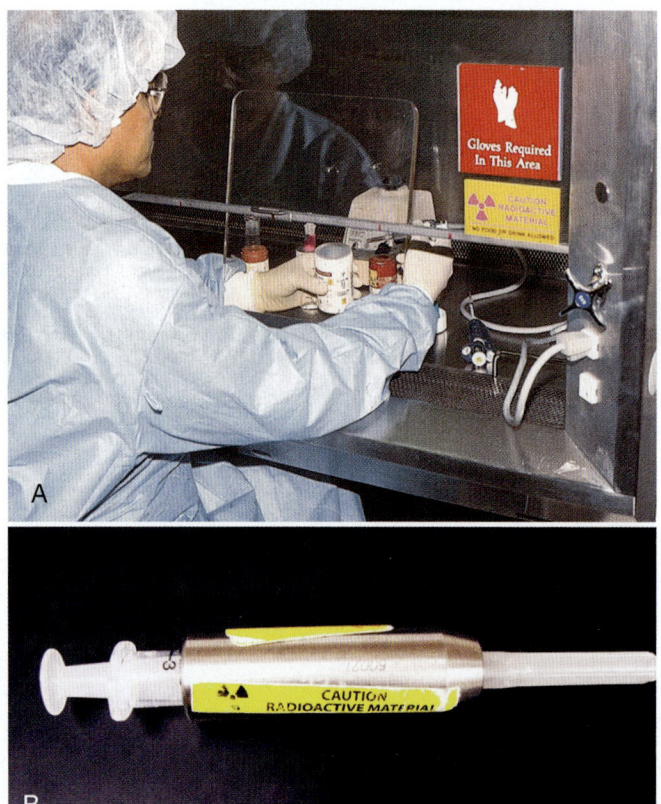

Fig. 29.8 (**A**) Fume hood located in a radiopharmacy where doses of radiopharmaceuticals are prepared in a clean and protected environment. (**B**) Syringe shields are used to protect the nuclear medicine technologist from excess radiation emitted from the radioisotope. They come in many shapes and sizes but are usually made out of lead, leaded glass, or tungsten.

(B, from Mettler FA Jr, Guiberteau MJ: *Essentials of nuclear medicine and molecular imaging.* ed 7. Philadelphia: Elsevier, 2019.)

Instrumentation in Nuclear Medicine

MODERN-DAY GAMMA CAMERA

The term *scintillate* means to emit light photons. Becquerel discovered that ionizing radiation caused certain materials to glow. A scintillation material is a sensitive element that emits light photons after being exposed to ionizing radiation. When a light-sensitive device is affixed to this material, the flash of light can be converted into small electrical impulses. Together, this is known as a *scintillation detector*. The electrical impulses are amplified and counted to determine the amount and nature of radiation striking the scintillating materials. Scintillation detectors were used in the development of the first-generation nuclear medicine scanner—the rectilinear scanner—which was built in 1950.

Scanners have evolved into complex imaging systems known today as *gamma cameras* (because they detect gamma rays). The gamma camera has many components that work together to produce an image (Fig. 29.9). These cameras are scintillation detectors that use a thallium-activated sodium iodide crystal to detect and transform radioactive emissions into light photons. Through a complex process, these light photons are amplified, and their locations are electronically recorded to produce an image that is displayed on computer output systems. Scintillation cameras today use single or multiple crystals.

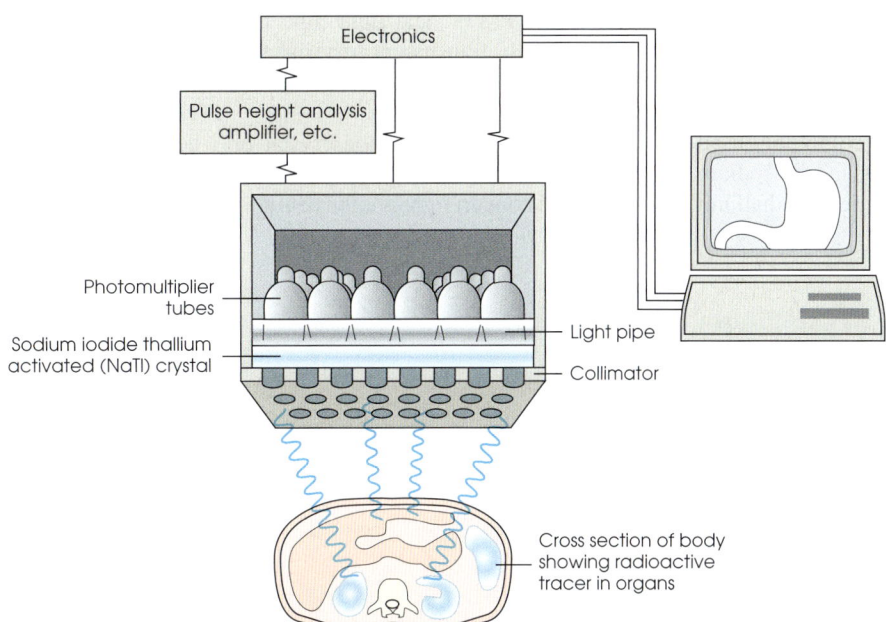

Fig. 29.9 Typical gamma camera system, which includes a processing station and electronic mechanical components for acquiring nuclear medicine images.

Collimator

Located at the face of the detector, where photons from radioactive sources first enter the camera, is the *collimator*. The collimator is used to filter gamma rays not perpendicular to the camera and keep scattered rays from reaching the scintillation crystal. *Resolution* and *sensitivity* are terms used to describe the physical characteristics of collimators. Collimator sensitivity is determined by the fraction of photons that are transmitted through the collimator and strike the face of the camera crystal. Spatial resolution refers to the system's ability to separate two points on an image.

Collimators are usually made of a material with a high atomic number, such as lead, which absorbs scattered gamma rays. Depending on the desired level of sensitivity and resolution, different collimators are used for different types of examinations (Fig. 29.10).

Crystal, light pipe, and PMT

The scintillation crystals commonly used in gamma cameras are made of sodium iodide with trace quantities of thallium added to increase light production. This crystal composition is effective for stopping most common gamma rays emitted from the radiopharmaceuticals used in nuclear medicine.

The thickness of the crystal varies from 0.6 to 1.3 cm (0.25–0.5 inch). Thicker crystals are better for imaging radiopharmaceuticals with higher energies (>180 keV) but have decreased resolution because of the decreased ability of the electronics to localize the exact location of the photon absorption within the thicker crystal. Thinner crystals provide improved resolution but cannot efficiently image photons with a higher kiloelectron voltage (keV) because of the inability of the thinner crystals to stop the higher-energy photons from passing through the crystal without being absorbed.

A *light pipe* may be used to attach the crystal to the PMTs. The light pipe is a disk of optically transparent material that helps direct photons from the crystal into the PMTs.

Attached to the back of the crystal or light pipe is an array of PMTs that are used to detect and convert light photons emitted from the crystal into an electronic signal. The PMT also amplifies the original photon signal by a factor of up to 10^7. A typical gamma camera detector head contains 80 to 100 PMTs. The PMTs send the detected signal through a series of processing steps, which include determining the location (x, y) of the original photon and its amplitude or energy (z). The x and y values are determined by where the photon strikes the face of the crystal. Electronic circuitry, known as a *pulse height analyzer,* is used to eliminate the z signals that are of the appropriate energy based on the particular radionuclide being used. It is also used for rejecting photons not within the desired energy range. This helps reduce scattered lower energy, unwanted photons ("noise") that generally would degrade the resolution of the image. When the information has been processed, the signals are transmitted to the display system.

Multihead gamma camera systems

The original gamma camera was a single detector that could be moved in various positions around the patient. Today, gamma camera systems may include up to

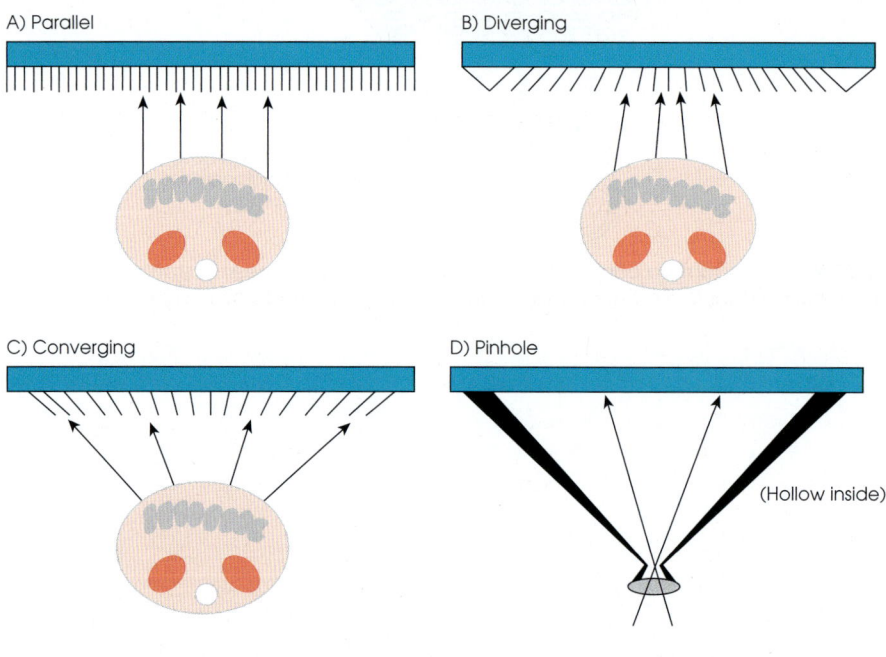

Fig. 29.10 Collimator designs: **(A)** Parallel collimators are used to visualize organs as is, usually with no or very little zoom. **(B)** Diverging collimators are used to shrink or minimize large organs or organ systems. **(C and D)** Converging and pinhole collimators magnify small organs so they can be better visualized.

three detectors (heads). Dual-head gamma camera systems are the most common, allowing for simultaneous anterior and posterior planar imaging, and are ideal for SPECT. Triple-head systems are not as popular as dual-head systems and are generally used for brain and heart studies. Although the triple-head systems are primarily suited for SPECT, they can also provide multiplanar images (see the section on imaging methods presented later in this chapter).

PROCESSING SYSTEMS

Processing systems have become an integral part of the nuclear medicine imaging structure. These systems are used to acquire and process data from gamma cameras. They allow data to be collected over a specific time frame or to a specified number of counts; the data can be analyzed to determine functional changes occurring over time (Fig. 29.11A and B). A common example is the renal study, in which the radiopharmaceutical that is administered is cleared by normally functioning kidneys in about 20 minutes. The computer can collect several images of the kidney during this period and analyze them to determine how effectively the kidneys clear the radiopharmaceutical. It does this by creating a time activity curve (Fig. 29.11C through E). The computer also allows the operator to enhance a particular structure by adjusting the contrast and brightness of the image.

Processing systems are necessary to acquire and process SPECT images (see the next section). SPECT uses a scintillation

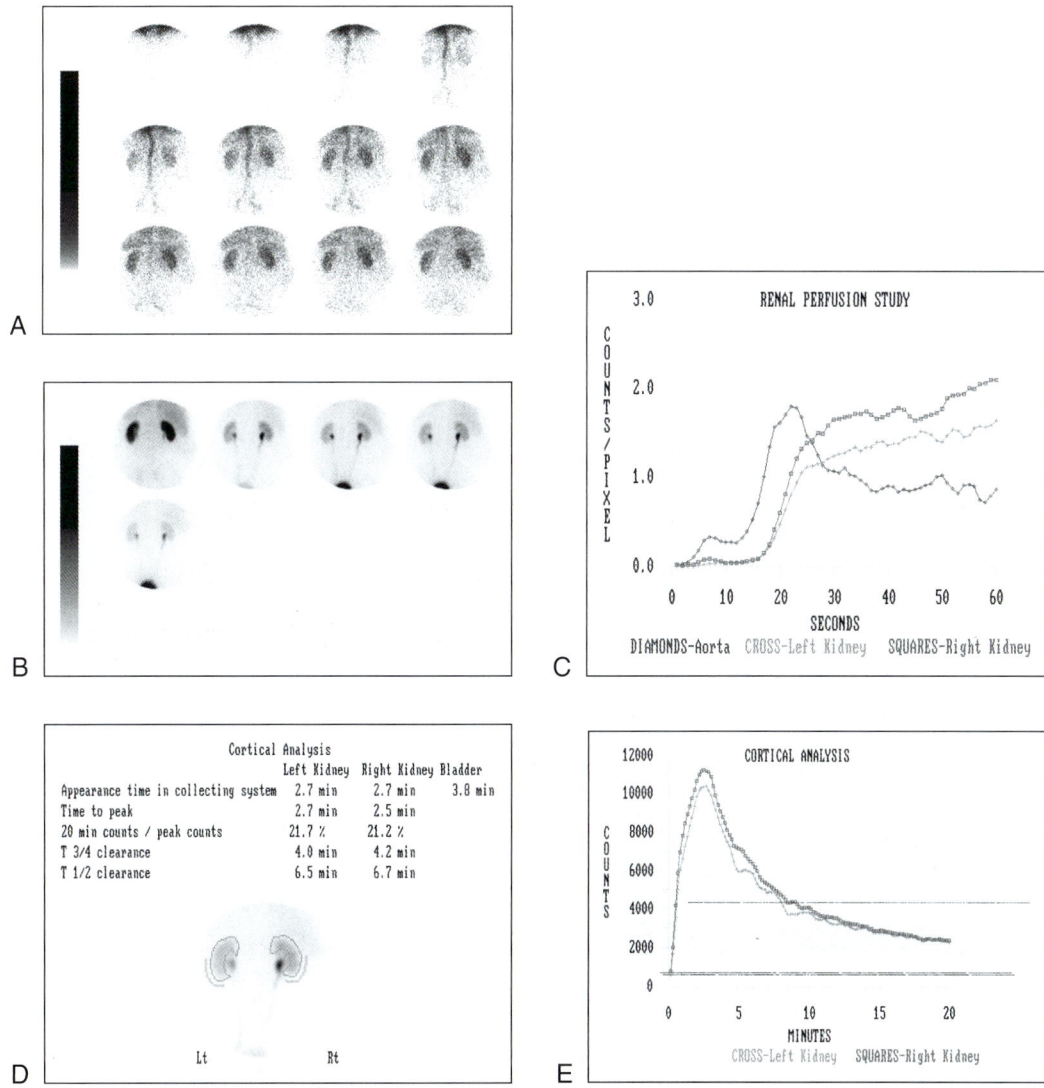

Fig. 29.11 (**A**) Posterior renal blood flow in an adult patient using 10 mCi of ^{99m}Tc with diethylenetriamine pentaacetic acid (DTPA) imaged at 3 seconds per frame. The image in the *lower right corner* is a blood-pool image taken immediately after the initial flow sequence. Together the images show normal renal blood flow to both kidneys. (**B**) Normal, sequential dynamic 20-minute ^{99m}Tc with mertiatide (MAG3) images. (**C**) Renal arterial perfusion curves showing minor renal blood flow asymmetry. (**D**) Renal cortical analysis curves showing rapid uptake and prompt parenchymal clearance. (**E**) Quantitative renal cortical analysis indices showing normal values.

camera that moves around the patient to obtain images from multiple angles for tomographic image reconstruction. SPECT studies are complex and, similar to MRI studies, require a great deal of computer processing to create images in transaxial, sagittal, and coronal planes. Rotating three-dimensional images can also be generated from SPECT data (Fig. 29.12).

Computer networks are an integral part of the way a department communicates information within and among institutions. In a network, several or many computers are connected so that they all have access to the same files, programs, and printers. Networking allows the movement of image-based and text-based data to any computer or printer in the network. Networking improves the efficiency of a nuclear medicine department. A computer network can serve as a vital component, reducing the time expended on menial tasks while allowing retrieval and transfer of information. Consolidation of all reporting functions in one area eliminates the need for the nuclear medicine physician to travel between departments to read studies. Centralized archiving, printing, and retrieval of most image-based and non–image-based data have increased the efficiency of data analysis, reduced the cost of image hard copy, and permitted more sophisticated analysis of image data than would routinely be possible.

Electronically stored records can decrease the reporting turnaround time, the physical image storage requirements, and the use of personnel for record maintenance and retrieval. Long-term computerized records can also form the basis for statistical analysis to improve testing methods and predict disease courses. Most institutions now use some form of picture archiving and communication systems (PACS) to organize all of the imaging that is done. PACS are the foundation of a digital department, allowing for easy transfer, retrieval, and archiving of all imaging done in the nuclear medicine department.

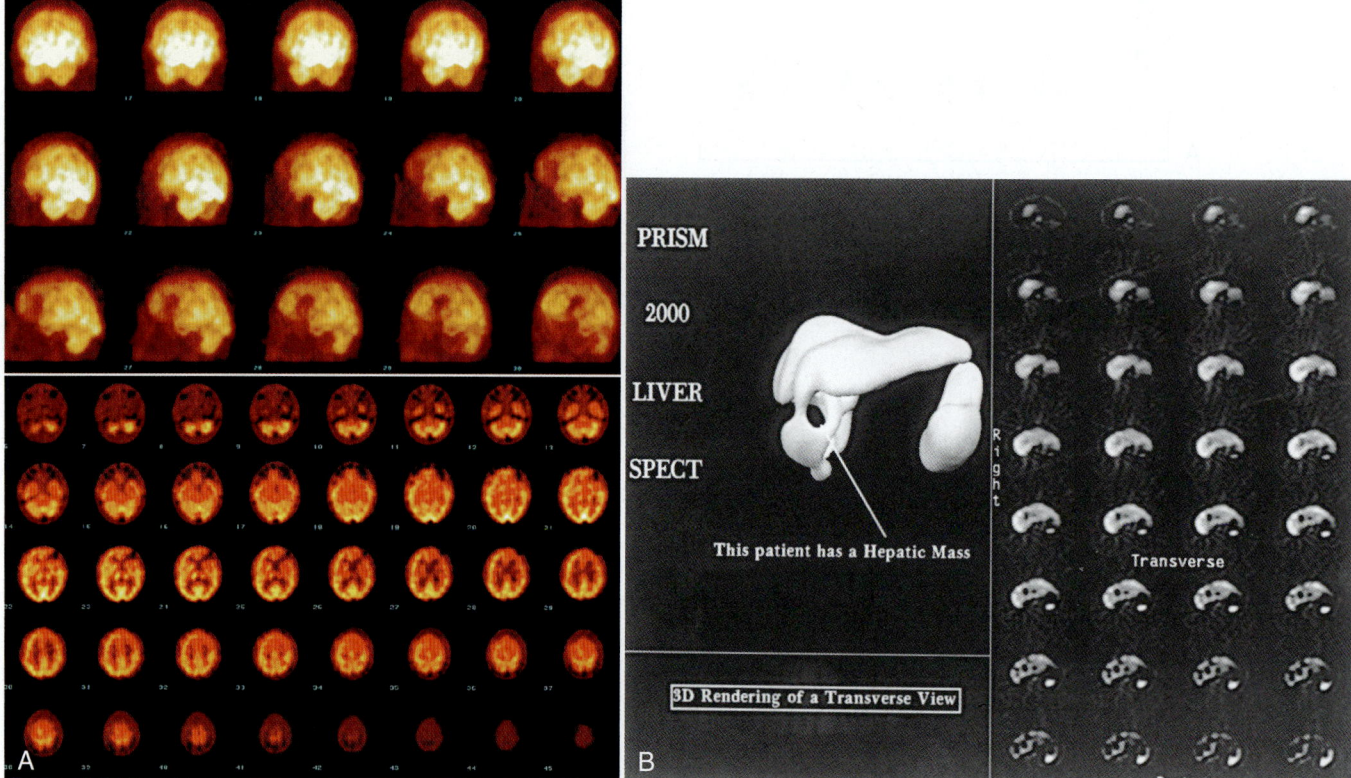

Fig. 29.12 (A) Three-dimensional SPECT brain study using 20 mCi of ^{99m}Tc ethylcysteinate dimer showing a patient with a left frontal lobe brain infarct *(top)*. Baseline and Diamox challenge transaxial, coronal, and sagittal images of the same patient, showing the left frontal lobe brain infarct *(bottom)*. (B) Three-dimensional SPECT liver study using 8 mCi of ^{99m}Tc sulfur colloid. A mass is seen on the three-dimensional image *(left)* and transaxial images *(right)*.

QUANTITATIVE ANALYSIS

Many nuclear medicine procedures require some form of quantitative analysis to provide physicians with numeric or statistical results based on and depicting organ function. Specialized software allows computers to collect, process, and analyze functional information obtained from nuclear medicine imaging systems. Cardiac left ventricular ejection fraction is a common quantitative study (Fig. 29.13). In this dynamic study of the heart's contractions and expansions, the computer accurately determines the ejection fraction, or the percent of blood pumped out of the left ventricle with each contraction.

Imaging Methods

A wide variety of diagnostic imaging examinations are performed in nuclear medicine. These examinations can be described on the basis of the imaging method used: static/planar, whole-body, dynamic, SPECT, and PET.

STATIC/PLANAR IMAGING

Static imaging is the acquisition of a single two-dimensional image of a particular structure. This image can be thought of as a snapshot of the radiopharmaceutical distribution within the body. Examples of static imaging used in general nuclear medicine include lung scans, limited bone scans, and thyroid imaging. Static images are usually obtained in various orientations around a particular structure to show multiple aspects of the region in question. Anterior, posterior, and oblique images are often obtained.

In static imaging, low radiopharmaceutical activity levels are used to minimize radiation exposure to the patients. Because of these low activity levels, images must be acquired for a preset time or a minimum number of counts or radioactive emissions. This time frame may vary from a few seconds to several minutes to acquire 100,000 to more than 1 million counts.

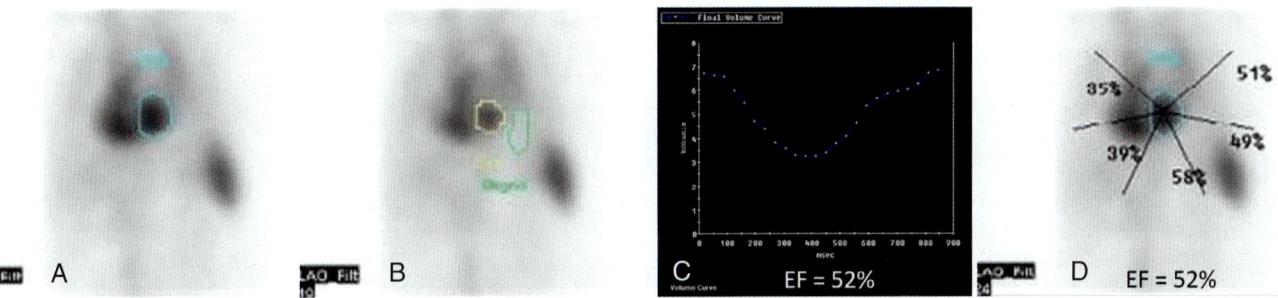

Fig. 29.13 Normal multigated acquisition scan. (**A**) Left anterior oblique (LAO) image of the left ventricle at end-diastole (relaxed phase) with a region of interest drawn around the left ventricle. (**B**) Same view showing end-systole (contracted phase). (**C**) Curve representing the volume change in the left ventricle of the heart before, during, and after contraction. This volume change is referred to as the ejection fraction (EF); normal value is approximately 52%. (**D**) LAO view with regional ejection fractions displayed.

WHOLE-BODY IMAGING

Whole-body imaging uses a specially designed moving detector system to produce an image of the entire body or a large body section. In this type of imaging, the gamma camera collects data as it passes over the body. Earlier detector systems were smaller and required two or three incremental passes to encompass the entire width of the body. Others took multiple static images and "zipped" them together to form one whole-body image.

Nearly all camera systems used for whole-body imaging incorporate a dual-head design for simultaneous anterior and posterior acquisitions. Whole-body imaging systems are used primarily for whole-body bone, tumor, or infection imaging along with other clinical and research applications (Fig. 29.14).

DYNAMIC IMAGING

Dynamic images display the distribution of a particular radiopharmaceutical over a specific period of time. Very similar to filming a movie, a series of sequential images is collected and aligned together to show function over time. A dynamic or "flow" study of a particular structure is generally used to evaluate blood perfusion to the tissue. Images may be acquired and displayed in time sequences from one-tenth of a second to longer than 10 minutes per image. Dynamic imaging is commonly used for three-phase bone scans, hepatobiliary studies, and renal exams (Fig. 29.15).

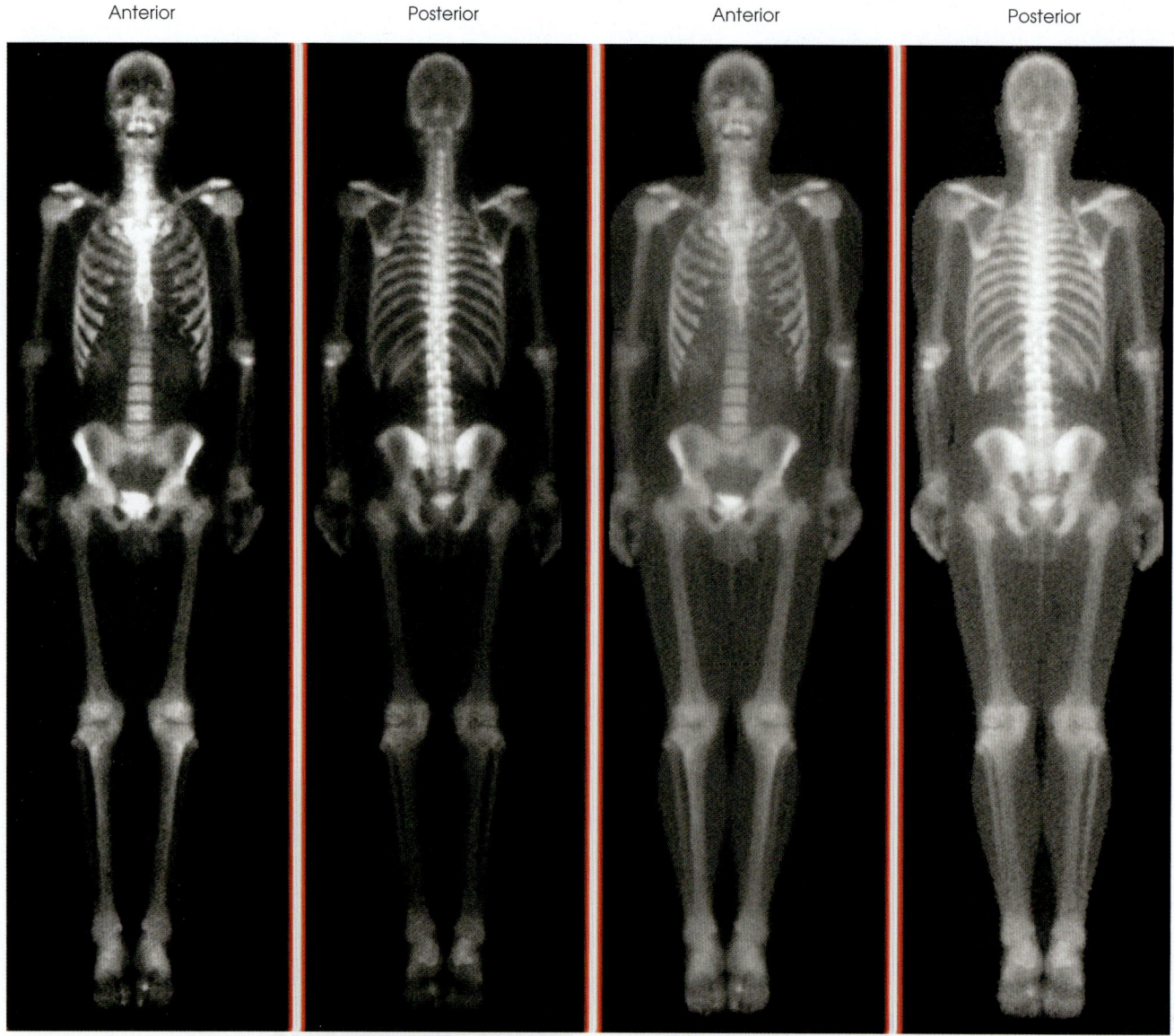

Fig. 29.14 Whole-body scan performed using 25 mCi ^{99m}Tc HDP in a 25-year-old man. The study was normal. (**A**) Anterior and posterior whole-body view in linear grayscale. (**B**) Anterior and posterior whole-body view in square-root grayscale to enhance soft tissue.

(Courtesy General Electric.)

SPECT IMAGING

With SPECT, typically, two gamma detectors are used to produce tomographic images (Fig. 29.16). Tomographic systems are designed to allow the detector heads to rotate 360 degrees around a patient's body to collect "projection" image data. The image data is restructured by a computer using reconstruction algorithms that populate all acquired projections to display the radiopharmaceutical distribution of the object into several formats, including transaxial, sagittal, coronal, planar, and three-dimensional representations.

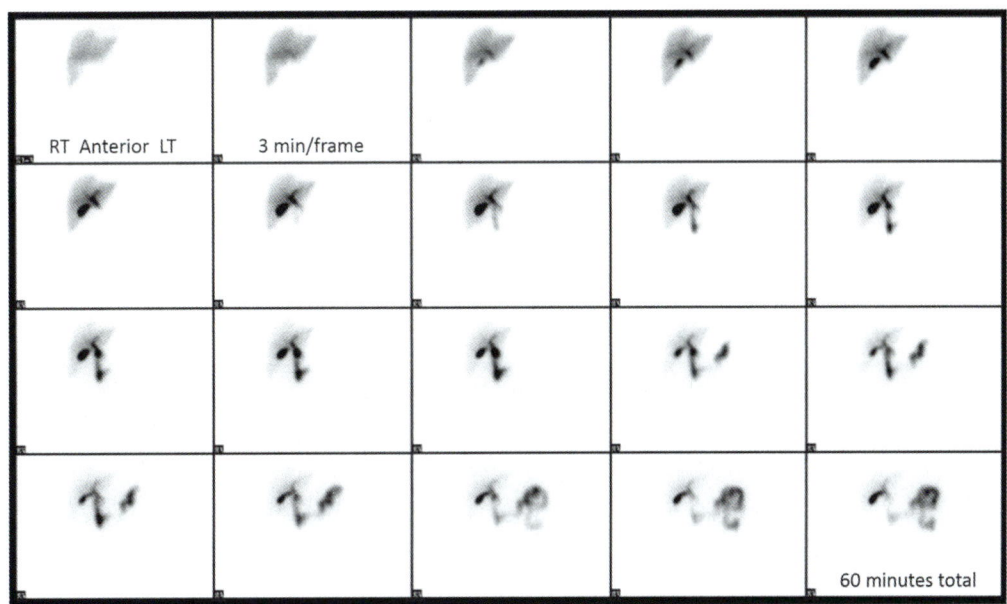

Hepatobiliary Scan, 5 mCi Mebrofenin

Fig. 29.15 Example of a dynamic hepatobiliary scan using 5 mCi of ^{99m}Tc mebrofenin. Imaging was acquired for 60 minutes and displayed over 20 frames (3 minutes/frame). Normal visualization of the liver, gallbladder, and small bowel is seen within the allotted time.

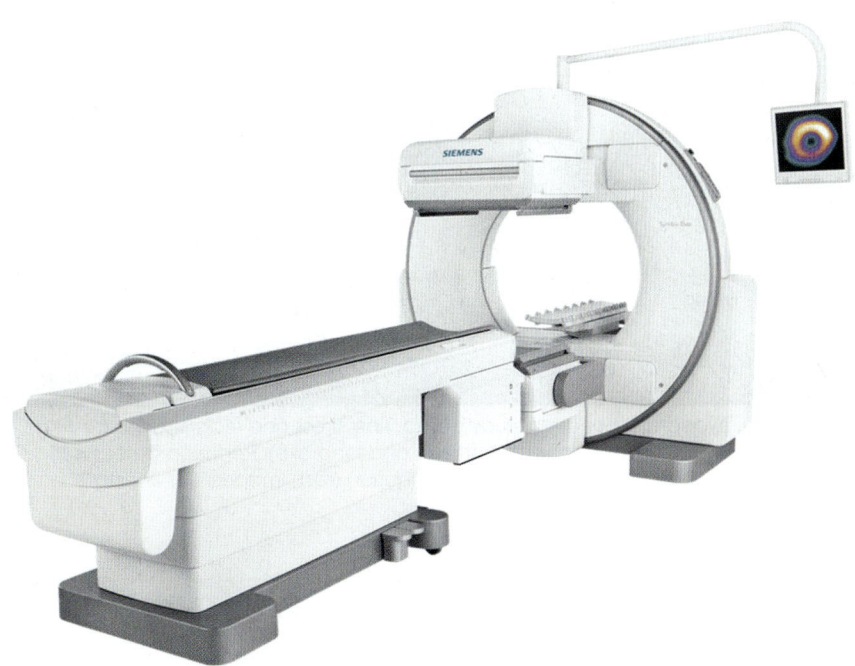

Fig. 29.16 Dual-headed SPECT camera system.

(Courtesy of Siemens Medical Solutions USA, Inc.)

The reconstruction of SPECT data produces image projections similar to those obtained by CT or MRI. This reconstruction technique is used to create thin slices through a particular organ from different angles or planes to help delineate small lesions within tissues. These images can be created for virtually any structure or organ that is acquired using SPECT. Improved clinical results with SPECT are due to improved target-to-background ratios. Planar images record and show all radioactive emissions from the patient within the region of interest (ROI), as well as above and below the ROI, causing degradation of the image. In contrast, SPECT eliminates unnecessary information.

The most common uses of SPECT include cardiac perfusion, brain, liver (see Fig. 29.12B), tumor, and bone studies. An example of a SPECT study is the myocardial perfusion thallium (^{201}Tl) study, which is used to identify perfusion defects in the left ventricular wall. The ^{201}Tl is injected intravenously while the patient is being physically stressed on a treadmill or is being infused with a vasodilator. The radiopharmaceutical is distributed in the heart muscle in the same fashion as blood flowing to the tissue. An initial set of images is acquired immediately after the stress test. A second set is obtained several hours later when the patient is rested (when the ^{201}Tl has redistributed to viable tissue) to determine whether any blood perfusion defects seen on the initial images have resolved. By comparing the two image sets, the physician may be able to tell whether the patient has damaged heart tissue resulting from a myocardial infarction or ischemia (Fig. 29.17).

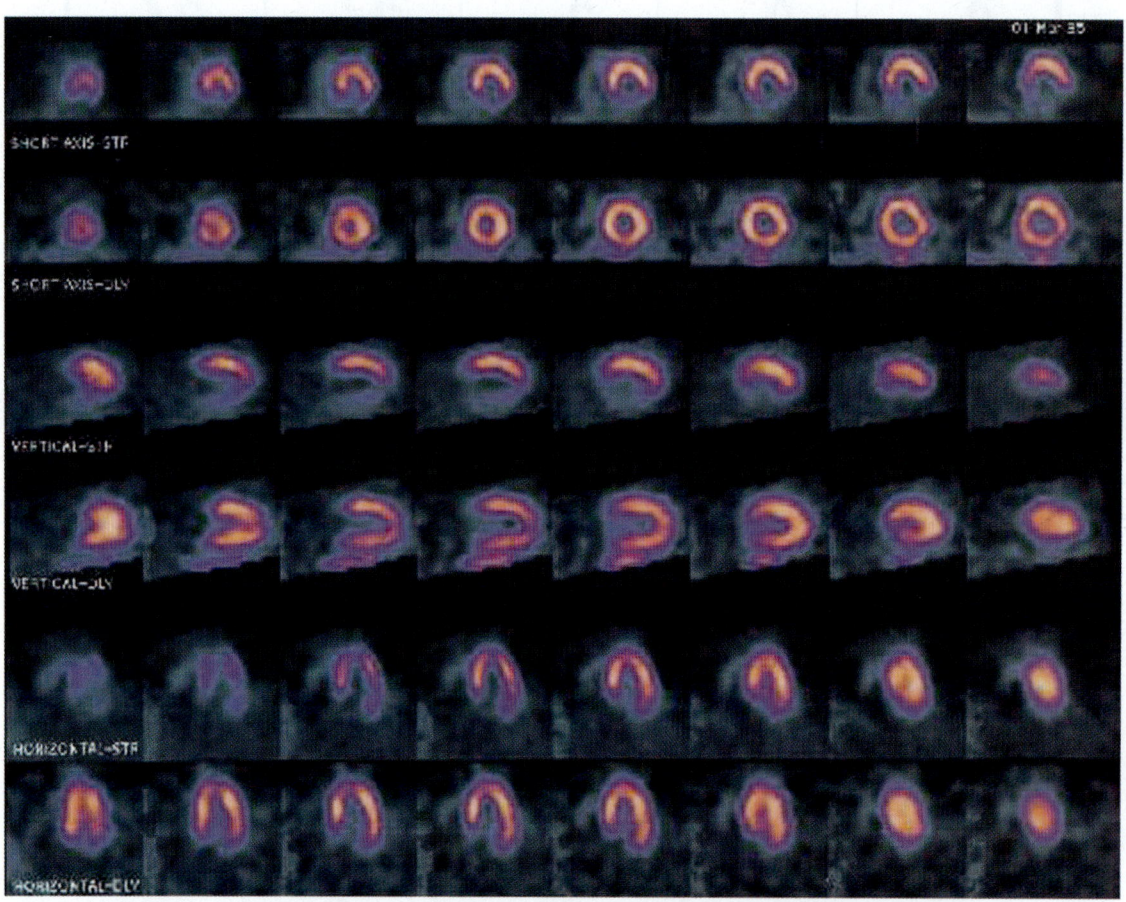

Fig. 29.17 ^{201}Tl myocardial perfusion study comparing stress and redistribution (resting) images in various planes of the heart (short axis and long axis). Perfusion defect is identified in stress images but not seen in redistribution (rest) images. This finding is indicative of ischemia.

COMBINED SPECT AND CT IMAGING

By merging or "fusing" the functional imaging of SPECT with the anatomic landmarks of CT, more powerful diagnostic information is obtainable (Fig. 29.18). This combination has a significant impact on diagnosing and staging malignant disease and on identifying and localizing metastases. This new technology can also be used for AC. According to manufacturers, statistics show that adding CT (for AC and anatomic definition) changes the patient course of treatment 25% to 30% of the time when compared to medical management based on interpreting the functional image alone. SPECT/CT is discussed further later in this chapter.

Clinical Nuclear Medicine

The term *in vivo* means "within the living body." Because all diagnostic nuclear medicine imaging procedures are based on the distribution of radiopharmaceuticals within the body, they are classified as in vivo examinations.

Patient preparation for nuclear medicine procedures is minimal, with most tests requiring no special preparation. Patients usually remain in their own clothing. All metal objects outside or inside the clothing must be removed because they may attenuate anatomic or pathologic conditions on nuclear medicine imaging. The waiting time between dose administration and imaging varies with each study. After completion of a routine procedure, patients may resume all normal activities.

Technical summaries of commonly performed nuclear medicine procedures follow. After each procedure summary is a list, by organ or system, of many common studies that may be done in an average nuclear medicine department.

BONE SCINTIGRAPHY

Bone scintigraphy is generally a survey procedure to evaluate patients with malignancies, diffuse musculoskeletal symptoms, abnormal laboratory results, osteomyelitis, and hereditary or metabolic disorders. Tracer techniques have been used for many years to study the exchange between bone and blood. Radionuclides have played an important role in understanding normal bone metabolism and the metabolic effects of pathologic involvement of bone. Radiopharmaceuticals used for bone imaging can localize in bone and in soft tissue structures. Skeletal areas of increased uptake are commonly a result of tumor, infection, or fracture.

Bone scan
Principle

^{99m}Tc-labeled diphosphonates are incorporated into bone at the molecular level based upon regional blood flow, osteoblastic activity, and extraction efficiency. In areas where osteoblastic activity is increased, active hydroxyapatite crystals with large surface areas adhere to the diphosphonate portion of the radiopharmaceutical.

Radiopharmaceutical

Adult dose (intravenous injection):
- 20 mCi (740 MBq) of ^{99m}Tc hydroxymethylene diphosphonate (HDP) or
- 20 mCi (740 MBq) of ^{99m}Tc methylene diphosphonate (MDP)

Pediatric dose (weight-based intravenous injection) (see Fig. 29.7):
- 0.25 mCi/kg (9.3 MBq/kg) of ^{99m}Tc MDP

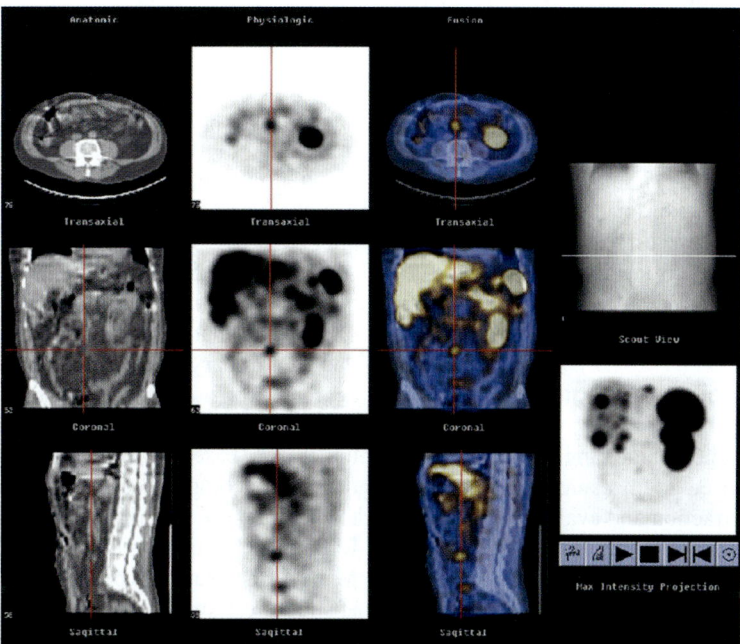

Fig. 29.18 ^{111}In-octreotide SPECT/CT fusion images showing numerous foci of increased uptake within the liver. This is consistent with the patient's known hepatic metastases. Very small focus of increased uptake is also seen in the inferior abdomen, near midline, anterior to the lumbar spine, and is consistent with nodal metastasis. These findings are indicative of somatostatin-avid hepatic and probable nodal metastases.

Scanning

A routine survey (whole-body, static views, or SPECT) begins about 3 hours after radiopharmaceutical injection and takes 30 to 60 minutes. A flow study would begin immediately after the injection, and extremity imaging may be needed 4 to 5 hours later. The number of camera images acquired depends on the indication for the examination.

Bone (skeletal) studies

Skeletal studies include bone scans, three-phase bone scans, and bone marrow scans.

NUCLEAR CARDIOLOGY

Nuclear cardiology has experienced rapid growth and currently constitutes a significant portion of daily nuclear medicine procedures. These noninvasive studies assess cardiac performance, evaluate myocardial perfusion, and measure viability and metabolism. Advances in camera technology have facilitated the development of a quantitative cardiac evaluation unequaled by any other noninvasive or invasive methods. Stress tests can be performed through exercise (i.e., treadmill or stationary bike) or by infusing a pharmacologic stress agent. Exercise is the gold standard because it provides a true representation of the body's response to stress. However, some patients cannot exercise because of peripheral vascular disease, neurologic problems, or musculoskeletal abnormalities. In these cases, a pharmacologic intervention can be used in place of the exercise stress test to alter the blood flow to the heart in a way that simulates exercise, allowing the detection of myocardial ischemia. Once the stress test has begun, the patient's heart rate, electrocardiogram (ECG), blood pressure, and symptoms are continuously monitored and recorded.

Radionuclide angiography
Principle

Gated radionuclide angiography (RNA) can be used to measure left ventricular ejection fraction and evaluate left ventricular regional wall motion. RNA requires that the blood be labeled with an appropriate tracer such as ^{99m}Tc. The technique is based on using a multigated acquisition (MUGA) format. During a gated acquisition, the cardiac cycle is divided into 16 to 20 frames. The R wave of each cycle resets the gate so that each count is added to each frame until there are adequate count statistics for analysis. RNA requires simultaneous acquisition of the patient's ECG and images of the left ventricle. The *ejection fraction* and wall motion analysis are measured at rest (see Fig. 29.13). In some cases RNA can be performed under stress conditions when clinically indicated.

Radiopharmaceutical

Adult dose (intravenous injection):
- 25 to 30 mCi (925–1110 MBq) of ^{99m}Tc-labeled red blood cells

Pediatric dose (weight-based intravenous injection) (see Fig. 29.7):
- 0.32 mCi/kg (11.8 MBq/kg) of ^{99m}Tc-labeled red blood cells

Scanning

Imaging can begin immediately after the injection and takes about 1 hour. For a rest MUGA, imaging of the heart should be obtained in the anterior, left lateral, and left anterior oblique positions. For an ejection fraction-only MUGA, only the left anterior oblique is necessary.

Myocardial perfusion imaging (MPI) using SPECT (imaging agents technetium-99m sestamibi and technetium-99m tetrofosmin)
Principle

^{99m}Tc sestamibi and ^{99m}Tc tetrofosmin are radiopharmaceuticals that both have favorable biologic properties for myocardial perfusion imaging (MPI). They are used to assess myocardial salvage resulting from therapeutic intervention in acute infarction, to determine the myocardial blood flow during periods of spontaneous chest pain, and to diagnose coronary artery disease. Both ^{99m}Tc sestamibi and ^{99m}Tc tetrofosmin localize in the heart wall based on regional blood flow. Thus, areas of the heart that suffer from reduced flow due to coronary artery disease will have decreased or no activity (photopenia) on the images. Injecting and imaging patients under rest (baseline) and stress (treadmill or pharmacologic) conditions can help to illustrate the severity of their situation (normal/ischemic/infarct). Gating (refer to MUGA) the exam can be performed either at stress, rest, or both to obtain an ejection fraction and evaluate wall motion.

Radiopharmaceutical

Adult dose (intravenous injection):
- At peak stress: 20 to 30 mCi (740–1110 MBq) for 2-day MPI and 30 to 36 mCi (1110–1332 MBq) for 1-day MPI
- At rest: 8 to 12 mCi (296–444 MBq) for a 1-day MPI and 20 to 30 mCi (740–1110 MBq) for a 2-day MPI

Scanning

SPECT imaging at 180 degrees (45 degrees right anterior oblique to 45 degrees left posterior oblique) is normally performed 30 to 60 minutes after the injection of the radiotracer for both stress and rest studies. When needed, delayed images can be obtained up to 4 to 6 hours after injection based on the tracer used. A 2-day protocol provides optimal image quality, but the 1-day protocol is more convenient for patients, technologists, and physicians.

Thallium-201 MPI and viability studies
Principle

^{201}Tl is sometimes used in MPI studies and has a high sensitivity (about 90%) and specificity (about 75%) for the diagnosis of coronary artery disease, but currently, sestamibi and tetrofosmin are used more often due to their better imaging properties. ^{201}Tl also has been useful for assessing myocardial viability in patients with known coronary artery disease and for evaluating patients after revascularization.

^{201}Tl is an analog of potassium and has a high rate of extraction by the myocardium over a wide range of metabolic and physiologic conditions. It is distributed in the myocardium in proportion to regional blood flow and myocardial cell viability. Regions of the heart that are infarcted or hypoperfused at the time of injection appear as areas of decreased activity (photopenia). Over time ^{201}Tl can perfuse into viable areas of the heart that may not exactly have adequate blood flow. Patients who have inadequate blood flow but viable tissue are excellent candidates for revascularization.

Radiopharmaceutical

Adult MPI dose (intravenous injection):
- At peak stress: 3 mCi (111 MBq) of ^{201}Tl thallous chloride
- At rest: 1 mCi (37 MBq) of ^{201}Tl thallous chloride (generally 3–4 hours after stress)

Adult viability dose (intravenous injection):
- One dose given at rest: 4 mCi (148 MBq) of ^{201}Tl thallous chloride

NOTE: In obese patients, ^{99m}Tc sestamibi (adult peak stress dose) can be used in place of ^{201}Tl so that a higher dose may be administered for clearer imaging results.

Scanning

Imaging for a ^{201}Tl MPI study includes a 180-degree SPECT study (45 degrees right anterior oblique to 45 degrees left posterior oblique) approximately 10 minutes after the peak stress injection has occurred. Due to ^{201}Tl's high redistribution rate, the patient must be scanned very close to their injection time. Rest 180-degree SPECT imaging usually takes place 4 hours after stress imaging and 15 to 30 minutes after the rest injection.

For a viability study, a 180-degree SPECT imaging usually takes place 15 minutes postinjection and 4 to 6 hours postinjection. The delay of 4 to 6 hours allows the ^{201}Tl to redistribute to regions of the heart that do not have direct blood flow but are viable.

Cardiovascular studies

Cardiovascular studies include cardiac shunt study, MUGA (dobutamine, exercise, and rest), MPI (^{99m}Tc sestamibi, ^{99m}Tc tetrofosmin, ^{201}Tl thallous chloride), viability imaging (^{99m}Tc sestamibi and ^{201}Tl thallous chloride), and ^{99m}Tc pyrophosphate (PYP) myocardial infarct scan.

CENTRAL NERVOUS SYSTEM IMAGING

The central nervous system consists of the brain and spinal cord. For patients with diseases of the central or peripheral nervous systems, nuclear medicine techniques can be used to assess the effectiveness of surgery or radiation therapy, document the extent of a tumor(s) or metastatic disease, and determine the progression or regression of lesions in response to different forms of treatment. Brain perfusion imaging is useful in the evaluation of patients with stroke, transient ischemia, and other neurologic disorders, such as Alzheimer disease (AD), epilepsy, and Parkinson disease. Radionuclide cisternography is particularly useful in facilitating the diagnosis of cerebrospinal fluid leakage after trauma or surgery and normal-pressure hydrocephalus. More recent studies indicate that documented lack of cerebral blood flow should be the criterion of choice to confirm brain death when clinical criteria are equivocal, when a complete neurologic examination cannot be performed, or when patients are younger than 1 year.

Brain SPECT study
Principle

Some imaging agents are capable of penetrating the intact *blood-brain barrier*. After a radiopharmaceutical crosses the blood-brain barrier, it becomes trapped inside the brain. The regional uptake and retention of the tracer are related to the regional perfusion.

Radiopharmaceutical

Adult dose (intravenous injection):
- 20 mCi (740 MBq) of ^{99m}Tc ethylcysteinate dimer (ECD) or
- 20 mCi (740 MBq) of ^{99m}Tc hexamethylpropyleneamine oxime (HMPAO)

Pediatric dose (weight-based intravenous injection) (see Fig 29.7)
- 0.3 mCi/kg (11.1 MBq/kg), minimum of 5 mCi (185 MBq)

Scanning

Before the tracer is injected, the patient is placed in a quiet, darkened area and instructed to close their eyes. These measures are helpful in reducing uptake of the tracer in the visual cortex (occipital lobe). Imaging begins 30 to 90 minutes after ^{99m}Tc ECD injection or ^{99m}Tc HMPAO injection. Tomographic images of the brain are obtained.

Dopamine transporter study
Principle

A reduction of dopaminergic neurons in the striatal region of the brain is a characteristic of Parkinson disease, parkinsonian syndromes, multiple system atrophy, and progressive supranuclear palsy. ^{123}I ioflupane has a high binding affinity for presynaptic dopamine transporters in the striatal region of the brain. This allows for the assessment of functionality in the brain.

Radiopharmaceutical

Adult dose (intravenous injection):
- A slow infusion of 3 to 5 mCi (111–185 MBq) of ^{123}I ioflupane

Scanning

Prior to the administration of ^{123}I ioflupane, a thyroid blocking agent such as Lugol solution should be given to the patient. This will prevent the iodine from being absorbed by the thyroid, thus protecting it from any unnecessary exposure. Imaging begins 3 to 6 hours after injection. Tomographic images of the brain are obtained.

Central nervous system studies

Central nervous system studies include brain perfusion imaging-SPECT study, brain imaging-acetazolamide challenge study, central nervous system shunt patency, cerebrospinal fluid imaging-cisternography/ventriculography, and ^{99m}Tc HMPAO scan for determination of brain death.

ENDOCRINE SYSTEM IMAGING

The endocrine system is located throughout the body. Its primary role is to secrete hormones into the bloodstream, helping maintain a homeostasis throughout the body. Hormones have profound effects on overall body function and metabolism. The endocrine system consists of the thyroid, parathyroid, pituitary, adrenal glands, the islet cells of the pancreas, and the gonads. Nuclear medicine procedures have played a significant part in the current understanding of the function of the endocrine glands and their role in health and disease. These procedures are useful for monitoring the treatment of endocrine disorders, especially in the thyroid gland.

Thyroid scan
Principle

Thyroid imaging is performed to evaluate the size, shape, nodularity, and functional status of the thyroid gland. Imaging is used to determine the relative function in different regions within the thyroid, to screen for thyroid cancer, and to differentiate hyperthyroidism, nodular goiter, solitary thyroid nodule, and thyroiditis. Scanning can also determine the presence and site of thyroid tissue in unusual areas of the body, such as the tongue and anterior chest (ectopic tissue).

^{99m}Tc pertechnetate or ^{123}I can be used to image the thyroid gland. ^{99m}Tc pertechnetate is trapped by the thyroid gland, but in contrast to ^{123}I, is not *organified*. ^{123}I is organified into the gland and trapped until it is metabolized into thyroid hormones. These agents offer the advantages of a low radiation dose to the patient and well-resolved images.

Radiopharmaceutical

Adult dose:
- 5 mCi (185 MBq) of ^{99m}Tc pertechnetate (intravenous injection)
- 0.2 to 0.3 mCi of ^{123}I (administered orally, pill)

Pediatric dose (see Fig. 29.7):
- 0.03 mCi/kg (1.1 MBq/kg) of ^{99m}Tc pertechnetate (weight-based intravenous injection), minimum of 2.5 mCi (93 MBq)
- 0.0075 mCi/kg (0.28 MBq/kg) of ^{123}I (weight based, administered orally, pill), minimum of 0.027 mCi (1 MBq)

NOTE: Uptake may be affected by thyroid medication, certain foods, and/or drugs, including some iodine-containing contrast agents.

Scanning

Imaging should start 20 minutes after the injection of ^{99m}Tc pertechnetate, or 24 hours after the administration of ^{123}I. A gamma camera with a pinhole collimator is used to obtain anterior, left anterior oblique, and right anterior oblique statics of the thyroid. The pinhole collimator is a thick, conical collimator that allows for magnification of the thyroid (see Fig. 29.10).

Iodine-123 thyroid uptake measurement
Principle

Radioiodine is concentrated by the thyroid gland in a manner that reflects the ability of the gland to handle stable dietary iodine. ^{123}I uptake is used to estimate the function of the thyroid gland by measuring its avidity for administered radioiodine. The higher the uptake of ^{123}I, the more active the thyroid; conversely, the lower the uptake, the less functional the gland. Uptake conventionally is expressed as the percentage of the dose in the thyroid gland at a given time after administration. Measurement of ^{123}I uptake is valuable in distinguishing between thyroiditis (significantly reduced uptake) and Graves disease and toxic nodular goiter (Plummer disease), which have an increased uptake. It is also used to determine the appropriateness of a therapeutic dose of ^{131}I in patients with Graves disease.

Radiopharmaceutical

The adult and pediatric doses are the same as listed earlier in the Thyroid Scan section. A standard dose is counted with the thyroid probe the morning of the procedure and is used as the 100% uptake value. The patient's total count is compared with the standard count to obtain the patient percent uptake.

Measurements are obtained using an uptake probe consisting of a 5 × 5 cm (2 × 2 inch) sodium iodide/PMT assembly fitted with a flat-field lead collimator (Fig. 29.19). Uptake readings are generally acquired at 6 hours, at 24 hours, or both.

Total-body iodine-123/ iodine-131 scan
Principle

A total-body ^{123}I/^{131}I (TBI) scan is recommended for locating residual thyroid tissue or recurrent thyroid cancer cells in patients with thyroid carcinoma. Most follicular or papillary thyroid cancers concentrate radioiodine; other types of thyroid cancer do not. A TBI scan is usually performed 1 to 3 months after a thyroidectomy to check for residual normal thyroid tissue and the metastatic spread of the cancer before ^{131}I ablation therapy. After the residual thyroid tissue has been ablated (destroyed), another ^{123}I/^{131}I TBI scan may be performed to check for residual disease.

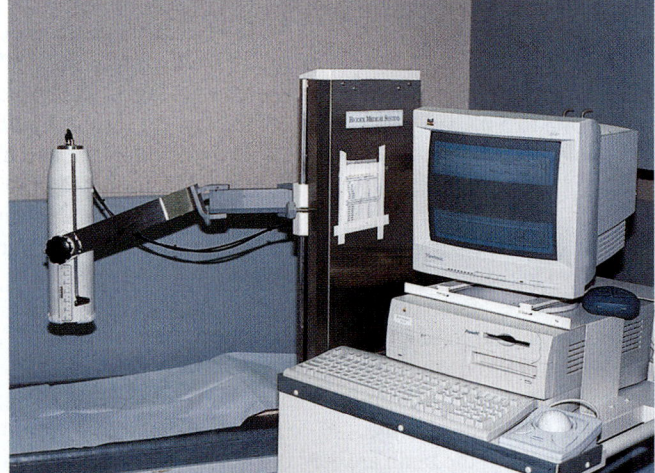

Fig. 29.19 Uptake probe used for thyroid uptake measurements over the extended neck area.

Radiopharmaceutical

Adult dose (administered orally):
- 2 to 5 mCi (74–185 MBq) of ^{123}I

Scanning

Total-body imaging begins 24 to 72 hours after dose administration (depending on the radiopharmaceutical used). Images are obtained of the anterior and posterior whole body. SPECT imaging can also be performed to localize any specific areas of interest.

Endocrine studies

Endocrine studies include the adrenal scan (^{131}I or ^{123}I-labeled MIBG), ectopic thyroid scan (^{131}I or ^{123}I), thyroid scan (^{123}I or ^{99m}Tc pertechnetate), thyroid uptake measurement (^{131}I or ^{123}I), thyroid uptake/scan (^{123}I), total-body iodine scan (^{131}I or ^{123}I), parathyroid scan, and ^{111}In pentetreotide scan (Fig. 29.20).

IMAGING OF THE GASTROINTESTINAL SYSTEM

The gastrointestinal system, or alimentary canal, consists of the mouth, oropharynx, esophagus, stomach, small bowel, colon, and several accessory organs (salivary glands, pancreas, liver, and gallbladder). The liver is the largest internal organ of the body. The portal venous system brings blood from the stomach, bowel, spleen, and pancreas to the liver.

Liver and spleen scan
Principle

Liver and spleen imaging is used to evaluate the liver for functional disease (e.g., cirrhosis, hepatitis, metastatic disease) and to search for residual splenic tissue after splenectomy or traumatic event. Imaging techniques, such as ultrasound, CT, and MRI, provide excellent information about the anatomy of the liver, but nuclear medicine studies can assess the *functional* status of this organ. Liver and spleen scintigraphy is also useful for detecting hepatic lesions and evaluating hepatic morphology, perfusion, and function. It is also used to determine whether certain lesions found with other methods may be benign (e.g., focal nodular hyperplasia), obviating the need for biopsy. Uptake of a radiopharmaceutical in the liver, spleen, and bone marrow depends on blood flow and the functional capacity of the phagocytic cells. In normal patients, 80% to 90% of the radiopharmaceutical is localized in the liver, 5% to 10% is localized in the spleen, and the rest is localized in the bone marrow.

Radiopharmaceutical

Adult dose (intravenous injection):
- 6 mCi (222 MBq) of ^{99m}Tc sulfur colloid

Scanning

Imaging sometimes begins with a flow study based on the indication, but usually planar images (anterior, posterior, right and left anterior oblique, right and left lateral, right posterior oblique, and a marker view) are obtained, followed by SPECT if necessary.

Gastrointestinal studies

Gastrointestinal studies include esophageal scintigraphy, gastroesophageal reflux study, gastric emptying study, hepatic artery perfusion scan, hepatobiliary scan, hepatobiliary scan with gallbladder ejection fraction, liver and spleen scan, liver hemangioma study, Meckel diverticulum study, and salivary gland study.

GENITOURINARY NUCLEAR MEDICINE

Genitourinary nuclear medicine studies are recognized as reliable noninvasive procedures for evaluating the anatomy and function of the renal system (kidneys, ureters, bladder, and urethra). These studies can be accomplished with minimal risk of allergic reactions, unpleasant side effects, or excessive radiation exposure to the organs.

Dynamic renal scan
Principle

Renal imaging is used to assess renal perfusion and function, particularly in renal failure and renovascular hypertension and after renal transplantation. ^{99m}Tc mertiatide (MAG3) is secreted primarily by the proximal renal tubules and is not retained in the parenchyma of normal kidneys.

Radiopharmaceutical

Adult dose (intravenous injection):
- 10 mCi (370 MBq) of ^{99m}Tc MAG3
Pediatric dose (weight-based intravenous injection) (see Fig. 29.7):
- Without flow study: 0.10 mCi/kg (1.85 MBq/kg), minimum of 1.0 mCi (37 MBq)
- With flow study: 0.15 mCi/kg (5.55 MBq/kg)

Scanning

Dynamic imaging is initiated immediately after radiopharmaceutical injection. Because radiographic contrast media may interfere with kidney function, renal scanning is usually delayed for 24 hours after contrast studies. Images are often taken over the posterior lower back, centered at the level of the 12th rib. Transplanted kidneys are imaged in the anterior pelvis. Patients need to be well hydrated before all renal studies.

Genitourinary studies

Genitourinary studies include dynamic renal scan (baseline or no pharmaceutical intervention, with furosemide, or with captopril), ^{99m}Tc dimercaptosuccinic acid (DMSA) renal scan, residual urine determination, testicular scan, and voiding cystography.

IMAGING FOR INFECTION

Imaging for infection is another useful nuclear medicine diagnostic tool. Inflammation, infection, and abscess may be found anywhere within the body. ^{67}Ga scans and ^{111}In-labeled white

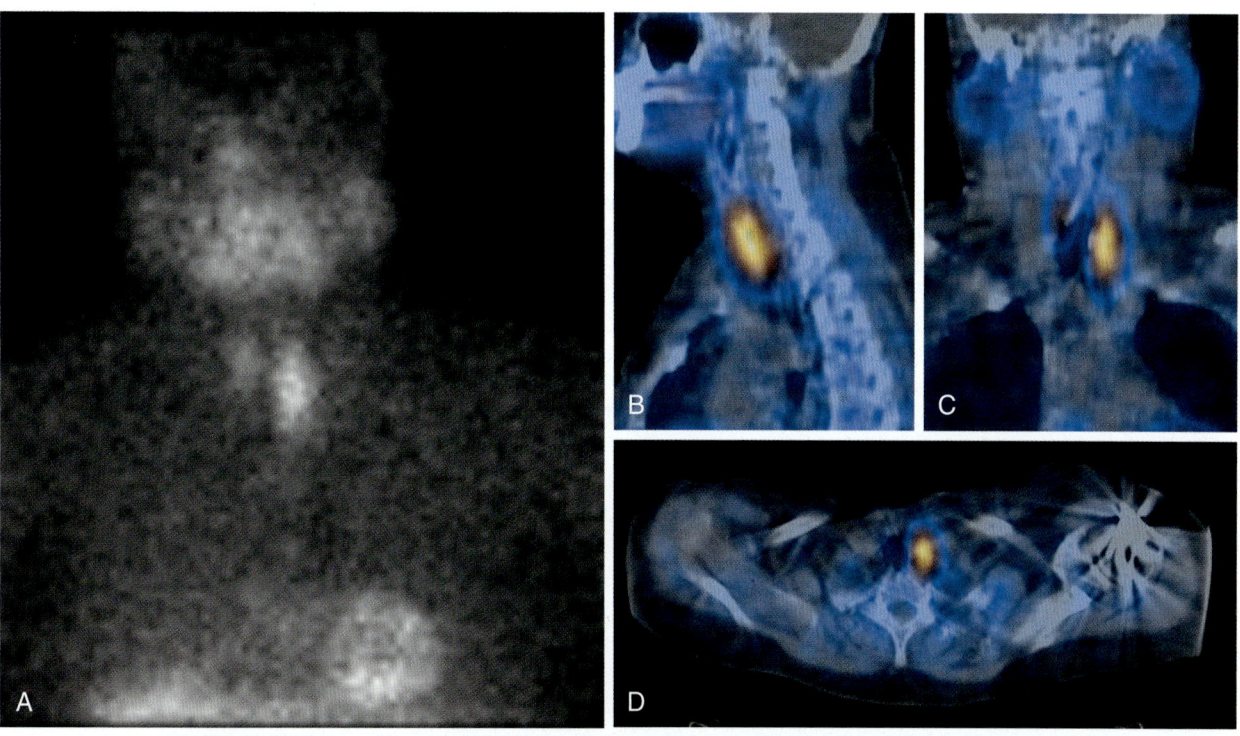

Fig. 29.20 ^{99m}Tc parathyroid SPECT/CT fused imaging. Increased uptake/activity in the left lower lobe. Results are indicative of an adenoma. (**A**) A 60-minute static delay of the neck and chest (tracer activity only). (**B**) Sagittal plane (SPECT/CT fused imaging). (**C**) Coronal plane (SPECT/CT fused imaging). (**D**) Axial plane (SPECT/CT fused imaging).

blood cell scans are useful for diagnosis and localization of infection and inflammation.

Infection studies

Infection studies include ^{67}Ga gallium scan, ^{111}In white blood cell scan, ^{99m}Tc HMPAO, and phase bone scans in conjunction with bone marrow exams following joint replacement surgeries.

RESPIRATORY IMAGING

Respiratory imaging commonly involves the comparison of pulmonary perfusion (using limited, transient capillary blockade) and pulmonary ventilation (using an inhaled radioactive gas or aerosol). Lung imaging is most commonly performed to evaluate acute and chronic pulmonary emboli in patients unable to undergo a CT angiography (CTA). It is also used for lung transplant evaluation.

Xenon-133 lung ventilation scan
Principle

Lung ventilation scans are used in combination with lung perfusion scans. The gas used for a ventilation study must be absorbed significantly by the lungs and diffuse easily. ^{133}Xe has adequate imaging properties, and the body usually absorbs less than 15% of the gas.

Radiopharmaceutical

Adult dose (inhalation):
- 15 to 30 mCi (555–1110 MBq) of ^{133}Xe gas

Scanning

Imaging begins immediately after inhalation of the ^{133}Xe gas within a closed rebreathing system to which oxygen is added and carbon dioxide is withdrawn. For optimal imaging, the ventilation study must precede the ^{99m}Tc perfusion scan. Anterior and posterior images are obtained for the first breath, equilibrium, and *washout*. If possible, left and right posterior oblique images should be obtained between the first breath and equilibrium.

Technetium-99m MAA lung perfusion scan
Principle

^{99m}Tc MAA is a collection of small radioactive particles (~400,000–600,000 in a standard dose) that become trapped in the arterioles of the lungs based on blood flow. If a region (lobe or wedge) of the lung is blocked via emboli, the area will not be perfused by the radiotracer, creating a photopenic area on the images. The lungs contain millions of arterioles; thus there are no side effects due to the blockade.

Radiopharmaceutical

Adult dose (intravenous injection):
- 5 mCi (185 MBq) of ^{99m}Tc MAA

Pediatric dose (weight-based intravenous injection) (see Fig. 29.7):
- If ^{133}Xe was used for the ventilation: 0.03 mCi/kg (1.11 MBq/kg), minimum of 0.4 mCi (14.8 MBq)
- If ^{99m}Tc was used for the ventilation: 0.07 mCi/kg (2.59 MBq/kg)

Scanning

Imaging starts approximately 5 minutes after radiopharmaceutical injection. Eight images are obtained: anterior, posterior, right and left lateral, right and left anterior oblique, and right and left posterior oblique. All patients should have a chest radiograph within 24 hours of the lung scan. The chest radiograph is required for accurate interpretation of the lung scans so as to determine the probability of pulmonary embolism.

Respiratory studies

Respiratory studies include the ^{133}Xe lung ventilation scan, ^{99m}Tc MAA lung perfusion scan, and ^{99m}Tc diethylenetriamine pentaacetic acid (DTPA) lung aerosol scan.

SENTINEL NODE IMAGING

Many tumors metastasize via lymphatic channels. Defining the anatomy of lymph nodes that drain from a primary tumor site helps guide surgeons resecting the nodes during surgery. Sentinel node imaging does just this; it maps the routes of lymphatic drainage and permits more effective surgical or radiation treatments. Radionuclide lympho-scintigraphy has been useful in patients in whom the channels are relatively inaccessible. This method is indicated for patients with melanoma and breast cancer.

Principle

Colloidal particles injected intradermally or subcutaneously adjacent to a tumor site show a drainage pattern similar to that of the tumor. Colloidal particles in the 10- to 50-nm range seem to be the most effective for this application. The colloidal particles drain into the sentinel lymph node, where they are trapped by phagocytic activity; this aids in the identification of the lymph nodes most likely to be sites of metastatic deposits from the tumor.

Radiopharmaceutical

Adult dose (intradermal/subcutaneous injection):
- 100 μCi (3.7 MBq) of ^{99m}Tc filtered sulfur colloid in a volume of 0.1 mL per injection site (up to four injection sites)

Scanning

Patients with malignant melanoma should be positioned supine or prone on the imaging table based on tumor location, and patients with breast cancer should be positioned supine with their arms extended over their head. Images are acquired immediately after injection, and then every few minutes for the first 15 minutes followed by every 5 minutes for 30 minutes. Additional lateral and oblique views are required after visualization of the sentinel node.

THERAPEUTIC NUCLEAR MEDICINE

The potential that radionuclides have for detecting and treating cancer has been recognized for a long time. The most common nuclear medicine therapies use radioiodine (^{131}I) to treat Graves disease. High-dose ^{131}I therapy (≥30 mCi) can be used in patients with residual thyroid cancer or thyroid metastases. ^{131}I is also labeled with monoclonal antibodies (^{131}I-MoAb) to target specific cancers such as non-Hodgkin lymphoma. ^{90}Yttrium (^{90}Y-MoAb) can also be labeled in a similar manner to treat the same cancer. Skeletal metastases occur in more than 50% of patients with breast, lung, or prostate cancer in the end stages of the disease. ^{89}Sr (strontium-89) or ^{153}Sm (samarium-153) ethylene diamine tetramethylene phosphate (EDTMP) is often useful for managing patients with bone pain from metastases when other treatments have failed. ^{90}Y microspheres are a new treatment in nuclear medicine. This therapy involves the embolization of radioactive ^{90}Y microspheres straight into the liver's arterial supply, directly delivering them into primary and secondary hepatic tumors. New radiopharmaceuticals are being developed every day to target inoperable/treatable cancers.

SPECIAL IMAGING PROCEDURES

Special imaging procedures include dacryoscintigraphy, the LeVeen shunt patency test, and lymphoscintigraphy of the limbs.

TUMOR IMAGING

Octreoscan

Principle

Somatostatin is a neuroregulatory peptide known to localize on many cells of neuroendocrine origin. Cell membrane receptors with a high affinity for somatostatin have been shown to be present in most neuroendocrine tumors, including carcinoids, islet cell carcinomas, and gonadotropin hormone–producing pituitary adenomas. ^{111}In pentetreotide (OctreoScan) is a radiolabeled analog of the neuroendocrine peptide somatostatin. This allows it to localize in somatostatin receptor–rich tumors and aid in identifying questionable masses.

Radiopharmaceutical

Adult dose (intravenous injection):
- 6 mCi (222 MBq) of ^{111}In pentetreotide

Scanning

At 4 to 6 hours after injection, anterior and posterior whole-body images should be acquired. At 24 hours, whole-body images should be obtained once more along with anterior and posterior spot views of the chest and abdomen. SPECT imaging is most helpful in the localization of intraabdominal tumors. SPECT/CT can assist in lesion localization. Additional imaging at 48 and 72 hours is at the discretion of the radiologist interpreting the exam. Images of an octreotide scan can be seen in Fig. 29.18.

Tumor studies

Tumor studies include ^{67}Ga tumor scan, ^{99m}Tc sestamibi breast scan, ^{111}In capromab pendetide (ProstaScint) scan, ^{99m}Tc nofetumomab merpentan (Verluma), and ^{111}In OctreoScan.

Principles and Facilities in Positron Emission Tomography (PET)

PET is a noninvasive nuclear imaging technique that involves the administration of a positron-emitting radioactive tracer followed by subsequent imaging of its physiologic distribution. PET radiotracers use extremely small molar amounts of the radiopharmaceutical per dose, which means equilibrium conditions within the body are not altered. Currently, PET is used to image multiple organs in the body (heart, brain, lungs, and prostate).

Three important factors distinguish PET from all radiologic procedures and from other nuclear imaging procedures. First, the results of the data acquisition and analysis techniques yield an image related to a particular physiologic parameter, such as blood flow or metabolism. The ensuing image is aptly called a *functional* or *parametric image*. Second, the images are created by the simultaneous detection of a pair of *annihilation photons* that result from *positron* decay (Fig. 29.21). The third factor that distinguishes PET is the chemical and biologic form of the radiopharmaceutical. The radiotracer is specifically chosen for its similarity to naturally occurring biochemical constituents of the human body. For example, if the radiopharmaceutical is a form of sugar, it behaves much like the natural sugar used by the body. The kinetics or the movement of the radiotracer (such as sugar) within the body is followed by using the PET scanner to acquire multiple images that measure the distribution of the *radioactivity concentration* as a function of time. From this measurement, the local tissue metabolism may be deduced by converting a temporal sequence of images into a single parametric image. PET is a multidisciplinary technique that involves four major processes: radionuclide production, radiopharmaceutical production, data acquisition (PET scanner or tomograph), and image reconstruction and processing. This section of the chapter is focused on these major categories within PET.

POSITRONS

Positrons (β^+) are the result of a radiation decay process (positron decay) in which an unstable *proton-rich* nucleus is attempting to reach its ground state. As the number of protons increases within a nucleus, so does the net positive charge and its instability. Based on *Coulomb forces* inside the nucleus, protons continuously try to push away from one another. To help stabilize these atoms, the nucleus spontaneously converts a proton into a neutron. This then lowers the net positive charge of the nucleus by one, and the neutron acts as a buffer among the remaining protons. To account for the loss of the positive charge and energy, a positron is emitted from the nucleus. Positrons are identical to electrons with the exception that they possess a positive charge instead of a negative one. The characteristics of positrons are listed in Table 29.3.

For the positron decay process to occur, the nucleus must possess at least an excess of energy greater than 1.022 MeV (equivalent to the mass of two electrons). Positrons are emitted from the nucleus with high velocity and kinetic energy. As mentioned in the Basic Nuclear Physics section of this chapter, each radioisotope releases its own defined amount of energy per decay and decay process (like a fingerprint). This means different radioisotopes that decay by positron emission emit positrons with different energies. Based on their energy, positrons from different elements can travel farther from the nucleus than others (Fig. 29.22A).

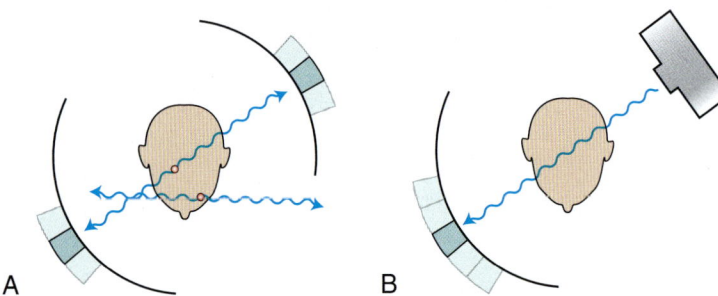

Fig. 29.21 (A) PET relies on the simultaneous detection of a pair of annihilation radiations emitted from the body. (B) In contrast, CT depends on the detection of x-rays transmitted through the body.

TABLE 29.3
Positron characteristics

Definition	Positively charged electron
Origin	Proton-rich nuclei
Production	Accelerators and cyclotrons
Nuclide decay	$p = n + \beta^+$ neutrino
Positron decay	Annihilation to two 0.511-MeV photons
Number	About 240 known
Range	Proportional to kinetic energy of β^+
Routine PET nuclides	^{11}C, ^{13}N, ^{15}O, ^{18}F, ^{82}Rb

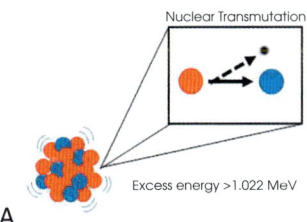

A

An unstable radioactive proton-rich nucleus goes through positron decay by converting a proton into a neutron and emitting a positron. For this decay process to occur the unstable nucleus must contain an excess of energy greater than 1.022 MeV.

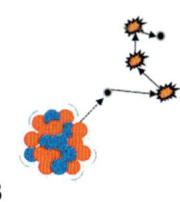

B

The emitted positron interacts with surrounding matter (attenuators), slowing it down.

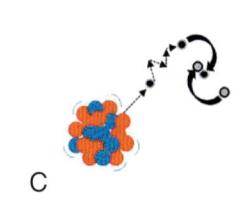

C

As the positron approaches a resting state, the more likely it is to interact with an electron due to the attractive forces between the two. These forces pull them toward one another in a spiraling manner.

Proton (+)
Neutron (0)
Electron (−)
Positron (β⁺)

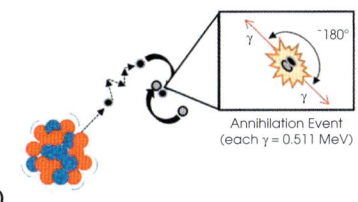

D

The positron and electron eventually collide and annihilate. *Annihilation* is a process that consists of a positron and an electron combining and transforming their collective masses completely into energy. The energy is released in the form of 2 gamma rays emitted ~180° apart from one another.

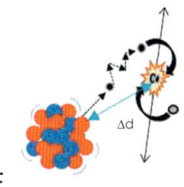

E

The distance between where the positron was emitted and where the annihilation takes place is known as the *range* (Δd). The range is based on a positron's energy at the time of emission. The more energy, the larger the range. Smaller ranges are better for imaging.

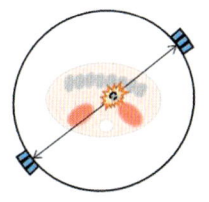

F

Within the PET camera, annihilation photons almost simultaneously strike the Detectors on opposing sides. When both photons of a single annihilation are detected by the camera it is called a *coincidence event*. Calculations are then made to localize where the event took place. The summation of thousands to millions of events are used to construct an image.

Fig. 29.22 The positron decay process.

Once the positron has been emitted, it begins to rapidly slow due to interactions with surrounding matter (attenuators) (Fig. 29.22B). As it decreases in speed, the positron becomes more likely to interact with a nearby electron (Coulomb forces, opposite charges attract). When the attraction between the two particles is strong enough to pull them away from their original path, they begin to spiral toward one another (like water circling a drain) (Fig. 29.22C). Eventually, the particles collide and totally *annihilate* or disintegrate. During the annihilation process, the combined positron-electron mass (1.022 amu) is completely transformed into two equal-energy photons of 0.511 MeV (annihilation photons/total energy 1.022 MeV), which are emitted approximately 180 degrees (±0.3 degrees) from one another (Fig. 29.22D). The average distance a positron travels after being ejected from the nucleus to where the annihilation takes place is known as the positron's *range* (Fig. 29.22E). Specific isotope properties can be reviewed in Table 29.4. The resulting annihilation photons behave like gamma and x-rays: they have sufficient energy to traverse body tissues with only modest attenuation, and they can be detected externally (Fig. 29.22F).

The positron-emitting radioisotopes currently being used in PET are carbon-11 (^{11}C), nitrogen-13 (^{13}N), oxygen-15 (^{15}O), rubidium-82 (^{82}Rb), and fluorine-18 (^{18}F). ^{18}F is the most commonly used radioisotope because it can be used as a hydrogen substitute in many compounds. This substitution of ^{18}F for hydrogen is successfully accomplished because of its small size and strong bond with carbon. Copper and gallium agents are currently being researched.

TABLE 29.4
Characteristics of common PET radionuclides

Nuclide (decay product)	Physical half-life	Decay mode	Maximal and average positron energy (keV)	Maximum and mean range in water (mm)	Production reaction
Carbon-11 (Boron-11)	20.3 min	99.8% positron 0.2% electron capture	960, 320	4.1, 1.1	^{14}N(p,alpha)^{11}C^a
Nitrogen-13 (Carbon-13)	10 min	100% positron	1198, 432	5.1, 1.5	^{16}O(p,alpha)^{13}N ^{13}C(p,n)^{13}N
Oxygen-15 (Nitrogen-15)	124 s	99.9% positron	1732, 696	7.3, 2.5	^{15}N(p,n)^{15}O ^{14}N(d,n)^{15}O
Fluorine-18 (Oxygen-18)	110 min	97% positron 3% electron capture	634, 202	2.4, 0.6	^{18}O(p,n)^{18}F ^{20}Ne(d,alpha)^{18}F ^{16}O(^{3}He,alpha)^{18}F
Rubidium-82	1.27 min (75 s)	96% positron 4% electron capture	3356, 1385	14.1, 5.9	^{82}Sr generator (T$_{1/2}$ 25.3 days)

^{a}This symbolism means that a proton is accelerated into an atom of nitrogen-14, causing ejection of an alpha particle from the nucleus to produce an atom of carbon-11.
From Mettler FA, Guiberteau MJ: *Mettler's essentials of nuclear medicine imaging*, ed 6. Philadelphia, 2012, Elsevier.

RADIONUCLIDE PRODUCTION

Radionuclides used in PET exams are produced using a *nuclear particle accelerator* or cyclotron to bombard appropriate nonradioactive *target* atoms with accelerated charged particles. High energies are necessary to overcome the electrostatic and nuclear forces of the target nuclei so that a nuclear reaction can occur. An example is the production of ^{15}O. *Deuterons* (d), or heavy hydrogen ions, are accelerated to approximately 7 MeV. The target material is stable nitrogen gas (N_2). The resultant nuclear reaction yields a neutron and a ^{15}O atom, which can be written in the following form: ^{14}N(d,n)^{15}O (^{14}N is the target material, the deuteron (d) is the bombarding charged particle, the neutron (n) is emitted from the nucleus, and ^{15}O is the product). The ^{15}O atom quickly associates with a stable ^{16}O atom that has been intentionally added to the target gas to produce a radioactive ^{15}O-^{16}O molecule in the form of O_2 (oxygen is a diatomic element).

When the unstable or radioactive ^{15}O atom decays via positron emission, the ^{15}O atom becomes a stable ^{15}N atom and forces the O_2 molecule to break apart. This process is shown in Fig. 29.23, and the decay schemes for the four routinely produced PET radionuclides are depicted in Fig. 29.24. The common reactions used for the production of positron-emitting forms of carbon, nitrogen, oxygen, and fluorine are given in Table 29.4.

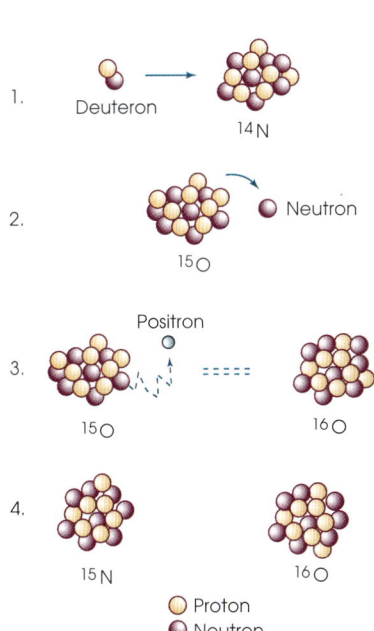

Fig. 29.23 Typical radionuclide production sequence. The ^{14}N(d,n)^{15}O reaction is used for making ^{15}O-^{16}O molecules. *1*, A deuteron ion is accelerated to high energy (7 MeV) by a cyclotron and impinges on a stable ^{14}N nucleus. *2*, As a result of the nuclear reaction, a neutron is emitted, leaving a radioactive nucleus of ^{15}O. *3*, ^{15}O atom quickly associates with ^{16}O atom to form O_2 molecule. Later, unstable ^{15}O atom emits a positron. *4*, As a result of positron decay (i.e., positron exits nucleus), ^{15}O atom is transformed into stable ^{15}N atom, and O_2 molecule breaks apart.

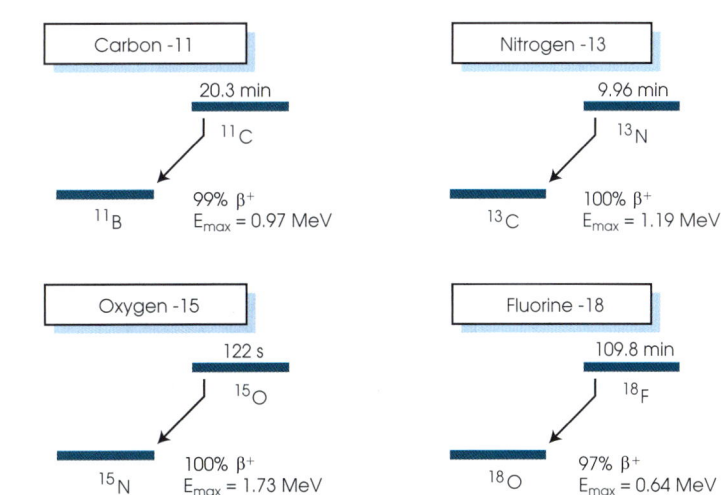

Fig. 29.24 Decay schemes for ^{11}C, ^{13}N, ^{15}O, and ^{18}F. Each positron emitter decays to a stable nuclide by ejecting a positron from the nucleus. E_{max} represents the maximum energy of the emitted positron. Electron capture is a competitive process with positron decay; positron decay is not always 100%.

Because of the very short half-lives of the routinely used positron-emitting radionuclides of oxygen, nitrogen, rubidium, and carbon, nearby access to a nuclear particle accelerator, cyclotron, or generator is necessary to produce sufficient quantities for diagnostic testing. The most common device to achieve nuclide production within reasonable space (223 m² [250 ft²]) and energy (150 kW) constraints is a compact medical cyclotron (Fig. 29.25).

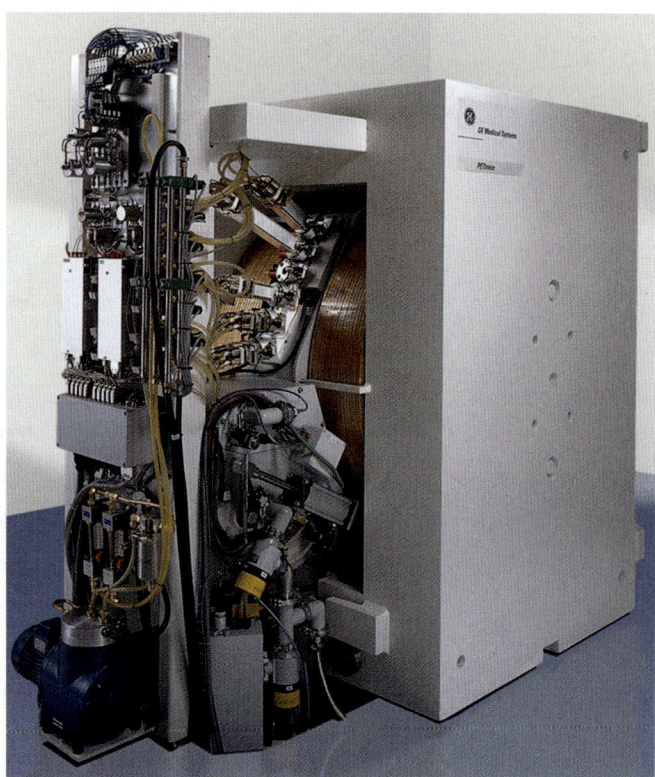

Fig. 29.25 Compact cyclotron (2.2 m high × 1.5 m wide × 1.5 m deep) used for routine production of PET isotopes. Cyclotron can be located in a concrete vault, or it can be self-shielded. Particles are accelerated in vertical orbits and impinge on targets located near the top center of the machine. This is an example of a negative-ion cyclotron.

(Courtesy GE Medical Systems, Milwaukee, WI.)

RADIOPHARMACEUTICAL PRODUCTION

Living organisms are composed primarily of compounds that contain the elements hydrogen, carbon, nitrogen, and oxygen. In PET, radiotracers are made by synthesizing compounds with radioactive isotopes of these elements. Chemically, the radioactive isotope is indistinguishable from its equivalent stable isotope.

Radiopharmaceuticals are synthesized from radionuclides derived from the target material. These agents may be simple, such as the ^{15}O-^{16}O molecules described earlier, or they may be much more complex. Regardless of the chemical complexity of the radioactive molecule, all radiopharmaceuticals must be synthesized rapidly. This entails specialized techniques not only to create the labeled substance but also to verify the purity (chemical, radiochemical, and radionuclide) of the radiotracer.

One of the simplest radiopharmaceuticals used in PET studies is ^{15}O-water ($[^{15}$O]-H_2O), which is produced continuously from the ^{14}N(d,n)^{15}O nuclear reaction or in batches from the ^{15}N(p,n)^{15}O nuclear reaction. As previously discussed, the radioactive oxygen quickly combines with a stable ^{16}O atom, which has been added to the stable N_2 target gas, to form an oxygen molecule (O_2). The ^{15}O-^{16}O molecule is reduced over a platinum catalyst with small amounts of stable H_2 and N_2 gas. Radioactive water vapor ($[^{15}$O]-H_2O) is produced and collected in sterile saline for injection. It is used primarily for the determination of local cerebral blood flow (LCBF). PET LCBF images from one subject using two different techniques are shown in Fig. 29.26. Blood flow to tumor, heart, kidney, or other tissues can also be measured using $[^{15}$O]-H_2O.

The most common and widely used PET radiopharmaceutical for clinical PET imaging is a little more complex than labeled water and employs ^{18}F-labeled fluoride ions (F–) to form a sugar analog called $[^{18}$F]-2-fluoro-2-deoxy-G-glucose (^{18}F-FDG). This agent is used to determine the local metabolic rate of glucose use in tumor, brain, heart, or other tissues that use glucose at an increased rate. The glucose obtained from food is metabolized by the body's cells via the first stage of cellular respiration (glycolysis) and continues to be broken down, creating large quantities of adenosine triphosphate (ATP). However, in contrast to glucose, ^{18}F-FDG cannot be completely metabolized. Once ^{18}F-FDG is phosphorylated into fluorodeoxyglucose-6-phosphate ($[^{18}$F]-FDG-6-PO_4), the cell can no longer process it. The cell then retains the newly formed $[^{18}$F]-FDG-6-PO_4 for a few hours before breaking it down and filtering it out. This period of retention allows for imaging. These pathways for glucose and ^{18}F-FDG are shown schematically in Fig. 29.27.

The total time for FDG production, which includes target irradiation (60–90 minutes), radiochemical synthesis (30–60 minutes), and purity certification (15 minutes), is approximately 2 to 3 hours (depending on the exact synthesis method used). Because of the short half-life of most positron-emitting radioisotopes, radiopharmaceutical production must be closely tied to the clinical patient schedule. Injected doses of ^{18}F-FDG range from 5 to 20 mCi; a standard dose is 15 to 20 mCi. FDG is dissolved in a few milliliters of isotonic saline and is administered intravenously.

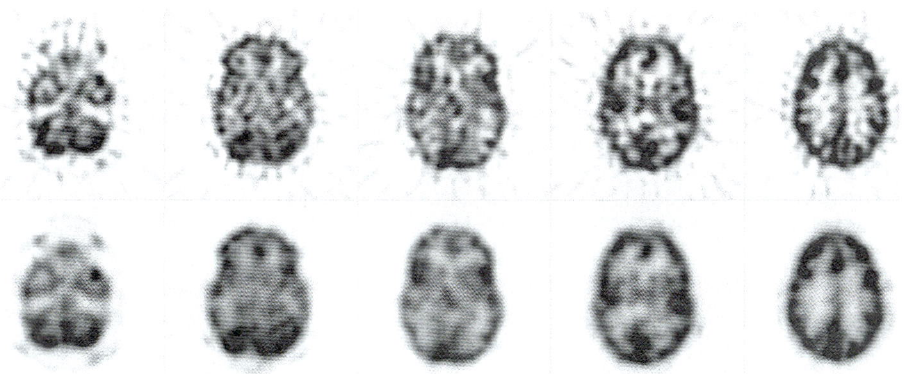

Camera design

Scintillators used in PET cameras can be constructed from various materials. Each material has a different set of characteristics that may improve or degrade the quality of the system. The optimal scintillator would have a short decay time, high light output, high-energy resolution, and high stopping power. Characteristics of commercial materials available are listed

Fig. 29.26 PET local cerebral blood flow images. Images in the *top row* were created using a standard filtered back-projection reconstruction technique. An iterative reconstructive method was used to create images in the *bottom row* from the same raw data that were used for upper images. In all images, *dark areas* correspond to high brain blood flow. There is about an 8-mm separation between each brain slice within a row.

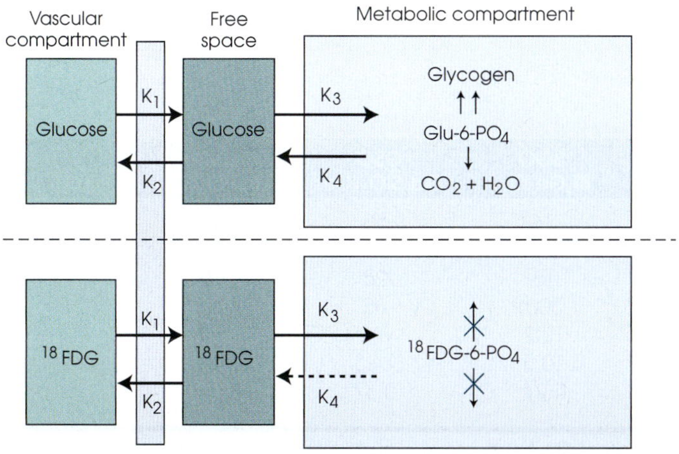

Fig. 29.27 Glucose compartmental model *(above dashed line)* compared with the ^{18}F-FDG model *(below dashed line)*. ^{18}F-FDG does not go to complete storage (glycogen) or metabolism (CO_2 + H_2O) as does glucose. The constants (K) refer to reaction rates for moving substances from one compartment to another. *Dashed arrow* refers to extremely small K value that can usually be neglected.

in Table 29.5. The newest scintillator, lutetium orthosilicate (Lu_2SiO_5:Ce), has a higher light output (approximately four times that of bismuth germanate [BGO]) and faster photofluorescent decay (approximately 7.5 times that of BGO). Scintillator dimensions are also being reduced to improve resolution. At the present time, the resolution within the image plane for PET scanners is between 3 mm and 5 mm full width at half maximum. This means an image of a point source of radioactivity appears to be 3 to 5 mm wide at half the maximum intensity of the source image.

The basic component of the PET scanner is the block. A block is composed of a scintillation crystal coupled with four PMTs. The crystal is cut into a matrix (6 × 6, 7 × 8, or 8 × 8) of small rectangular boxes (3–6 mm long, 3–6 mm wide) with varying depths (10–30 mm deep) (Fig. 29.28). These blocks are then organized into a row to form detector modules. Next, the modules are aligned side by side to construct a ring (Fig. 29.29), and to increase the imaging field (z), several rings are combined. Typical new scanners have 800 to 1000 detectors per ring.

The average bore width (x, y) of these scanners is approximately 70 cm, with newer scanners being slightly larger in diameter. The radial field of view (FOV) or the imaging dimension parallel to the detector rings for these scanners is approximately 25 cm (10 inches) and 55 cm (22 inches) (Fig. 29.30). The z-axis, or dimension perpendicular to the detector rings, is 15 to 50 cm (6–20 inches). An actual PET/CT scanner can be seen in Fig. 29.31.

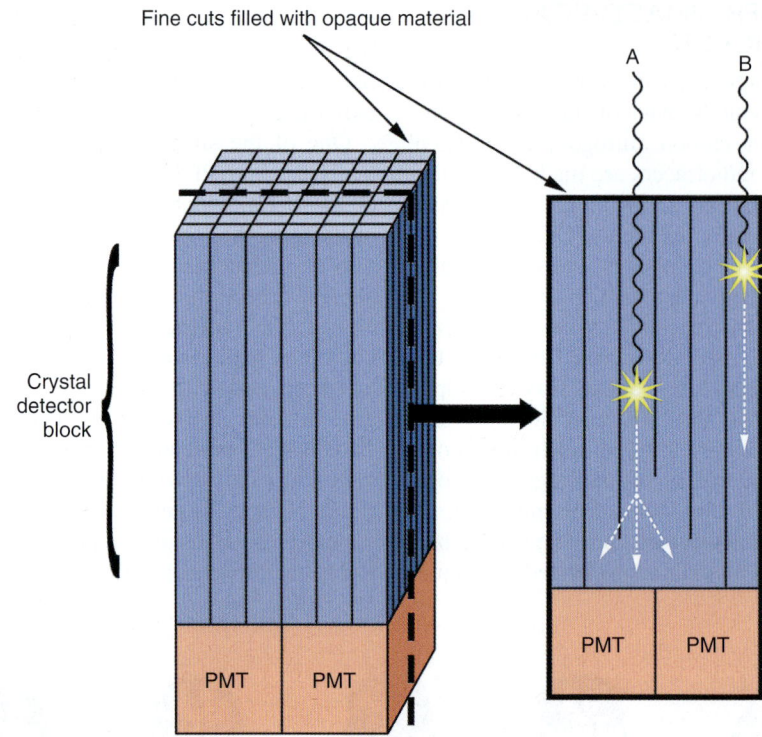

Fig. 29.28 PET scintillation block detector. Many crystal detectors are made from a single block of material and have cuts made to different depths and filled with opaque material. There are often 8 × 8 detector elements made, and the different depths of cuts allow localization with only four photomultiplier tubes (*PMTs*). *A,* If a photon interacts with a central detector element, the shallow cut allows the light from the scintillation to be localized by several PMTs. *B,* A photon interacting with a detector element near the edge of the block may have light that is seen by one PMT only.

(From Mettler FA, Guiberteau MJ. *Mettler's essentials of nuclear medicine imaging*, ed 6, Philadelphia: Elsevier; 2012.)

TABLE 29.5
Properties of PET scintillator materials

Property	NaI	BGO $Bi_4Ge_3O_{12}$	GSO Gd_2SiO_5(Ce)	LSO Lu_2SiO_5(Ce)	LYSO $Lu_{2(1-x)}Y_{2x}SiO_5$(Ce)
Z (atomic number) stopping power	50	74	58	66	65
Density (g/cm³)	3.7	7.1	6.7	7.4	7.1
Light yield	100	15	26	75	80
Decay constant (ns)	230	300	65	40	41
Energy resolution @ 511 keV (%)	6.6	10.2	8.5	10	14
Attenuation length (mm) for 511 keV photons	28.8	10.5	14.3	11.6	12
Attenuation coefficient (cm⁻¹) @ 511 keV	0.34	0.94	0.67	0.87	0.83

BGO, Bismuth germanium oxide; *GSO*, gadolinium oxyorthosilicate; *LSO*, lutetium oxyorthosilicate; *LYSO*, lutetium yttrium orthosilicate; *NaI*, sodium iodide.

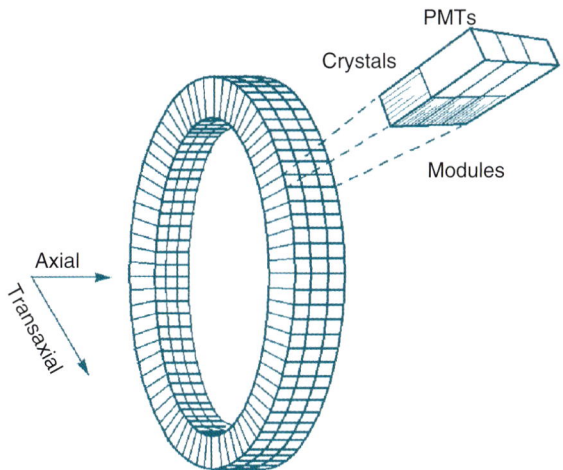

Fig. 29.29 Detector blocks, or modules, are used to construct a ring of detectors around the patient. Hundreds of blocks are used to create 18 to 40 consecutive rings of detectors that form a cylindrical field of view approximately 5 cm long and that can acquire many slices of coincidence data at one time. *PMTs,* Photomultiplier tubes.

(From Waterstram-Rich K, Gilmore D. *Nuclear medicine and PET/CT: technology and techniques,* ed 8, Philadelphia: Elsevier; 2017.)

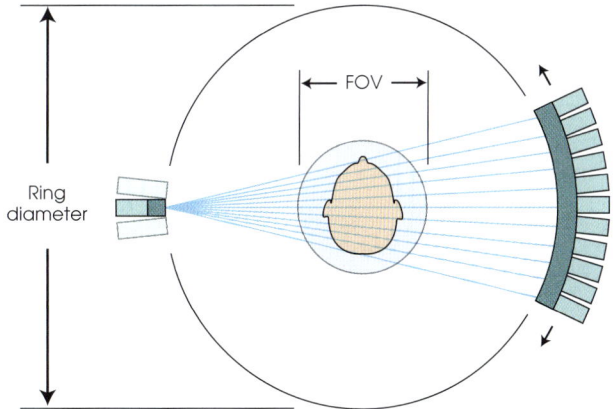

Fig. 29.30 Detector arrangement in neurologic PET ring (head-only scanner). Rays from opposed detector pairs (*lines* between detectors) depict possible coincidence events. The useful field of view *(FOV)* is delineated by the *central circle*.

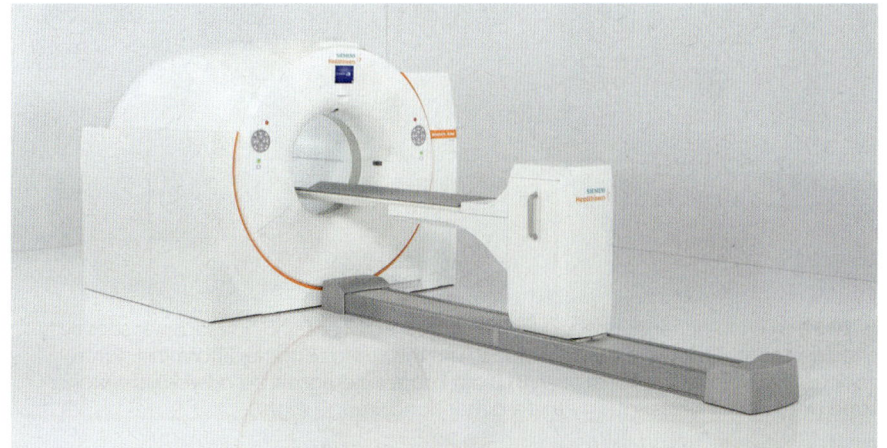

Fig. 29.31 The Siemens Biograph Vision Quadra is a whole-body PET/CT scanner. The bed is capable of moving in and out of the unit to measure the distribution of PET radiopharmaceuticals throughout the entire body.

(Courtesy of Siemens Medical Solutions USA, Inc.)

The sensitivity of a PET camera has contributed to not only the scintillator being used but also whether or not the camera is using *septa*. PET collimation is the addition of thin lead or tungsten attenuators placed between the detector elements. The collimation is designed to block annihilation photons not directly in line with the detector. This reduces the sensitivity greatly, requires higher radiopharmaceutical doses to be administered, and requires longer imaging times, but increases the camera's resolution. PET cameras with septa installed are known as *2-dimensional (2D)* PET Scanners. With improvements in software reconstruction techniques, current PET scanners have eliminated septa between detector components. These cameras are referred to as *3-dimensional (3D)* PET scanners. 3D systems allow for first, second, third, fourth, and upward adjacent planes (rings) to be used to produce images all at one time (Fig. 29.32). With the inclusion of the additional cross-plane information, the PET scanner's *sensitivity* is greatly increased. Thus, injected doses of radiopharmaceutical are significantly reduced (50%–90% less radioactivity given) to yield PET images with a quality equivalent to that of images obtained from the original dose levels used in 2D PET scanners.

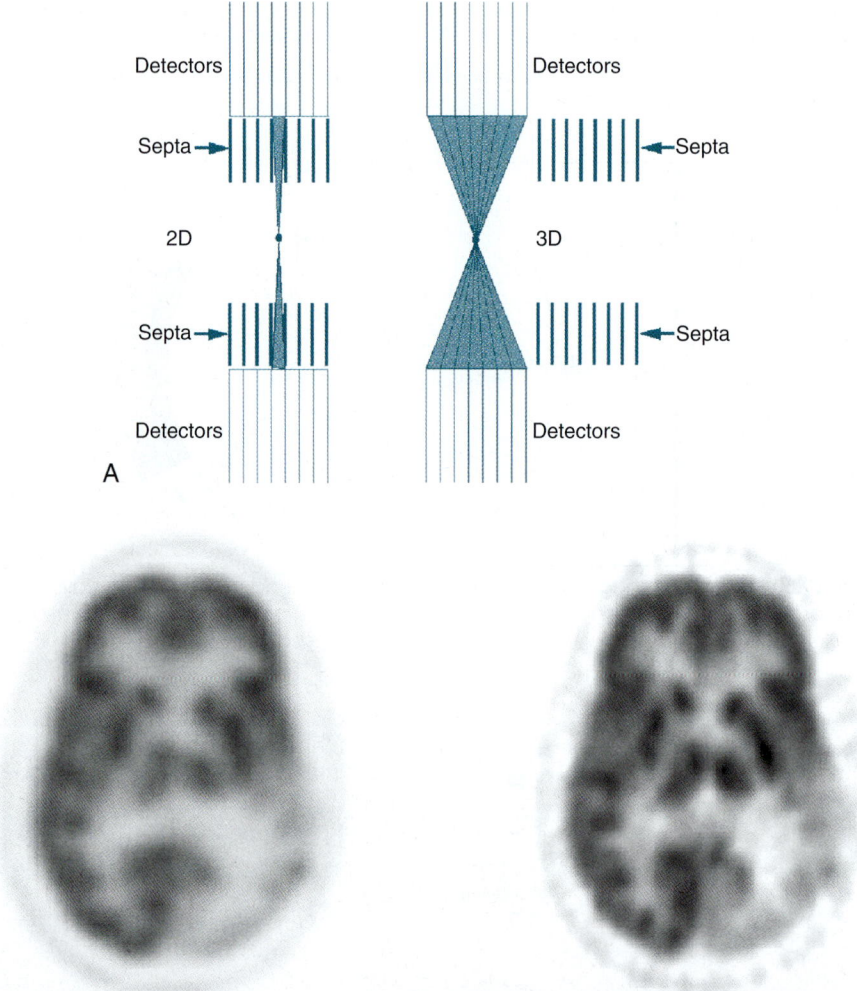

Fig. 29.32 (**A**) Two-dimensional acquisition with septa in position has scanner sensitivity limited by septa. Three-dimensional mode with the septa retracted from the gantry significantly increases the sensitivity. (**B**) Brain images demonstrate a two-dimensional image *(left)* and a higher-quality three-dimensional image *(right)*.

(From Waterstram-Rich K, Gilmore D. *Nuclear medicine and PET/CT: technology and techniques,* ed 8, Philadelphia: Elsevier; 2017.)

DATA AND IMAGE ACQUISITION

The ring design described above is engineered to capture annihilation photons after they are produced. When two identical or isoenergetic photons are emitted at almost exactly 180 degrees from one another, the nearly simultaneous detection of both photons can define a straight line that passes through the body. The detection of the two annihilation photons is called a *coincidence event*, and the theoretical line that was created is known as the *line-of-response* (LOR). For a coincidence event to occur and be deemed real, the photons must reach the detectors within a specific time frame or the *coincidence time window* (6–12 ns). If one photon is detected and no other photon is observed during that time window, the original event is discarded. This is defined as electronic collimation. If both photons strike opposing detectors, it is referred to as a *true* coincidence event, a LOR is generated, and it is used to identify the location of the annihilation. Because each photon travels at the speed of light, coincidence electronics can use simple math to deduce where the event took place based on the time it took each photon to reach the detectors. Multiple true events are summed to formulate an image.

Coincidence events fall into one of three categories: true events, scattered events, or random events. A true event is when the annihilation photon pair, unaffected by any attenuation or scatter, strikes the detectors within the resolving time and is registered as a single count. Scattered events are those in which one of the photons from the annihilation is deflected but not slowed enough to fall outside of the coincidence time frame. This creates a false LOR and increases background noise in the image. A random event is two annihilations taking place in two separate locations, and a single photon from each pair strikes opposing detectors within the coincidence timing window. Again, a false LOR is created, degrading the images. Refer to Fig. 29.33 to get a better understanding of these events.

PET scanners must operate with a high sensitivity; as a result, scanners must also be able to handle very high count rates with minimum *deadtime* losses. Coincidence events are collected not only for detector pairs within each ring (direct-plane information) but also between adjacent rings (cross-plane information), as shown in Fig. 29.34. However, not all photons emitted from the patient can be detected. The emission process is *isotropic*, which means that the annihilation photons are emitted with equal probability in all directions so that only a small fraction of the total number of photons emitted from the patient actually strike two opposing detectors (Fig. 29.35). In most cases, almost 99% of annihilation events are missed or discarded by the camera.

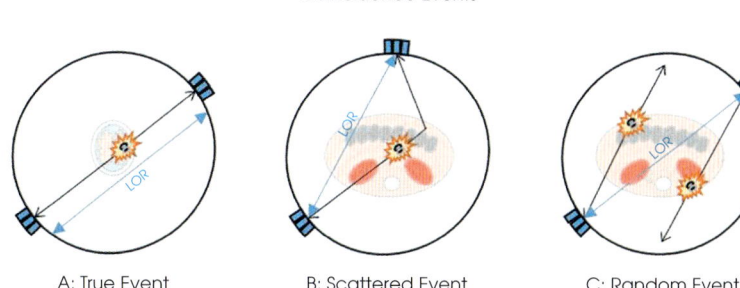

Fig. 29.33 (**A**) A *true event* is when annihilation photons from a single annihilation event are detected ~180 degrees apart within the coincidence timing window. This creates correct LOR, increasing the target to background ratio. (**B**) A *scattered event* occurs due to attenuation deflecting the photon. This results in an incorrect LOR and degrades the image. (**C**) A *random event* is the resultant of two separate annihilation events striking detectors on opposite sides of the gantry within the same coincidence timing window. This also creates a false LOR and decreases the target to background ratio. *Remember,* all coincidence events are detected and are potentially applied to the final image.

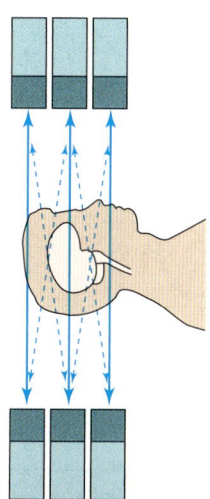

Fig. 29.34 Side-view schematic of a small portion of a multiring PET scanner. *Darker green squares* indicate the scintillator-matrix, which is attached to multiple photomultiplier tubes. *Solid lines* indicate the direct planes, and *dashed lines* depict the cross planes. Improvements in PET scanner instrumentation not only permit cross-plane information between adjacent rings to be acquired but also allow for expansion to the second, third, fourth, and fifth neighboring rings. This significantly enhances overall scanner sensitivity.

Imaging

The *z*-axis, or the imaging dimension parallel to the detector rings for these scanners, is approximately 15 to 50 cm (6–20 inches). When imaging a patient, the length of the *z*-axis is referred to as the bed. Depending on the imaging being performed, one to several beds may be required. To obtain enough counts to form a diagnostic PET image, the patient must remain in one bed position for a set period of time (~2–4 minutes). Once adequate counts have been gathered, the scanner table moves the patient in/out to scan the next section of their body. Because the resolution and sensitivity of PET cameras become increasingly poor as it approaches the edges of the FOV, motion increments are designed to overlap by a few centimeters. This allows for sufficient axial sampling achieved for all but the first and last bed positions. Fig. 29.36 illustrates bed and patient positioning.

In PET there are three types of scans. The first type is brain and cardiac imaging, which only requires one bed. Imaging times vary due to the attenuation (skull) and radiopharmaceutical doses. Brain scans can take up to 10 minutes, while only 5 minutes are required for most heart scans. The second type is known as "eye-to-thigh" imaging. Eye-to-thigh imaging is just that; images are obtained from a patient's orbitals to their midthighs. A scout or low-grade x-ray image (similar to CT) is taken of the patient to identify these anatomic structures so that the technologist can adjust the beginning and ending points. The average eye-to-thigh exam is composed of about seven beds, at 3 minutes per bed. The third type of scan is the whole-body scan. A whole-body scan is used in patients with melanoma or cancers that are known to metastasize anywhere in the body. These scans are begun at the top of the head and continued all the way to the tip of the toes. Due to most table constraints, the patients' legs must be scanned separately. Whole-body scans consist of nine to 12 beds, at 1 to 3 minutes per bed.

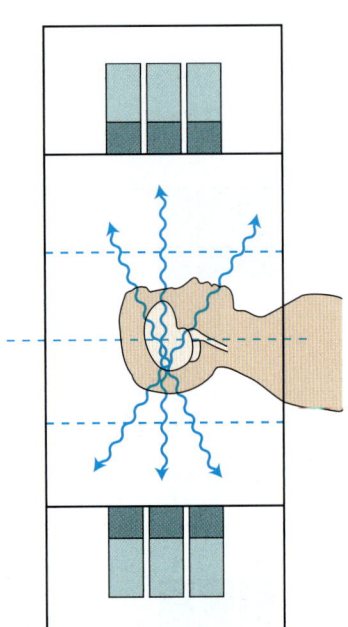

Fig. 29.35 Side view of PET scanner, illustrating possible photon directions. Only 15% of the total number of emitted photons from the patient can be detected in a whole-body tomograph (ring diameter 100 cm (39 inches)). This is increased to 25% for a head tomograph (ring diameter 60 cm (24 inches)). For these estimates, axis coverage was considered to be 15 cm (6 inches). The actual number of detected coincidences would be less than either the 15% or 25% estimate because the detector efficiency is not 100% (typical efficiency 30%).

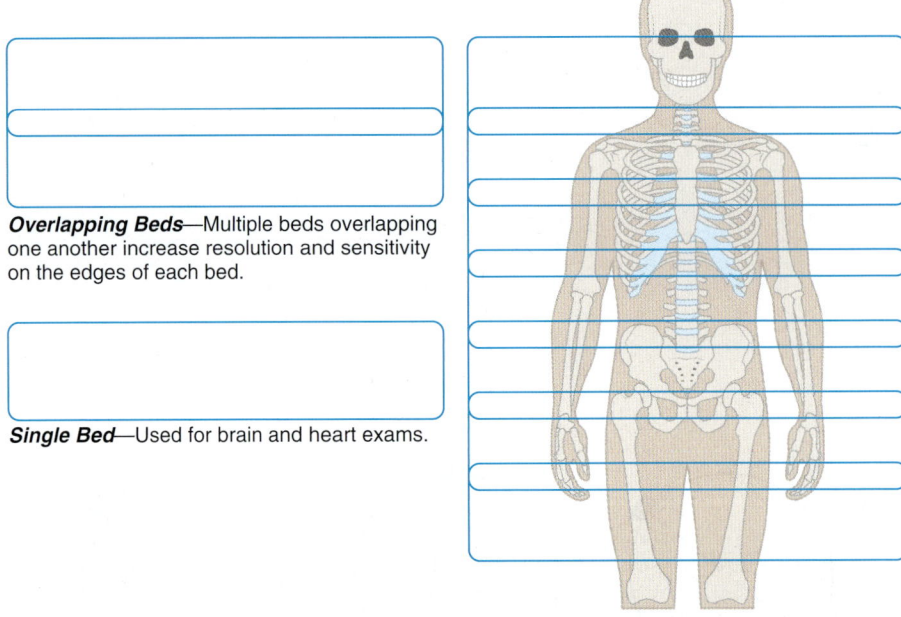

Overlapping Beds—Multiple beds overlapping one another increase resolution and sensitivity on the edges of each bed.

Single Bed—Used for brain and heart exams.

Example of "eye-to-thigh" exam. The patient is positioned in a manner to be scanned from their orbitals to their midthighs.

Fig. 29.36 Bed positions during a typical PET scan.

IMAGE RECONSTRUCTION AND IMAGE PROCESSING

Array processors are used to perform the maximum likelihood (iterative) reconstruction that converts the raw *sinogram* data into PET images. This technique is similar to the technique employed for CT image reconstruction. Faster and less costly desktop computers are replacing array processor technology and greatly simplifying software requirements for image reconstruction. A simplified block diagram for a single coincidence circuit is shown in Fig. 29.37.

Three important corrections need to be made during image reconstruction to ensure an accurate and interpretable scan. First, the disintegration of radionuclides follows Poisson statistics. As discussed earlier, random and scattered events are registered by the PET scanner as coincidence events, which degrade the overall image quality. A simple approximation allows for the subtraction of the random events after image acquisition and is based on the individual count rates for each detector and the coincidence resolving time (8–12 ns) of the tomograph electronics.

Second, photons traversing biologic tissues also undergo absorption and scatter. As shown in Fig. 29.38, an AC is applied to account for photons that should have been detected but were not. AC also identifies events that were registered outside the body and subtracts them from the final images. In the past, the correction was typically based on a transmission scan acquired under computer control using a radioactive rod or pin source of ^{68}Ge (germanium; 271-day half-life) that circumscribed the portion of the patient's body within the PET scanner. At the present time, PET/CT scanners use the CT data to correct for attenuation more accurately (Fig. 29.39).

Lastly, count rates from the detectors also need to be corrected for deadtime losses. At high count rates, detector electronics cannot handle every incoming event; some events are lost because the electronics are busy processing prior events. Measuring the tomograph response to known input count rates allows empiric formulations for the losses to be determined and applied to the reconstructed image data. Valid corrections for deadtime losses can approach 100%.

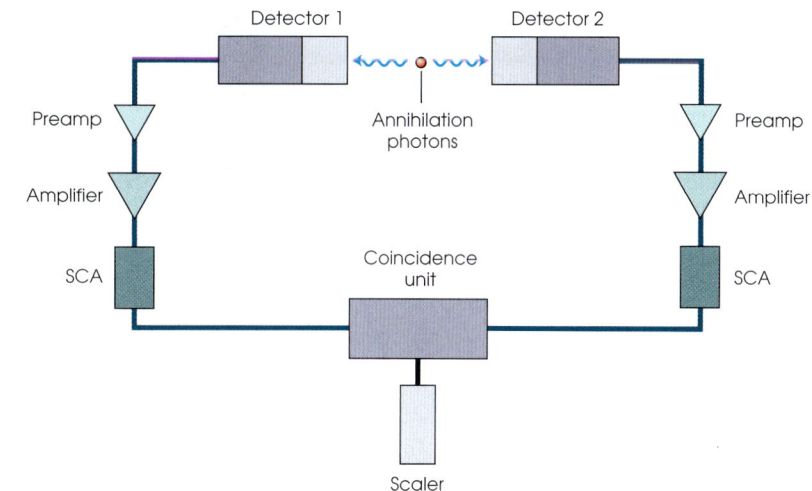

Fig. 29.37 Simplified coincidence electronics for one pair of detectors in a PET tomograph. A single-channel analyzer *(SCA)* is used to measure and verify the amplitude of the pulse received by the detector (e.g., 511 keV). Different radioisotopes present the PET unit with different photo-peaks. Photo-peaks that fall outside that of the radioisotope being used are discarded.

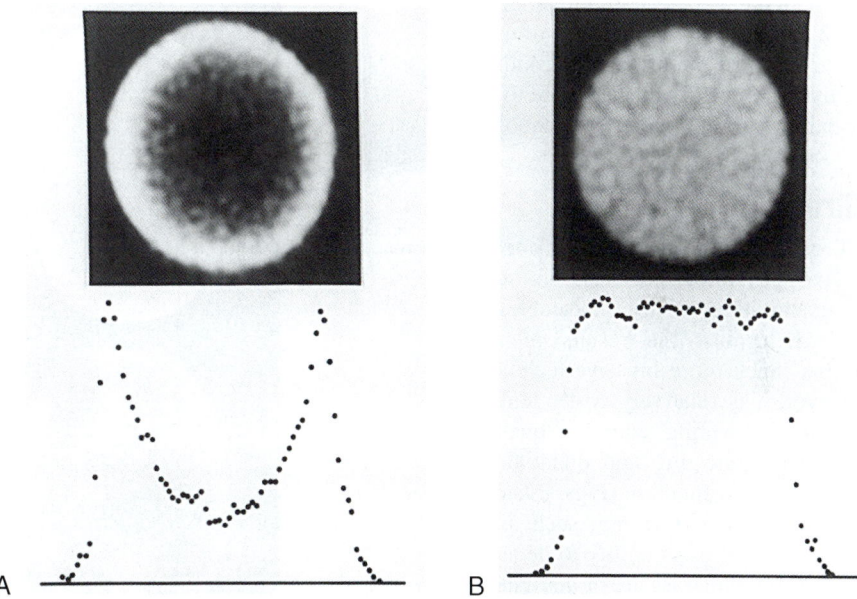

Fig. 29.38 (**A**) Uncorrected image of a phantom homogeneously filled with water-soluble PET nuclide of ^{68}Ga or ^{18}F. (**B**) Attenuation-corrected image of same phantom. Cross-sectional cuts through the center of each image are shown in *lower panels*. The attenuation correction for a phantom with a diameter of 20 cm (8 inches) can be 70% in the center of the object.

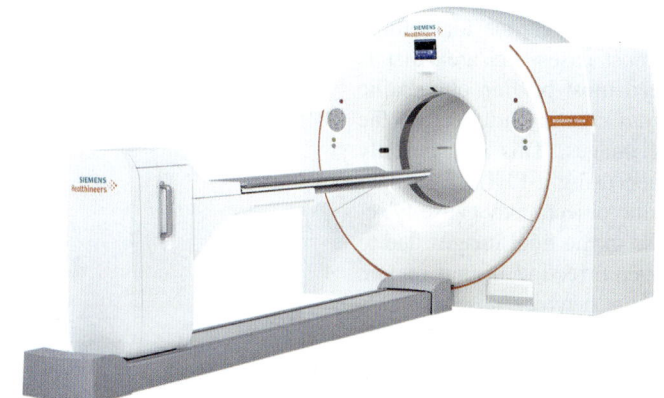

Fig. 29.39 The Siemens Biograph Vision is an example of a PET/CT scanner capable of both PET and CT imaging. The CT data can be used to create an attenuation map to help improve the accuracy of the PET data. The end result is a better image for the radiologist and better outcomes for the patient.

(Courtesy of Siemens Medical Solutions USA, Inc.)

For PET procedures, data acquisition is not limited to images of tomographic count rates. The creation of *quantitative parametric* images for the measurement of glucose metabolism is used to identify the locations of potential metastases. Cancers known to have high metabolic activity tend to absorb ^{18}F-FDG at a higher rate. By identifying the absorption rates of normal tissues to those of potentially abnormal ones, the physician can gain a better understanding of a patient's condition. This begins with the assessment of the radioactive concentration (mCi/mL) within a specific volume or voxel (cubic pixel) of tissue. This information is then applied to calculate the *standardized uptake value* (SUV). The SUV is a semiquantitative index used to identify tissues that are likely cancerous. On average, when the SUV is found to be greater than 2.5, the tissue is suggestive of malignancy. SUVs of the brain, heart, kidneys, and liver are already elevated due to their normal high level of glucose metabolism.

Clinical PET

PET is unique in its ability to measure in vivo physiology because its results are quantitative, easily repeatable, and validated against the results of accurate but much more invasive techniques. However, it is relatively costly and best used for answering complex questions that involve locating and quantitatively assessing tissue function (Figs. 29.40 and 29.41). Anatomic imaging, such as CT, is often limited in its ability to determine whether found masses are of malignant or benign etiology. Because PET is a functional modality, it can often be used to determine malignancy, even in very small nodes or masses.

Patient preparation for PET studies can be detailed and is imperative for optimal imaging. In most cases, the area that is to be examined must be free of metallic objects to avoid creating artifacts on the reconstructed images. This is especially important when using a PET/CT scanner because metallic objects may cause false-positive results in the final images due to attenuation overcorrection in that region. The waiting time between dose administration and imaging varies with each study, as does the total imaging time. After completion, patients may resume all normal activities. Technical summaries of commonly performed PET procedures follow.

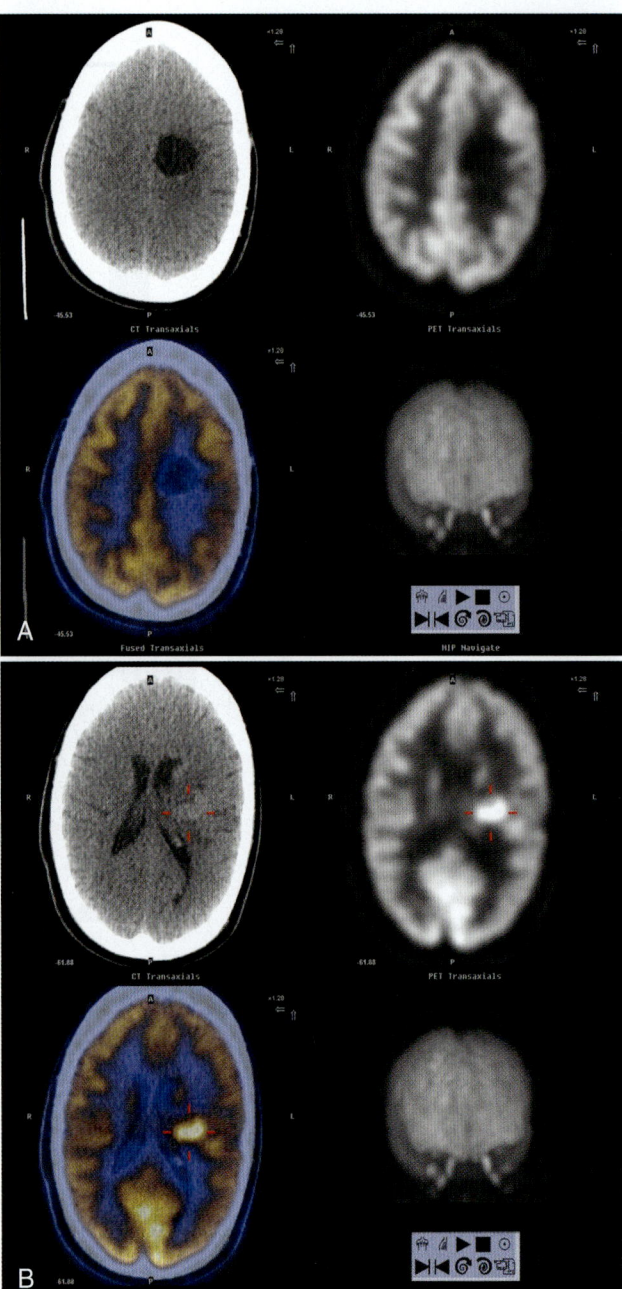

Fig. 29.40 (**A**) PET FDG brain imaging with CT fusion shows left subcortical resection site consistent with prior tumor resection. (**B**) At inferior and lateral margins of resection site, in the adjacent white matter, a hypermetabolic mass is identified. This case represents recurrent high-grade malignancy located in the left periventricular white matter at the frontoparietal junction adjacent to previous resection site.

PET ONCOLOGY IMAGING

Clinically, 70% to 80% of PET scans are done to diagnose, stage, or restage cancer (Fig. 29.42). ^{18}F-FDG is the radiopharmaceutical of choice. PET plays an important role in differentiating benign from malignant processes and is used for image-guided biopsies. PET is an important modality for detecting cancer recurrence in patients who have undergone surgery, chemotherapy, or radiation treatments. It is also very effective in monitoring therapeutic interventions by rapidly yet noninvasively assessing the metabolic response of the tissues to drugs.

With new reimbursement policies in effect, most malignant tumors are being imaged with ^{18}F-FDG in PET. The most common cancers imaged include lung, colorectal, head and neck, lymphoma, thyroid, esophageal, ovarian, and melanoma.

^{18}F-FDG ONCOLOGIC STUDY
Principle

Even though ^{18}F-FDG is currently the prevailing radiopharmaceutical in tumor PET imaging, it was initially developed as a tracer to study glucose metabolism in the brain. In the late 1980s, successful reports of ^{18}F-FDG tumor imaging began to surface. It became apparent that certain tumors had a much greater uptake of ^{18}F-FDG than surrounding tissues. Tumor cells tend to have a much greater affinity for glucose than cells of surrounding tissues because of their higher glucose metabolism. This distinction is paramount in understanding how ^{18}F-FDG PET is able to detect metastatic disease.

Although there are many considerations to take into account when performing ^{18}F-FDG PET, the most important is in the regulation of the patient's blood glucose. Generally, a blood glucose level of <180 mg/dL is required for optimal imaging and can be achieved with a 4-hour fast. Patients with high glucose levels generally have poor ^{18}F-FDG uptake because of the already overabundant presence of glucose in their blood. In cases in which the glucose level is <150 mg/dL, it is still important to have the patient fasting for approximately 4 hours before the injection of ^{18}F-FDG because postprandially the insulin response is still strong enough to push the ^{18}F-FDG into more soft tissue than is normally seen in a fasting patient. The result is an image that appears to have a low target-to-background ratio. There are several other protocols that various

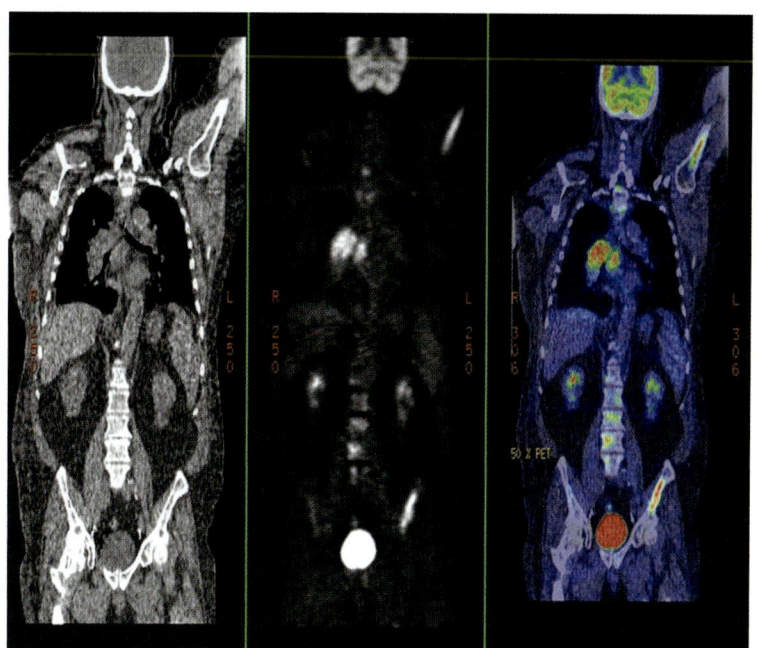

Fig. 29.41 PET FDG image with CT fusion shows large hypermetabolic right lung mass. Many PET FDG studies are done for lung cancer because of its high glucose metabolism.

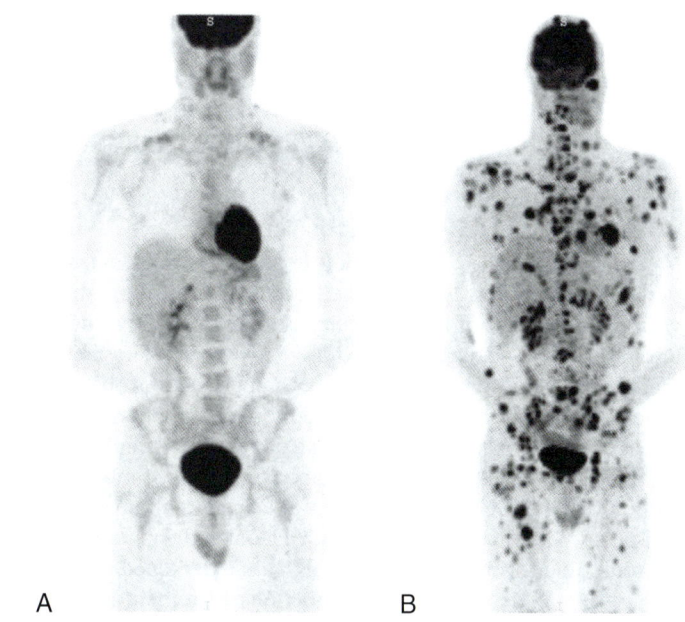

Fig. 29.42 (**A**) PET image to evaluate a patient with a history of melanoma on the scalp. Scan shows no definite evidence for recurrence. (**B**) Image 6 months later shows profound and widely disseminated hypermetabolic metastases throughout the body.

institutions follow to increase ^{18}F-FDG uptake by the tumor, including having the patient eat low-carbohydrate meals the day before and the day of the scan.

^{18}F-FDG studies require a 60- to 90-minute uptake period after injection for the incorporation of the radiopharmaceutical into the body. Some protocols suggest that imaging tumors after 90 minutes of ^{18}F-FDG incorporation may lead to significantly better signal-to-noise values in the tumor compared with surrounding tissues. During the uptake phase of the protocol, it is important that the patient be still and relaxed. Any motion, especially in the area of interest, would cause the muscles in that area to accumulate FDG and make interpretation of the images difficult. No reading, talking on the phone, or other activity is allowed. The patient also must be kept warm. If the patient develops a shiver, muscle uptake can be increased.

Radiopharmaceutical
Adult dose (intravenous injection):
- 0.214 mCi/kg (7.9 MBq/kg) of ^{18}F-FDG, minimum 10 mCi (370 MBq), maximum 20 mCi (740 MBq)

Pediatric dose (weight-based intravenous injection) (see Fig. 29.7):
- 0.10 to 0.14 mCi/kg (3.7–5.2 MBq/kg) of ^{18}F-FDG, minimum of 0.7 mCi (27 MBq)

Scanning
Most oncologic PET exams are eye-to-thigh studies with the exception of melanoma and thyroid cancer (whole-body imaging). Depending on the dose injected and PET scanner sensitivity, approximately 3 minutes per bed position are required for the emission scan to measure the distribution of ^{18}F-FDG glucose metabolism in tissue. When using a CT scan for AC, the total time for the scan is about 25 minutes.

PET NEUROLOGIC IMAGING
Metabolic neurologic study
Principle
Because the brain uses about 25% of the body's total metabolic energy, it provides an excellent gateway for functional imaging of glucose metabolism using ^{18}F-FDG, and this is why most clinical PET brain imaging is currently done with ^{18}F-FDG. PET brain scanning is done to differentiate necrotic tissue from recurrent disease, to facilitate a diagnosis of cognitive status, and to monitor cerebrovascular disease. Another use that is proving to be beneficial is using PET imaging in patients with temporal lobe epilepsy. The identification and location of brain tumors are difficult to assess with ^{18}F-FDG, because of the high metabolic uptake of ^{18}F-FDG in the brain.

When using a PET/CT system, the anatomic information provided by the CT scan can be especially helpful in determining the effects of therapy. The guiding principle in ^{18}F-FDG PET brain imaging is that the healthy brain has high glucose metabolism and high blood flow to the cerebral cortex, which demonstrates the concentration of ^{18}F-FDG within the brain. PET is also routinely used in monitoring the response to therapy and the progression of cognitive disease. With the progression of cognitive decline, glucose metabolism in the brain declines. ^{18}F-FDG assesses temporal lobe epilepsy by evaluating the brain's blood flow.

Radiopharmaceutical
Adult dose (intravenous injection):
- 5 to 10 mCi (185–370 MBq) of ^{18}F-FDG

Pediatric dose (weight-based intravenous injection) (see Fig. 29.7):
- 0.10 mCi/kg (3.7 MBq/kg) of ^{18}F-FDG, minimum 0.37 mCi (14 MBq)

Scanning
Before and after injection with ^{18}F-FDG, the patient should follow the same procedure as though undergoing an ^{18}F-FDG whole-body scan. The main difference is the importance of having no visual or auditory stimulation if possible. The visual cortex has a high rate of glucose metabolism during stimulation, which can make the images more difficult to interpret. Generally, the patient is injected with ^{18}F-FDG in a darkened room and is given instructions to remain still and to try to stay awake for a 30-minute uptake period. At the end of this period, the scan is performed in three-dimensional mode, with a bed time of 8 to 10 minutes. The transmission is generally done for 5 minutes unless an elliptic or contoured AC is done. When done on a PET/CT scanner, the CT scan is used to determine positioning of the brain and for the attenuation map. The time savings of using the CT scan for the AC can be very helpful, especially in pediatric or claustrophobic patients, who may have difficulty staying still for any length of time.

Amyloid neurologic study
Principle
β-Amyloid protein is a protein that forms in patients with AD along with other cognitive disorders. Thioflavin binds to beta-amyloid histologically and fluoresces. Amyloid radiotracers are thioflavin derivatives. Patients with AD tend to have a buildup of beta-amyloid proteins between nerve cells that form plaques. Amyloid radiotracers target these plaques and identify their presence. Patients with AD will have increased uptake of ^{18}F-florbetapir as it targets beta-amyloid plaque.

Radiopharmaceutical
Adult dose (intravenous injection):
- 10 mCi (370 MBq) of ^{18}F-florbetapir (total volume of 10 mL or less)

Scanning
Because ^{18}F-florbetapir does not rely on glucose metabolism for distribution, blood glucose does not need to be assessed. A 10-minute, dynamic acquisition should be acquired after a 30- to 50-minute uptake period with the patient lying supine and their head positioned in a head holder to help eliminate movement. The FOV should include the entire brain.

Other brain studies
Other brain imaging is now being done for Parkinson disease with ^{18}F-fluorodopa, which traces dopamine synthesis in the brain. There are also a few ^{15}O radiotracers in use, such as H$_2$^{15}O, which are employed to assess cerebral blood flow quantitatively.

PET CARDIOLOGY IMAGING
PET is a highly valuable diagnostic tool in the determination of myocardial viability and coronary flow reserve. Because of its higher temporal and spatial resolution and its built-in AC, PET is able to offer higher diagnostic accuracy than conventional nuclear medicine techniques. Because PET tracers emit higher energy gamma rays (511 keV) compared with conventional nuclear tracers (^{201}Tl at 80 keV and ^{99m}Tc sestamibi at 140 keV), PET is able to measure tracer uptake in the body more accurately. Currently, the clinical application of PET imaging in cardiology can be divided into two main categories: the detection of myocardial viability and the assessment of coronary flow reserve.

Cardiac Viability
Principle
PET imaging for cardiac viability is an invaluable tool in the assessment of viable tissue in the left ventricle. The use of ^{18}F-FDG as an indicator of glucose metabolism allows the clinician to assess the likelihood of successful coronary revascularization. Patients with moderate to severe left ventricular dysfunction, yet high myocardial viability are the most likely to benefit from revascularization. Patients who are found to have minimally viable tissue would not benefit from revascularization and may undergo the procedure needlessly if no noninvasive testing is done. Normal protocols stipulate that patients undergo a resting cardiac perfusion scan before cardiac ^{18}F-FDG PET. Traditional patterns of myocardial viability include decreased resting blood perfusion in the presence of enhanced metabolic uptake.

Radiopharmaceutical
Adult dose (intravenous injection):
- Viability imaging:
  - 10 mCi of ^{18}F-FDG
- Perfusion (rest imaging):
  - 20 mCi (740 MBq) of ^{13}N-ammonia
  - 30 to 60 mCi (1110–2220 MBq) of ^{82}Rb

Scanning
The patient preparation for PET cardiac viability scans is very important in obtaining accurate images. On the day of the scan, all patients are to fast and refrain from caffeine and nicotine intake. Upon arrival, patients have two intravenous lines placed, one in each arm. One line is for the radiopharmaceutical injection; the other is for the insulin and dextrose infusion. A rest perfusion scan with ^{13}N-ammonia or ^{82}Rb is usually performed first. After completion of the scan, the patient is given a combination of dextrose and insulin intravenously to increase the levels of glucose in the bloodstream. This converts the heart from using fatty acids as its primary source of energy to glucose. When the patient's blood glucose level reaches an optimal level, ^{18}F-FDG is injected. Approximately 30 minutes after injection, the patient is moved onto the scanner and positioned for the transmission scan. A transmission scan of 10 to 15 minutes ensues with a 5 to 10 minute emission scan to follow. When the scan is completed, patients are fed a light lunch, and their blood glucose levels are monitored until they reach normal levels.

Coronary flow reserve
Principle
PET is now commonly used to facilitate diagnoses of coronary artery disease and to assess coronary flow reserve. It is especially helpful in differentiating between stress-induced coronary ischemia and necrosis. These studies are most often done using ^{13}N-ammonia, but the advantages of other radioisotopes, such as ^{82}Rb and ^{15}O, are making their use more common. The advantage of ^{82}Rb is that it is generator-produced and acts as a potassium analog, similar to ^{201}Tl, but it is expensive and requires a large patient load to make it cost effective. The benefit of ^{15}O is that it is freely diffusible into the myocardium and is independent of metabolism, making it an excellent choice for quantitative studies. However, it does present other problems because its short half-life and short imaging time can lead to grainy images, making it a poor choice for qualitative studies. The use of ^{13}N-ammonia is most common because of its relatively short half-life (10 minutes) and because it is trapped by the myocardium by means of the glutamine synthesis reaction.

Radiopharmaceutical
Adult dose (intravenous injection):
- 10 to 20 mCi (370–740 MBq) of ^{13}N-ammonia
- 30 to 60 mCi (1110–2220 MBq) of ^{82}Rb

NOTE: Rest and stress doses are the same.

Scanning
Patients are asked to eat a light meal approximately 2 hours before the test and to avoid caffeine and nicotine products for 24 hours before the test. This is because caffeine may affect the pharmacologic stress agent used for PET coronary flow reserve studies. The test consists of two portions: rest imaging and stress imaging. The rest imaging is initiated by using the transmission scan to locate and position the heart in the center of the FOV. If the imaging is being done on a PET/CT system, this is done using the CT scan as a scout. When the heart is centered, a transmission scan of 10 to 15 minutes, based on patient girth, is performed for attenuation purposes. On completion of the transmission scan, ^{13}N-ammonia may be injected. The emission scan generally takes 10 to 15 minutes, and may be done as a gated acquisition if desired. After approximately 50 minutes (five ^{13}N half-lives), the stress study may begin. The stress agent is infused over the appropriate time and ^{13}N-ammonia is injected based on the department protocol. Emission imaging should begin immediately. On completion of the examination, the patient may be discharged and allowed to resume normal activity.

Future of Nuclear Medicine
RADIOIMMUNOTHERAPY
Several radioimmunotherapy protocols have come into clinical use in recent years. Monoclonal antibodies specifically designed to localize on the surface of different types of cancer cells can now be tagged with a radioisotope and then imaged. If the monoclonal antibody successfully localizes on the tumor site, the radioisotope may be replaced with a beta-emitting therapeutic radioisotope such as ^{131}I or ^{90}Y. Current studies are looking to treat refractory low-grade transformed B-cell non-Hodgkin lymphoma with ^{90}Y-ibritumomab tiuxetan (Zevalin) or ^{131}I-tositumomab (Bexxar). Other cancers in which specific gene expression is present are also targets using this type of treatment. These studies provide convincing evidence that more diseases may be treatable in the future using radioimmunotherapy.

HYBRID IMAGING
Considerable research into the fusion of functional (SPECT and PET) and anatomic (CT and MRI) imaging has led to the introduction of dual-modality, or hybrid, imaging systems. This is one of the most exciting developments in the field of nuclear medicine. The combined PET/CT camera shown in Fig. 29.39 couples the functional imaging capabilities of PET with the superb anatomic imaging of CT. Images from each modality are coregistered during the acquisition process and in near-simultaneity. Because the images can be overlaid one on another, the position of suspected tumors can be recognized more easily. Suspicious metabolically active areas can now be identified anatomically from the CT information. These features have improved the reliability of SPECT and PET interpretation. Metabolic and anatomic evaluation after therapy can now be accomplished in one imaging session. For all these reasons, SPECT/CT and PET/CT are becoming among the most useful diagnostic procedures for staging disease and

evaluating the treatment of cancer. All of the advantages of the integration between PET and MRI have not yet been identified. Continued research utilizing PET/MRI in the areas of oncology, neurology, and cardiology will lead radiologic imaging into a new era. With the hybridization of PET/CT and PET/MRI, molecular imaging has made tremendous advancements toward improving diagnostic care for all patients.

PET

PET technology is advancing on many fronts. ^{18}F-FDG is routinely being produced in distribution centers throughout the United States and Europe. One or more cyclotrons at each distribution site are continuously producing ^{18}F-fluoride for incorporation into ^{18}F-FDG. Unit doses are shipped via common commercial carriers, which also include chartered air and special ground couriers from a network of registered pharmacy distribution centers, to individual PET centers that do not have cyclotrons. Clinical PET imaging no longer requires the high financial commitment to own and operate a nuclear accelerator to produce PET radiopharmaceuticals at a local site.

New radiopharmaceuticals are also being developed. As PET radiopharmaceutical distribution centers expand and are able to handle the daily demands of providing ^{18}F-FDG to the existing and new PET centers, production of more ^{18}F-labeled radiopharmaceuticals specifically for tumor imaging is likely to become available. FDA approval would be required before clinical imaging, but several PET radiopharmaceutical manufacturers are sponsoring drug clinical trials to accelerate the deployment of new and viable clinical PET imaging agents. Radiolabeled choline, thymidine, fluorodopa, estrogen receptors, and numerous other biomolecules are likely candidates for new PET clinical tracers.

Mobile PET units are a reality, as shown in Figs. 29.43 and 29.44. PET scanner technology has matured to the point that the original frailty of the electronics and detector systems has been eliminated. Robust mobile units travel to community hospitals that need PET imaging but not at the level that necessitates a dedicated in-house PET scanner. By spending 1 or 2 days/week at several different hospitals in smaller communities or rural settings, the mobile PET camera best serves the needs of their oncology patients. The ^{18}F-FDG distribution centers are necessary in this scenario because the mobile PET camera unit needs a supply of radiotracer to carry out PET imaging studies. Until nationwide ^{18}F-FDG distribution centers became a reality, as they now are, the use of mobile PET was extremely limited.

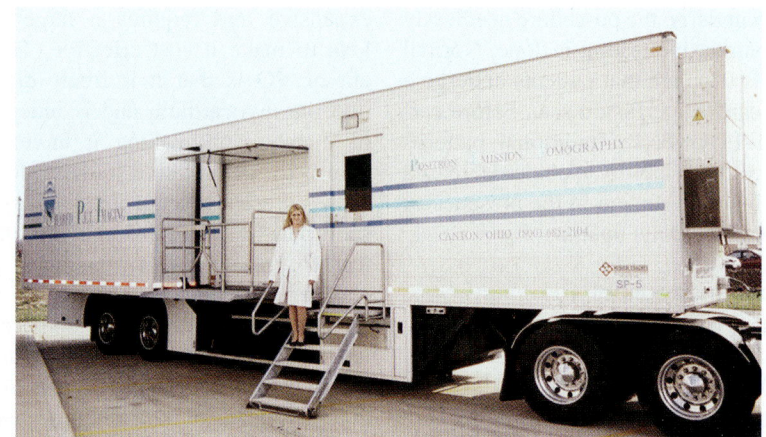

Fig. 29.43 A mobile PET coach showing operator on staff stairs and an elevator platform in the elevated position. The elevator is used to transport patients from the ground level to the floor level of the PET scanner unit.

(Courtesy Shared PET Imaging, LLC.)

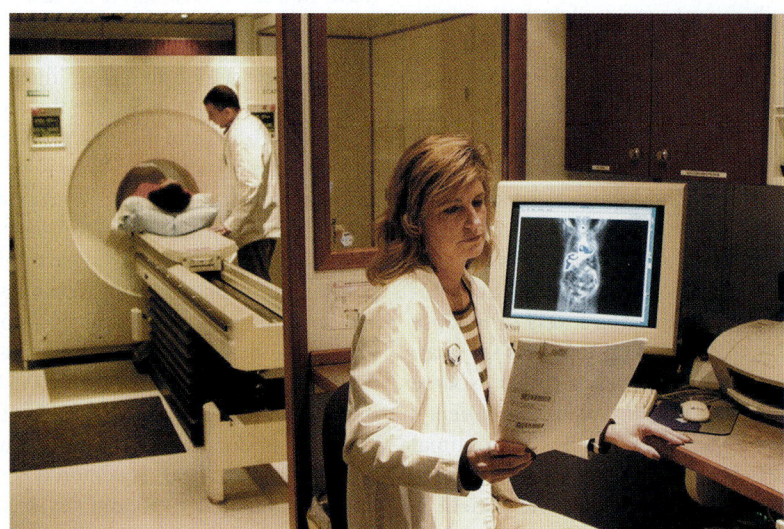

Fig. 29.44 Interior of mobile coach showing PET workstation (*foreground*) and PET scanner (*background*).

(Courtesy Shared PET Imaging, LLC.)

Best Practices

Every patient and/or procedure presents its own set of challenges and obstacles to completion of an exam. In nuclear medicine, best practices include performing the "8 Rights" on every patient. These rights include the following.

1. *Right patient preparation:* Nuclear medicine is founded on appropriate patient preparation due to the physiologic limitations each exam can potentially bring. Things like NPO status and underlying medications are essential to making sure correct radiopharmaceutical localization occurs. For example, something as simple as a multivitamin can drastically change a patient's thyroid uptake percentage due to the potential amounts of iodine in the vitamin. This would decrease the patient's radioactive iodine uptake, making it appear as if the patient has a hypofunctioning thyroid. Proper and consistent patient preparation will lead to quality imaging and accurate data collection.
2. *Right patient education:* Patient education is one of the best weapons a nuclear medicine technologist can have. These exams are long and boring for most patients. Patients tend to become uncomfortable, fidgety, and anxious while in the scanner. By educating the patient on what to expect during the exam, informing the patient of what they can and can't do during the exam, and providing answers to their questions, a technologist can calm a patient before anything has even been started. This leads to less patient motion and anxiety, which ultimately leads to better imaging.
3. *Right radiopharmaceutical:* Identifying the correct radiopharmaceutical for each exam is essential in the success of the study. The wrong selection will lead to incorrect physiologic distribution.
4. *Right dose:* Radiopharmaceutical dose ranges are set to not only enhance image quality but also to reduce radiation to the patient. Administering a dose that is too low causes low counts within the images, which increase scan times. This leads to patient motion and image distortion. A dose that is too high can lead to not only imaging problems but also potential overexposure of patients to unnecessary radiation.
5. *Right patient positioning:* Imaging is only as good as the positioning of the patient. Although most imaging in nuclear medicine is taken in the prone position, there are little details that have to be considered, such as arm and leg positioning for a procedure. Due to the limitations of the gamma camera, arms and feet can be clipped during initial whole-body imaging. In other exams, limbs can attenuate and create artifacts. Technologists need to be aware of potential issues and know how to maximize imaging in these situations.
6. *Right timing:* Once a radiopharmaceutical is administered, it is vital to obtain imaging at the right time. Some studies require immediate imaging following injections, and others can require delays of up to 5 to 10 days. Timing is also used to set up appropriate uptake times, which increases image quality. For example, in parathyroid imaging, the radiopharmaceutical is localized by both the thyroid and parathyroid. The thyroid processes the radiotracer faster than the parathyroid. This means that if the technologist performs images too early, the images would include both organs without separation, and if too late, the tracer may have washed completely out. In both cases, an adenoma may be missed. Maintaining consistency and standardized imaging times within protocols is very important in establishing best practices.
7. *Right imaging:* As discussed before, there is not only one kind of imaging in nuclear medicine. A study may require a blood flow, static(s), whole body, or SPECT imaging. Identifying what type of imaging will provide the most information in regard to the exam's indication drives best practices.
8. *Right documentation:* A large part of a radiologist's dictation is the alignment with regulatory agencies. This includes a list of documentation requirements relevant to each exam. Documentation in some studies is as simple as the radiopharmaceutical, the dose, and the technologist who performed the procedure. Others require dose sheets, public exposure notifications, and even planned diets. Verifying the right documentation is important before completing the exam.

Each of the eight rights is a cornerstone of effective nuclear medicine imaging and patient care. When performed correctly, these rights come together like a puzzle, allowing every exam to be considered a best practice.

Conclusion

Nuclear medicine technology is a multidisciplinary field in which medicine is linked to quantitative sciences, including chemistry, radiation biology, physics, and computer technology. Since the early 20th century, nuclear medicine has expanded to include molecular nuclear medicine, in vivo and in vitro chemistry, and physiology. The spectrum of nuclear medicine technology skills and responsibilities varies. The scope of nuclear medicine technology includes patient care, quality control, diagnostic procedures, computer data acquisition and processing, radiopharmaceuticals, radionuclide therapy, and radiation safety. Many clinical procedures are performed in nuclear medicine departments across the United States and throughout the world. Nuclear medicine procedures complement other imaging methods in radiology and pathology departments. This complementation drastically increases exam specificity and accuracy.

The evolution of PET has provided the nuclear medicine department with complex diagnostic imaging procedures. PET is a useful clinical and research tool that requires the multidisciplinary support of the physician, physicist, physiologist, chemist, engineer, software programmer, and radiographer. This imaging procedure allows numerous biologic parameters in the working human body to be examined without disturbing normal-equilibrium physiology. PET measures regional function that cannot be determined by any other means, including CT and MRI. Current PET studies of the brain involve the imaging of patients with epilepsy, Huntington disease, stroke, schizophrenia, brain tumors, AD, and other disorders of the central nervous system. PET studies of the heart are providing routine diagnostic information on patients with coronary artery disease by identifying viable myocardium for revascularization. The greatest impact PET has made is the ability to identify highly metabolic tumors. PET scanning is critically involved in the determination of the effects of therapeutic drug regimens on tumors and the differentiation of necrosis from viable tumor. Nearly 80% of all PET imaging today is directed at tumor detection and the evaluation of therapeutic intervention. Overall, human physiology will become better understood as the technology advances, yielding higher resolution instruments, new radiopharmaceuticals, and improved analysis of PET data.

The future of nuclear medicine may lie in its unique ability to identify functional or physiologic abnormalities. With the continued development of new radiopharmaceuticals and imaging technology, nuclear medicine will continue to be a unique and valuable tool for diagnosing and treating disease.

Definition of Terms

alpha particle: Nucleus of a helium atom, consisting of two protons and two neutrons, having a positive charge of 2.

analog: Radiopharmaceutical biochemically equivalent to a naturally occurring compound in the body.

annihilation: Total transformation of matter into energy; occurs after the antimatter positron collides with an electron. Two photons are created; each equals the rest mass of the individual particles.

attenuation coefficient: Number that represents the statistical reduction in photons that exit a material (N) from the value that entered the material (N_o). The reduced flux is the result of scatter and absorption, which can be expressed in the following equation: $N = N_o e - \mu\chi$, where μ is the attenuation coefficient and l is the distance traversed by the photons.

becquerel (Bq): Unit of activity in the International System of Units; equal to 1 disintegration per second (dps): 1 Bq = 1 dps.

beta particle: Electron whose point of origin is the nucleus; electron originating in the nucleus by way of decay of a neutron into a proton and an electron.

blood-brain barrier: Anatomic and physiologic features of the brain thought to consist of walls of capillaries in the central nervous system and surrounding glial membranes. The barrier separates the parenchyma of the central nervous system from blood. The blood-brain barrier prevents or slows the passage of some drugs and other chemical compounds, radioactive ions, and disease-causing organisms, such as viruses from the blood, into the central nervous system.

coincidence event: The result of two annihilation photons striking opposing detectors in a PET scanner.

coincidence time window: The time span within which annihilation photons must strike opposing detectors to be considered coincidence events (6–12 nanoseconds).

cold spot: Lack of radiation being received or recorded, not producing any image and resulting in an area of no, or very light, density; may be caused by disease or artifact.

collimator: Shielding device used to limit the angle of entry of radiation; usually made of lead.

Coulomb forces: Forces exerted upon objects with charge. When the charges are the same, the forces repel one another (+, +). If the charges are opposite, the forces attract one another (+, –). Particles without charge (neutrons) are unaffected by these forces.

curie: Standard of measurement for radioactive decay; based on the disintegration of 1 g of radium at 3.731010 disintegrations per second.

cyclotron: Device for accelerating charged particles to high energies using magnetic and oscillating electrostatic fields. As a result, particles move in a spiral path with increasing energy.

daughter: Element that results from the radioactive decay of a parent element.

deadtime: Time when the system electronics are already processing information from one photon interaction with a detector and cannot accept new events to be processed from other detectors.

decay: Radioactive disintegration of the nucleus of an unstable nuclide.

detector: Device that is a combination of a scintillator and photomultiplier tube; used to detect x-rays and gamma rays.

deuteron: Ionized nucleus of heavy hydrogen (deuterium), which contains one proton and one neutron.

dose: Measure of the amount of energy deposited in a known mass of tissue from ionizing radiation. Absorbed dose is described in units of rads; 1 rad is equal to 10^{-2} J/kg or 100 ergs/g.

ejection fraction (cardiac): Percent of the total volume of blood of the left ventricle ejected per contraction.

electron capture: Radioactive decay process in which a nucleus with an excess of protons brings an electron into the nucleus, converting a proton into a neutron. The resulting atom is often unstable and gives off a gamma ray to achieve stability.

external radiation detector: Instrument used to determine the presence of radioactivity from the exterior.

^{18}F-FDG: Radioactive analog of naturally available glucose. It follows the same biochemical pathways as glucose; however, in contrast to glucose, it is not totally metabolized to carbon dioxide and water.

fission: Splitting of a nucleus into two or more parts with the subsequent release of enormous amounts of energy.

functional image: See *parametric image*.

gamma camera: Device that uses the emission of light from a crystal struck by gamma rays to produce an image of the distribution of radioactive material in a body organ.

gamma ray: High-energy, short-wavelength electromagnetic radiation emanating from the nucleus of some nuclides.

generator system: A piece of equipment used in radiopharmacies to quantitatively separate technetium-99m from its parent radionuclide molybdenum-99.

ground state: State of lowest energy of a system.

half-life (T½): Term used to describe the time elapsed until some physical quantity has decreased to half of its original value.

homeostasis: State of equilibrium of the body's internal environment.

hot lab: Location in a nuclear medicine department or radiopharmacy where radioisotopes are stored before use or compounding.

image coregistration: Computer technique that permits realignment of images that have been acquired from different modalities and have different orientations and magnifications. With realignment, images possess the same orientation and size. Images can then be overlaid, one on the other, to show similarities and differences between the images.

in vitro: Outside a living organism.

in vivo: Within a living organism.

isotope: Nuclide of the same element with the same number of protons but a different number of neutrons.

isotropic: Referring to uniform emission of radiation or particles in three dimensions.

kinetics: Movement of materials into, out of, and through biologic spaces. A mathematic expression is often used to describe and quantify how substances traverse membranes or participate in biochemical reactions.

light pipe: Tube-like structure attached to the scintillation crystal to convey the emitted light to the photomultiplier tube.

line-of-response (LOR): Theoretical line created by the detection of a coincidence event on opposing sides of the PET camera (see Fig. 29.33).

magnetic resonance imaging (MRI): Technique of nuclear magnetic resonance (NMR) as it is applied to medical imaging. Magnetic resonance is abbreviated *MR*.

metastable: Describes the excited state of a nucleus that returns to its ground state by emission of a gamma ray; has a measurable lifetime.

nuclear particle accelerator: Device to produce radioactive material by accelerating ions (e.g., electrons, protons, deuterons) to high energies and projecting them toward stable materials. Accelerators include linac, cyclotron, synchrotron, Van de Graaff accelerator, and betatron.

nuclear reactor: Device that under controlled conditions is used for supporting a self-sustained nuclear reaction.

nuclide: General term applicable to all atomic forms of an element.

organified: The ability of the thyroid to absorb and incorporate iodine into thyroid hormone.

parametric image: Image that relates anatomic position (the *x* and *y* position on an image) to a physiologic parameter such as blood flow (image intensity or color). It may also be referred to as a functional image.

parent: Radionuclide that decays to a specific daughter nuclide either directly or as a member of a radioactive series.

particle accelerator: Device that provides the energy necessary to enable a nuclear reaction.

pharmaceutical: Relating to a medicinal drug.

photomultiplier tube (PMT): Electronic tube that converts light photons to electrical pulses.

photopenia: See *cold spot*.

pixel (picture element): Smallest indivisible part of an image matrix for display on a computer screen. Typical images may be 128 × 128, 256 × 256, or 512 × 512 pixels.

positron: Positively charged particle emitted from neutron-deficient radioactive nuclei.

positron emission tomography (PET): Imaging technique that creates transaxial images of organ physiology from the simultaneous detection of positron annihilation photons.

pulse height analyzer: Instrument that accepts input from a detector and categorizes the pulses on the basis of signal strength.

pyrogen-free: Free of a fever-producing agent of bacterial origin.

quantitative: Type of PET study in which the final images are not simply distributions of radioactivity but rather correspond to units of capillary blood flow, glucose metabolism, or receptor density. Studies between individuals and repeat studies in the same individual permit comparison of pixel values on an absolute scale.

radiation: Emission of energy; rays of waves.

radioactive: Exhibiting the property of spontaneously emitting alpha, beta, and gamma rays by disintegration of the nucleus.

radioactivity: Spontaneous disintegration of an unstable atomic nucleus resulting in the emission of ionizing radiation.

radioisotope: Synonym for radioactive isotope. Any isotope that is unstable undergoes decay with the emission of characteristic radiation.

radionuclide: Unstable nucleus that transmutes via nuclear decay.

radiopharmaceutical: Refers to a radioactive drug used for diagnosis or therapy.

radiotracer: Synonym for *radiopharmaceutical*.

random event: When two annihilations take place in two separate locations and a single photon from each pair strikes opposing detectors within the coincidence timing window, a false LOR is created, degrading PET images.

ray: Imaginary line drawn between a pair of detectors in the PET scanner or between the x-ray source and detector in a CT scanner.

reconstruction: Mathematic operation that transforms raw data acquired on a PET tomograph (sinogram) into an image with recognizable features.

region of interest (ROI): Area that circumscribes a desired anatomic location on a PET image. Image-processing systems permit drawing of ROI on images. The average parametric value is computed for all pixels within the ROI and returned to the radiographer.

resolution: Smallest separation of two point sources of radioactivity that can be distinguished for PET or SPECT imaging.

scattered event: The result of a photon from an annihilation being deflected but not slowed enough to fall outside of the coincidence time frame.

scintillation camera: See *gamma camera*.

scintillation detector: Device that relies on the emission of light from a crystal subjected to ionizing radiation. The light is detected by a photomultiplier tube and converted to an electronic signal that can be processed further. An array of scintillation detectors is used in a gamma camera.

scintillator: Organic or inorganic material that transforms high-energy photons such as x-rays or gamma rays into visible or nearly visible light (ultraviolet) photons for easy measurement.

sensitivity: Term used when describing the percentage of photons striking the detector versus those being attenuated by collimation.

septa: High-density metal collimators that separate adjacent detectors on a ring tomograph to reduce scattered photons from degrading image information.

single photon emission computed tomography (SPECT): Nuclear medicine scanning procedure that measures conventional single photon gamma emissions (^{99m}Tc) with a specially designed rotating gamma camera.

sonogram: Two-dimensional raw data format that depicts coincidence detectors against possible rays between detectors. For each coincidence event, a specific element of the sinogram matrix is incremented by 1. The sum of all events in the sinogram is the total number of events detected by the PET scanner minus any corrections that have been applied to the sinogram data.

target: Device used to contain stable materials and subsequent radioactive materials during bombardment by high-energy nuclei from a cyclotron or other particle accelerator. The term is also applied to the material inside the device, which may be solid, liquid, or gaseous.

tracer: Radioactive isotope used to allow a biologic process to be seen. The tracer is introduced into the body, binds with a specific substance, and is followed by a scanner as it passes through various organs or systems in the body.

transmission scan: Type of PET scan that is equivalent to a low-resolution CT scan. Attenuation is determined by rotating a rod of radioactive 68Ge around the subject. Photons that traverse the subject either impinge on a detector and are registered as valid counts or are attenuated (absorbed or scattered). Ratio of counts with and without the attenuating tissue in place provides the factors to correct PET scans for the loss of counts from attenuation of the 0.511-MeV photons.

true event: The result when an annihilation photon pair, unaffected by any attenuation or scatter, strikes PET detectors within the coincidence time window and is registered as a single count.

washout: End of the radionuclide procedure, during which time the radioactivity is eliminated from the body.

Selected bibliography

Christian PE, Waterstram-Rich KM. *Nuclear Medicine and PET/CT: Technology and Techniques*. 7th ed. St Louis: Elsevier; 2012.

Mettler FA, Guiberteau MJ. *Essentials of Nuclear Medicine Imaging*. 6th ed. St Louis: Elsevier; 2012.

Steves AM. *Review of Nuclear Medicine Technology*. Reston, VA: Society of Nuclear Medicine; 2004.

Waterstram-Rich KM, Gilmore D. *Nuclear Medicine and PET/CT: Technology and Techniques*. 8th ed. St Louis: Elsevier; 2017.

Wieler HJ, Coleman RE. *PET in Clinical Oncology*. Darmstadt: Steinkopff Verlag; 2000.

30
RADIATION ONCOLOGY
MACHELE D. MICHELS

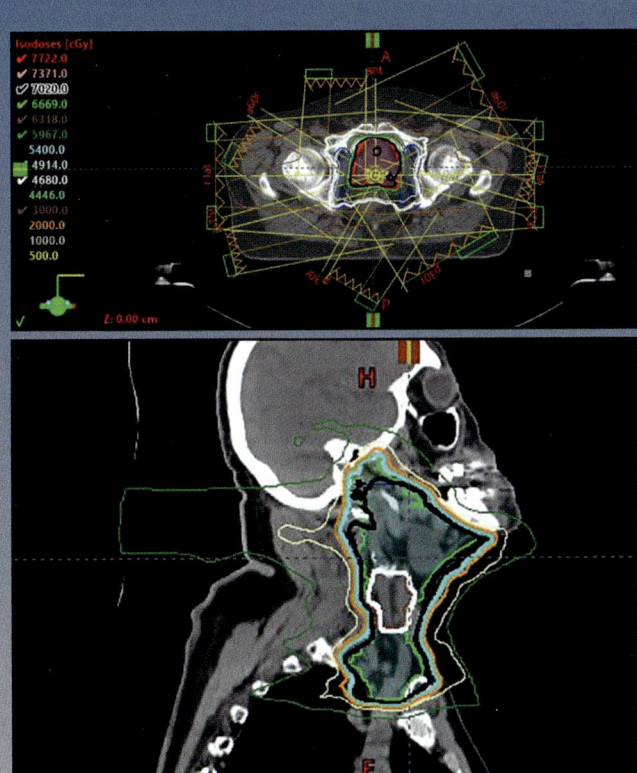

OUTLINE

Principles of Radiation Oncology, 482
Historical Development, 483
Cancer, 483
Theory, 486
Technical Aspects, 487
Steps in Radiation Oncology, 491
Proton Therapy, 502
Best Practices, 504
Clinical Applications, 505
Future Trends, 508
Conclusion, 508
Definition of Terms, 508

Used with permission of Mayo Foundation for Medical Education and Research, all rights reserved.

Principles of Radiation Oncology

Radiation oncology,[a] or *radiation therapy*, is one of four principal modalities used in the treatment of cancer, with chemotherapy, surgery, and *immunotherapy* comprising the other three. In radiation therapy for malignancies, *tumors* or *lesions* are treated with *cancericidal doses* of ionizing radiation as prescribed by a *radiation oncologist*, a physician who specializes in the treatment of malignant disease with radiation. The goals of the treatment are to deliver a cancericidal dose of radiation precisely to the tumor, while limiting as much radiation dose as possible received by normal, noncancerous tissues. These dual tasks make this form of treatment complex and often challenging. Input from all members of the radiation oncology team is crucial in developing the optimal treatment plan or approach for a patient.

Cancer treatment requires a multidisciplinary approach from various departments. First, diagnostic radiologic studies, including radiographs, computed tomography (CT) scans, magnetic resonance imaging (MRI), positron emission tomography (PET) scans, and sonograms are obtained to acquire information about the location and anatomic extent of the tumor. Second, a tissue specimen (*biopsy*) is removed surgically. A *pathologist* examines the tissue to determine whether the lesion is cancerous. Once cancer is officially diagnosed, the best treatment approach is determined through consultation with various *oncology* specialists (e.g., surgical *oncologist*, radiation oncologist, medical oncologist).

[a] Almost all italicized words on the succeeding pages are defined at the end of the chapter.

Although radiation oncology may be used as the only method of treatment for malignant disease, a more common approach is to use it in conjunction with surgery, chemotherapy, or immunotherapy, or in some combination of the four modalities. Some patients with cancer may be treated only with surgery or chemotherapy; however, more than half of all diagnosed cancer patients can benefit from radiation therapy. The choice of treatment can depend on many patient variables, such as the patient's overall physical and emotional condition, the histologic type of the disease, and the extent and anatomic position of the tumor. If a tumor is small and its margins are well defined, a surgical approach alone may be prescribed. If the disease is *systemic*, a chemotherapeutic approach may be chosen. However, most tumors exhibit degrees of size, invasion, and spread and require variations in the treatment approach, which is likely to include radiation treatments administered as an adjunct to or in conjunction with surgery or chemotherapy.

Radiation is generally used after surgery when a patient is deemed to be at high risk for tumor recurrence in the *surgical bed*. The risk of recurrence is considered to be increased in the following situations:

- When the surgical margin between normal tissue and cancerous tissue is minimal (<2 cm)
- When the margin is positive for cancer (i.e., when cancerous tissue is not completely removed)
- When the tumor is incompletely resected because of its large size, its relationship with normal vital structures, or both
- When the cancer has spread to adjacent lymph nodes

Radiation can be used as the definitive (primary) cancer treatment or as an adjuvant treatment (i.e., in combination with another form of therapy). It can also be used for *palliation*.

Radiation treatments most often are delivered on a daily basis, Monday through Friday, for 2 to 8 weeks. The length of time and the total dose of radiation delivered depend on the type of cancer being treated and the purpose of treatment (*cure* or palliation). Prescribed dosages of radiation can range from 800 centigray (cGy) for palliation to 8000 cGy for curative intent (total doses). The delivery of a small amount of radiation per day (180–200 cGy) for a certain number of treatments, instead of one large dose, is termed *fractionation*. Because these smaller doses of radiation are more easily tolerated by normal tissue, fractionation can help minimize the acute toxic effect a patient experiences during treatment and the possible long-term side effects of treatment.

The precision and accuracy necessary to administer high doses of radiation to tumors while not harming normal tissue require the combined effort of all members of the radiation oncology team. Members of this team include radiation oncologists, physicists, dosimetrists, radiation therapists, and oncology nurses.

The radiation oncologist prescribes the quantity of radiation and determines the anatomic region or regions to be treated. The *medical physicist* is responsible for calibration and maintenance of the radiation-producing equipment. The physicist also advises the physician about dosage calculations and complex treatment techniques. The *medical dosimetrist* devises a plan for delivering the treatments in a manner to best meet the physician's goals of irradiating the tumor while protecting normal vital structures. The *radiation therapist* is responsible for obtaining radiographs or CT scans that localize the area to be treated, administering the treatments, keeping accurate records of the dose delivered each day, and monitoring the patient's physical and emotional well-being. Educating patients about potential radiation side effects and assisting patients with the management of these side effects are often the responsibilities of the oncology nurse.

The duties and responsibilities of the radiation therapist are more thoroughly described later in this chapter. In addition, more information is provided about the circumstances in which radiation is used to treat cancer. The steps necessary to prepare a patient for treatment are also described. These steps include (1) simulation, (2) development of the optimal treatment plan in dosimetry, and (3) treatment delivery. Current techniques and future trends are also discussed.

Historical Development

Ionizing radiation was originally used to obtain a radiographic image of internal anatomy for diagnostic purposes. The resultant image depended on many variables, including the energy of the beam, the processing techniques, the material on which the image was recorded, and, most importantly, the amount of energy absorbed by the various organs of the body. The transfer of energy from the beam of radiation to the biologic system and the observation of the effects of this interaction became the foundation of radiation oncology.

Two of the most obvious and sometimes immediate biologic effects observed during the early diagnostic procedures were epilation (loss of hair) and erythema (reddening of the skin). Epilation and erythema result primarily from the great amount of energy absorbed by the skin during radiographic procedures. These short-term, radiation-induced effects afforded radiographic practitioners an opportunity to expand the use of radiation to treat conditions ranging from relatively benign maladies such as hypertrichosis (excessive hair), acne, and boils to grotesque and malignant diseases such as lupus vulgaris and skin cancer.

Ionizing radiation was first applied for the treatment of a more in-depth lesion on January 29, 1896, when Emil Grubbé is reported to have irradiated a woman with carcinoma of the left breast. This event occurred only 3 months after the discovery of x-rays by Wilhelm Röntgen (Table 30.1). Although Grubbé neither expected nor observed any dramatic results from the irradiation, the event is significant simply because it occurred.

In January 1902, in New Haven, Connecticut, Clarence Skinner performed the first reported curative treatment using ionizing radiation. Skinner treated a woman who had a diagnosed malignant fibrosarcoma. Over the next 2 years and 3 months, the woman received 136 applications of the x-rays. In April 1909, 7 years after the initial application of the radiation, the woman was free of disease and considered "cured."

As data were collected, the interest in radiation therapy increased. More sophisticated equipment, a greater understanding of the effects of ionizing radiation, an appreciation for time-dose relationships, and numerous other related medical breakthroughs gave impetus to the interest in radiation therapy, which led to the evolution of a distinct medical specialty—radiation oncology.

Cancer

Cancer is a disease process that involves an unregulated, uncontrolled replication of cells; put more simply, the cells do not know when to stop dividing. These abnormal cells grow without regard to normal tissue. They invade adjacent tissues, destroy normal tissue, and create a mass of tumor cells. Cancerous cells can spread further by invading the lymph or blood vessels that drain the area. When tumor cells invade the lymphatic or vascular system, they are transported by that system until they become caught or lodged within a lymph node or an organ such as the liver or lungs, where secondary tumors form. The spread of cancer from the original site to different, remote parts of the body is termed *metastasis*. When cancer has spread to a distant site via blood-borne metastasis, the patient is considered incurable. Early detection and diagnosis are the keys to curing cancer.

For the year 2023, the estimated number of new cancer cases in the United States was over 1.9 million, and the estimated number of deaths from cancer was over 600,000. Data based on cases reported between 2013 and 2017 indicated that the rate of new cancer cases was 403 per 100,000 men and women and that cancer was diagnosed most frequently among persons aged 65 to 74 years. The most common cancers that occur in the United States are lung, prostate, breast, and colorectal cancer. Prostate cancer is the most common malignancy in men, and

TABLE 30.1
Significant developments in radiation therapy

Date	Person	Event
1895	Röntgen	Discovery of x-rays
1896	Grubbé	First use of ionizing radiation in treatment of cancer
	Becquerel	Discovery of radioactive emissions by uranium compounds
1898	M. and P. Curie	Discovery of radium
1902	Skinner	First documented case of cancer "cure" using ionizing radiation
1906	Bergonié and Tribondeau	Postulation of first law of radiosensitivity
1932	Lawrence	Invention of cyclotron
1934	Joliot and Joliot-Curie	Production of artificial radioactivity
1939	Lawrence and Stone	Treatment of cancer patient with neutron beam from cyclotron
1940	Kerst	Construction of betatron
1951		Installation of first cobalt-60 teletherapy units
1952		Installation of first linear accelerator (Hammersmith Hospital, London)

breast cancer is the most common malignancy in women. The second and third most common cancers in men and women are lung and colorectal cancer (Table 30.2). Overall, cancer incidence rates are higher among men than women. Health disparities are a large public health challenge in the United States. For example, the American Indian and Alaskan Native population has an 80% higher incidence rate of kidney cancer as compared to the Caucasian population, and the black population has more than double the mortality rate of multiple myeloma. In 2019, heart disease was the first leading cause of death, followed by cancer for the non-Hispanic white, non-Hispanic black, and non-Hispanic American Indian or Alaska Native populations. However, cancer surpassed heart disease as the first leading cause of death for the non-Hispanic Asian or Pacific Islander and Hispanic populations.

RISK FACTORS
External factors

Many factors can contribute to a person's potential for the development of a *malignancy*. These factors can be external exposure to chemicals, viruses, or radiation within the environment or internal factors such as hormones, genetic mutations, and disorders of the immune system. Cancer is commonly the result of exposure to a *carcinogen*, which is a substance or material that causes cells to undergo malignant transformation and become cancerous. Some known carcinogenic agents are listed in Table 30.3. Cigarettes and other tobacco products are the principal cause of cancers of the lung, esophagus, oral cavity and pharynx, and bladder. Cigarette smokers are 25 times more likely to develop lung cancer than nonsmokers. Occupational exposure to chemicals such as chromium, nickel, or arsenic can also cause lung cancer. A person who smokes and works with chemical carcinogens is at even greater risk for developing lung cancer than a nonsmoker. In other words, risk factors can have an additive effect, acting together to initiate or promote the development of cancer. Other risk factors that have been identified are obesity, physical inactivity, and poor nutrition.

The human papillomavirus (HPV) is associated with the development of cancer of the uterine cervix, oropharynx, and anus. Infection with the hepatitis B virus (HBV) or hepatitis C virus (HCV) increases one's risk for the development of hepatocellular carcinoma of the liver. Vaccines do exist to prevent infection with HPV or HBV.

Another carcinogen is *ionizing radiation*. It was responsible for the development of osteogenic sarcoma in radium-dial painters in the 1920s and 1930s, and it caused the development of skin cancers in pioneer radiologists. Early radiation therapy equipment used in the treatment of cancer often induced a second malignancy in the bone. The low-energy x-rays produced by this equipment were within the photoelectric range of interactions with matter, resulting in a 3:1 preferential absorption in bone compared with soft tissue. Some patients with breast cancer who were irradiated developed an osteosarcoma of their ribs after a 15- to 20-year latency period. With advances in diagnostic and therapeutic equipment and improved knowledge of radiation physics, radiobiology, and radiation safety practices, radiation-induced malignancies have become relatively uncommon, although the potential for their development still exists. In keeping with standard radiation safety guidelines, any dose of radiation, no matter how small, significantly increases the chance of a genetic mutation.

Internal factors

Internal factors are causative factors over which persons have no control. Genetic mutations on individual genes and *chromosomes* have been identified as predisposing factors for the development of cancer. Mutations can be sporadic or hereditary, as in colon cancer. Chromosomal defects have also been identified in other cancers, such as leukemia, Wilms tumor, retinoblastoma, and breast cancer. Because of their familial pattern of occurrence, breast, ovarian, and colorectal cancer are three major areas currently under study to obtain an earlier diagnosis, which increases the cure rate. Patients with a family history of breast or ovarian cancer can be tested to see whether they have inherited the altered *BRCA-1* and *BRCA-2* genes. Patients with these altered genes are at a significantly higher risk of developing breast and ovarian cancer. Women identified as carriers of the altered genes can benefit from more intensive and early screening programs in which breast cancer may be diagnosed at a much earlier and more curable stage. These patients also have the option of *prophylactic surgery* to remove the breasts or ovaries. Some women still develop cancer, however, in the remaining tissue after surgery.

TABLE 30.2

Top five most common cancers in men and women

Men	Women
1. Prostate	1. Breast
2. Lung and bronchus	2. Lung and bronchus
3. Colon and rectum	3. Colon and rectum
4. Bladder	4. Uterus (endometrium)
5. Melanoma	5. Thyroid

TABLE 30.3

Carcinogenic agents and the cancers they cause

Carcinogen	Resultant cancer
Cigarette smoking	Cancers of lung, esophagus, bladder, and oral cavity/pharynx
Arsenic, chromium, nickel, hydrocarbons	Lung cancer
Ultraviolet light	Melanoma and nonmelanomatous skin cancers
Benzene	Leukemia
Ionizing radiation	Sarcomas of bone and soft tissue, skin cancer, and leukemia

Familial adenomatous polyposis

Familial adenomatous polyposis is a hereditary condition in which the lining of the colon becomes studded with hundreds to thousands of polyps by late adolescence. A mutation in a gene identified as the adenomatous polyposis coli *(APC)* gene is considered the cause of this abnormal growth of polyps. Virtually all people with this condition eventually develop colon cancer. These individuals develop cancer at a much earlier age than the normal population. Treatment involves the removal of the entire colon and rectum.

Hereditary nonpolyposis colorectal cancer syndrome

Hereditary nonpolyposis colorectal cancer syndrome develops in the proximal colon in the absence of polyps or with fewer than five polyps. It has a familial distribution, occurring in three first-degree relatives in two generations, with at least one person being diagnosed before age 50. Hereditary nonpolyposis colorectal cancer syndrome, also known as Lynch syndrome, has also been associated with the development of cancers of the breast, endometrium, pancreas, and biliary tract.

Familial cancer research

Current research to identify the genes responsible for cancer can assist in detecting cancers at a much earlier stage in high-risk patients. Many institutions have familial cancer programs to provide genetic testing and counseling for persons with strong family histories of cancer. Experts assist in educating individuals about their potential risk for developing cancer and the importance of screening and early detection. Genetic testing remains the patient's option, and many patients prefer not to be tested.

TISSUE ORIGINS OF CANCER

Cancers may arise in any human tissue. Tumors are usually categorized under six general headings according to their tissue of origin (Table 30.4). Of cancers, 80 to 90% arise from *epithelial tissue* and are classified as *carcinomas*. Epithelial tissue lines the free internal and external surfaces of the body. Carcinomas are subdivided further into squamous cell carcinomas and adenocarcinomas based on the type of epithelium from which they arise. A squamous cell carcinoma arises from the surface (squamous) epithelium of a structure. Examples of surface epithelium include the oral cavity, pharynx, bronchus, skin, and cervix. An adenocarcinoma is a cancer that develops in glandular epithelium, such as in the prostate, colon and rectum, lung, breast, or endometrium.

To facilitate the exchange of patient information from one physician to another, the International Union Against Cancer and the American Joint Committee on Cancer (AJCC) Staging and End Results Reporting designed a system for classifying tumors based on anatomic and histologic considerations. The AJCC TNM classification (Table 30.5) describes a tumor according to the size of the primary lesion or tumor (T), the involvement of the regional lymph nodes (N), and the occurrence of metastasis (M).

TABLE 30.4

Categorization of cancers by tissue of origin

Tissue of origin	Type of tumor
Epithelium	
Surface epithelium	Squamous cell carcinoma
Glandular epithelium	Adenocarcinoma
Connective tissue	
Bone	Osteosarcoma
Fat	Liposarcoma
Lymphoreticular-hematopoietic tissue	
Lymph nodes	Lymphoma
Plasma cells	Multiple myeloma
Blood cells/bone marrow	Leukemia
Nerve tissue	
Glial tissue	Glioma
Neuroectoderm	Neuroblastoma
Tumors of more than one tissue	
Embryonic	Nephroblastoma kidney
Tumors that do not fit into above categories	
Testis	Seminoma
Thymus	Thymoma

TABLE 30.5

Application of TNM classification system

Classification	Description of tumor
Stage 0—$T_0N_0M_0$	Occult lesion; no evidence clinically
Stage I—$T_1N_0M_0$	Small lesion confined to organ of origin with no evidence of vascular and lymphatic spread or metastasis
Stage II—$T_2N_1M_0$	Tumor of <5 cm invading surrounding tissue and first-station lymph nodes but no evidence of metastasis
Stage III—$T_3N_2M_0$	Extensive lesion >5 cm with fixation to deeper structure and lymph invasion but no evidence of metastasis
Stage IV—$T_4N_3M_1$	More extensive lesion than above with invasion of bone or other adjacent structures or with distant metastasis (M_1)

Note: This is a generalization. Variations of the staging system exist for each tumor site.

Theory

The biologic effectiveness of ionizing radiation in living tissue depends partially on the amount of energy that is deposited within the tissue and partially on the condition of the biologic system. The terms used to describe this relationship are *linear energy transfer* (LET) and *relative biologic effectiveness* (RBE).

LET values are expressed in thousands of electron volts deposited per micron of tissue (keV/μm) and vary depending on the type of radiation being considered. Because of their mass and possible charge, particles tend to interact more readily with the material through which they are passing and have a greater LET value. A 5-MeV (megaelectron volt) alpha particle has an LET value of 100 keV/mm in tissue; nonparticulate radiations such as 250-kilovolt (peak) (kVp) x-rays and 1.2-MeV gamma rays have much lower LET values: 2.0 and 0.2 keV/mm.

RBE values are determined by calculating the ratio of the dose from a standard beam of radiation to the dose required of the radiation beam in question to produce a similar biologic effect. The standard beam of radiation is 250-kVp x-rays, and the ratio is set up as follows:

$$\text{RBE} = \frac{\text{Standard beam does to obtain effect}}{\text{Similar effect using beam in question}}$$

As the LET increases, so does the RBE. RBE and LET values are listed in Table 30.6.

The effectiveness of ionizing radiation on a biologic system depends not only on the amount of radiation deposited but also on the state of the biologic system. One of the first laws of radiation biology, postulated by Bergonié and Tribondeau, stated in essence that the *radiosensitivity* of a tissue depends on the number of *undifferentiated* cells in the tissue, the degree of mitotic activity of the tissue, and the length of time that cells of the tissue remain in active proliferation. Although exceptions exist, the preceding is true in most tissues. The primary target of ionizing radiation is the DNA molecule, and the human cell is most radiosensitive during mitosis. Current research tends to indicate that all cells are equally radiosensitive; however, the manifestation of the radiation injury occurs at different time frames (i.e., acute versus late effects).

Because tissue cells are composed primarily of water, most of the *ionization* occurs with water molecules. These events are called *indirect effects* and result in the formation of free radicals such as OH, H, and HO_2. These highly reactive free radicals may recombine with no resultant biologic effect, or they may combine with other atoms and molecules to produce biochemical changes that may be deleterious to the cell. The possibility also exists that the radiation may interact with an organic molecule or atom, which may result in the inactivation of the cell; this reaction is called the *direct effect*. Because ionizing radiation is nonspecific (i.e., it interacts with normal cells as readily as with tumor cells), cellular damage occurs in normal and abnormal tissue. The deleterious effects are greater in the tumor cells, however, because a greater percentage of these cells are undergoing mitosis, tumor cells also tend to be more poorly *differentiated*. In addition, normal cells have a greater capability for repairing sublethal damage than tumor cells. Greater cell damage occurs to tumor cells than to normal cells for any given increment of dose. The effects of the interactions in either normal or tumor cells may be expressed by the following descriptions:
- Loss of reproductive ability
- Metabolic changes
- Cell transformation
- Acceleration of the aging process
- Cell mutation

As the number of interactions increases, so does the possibility of cell death.

The preceding information leads to a categorization of tumors according to their radiosensitivity:
1. Very radiosensitive
   - Gonadal germ cell tumors (seminoma of testis, dysgerminoma of ovary)
   - Lymphoproliferative tumors (Hodgkin and non-Hodgkin lymphomas)
   - Embryonal tumors (Wilms tumor of the kidney)
2. Moderately radiosensitive
   - Epithelial tumors (squamous and basal cell carcinomas of skin)
   - Glandular tumors (adenocarcinoma of prostate)
3. Relatively radioresistant
   - Mesenchymal tumors (sarcomas of bone and connective tissue)
   - Nerve tumors (glioma)

As cellular function are increasingly understood, supplemental therapy with drugs or simply oxygen has continuously been found to enhance the effectiveness of radiation treatments.

TABLE 30.6

Relative biologic effectiveness and linear energy transfer values for certain forms of radiation

Radiation	RBE	LET
250-kV x-rays	1	2.0
^{60}Co gamma rays	0.85	0.2
14-MeV neutrons	12	75
5-MeV alpha particles	20	100

LET, Linear energy transfer; *RBE*, relative biologic effectiveness.

Technical Aspects

EXTERNAL-BEAM THERAPY AND BRACHYTHERAPY

Two major categories for the application of radiation for cancer treatment are external-beam therapy and brachytherapy. For *external-beam treatment*, the patient lies underneath a machine that emits radiation or generates a beam of x-rays. Most cancer patients are treated in this fashion. Some patients may also be treated with *brachytherapy*, a technique in which the radioactive material is placed within the patient.

The theory behind brachytherapy is to deliver low-intensity radiation over an extended period to a relatively small volume of tissue. The low-intensity isotopes are placed directly into a tissue or cavity, depositing radiation only a short distance, covering the tumor area but sparing surrounding normal tissue. This technique allows a higher total dose of radiation to be delivered to the tumor than is achievable with external-beam radiation alone. Brachytherapy may be accomplished in any of the following ways:

1. Mold technique—placement of a *radioactive* source or sources on or in close proximity to the lesion
2. Intracavitary implant technique—placement of a radioactive source or sources in a body cavity (i.e., uterine canal and vagina)
3. Interstitial implant technique—placement of a radioactive source or sources directly into the tumor site and adjacent tissue (i.e., sarcoma in a muscle)

Most brachytherapy applications tend to be temporary in that the sources are left in the patient until a designated tumor dose has been attained. Two different brachytherapy systems exist. They are *low-dose-rate* (LDR) and *high-dose-rate* (HDR). LDR brachytherapy has been the standard system for many years. A low-activity isotope is used to deliver a dose of radiation at a slow rate of 40 to 500 cGy per hour. This therapy requires that a patient be hospitalized for 3 to 4 days until the desired dose is delivered.

HDR systems are the current standard method of brachytherapy. This system uses a high-activity isotope capable of delivering greater than 1200 cGy per hour. The HDR system allows the prescribed dose to be delivered in minutes, which means that this treatment can occur on an outpatient basis. Gynecologic tumors are one of the most common sites to be treated with HDR brachytherapy. HDR systems use a high-activity iridium-192 source.

Permanent implant therapy may also be accomplished. This is the most common type of LDR brachytherapy in practice today. An example of a permanent implant nuclide is iodine-125 and palladium-103 seeds. Permanent implant nuclides have relatively short *half-lives* of days and are indefinitely left in the patient. The amount and distribution of the radionuclide implanted in this manner depends on the total dose that the radiation oncologist is trying to deliver. Early-stage prostate cancer is commonly treated with this technique alone. In some cases of brachytherapy implantation, the implant is applied as part of the patient's overall treatment plan and may be preceded by or followed by additional external-beam radiation therapy.

EQUIPMENT

Most radiation oncology departments use linear accelerators (linacs) as their main treatment unit. Following are treatment units that may be found in a radiation oncology department:

- 120-kVp superficial x-ray unit for treating lesions on or near the surface of the patient
- 250-kVp orthovoltage x-ray unit for moderately superficial tissues
- ^{60}Co (cobalt-60) *gamma ray* source with an average energy of 1.25-MeV; Gamma Knife Unit
- 6-MV to 35-MV *linear accelerator* to serve as a source of high-energy (megavoltage) electrons and x-rays
- TomoTherapy
- CyberKnife
- Proton therapy

The dose depositions of these units are compared in Fig. 30.1.

The penetrability, or energy, of an x-ray or gamma ray totally depends on its wavelength: The shorter the wavelength, the more penetrating the photon; conversely, the longer the wavelength, the less penetrating the photon. A low-energy beam ($\leq$120 kVp) of radiation tends to deposit all or most of its energy on or near the surface of the patient and is suitable for treating lesions on or near the skin surface. In addition, with the low-energy beam, a greater amount of absorption or dose deposition occurs in bone than in soft tissue.

A high-energy beam of radiation ($\geq$1 MeV) tends to deposit its energy throughout the entire volume of tissue irradiated, with a greater amount of dose deposition occurring at or near the entry port than at the exit port. In this energy range, the dose is deposited about equally in soft tissue and bone. The high-energy (megavoltage) beam is most suitable for tumors deep beneath the body surface.

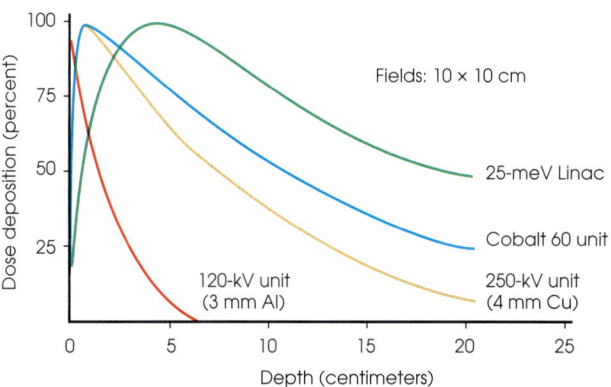

Fig. 30.1 Plot of percent of dose deposition in relation to depth in centimeters of tissue for various energies of photon beams.

The *skin-sparing* effect, a phenomenon that occurs as the energy of a beam of radiation is increased, is valuable from a therapeutic standpoint. In the superficial and orthovoltage energy range, the maximum dose occurs on the surface of the patient, and the deposition of the dose decreases as the beam traverses the patient. As the energy of the beam increases into the megavoltage range, the maximum dose absorbed by the patient occurs at some point below the skin surface. The skin-sparing effect is important clinically because the skin is a radiosensitive organ. Excessive dose deposition to the skin can damage the skin, requiring treatments to be stopped and compromising treatment for the underlying tumor. The greater the energy of the beam, the more deeply the maximum dose is deposited (Fig. 30.2).

Cobalt-60 units

The cobalt-60 (^{60}Co) unit was the first skin-sparing machine. It replaced the orthovoltage unit in the early 1950s because of its greater ability to treat tumors located deeper within tissues. ^{60}Co is an artificially produced *isotope* formed in a nuclear *reactor* by the bombardment of stable cobalt-59 with neutrons. ^{60}Co emits two gamma-ray beams with an energy of 1.17 and 1.33 MeV. The unit was known as a "workhorse" because it was extremely reliable, was mechanically simple, and had little downtime. It was the first radiation therapy unit to rotate 360 degrees around a patient. A machine that rotates around a fixed point, or axis, and maintains the same distance from the source of radiation is called an *isocentric machine*. All modern therapeutic units are isocentric machines. This type of machine allows the patient to remain in one position, lessening the chance for patient movement during treatment. Isocentric capabilities also assist in directing the beam precisely at the tumor while sparing normal structures.

Because ^{60}Co is a radioisotope, it constantly emits radiation as it *decays* in an effort to return to a stable state. It has a half-life of 5.26 years (i.e., its activity is reduced by 50% at the end of 5.26 years). Because the source decays at a rate of 1% per month, the radiation treatment time must be adjusted, resulting in longer treatment times as the source decays.

The use of ^{60}Co units has declined significantly since the 1980s, and ^{60}Co is rarely used for conventional external-beam radiation therapy today. This decline has been basically attributed to the introduction of the more sophisticated linac, which has greater skin-sparing capabilities and more sharply defined radiation *fields*. The radiation beam, or field, from a ^{60}Co unit also has large penumbra, which results in fuzzy field edges, another undesirable feature. ^{60}Co is still used in radiation oncology as part of a special procedure called stereotactic radiosurgery (SRS). The treatment unit is called the Gamma Knife. The Gamma Knife consists of 192 to 201 ^{60}Co sources arranged in a hemispherical array with all sources converging at a single

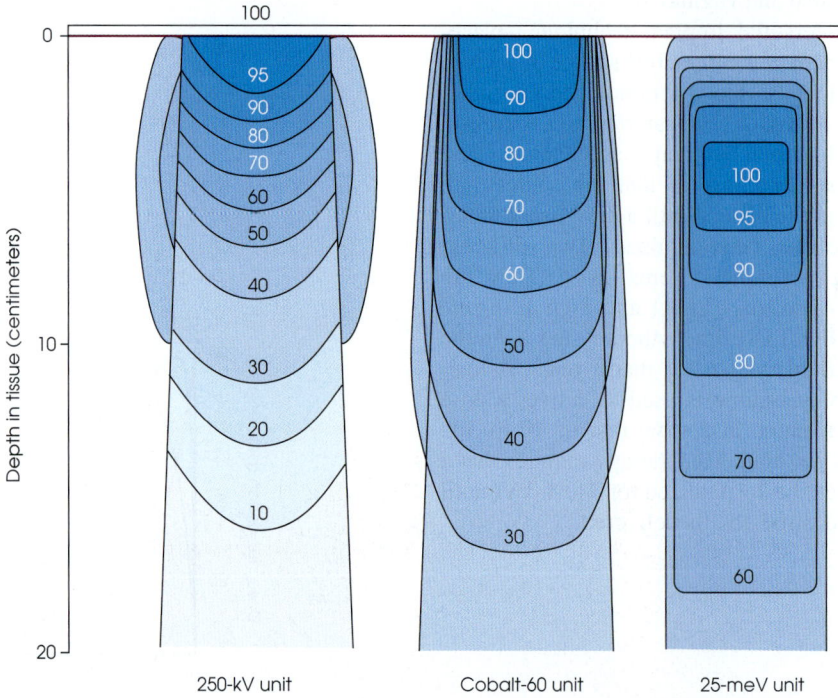

Fig. 30.2 Three isodose curves showing comparison of percent of dose deposition from three x-ray units of different energies. As the energy of the beam increases, the percentage of dose deposited on the surface of the patient decreases.

point (Fig. 30.3). The point where the beams converge forms a treatment area of 4 to 18 mm in diameter.

The Gamma Knife is primarily used to treat small benign or malignant lesions located deep within the brain, employing an external rigidly fixed stereotactic head frame. The Gamma Knife does not involve surgery. It is called radiosurgery because the radiation is delivered in such a precise, focused manner that the lesion is ablated as if removed surgically. Adjacent normal tissues receive minimal radiation and are unharmed. The stereotactic head frame provides a coordinate system that allows the lesion to be three-dimensionally localized on MRI, CT scan, or angiography so that the radiation can be planned and targeted directly to the involved area. The Gamma Knife delivers a large dose of radiation in a single treatment to one or more areas in the brain. The types of conditions treated with the Gamma Knife include benign conditions such as acoustic neuromas, pituitary adenomas, arteriovenous malformations, and trigeminal neuralgia. Malignant lesions treated with the Gamma Knife include gliomas, meningiomas, chordoma, and solitary brain metastasis.

Gamma Knife radiosurgery has many advantages over conventional neurosurgery. First, the patient does not have to undergo an invasive surgical procedure. The procedure can be done as an outpatient or may require an overnight stay in the hospital. The Gamma Knife procedure requires no major recuperation period. The cost of Gamma Knife radiosurgery is much less than the cost of neurosurgery. The Gamma Knife is considered a very effective treatment for small intracranial lesions. One disadvantage of the Gamma Knife is that it can be used only for intracranial lesions. Another disadvantage is that the effects of radiation on the lesion are not immediate but occur over a period of weeks.

Linear accelerators

Linacs are the most commonly used machines for cancer treatment. The first linac was developed in 1952 and first used clinically in the United States in 1956. A linac is capable of producing high-energy beams of photons (x-rays) or electrons in the range of 4 million to 35 million volts. These megavoltage photon beams allow a better distribution of dose to deep-seated tumors with better sparing of normal tissues than their earlier counterparts—the orthovoltage or ^{60}Co units.

The photon beam is produced by accelerating a stream of electrons toward a target. When the electrons hit the target, a beam of x-rays is produced. By removing the target, the linac can also produce a beam of electrons of varying energies.

Typically, a linear accelerator is equipped with two photon energies consisting of one low-energy (6-MeV) and one high-energy (18-MeV) photon beam plus a range of electron energies (Fig. 30.4). The dual photon energy machine gives the radiation oncologist more options in prescribing radiation treatments. As the energy of the beam increases, so does its penetrating power. A lower-energy beam is used to treat tumors in thinner parts of the body, whereas high-energy beams are prescribed for tumors in thicker parts of the body. A brain tumor or a tumor in a limb would most likely be treated with a 6-MeV beam; conversely, a pelvic malignancy would be better treated with an 18-MeV beam.

Electrons are advantageous over photons in that they are a more superficial form of treatment. Electrons are energy dependent, which means that they deposit their energy within a given depth of tissue and go no deeper, depending on the energy selected. An 18-MeV beam has a total penetration depth of 9 cm (3.5 inches). Any structure located deeper than 9 cm (3.5 inches) would not be appreciably affected. This is important when the radiation oncologist is trying to treat a tumor that overlies a critical structure.

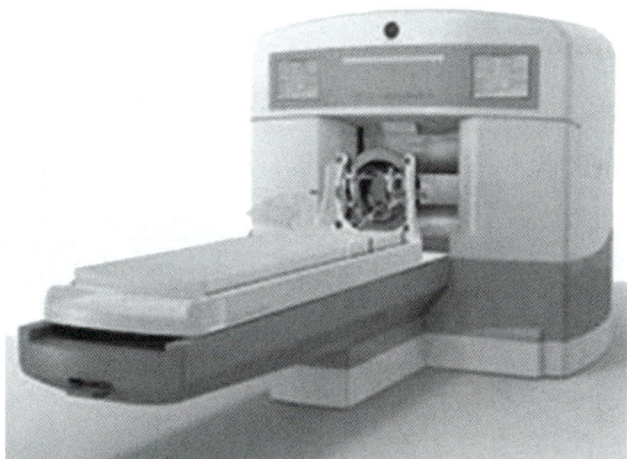

Fig. 30.3 Gamma Knife unit without a patient on the treatment table.

(From Washington CM, Leaver DT, eds. *Principles and practice of radiation therapy*, 3rd ed. St Louis: Elsevier; 2010.)

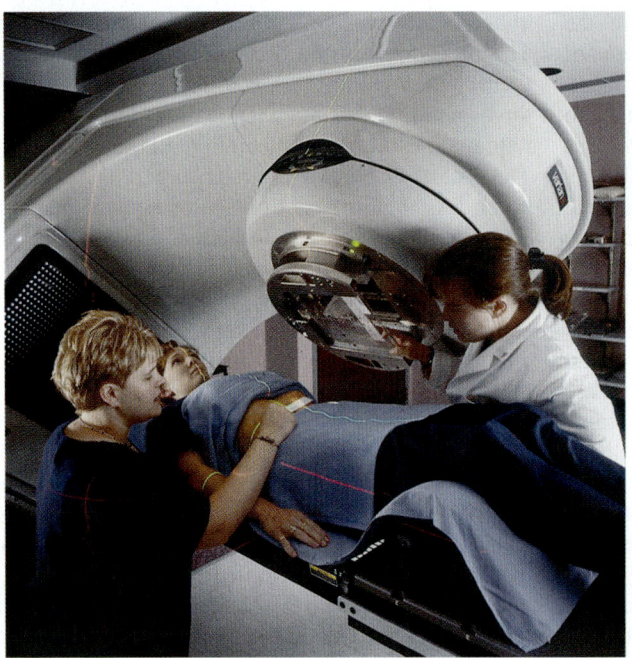

Fig. 30.4 Radiation therapists shown aligning the patient and shielding block in preparation for treatment using a modern linac. X-ray beams of 6 to 25 million V may be produced to treat tumors in the body.

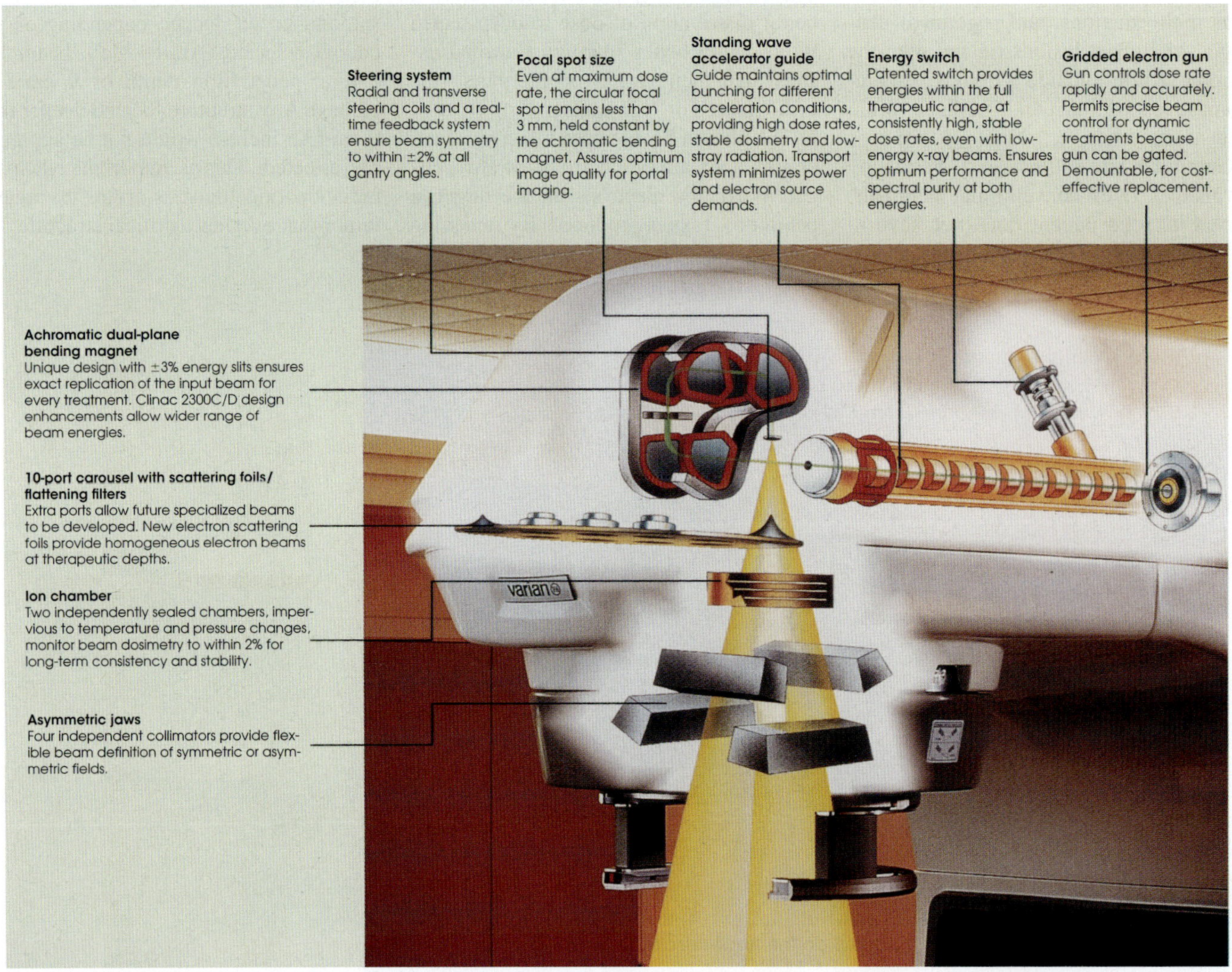

Steering system
Radial and transverse steering coils and a real-time feedback system ensure beam symmetry to within ±2% at all gantry angles.

Focal spot size
Even at maximum dose rate, the circular focal spot remains less than 3 mm, held constant by the achromatic bending magnet. Assures optimum image quality for portal imaging.

Standing wave accelerator guide
Guide maintains optimal bunching for different acceleration conditions, providing high dose rates, stable dosimetry and low-stray radiation. Transport system minimizes power and electron source demands.

Energy switch
Patented switch provides energies within the full therapeutic range, at consistently high, stable dose rates, even with low-energy x-ray beams. Ensures optimum performance and spectral purity at both energies.

Gridded electron gun
Gun controls dose rate rapidly and accurately. Permits precise beam control for dynamic treatments because gun can be gated. Demountable, for cost-effective replacement.

Achromatic dual-plane bending magnet
Unique design with ±3% energy slits ensures exact replication of the input beam for every treatment. Clinac 2300C/D design enhancements allow wider range of beam energies.

10-port carousel with scattering foils/ flattening filters
Extra ports allow future specialized beams to be developed. New electron scattering foils provide homogeneous electron beams at therapeutic depths.

Ion chamber
Two independently sealed chambers, impervious to temperature and pressure changes, monitor beam dosimetry to within 2% for long-term consistency and stability.

Asymmetric jaws
Four independent collimators provide flexible beam definition of symmetric or asymmetric fields.

Fig. 30.5 Asymmetric jaws. Note the four independent collimators.

(Courtesy Varian Associates, Palo Alto, CA.)

As with a diagnostic x-ray machine, the irradiated field of a linac is defined by a light field projected onto the patient's skin. This corresponding square or rectangle equals the length and width setting of the x-ray *collimators*. A modern linac is equipped with *asymmetric (independent) jaws;* this allows each of the four collimator blades that define length or width to move independently (Fig. 30.5). The jaw that defines the superior extent of the field may be 7 cm (2.75 inches) from the central axis, whereas the inferior region may be at 10 cm (4 inches). The total length would equal 17 cm (6.75 inches), but it is not divided equally because it is in a diagnostic x-ray collimator. The radiation oncologist is able to design a field that optimally covers the area of interest while sparing normal tissue. Independent collimation can also assist in reducing the total weight of lead shielding blocks generally constructed to protect normal tissues.

Multileaf collimation

Multileaf collimation (MLC) is the newest and most complex beam-defining system. Within the head of the linac, 45 to 80 individual collimator blades, 1 to 2 cm wide (about 0.4–0.75 inch), are located and can be adjusted to shape the radiation field to conform to the target volume (Fig. 30.6). The design of the field is digitized from a radiograph into a computer software program, which is transferred to the treatment room. The MLC machine receives a code that tells it how to position the individual leaves for the treatment field. Before MLC, custom-made lead blocks, or *Cerrobend* blocks, were constructed to shape radiation fields and shield normal tissues from the beam of radiation. Heavy Cerrobend blocks were placed within the head of the linac for each treatment field. Linacs equipped with the MLC package receive a custom-designed field at the stroke of a computer keyboard. Multileaf collimators are programmed to move across the radiation field during a treatment to alter the intensity of the radiation beam. Altering the beam intensity across the radiation field allows a lower dose to be delivered to normal structures and tissues and ensures that the tumor or target receives the prescribed dose. This technique is called *intensity-modulated radiation therapy* (IMRT). IMRT allows the dose of radiation to be more tightly conformed to the target areas and has greatly reduced the dose to normal tissues and structures. IMRT is widely used and has replaced the conventional treatment field approach for most cancers, such as prostate and gynecologic cancers in the pelvis and cancers of the head and neck. IMRT can be used for any anatomic site.

Steps in Radiation Oncology
SIMULATION

The first step of radiation therapy involves determining the volume of tissue that needs to be encompassed within the radiation field. This is done with a *CT simulator*. During simulation, the radiation oncologist uses the patient's CT images or MRI to determine the tumor's precise location and to design a treatment volume or area. The treatment volume often includes the tumor plus a small margin, the draining lymphatics that are at risk for involvement, and a rim of normal tissue to account for patient movement.

Most centers perform virtual simulations using a CT scanner equipped with radiation oncology software tools (Fig. 30.7). CT simulation is to position the patient in a manner that is stable and reproducible for each of the prescribed radiation treatments, which can range from 1 to 68 treatments (most commonly 25 to 40). Therapists are responsible for constructing immobilization devices to help patients hold their position. It is crucial for a patient to hold still and maintain the same position. If the patient does not maintain the planned position, critical normal tissues may be irradiated, or the tumor may not be irradiated.

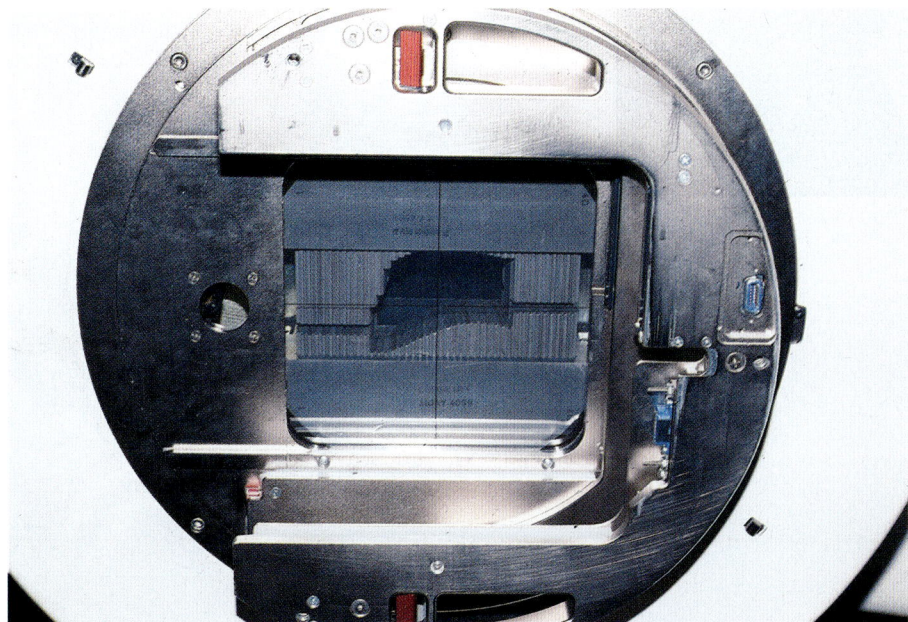

Fig. 30.6 Multileaf collimation system on the treatment head.

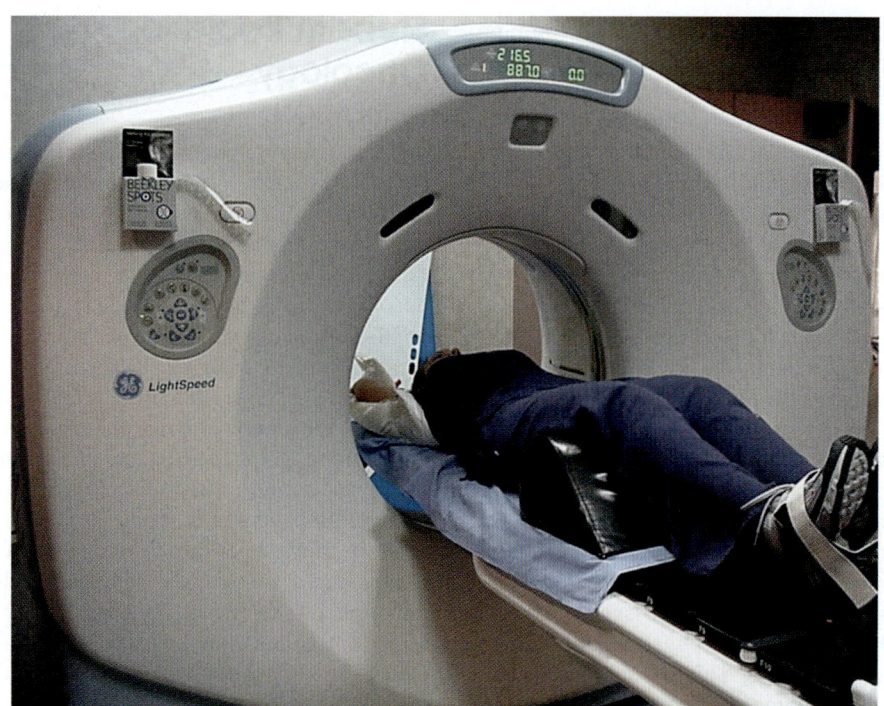

Fig. 30.7 CT simulator.

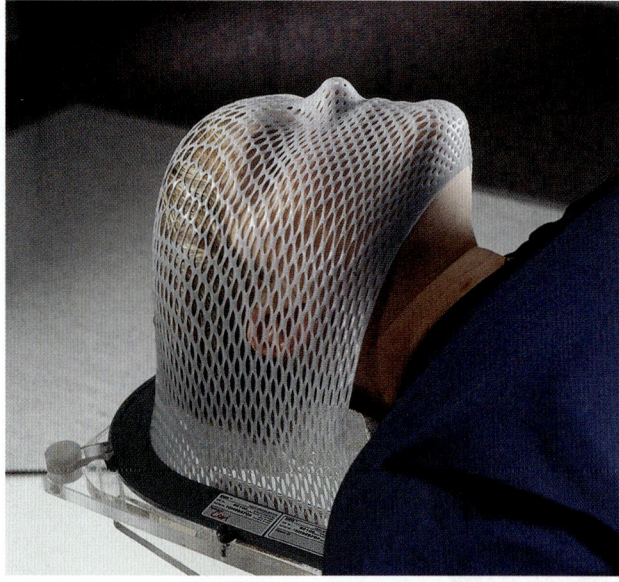

Fig. 30.8 Aquaplast mask.

Immobilization devices greatly assist the radiation therapist in correctly aligning the patient for each treatment, and many patients feel more secure when supported by these devices. Immobilization devices can be constructed for any part of the body but are most important for more mobile parts, such as the head and neck region or the limbs. Many different types of immobilization systems exist. Fig. 30.8 shows a thermoplastic device that secures the head and neck against rotation or flexion-extension. Fig. 30.9 shows a vacuum bag device that may be used to secure the upper body or lower extremities.

Contrast material is often administered before or during a simulation to localize the area that needs to be treated or to identify vital normal structures that are to be shielded. A small amount of meglumine diatrizoate (Gastrografin or Gastroview) for CT simulation is injected into the rectum of a patient with rectal cancer to assist in localizing the rectum on the simulation images. Contrast material in the bladder is used to assist in localizing the prostate gland, which lies directly inferior to the bladder. Rectal contrast material is used to show the relationship of the rectum to the prostate to monitor and minimize the dose the rectum receives (Fig. 30.10).

When a CT simulation is performed, a reference isocenter is marked on the patient, and a pilot or scout scan is obtained. The radiation oncologist uses the scout or pilot image to determine the superior and inferior extent of the area to be scanned. The CT data are transferred to the virtual simulation computer workstation. From this limited scan, the physician reviews the CT images and uses imaging tools to outline the target volume and critical normal structures. The physician establishes the actual treatment isocenter. The computer software determines the change in location from the coordinates associated with the reference marks to the newly established treatment isocenter. The radiation therapist adjusts the couch and uses the laser marking system to apply these shifts to mark the treatment isocenter on the patient. The radiation therapist records all details regarding the patient's position in the treatment chart, and the patient is dismissed.

The physician, physicist, or dosimetrist creates treatment fields (length and width) electronically with the CT virtual simulation software (Fig. 30.11). The CT simulation data are transferred to the treatment planning system. In complex cases, the physician communicates preferences for treatment goals to the dosimetrist, who then designs the beam's eye view treatment fields and beam arrangement as part of the three-dimensional planning. A digitally reconstructed radiograph (DRR) for each treatment field is produced. The DRR is analogous to the radiograph taken in the conventional simulator (Fig. 30.12).

Precise measurements and details about the field dimensions, machine position, and patient positioning are recorded in the treatment chart. In some centers, the treatment parameters, such as field length, width, couch, and gantry positions, are electronically captured and transferred to the treatment unit. Recording of this information is crucial so that the radiation therapist performing the treatment can precisely reproduce the exact information.

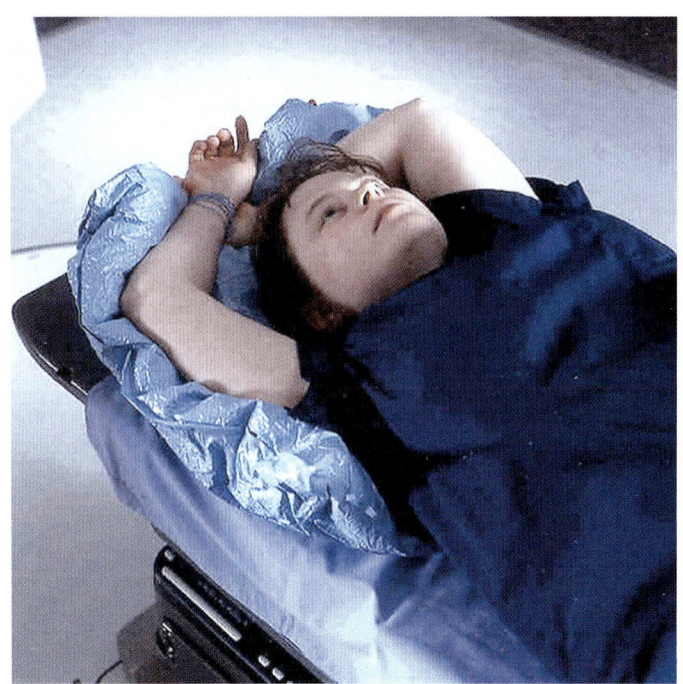

Fig. 30.9 Vacuum bag immobilization device.

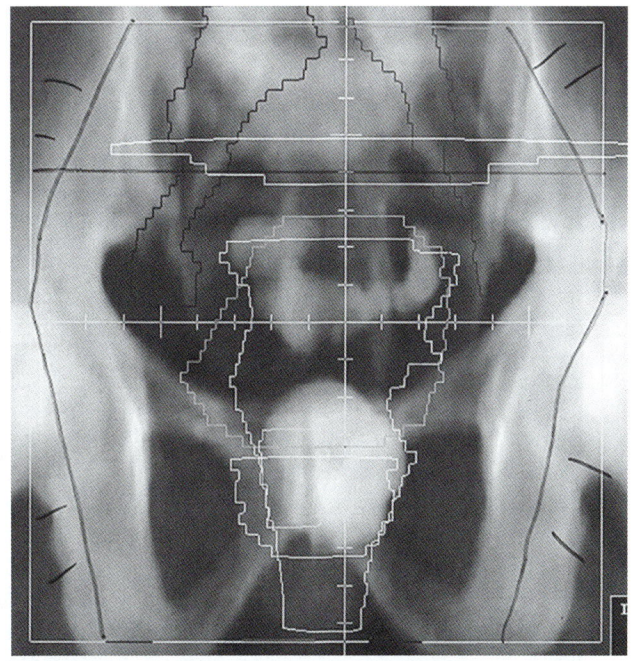

Fig. 30.10 CT simulation digitally reconstructed radiograph of standard PA field.

(From Washington CM, Leaver DT, eds. *Principles and practice of radiation therapy*, 4th ed. St Louis: Elsevier; 2016.)

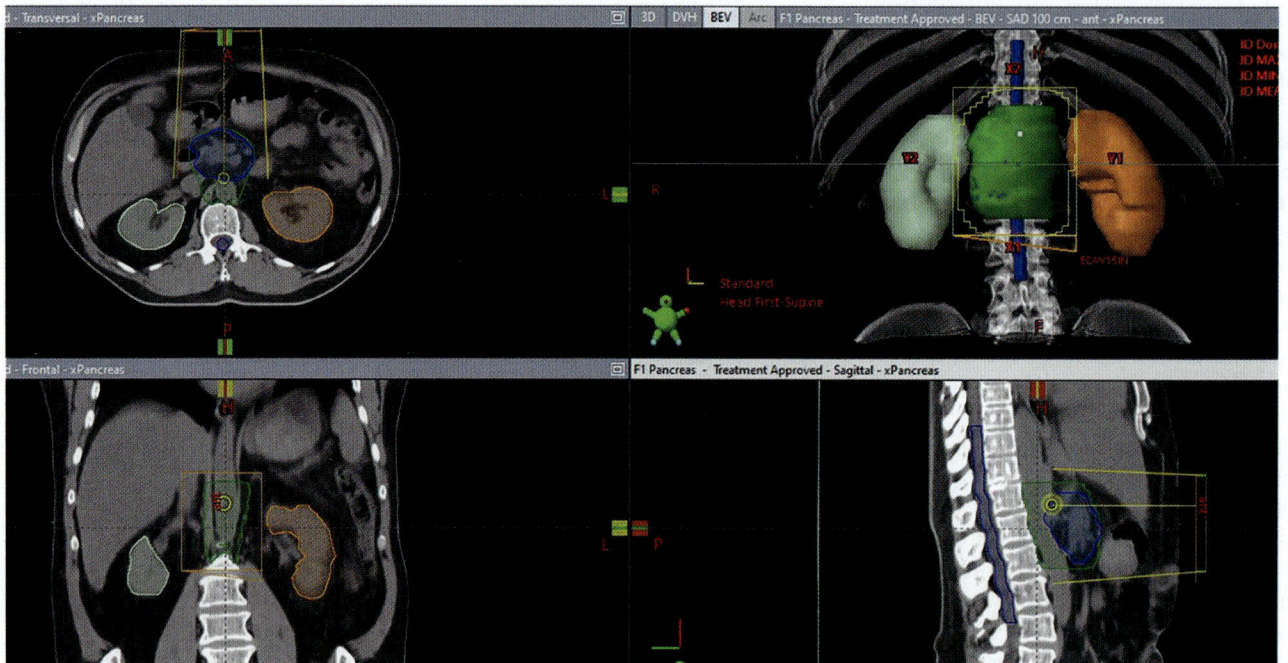

Fig. 30.11 Virtual CT simulation. Note divergent radiation beam lines indicating the path of the beam. Target volume (the pancreas), kidneys, and spinal cord have been outlined on CT axial image and reconstructed sagittal and coronal images. Treatment field outline is seen on DRR and coronal image.

(Used with permission of Mayo Foundation for Medical Education and Research, all rights reserved.)

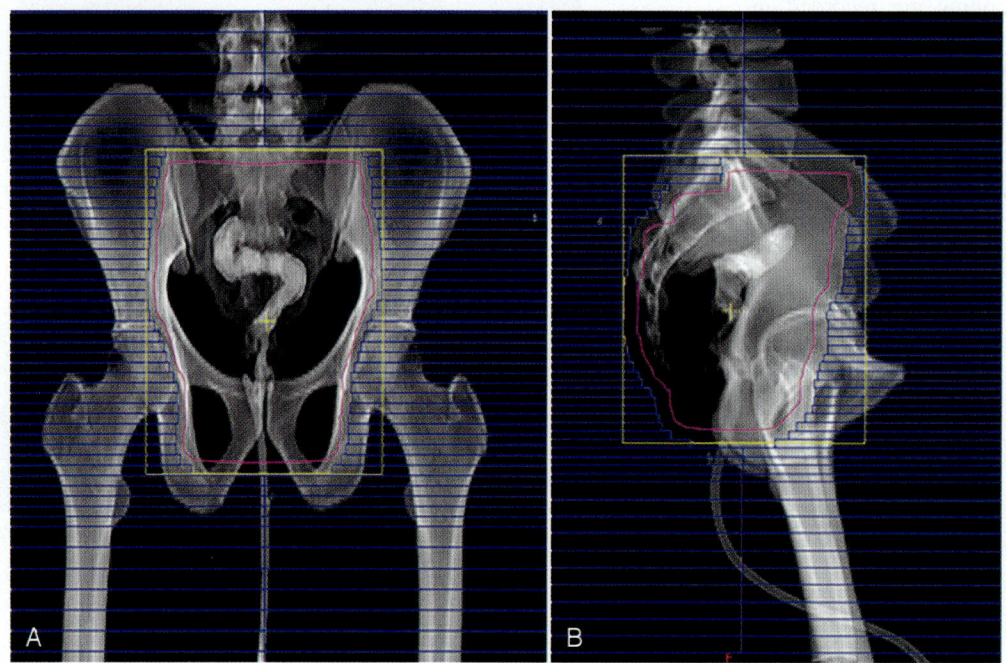

Fig. 30.12 DRR PA (**A**) and lateral (**B**) pelvis with rectal contrast. Note outline of treatment field.

DOSIMETRY

Dosimetry refers to the measurement of radiation dose, and it shows how the radiation is distributed or *attenuated* throughout the patient's body (absorbing medium). The dosimetrist devises a treatment plan that best fulfills the physician's prescription for the desired dose to the *tumor/target volume* while minimizing the amount of radiation to critical normal structures or tissues.

Each organ of the body has a tolerance dose to radiation that limits the amount it can receive and still function normally. If an organ receives an excess of the tolerance dose, the organ can fail, resulting in a fatal complication. The kidneys are among the more radiosensitive structures of the body (Table 30.7). A dose greater than 2500 cGy can result in fatal radiation nephritis. The spinal cord has a higher tolerance dose, but many tumors require even higher doses for treatment to be effective.

Precise localization of dose-limiting structures and their relationship with the target volume is crucial for adequate planning. The dosimetrist must devise a plan that delivers a homogeneous dose to the tumor, while not exceeding the tolerance dose of a specific organ. This task can be quite challenging. The radiation oncologist might prescribe 6000 cGy to treat lung cancer located in the mediastinum directly over the spine but must limit the spinal cord dose to 4500 cGy to prevent irreparable damage, which could result in paralysis. The dosimetrist must devise a plan that enables combined treatment and protection to be accomplished.

Historically, the first step in dosimetry is to obtain a contour or CT scan of the patient in treatment position. A *contour* is an outline of the external surface of the patient's body at the level of the central axis (center of treatment field). This contour is typically performed in the transverse plane, but other planes may be used. Then the tumor volume and critical dose-limiting internal structures are transferred from the simulation radiographs and drawn onto the contour. CT scans from a CT simulator are almost exclusively used today rather than contours. With CT scanning, the tumor and internal structures and their relationships are directly visible. These images are interfaced with the treatment planning computer system for the development of the plan.

PET and MRI with the patient in treatment position are also obtained sometimes to facilitate the planning process. Fusion of MRI or PET images onto the CT simulation dataset allows a more precise delineation of the tumor volume than what would be seen on CT alone. To obtain an even distribution of radiation to the target volume, radiation is delivered from various angles focused on the area of interest. Three-dimensional treatment planning allows for the design of a beam that exactly conforms to the shape of the tumor at any plane within the body. The treatment planning system can digitally reconstruct the anatomy, which allows the dosimetrist to manipulate the image to view the tumor from any angle or plane. Important critical anatomic structures such as the kidneys and spinal cord are also more readily identified. Such a system allows the dosimetrist to plan and design beams that are coplanar and non-coplanar, tightly conforming to the target or tumor volume. This is known as *three-dimensional conformal radiotherapy* (CRT). The beam's eye view obtained by three-dimensional beams allows higher doses of radiation to be administered more safely by treating the cancer through multiple fields (more than four) on different planes, which reduces the amount of dose that normal tissues receive (Fig. 30.13).

The standard approach for a tumor located in the pelvis, such as rectal cancer, is the use of three fields—posteroanterior (PA), right lateral, and left lateral. Using the treatment parameters established in the simulator, the dosimetrist enters this information into the treatment planning system, designs beam's eye view conformal fields, and obtains an isodose distribution, which shows how the radiation is being deposited. An *isodose line/curve* is a summation of areas of equal radiation dosage and may be stated as percentages of the total prescribed dose or as actual radiation dosages in *gray* (Gy) units.

TABLE 30.7
Tolerance doses to radiation

Structure	Tolerance dose (cGy)
Testes	500
Ovary	500
Lung (whole lung)	1800
Kidney (whole organ)	2300
Liver (whole organ)	3000
Spinal cord (5 cm^3)	4500

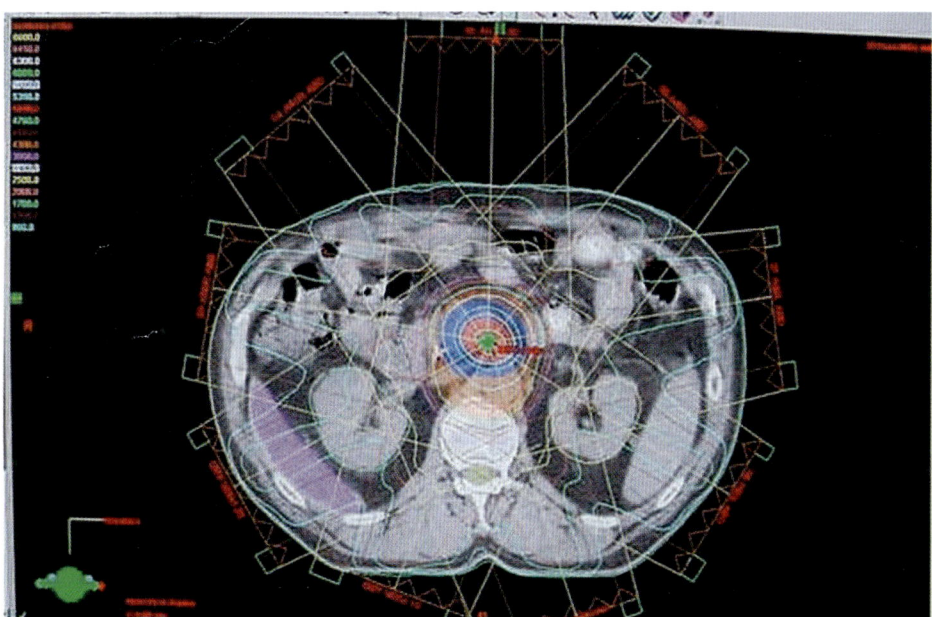

Fig. 30.13 Dosimetry plan showing nine different radiation fields used to treat pancreatic tumor.

The dosimetrist optimizes the plan by eliminating any areas of dose inhomogeneity (e.g., hot spots). A *hot spot* is an area of excessive radiation dose. One method to adjust for hot spots is to add a *wedge filter*. This wedge-shaped device is made of lead and is placed within the radiation beam to absorb the radiation preferentially, altering the shape of the isodose curve (Fig. 30.14). Another method of reducing hot spots is to change the weighting of the radiation beams by delivering a greater dose of radiation from a particular field (i.e., a greater dose from the anterior field than from the posterior field).

Another major task of the dosimetrist is to monitor the dose that critical structures are receiving and to keep the dose within the established guidelines dictated by the physician. To avoid treating the spinal cord in the aforementioned example, the dosimetrist may angle the entry points of the radiation beams to include the target volume while not irradiating the spinal cord. The resultant fields might be right anterior oblique and left posterior oblique (RAO/LPO) fields. The dosimetrist evaluates the dose distribution after each modifier is added and looks at different combinations of wedges, beam weighting, and beam entry points until an acceptable plan is produced. This technique is called *forward planning*. The final plan directs the radiation therapist, who treats the patient, how to proceed. For the example presented previously (i.e., lung cancer in the mediastinum directly over the spine), the plan might consist of the following specifications:

1. Deliver 25 treatments anteroposterior (AP) and PA fields, RAO and LPO, 30 degrees off vertical.
2. Reduce field size to 12 cm long; deliver five more treatments AP, PA, RAO, and LPO, 30 degrees off vertical.

When the plan is complete, treatment of the patient can begin.

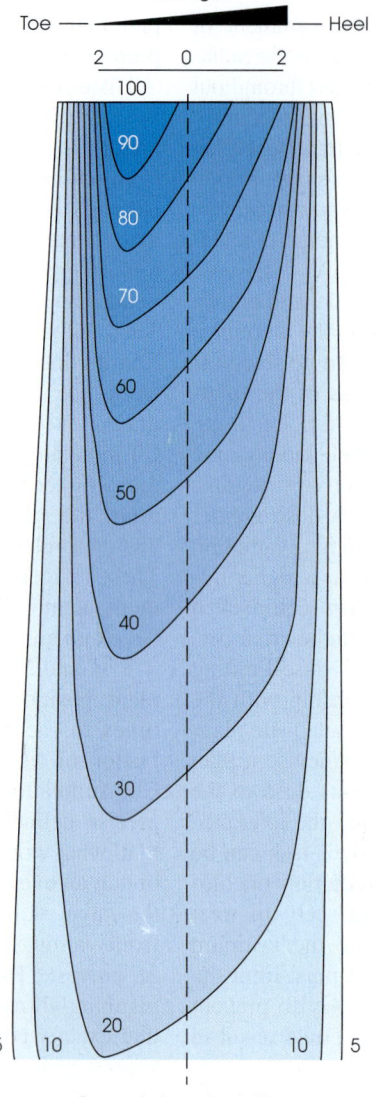

Fig. 30.14 Isodose curve obtained from ^{60}Co unit, with wedge placed between the source and absorbing material.

Another type of three-dimensional treatment planning is IMRT. The planning process begins as previously described—the physician identifies the target volume and critical structures. Treatment fields are designed and arranged so that the target receives the prescribed dose, and the dose to critical structures is limited. The optimization of the dose distribution is not done, however, by trying different combinations of wedges or dose weighting, as in conventional forward planning. IMRT uses a method called *inverse planning*. The prescribed dose to the target and the dose limit assigned to each critical structure are entered into the inverse planning system. A sophisticated mathematic algorithm creates a dose distribution that conforms to the target area while sparing critical normal structures. This is achieved by modifying the intensity of radiation within the treatment field and moving the individual leaves of the multileaf collimator across the radiation field during a treatment from open to closed position, modulating the intensity of a beam to obtain the desired dose. The plan is computed by dividing the treatment field beam into hundreds of beamlets. Each beamlet can have an intensity level that measures from 0% to 100%. The intensity of a beamlet is changed by maintaining the multileaf collimator open at a certain position for a specific amount of time and then closing it.

The IMRT planning process is time intensive and requires a comprehensive physics quality assurance check of multileaf collimator movement and dose verification before treatment is administered for the first time. IMRT has proven to be better at minimizing the dose to normal structures than conventional three-dimensional CRT and has allowed higher doses to be delivered to the target or tumor volume. IMRT was initially used for prostate cancer and cancers of the head and neck region. In prostate cancer treatment, IMRT optimized the dose to the prostate, while substantially minimizing the dose to the rectum and bladder. When treating cancer in the head and neck region (e.g., nasopharynx), IMRT significantly reduced the dose to the parotid glands, larynx, oral cavity, and spinal cord. IMRT is also used in the treatment of brain tumors and gastrointestinal, gynecologic, lung, breast, and soft tissue sarcomas.

The advantages of IMRT are well known—a method to deliver a highly conformal dose of radiation to the tumor while reducing the dose received by normal tissues. One disadvantage of IMRT is the total time it takes to deliver the daily session of radiation therapy. With the traditional IMRT stationary technique (static IMRT), a patient with head and neck cancer might be on the table for 30 minutes each day to deliver 10 to 18 different radiation fields. The patient might move between or during the time the radiation beam is on. The current and more common method of delivering IMRT treatment is called volumetric modulated arc therapy (VMAT). This method involves the linac rotating around the patient while the radiation beam is on and while the MLC leaves are dynamically moving for the IMRT delivery. With VMAT, the dose to the target and normal tissues is customized by altering the speed of the rotation, altering the dose rate of the linac, and simultaneously moving the MLC leaves. VMAT results in the delivery of the same highly conformal dose to the target while sparing normal tissues but in about half the time of a traditional IMRT stationary field technique. VMAT is also being used for prostate, lung, gynecologic, gastrointestinal, breast, and brain cancers. VMAT is widely utilized and is a very common form of treatment delivery today and has replaced static field IMRT in many cases.

TREATMENT

On completion of the planning stage, including simulation and dosimetry, patient treatment can begin. The radiation therapist positions the patient and aligns the skin marks according to what was recorded in the treatment chart at the time of simulation. Accuracy and attention to detail are crucial for the precise administration of the radiation to the patient. The radiation therapist is responsible for interpreting the radiation oncologist's prescription and calculating the correct monitor units to achieve a desired dose of radiation for each treatment field. This responsibility also involves recording the daily administration of the radiation and the cumulative dose to date.

Precision in positioning the machine, the proper selection of the treatment field and MLC, accurate placement of Cerrobend blocks or wedges, and implementation of any change in a patient's treatment plan are crucial for ensuring optimal treatment. Failure to do any of these may result in an overdose to normal tissue, causing long-term side effects, or an underexposure of the tumor, reducing the patient's chance for cure. Most radiation oncology departments use an electronic radiation oncology medical record and computer verification system that ensures a patient's treatment parameters are correct before treatment may begin. The complexity of three-dimensional CRT, IMRT, and VMAT treatments with the numerous positions of the treatment couch, gantry, or collimator necessitates the use of a verification system. The computer verification system compares the machine settings with the information in the patient's electronic radiation chart. If there is a mismatch between any of the parameters in the electronic chart and what is being set up for treatment, the radiation therapist would be unable to initiate treatment. When a mismatch occurs, a computer prompt appears, highlighting the areas of disagreement. The radiation therapist must double-check parameters and patient setup, making corrections before treatment may occur. The verification and record system also records and adds the cumulative radiation doses.

Almost all linacs are now equipped with electronic portal imaging devices (EPIDs) and a kilovolt (kV) imager. These retractable imaging devices produce digital images that are displayed immediately on a computer screen adjacent to the linac computer console. The EPID imager uses the 6-MV beam of the linac to obtain an image. Most radiation oncology departments have linacs equipped with a kV x-ray tube and flat-panel image detector in addition to EPID. The kV imager, called an onboard imager (OBI), provides a better diagnostic quality image with improved skeletal to soft tissue contrast compared with the megavoltage EPID imagers. These images can be viewed before treatment, and adjustments can be made to the table or patient position before delivering radiation, ensuring accurate and precise treatment. Most systems have computer software that compares the CT simulation image with the EPID or kV image, using a registration algorithm. The computer automatically calculates the necessary adjustments (e.g., shift in couch position) to be made. The radiation therapist makes the adjustments and begins treatment.

When this treatment is used in cases of prostate cancer, gold seed markers are injected into the prostate gland before simulation. After the CT simulation is performed, the patient's treatment plan is completed, and treatment begins. The radiation therapist positions the patient, aligns the treatment machine, and takes an anterior and lateral or oblique kV image. The images are analyzed, and the computer generates any necessary shifts. These adjustments in the couch or collimator position are made before initiating treatment. This process is done daily. Many treatment systems or situations also require the radiation therapist to analyze the kV images, compare skeletal anatomy to CT simulation DRR, and make adjustments to the couch position before treating the patient (Fig. 30.15).

If the patient has been positioned correctly, why do these changes or errors in the treatment field position occur? Patient movement during treatment has always been a major constraint in providing accurate and precise delivery of radiation treatments. Improvements in immobilization devices have been made; however, they do not prevent internal organ movement. The prostate may move and be in a different position within the treatment field from day to day or even during treatment because of the filling of the rectum or bladder. Tumor or organ movement can also occur because of normal respiration. This movement can result in a geographic miss of the tumor or irradiation of critical normal structures.

Because movement of internal structures does occur, many technologic innovations are being developed to address this issue. Obtaining daily kV or EPID images before treatment is one method. The process of using images such as EPID or kV to verify the treatment field position daily before treatment is known as *image-guided radiation therapy* (IGRT). Other methods of IGRT involve the use of a CT scan, an infrared camera system, or a sophisticated tracking system that uses two x-ray tubes mounted 90 degrees apart. In addition, there are two alternative developed treatment units, TomoTherapy and the CyberKnife, which combine IGRT and innovative treatment delivery. These various IGRT methods are discussed subsequently.

The use of a CT scan before treatment as a means of IGRT is very common. A CT scan is obtained with the patient in treatment position immediately before treatment to verify target, isocenter, and patient position. This method is accomplished in one of two ways. One approach is to equip the linac with a kV x-ray tube and panel detector that obtains a cone-beam CT image when the accelerator gantry rotates a complete 360 degrees. The kV x-ray tube also provides a means of obtaining diagnostic quality images for treatment and patient position verification as previously discussed (Fig. 30.16). Another technique is using the linac's megavoltage beam and EPID imager to acquire a cone-beam CT image. The cone-beam CT image is obtained in the same fashion by rotating the linac 360 degrees. The kV cone-beam CT image provides better contrast and soft tissue delineation than megavoltage CT and has proved advantageous to evaluate rectum or bladder filling consistency for prostate patients. The megavoltage CT images are of a high enough quality to compare target position and related bony anatomy to determine whether any adjustments in patient or couch position are necessary before treatment. Another method of CT image guidance is to have a CT scanner located in the actual treatment

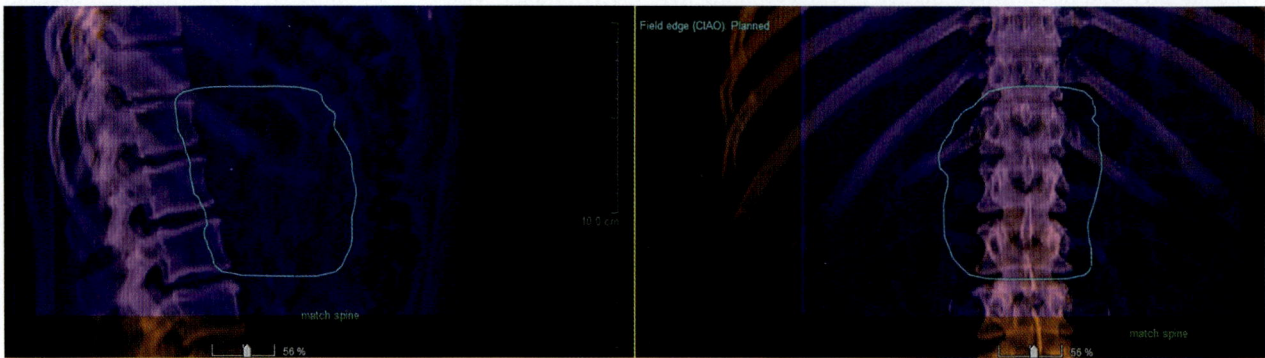

Fig. 30.15 OBI kV image overlaid on CT DRR; therapists shift couch to match skeletal anatomy.

(Used with permission of Mayo Foundation for Medical Education and Research, all rights reserved.)

room opposite the linac, near the foot end of the treatment couch. The scanner can be moved into position to obtain a CT scan with the patient positioned for treatment. The most common method is the use of the linac to obtain a cone-beam CT image.

The infrared camera is a complex system that detects respiratory motion during simulation and treatment. This is a technique called *respiratory gating*. A reflective marker box is placed on the external surface of the patient's abdomen during simulation. The infrared camera detects the marker box, and a special computer software program connected to the infrared camera monitors the marker box movement (Fig. 30.17). The movement of the reflective marker is correlated with the patient's diaphragm position during the CT simulation. The respiratory cycle is evaluated relative to the treatment target volume and diaphragm movement. A specific portion of the respiratory cycle that has the least amount of motion is selected as the gated interval. This information is saved as a tolerance or standard to use during treatment. When the patient is treated, the reflective marker box is placed on the same place on the abdomen, and an infrared camera is used to monitor the movement of the box. Pretreatment portal images (AP and lateral) to verify patient position, isocenter location, and gating interval are obtained with the EPID or kV imager. When approved, the radiation therapist initiates treatment. The respiratory gating computer monitors the marker box movement and automatically turns off the radiation beam if the marker moves out of the acceptable gated interval. Treatment automatically begins again when the marker box returns to the acceptable position. Respiratory gating has been done in various ways. One method is to have patients breathe freely, whereas another method is to have patients exhale and hold their breath.

The ExacTrac by Brainlab AG (Heimstetten, Germany) is a system that uses two kV x-ray tubes mounted in the floor 90 degrees apart that project a beam at 45-degree angles to the patient through the linac isocenter. The flat-panel detectors are located in the ceiling. This sophisticated system is able to analyze the stereoscopic images and compare bony anatomy or implanted fiducial markers with the digital radiographs from simulation. The computer system calculates shifts in six dimensions rather than using the typical three-dimensional imaging. When the radiation therapist has acknowledged the recommended shifts, the information is sent to the robotic couch, and the adjustments are made automatically from outside the treatment room. The ExacTrac system may be used to take images anytime during treatment for real-time tracking of target motion during treatment as in respiratory gating. ExacTrac is commonly used for the treatment of head and neck cancers, prostate cancer, lung cancer, and small centrally located brain tumors and for stereotactic radiation therapy (SRT).

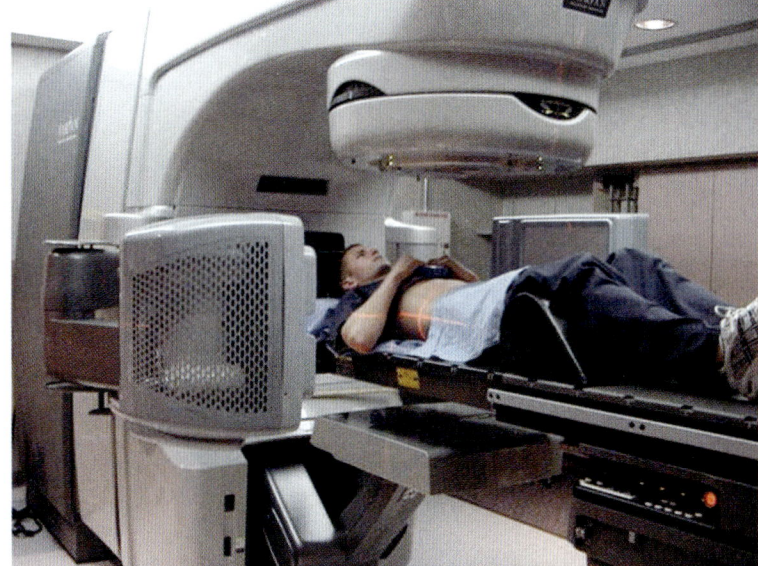

Fig. 30.16 Linac equipped with kV x-ray tube and flat-panel detector. EPID is extended underneath the patient.

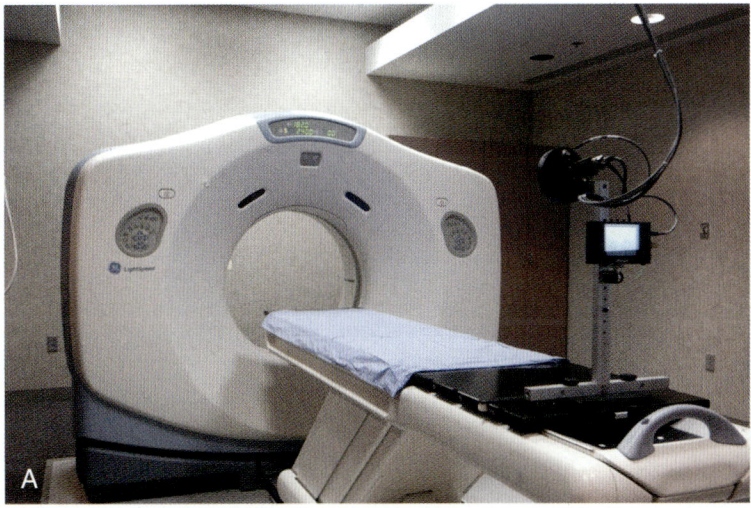 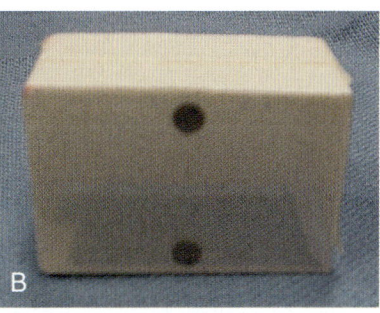

Fig. 30.17 (**A**) Infrared camera system attached to CT simulator. (**B**) Reflective marker box.

SRT is similar to SRS in that the area being treated is small and surrounded by critical structures. The difference is that SRS is a large dose delivered in one treatment and is typically used for intracranial lesions. SRT is a conventional dose delivered in a fractionated manner using very focused small beams while the patient is rigidly immobilized. This technique is typically for intracranial lesions. SRT has been expanded to include tumors within the body. The treatment involves delivering larger doses of radiation per treatment than conventional treatment with a smaller number of total treatments. A patient may receive only one to five total treatments, but the dose may be similar to that of conventional treatment. This increasingly more common technique is called stereotactic body radiation therapy (SBRT). SBRT is being used for small lesions in the lung, liver, pancreas, prostate, other bone metastasis, and spine patients who cannot undergo surgery.

TomoTherapy

TomoTherapy is a treatment unit developed at the University of Wisconsin in 2001 that first treated patients clinically in 2004, providing precise and conformal radiation treatment. The system delivers radiation slice by slice ("tomo"), combining the principles of helical CT scanning with a 6-MV linac, and is one of the first devices capable of providing daily image guidance. The TomoTherapy unit contains a CT scanner geometry with a detector system originally utilizing kV imaging; however, current models use only MV imaging. The 6-MV gantry rotates in a continuous full circle while the couch and patient simultaneously move slowly through the aperture of the machine (Fig. 30.18). The TomoTherapy unit is equipped with computer-controlled multileaf collimators that move to modulate the radiation beam intensity. TomoTherapy provides IMRT in a helical pattern, delivering highly conformal radiation to the specific prescribed anatomic regions while sparing normal structures. Before initiating treatment, megavoltage CT of the patient is obtained and is compared against the initial CT image used in treatment planning to verify patient position. Any necessary shifts to match isocenter location are made before treatment is delivered. Tomotherapy is an excellent routine application for sites such as prostate, head and neck, and brain.

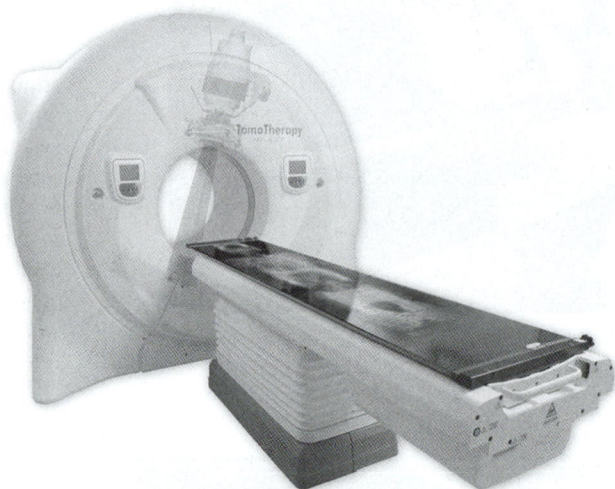

Fig. 30.18 TomoTherapy Hi-Art imaging and treatment system, which uses a megavoltage source for CT and for treatment.

(Courtesy TomoTherapy Incorporated. From Washington CM, Leaver DT, eds. *Principles and practice of radiation therapy*, 3rd ed. St Louis: Elsevier; 2010.)

CyberKnife

The CyberKnife (Accuray Inc., Sunnyvale, CA) is an SRS system that uses continuous image guidance for delivering radiation treatments with submillimeter precision. The treatments are delivered in a single fraction or in two to five fractions termed hypofractionated radiotherapy. The CyberKnife is a 6-MV linac housed within a robotic arm containing six different joints, or axes, that allow thousands of beam angle options from essentially any direction around the patient (Fig. 30.19), providing excellent tumor coverage with steep dose fall-off outside of the target. The beams are collimated to range in diameter from 5 to 60 mm, allowing dose to conform tightly to the target while sparing normal surrounding tissue, thereby achieving higher doses safely.

The image guidance system consists of two diagnostic x-ray tubes mounted in the ceiling at 45-degree angles, offset 90 degrees from one another, with two opposing amorphous silicon detectors located in the floor. The imaging system continually takes a set of images at each treatment angle and analyzes the images during treatment to track target and patient motion. The robotic arm is automatically adjusted to correct for any motion it detects, resulting in treatment times that range from 30 to 90 minutes. CyberKnife was the first system to use real-time tracking of target motion during treatment and is used to treat cancers of the lung, pancreas, brain, head and neck, spine, and prostate.

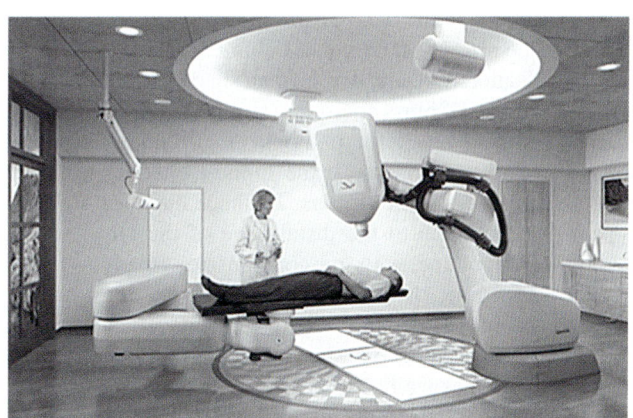

Fig. 30.19 Accelerator on a robotic arm. Two ceiling-mounted x-ray tubes are clearly shown.

(From Washington CM, Leaver DT, eds. *Principles and practice of radiation therapy*, 3rd ed. St Louis: Elsevier; 2010.)

Proton Therapy

The first use of a proton beam was in 1954 at the University of California in Berkeley; however, owing to the complexity, cost, and size of a cyclotron or synchrotron facility, protons were not widely implemented at that time but are increasingly common today with over 40 proton centers in the United States. Characteristic properties of the proton beam create dosimetrical advantages that allow treatment for challenging tumors, such as higher doses to volumes adjacent to critical structures and for nonresectable volumes in patients who are not ideal surgical candidates. Protons are especially useful for patients with recurrences or secondary malignancies in which specific organs at risk have been previously irradiated; therefore, the patients have lower radiation thresholds. Therapeutic proton energies range between 70 and 250 MeV, which deposit minimal scatter and little energy as the beam first traverses tissue as it enters the body (termed entrance dose). In a uniform medium, monoenergetic protons will increasingly lose energy as they slow down before coming to a stop and depositing their dose at the predetermined depth.

This burst of energy deposited at a specific depth is termed the *Bragg peak* (Fig. 30.20). The depth at which this peak dose deposition occurs can be adjusted by changing the energy of the proton beam and adding beam modifiers. The proton beam can be precisely controlled to deliver the Bragg peak dose at a prescribed depth, providing the principle advantage of sparing surrounding normal tissues at risk. The rapid fall-off of the beam allows treatment of the tumor volume while sparing critical structures located within millimeters of the target (Fig. 30.21).

Proton therapy units can have various treatment unit designs, and most centers utilize more than one type. The most common types include a fixed horizontal beam, a fixed vertical beam, a 360-degree gantry, or a partial 185-degree gantry. The two main ways to deliver proton therapy treatments are passively scattered particle therapy and pencil beam scanning (PBS). *Passively scattered particle therapy* involves the use of specific devices intended to spread the proton beam out laterally and longitudinally. Two scattering foils of high Z materials are placed in the path of the pencil-thin beam to spread the beam out laterally to a useful treatment field size. A device within the machine called a range modulator wheel *spreads out the Bragg peak* (SOBP) longitudinally to allow the high-energy beam to treat from the distal extent of the tumor to the most proximal aspect of the tumor. To shape the dose distribution laterally to the size of the targeted volume, passively scattered beams are further shaped using blocks of brass apertures (similar to a Cerrobend block for photons) thick enough (2–8 cm) to absorb the highest energies of the incident protons. To shape the dose distribution to the distal edge of the target volume, a tissue compensator (made of acrylic or wax) is used to degrade the beam energy to further conform and adjust for variation in the patient's external shape, as well as internal tissue heterogeneity or density differences.

PBS is the most current method of proton beam delivery that does not require custom-made apertures or compensators and that allows for more flexibility and control for conformality of the dose distribution to the target. The positively charged proton beamlet is directed by magnets to deliver the beam in an alternating scanning fashion to paint the tumor across the intended treatment volume in layers. Once the protons reach the required energy, they are extracted via the "beamline" to the treatment room and used to treat varying depths in tissue (Fig. 30.22). Typically, the deepest layer is painted first, using the highest energy, followed by the next layer per energy level, moving upward until the entire tumor is treated. PBS delivers a more conformal dose distribution to the tumor than passively scattered particle therapy and also allows for modulation of the intensity of the proton beam or intensity-modulated proton therapy (IMPT). This is a similar principle to IMRT for photons and the standard delivery in new proton centers. Characteristic differences, as well as main planning considerations between photon and proton characteristics, are noteworthy.

Proton beam therapy is the preferred modality of treatment for pediatric malignancies since there is virtually no exit dose, thus delivering lower dosage to normal tissues and decreasing the risk of secondary malignancies due to radiation. The use of proton therapy has expanded to treat essentially any anatomic site where clinically significant reduction of doses can be achieved, such as craniospinal volumes, prostate, brain, head and neck, breast, lung, gastrointestinal, and gynecologic malignancies.

With new and emerging technological advancements, it is imperative that

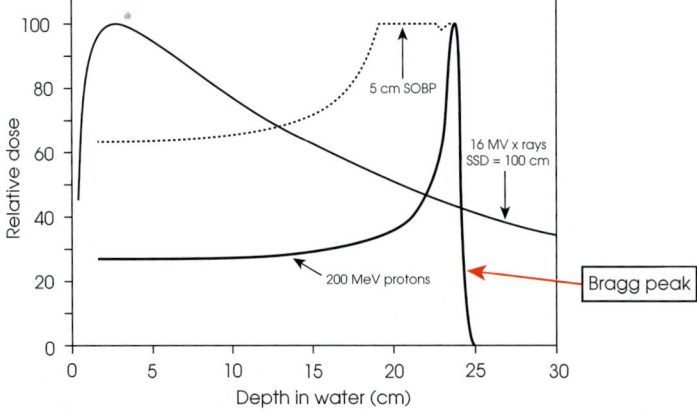

Fig. 30.20 Depth-dose curves for a 200-MeV proton beam: both unmodulated and with a 5-cm spread-out Bragg peak *(SOBP)*, compared with a 16-MV x-ray beam (for 10 × 10 cm² fields). The curves are normalized in each case to 100 at maximum dose.

(Adapted from Jones DTL. Present status and future trends of heavy particle radiotherapy. In: Baron E, Lieuvin M, eds. *Cyclotrons and their applications 1998*. Bristol: Institute of Physics Publishing; 1999:13–20.)

the radiation therapist does not become complacent or dependent on automated equipment. The therapist must still use critical thinking skills to analyze why couch parameters are being adjusted and to evaluate all aspects of the patient's setup before automatically implementing shifts to the table or patient position. The therapist should consider whether the computer-generated shifts are excessive or abnormal for this particular patient. If it is an outlier, further questioning should be performed and assessed.

The radiation therapist is also responsible for monitoring the patient's physical and emotional well-being. The radiation therapist is generally the only member of the radiation oncology team who sees the patient on a daily basis. The radiation therapist monitors the patient's progress and assists in the management of any side effects. Acting as a liaison between the patient and the physician, the radiation therapist must know when to withhold treatment and refer the patient to be seen by the physician or oncology nurse for further evaluation. The daily interaction with the patient is generally the most rewarding aspect of the radiation therapist's job. Putting the patient at ease and making a cancer diagnosis and subsequent treatment a less traumatic experience is a satisfying aspect of the career. Patients often express their gratitude to radiation therapists for their care and support.

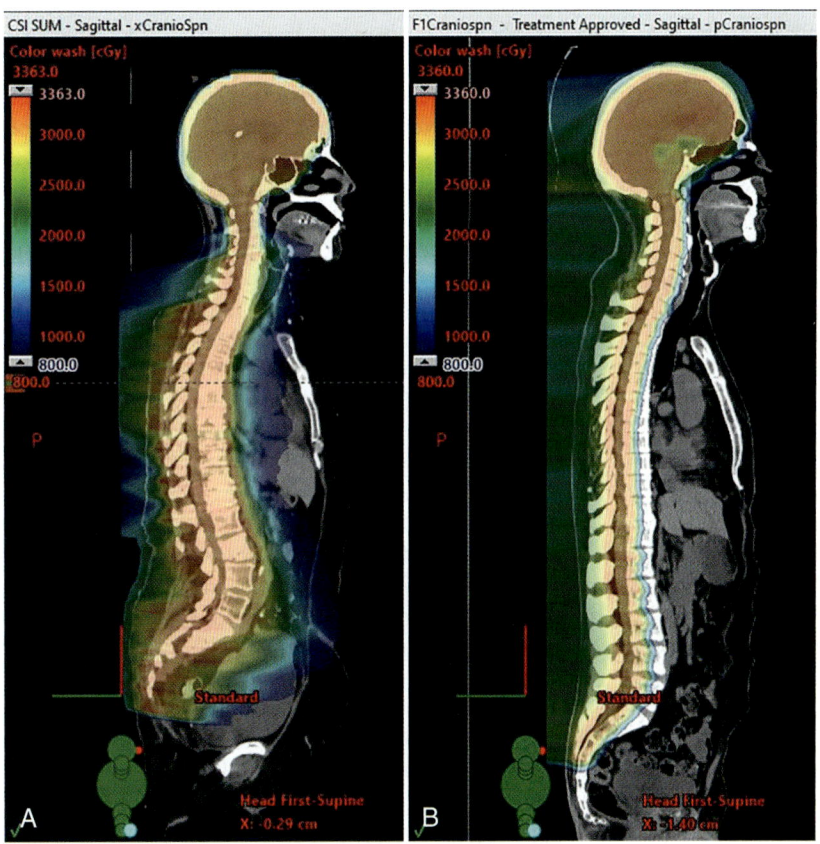

Fig. 30.21 (A) Single-beam photon compared to (B) single beam of protons. Note no exit dose and sparing of normal tissues with proton beam in the anterior abdomen.

(Used with permission of Mayo Foundation for Medical Education and Research, all rights reserved.)

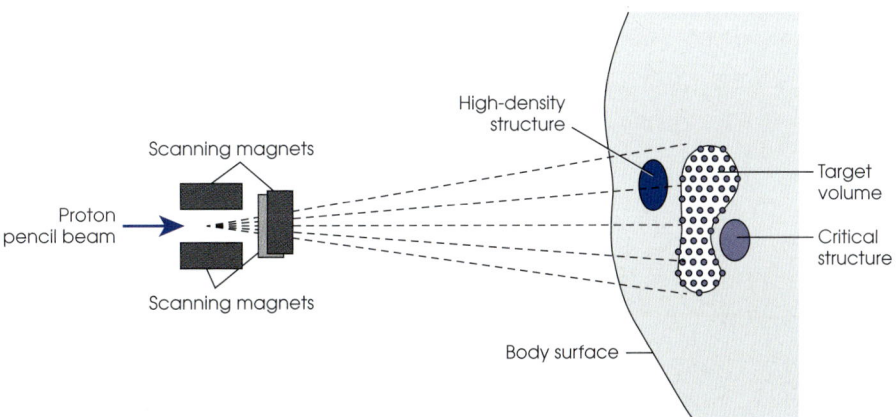

Fig. 30.22 Pencil beam scanning note magnet for directing the beam to spot paint the dose in the target volume.

(Courtesy MD Anderson Cancer Center website.)

Best Practices

The following best practices adhere to professional ethics and standards of practice established by national guidelines. All oncology team members should embrace a culture that supports professionalism and ensures patient safety on all levels.

1. *Staffing:* A minimum of two radiation therapists per linear accelerator is recommended, with potentially more, depending on a facility's number of new patients and procedures performed annually. As technology advances and complicated treatments are more commonly used as the standard of delivery, the complexity of plan review, image review, and margin of error also increases demands for the radiation therapists. These challenges should be considered for staffing purposes.

2. *Accuracy:* Since cancer cells divide rapidly, making them particularly susceptible to radiation, accuracy is crucial to effective treatment. Too little radiation to the treatment volume will allow cancer cells to regrow while too much (or missed targets) will harm surrounding organs at risk, harming the patient. Image guidance assists in delivering accurate treatments to the intended target volumes; however, therapists should verify that all shifts make sense to ensure that accuracy is maintained.

3. *Attention to detail:* This is especially important in radiation therapy as even minor inconsistencies can have major effects, such as a shift in the wrong direction, incorrectly recorded treatment doses, or immobilization or treatment devices misplaced or not used. All of these finite details play an important role in delivering the correct dose to the correct volume and can be detrimental for the patient if directions are not followed correctly or are missed.

4. *Speed:* As accuracy and attention to detail demand being thorough and taking time for critical thinking, speed is also very important for effective treatment. Many patients requiring radiation are under an intense amount of pain, making it difficult to hold a specific position to be treated for very long. If the patient is unable to maintain the correct position verified by the therapists using image guidance, a geometric miss can occur. If treatment cannot be delivered in a reasonable time frame, patient motion, breathing motion, and time between image matching verification increasingly introduce higher risks of missing the target volume.

5. *Patient care:* As stated earlier, the radiation therapist is often the only member of the oncology team that interacts with the patient on a daily basis. A change in routine for the patient, such as dietary restrictions or any new symptom or side effect, can also have an effect on the patient's radiation treatment. Diet or stress can affect weight gain or loss or the displacement of internal organs (e.g., the bowel or stomach), therefore possibly changing position from the treatment plan intent and dose distribution. Communication between the patient and therapist minimizes unexpected circumstances that could alter these variabilities.

6. *Receptive/questioning workplace culture:* Error reporting and prevention are top priorities in radiation therapy. National guidelines specify criteria for reporting purposes, and facilities should use these guidelines, as well as have processes in place for "near misses" and error prevention. Administration should provide the tools, training, sufficient staff, and time to ensure that these processes are completed. All members of the team should feel comfortable in questioning any aspect of the patient's treatment at any time without fear of reprimand or consequence. Physicians, physicists, dosimetrists, and therapists should all be open to a questioning and receptive environment, as well as encourage this type of workplace culture.

7. *Professionalism:* Part of professionalism in radiation therapy is to minimize distractions during patient treatment. Monitoring patients and focusing on their needs during treatment are the top priorities during beam delivery, and therapists should feel open to remind colleagues if these priorities are not being followed. Therapists report that crowded workspaces commonly contribute to distractions, as well as interruptions from oncology nurses, physicians, and fellow therapists.

8. *Proper training:* Rapidly changing technological advancements within the field introduce reliance on complex new equipment without previous and thorough training. Proper skills assessments should be performed and evaluated before equipment is put into clinical use and periodically to avoid complacency. Work environments should embrace a lifelong learning approach and process improvement.

Clinical Applications

The amount of radiation prescribed depends on the type of tumor and the extent of the disease. The following are brief summaries of radiation therapy techniques used in the management of common forms of cancer.

LUNG CANCER

Treatment of lung cancer varies by type and stage. Radiation therapy is often used in conjunction with surgery and chemotherapy. A dose of 5000 to 6000 cGy of 10-MeV photons is often applied via a combination of AP, PA, and off-cord oblique fields. The primary tumor plus draining lymphatics are generally included in the treatment volumes (Fig. 30.23). The use of multiple oblique IMRT fields, VMAT, or a hybrid technique that incorporates both static fields and VMAT is used to treat lung cancer. These techniques provide a more conformal dose to the target volume while delivering a lower dose to normal lung and spinal cord than the traditional static AP-PA and oblique fields. SBRT is used for the treatment of medically inoperable patients with stage I non–small-cell lung cancers. One to five treatments with doses in the range of 1000 to 2000 cGy per treatment may be given for a total dose of 5000 to 6000 cGy.

PROSTATE CANCER

Definitive radiation therapy is a standard treatment for prostate cancer. Surgical removal of the prostate gland is another common approach to the management of this disease. Traditionally, a four-field technique of AP, PA, and right and left lateral ports using a megavoltage beam of 10 MV or more is used to deliver a dose of 7000 to 7600 cGy to the prostate gland. A series of six to eight oblique fields delivered with IMRT or VMAT to a dose of 7600 cGy is a common method of treatment for prostate cancer. Another method of treating limited, early-stage prostate cancer is a brachytherapy procedure known as prostate seed implant. This procedure involves the permanent implantation of 100 or more seeds of the radioisotope iodine-125 or palladium-103 into the prostate gland. A dose of 145 Gy is delivered with iodine-125, and a dose of 125 Gy is delivered with palladium-103.

HDR brachytherapy is another method for treating early-stage prostate cancer. This procedure is done on an outpatient basis and is a temporary implant. The patient has four HDR brachytherapy treatments. The interstitial needles are inserted early in the morning; then the patient has a morning and afternoon treatment. The patient comes back 2 to 3 weeks later for another two HDR treatments. Prostate cancer is a common anatomic site that may be treated with protons.

HEAD AND NECK CANCERS

Numerous approaches may be used to treat head and neck cancers, depending on the location, size, and extent of the tumor. The most common method of treating head and neck cancer is with VMAT. VMAT allows a significant reduction in the dose to the parotid gland and spinal cord, while allowing a greater dose to be delivered to the target area. VMAT treatments are shorter in duration than the traditional IMRT technique for head and neck cancer. This makes the treatment more tolerable for the patient, who is held in place on the table by a thermoplastic mask. VMAT is the standard IMRT method for delivering radiation to head and neck cancers.

CERVICAL CANCER

Early diagnosed cervical cancers can be treated with either surgery or radiation therapy. Historically, a four-field technique of AP, PA, and right and left lateral ports using a megavoltage unit, preferably 10 MV or greater, delivers 4500 to 5000 cGy in 5 weeks to an area of the primary and regional lymph nodes (Fig. 30.24). IMRT and VMAT are two common standard methods of treating cervical cancer. An intracavitary HDR implant is also included in the standard treatment of cervical cancer.

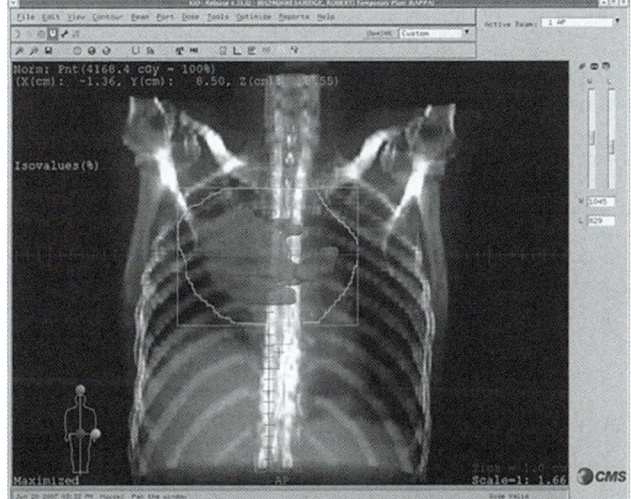

Fig. 30.23 Digitally reconstructed radiograph for parallel-opposed fields for right lung tumor with extension across the midline.

(Courtesy Bayhealth Medical Center at Kent General Hospital, Dover, DE.)

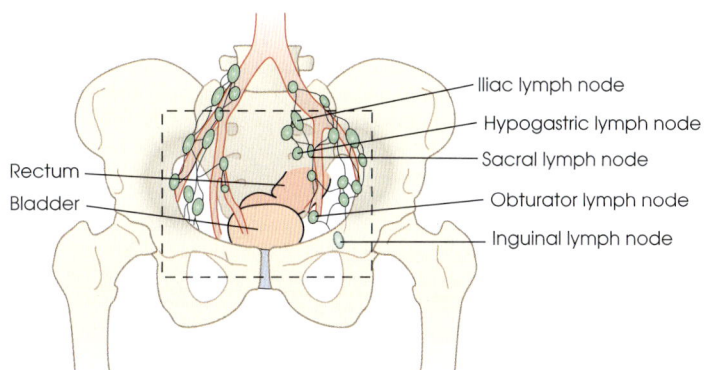

Fig. 30.24 Field used for irradiation of primary tumor and adjacent lymph nodes.

HODGKIN LYMPHOMA

The age of the patient and extent of the disease may determine treatment and prognosis for Hodgkin lymphoma. Involved field lymph node irradiation after chemotherapy is more commonly used than extended field therapy that included the lymphatic chain above or below the diaphragm. Treatment consists of chemotherapy followed by 2000 to 3000 cGy delivered through AP-PA fields or IMRT fields using a megavoltage unit. Chemotherapy may also be indicated for more advanced cases.

BREAST CANCER

Using two tangential fields to the chest wall or intact breast, megavoltage radiation delivers 5000 cGy in 5 weeks (Fig. 30.25). An electron boost to the site of initial lumpectomy adds an additional 1000 cGy. Irradiation of the axillary, supraclavicular, and internal mammary nodes to a dose of 5000 cGy is indicated for patients with a large primary tumor or node-positive disease. IMRT may also be used for the treatment of breast cancer. The breast is one location, so respiratory gating may be utilized. A patient's breathing is monitored, and patients are instructed to hold their breath to limit internal organ motion during treatment delivery. Respiratory gating limits the dose to the heart in patients with left-sided breast cancer.

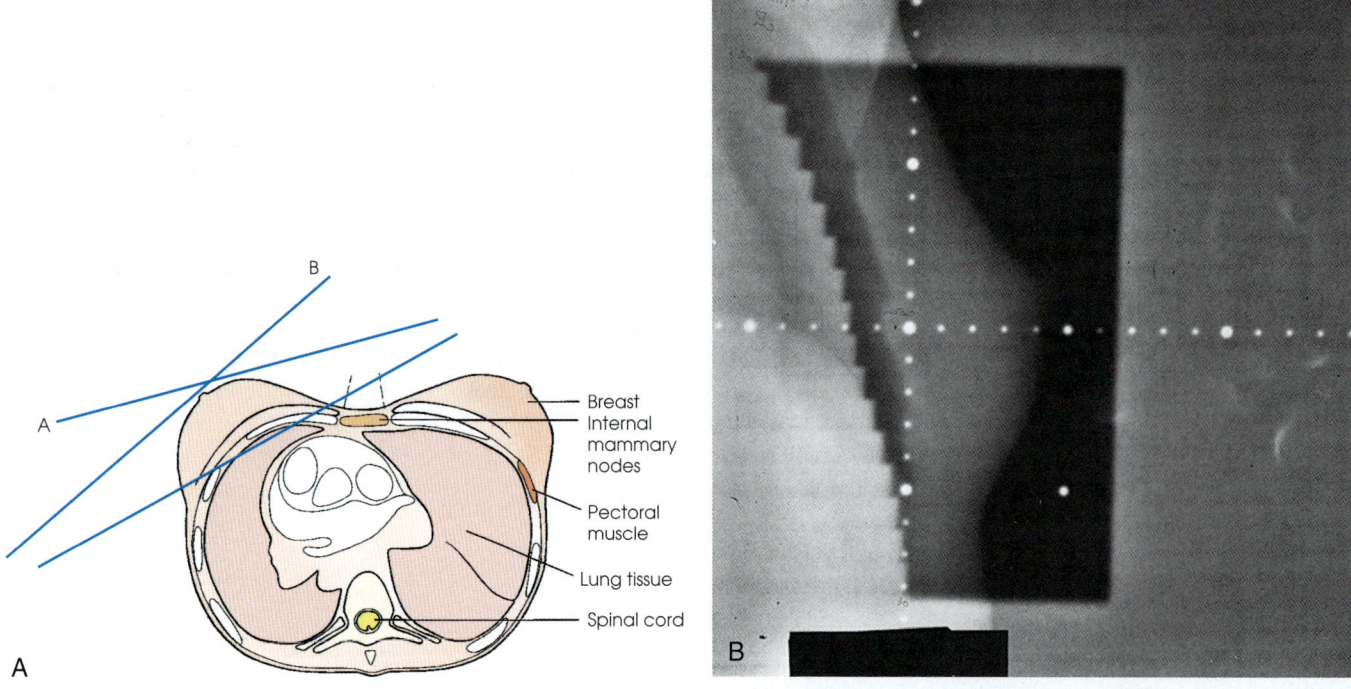

Fig. 30.25 (**A**) Cross section of thorax showing field arrangements to irradiate the intact breast tangentially while sparing the lung (*lines A* and *B*). (**B**) Port image of tangential breast field. Note sparing of lung tissue.

Accelerated partial-breast irradiation (APBI) is a breast conservation method being studied as an alternative to whole breast irradiation. This treatment option may be offered to a subset of women who are older than 50 years of age with tumors of less than 3 cm located in the outer quadrant of the breast. The patient must have negative surgical margins and no lymph nodes involved. *Accelerated* is the term used because the treatment is delivered in 1 week with twice-a-day treatments using external beam or brachytherapy. The two commonly used brachytherapy applicators are MammoSite and strut adjusted volume implant applicator (SAVI). Both applicators are placed in the lumpectomy site. The MammoSite applicator is a balloon catheter that is placed in the lumpectomy cavity. The SAVI has individual catheters in the shape of an eggbeater and is placed in the cavity created by the lumpectomy. The applicator used is hooked up to the HDR unit for treatment delivery. A total dose of 3400 cGy is delivered in the 1-week period. Chemotherapy, hormonal therapy, or both are also commonly used to treat breast cancer.

LARYNGEAL CANCER

Cancer of the larynx is best treated with megavoltage radiation. Tumors that are confined to the true vocal cord, with normal cord mobility, have a 90% 5-year cure rate; in addition, the voice remains useful. The method of treatment is usually accomplished by using small 5 × 5-cm (2 × 2-inch) opposing lateral wedged fields and delivering a dose of 6300 to 6500 cGy over a 6-week period.

SKIN CANCER

Carcinomas of the skin are usually squamous cell or basal cell lesions that may be treated with superficial radiation or surgery. Cure rates tend to be 80% to 90%, and basal cell lesions less than 1 cm (0.4 inch) in diameter have a cure rate of almost 100%. The method of treatment is usually a single-field approach, with attention given to shielding the uninvolved skin and delivering 4000 to 5000 cGy in a 3- to 4-week period.

MEDULLOBLASTOMA

Children with medulloblastoma are usually referred to the radiation oncology department after a biopsy and shunt procedure. The tumor is radiosensitive, and patients who have had treatment of the entire cerebrospinal axis have a 5-year cure rate of greater than 60%. The therapeutic approach tends to be complicated because the entire brain is irradiated with 3600 cGy, the spinal cord receives a dose of 2340 to 3600 cGy, and the cerebellum receives an additional dose of radiation to bring the total up to 5500 cGy (Fig. 30.26). This irradiation is usually accomplished with parallel opposed fields to the cranial vault and an extended single field to the spinal cord. The boost dose of 2000 cGy to the posterior fossa may be given with IMRT to provide better dose optimization to the target and a lower dose to critical structures. A megavoltage unit is used, with extreme care given to the areas of abutting fields. Proton therapy has also proven very beneficial for medulloblastoma.

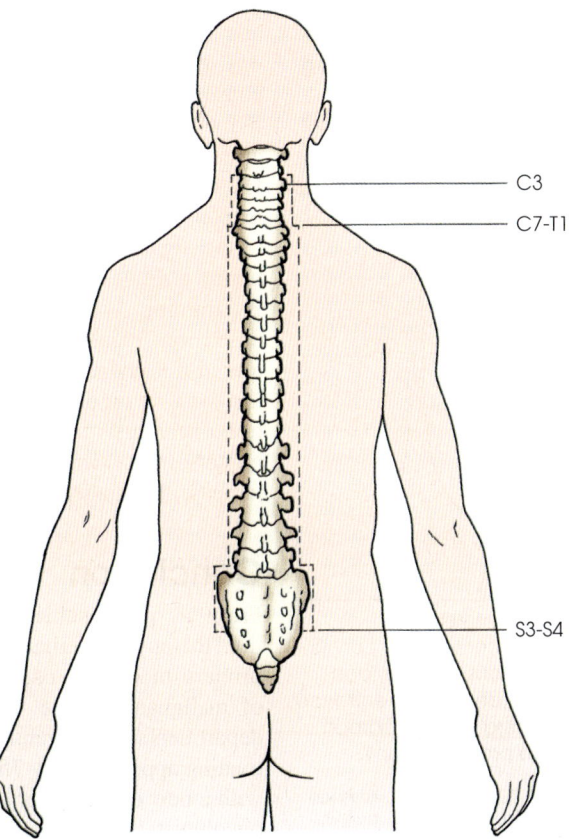

Fig. 30.26 Spinal treatment portal for medulloblastoma.

Future Trends

Radiation therapy has entered the electronic age, with increased technologic advancement in the areas of simulation, dosimetry, and treatment delivery. Most institutions use computer-interfaced accelerators with treatment verification software packages to ensure accurate treatment. Paperless treatment charting and filmless departments are the standard design of a facility. VMAT and IMRT are standard treatment techniques used in most facilities to treat various tumor types. Developments will continue to occur in the use of IGRT. Refinements in the application of linac cone-beam CT and other modalities, such as PET, to verify target, isocenter, and patient position prior to treatment will occur more routinely. Advancements and implementation of respiratory gating will permit better delineation of three-dimensional conformal target volumes, lessen the chance of a geographic miss of the target volume, and further minimize the dose to normal structures. The use of gating may permit higher doses to be prescribed and result in greater control and cure rates. The increasing use of SBRT and hypofractionation is continuously expanding into other anatomic disease sites in the body. The current treatment methods for radiation therapy are constantly advancing and being upgraded to ensure that the most effective and up-to-date techniques are being utilized.

Along with the progression of proton therapy as a more common approach for cancer treatment, carbon ion therapy is emerging with promising safety and efficacy data. Its radiobiologic properties exhibit an increased linear energy transfer (LET) compared to photons and protons (Fig. 30.27), leading to higher biologic effectiveness, which ultimately has the potential to safely deposit higher doses to traditionally radioresistant tumors while maintaining minimal irradiation to normal surrounding tissue and organs at risk (OARs). There are currently 13 operating carbon ion centers, with a few more under construction, all of which are in Europe and Asia, with the first center for North America currently in the planning stages.

Artificial intelligence is steadily advancing and rapidly transforming health care with the ability to forecast future outcomes, identify patterns as well as outliers in data, and execute actions to achieve objectives. The machine learning and computer vision of AI hold limitless possibilities for EHR systems, physician efficiency, and personalized care. The systems must be trained to recognize patterns, understand relationships between diagnosis and treatment, and provide accurate, personalized recommendations tailored to individuals. This learning takes time to safely integrate the potential advantages with its widespread popularity and implementation. In radiation oncology, the use of AI has streamlined time-consuming processes such as contouring individual normal tissue organs at risk, affecting decisions in treatment planning. Historically, radiation oncologists are responsible for providing accurate normal tissue organ contours adjacent to or near tumor volumes for dosimetry planning. By training AI recognition and patterns based on hundreds of manually contoured CT images, this process has made the work so productive as to allow radiation oncologists to allocate their time for higher-priority demands and ultimately to increase the quality of patient care.

Conclusion

From a questionable beginning, radiation therapy has emerged as one of the primary modalities used in the treatment of malignant disease. Radiation therapy departments are currently examining and treating approximately 75% of all patients with a new diagnosis of cancer. Radiation oncologists and radiation therapists are integral members of the health care team that discusses and selects the appropriate treatment regimens for all cancer patients.

As the factors that initiate cellular change, growth, and spread become better understood, radiation treatments for cancer are expected to become even more effective. The irradiation techniques presently used may change dramatically based on this new information. In addition, new, more sophisticated radiation-producing equipment is currently under design and may lead to the reevaluation of presently accepted therapeutic techniques and dose levels. Finally, new chemotherapeutic agents are being produced that, when used by themselves or with other drugs, may enhance tumor sensitivity when used in conjunction with irradiation.

Definition of Terms

absorbed dose: Amount of ionizing radiation absorbed per unit of mass of irradiated material.

accelerator (particle): Device that accelerates charged subatomic particles to great energies. These particles or rays may be used for direct medical irradiation and basic physical research. Medical units include linear accelerators, betatrons, and cyclotrons.

asymmetric jaws: Four independent x-ray collimators that are used to define the radiation treatment field.

attenuation: Removal of energy from a beam of ionizing radiation when it traverses matter, accomplished by disposition of energy in matter and by deflection of energy out of the beam.

betatron: Electron accelerator that uses magnetic induction to accelerate electrons in circular path; also capable of producing photons.

biopsy: Removal of a small piece of tissue for examination under the microscope.

brachytherapy: Placement of radioactive nuclide or nuclides in or on a neoplasm to deliver a cancericidal dose.

cancer: Term commonly applied to malignant disease; abnormal growth of cells; *neoplasm* (new growth) or *-oma* (tumor).

cancericidal dose: Dose of radiation that results in the death of cancer cells.

carcinogen: Any cancer-producing substance or material, such as nicotine, radiation, or ingested uranium.

carcinoma: Cancer that arises from epithelial tissue—either glandular or squamous epithelium.

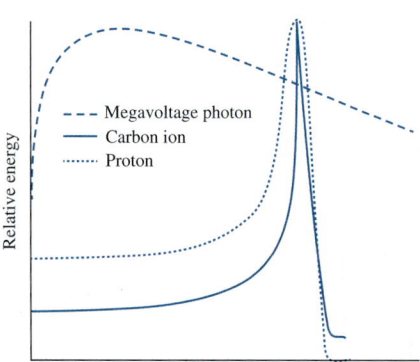

Fig. 30.27 Depth dose comparison curves for megavoltage photons, protons, and carbon ions. Note the decreased entrance dose and sharper Bragg peak of carbon ions as compared to proton therapy.

(Redrawn from Malouff TD, Mahajan A, Krishnan S, et al. Carbon ion therapy: a modern review of an emerging technology. *Front Oncol.* 2020; 10:82.)

Cerrobend block: Beam-shaping device made of a lead alloy that attenuates the x-ray beam, preventing exposure of normal tissue.

chromosome: Unit of genetic information that guides cytoplasmic activities of the cell and transmits hereditary information.

cobalt-60: Radioisotope with half-life of 5.26 years, average gamma ray energy of 1.25 MeV (range 1.17–1.33 MeV), and ability to spare skin with buildup depth in tissue of 0.5 cm.

collimator: Diaphragm or system of diaphragms made of radiation-absorbing material that defines dimension and direction of beam.

conformal radiation: Treatment designed to deliver radiation to the exact target volume as seen on any plane (e.g., transverse, sagittal, vertex views); requires a three-dimensional treatment planning system.

contour: Reproduction of an external body shape, typically in the transverse plane at the level of the central axis of the beam; facilitates planning of radiation treatment. Other planes of interest may also be obtained.

cure: Usually a 5-year period after completion of treatment during which time the patient exhibits no evidence of disease.

decay or disintegration: Transformation of radioactive nucleus, resulting in emission of radiation.

differentiation: Acquisition of cellular function and structure that differ from that of the original cell type.

direct effect: Radiation that interacts with an organic molecule such as DNA, RNA, or a protein molecule. This interaction may inactivate the cell.

dosimetry: Measurement of radiation dose in an absorbing medium.

epithelial tissue: Cells that line the surfaces of serous and mucous membranes, including the skin.

etiology: Study of causes of diseases.

external-beam treatment: Delivery of radiation to a patient from a unit such as a linear accelerator in which the radiation enters the patient from the external surface of the body.

field: Geometric area defined by collimator or radiotherapy unit at skin surface.

fractionation: Division of total planned dose into numerous smaller doses to be given over a longer period. Consideration must be given to biologic effectiveness of smaller doses.

gamma ray: Electromagnetic radiation that originates from radioactive nucleus and causes ionization in matter; identical in properties to x-ray.

gray (Gy): International unit for the quantity of radiation received by the patient; previously rad; 1 cGy = 1 rad.

grenz rays: X-rays generated at 20 kVp or less.

half-life: Time (specific for each radioactive substance) required for radioactive material to decay to half its initial activity; types are biologic and physical.

half-value layer: Thickness of attenuating material inserted in beam to reduce beam intensity to half of the original intensity.

hypofractionation: Higher doses of radiation delivered in a shorter period of time as compared to standard fractionation.

high-dose-rate brachytherapy: Use of a high-activity radionuclide placed within the body for the treatment of cancer. Delivers more than 1200 cGy per hour.

image-guided radiation therapy (IGRT): Use of images to verify treatment isocenter, target, and patient positioning before initiating radiation treatment.

immunotherapy: Type of biologic therapy using substances from living organisms such as white blood cells, organs, and lymph system tissue to help the immune system fight infections, diseases, and cancer.

independent jaws: X-ray collimator with four individual blades that can be moved independently of one another (see *asymmetric jaws*).

indirect effect: Interaction of radiation with water molecules within the cell; results in the formation of free radicals OH, H, and HO_2, which can damage the cell.

intensity-modulated radiation therapy (IMRT): Modification of beam intensity to deliver nonuniform exposure across radiation field.

ionization: Process in which one or more electrons are added to or removed from atoms, creating ions; can be caused by high temperatures, electrical discharges, or nuclear radiations.

ionizing radiation: Energy emitted and transferred through matter that results in the removal of orbital electrons (e.g., x-rays or gamma rays).

isocentric: Refers to rotation around a fixed point.

isodose line curve: Curve or line drawn to connect points of identical amounts of radiation in a given field.

isotope: Atoms that have the same atomic number but different mass numbers.

lesion: Morbid change in tissue; mass of abnormal cells.

linear accelerator (linac): Device for accelerating charged particles, such as electrons, to produce high-energy electron or photon beams.

linear energy transfer (LET): Rate at which energy is deposited as it travels through matter.

low-dose-rate brachytherapy: Use of a low-activity radionuclide placed within the body for treatment of cancer. Dose is slowly delivered, 40 to 500 cGy per hour, to a small volume of tissue over a period of days.

malignancy: Cancerous tumor or lesion.

medical dosimetrist: Person responsible for calculation of proper radiation treatment dose who assists the radiation oncologist in designing individual treatment plans.

medical physicist: Specialist in the study of the laws of ionizing radiation and their interactions with matter.

metastasis: Transmission of cells or groups of cells from primary tumor to sites elsewhere in body.

multileaf collimator (MLC): Individual collimator rods within the treatment head of the linear accelerator that can slide inward to shape radiation field.

oncologist: Physician specializing in the study of tumors.

oncology: Study of tumors.

palliation: To relieve symptoms; not for cure.

passively scattered particle therapy: Involves the use of special devices to spread the proton beam out laterally and distally.

pathologist: Specialist in the study of the microscopic nature of disease.

pencil beam scanning: Method of proton beam delivery. The positively charged thin proton beamlet is directed by two magnets to deliver the beam in an alternating scanning fashion to paint the tumor with dose.

prophylactic surgery: Preventive surgical treatment.

radiation oncologist: Physician who specializes in the use of ionizing radiation in treatment of disease.

radiation oncology: Medical specialty involving the treatment of cancerous lesions using ionizing radiation.

radiation therapist: Person trained to assist and take directions from the radiation oncologist in the use of ionizing radiation for treatment of disease.

radiation therapy: Older term used to define the medical specialty involving treatment with ionizing radiation.

radioactive: Pertaining to atoms of elements that undergo spontaneous transformation, resulting in emission of radiation.

radiocurable: Susceptibility of neoplastic cells to cure (destruction) by ionizing radiation.

radiosensitivity: Responsiveness of cells to radiation.

radium (Ra): Radionuclide (atomic number 88, atomic weight 226, half-life 1622 years) used clinically for radiation therapy. In conjunction with its subsequent transformations, radium emits alpha and beta particles and gamma rays. In encapsulated form, it is used for various intracavitary radiation therapy applications (e.g., for cervical cancer).

reactor: Cubicle in which isotopes are artificially produced.

relative biologic effectiveness (RBE): Compares radiation beams with different LETs and their ability to produce a specific biologic response. Dose in gray from 250 kVp beam of x-rays/dose from another type of radiation to produce the same effect.

simulator: Diagnostic x-ray machine that has the same geometric and physical characteristics as a radiation therapy treatment unit.

skin sparing: In megavoltage beam therapy, reduced skin injury per centigray (cGy) exposure because electron equilibrium occurs below skin; occurs 0.6 to 5 cm (0.25–2 inches) deep, depending on energy.

spread out Bragg peak: Individual Bragg peaks are spread across the various depths of the tumor, providing a more useful beam.

stereotactic radiation therapy: Use of small, focused radiation beams to treat small extracranial or intracranial lesions; delivered with conventional fractionation or in two to five treatments instead of a single treatment as in stereotactic radiosurgery. Rigid immobilization of the patient is required.

stereotactic radiosurgery: Use of multiple, narrow, highly focused radiation beams to deliver a large dose in a single treatment to a small intracranial lesion. The patient is immobilized with a fixed stereotactic head frame.

surgical bed: Area of excision and adjacent tissues manipulated during surgery.

systemic: Throughout the human body.

teletherapy: Radiation therapy technique for which the source of radiation is at some distance from the patient.

treatment field: Anatomic area outlined for treatment (e.g., AP or RL pelvis).

tumor/target volume: Portion of anatomy that includes tumor and adjacent areas of invasion.

undifferentiation: Lack of resemblance of cells to cells of origin.

wedge filter: Wedge-shaped beam attenuating device used to absorb beam preferentially to alter the shape of the isodose curve.

Selected bibliography

Accuray. Available at: www.accuray.com. (Accessed August 5, 2024.)

American Cancer Society. *Cancer Facts and Figures 2017*. Atlanta: American Cancer Society; 2013.

Barker C, Lowe M, Radhakrishna G. An introduction to proton beam therapy. *Br J Hosp Med (Lond)*. 2019;80(10):574–578.

Berson AM, Emery R, Rodriguez L, et al. Clinical experience using respiratory gated radiation therapy: comparison of free-breathing and breath-hold techniques. *Int J Radiat Oncol Biol Phys*. 2004;60(2):419–426.

Boyer AL. The physics of intensity-modulated radiation therapy. *Phys Today*. 2002;55(9):38–43.

BrainLab. Available at: www.BrainLab.com. (Accessed August 5, 2024.)

Brenner DJ. Dose, volume, and tumor-control predictions in radiotherapy. *Int J Radiat Oncol Biol Phys*. 1993;26(1):171–179.

Centers for Disease Control and Prevention. *Leading Causes of Death*; 2023. Available at https://www.cdc.gov/nchs/fastats/leading-causes-of-death.htm. (Accessed August 5, 2024.)

Chan OSH, Lee MCH, Hung AWM, et al. The superiority of hybrid-volumetric arc therapy (VMAT) technique over double arcs VMAT and 3D-conformal technique in the treatment of locally advanced non-small cell lung cancer—a planning study. *Radiother Oncol*. 2011;101(2):298–302.

Chang J, Sillanpaa J, Ling CC, et al. Integrating respiratory gating into a megavoltage cone-beam CT system. *Med Phys*. 2006;33(7):2354–2361.

Chang JY, Dong L, Liu H, et al. Image-guided radiation therapy for non-small cell lung cancer. *J Thorac Oncol*. 2008;3(2):177–186.

Chang SD, Main W, Martin DP, et al. An analysis of the accuracy of the CyberKnife: a robotic frameless stereotactic radiosurgical system. *Neurosurgery*. 2003;52(1):140–147.

Cheng JC, Chao KS, Low D. Comparison of intensity modulation radiation therapy (IMRT) treatment techniques for nasopharyngeal carcinoma. *Int J Cancer*. 2001;96(2):126–131.

Chirag S, Vicini F, Wazer DE, et al. The American Brachytherapy Society consensus statement for accelerated partial breast irradiation. *Brachytherapy*. 2013;12(4):267–277.

Chuong MD, Springett GM, Freilich JM, et al. Stereotactic body radiation therapy for locally advanced and borderline resectable pancreatic cancer is effective and well tolerated. *Int J Radiat Oncol Biol Phys*. 2013;86(3):516–522.

Coleman A. Treatment procedures. In: Washington CM, Leaver DT, eds. *Principles and Practices of Radiation Therapy*. 3rd ed. St Louis: Elsevier; 2010.

Das IJ, Cheng CW, Chopra KL, et al. Intensity-modulated radiation therapy dose prescription, recording, and delivery: patterns of variability among institutions and treatment planning systems. *J Natl Cancer Inst*. 2008;100(5):300–307.

Dawson LA, Jaffray DA. Advances in image-guided radiation therapy. *J Clin Oncol*. 2007;25(8):938–946.

Dieterich SP, Pawlicki TP. Cyberknife image-guided delivery and quality assurance. *Int J Radiat Oncol Biol Phys*. 2008;71(1 Suppl):S126–S130.

Dische S. Radiotherapy in the nineties: increase in cure, decrease in morbidity. *Acta Oncol*. 1992;31(5):501–511.

Furlow B. Three-dimensional conformal radiation therapy. *Radiat Therapist*. 2003;12(131).

Gierga DP, Brewer J, Sharp GC, et al. The correlation between internal and external markers for abdominal tumors: implications for respiratory gating. *Int J Radiat Oncol Biol Phys*. 2005;61(5):1551–1558.

Gillin MT. Special procedures. In: Washington CM, Leaver DT, eds. *Principles and Practices of Radiation Therapy*. 3rd ed. St Louis: Elsevier; 2010.

Goitein M, Lomax AJ, Pedroni ES. Treating cancer with protons. *Phys Today*. 2002;55(9):45–50.

Greenlee RT, Hill-Harmon MB, Murray T, et al. Cancer statistics, 2001. *CA Cancer J Clin*. 2001;51(1):15–36.

Heron M, Anderson RN. Changes in the leading cause of death: recent patterns in heart disease and cancer mortality. *NCHS Data Brief*. 2016;(254):1–8.

Howington JA, Blum MG, Chang AC, et al. Treatment of stage I and II non-small cell lung cancer. *Chest*. 2013;143(5 Suppl):e278S–e313S.

Jaffray DA, Siewerdsen JH, Wong JW, et al. Flat-panel cone-beam computed tomography for image-guided radiation therapy. *Int J Radiat Oncol Biol Phys.* 2002;53(5):1337–1349.

Jessup JM, Menck HR, Fremgen A, et al. Diagnosing colorectal carcinoma: clinical and molecular approaches. *CA Cancer J Clin.* 1997;47(2):70–92.

Khan F. Proton beam therapy. In: *The physics of radiation therapy*. Philadelphia: Lippincott, Williams and Wilkins; 2010.

Leaver D. Intensity modulated radiation therapy: part 2. *Radiat Therapist.* 2003;12(17).

Leaver D, et al. Simulation procedures. In: Washington CM, Leaver DT, eds. *Principles and Practices of Radiation Therapy*. 3rd ed. St Louis: Elsevier; 2010.

Lipa LA, Mesina CF. Virtual simulation in conjunction with 3-D conformal therapy. *Radiat Therapist.* 1995;2:99.

Marks JE, Armbruster JS. Accreditation of radiation oncology in the United States. *Int J Radiat Oncol Biol Phys.* 1992;24(5):857–860.

Mell LK, Roeske JC, Mundt AJ. A survey of intensity-modulated radiation therapy use in the United States. *Cancer.* 2003;98(1):204–211.

McDermott P, Orton C. *Special Modalities in Radiation Therapy. The Physics & Technology of Radiation Therapy*. Madison, WI: Medical Physics; 2010.

Mohan R, Das IJ, Ling CC. Empowering intensity modulated proton therapy through physics and technology: an overview. *Int J Radiat Oncol Biol Phys.* 2017;99(2):304–316.

Mohan R, Grosshans D. Proton therapy – present and future. *Adv Drug Deliv Rev.* 2017;109:26–44.

Morgan HM. Quality assurance of computer controlled radiotherapy treatments. *Br J Radiol.* 1992;65(773):409–416.

National Association for Proton Therapy. Available at http://www.proton-therapy.org. (Accessed August 5, 2024.)

National Cancer Institute. *Genetic Testing for Breast Cancer Risk: It's Your Choice*. Washington, DC: National Cancer Institute; 1997.

National Cancer Institute. *Radiation Therapy to Treat Cancer*; 2019. Available at: https://www.cancer.gov/about-cancer/treatment/types/radiation-therapy. (Accessed August 5, 2024.)

Navarria P, Ascolese AM, Mancosu P, et al. Volumetric modulated arc therapy with flattening filter free (FFF) beams for stereotactic body radiation therapy (SBRT) in patients with medically inoperable early stage non small cell lung cancer (NSCLC). *Radiother Oncol.* 2013;107(3):414–418.

Order SE. Training in systemic radiation therapy. *Int J Radiat Oncol Biol Phys.* 1992;24(5):895–896.

Otto K. Volumetric modulated arc therapy: IMRT in a single gantry arc. *Med Phys.* 2008;35(1):310–317.

Palma DA, Verbakel WFAR, Otto K, et al. New developments in arc radiation therapy: a review. *Cancer Treat Rev.* 2010;36(5):393–399.

Palma D, Vollans E, James K, et al. Volumetric modulated arc therapy for delivery of prostate radiotherapy: comparison with intensity-modulated radiotherapy and three-dimensional conformal radiotherapy. *Int J Radiat Oncol Biol Phys.* 2008;72(4):996–1001.

Palmer M. Particle therapy. In: Washington CM, Leaver DT, eds. *Principles and Practices of Radiation Therapy*. 4th ed. St Louis: Elsevier; 2016.

Perez CA. Quest for excellence: the ultimate goal of the radiation oncologist: ASTRO Gold Medal Address, 1992. *Int J Radiat Oncol Biol Phys.* 1993;26(4):567–580.

Prado K, Prado C. Dose distributions. In: Washington CM, Leaver DT, eds. *Principles and Practices of Radiation Therapy*. 3rd ed. St Louis: Elsevier; 2010.

Qi XS, Hu AY, Lee SP, et al. Assessment of interfraction patient setup for head-and-neck cancer intensity modulated radiation therapy using multiple computed tomography-based image guidance. *Int J Radiat Oncol Biol Phys.* 2013;86(3):432–439.

Ramsey CR, Langen KM, Kupelian PA, et al. A technique for adaptive image-guided helical tomotherapy for lung cancer. *Int J Radiat Oncol Biol Phys.* 2006;64(4):1237–1244.

Rietzel E, Chen GTY, Choi NC, et al. Four-dimensional image-based treatment planning: target volume segmentation and dose calculation in the presence of respiratory motion. *Int J Radiat Oncol Biol Phys.* 2005;61(5):1535–1550.

Roberge SL. Virtual reality: radiation therapy treatment planning of tomorrow. *Radiat Therapist.* 1996;2:113.

Shimizu S, Matsuura T, Umezawa M, et al. Preliminary analysis for integration of spot-scanning proton beam therapy and real-time imaging and gating. *Phys Med.* 2014;30(5):555–558.

Simone CB 2nd, Wildt B, Haas AR, et al. Stereotactic body radiation therapy for lung cancer. *Chest.* 2013;143(6):1784–1790.

Torre LA, Siegel RL, Jemal A. Lung cancer statistics. *Adv Exp Med Biol.* 2016;893:1–19.

Vlachaki MT, Teslow TN, Amosson C, et al. IMRT versus conventional 3DCRT on prostate and normal tissue dosimetry using an endorectal balloon for prostate localization. *Med Dosim.* 2005;30(2):69–75.

Wagner LK. Absorbed dose in imaging: why measure it? *Radiology.* 1991;178(3):622–623.

Washington CM, Leaver DT, eds. *Principles and Practice of Radiation Therapy*. 4th ed. St Louis: Elsevier; 2016.

Weber DC, Zilli T, Vallee JP, et al. Intensity modulated proton and photon therapy for early prostate cancer with or without transperineal injection of a polyethylene glycol spacer: a treatment planning comparison study. *Int J Radiat Oncol Biol Phys.* 2012;84(3):e311–e318.

Wilkinson JB, Beitsch PD, Shah C, et al. Evaluation of current consensus statement recommendations for accelerated partial breast irradiation: a pooled analysis of William Beaumont Hospital and American Society of Breast Surgeons MammoSite registry trial data. *Int J Radiat Oncol Biol Phys.* 2013;85(5):1179–1185.

Yamada Y, Lovelock DM, Bilsky MH. A review of image-guided intensity-modulated radiotherapy for spinal tumors. *Neurosurgery.* 2007;61(2):226–235.

Yashar CM, Scanderbeg D, Kuske R, et al. Initial clinical experience with the Strut-Adjusted Volume Implant (SAVI) breast brachytherapy device for accelerated partial-breast irradiation (APBI): first 100 patients with more than 1 year of follow-up. *Int J Radiat Oncol Biol Phys.* 2011;80(3):765–770.

INDEX

A
Abbreviations
 for contrast arthrography, **2:**143*b*
 for cranium, **2:**28*b*
 for digestive system, **2:**187*b*
 for general anatomy and radiographic positioning terminology, **1:**80*b*
 for lower extremity, **1:**281*b*
 for pelvis and hip, **1:**378*b*
 for preliminary steps in radiography, **1:**44*b*
 for reproductive system, **2:**335*b*
 for shoulder girdle, **1:**224*b*
 for trauma radiography, **2:**115*b*
 for upper extremity, **1:**151*b*
 for urinary system, **2:**281*b*
 for vertebral column, **1:**423*b*
Abdomen, **1:**125–140
 abbreviations for, **1:**130*b*
 anatomy of, **1:**127, **1:**127*f*–128*f*, **1:**129*b*
 AP projection of, **1:**133*f*, **1:**134–135, **1:**135*f*
  central ray in, **1:**134
  collimation in, **1:**134
  evaluation criteria in, **1:**136*b*–138*b*
  in left lateral decubitus position, **1:**136–137, **1:**136*f*–137*f*
  position of part of, **1:**134
  respiration in, **1:**134
  structures in, **1:**135, **1:**135*f*
  in supine position, **1:**132, **1:**134*f*
  upright, **1:**134*f*
 in children, **3:**84–88
  image assessment for, **3:**96*t*
  with intussusception, **3:**87, **3:**87*f*
  with pneumoperitoneum, **3:**88, **3:**88*f*
  positioning and immobilization for, **3:**86, **3:**86*f*
 diagnostic medical sonography of, **3:**414–419, **3:**414*f*–415*f*
 divisions of, **1:**50, **1:**50*f*
  surface landmarks, **1:**51, **1:**51*f*, **1:**51*t*
 exposure technique for, **1:**131, **1:**131*f*
 immobilization for, **1:**131, **1:**132*f*
 lateral projection of, **1:**138–139
  evaluation criteria for, **1:**138*b*–139*b*
  right or left dorsal decubitus position, **1:**139, **1:**139*f*
  in right or left position, **1:**138, **1:**138*f*
 mobile radiography of, **2:**14–17
  AP or PA projection, in left lateral decubitus position, **2:**16–17, **2:**16*f*–17*f*, **2:**17*b*
  AP projection, **2:**14–17, **2:**14*b*, **2:**14*f*–15*f*
 MRI of, **3:**295–297, **3:**295*f*–297*f*
 PA projection of, **1:**136
  upright position in, **1:**136–137, **1:**136*f*
 positioning protocols in, **1:**132
 radiographic projections in, **1:**132
 recommended sequence for, **1:**132–139, **1:**132*f*–133*f*
 regions of, **1:**50, **1:**50*f*
 sample exposure technique chart for, **1:**130*t*
 scout or survey image of, **1:**132
 summary of pathology of, **1:**129*t*
 summary of projections in, **1:**126, **1:**126*t*
 supine position, **1:**134, **1:**134*f*–135*f*
 three-way series of, **1:**132
 trauma radiography of
  AP projection of, **2:**122–124, **2:**122*f*

Abdomen *(Continued)*
 in left lateral decubitus position, **2:**123, **2:**123*f*
 lateral projection of, **2:**124, **2:**124*f*
 upright position, **1:**132, **1:**133*f*–135*f*, **1:**134
Abdominal aorta
 MRA of, **3:**302*f*
 sectional anatomy of, **3:**192, **3:**193*f*
  on axial plane
   at level A, **3:**194*f*
   at level B, **3:**195, **3:**195*f*
   at level C, **3:**196–197, **3:**196*f*
   at level D, **3:**197, **3:**197*f*
   at level E, **3:**197–199, **3:**198*f*–199*f*
   at level F, **3:**200, **3:**200*f*
   at level G, **3:**200, **3:**201*f*
  on coronal plane, **3:**203*f*
  on sagittal plane, **3:**202*f*
Abdominal aortic aneurysm (AAA), **1:**129*t*, **3:**358–359
 endografts for, **3:**358–360, **3:**358*f*–359*f*
 three-dimensional CT of, **3:**239*f*
Abdominal aortography, **3:**335, **3:**335*f*
Abdominal cavity
 general anatomy of, **1:**49, **1:**49*f*, **1:**127
 sectional anatomy of, **3:**205
Abdominal circumference, fetal ultrasound for, **3:**426, **3:**426*f*
Abdominal duplex examinations, **3:**428
Abdominal fistulae and sinuses, **2:**270, **2:**270*f*
Abdominal viscera, **1:**127*f*
Abdominal wall, diagnostic medical sonography of, **3:**420
Abdominopelvic cavity, **1:**49, **1:**49*f*, **1:**127, **1:**127*f*, **1:**129*f*
Abdominopelvic region, sectional anatomy of, **3:**204–221, **3:**204*f*, **3:**206*f*
 on axial plane
  at level A, **3:**207*f*
  at level B, **3:**208*f*
  at level C, **3:**209*f*
  at level D, **3:**210*f*
  at level E, **3:**211*f*
  at level F, **3:**212*f*
  at level G, **3:**213*f*
  at level H, **3:**214*f*
  at level I, **3:**215*f*
  at level J, **3:**216*f*
  at level K, **3:**217*f*–218*f*
 on coronal plane, **3:**220*f*–221*f*
 on midsagittal plane, **3:**219*f*
Abduction, **1:**78, **1:**78*f*
Ablation, **3:**402
Abscess, in breast, **2:**376*t*–377*t*
Absorbed dose, **3:**508
Acanthion, **2:**18, **2:**18*f*–19*f*, **2:**29*f*
Acanthioparietal projection, of facial bones, **2:**64*b*, **2:**64*f*–65*f*, **2:**65, **2:**132, **2:**132*f*
Acanthoparietal projection, **1:**70*t*
Accelerator (particle), **3:**508
Accessory glands, of digestive system, **2:**171, **2:**171*f*
Accessory process, **1:**419
Accuracy
 for mobile radiography, **2:**26
 for trauma radiography, **2:**113
Acetabulum
 anatomy of, **1:**371, **1:**371*f*, **1:**374*f*, **1:**376*f*
 AP oblique projection of, Judet method for, **1:**400, **1:**400*b*–401*b*, **1:**400*f*–401*f*
  modified, **1:**400, **1:**401*f*
 comminuted fracture of, **2:**19*f*
 PA axial oblique projection of, Teufel method for, **1:**398–399, **1:**398*f*–399*f*, **1:**399*b*
 sectional anatomy of, **3:**216

Achalasia, **2:**190*t*–191*t*
Acinus, of breast, **2:**360
Acoustic impedance, **3:**410, **3:**410*f*
Acoustic nerve tumor, **3:**293*f*
Acoustic neuroma, **2:**26*t*
Acoustic window, in transabdominal ultrasonography, **3:**423, **3:**433
Acquisition rate, **3:**402
Acromial extremity, of clavicle, **1:**219, **1:**219*f*
Acromioclavicular (AC) articulations, **1:**249–252
 Alexander method for, AP axial projection of, **1:**251–252, **1:**251*f*–252*f*, **1:**252*b*
 anatomy of, **1:**224, **1:**224*b*, **1:**224*f*
 Pearson method for, bilateral AP projection of, **1:**249–250, **1:**249*f*–250*f*, **1:**250*b*
 sectional anatomy of, **3:**192
Activated clotting time (ACT), **3:**402
Active shielding, in MRI, **3:**306
ACTM. *See* Automatic tube current modulation
Acute abdomen series, **1:**132
Adam's apple, **1:**89, **2:**176
Adduction, **1:**78, **1:**78*f*
Adductor tubercle, of femur, **1:**274*f*, **1:**275
Adenocarcinoma, **3:**485
Adenoids, **1:**88, **2:**174
Adenomatous polyposis coli *(APC)* gene, **3:**485
Adhesion, **2:**335*t*
Adipose capsule, **2:**276
Adolescent, development of, **3:**76
Adolescent kyphosis, **1:**424*t*
Adrenal glands
 anatomy of, **2:**275, **2:**275*f*
 diagnostic medical sonography of, **3:**414*f*
Adrenaline, **2:**316*c*
Advanced clinical practice, **1:**3
Advanced visualization, for sectional anatomy, **3:**222–223, **3:**222*f*–224*f*
Adventitia, **3:**402
AEC. *See* Automatic exposure control
Afferent arteriole, of kidney, **2:**277, **2:**277*f*
Afferent lymph vessels, **3:**318, **3:**402
Age-based development, **3:**73–76
 of adolescent, **3:**76
 of infant, **3:**74
 of neonate, **3:**73
 of premature infants, **3:**73
 of preschooler, **3:**74–76, **3:**74*f*–75*f*
 of school-age children, **3:**76
 of toddler, **3:**74
Age-related competencies, in older adults, **3:**162
Age-specific competencies, **1:**8–9, **1:**9*b*, **1:**9*t*
Aging. *See also* Older adults
 concept of, **3:**150, **3:**150*f*
 demographics and social effects of, **3:**148–168, **3:**148*f*, **3:**150*f*
 physical, cognitive, and psychosocial effects of, **3:**152–154, **3:**153*b*, **3:**153*f*
 physiology of, **3:**154–159
  endocrine system disorders in, **3:**159
  gastrointestinal system disorders in, **3:**157, **3:**157*f*
  genitourinary system disorders in, **3:**159
  hematologic system disorders in, **3:**159
  immune system decline in, **3:**158
  integumentary system disorders in, **3:**154, **3:**155*f*
  musculoskeletal system disorders in, **3:**156, **3:**156*f*–157*f*
  nervous system disorders in, **3:**154–155
  respiratory system disorders in, **3:**158, **3:**158*f*
  sensory system disorders in, **3:**155
  summary of, **3:**159

Page numbers followed by "*f*" indicate figures, "*t*" indicate tables, and "*b*" indicate boxes. Boldface numbers indicate the volume.

I-1

Index

Air calibrations, for CT, **3:**255, **3:**265
Air cells, **2:**8*f*
Air-contrast study, of large intestine, **2:**234
Airway foreign body, in children, **3:**112, **3:**112*f*
Ala
  of ilium, **1:**371*f*, **1:**372, **1:**382*f*
  of sacrum, **1:**421
ALARA. *See* As low as reasonably achievable
Alert value, for CT, **3:**256
Alexander method, for AP axial projection, of acromioclavicular articulation, **1:**251–252, **1:**251*f*–252*f*, **1:**252*b*
Algorithm, in CT, **3:**228, **3:**265
Alimentary canal, **2:**171, **2:**171*f*. *See also* Digestive system
Alpha particle, **3:**478
Alveolar ducts, **1:**84*f*, **1:**85
Alveolar process, **2:**18, **2:**19*f*
  sectional anatomy of, **3:**175
Alveolar sacs, **1:**84*f*, **1:**85
Alveolus, of lung, **1:**84*f*, **1:**85, **2:**361*f*
Alzheimer disease, **3:**153, **3:**160*t*
  performing radiography with, **3:**162–163
  stages and symptoms of, **3:**163*t*
American Association of Physicists in Medicine (AAPM), **1:**20
American Registry of Radiologic Technologists (ARRT), **1:**65
  Code of Ethics, **1:**2
American Society of Radiologic Technologists (ASRT), **1:**2
Amnion, **2:**331
Amniotic cavity, diagnostic medical sonography of, **3:**424, **3:**425*f*
Amphiarthroses, **1:**61
Ampulla
  of breast, **2:**361*f*
  of ductus deferens, **2:**332, **2:**333*f*
  of uterine tube, **2:**329, **2:**329*f*
Amyloid neurologic study, **3:**474
Anal canal
  anatomy of, **2:**182*f*–183*f*, **2:**183
  defecography of, **2:**262, **2:**262*f*
Analog, radioactive, **3:**439–440, **3:**478
Anaphylactic reaction, **2:**325
Anastomose, **3:**353, **3:**402
Anatomic body parts, in mobile radiography, **2:**26
Anatomic markers, **1:**27–28, **1:**27*f*, **1:**28*b*
Anatomic neck, of humerus, **1:**146–147, **1:**146*f*
Anatomic programmers, **1:**20, **1:**22*f*
Anatomically programmed radiography (APR) systems, for obese patients, **1:**42
Anatomy
  anatomic relationship terms in, **1:**65
  of bones
    appendicular skeleton in, **1:**55, **1:**55*f*, **1:**55*t*
    axial skeleton in, **1:**55, **1:**55*f*, **1:**55*t*
    classification of, **1:**59, **1:**59*f*
    development in, **1:**57–58
    fractures of, **1:**64, **1:**64*f*
    general features in, **1:**56, **1:**56*f*
    markings and features of, **1:**64
    vessels and nerves in, **1:**57, **1:**57*f*
  defined, **1:**46
  general, **1:**46–80
    of body cavities, **1:**49, **1:**49*f*
    body habitus in, **1:**52–54, **1:**52*f*, **1:**53*b*
    body planes in, **1:**46–47, **1:**46*f*
    divisions of abdomen, **1:**50, **1:**50*f*
    special planes in, **1:**48, **1:**48*f*
  of joints, **1:**60
    cartilaginous, **1:**60*t*, **1:**61, **1:**61*f*
    fibrous, **1:**60*t*, **1:**61
    functional classification of, **1:**61
    structural classification of, **1:**60*t*, **1:**61–62
    synovial, **1:**60*t*, **1:**62, **1:**62*f*–63*f*
  sectional. *See* Sectional anatomy
Andren-von Rosén approach, for congenital dislocation of hip, **1:**389
Anechoic structure/mass, **3:**412, **3:**413*f*, **3:**433
Anemia, in older adults, **3:**159
Anencephaly, **3:**427*f*
Anesthesia provider, **3:**32
Aneurysm, **3:**320, **3:**402
  aortic, abdominal, **1:**129*t*, **3:**358–359
    endografts for, **3:**358–360, **3:**358*f*–359*f*
    three-dimensional CT of, **3:**239*f*

Aneurysmal bone cyst (ABC), **3:**136, **3:**136*f*
Angina pectoris, **3:**402
Angiocatheters, **2:**318*f*, **2:**319
Angiography, **3:**320–332, **3:**402–403
  aortic arch (cranial vessels), **3:**348, **3:**348*f*
  aortography as, **3:**334–341
    abdominal, **3:**335, **3:**335*f*
    thoracic, **3:**334, **3:**334*f*
  arteriography. *See* Arteriography
  catheterization for, **3:**327–332, **3:**328*f*, **3:**330*f*–332*f*
  cerebral. *See* Cerebral angiography
  contrast media for, **3:**322
  coronary, **3:**372, **3:**373*t*
  CT. *See* Computed tomography angiography
  digital subtraction. *See* Digital subtraction angiography
  external carotid, **3:**348–349
  guidewires for, **3:**329, **3:**329*f*
  historical development of, **3:**312
  imaging equipment for, **3:**324–326
  indications for, **3:**320–332
  injection technique for, **3:**323
  introducer sheaths for, **3:**331–332, **3:**332*f*
  magnetic resonance, **3:**302, **3:**302*f*
  magnification in, **3:**325
  micropuncture access sets for, **3:**330, **3:**330*f*
  patient care for, **3:**326
  peripheral, **3:**340–341
    lower limb arteriograms, **3:**340, **3:**340*f*
    lower limb venograms, **3:**353, **3:**354*f*
    upper limb arteriograms, **3:**341, **3:**341*f*
    upper limb venograms, **3:**353, **3:**353*f*
  postprocedure for, **3:**332, **3:**333*f*
  preparation of procedure room for, **3:**321, **3:**321*f*
  preprocedure for, **3:**327
  procedures for, **3:**326–332
  radiation protection for, **3:**322
  team for, **3:**321
  three-dimensional intraarterial, **3:**326, **3:**326*f*
  vascular access needles for, **3:**329
  venography. *See* Venography
  vertebral arteriography, **3:**348–349
Angular notch, of stomach, **2:**178, **2:**178*f*
Anisotropic spatial resolution, **3:**265
Ankle, **1:**319–329
  with antibiotic beads, mobile radiography procedures for, in operating room, **3:**62*f*
  AP projection of, **1:**319*f*, **1:**319–323, **1:**319*f*
    evaluation criteria for, **1:**319*b*, **1:**328*b*
    in lateral rotation, **1:**326, **1:**326*b*, **1:**326*f*
    in medial rotation, **1:**323, **1:**323*f*
    in neutral position, **1:**327*f*
    stress method for, **1:**327, **1:**327*f*
    weight-bearing method for, **1:**328, **1:**328*b*, **1:**328*f*
  evaluation criteria for, **1:**319*b*
  lateral projection of
    evaluation criteria for, **1:**329*b*
    lateromedial, **1:**302, **1:**322, **1:**322*b*, **1:**322*f*
    mediolateral, **1:**300, **1:**320, **1:**320*b*, **1:**320*f*–321*f*
    weight-bearing method for, **1:**329, **1:**329*b*, **1:**329*f*
  mortise joint of
    anatomy of, **1:**272*f*, **1:**278*t*
    AP oblique projection in, medial rotation of, **1:**324–325, **1:**324*f*–325*f*
  MRI of, **3:**300*f*
Ankle fracture, mobile radiography procedures for, in operating room, **3:**61*f*
Ankle joint, AP oblique projection in medial rotation of, **1:**323, **1:**323*b*, **1:**323*f*
Ankle mortise
  anatomy of, **1:**272*f*, **1:**278*t*
  AP oblique projection in medial rotation of, **1:**324–325, **1:**324*f*–325*f*
Ankle/brachial index (ABI), **3:**429, **3:**433
Ankylosing spondylitis, **1:**379*t*, **1:**424*t*
Annihilation photons, **3:**460, **3:**461*f*, **3:**478
Annotation, **1:**34
Annulus fibrosus
  anatomy of, **1:**413
  sectional anatomy of, **3:**191–192
Anode heel effect, in mobile radiography, **2:**5, **2:**5*t*
Anomaly, **3:**402
Antegrade femoral nailing, **3:**48
Antenna, in MRI, **3:**271, **3:**306
Anterior, definition of, **1:**65
Anterior arches, anatomy of, **2:**172, **2:**172*f*

Anterior cerebral arteries
  CT angiography of, **3:**251*f*
  MRI of, **3:**302*f*
  sectional anatomy of, **3:**176, **3:**179–180, **3:**179*f*–181*f*
Anterior cervical diskectomy, **3:**43, **3:**43*b*, **3:**43*f*
Anterior circulation, cerebral angiography of, **3:**349–351
  AP axial oblique projection, **3:**351, **3:**351*f*
  AP axial projection, **3:**350, **3:**350*f*
  lateral projection for, **3:**349, **3:**349*b*, **3:**349*f*
Anterior clinoid process, **2:**4*f*, **2:**10*f*–11*f*, **2:**11, **3:**182*f*
Anterior communicating artery
  anatomy of, **3:**344
  CT angiography of, **3:**251*f*
Anterior cranial fossa, **2:**6
Anterior crest of tibia, **1:**272*f*
Anterior cruciate ligament, **1:**276*f*
Anterior fat pad, of elbow, **1:**149, **1:**149*f*
Anterior fontanel, **2:**6, **2:**6*f*
Anterior horn, **2:**154, **2:**154*f*
Anterior inferior iliac spine, **1:**371*f*, **1:**377*f*, **1:**382*f*
Anterior nasal spine, **2:**18, **2:**18*f*–19*f*
Anterior superior iliac spine, **1:**371*f*, **1:**374*f*, **1:**377, **1:**382*f*, **1:**390*f*
  as bony landmark, **1:**377*f*
  sectional anatomy of, **3:**215
  as surface landmark, **1:**51*f*
Anterior tubercle, of tibia, **1:**273, **1:**273*f*
Anteroposterior (AP) axial oblique projection, **1:**67*t*
Anteroposterior (AP) axial projection, **1:**67*t*
Anteroposterior (AP) oblique projection, **1:**67*t*
Anteroposterior (AP) projection, **1:**47, **1:**66, **1:**66*f*, **1:**67*t*
Anthracosis, **1:**93*t*
Anthropomorphic, definition of, **2:**491
Anticipation, for trauma radiography, **2:**113
Antisepsis, **3:**69
Anus
  anatomy of, **2:**171, **2:**182*f*–183*f*, **2:**183
  diagnostic medical sonography of, **3:**422*f*
Aorta, **1:**92*f*, **1:**110*f*
  abdominal. *See* Abdominal aorta
  anatomy of, **2:**275*f*
  diagnostic medical sonography of, **3:**414*f*, **3:**417*f*
  lateral view of, **2:**177*f*
  sectional anatomy of
    ascending, **3:**192, **3:**193*f*, **3:**197–199, **3:**198*f*
    on axial plane
      at level A, **3:**207, **3:**207*f*
      at level B, **3:**207, **3:**208*f*–209*f*
      at level D, **3:**210, **3:**210*f*
      at level E, **3:**211, **3:**211*f*
      at level F, **3:**212, **3:**212*f*
      at level G, **3:**213, **3:**213*f*
    on coronal plane, **3:**220–221, **3:**221*f*
    descending, **3:**192, **3:**193*f*, **3:**197–199, **3:**198*f*, **3:**220*f*
  sectional image of, **2:**187*f*
Aortic aneurysm, abdominal, **3:**358–359
  endografts for, **3:**358–360, **3:**358*f*–359*f*
  three-dimensional, CT of, **3:**239*f*
Aortic arch
  angiogram, **3:**348, **3:**348*f*
  MRA of, **3:**302*f*
  sectional anatomy of, **3:**192, **3:**197, **3:**197*f*
Aortic dissection, **3:**402
Aortic valve, **3:**317, **3:**317*f*
Aortobronchial constriction, **2:**176
Aortofemoral arteriography, **3:**340
Aortography, **3:**334–341, **3:**402–403
  abdominal, **3:**335, **3:**335*f*
  thoracic, **3:**334, **3:**334*f*
APC (adenomatous polyposis coli) gene, **3:**485
Aperture, in CT, **3:**236, **3:**265
Appendicitis, **2:**190*t*–191*t*
Appendicular skeleton, **1:**55, **1:**55*f*, **1:**55*t*
Appendix, anatomy of, **2:**184*f*
Apple method, for AP oblique projection, of glenoid cavity, **1:**231–232, **1:**231*f*–232*f*, **1:**232*b*
Aquaplast mask, **3:**492*f*
Arachnoid
  anatomy of, **2:**153
  defined, **2:**167
  sectional anatomy of, **3:**175
Architectural distortions (AD), of breast, **2:**375, **2:**375*f*
Archiving, for CT, **3:**235, **3:**265
Arcuate eminence, **2:**15*f*
Arcuate line, **1:**371*f*, **1:**372, **1:**376*f*

Areal technique, **2:**491
Areola, **2:**360, **2:**361*f*
Array-beam techniques, for DXA, **2:**468–471, **2:**468*f*, **2:**491
Arrhythmia, **3:**402
Arteries, **3:**403
　coronary, **3:**317*f*, **3:**318
　systemic, **3:**315
Arteriography, **3:**320
　femoral/tibial, **3:**54*b*, **3:**55–56, **3:**55*f*–56*f*, **3:**56*b*
　peripheral, **3:**340–341
　　lower limb, **3:**340, **3:**340*f*
　　upper limb, **3:**341, **3:**341*f*
　pulmonary, **3:**339, **3:**339*f*
　visceral, **3:**336–339, **3:**336*f*
　　celiac, **3:**336, **3:**336*f*
　　hepatic, **3:**337, **3:**337*f*
　　inferior mesenteric, **3:**338, **3:**338*f*
　　other, **3:**339
　　renal, **3:**339, **3:**339*f*
　　splenic, **3:**337, **3:**337*f*
　　superior mesenteric, **3:**338, **3:**338*f*
Arterioles, **3:**315, **3:**403
Arteriotomy, **3:**403
Arteriovenous malformation, **3:**403
Arthritis, rheumatoid, **1:**151*t*, **1:**225*t*
Arthrography, **1:**62
　contrast. *See* Contrast arthrography
Arthrology, **1:**60–62
　of cartilaginous joints, **1:**61, **1:**61*f*
　defined, **1:**60
　of fibrous joints, **1:**60*f*, **1:**60*t*, **1:**61
　functional classification of joints in, **1:**61
　structural classification of joints in, **1:**60*t*, **1:**61–62
　of synovial joints, **1:**60*t*, **1:**62*f*–63*f*
Arthroplasty, in older adults, **3:**156, **3:**157*f*
Articular capsule, **1:**62*f*
Articular cartilage, **1:**56, **1:**56*f*, **1:**62*f*, **1:**413
Articular pillars, **1:**415
Articular processes, of vertebral arch, **1:**413
Articular surface, **1:**372*f*
Articular tubercle, **2:**14, **2:**14*f*
　axiolateral oblique projection of, **2:**88*f*
Artifacts
　in CT, **3:**245, **3:**245*f*, **3:**265
　in diagnostic medical sonography, **3:**412, **3:**413*f*
　in digital radiography, **3:**82–83, **3:**82*f*–83*f*
　in MRI, **3:**293, **3:**306
As low as reasonably achievable (ALARA), **1:**2, **2:**491
Asbestosis, **1:**93*t*
Ascites, **1:**129*t*
Asepsis, **3:**69
　in mobile radiography, **2:**9
Aseptic technique, **3:**69
　for minor surgical procedures, in radiology department, **1:**5, **1:**5*f*
　principles of, **3:**36*b*
Aspiration pneumonia, **1:**93*t*
Asterion, **2:**4*f*
Asthenic body habitus, **1:**52*f*, **1:**53*b*, **1:**54
　gallbladder and, **2:**186, **2:**186*f*
　skull radiography with, **2:**32*f*
　stomach and duodenum and, **2:**179, **2:**179*f*
　thoracic viscera and, **1:**83*f*
Asymmetric jaws, of linear accelerators, **3:**490*f*, **3:**508
Atelectasis, **1:**93*t*
Atherectomy, **3:**388–389, **3:**388*f*–389*f*, **3:**403
Atheromatous plaque, **3:**372, **3:**403
Atherosclerosis, **3:**320, **3:**403
　echocardiography of, **3:**430
　in older adults, **3:**156, **3:**160*t*
Atlantoaxial joint, **1:**422
Atlantooccipital articulation, **1:**422
Atlantooccipital joint, **2:**12*f*, **2:**21*t*
Atlas
　anatomy of, **1:**414, **1:**414*f*
　AP projection (open-mouth) of, **1:**428–429, **1:**428*f*–429*f*, **1:**429*b*
　lateral projection of, **1:**430–431, **1:**430*f*–431*f*, **1:**431*b*
Atrial septal defect closure, **3:**396
Atrium
　anatomy of, **1:**92*f*, **3:**316, **3:**317*f*, **3:**403
　sectional anatomy of, **3:**192, **3:**193*f*
　　left, **3:**200, **3:**200*f*
　　right, **3:**200, **3:**200*f*

Atropine sulfate (Atropine), **2:**316*t*
Attenuation
　in CT, **3:**265
　in diagnostic medical sonography, **3:**433
　MRI *vs.* conventional radiography, **3:**270, **3:**306
　in radiation oncology, **3:**508
Attenuation coefficients, **3:**438, **3:**478
Atypia, papilloma with, **2:**376*t*–377*t*
Atypical ductal hyperplasia (ADH), **2:**376*t*–377*t*
Atypical lobular hyperplasia, **2:**376*t*–377*t*
Auditory ossicles, **2:**15*f*, **2:**16, **2:**17*f*
Auditory (eustachian) tube, **2:**16, **2:**17*f*
Augmented breast, routine projections of, **2:**400–401, **2:**401*f*
　complications of, **2:**400–401
　craniocaudal projection
　　with full implant, **2:**402–408, **2:**402*b*, **2:**402*f*
　　with implant displaced, **2:**403–404, **2:**403*f*–404*f*, **2:**404*b*
　mediolateral oblique projection
　　with full implant, **2:**405, **2:**405*b*
　　with implant displaced, **2:**406, **2:**406*b*
　MRI and, **2:**400–401
　ultrasonography and, **2:**401
Auricle, **3:**316
　of ear, **2:**16, **2:**17*f*
　as lateral landmark, **2:**29*f*
Auricular surface
　of ilium, **1:**371*f*, **1:**372
　of sacrum, **1:**421
Autism spectrum disorders (ASDs), **3:**77–79, **3:**77*b*
Automatic collimation, **1:**25
Automatic exposure control (AEC), **1:**20
　for mammography, **2:**391
　for obese patients, **1:**42
Automatic tube current modulation (ATCM), **3:**257, **3:**258*f*
Axial image, in CT, **3:**228, **3:**229*f*, **3:**265
Axial plane, **1:**46, **1:**46*f*
　in sectional anatomy, **3:**172
Axial projection, **1:**67*t*, **1:**68, **1:**68*f*
Axial resolution, in diagnostic medical sonography, **3:**433
Axial skeletal measurements, **2:**483–485, **2:**483*f*–485*f*
Axial skeleton, **1:**55, **1:**55*f*, **1:**55*t*
Axilla, labeling codes for, **2:**385*t*–390*t*
Axillary arteries, **3:**192
Axillary fossa, anatomy of, **2:**360, **2:**360*f*
Axillary lymph nodes
　anatomy of, **2:**360, **2:**361*f*
　pathologic and mammographic findings of, **2:**368
Axillary prolongation, **2:**360
Axillary tail (AT)
　anatomy of, **2:**360, **2:**360*f*
　axilla projection for, **2:**431, **2:**431*f*
　labeling codes for, **2:**385*t*–390*t*
　mediolateral oblique projection for, **2:**429–430, **2:**429*f*
Axillary vein, **3:**195, **3:**195*f*
Axiolateral oblique projection, **1:**70*t*
Axiolateral projection, **1:**69, **1:**70*t*
Axis
　anatomy of, **1:**414, **1:**414*f*
　AP projection (open-mouth) of, **1:**428–429, **1:**428*f*–429*f*, **1:**429*b*
　lateral projection of, **1:**430–431, **1:**430*f*–431*f*, **1:**431*b*
Azygos vein, **3:**200, **3:**201*f*

B
Baby box device, **3:**92, **3:**93*f*
　for abdominal imaging, **3:**84, **3:**84*f*–85*f*
Backboard, in trauma radiography, **2:**109, **2:**109*f*
Bacterial pneumonia, **1:**93*t*
Ball and socket (spheroid) joint, **1:**62
Balloon angioplasty, **3:**312
Balloon aortic valvuloplasty (BAV), **3:**393, **3:**403
Balloon kyphoplasty, **2:**463, **2:**463*f*
Balloon mitral valvuloplasty (BMV), **3:**393, **3:**403
Balloon septostomy, **3:**396
Balloons, for cardiac catheterization, **3:**376
Bare metal stent, **3:**403
Barium enema (BE)
　double-contrast method for, **2:**234, **2:**234*f*
　　single-stage, **2:**234, **2:**240–241, **2:**240*f*–241*f*
　　two-stage, **2:**234, **2:**240
　insertion of enema tip for, **2:**238
　preparation and care of patient for, **2:**238
　preparation of barium suspension for, **2:**238

Barium enema (BE) *(Continued)*
　single-contrast, **2:**234, **2:**234*f*, **2:**239, **2:**239*f*
　standard barium enema apparatus for, **2:**236–237, **2:**236*f*–237*f*
Barium studies, of heart
　lateral projection for, **1:**107
　PA oblique projection for, **1:**111
　PA projection for, **1:**105
Barium sulfate
　for alimentary canal imaging, **2:**203, **2:**203*f*
　high-density, **2:**234
Barium sulfate suspension
　for alimentary canal imaging, **2:**203, **2:**203*f*–204*f*
　for barium enema, **2:**238
　for gastrointestinal examinations, **2:**212
Barrett esophagus, **2:**190*t*–191*t*
Basal fracture, of cranium, **2:**26*t*
Basal ganglia, **3:**175–176
Basal nuclei, **3:**175–176
Basal segmental bronchus, **1:**92*f*
Base, of lungs, **1:**85–86, **1:**85*f*
Basilar artery
　CT angiography of, **3:**251*f*
　MRI of, **3:**302*f*
　sectional anatomy of, **3:**176, **3:**181*f*, **3:**184*f*
Basilar portion, of occipital bone, **2:**12–13, **2:**12*f*–13*f*
Beam collimation, in CT, **3:**258, **3:**258*t*
Beam hardening
　artifact, in CT, **3:**245, **3:**245*f*
　in energy-switching systems, **2:**466
Beam shaping filters, for CT, **3:**255–256, **3:**255*f*
Béclère method, for AP axial projection of intercondylar fossa, **1:**348, **1:**348*b*, **1:**348*f*
Becquerel (Bq), **3:**442, **3:**478
Benadryl (diphenhydramine hydrochloride), **2:**316*t*
Benign prostatic hyperplasia (BPH), **2:**280*t*
　in older adults, **3:**159, **3:**160*t*
Bennett fracture, **1:**151*t*
Beta particle, **3:**439, **3:**478
Betatron, **3:**508
Bezoar, **2:**190*t*–191*t*
Bicipital groove
　anatomy of, **1:**221, **1:**221*f*
　Fisk modification for, tangential projection of, **1:**247–248, **1:**247*f*–248*f*, **1:**248*b*
Bicornuate uterus, **2:**337*f*
Bifurcation, **3:**403
Bile, **2:**184
Bile ducts, **2:**185, **2:**185*f*
Biliary drainage procedure, **2:**265, **2:**265*f*
Biliary ducts, anatomy of, **2:**184*f*
Biliary stenosis, **2:**190*t*–191*t*
Biliary tract, **2:**263–267
　biliary drainage procedure and stone extraction for, **2:**265, **2:**265*f*
　cholangiography of
　　percutaneous transhepatic, **2:**264–265, **2:**264*f*
　　postoperative (T-tube), **2:**266–267, **2:**266*f*–267*f*
　diagnostic medical sonography of, **3:**411*f*, **3:**415–416, **3:**416*f*
　endoscopic retrograde cholangiopancreatography of, **2:**268, **2:**268*f*–269*f*
　prefixes associated with, **2:**263, **2:**263*t*
　radiographic techniques for, **2:**263
Biochemical markers, of bone turnover, **2:**462, **2:**491
Biometric measurements, fetal ultrasound for, **3:**426, **3:**426*f*
Biopsy, **3:**508
Biparietal diameter (BPD), **3:**426, **3:**426*f*, **3:**433
Biplane, **3:**324, **3:**324*f*, **3:**403
Bisphosphonates, for osteoporosis, **2:**462*t*
Bit depth, in CT, **3:**234
Black lung, **1:**93*t*
Bladder carcinoma, **2:**280*t*
Bloch, Felix, **3:**270
Blood oxygen level-dependent (BOLD) imaging, **3:**305
Blood-brain barrier, **3:**455, **3:**478
Blood-vascular system, **3:**314–318, **3:**314*f*, **3:**403
　arteries in, **3:**315–318
　　coronary, **3:**317*f*, **3:**318
　　systemic, **3:**315
　arterioles in, **3:**315
　capillaries in, **3:**315
　complete circulation of blood through, **3:**318
　heart in, **3:**315, **3:**315*f*
　main trunk vessels in, **3:**315

Blood-vascular system *(Continued)*
  portal system in, **3:**315, **3:**315*f*
  pulmonary circulation in, **3:**315, **3:**315*f*
  systemic circulation in, **3:**315, **3:**315*f*
  veins in
    coronary, **3:**317, **3:**317*f*
    systemic, **3:**316
  venules in, **3:**315
Blowout fracture, of cranium, **2:**26*t*
Blunt trauma, **2:**105
Body cavities, **1:**49, **1:**49*f*
Body composition, **2:**491
Body fluids, containing pathogenic microorganisms, **1:**4*b*
Body habitus, **1:**52–54, **1:**52*f*, **1:**53*b*
  body position and, for skull radiography
    in horizontal sagittal plane, **2:**32*f*
    in perpendicular sagittal plane, **2:**33*f*
  gallbladder and, **2:**186, **2:**186*f*
  stomach and duodenum and, **2:**179, **2:**179*f*
    PA projection of, **2:**215, **2:**216*f*
  thoracic viscera and, **1:**83–92, **1:**83*f*
Body mass index (BMI), **1:**34–35
Body mechanics, in mobile radiography, **2:**26
Body movement terminology, **1:**78–79
  abduction as, **1:**78, **1:**78*f*
  adduction as, **1:**78, **1:**78*f*
  circumduction as, **1:**79, **1:**79*f*
  deviation as, **1:**79, **1:**79*f*
  dorsiflexion as, **1:**79, **1:**79*f*
  evert/eversion as, **1:**78, **1:**78*f*
  extension as, **1:**78, **1:**78*f*
  flexion as, **1:**78, **1:**78*f*
  hyperextension as, **1:**78, **1:**78*f*
  hyperflexion as, **1:**78, **1:**78*f*
  invert/inversion as, **1:**78*f*, **1:**79
  plantar flexion as, **1:**79, **1:**79*f*
  pronate/pronation as, **1:**79, **1:**79*f*
  rotate/rotation as, **1:**79, **1:**79*f*
  supinate/supination as, **1:**79, **1:**79*f*
  tilt as, **1:**79, **1:**79*f*
Body planes, **1:**46–47
  coronal, **1:**46, **1:**46*f*
  in CT, **1:**47, **1:**47*f*
  horizontal, **1:**46, **1:**46*f*
  imaging in several, **1:**47, **1:**47*f*
  interiliac, **1:**48, **1:**48*f*
  midcoronal (midaxillary), **1:**46, **1:**46*f*
  midsagittal, **1:**46, **1:**46*f*
  in MRI, **1:**47, **1:**47*f*
  oblique, **1:**46*f*, **1:**47
  occlusal, **1:**48, **1:**48*f*
  sagittal, **1:**46, **1:**46*f*
  special, **1:**48
  transverse, **1:**46, **1:**46*f*
Body rotation method, for PA oblique projection, of sternoclavicular articulation, **1:**515, **1:**515*b*, **1:**515*f*
Bohr atomic model, **3:**439, **3:**439*f*
Bolus, for CT angiography, **3:**250, **3:**265–266
"Bolus chase," for digital subtraction angiography, **3:**323
Bone(s), **1:**55
  appendicular skeleton of, **1:**55, **1:**55*f*, **1:**55*t*
  axial skeleton in, **1:**55, **1:**55*f*, **1:**55*t*
  biology of, **2:**459–460
  classification of, **1:**59, **1:**59*f*
  cortical (or compact), bone densitometry and, **1:**459, **2:**459*t*
  development of, **1:**57–58
  flat, **1:**59, **1:**59*f*
  formation of. *See* Fracture(s)
  fractures of. *See* Fracture(s)
  general features in, **1:**56, **1:**56*f*
  irregular, **1:**59, **1:**59*f*
  long, **1:**59, **1:**59*f*
  markings and features of, **1:**64
  mass, **2:**491
  sesamoid, **1:**59, **1:**59*f*
  short, **1:**59, **1:**59*f*
  spongy, **1:**56, **1:**56*f*
  trabecular (or cancellous), bone densitometry and, **2:**459, **2:**459*t*
  vessels and nerves of, **1:**57, **1:**57*f*
Bone cyst, **1:**151*t*, **1:**282*t*
  aneurysmal, **3:**136, **3:**136*f*
Bone densitometry, **2:**455–494
  bone biology and remodeling in, **2:**459–460, **2:**459*f*–460*f*, **2:**459*t*

Bone densitometry *(Continued)*
  central (or axial) skeletal measurements in, **2:**483–485, **2:**483*f*–485*f*
  children from infancy to adolescence, skeletal health assessment in, **2:**487–488, **2:**487*f*
  conventional radiography in, **2:**457
  definition of, **2:**456, **2:**491
  dual energy x-ray absorptiometry in, **2:**457
    accuracy and precision of, **2:**469–471, **2:**469*f*
    anatomy, positioning, and analysis for, **2:**477–483
    computer competency for, **2:**474
    cross-calibration of, **2:**471
    of forearm, **2:**482–483, **2:**482*f*
    longitudinal quality control for, **2:**475–476, **2:**475*f*–476*f*
    of PA lumbar spine, **2:**478–480, **2:**478*f*–479*f*
    patient care and education for, **2:**473
    patient history for, **2:**473
    pencil-beam and array-beam techniques for, **2:**468–471, **2:**468*f*
    physical and mathematic principles of, **2:**465–467, **2:**465*f*–467*f*
    of proximal femur, **2:**480–481, **2:**480*f*–481*f*
    radiation protection for, **2:**472, **2:**472*t*
    reporting, confidentiality, record keeping, and scan storage for, **2:**474
    scanning, **2:**472–483
    serial scans in, **2:**477–478, **2:**477*f*
    T-scores of, **2:**471, **2:**472*t*
    Z-scores of, **2:**471
  dual photon absorptiometry in, **2:**458
  fracture risk models in, **2:**489–490
  history of, **2:**457–458
  osteoporosis and, **2:**456, **2:**461–464, **2:**462*t*
    bone health recommendations for, **2:**464, **2:**464*t*
    definition of, **2:**461
    fractures and falls in, **2:**463, **2:**463*f*
  peripheral skeletal measurements in, **2:**487, **2:**488*f*–489*f*
  principles of, **2:**456–492, **2:**456*f*
  quantitative computed tomography in, **2:**458
  radiogrammetry for, **2:**457
  radiographic absorptiometry for, **2:**457
  single photon absorptiometry in, **2:**458, **2:**458*f*
  total body and body composition in, **2:**485, **2:**486*f*
  trabecular bone score in, **2:**489–490
Bone health, recommendations for, **2:**464, **2:**464*t*
Bone marrow
  red, **1:**56
  yellow, **1:**56
Bone mass, **2:**460
Bone mineral content (BMC), **2:**456, **2:**491
Bone mineral density (BMD), **2:**456, **2:**491
Bone remodeling, **2:**459–460, **2:**459*f*, **2:**459*t*, **2:**491
Bone scan, **3:**453–454
Bone scintigraphy, in nuclear medicine, **3:**453–454
Bone studies, **3:**454
Bone turnover, biochemical markers of, **2:**462
Bony labyrinth, **2:**16
Bony thorax, **1:**495–526
  anatomy of, **1:**497–503
    anterior aspect of, **1:**497*f*
    anterolateral oblique aspect of, **1:**497*f*
    lateral aspect of, **1:**498*f*
    ribs in, **1:**497*f*–499*f*, **1:**498, **1:**517
    sternum in, **1:**497–498, **1:**497*f*
    summary of, **1:**503*b*
  articulations, **1:**499–503, **1:**499*f*
  body position for, **1:**503
  joints of, **1:**499*t*
  respiratory movement of, **1:**501, **1:**501*f*
    diaphragm in, **1:**502, **1:**502*f*
  ribs in. *See* Ribs
  sample exposure technique chart routine projections for, **1:**505*t*
  sternum in. *See* Sternum
  summary of pathology of, **1:**504*t*
  summary of projections for, **1:**496, **1:**496*t*
  trauma patients and, **1:**503
Bowel obstruction, **1:**129*t*
Bowel preparation, **1:**11
Bowing fractures, **3:**102
Bowman capsule, **2:**277, **2:**277*f*
Bowtie filter, for CT, **3:**255*f*
Boxer fracture, **1:**151*t*
Brachiocephalic artery, **3:**343
  sectional anatomy of, **3:**192, **3:**196–197

Brachiocephalic vein, sectional anatomy of, **3:**195, **3:**195*f*, **3:**197
  on coronal plane, **3:**202–203
Brachycephalic skull, **2:**30, **2:**30*f*
Brachytherapy, **3:**487, **3:**508
Bradyarrhythmia, **3:**403
Bradycardia, **3:**403
Bragg peak, **3:**502, **3:**502*f*, **3:**510
Brain, **2:**152–156
  anatomy of, **2:**152–156, **2:**152*f*
  CT angiography of, perfusion study for, **3:**250–252
  defined, **2:**167
  MR image of, **3:**177*f*–178*f*
  sectional anatomy of, **3:**175
  SPECT study of, **3:**455
  ventricular system of, **2:**154
Brain stem
  anatomy of, **2:**152, **2:**152*f*
  sectional anatomy of, **3:**176
Brain tissue scanner, **3:**231
BRCA1 genes, **2:**358–359, **3:**484
BRCA2 genes, **2:**358–359, **3:**484
Breast(s)
  abscess, **2:**376*t*–377*t*
  anatomy of, **2:**360–375, **2:**360*f*–361*f*
  augmented, **2:**402–408, **2:**402*f*
    complications of, **2:**400–401
    craniocaudal projection
      with full implant, **2:**402–408, **2:**402*b*, **2:**402*f*
      with implant displaced, **2:**403–404, **2:**403*f*–404*f*, **2:**404*b*
    mediolateral oblique projection
      with full implant, **2:**405, **2:**405*b*
      with implant displaced, **2:**406, **2:**406*b*
  connective tissue of, **2:**361*f*, **2:**363
  cushions, **2:**391, **2:**392*f*
  density of, **2:**364
  diagnostic medical sonography of, **3:**413*f*, **3:**420*f*
  diaphanography of, **2:**451
  digital breast tomosynthesis of, **2:**354–355, **2:**355*f*
  ductography of, **2:**436–437, **2:**436*f*–437*f*
  fat of, **2:**361*f*
  fatty tissue of, **2:**363
  glandular tissue of, **2:**363
  involution of, **2:**360
  during lactation, **2:**362*f*, **2:**364
  localization and biopsy of suspicious lesions of, **2:**438–448
    breast specimen radiography, **2:**446*f*–447*f*, **2:**449, **2:**449*f*
    for dermal calcifications, **2:**441
    material for, **2:**438*f*
    with specialized compression plate, **2:**438*f*–440*f*, **2:**439–441
    stereotactic imaging and biopsy procedures, **2:**442–448, **2:**448*f*
      equipment for, **2:**443, **2:**443*f*–444*f*
      images, **2:**442, **2:**443*f*, **2:**445*f*
      three-dimensional localization, **2:**442, **2:**442*f*
      X, Y, and Z coordinates, **2:**442, **2:**442*f*–443*f*
    tangential projection in, **2:**441, **2:**441*b*
  MRI of, **3:**294, **3:**294*f*, **2:**400–401, **2:**450
  oversized, **2:**382, **2:**383*f*
  pathologic and mammographic findings in, **2:**365–375
    architectural distortions as, **2:**375, **2:**375*f*
    calcifications as, **2:**370–375, **2:**370*f*–374*f*
    masses as, **2:**365–368, **2:**365*f*–369*f*
      circumscribed, **2:**365, **2:**366*f*
      density of, **2:**366, **2:**368
      indistinct, **2:**365
      interval change in, **2:**368, **2:**368*f*
      location of, **2:**368
      margins of, **2:**365
      palpable, **2:**391
      radiolucent seen on only one projection, **2:**366, **2:**367*f*, **2:**368, **2:**369*f*
      shape of, **2:**365
      spiculated, **2:**366, **2:**369*f*
  during pregnancy, **2:**364
  radiography of. *See* Mammography
  in radiography of sternum, **1:**506
  summary of, **2:**376*b*, **2:**376*t*–377*t*
  superolateral to inferomedial oblique projection of, **2:**434–435, **2:**434*f*–435*f*
  thermography of, **2:**451
  tissue variations in, **2:**362*f*–364*f*, **2:**363–375
  ultrasonography of, **2:**401

I-4

Breast cancer, **3:**509
 calcifications in, **2:**374*f*
 diagnostic medical sonography of, **3:**413*f*
 genetic factors in, **3:**484
 male, **2:**407
 prophylactic surgery for, **3:**484, **3:**509
 risk factors for, **2:**358–359
Breast cancer screening, **2:**357
 diagnostic mammography *vs.*, **2:**358
 high-risk, **2:**450
 risk *versus* benefit, **2:**357–358
Breast specimen radiography, **2:**446*f*, **2:**449, **2:**449*f*
Breastbone. *See* Sternum
Breathing
 chest radiographs and, **1:**100*f*, **1:**101
 diaphragm in, **1:**502, **1:**502*f*
 technique, **1:**14
Bregma, **2:**4*f*–5*f*
Bridge of nose, **2:**18
Bridgman method, for superoinferior axial inlet projection, of anterior pelvic bones, **1:**404, **1:**404*b*, **1:**404*f*
Broad ligaments, **1:**206
Broadband ultrasound attenuation (BUA), **2:**488
Bronchial tree, **1:**84, **1:**84*b*, **1:**84*f*
Bronchiectasis, **1:**93*t*
Bronchioles, **1:**84, **1:**84*f*
 terminal, **1:**84, **1:**84*f*
Bronchitis, **1:**93*t*
Bronchomediastinal trunk, **3:**318
Bronchopneumonia, **1:**93*t*
Bronchopulmonary segments, **1:**86
Bronchoscopy, **3:**42, **3:**42*b*, **3:**42*f*
Bronchus, **1:**113*f*
 mainstem, **1:**84*f*, **1:**92*f*, **1:**111*f*
 primary, **1:**84, **1:**84*f*
 secondary, **1:**84, **1:**84*f*
 tertiary, **1:**84, **1:**84*f*
Buckle fracture, **1:**151*t*
Bucky grid, for obese patients, **1:**17–18, **1:**17*f*, **1:**42, **1:**42*f*
Bulbourethral glands, **2:**332
"Bunny" method
 for limb radiography, **3:**99*f*
 for skull radiography, **3:**104, **3:**105*f*
Burman method, for AP projection, of CMC joints, **1:**162–163
 central ray for, **1:**162
 evaluation criteria for, **1:**163*b*
 position of part for, **1:**162, **1:**162*f*
 position of patient for, **1:**162
 structures shown on, **1:**163, **1:**163*f*
Bursae, **1:**62, **1:**222, **1:**222*f*
Bursitis, **1:**151*t*, **1:**225*t*
Butterfly sets, **2:**318*f*, **2:**319

C
Cadaveric sections, **3:**173
Calcaneal sulcus, **1:**271, **1:**271*f*
Calcaneocuboid joint, **1:**278*f*, **1:**278*t*
Calcaneus
 anatomy of, **1:**270–271, **1:**270*f*, **1:**278*f*
 axial projection of
  dorsoplantar, **1:**312–313, **1:**312*f*–313*f*, **1:**313*b*
  evaluation criteria for, **1:**311*b*
  plantodorsal, **1:**311, **1:**311*f*
  weight-bearing coalition (Harris-Beath) method for, **1:**313, **1:**313*f*
 lateromedial oblique projection (weight-bearing) of, **1:**315, **1:**315*b*, **1:**315*f*
 mediolateral projections of, **1:**314, **1:**314*b*, **1:**314*f*
Calcifications, of breast, **2:**370–375, **2:**370*f*–374*f*
 amorphous or indistinct, **2:**373
 arterial, **2:**376*t*–377*t*
 branching, **2:**373
 coarse, **2:**370*f*–372*f*
 linear, **2:**373
 male, **2:**408
 milk of calcium as, **2:**373, **2:**373*f*, **2:**376*t*–377*t*
 pleomorphic, **2:**373
 popcorn, **2:**370*f*–372*f*
 rim, **2:**376*t*–377*t*
 rod-like secretory, **2:**370*f*–372*f*
 round, **2:**370*f*–372*f*
 skin, **2:**376*t*–377*t*
 vascular, **2:**370*f*–372*f*
Calcitonins, for osteoporosis, **2:**462*t*

Calcium, osteoporosis and, **2:**461
Calculus, **2:**190*t*–191*t*
 renal, **2:**280*t*, **2:**282*f*
Caldwell method
 for PA axial projection
  of facial bones, **2:**66, **2:**66*f*–67*f*, **2:**67*b*
  of frontal and anterior ethmoidal sinuses, **2:**94–95, **2:**94*f*–95*f*, **2:**95*b*
  in children, **3:**108, **3:**109*f*
 for PA projection and PA axial projection of skull, **2:**37–39, **2:**37*f*–38*f*
  evaluation criteria for, **2:**39*b*
  position of part for, **2:**37–39
  position of patient for, **2:**37–39
  structures shown in, **2:**38*f*, **2:**39
Calvaria, **2:**3
Camera design, **3:**465–468, **3:**466*f*–467*f*, **3:**466*t*
Camp-Coventry method, for PA axial projection, of intercondylar fossa, **1:**346, **1:**346*b*, **1:**346*f*–347*f*
Canadian Association of Medical Radiation Technologists (CAMRT), **1:**3, **1:**65
 Member Code of Ethics and Professional Conduct, **1:**3
Cancellous bone, bone densitometry and, **2:**459, **2:**459*t*
Cancer, **3:**483–485
 breast. *See* Breast cancer
 common types of, **3:**483–484, **3:**484*t*
 defined, **3:**483, **3:**508
 metastasis of, **3:**483, **3:**509
 radiation oncology for. *See* Radiation oncology
 risk factors for, **3:**484–485, **3:**484*t*
 tissue origins of, **3:**485, **3:**485*t*
 TNM classification, **3:**485, **3:**485*t*
Cancericidal doses, **3:**482, **3:**508
Cannulated hip screws, **3:**46–47, **3:**46*f*–47*f*, **3:**47*b*
Capillaries, **3:**315
Capitate, **1:**143*f*–144*f*, **1:**144
Capitulum, **1:**146, **1:**146*f*, **1:**149*f*
Caps, **3:**33
Captured lesion projection, **2:**425, **2:**425*b*, **2:**425*f*–426*f*
 labeling codes for, **2:**385*t*–390*t*
Carbon, in nuclear medicine, **3:**442*t*
Carbon dioxide (CO_2), as contrast media, **3:**322
Carcinogens, **3:**484, **3:**484*t*, **3:**508
Carcinoma, **2:**190*t*–191*t*, **3:**485, **3:**508
Cardia of stomach, **2:**178, **2:**178*f*
Cardiac antrum, **2:**176, **2:**178*f*
Cardiac catheterization, **3:**372–405
 balloons for, **3:**376
 catheters for, **3:**375–376, **3:**375*f*
 complications of, **3:**374
 contraindications of, **3:**374
 contrast media for, **3:**376
 diagnostic cardiac procedures, **3:**379–385
  of left heart, **3:**379–381, **3:**380*f*–381*f*
  of right heart, **3:**381–384, **3:**384*f*
  selective coronary angiography, **3:**381, **3:**382*f*–383*f*
 equipment for, **3:**377
 guidewires for, **3:**375
 historical development of, **3:**312
 imaging for
  other equipment for, **3:**377*f*–378*f*, **3:**378*t*
  physiologic equipment for, **3:**377*f*
 indications for, **3:**372–373, **3:**372*t*
 interventional cardiac procedures, **3:**386–395
  percutaneous coronary intervention, **3:**386–387, **3:**386*f*–387*f*
 physiologic equipment for, **3:**377
 postcatheterization care, **3:**379
 precatheterization care for, **3:**379
 pressure injector for, **3:**376, **3:**376*f*
 risk of, **3:**374
 sheaths for, **3:**375, **3:**375*f*
 stents for, **3:**376
 supplies and equipment for, **3:**375–378
Cardiac cycle, **3:**316
Cardiac gating, for MRI, **3:**292, **3:**292*f*
Cardiac muscular tissue, motion and control of, **1:**13
Cardiac notch, **1:**85–86, **1:**85*f*, **2:**178, **2:**178*f*
Cardiac orifice, anatomy of, **2:**179
Cardiac output, **3:**403
Cardiac sphincter, **2:**178*f*, **2:**179
Cardiac studies, with barium
 lateral projection for, **1:**107
 PA oblique projection for, **1:**111
 PA projection for, **1:**105

Cardiac viability, **3:**475
Cardiomyopathies, **3:**403
 congestive, **3:**430
Cardiovascular studies, **3:**455
Cardiovascular system disorders, in older adults, **3:**156–157
Carina
 anatomy of, **1:**84, **1:**84*f*
 sectional anatomy of, **3:**192
C-arm
 dedicated, **2:**106*f*
 mobile fluoroscopic, **2:**106, **2:**107*f*
 in surgical radiography, **3:**37, **3:**37*f*
  of cervical spine (anterior cervical diskectomy and fusion), **3:**43, **3:**43*f*
  of chest (line placement, bronchoscopy), **3:**42, **3:**42*f*
  of femoral/tibial arteriogram, **3:**55, **3:**56*f*
  of femur nail, **3:**48–49, **3:**48*f*
  of hip (cannulated hip screws or hip pinning), **3:**46–47, **3:**46*f*–47*f*
  of humerus, **3:**53–54, **3:**53*f*
  of lumbar spine, **3:**44–45, **3:**44*f*
  for operative (immediate) cholangiography, **3:**40, **3:**40*f*
  radiation safety with, **3:**39, **3:**39*f*
  of tibia (nail), **3:**51, **3:**51*f*
Carotid arteries
 extracranial, duplex sonography of, **3:**428, **3:**428*f*
 MRA of, **3:**302*f*
Carotid canal, **2:**14, **2:**15*f*
Carotid sinus, sectional anatomy of, **3:**192
Carotid sulcus, **2:**10*f*, **2:**11
Carpal(s), anatomy of, **1:**143*f*, **1:**144
Carpal boss, **1:**176*b*, **1:**176*f*
Carpal bridge, tangential projection, **1:**187, **1:**187*b*, **1:**187*f*
Carpal canal, tangential projection, **1:**188–189, **1:**188*f*–189*f*, **1:**189*b*
Carpal sulcus, **1:**144–145, **1:**144*f*
Carpal tunnel, **1:**144–145
Carpometacarpal (CMC) joints, **1:**160
 anatomy of, **1:**148, **1:**148*f*
 Burman method for, AP projection of, **1:**162–163
  central ray for, **1:**162
  evaluation criteria for, **1:**163*b*
  position of part for, **1:**162, **1:**162*f*
  position of patient for, **1:**162
  structures shown on, **1:**163, **1:**163*f*
 Robert method for, AP projection of, **1:**160–161
  central ray for, **1:**161, **1:**161*f*
  collimation for, **1:**161
  evaluation criteria for, **1:**161*b*
  Lewis modification of, **1:**161, **1:**161*f*
  Long and Rafert modification of, **1:**161, **1:**161*f*
  position of part for, **1:**160, **1:**160*f*
  position of patient for, **1:**160, **1:**160*f*
  structures shown on, **1:**161, **1:**161*f*
Cartilaginous joints, **1:**161, **1:**161*f*
Cartilaginous symphysis joints, **1:**375, **1:**422, **1:**500
Cartilaginous synchondrosis, **1:**500
Cassette with film, **1:**14
Catheter, for cardiac catheterization, **3:**375–376, **3:**375*f*
Catheterization
 for angiography, **3:**327–332, **3:**328*f*, **3:**330*f*–332*f*
 cardiac. *See* Cardiac catheterization
Cauda equina
 anatomy of, **2:**153, **2:**153*f*
 defined, **2:**167
Caudad, definition of, **1:**65, **1:**65*f*
Caudate nucleus, sectional anatomy of, **3:**174*f*, **3:**179–181, **3:**180*f*
 on coronal plane, **3:**189*f*
 on sagittal plane, **3:**187*f*
Caudocranial projection, **2:**427–428, **2:**427*f*–428*f*
Cavernous sinus, **3:**184*f*, **3:**189–190
Cecum, anatomy of, **2:**181*f*–182*f*, **2:**182
Celiac arteriogram, **3:**336, **3:**336*f*
Celiac artery, sectional anatomy of, **3:**206
Celiac disease, **2:**190*t*–191*t*, **2:**491
Centers for Disease Control and Prevention (CDC), **1:**4
Central, definition of, **1:**65
Central nervous system (CNS), **2:**151–168
 anatomy of, **2:**152–156
  brain in, **2:**152–156, **2:**152*f*
  meninges in, **2:**153
  spinal cord in, **2:**153, **2:**153*f*

Central nervous system (CNS) *(Continued)*
 ventricular system in, **2:**154–155, **2:**154*f*
 definition of terms for, **2:**167
 interventional pain management, **2:**166, **2:**166*f*
 MRI of, **3:**293
  of brain, **3:**293, **3:**293*f*
  of spine, **3:**293
   lumbar, **3:**293*f*
   thoracic, **3:**293*f*
 myelography of., **2:**160–164
 nuclear medicine imaging, **3:**455
 plain radiographic examination of, **2:**159–167
 provocative diskography of, **2:**166, **2:**166*f*
 vertebral augmentation of, **2:**164–165, **2:**164*f*–165*f*
Central nervous system disorders, in older adults, **3:**154
Central nervous system studies, **3:**455
Central ray
 placement and direction of, **1:**24
 for trauma radiography, **2:**115
Central skeletal measurements, **2:**483–485, **2:**483*f*–485*f*
Cephalad, definition of, **1:**65, **1:**65*f*
Cerebellar peduncles, **3:**176, **3:**180*f*, **3:**181–182, **3:**187*f*
Cerebellar tonsils, **3:**186
Cerebellum, **2:**5*f*
 anatomy of, **2:**152, **2:**152*f*
 defined, **2:**167
 fossa for, **2:**13*f*
Cerebellum, sectional anatomy of, **3:**176, **3:**180*f*–181*f*, **3:**181–182
 on axial plane, **3:**182*f*, **3:**185*f*
 on coronal plane, **3:**190*f*
 inferior portions of, **3:**184, **3:**184*f*
 on midsagittal plane, **3:**187*f*
 on sagittal plane, **3:**187*f*
Cerebral anatomy, **3:**342–352, **3:**342*f*–345*f*
Cerebral angiography
 of anterior circulation, **3:**349–351
  AP axial oblique projection, **3:**351, **3:**351*f*
  AP axial projection, **3:**350, **3:**350*f*
  lateral projection for, **3:**349, **3:**349*b*, **3:**349*f*
 aortic arch (cranial vessels), **3:**348, **3:**348*f*
 cerebral anatomy and, **3:**342, **3:**342*f*–344*f*
 circulation time and imaging program for, **3:**346, **3:**346*f*–347*f*
 extracranial, **3:**348–349
 position of head for, **3:**347
 of posterior circulation, **3:**351–352
  axial projection, **3:**352, **3:**352*f*
  lateral projection, **3:**351–352, **3:**351*f*
 technique for, **3:**345–347
 vertebral arteriography, **3:**348–349
Cerebral aqueduct (of Sylvius)
 anatomy of, **2:**154, **2:**154*f*
 defined, **2:**167
 sectional anatomy of, **3:**176, **3:**180*f*, **3:**181–182
Cerebral arteries
 CT angiography of, **3:**251*f*
 MRA of, **3:**302*f*
Cerebral hemisphere, sectional anatomy of, **3:**178–179
Cerebral lobes, **3:**178–179
Cerebrospinal fluid (CSF)
 anatomy of, **2:**153
 defined, **2:**167
 sectional anatomy of, **3:**175
Cerebrum, **2:**5*f*
 anatomy of, **2:**152, **2:**152*f*
 defined, **2:**167
 fossa for, **2:**13*f*
 sectional anatomy of, **3:**175–176
Cerrobend blocks, **3:**491, **3:**509
Certified surgical technologist (CST), **3:**31
Cervical curve, **1:**411*f*
Cervical diskectomy, anterior, **3:**43, **3:**43*b*, **3:**43*f*
Cervical myelogram, **2:**163*f*
Cervical ribs, **1:**498
Cervical vertebrae, **1:**414–416
 anatomy of, **1:**411*f*
  atlas in, **1:**414, **1:**414*f*
  axis in, **1:**414, **1:**414*f*
  seventh vertebra in, **1:**415
 AP axial projection of, **1:**432–437, **1:**432*f*–433*f*, **1:**433*b*
 AP projection of (Ottonello method), **1:**442–443, **1:**442*f*–443*f*, **1:**443*b*
 body, **2:**174*f*
 dens of

Cervical vertebrae *(Continued)*
 anatomy of, **1:**414
 AP projection of (Fuchs method), **1:**427, **1:**427*f*
 fluoroscopic procedures for, **3:**43, **3:**43*b*, **3:**43*f*
 intervertebral foramina of
  anatomy of, **1:**413, **1:**415*f*–416*f*, **1:**416
  AP axial oblique projection of, **1:**438–440, **1:**438*b*–439*b*, **1:**438*f*–439*f*
  PA axial oblique projection of, **1:**440, **1:**440*b*, **1:**440*f*–441*f*
  positioning rotations needed to show, **1:**416*t*
 lateral projection of
  in flexion and extension, **1:**436–437, **1:**436*b*–437*b*, **1:**436*f*–437*f*
  Grandy method for, **1:**434, **1:**434*b*–435*b*, **1:**434*f*–435*f*
  swimmer's technique for, **1:**448–449, **1:**448*b*–449*b*, **1:**448*f*–449*f*
 mobile radiography of, **2:**24–27
  best practices in, **2:**26–27
  lateral projection, in right or left dorsal decubitus position, **2:**24–25, **2:**24*f*–25*f*, **2:**25*b*
  in operating room, **3:**57, **3:**57*b*, **3:**57*f*–58*f*
 sectional anatomy of, **3:**187*f*
 transverse foramina of, **1:**415
 trauma radiography of, **2:**116
  AP axial oblique projection in, **2:**119, **2:**119*b*, **2:**119*f*
  AP axial projection in, **2:**118–119, **2:**118*b*, **2:**118*f*
  lateral projection in, **2:**116, **2:**116*b*, **2:**116*f*
 typical, **1:**415–416, **1:**415*f*–416*f*
 vertebral arch
  anatomy of, **1:**413
  AP axial oblique projection of, **1:**446–447, **1:**446*f*–447*f*, **1:**447*b*
  AP axial projection of, **1:**444–445, **1:**444*b*–445*b*, **1:**444*f*–445*f*
 zygapophyseal joints of
  anatomy of, **1:**413, **1:**416, **1:**416*f*
  positioning rotations needed to show, **1:**416*t*
Cervicothoracic region, lateral projection of
 in dorsal decubitus position, for trauma, **2:**117, **2:**117*b*, **2:**117*f*
 swimmer's technique for, **1:**448–449, **1:**448*b*–449*b*, **1:**448*f*–449*f*
Cervix
 anatomy of, **2:**330, **2:**330*f*
 diagnostic medical sonography of, **3:**424*f*–425*f*
 sectional anatomy of, **3:**206
Channel, in CT, **3:**266
Charge-coupled device (CCD), **1:**14
Chemoembolization, **3:**362
Chest
 AP projection of, for trauma, **2:**121, **2:**121*f*
 fluoroscopic procedures for, **3:**42, **3:**42*b*, **3:**42*f*
 MRI of, **3:**294, **3:**294*f*
 PA projection of, **1:**32*f*
Chest radiographs
 breathing instructions for, **1:**100*f*, **1:**101
 in children, **3:**92–97
  with cystic fibrosis, **3:**125, **3:**125*f*
  image assessment for, **3:**96*t*
  image evaluation for, **3:**94, **3:**96*t*
  less than one year old, **3:**92–93, **3:**93*f*–94*f*
  more than one year old, **3:**93–94, **3:**95*f*
  Pigg-O-Stat, **3:**92, **3:**92*f*
  with pneumonia, **3:**137–138, **3:**138*f*
  3 to 18 years old, **3:**94–97, **3:**97*f*
 general positioning considerations for, **1:**99
  for lateral criteria, **1:**99, **1:**99*f*
  for oblique criteria, **1:**99
  for PA criteria, **1:**99, **1:**100*f*
  prone, **1:**99*f*
  upright, **1:**99*f*
 of geriatric patients, **3:**158
 grid technique for, **1:**101, **1:**102*f*
 limb radiography in, **3:**99–103
  with fractures, **3:**101–102
  preschool age, **3:**101, **3:**101*f*
  radiation protection for, **3:**101, **3:**101*f*
  school age, **3:**101
 of lungs and heart
  AP oblique projection for, **1:**112–113
   central ray for, **1:**113
   collimation for, **1:**113
   evaluation criteria for, **1:**113*b*
   position of part for, **1:**112, **1:**112*f*

Chest radiographs *(Continued)*
   position of patient for, **1:**112
   SID for, **1:**112
   structures shown on, **1:**113, **1:**113*f*
  AP projection for, **1:**114–115
   central ray for, **1:**114
   collimation for, **1:**114
   evaluation criteria for, **1:**115*b*
   position of part for, **1:**114, **1:**114*f*
   position of patient for, **1:**114
   respiration, **1:**114
   SID for, **1:**114
   structures shown on, **1:**115, **1:**115*f*
  lateral projection for, **1:**106–107
   cardiac studies with barium in, **1:**107
   central for, **1:**106
   collimation for, **1:**106
   evaluation criteria for, **1:**107*b*
   foreshortening in, **1:**106, **1:**107*f*
   forward bending in, **1:**106, **1:**107*f*
   with pleura, **1:**122*f*
   position of part for, **1:**106, **1:**106*f*–107*f*
   position of patient for, **1:**106
   SID for, **1:**106
   structures shown on, **1:**106–107, **1:**107*f*–108*f*
  PA oblique projection for, **1:**109–111
   barium studies in, **1:**111
   central ray for, **1:**109
   collimation for, **1:**109
   evaluation criteria for, **1:**111*b*
   LAO position for, **1:**109, **1:**109*f*–110*f*
   position of part for, **1:**109, **1:**109*f*
   position of patient for, **1:**109
   RAO position for, **1:**109–111, **1:**109*f*, **1:**111*f*
   SID for, **1:**109
   structures shown on, **1:**110–111
  PA projection for, **1:**99–115
   cardiac studies with barium in, **1:**105
   central ray for, **1:**104–105
   collimation for, **1:**104–105
   evaluation criteria for, **1:**105*b*
   with pleura, **1:**120–123, **1:**120*f*–121*f*
   position of part for, **1:**103, **1:**103*f*–104*f*
   position of patient for, **1:**103–105
   respiration, **1:**99–115, **1:**104*f*
   SID for, **1:**103
   structures shown on, **1:**105, **1:**105*f*
 of lungs and pleurae
  AP or PA projection for, **1:**120–123, **1:**120*f*–121*f*
   central ray, **1:**120
   collimation, **1:**120
   evaluation criteria, **1:**121*b*
   position of part, **1:**120
   position of patient in, **1:**120
   respiration, **1:**120
   structures shown, **1:**120–121
  lateral projection for, **1:**122–123, **1:**122*f*
   central ray, **1:**122
   collimation, **1:**122
   evaluation criteria, **1:**123*b*
   position of part, **1:**122
   position of patient, **1:**122
   respiration, **1:**122
   structures shown, **1:**122–123, **1:**123*f*
 mobile, **2:**10–13
  AP or PA projection, in right or left lateral decubitus position, **2:**12–13, **2:**12*f*–13*f*, **2:**13*b*
  AP projection, in upright or supine position, **2:**10–13, **2:**10*f*–11*f*, **2:**11*b*
 of pulmonary apices, **1:**116–119
  AP axial projection for, **1:**116–119, **1:**118*f*
  in lordotic position (Lindblom method), **1:**116–117, **1:**116*f*–117*f*
  PA axial projection for, **1:**119, **1:**119*b*, **1:**119*f*
  SID for, **1:**101, **1:**101*f*
  technical procedure for, **1:**101, **1:**101*f*–102*f*
Child abuse, **3:**127–131, **3:**128*f*–130*f*
Children, **3:**72
 abdominal radiography in, **3:**84
  with intussusception, **3:**87, **3:**87*f*
  with pneumoperitoneum, **3:**88, **3:**88*f*
  positioning and immobilization for, **3:**86, **3:**86*f*
 adult *versus*, **3:**80
 age-based development of, **3:**73–76
  of adolescent, **3:**76

I-6

Children (Continued)
 of infant, **3:**74
 of neonate, **3:**73
 of premature infants, **3:**73
 of preschooler, **3:**74–76, **3:**74*f*–75*f*
 of school age, **3:**76
 of toddler, **3:**74
aneurysmal bone cyst in, **3:**136, **3:**136*f*
artifacts with, **3:**82–83, **3:**82*f*–83*f*
with autism spectrum disorders, **3:**77–79, **3:**77*b*
chest radiograph in, **3:**92–97
 for children less than one year old, **3:**92–93, **3:**93*f*–94*f*
 for children more than one year old, **3:**93–94, **3:**95*f*
 image evaluation for, **3:**94, **3:**96*t*
 Pigg-O-Stat, **3:**92, **3:**92*f*
 with pneumonia, **3:**137–138, **3:**138*f*
 3 to 18 years old, **3:**94–97, **3:**97*f*
communication with, **3:**73
CT of, **3:**143–144, **3:**143*f*
cystic fibrosis in, **3:**125, **3:**125*f*
developmental dysplasia of hip in, **3:**126, **3:**126*f*
EOS system for, **3:**142, **3:**142*f*
Ewing sarcoma in, **3:**137, **3:**137*f*
foreign bodies in, **3:**112–114
 airway, **3:**112, **3:**112*f*
 ingested, **3:**112, **3:**113*f*
 inserted, **3:**114, **3:**114*f*
fractures in, **3:**101–102
 due to child abuse, **3:**127–131, **3:**127*f*–130*f*
 due to osteogenesis imperfecta, **3:**134, **3:**134*f*
 greenstick, **3:**102
 growth plate, **3:**103
 pathologic, **3:**135–137
 plastic or bow, **3:**102
 Salter-Harris, **3:**102, **3:**102*f*
 supracondylar, **3:**103, **3:**103*f*
 torus, **3:**102
gastrointestinal and genitourinary studies in, **3:**89–90, **3:**89*t*
 indications for, **3:**89*t*
 with vesicoureteral reflux, **3:**90, **3:**90*f*–91*f*
image assessment for, **3:**96*t*
imaging, **3:**72–83
immobilization techniques for
 for abdominal radiography, **3:**86, **3:**86*f*
 for chest radiography, **3:**92–97
 for gastrointestinal and genitourinary studies, **3:**89–90, **3:**89*t*
 for limb radiography, **3:**99–103, **3:**99*f*
 for pelvis and hip imaging, **3:**98
 for skull radiography, **3:**104–108, **3:**106*f*–107*f*
injections/needle sticks, **3:**79
interventional radiology in, **3:**144–145, **3:**144*f*–145*f*
limb radiography in, **3:**99–103, **3:**99*f*
 image evaluation for, **3:**96*t*
 immobilization for, **3:**99–103, **3:**99*f*–101*f*
MRI of, **3:**142–143, **3:**143*f*
noise of, **3:**78
nonaccidental trauma (child abuse) in, **3:**127–131, **3:**127*f*–130*f*
 imaging protocol for, **3:**131, **3:**131*b*, **3:**132*f*–133*f*
osteochondroma in, **3:**135, **3:**135*f*
osteoid osteoma in, **3:**136, **3:**136*f*
osteosarcoma in, **3:**137
pathologic fractures in, **3:**135–137
patient responses, **3:**78
pelvis and hip imaging in, **3:**98
 general principles of, **3:**98
 image evaluation for, **3:**96*t*
 initial images in, **3:**98
 positioning and immobilization for, **3:**93*f*, **3:**98
 preparation and communication for, **3:**98
personal space and body awareness in, **3:**78
pneumonia in, **3:**137–138, **3:**138*f*
progeria in, **3:**139, **3:**139*f*
providing adequate care and service for, **3:**73
radiation protection for, **3:**80–83, **3:**80*f*, **3:**81*t*
 holding as, **3:**82
radiography of, **3:**142*f*–143*f*
radiography protocols for, **3:**73
respect and dignity for, **3:**73
safety with, **3:**73
scoliosis in, **3:**139–141
 Cobb angle in, **3:**141, **3:**141*f*
 congenital, **3:**140

Children (Continued)
 estimation of rotation, **3:**141
 idiopathic, **3:**140
 imaging of, **3:**140, **3:**140*f*
 lateral bends with, **3:**141
 neuromuscular, **3:**140
 patterns of, **3:**141
 skeletal maturity with, **3:**141
 symptoms of, **3:**139*f*
 treatment options for, **3:**141
skull and paranasal sinus in, **3:**104–108, **3:**105*f*
skull radiography in, **3:**104–108, **3:**106*f*
 AP axial Towne projection for, **3:**106–108, **3:**106*f*, **3:**108*t*
 AP projection for, **3:**106–108, **3:**106*f*
 with craniosynostosis, **3:**104
 with fractures, **3:**104
 lateral projection for, **3:**106–108, **3:**109*f*
 summary of projections for, **3:**108*t*
soft tissue neck (STN) radiography in, **3:**110–111, **3:**110*f*–111*f*
with special needs, **3:**77–79
touch, **3:**78
ultrasound of, **3:**143
waiting room for, **3:**72, **3:**72*f*
Chloral hydrate (Noctec), **2:**316*t*
Cholangiography, **2:**263
 operative (immediate), **3:**39–41, **3:**40*f*, **3:**41*b*
 percutaneous transhepatic, **2:**264–265, **2:**264*f*
 postoperative (T-tube), **2:**266–267, **2:**266*f*–267*f*
Cholangiopancreatography
 endoscopic retrograde, **2:**268, **2:**268*f*–269*f*
 magnetic resonance, **3:**296*f*
Cholecystitis, **2:**190*t*–191*t*
 diagnostic medical sonography of, **3:**416*f*
Cholecystography, **2:**263
Cholecystokinin, **2:**186
Choledochal sphincter, **2:**185
Choledocholithiasis, **2:**190*t*–191*t*
Cholegraphy, **2:**263
Cholelithiasis, **2:**190*t*–191*t*
Chondrosarcoma, **1:**151*t*, **1:**225*t*, **1:**282*t*, **1:**379*t*, **1:**504*t*
Chorion, **2:**331
Chorion laeve, diagnostic medical sonography of, **3:**425*f*
Chorionic cavity, diagnostic medical sonography of, **3:**425*f*
Choroid plexuses, sectional anatomy of, **3:**176
Chromosomes, cancer and, **3:**484, **3:**509
Chronic bronchitis, in older adults, **3:**158
Chronic obstructive pulmonary disease, **1:**93*t*
 in older adults, **3:**158, **3:**158*f*, **3:**160*t*
Chronologic age, age-specific competencies by, **1:**8
Chyme, **2:**179
Cigarette smoking and cancer, **3:**484, **3:**484*t*
Cilia, of uterine tube, **2:**329
Cine mode, **3:**222
Cinefluorography, **3:**403
Circle of Willis
 anatomy of, **3:**344, **3:**344*f*
 CT angiography of, **3:**251*f*
 MRA of, **3:**302*f*
 sectional anatomy of, **3:**176, **3:**181*f*
Circulator, **3:**32
Circulatory system, **3:**314–318, **3:**314*f*
 blood-vascular system in, **3:**314
  arteries in, **3:**315–318
   coronary, **3:**317*f*, **3:**318
   systemic, **3:**315
  arterioles in, **3:**315
  capillaries in, **3:**315, **3:**403
  complete circulation of blood through, **3:**318
  heart in, **3:**315, **3:**315*f*
  main trunk vessels in, **3:**315
  portal system in, **3:**315, **3:**315*f*
  pulmonary circulation, **3:**315, **3:**315*f*
  systemic circulation, **3:**315, **3:**315*f*
  veins in
   coronary, **3:**317, **3:**317*f*
   systemic, **3:**316
  venules in, **3:**315
 lymphatic system in, **3:**314, **3:**318, **3:**319*f*
 venules in, **3:**315
Circumduction, **1:**79, **1:**79*f*
Cisterna chyli, **3:**318
Cisterna magna, **3:**175, **3:**184–185
Claudication, **3:**320, **3:**403

Claustrophobia, **3:**306
Claustrum, **3:**174*f*, **3:**180*f*, **3:**181
Clavicle, **1:**253–256
 anatomy of, **1:**219, **1:**219*f*
 AP axial projection of, **1:**254–255, **1:**254*b*–255*b*, **1:**254*f*–255*f*
 AP projection of, **1:**253–256, **1:**253*b*, **1:**253*f*
 PA axial projection of, **1:**256, **1:**256*f*
 PA projection of, **1:**256, **1:**256*f*
Clavicular notch, **1:**497–498
Clay shoveler's fracture, **1:**424*t*
Cleavage view, labeling codes for, **2:**385*t*–390*t*
Cleaves method
 for AP oblique projection, of proximal femora and femoral necks, **1:**386, **1:**386*b*
  bilateral, **1:**386, **1:**386*f*
  evaluation criteria for, **1:**387*b*
  position of part for, **1:**386
  position of patient for, **1:**386
  structures shown on, **1:**387, **1:**387*f*
  unilateral, **1:**386–387, **1:**386*f*
 for axiolateral projection, **1:**388–389, **1:**388*b*, **1:**388*f*
  evaluation criteria for, **1:**389*b*
  structures shown on, **1:**389, **1:**389*f*
Clements-Nakayama method
 for axiolateral projection, of hip, **1:**396–397, **1:**396*f*–397*f*, **1:**397*b*
 for PA axial oblique projection, of trapezium, **1:**186, **1:**186*b*, **1:**186*f*
Clinical history, **1:**10, **1:**10*f*
Clivus, **2:**4*f*–5*f*, **2:**11, **2:**11*f*, **2:**13
Closed fracture, **1:**64
Closed scanners, in MRI, **3:**275, **3:**275*f*
Clubfoot, congenital
 defined, **1:**282*t*
 evaluation criteria for, **1:**309*b*
 Kandel method for, dorsoplantar axial projection of, **1:**310, **1:**310*f*
 Kite method for, mediolateral projection of, **1:**308–309, **1:**308*f*–309*f*
CNS. *See* Central nervous system
Coagulopathy, **3:**403
Coal miner lung, **1:**93*t*
Coalition position, for axial projection of calcaneus, **1:**313, **1:**313*f*
Coat-hanger projection, **2:**425, **2:**425*b*, **2:**425*f*
 labeling codes for, **2:**385*t*–390*t*
Cobalt-60 (60Co) units, **3:**487–489, **3:**489*f*, **3:**509
Cobb angle, **3:**141, **3:**141*f*
Coccygeal cornua, **1:**421–422
Coccygeal vertebrae, **1:**411
Coccyx, **1:**371, **1:**411, **1:**422
 anatomy of, **1:**374*f*, **1:**376*f*–377*f*, **1:**411*f*
 AP axial and PA axial projections of, **1:**478–481, **1:**478*f*–479*f*, **1:**479*b*
 lateral projection of, **1:**480–481, **1:**480*f*–481*f*, **1:**481*b*
 as surface landmark, **1:**51*f*
Cochlea, **2:**15*f*, **2:**16, **2:**17*f*
Cochlear nerve, **2:**17*f*
"Code lift" process, **1:**37
Cognitive impairment, in older adults, **3:**153
Coils, in MRI, **3:**274, **3:**274*f*, **3:**290, **3:**306
Coincidence event, **3:**469, **3:**469*f*, **3:**478
Coincidence time window, **3:**469, **3:**469*f*, **3:**478
Cold spot, **3:**478
Colitis, **2:**190*t*–191*t*
Collecting ducts, **2:**277, **2:**277*f*
Collecting system, duplicate, **2:**280*t*
Colles fracture, **1:**151*t*
Collimation
 multileaf, **3:**491, **3:**491*f*, **3:**509
 with obese patients, **1:**40–41, **1:**41*f*
 of radiation field, **1:**25–26, **1:**25*f*–26*f*
 for trauma radiography, **2:**116
Collimator(s), **3:**478
 of gamma camera, **3:**446, **3:**446*f*
 for linear accelerators, **3:**491, **3:**509
Colloidal preparations, for large intestine contrast media studies, **2:**234
Colon
 anatomy of, **2:**182*f*, **2:**183
 AP axial projection of, **2:**249, **2:**249*b*, **2:**249*f*
 AP oblique projection of
  in LPO position, **2:**250, **2:**250*b*, **2:**250*f*
  in RPO position, **2:**251, **2:**251*b*, **2:**251*f*

Colon *(Continued)*
　in upright position, **2:**258, **2:**258*f*
　AP projection of, **2:**248, **2:**248*b*, **2:**248*f*
　　in left lateral decubitus position, **2:**255–256, **2:**255*f*–256*f*, **2:**256*b*
　　in right lateral decubitus position, **2:**253–254, **2:**253*f*–254*f*, **2:**254*b*
　　in upright position, **2:**258, **2:**258*f*
　ascending, anatomy of, **2:**181*f*–182*f*, **2:**183
　colostomy studies of, **2:**259
　contrast media studies of, **2:**234–251
　　contrast media for, **2:**234–235
　　double-contrast method for, **2:**234, **2:**234*f*, **2:**240–241, **2:**240*f*–241*f*
　　insertion of enema tip for, **2:**238
　　opacified colon in, **2:**239, **2:**242
　　preparation and care of patient for, **2:**238
　　preparation of barium suspension for, **2:**238
　　preparation of intestinal tract for, **2:**236, **2:**236*f*
　　single-contrast, **2:**234, **2:**234*f*, **2:**239, **2:**239*f*
　　standard barium enema apparatus for, **2:**236–237, **2:**236*f*–237*f*
　CT colonography (virtual colonoscopy) for, **2:**234, **2:**235*f*
　decubitus positions for, **2:**252–262
　defecography for, **2:**262, **2:**262*f*
　descending, **2:**182*f*, **2:**183
　　sectional anatomy of, on axial plane
　　　at level D, **3:**210, **3:**210*f*
　　　at level E, **3:**211, **3:**211*f*
　　　at level F, **3:**212, **3:**212*f*
　　　at level G, **3:**213, **3:**213*f*
　　　at level H, **3:**214, **3:**214*f*
　　　at level I, **3:**215, **3:**215*f*
　diagnostic enema for, **2:**259–260, **2:**259*f*
　lateral projection of
　　right or left position, **2:**247, **2:**247*b*, **2:**247*f*
　　right or left ventral decubitus position, **2:**257, **2:**257*b*, **2:**257*f*
　　in upright position, **2:**258
　opacified, **2:**239, **2:**242
　PA axial projection of, **2:**244, **2:**244*b*, **2:**244*f*
　PA oblique projection of
　　in LAO position, **2:**246, **2:**246*b*, **2:**246*f*
　　in RAO position, **2:**245, **2:**245*b*, **2:**245*f*
　PA projection of, **2:**242, **2:**242*b*, **2:**242*f*–243*f*
　　in left lateral decubitus position, **2:**255–256, **2:**255*f*–256*f*, **2:**256*b*
　　in right lateral decubitus position, **2:**253–254, **2:**253*f*–254*f*, **2:**254*b*
　　in upright position, **2:**258, **2:**258*f*
　sigmoid, **2:**182*f*–183*f*, **2:**183
　transverse
　　anatomy of, **2:**182*f*, **2:**183
　　sectional anatomy of, on axial plane
　　　at level D, **3:**210, **3:**210*f*
　　　at level E, **3:**211, **3:**211*f*
　　　at level F, **3:**212, **3:**212*f*
　　　at level G, **3:**213, **3:**213*f*
Colon cancer, familial adenomatous polyposis and, **3:**485
Colonography, CT, **2:**234, **2:**235*f*
Colonoscopy, virtual, **2:**234, **2:**235*f*, **3:**259, **3:**260*f*
Colorectal cancer syndrome, hereditary nonpolyposis, **3:**485
Color-flow Doppler, **3:**432–433
Colostomy studies, **2:**259
　colostomy enema equipment for, **2:**259
　preparation of intestinal tract for, **2:**259
　preparation of patient for, **2:**260, **2:**260*f*–261*f*
Comminuted fracture, **1:**64*f*
Common bile duct
　anatomy of, **2:**181*f*, **2:**185, **2:**185*f*
　sectional anatomy of, **3:**205
Common hepatic artery, **3:**206
Common hepatic duct, anatomy of, **2:**181*f*, **2:**185, **2:**185*f*
Common iliac arteries, sectional anatomy of, **3:**215
Common iliac vein, **3:**206
Communication
　with children, **3:**73
　　with autism spectrum disorders, **3:**78
　with obese patients, **1:**38
　with older adults, **3:**161
Compact bone, **1:**56, **1:**56*f*
　bone densitometry and, **2:**459, **2:**459*t*
Compact cyclotron, **3:**464*f*

Compensatory curves, **1:**412
Complete reflux examination, of small intestine, **2:**231, **2:**231*f*
Complex projections, **1:**69
Complex structure/mass, in diagnostic medical sonography, **3:**412, **3:**412*f*, **3:**433
Compound fracture, **1:**64*f*
Compression cone, for abdominal imaging, **2:**205, **2:**205*f*
Compression devices, for abdominal imaging, **2:**205, **2:**205*f*
Compression fracture, **1:**64*f*, **1:**424*t*
　in older adults, **3:**156, **3:**156*f*, **3:**160*t*
Compression paddle, for abdominal imaging, **2:**205, **2:**205*f*
Compression plate, breast lesion localization with, **2:**438*f*–440*f*, **2:**439–441
Computed axial tomography (CAT), **3:**228
Computed radiography, **1:**153
Computed tomography (CT), **3:**227–268
　of abdominal aortic aneurysm, **3:**239*f*
　advancements for, **3:**259, **3:**260*f*
　after shoulder arthrography, **2:**145, **2:**145*f*
　algorithm in, **3:**228
　aperture in, **3:**236
　archiving in, **3:**235
　artificial intelligence in, **3:**259, **3:**259*f*
　axial image in, **3:**228, **3:**229*f*
　best practices in, **3:**265
　bit depth, **3:**234
　body planes in, **1:**47, **1:**47*f*
　of children, **3:**143–144, **3:**143*f*
　contrast media for, **3:**242–244, **3:**242*f*, **3:**243*t*
　　intravenous, power injector for, **3:**243, **3:**243*f*
　contrast resolution and, **3:**229, **3:**229*f*
　conventional radiography and, **3:**228–229, **3:**228*f*
　cradle for, **3:**236
　CT numbers (Hounsfield units), **3:**234, **3:**234*t*
　curved planar reformations in, **3:**239, **3:**239*f*
　data acquisition system for, **3:**235
　data storage and retrieval for, **3:**235
　detector assembly for, **3:**228
　detectors in, **3:**231–232
　diagnostic applications of, **3:**239–240, **3:**240*f*–242*f*
　dual-energy source for, **3:**233, **3:**234*f*
　dynamic scanning with, **3:**247
　enteroclysis, **2:**231, **2:**232*f*
　examination protocols, **3:**262*f*–265*f*
　factors affecting image quality in, **3:**244–246
　　artifacts as, **3:**245, **3:**245*f*
　　contrast resolution as, **3:**244
　　noise as, **3:**244
　　patient factors as, **3:**245–246
　　scan diameter as, **3:**246
　　scan times as, **3:**246
　　spatial resolution as, **3:**244
　　temporal resolution as, **3:**244
　field of view in, **3:**234
　flat-panel, **3:**233
　fundamentals of, **3:**228*f*
　grayscale image in, **3:**237
　high-resolution scans in, **3:**245–246, **3:**246*f*
　historical development of, **3:**231
　image manipulation for, **3:**229, **3:**230*f*
　image misregistration in, **3:**247–249
　index in, **3:**236
　for interventional procedures, **3:**240, **3:**240*f*–242*f*
　matrix in, **3:**228, **3:**234
　of mediastinum, **1:**92*f*, **1:**93*t*
　multiplanar reconstruction in, **3:**239, **3:**239*f*
　new technologies for, **3:**260, **3:**261*f*
　number, **3:**266
　with PET, **3:**253–255, **3:**255*f*
　pixel in, **3:**234, **3:**234*f*
　post-processing technique in, **3:**252
　primary data in, **3:**228
　principles of, **3:**228–267
　projections (scan profiles), **3:**234
　quality control for, **3:**255
　quantitative
　　for bone densitometry, **2:**458, **2:**483, **2:**492
　　peripheral, **2:**487, **2:**492
　radiation dose in, **3:**255–257
　　estimating effective, **3:**257
　　factors affecting, **3:**257–258
　　　automatic tube current modulation (ATCM) as, **3:**257, **3:**257*f*–258*f*

Computed tomography (CT) *(Continued)*
　　beam collimation as, **3:**258, **3:**258*t*
　　patient size as, **3:**258
　　"selectable" filters as, **3:**257
　measurement of, **3:**256, **3:**256*f*
　reduction and safety, **3:**259
　reporting, **3:**256, **3:**256*f*–257*f*
　for radiation treatment planning, **3:**253, **3:**254*f*
　scanner generation classification in, **3:**231–234
　　fifth-generation, **3:**233, **3:**233*f*
　　first-generation, **3:**231–232, **3:**231*f*–232*f*
　　fourth-generation, **3:**232–233, **3:**233*f*
　　second-generation, **3:**232
　　sixth-generation, **3:**233, **3:**233*f*
　　third-generation, **3:**232, **3:**232*f*
　slice in, **3:**228
　special features of, **3:**247–255
　spiral or helical
　　multislice, **3:**233, **3:**249–250, **3:**249*f*–250*f*
　　single slice, **3:**233, **3:**247–249, **3:**247*f*–248*f*, **3:**267
　system components for, **3:**235–239, **3:**235*f*
　　computer as, **3:**235, **3:**235*f*
　　display monitor as, **3:**237–238, **3:**238*f*, **3:**238*t*
　　gantry and table as, **3:**235*f*, **3:**236
　　operator's console as, **3:**237, **3:**237*f*
　　workstation for image manipulation and multiplanar reconstruction, **3:**239
　technical aspects of, **3:**234
　of thoracic vertebrae, **1:**451*f*
　of thoracic viscera, **1:**92*f*, **1:**93*t*
　three-dimensional imaging with, **3:**252–253
　　maximum intensity projection for, **3:**252
　　shaded surface display for, **3:**252
　　volume rendering for, **3:**252–253
　for trauma, **2:**106, **2:**137–139
　of urinary system, **2:**282, **2:**282*f*
　volume, **3:**233
　voxel in, **3:**234, **3:**234*f*
Computed tomography angiography (CTA), **3:**250–252, **3:**266
　advantages of, **3:**250
　bolus in, **3:**250
　of brain, perfusion study for, **3:**250–252, **3:**252*f*
　cardiac, **3:**250–252, **3:**251*f*–252*f*
　gated, **3:**252*f*
　scan duration in, **3:**250
　steps in, **3:**250
　table speed in, **3:**250
　uses of, **3:**250
Computed tomography (CT) colonography, **2:**234, **2:**235*f*
Computed tomography dose index (CTDI), **3:**256, **3:**266
Computed tomography dose index$_{100}$ (CTDI$_{100}$), **3:**266
Computed tomography dose index$_{vol}$ (CTDI$_{vol}$), **3:**266
Computed tomography dose index$_w$ (CTDI$_w$), **3:**266
Computed tomography (CT) simulator, for radiation oncology, **3:**491, **3:**491*f*
Computer competency, in DXA, **2:**474
Computer-aided design (CAD), **3:**225
Computer-aided detection (CAD), **2:**356–359, **2:**356*f*
Computerized planimetry, for evaluation of left ventricular ejection fraction, **3:**379–381, **3:**381*f*
Computers, for CT, **3:**235, **3:**235*f*
Concha, **2:**16, **2:**17*f*
Condylar canals, **2:**12*f*, **2:**13
Condylar process, **2:**20, **2:**20*f*
Condyle, **2:**20, **2:**20*f*, **1:**64
　AP axial projection of, **2:**84*f*
　for articulation with atlas, **2:**13*f*
　axiolateral oblique projection of, **2:**88*f*
　axiolateral projection of, **2:**81*f*
　PA axial projection of, **2:**78*f*
　PA projection of, **2:**75*f*
　submentovertical projection of, **2:**82*f*
Condyloid process, **3:**175
Cones, **2:**53
Confluence of sinuses, **3:**183
Conformal radiotherapy (CRT), **3:**495, **3:**509
Congenital aganglionic megacolon, **2:**190*t*–191*t*
Congenital defects, cardiac catheterization for, **3:**396, **3:**396*f*
Congenital hip dysplasia, **1:**379*t*
Congestive heart failure, in older adults, **3:**156–157, **3:**160*t*
Conjunctiva, **2:**52, **2:**52*f*–53*f*
Connective tissue, cancer arising from, **3:**485*t*
Console, for MRI, **3:**273, **3:**273*f*

Construction, in three-dimensional imaging, **3:**252
Contamination, **3:**69
Contamination control, **1:**4
   in minor surgical procedures, in radiology department, **1:**5, **1:**5*f*
   in operating room, **1:**6, **1:**6*f*–7*f*
   outside radiology department, **1:**6
   standard precautions in, **1:**4*b*, **1:**4*f*, **1:**5
Continuous wave transducers, for diagnostic medical sonography, **3:**410
Continuous wave ultrasound, **3:**433
Contour, in radiation oncology, **3:**495, **3:**509
Contractures, in older adults, **3:**160*t*
Contralateral, definition of, **1:**65
Contrast, **3:**306
Contrast agent administration, in older adults, **3:**162
Contrast arthrography, **2:**141–150
   abbreviations for, **2:**143*b*
   of hip, **2:**148, **2:**148*f*–149*f*
     AP, **2:**149*f*
     axiolateral "frog,", **2:**148*f*
     with congenital dislocation, **2:**148*f*
     digital subtraction technique for, **2:**148, **2:**149*f*
   of knee, **2:**146
     double-contrast, **2:**147, **2:**147*f*
     vertical ray method for, **2:**146, **2:**146*f*
   of other joints, **2:**150, **2:**150*f*
   overview of, **2:**142–150, **2:**142*f*
   of shoulder, **2:**144–145
     CT after, **2:**145, **2:**145*f*
     double-contrast, **2:**144, **2:**144*f*–145*f*
     MRI *vs*., **2:**145*f*
     single-contrast, **2:**144, **2:**144*f*–145*f*
   summary of pathology found on, **2:**143*t*
Contrast media
   for alimentary canal, **2:**203–204, **2:**203*f*–204*f*
   angiography, **3:**322
   for cardiac catheterization, **3:**376
   for CT, **3:**242–244, **3:**242*f*, **3:**243*t*
     intravenous, power injector for, **3:**243, **3:**243*f*
   for MRI, **3:**291–292, **3:**291*f*–292*f*
   for myelography, **2:**160–161, **2:**160*f*
   for simulation in radiation oncology, **3:**492
Contrast media studies
   of esophagus, **2:**207–209, **2:**207*f*
     barium administration and respiration for, **2:**211, **2:**211*f*
     barium sulfate mixture for, **2:**207
     double-contrast, **2:**207, **2:**209, **2:**209*f*
     examination procedures for, **2:**208–209, **2:**208*f*–209*f*
     single-contrast, **2:**207, **2:**208*f*–209*f*
   of large intestine
     contrast media for, **2:**234–235
     double-contrast method for, **2:**234, **2:**234*f*, **2:**240–241, **2:**240*f*–241*f*
     insertion of enema tip for, **2:**238
     opacified colon in, **2:**239, **2:**242
     preparation and care of patient for, **2:**238
     preparation of barium suspension for, **2:**238
     preparation of intestinal tract for, **2:**236, **2:**236*f*
     single-contrast, **2:**234, **2:**234*f*, **2:**239, **2:**239*f*
     standard barium enema apparatus for, **2:**236–237, **2:**236*f*–237*f*
   of stomach, **2:**213–214
     barium sulfate suspension for, **2:**203, **2:**203*f*–204*f*
     biphasic, **2:**214
     double-contrast, **2:**214, **2:**214*f*
     single-contrast, **2:**213, **2:**213*f*
     water-soluble, iodinated solution for, **2:**203, **2:**203*f*–204*f*
Contrast resolution, for CT, **3:**229, **3:**229*f*, **3:**266
Contrecoup fracture, of cranium, **2:**26*t*
Conus medullaris
   anatomy of, **2:**153, **2:**153*f*
   defined, **2:**167
Conus projection, **2:**162
Conventional radiography, DXA and, **2:**457
Convolutions, **3:**178–179
Cooper's ligaments, **2:**360, **2:**361*f*
Coracoid process
   defined, **1:**64
   sectional anatomy of, **3:**192
Cornea, **2:**52*f*–53*f*, **2:**53
Corona radiata, **3:**175–176, **3:**178–179
Coronal image plane, in diagnostic medical sonography, **3:**433

Coronal plane, **1:**46, **1:**46*f*
Coronal suture, **2:**4*f*, **2:**5, **2:**21*t*
   lateral projection of, **2:**36*f*
Coronary angiography, **3:**372, **3:**373*t*
Coronary arteries
   anatomy of, **3:**317*f*, **3:**318
   sectional anatomy of, **3:**192
Coronary flow reserve, **3:**475, **3:**475*b*
Coronary veins, **3:**317*f*
Coronoid fossa, **1:**146, **1:**146*f*
Coronoid process, **2:**19*f*–20*f*, **2:**20
   anatomy of, **1:**145, **1:**145*f*
   axiolateral oblique projection of, **2:**80*f*
   Coyle method for, axiolateral projection of, **1:**204–206
     central ray for, **1:**205
     collimation for, **1:**205
     evaluation criteria for, **1:**206*b*
     position of part for, **1:**204, **1:**204*f*–205*f*
     position of patient for, **1:**204
     structures shown on, **1:**206, **1:**206*f*
   defined, **1:**64
   PA axial projection of, **2:**78*f*
   radiography of, **1:**204–206
   sectional anatomy of, **3:**175
   submentovertical projection of, **2:**82*f*
Corpora quadrigemina, **3:**176, **3:**181–182, **3:**186
Corpus callosum
   anatomy of, **2:**152, **2:**152*f*
   genu of, **3:**180*f*
   at level A, **3:**178*f*
   sectional anatomy of, **3:**175–176, **3:**178–179
     on coronal plane, **3:**189*f*–190*f*
     on midsagittal plane, **3:**187*f*
   splenium of, **3:**174*f*, **3:**180*f*
Cortex of brain
   anatomy of, **2:**152
   defined, **2:**167
   sectional anatomy of, **3:**178–179
Cortical bone, **2:**491
   bone densitometry and, **2:**459, **2:**459*t*
Costal cartilage, **1:**498
Costal facets, of thoracic vertebrae, **1:**417, **1:**418*t*
Costal groove, **1:**498
Costochondral articulations, **1:**500
Costophrenic angle
   anatomy of, **1:**85–86, **1:**85*f*–86*f*
   sectional anatomy of, **3:**192
Costotransverse joints, **1:**422, **1:**500
   sectional anatomy of, **3:**191–192, **3:**194, **3:**194*f*
   in thoracic spine, **1:**417*f*
Costovertebral joints, **1:**417*f*, **1:**422, **1:**500
Coulomb forces, **3:**460, **3:**478
Coyle method, for axiolateral projection, of radial head and coronoid fossa, **1:**204–206, **1:**204*b*
   central ray for, **1:**205
   collimation for, **1:**205
   evaluation criteria for, **1:**206*b*
   position of part for, **1:**204, **1:**204*f*–205*f*
   position of patient for, **1:**204
   structures shown on, **1:**206, **1:**206*f*
CR angulation method, for PA oblique projection, of sternoclavicular articulation, **1:**516, **1:**516*b*, **1:**516*f*
Cradle, for CT, **3:**236
Cragg, Andrew, **3:**312–313
Cranial base, submentovertical projection of (Schüller method)
   central ray of, **2:**49
   position of part in, **2:**48–49, **2:**48*f*
   position of patient in, **2:**48
   structures shown in, **2:**49, **2:**49*b*, **2:**49*f*
Cranial bones
   anatomy of, **2:**7–14
   ethmoid bone as, **2:**8, **2:**8*f*–9*f*
     location of, **2:**3*f*–5*f*
   frontal bone as
     anatomy of, **2:**7, **2:**7*f*, **2:**53*f*
     location of, **2:**3*f*–5*f*
     lateral aspect of, **2:**5*f*–6*f*
   occipital bone, **2:**4*f*–5*f*, **2:**12–13, **2:**12*f*–13*f*
   parietal bones as, **2:**3*f*–5*f*, **2:**9, **2:**9*f*
   sectional anatomy of, **3:**174
   sphenoid bones in, **2:**3*f*–4*f*, **2:**10–12, **2:**10*f*–11*f*
   superior aspect, **2:**6*f*
   temporal bones as, **2:**3*f*–4*f*, **2:**14, **2:**14*f*–15*f*
     location of, **2:**3*f*

Cranial bones *(Continued)*
     petromastoid portion of, **2:**14, **2:**17*f*
     petrous portion of, **2:**5*f*, **2:**14*f*–15*f*
     squamous portion ot, **2:**5*f*, **2:**14, **2:**14*f*–15*f*
     tympanic portion of, **2:**14, **2:**14*f*
Cranial nerves, **2:**156, **2:**156*f*–158*f*
Cranial region, sectional anatomy of, **3:**174–190
   on cadaveric image, **3:**174, **3:**174*f*
   at level A, **3:**179*f*
   at level B, **3:**179*f*
   at level E, **3:**183*f*
Cranial suture synostosis, premature, **3:**104
Cranial-caudal view, labeling codes for, **2:**385*t*–390*t*
Craniocaudal projection, **1:**70*t*
Craniosynostosis, **3:**104
Cranium, **2:**1–102, **2:**28*b*
   abbreviations for, **2:**28*b*
   anatomy of, **2:**3–23, **2:**24*b*–25*b*
   anterior aspect of, **2:**3*f*
   cleanliness in imaging of, **2:**32
   deviation from, **2:**6
   general body position, **2:**31–32, **2:**31*f*–33*f*
   lateral aspect of, **2:**4*f*
   of newborn, **2:**6, **2:**6*f*
   normal size of, **2:**6
   radiation protection for, **2:**33
   sample exposure technique chart routine projections for, **2:**27*t*–28*t*
   summary of pathology of, **2:**26*t*
   summary of projections, **2:**2, **2:**2*t*
   superior aspect of, **2:**4*f*
   technical considerations for radiography of, **2:**31–32
Crest, **1:**64
Cribriform plate, **2:**4*f*, **2:**8, **2:**8*f*–9*f*
   sectional anatomy of, **3:**174, **3:**183
Crista galli, **2:**4*f*–5*f*, **2:**8, **2:**8*f*–9*f*
   PA axial projection of, **2:**5*f*, **2:**38*f*
   sectional anatomy of, **3:**174, **3:**185–186
Crohn disease, **3:**190*t*–191*t*
Cross-calibration, of DXA, **2:**471, **2:**491
The Crosser, **3:**378*t*
Cross-sectional plane, **1:**46, **1:**46*f*
Cross-table projections, with obese patients, **1:**40
Crosswise position, **1:**22, **1:**23*f*
Cryoablation, **3:**399, **3:**399*f*, **3:**403
Cryogenic magnets, MRI, **3:**274, **3:**306
Cryptorchidism, **2:**335*t*
Crystalline lens, **2:**52*f*–53*f*
CSF. *See* Cerebrospinal fluid
CT. *See* Computed tomography
CT number. *See* Hounsfield units
CTA. *See* Computed tomography angiography
CTDI. *See* Computed tomography dose index
Cuboid bone, **1:**271
Cuboidonavicular joint, **1:**278*f*, **1:**278*t*
Cuneiforms, **1:**271, **1:**292*f*
Cuneocuboid joint, **1:**278*f*, **1:**278*t*
Cure, definition of, **3:**509
Curie (Ci), **3:**442, **3:**478
Curved planar reformations, in CT, **3:**239, **3:**239*f*, **3:**266
Cutting balloon, **3:**387, **3:**403
CyberKnife, **3:**501, **3:**501*f*
Cyclotron, **3:**436, **3:**478
Cyst
   bone, **1:**151*t*
     aneurysmal, **3:**136, **3:**136*f*
   breast, **2:**376*t*–377*t*
   dermoid, **2:**335*t*
   oil, **2:**367*f*
   ovarian
     CT of, **3:**241*f*
     diagnostic medical sonography of, **3:**413*f*, **3:**424
   renal, **2:**302*f*
   retroareolar, **2:**366*f*
Cystic duct, anatomy of, **2:**181*f*, **2:**185–186, **2:**185*f*
Cystic fibrosis (CF), **1:**93*t*, **3:**125, **3:**125*f*
Cystitis, **2:**280*t*
Cystography, **2:**284*f*, **2:**285, **2:**306
Cystoureterography, **2:**285, **2:**285*f*, **2:**306
Cystourethrography, **2:**285, **2:**285*f*
   female, **2:**314, **2:**314*f*
   male, **2:**313, **2:**313*f*
   voiding, **2:**307*f*, **2:**314*f*
     in children, **3:**90, **3:**90*f*–91*f*

D

Damadian, Raymond, **3:**270
Danelius-Miller method, for axiolateral projection, of hip, **1:**394–395, **1:**394*f*–395*f*, **1:**395*b*
Data acquisition, in 3D printing, **3:**224
Data acquisition system (DAS), for CT, **3:**235, **3:**266
Data storage and retrieval, for CT, **3:**235
Daughter nuclide, **3:**439, **3:**478
Deadtime, **3:**469, **3:**478
Decay
  in radiation oncology, **3:**488, **3:**509
  radionuclides, **3:**439, **3:**478
Decidua capsularis, diagnostic medical sonography of, **3:**425*f*
Decidua parietalis, diagnostic medical sonography of, **3:**425*f*
Decidual basalis, diagnostic medical sonography of, **3:**425*f*
Decubitus position, **1:**66*f*, **1:**76, **1:**76*f*
Decubitus ulcers, in older adults, **3:**161
Deep, definition of, **1:**65
Deep vein thrombosis, diagnostic medical sonography of, **3:**429, **3:**429*f*
Defecography, **2:**262, **2:**262*f*
Degenerative joint disease, **1:**151*t*, **1:**225*t*, **1:**282*t*, **1:**379*t*
  in older adults, **3:**156
  vertebrae and, **1:**424*t*
Delayed cholangiography, **2:**266–267, **2:**266*f*–267*f*
Dementia, **3:**153, **3:**160*t*
  in Alzheimer disease, **3:**153
  multi-infarct, **3:**155
Demerol (meperidine hydrochloride), **2:**316*t*
Demifacet, of thoracic vertebrae, **1:**417, **1:**418*t*
Dens
  anatomy of, **1:**414
  AP projection of (Fuchs method), **1:**427, **1:**427*f*
  submentovertical projection of, **2:**49*f*
Depressed fracture, of cranium, **2:**26*t*
Depressions, in bone, **1:**64
Dermoid cyst, **2:**335*t*
Detail resolution, in diagnostic medical sonography, **3:**410, **3:**433
Detector(s)
  for CT, **3:**231–232, **3:**266
  for PET, **3:**436–437, **3:**478
Detector array, for CT, **3:**266
Detector assembly, in CT, **3:**266
Deuteron, **3:**463, **3:**478
Development, age-based, **3:**73–76
  of adolescent, **3:**76
  of infant, **3:**74
  of neonate, **3:**73
  of premature infants, **3:**73
  of preschooler, **3:**74–76, **3:**74*f*–75*f*
  of school-age children, **3:**76
  of toddler, **3:**74
Developmental dysplasia of hip (DDH), **3:**126, **3:**126*f*, **2:**143*t*
Deviation, **1:**79, **1:**79*f*
Diabetes mellitus, in older adults, **3:**159
Diagnosis, radiographer and, **1:**10
Diagnostic enema, through colostomy stoma, **2:**259–260, **2:**259*f*
Diagnostic mammography, **2:**358
Diagnostic medical sonography, **3:**407–434
  of abdomen and retroperitoneum, **3:**414–419, **3:**414*f*–415*f*
  anatomic relationships and landmarks for, **3:**411, **3:**411*f*
  artifacts in, **3:**412, **3:**413*f*
  of breast, **3:**413*f*, **3:**420, **3:**420*f*
  cardiologic applications of, **3:**430–432
    cardiac pathology in, **3:**430–432, **3:**432*f*
    for congenital heart lesions, **3:**432
    procedure for echocardiography in, **3:**430, **3:**431*f*
  characteristics of, **3:**408, **3:**408*f*
  defined, **3:**408
  of gallbladder and biliary tree, **3:**411*f*, **3:**415–416, **3:**416*f*
  gynecologic applications of, **3:**422–424
    anatomic features and, **3:**422, **3:**422*f*
    endovaginal transducers for, **3:**413*f*, **3:**424, **3:**424*f*, **3:**433
    indication for, **3:**423–424
    of ovaries, **3:**411*f*, **3:**413*f*, **3:**424, **3:**425*f*
    transabdominal, **3:**423, **3:**423*f*
    of uterus, **3:**423*f*–425*f*, **3:**424
  historical development of, **3:**409

Diagnostic medical sonography *(Continued)*
  of kidneys and bladder, **3:**418–419, **3:**418*f*–419*f*
  of liver, **3:**411*f*–412*f*, **3:**415–416, **3:**416*f*
  of musculoskeletal structures, **3:**419, **3:**419*f*
  obstetric applications of, **3:**424–427
    in first trimester, **3:**424, **3:**425*f*–426*f*
    history of, **3:**409
    in second trimester, **3:**426, **3:**426*f*–427*f*
    in third trimester, **3:**426–427
  of pancreas, **3:**415*f*, **3:**417, **3:**417*f*
  for pediatric sonography, **3:**421, **3:**421*f*
  personnel for, **3:**408, **3:**408*f*
  principles of, **3:**408–434
  properties of sound waves in, **3:**410, **3:**410*f*
  resource organizations for, **3:**409
  sonographic image in, **3:**412, **3:**412*f*–413*f*
  of spleen, **3:**414*f*, **3:**418, **3:**418*f*
  of superficial structures, **3:**420, **3:**420*f*
  transducer selection for, **3:**410, **3:**410*f*
  vascular applications of, **3:**428–429, **3:**428*f*–429*f*
  volume scanning and three-dimensional and four-dimensional imaging in, **3:**410
Diagnostic reference levels (DRLs), for CT, **3:**256
Diagonal position, **1:**22, **1:**23*f*
Diaper rash ointments, **1:**11
Diaphanography, of breast, **2:**451
Diaphragm, **1:**54*f*
  anatomy of, **1:**83, **1:**83*f*, **1:**107*f*, **1:**113*f*, **2:**177*f*
  hiatal hernia of
    AP projection of, **2:**224, **2:**225*f*
    PA oblique projection of (Wolf method), **2:**226, **2:**226*b*–227*b*, **2:**226*f*–227*f*
    upright lateral projection of, **2:**225*f*
  in respiratory movement, **1:**502, **1:**502*f*
  sectional anatomy of, in abdominopelvic region
    on axial plane, **3:**207, **3:**207*f*–209*f*
    on coronal plane, **3:**220*f*
Diaphragmatic constriction, **2:**176
Diaphysis, **1:**57, **1:**57*f*
Diarthroses, **1:**61
Diastole, **3:**403
Diazepam (Valium), **2:**316*t*
DICOM file conversion to 3D MESH file, **3:**225
Differentiation, **3:**509
Diffusion study, in MRI, **3:**303, **3:**303*f*, **3:**306
Digestive system, **2:**169–272
  abbreviations for, **2:**187*b*
  abdominal fistulae and sinuses in, **2:**270, **2:**270*f*
  anatomy of, **2:**171–186, **2:**171*f*
    esophagus, **2:**171, **2:**171*f*, **2:**176, **2:**177*f*, **2:**184*f*
    gallbladder in, **2:**184*f*–186*f*, **2:**186
    large intestine in, **2:**171, **2:**171*f*, **2:**182–183, **2:**182*f*–184*f*
    liver in, **2:**171, **2:**184–186, **2:**184*f*–186*f*
    pancreas and spleen in, **2:**171, **2:**171*f*, **2:**181*f*, **2:**184*f*–185*f*, **2:**186, **2:**187*f*
    small intestine in, **2:**171, **2:**171*f*, **2:**180, **2:**181*f*, **2:**184*f*
    stomach in, **2:**171, **2:**171*f*, **2:**178–179, **2:**178*f*–179*f*, **2:**181*f*
    summary of, **2:**189*b*
  biliary tract and gallbladder in, **2:**263–267
    biliary drainage procedure and stone extraction for, **2:**265, **2:**265*f*
    endoscopic retrograde cholangiopancreatography of, **2:**268, **2:**268*f*–269*f*
    percutaneous transhepatic cholangiography of, **2:**264–265, **2:**264*f*
    postoperative (T-tube) cholangiography of, **2:**266–267, **2:**266*f*–267*f*
    prefixes associated with, **2:**263, **2:**263*t*
    radiographic techniques for, **2:**263
  contrast media for, **2:**203–204, **2:**203*f*–204*f*
  esophagus in
    anatomy of, **2:**171, **2:**171*f*, **2:**176, **2:**177*f*, **2:**184*f*
    AP, PA, oblique, and lateral projections of, **2:**210, **2:**210*b*–211*b*, **2:**210*f*
    contrast media studies of, **2:**207–209, **2:**207*f*
    opaque foreign bodies in, **2:**209, **2:**209*f*
    PA oblique projection of (Wolf method), position of part for, **2:**226, **2:**226*b*, **2:**226*f*
  examination procedure for, **2:**202–206
  exposure time for, **2:**206
  gastrointestinal transit in, **2:**202
  preparation of examining room for, **2:**206
  radiation protection for, **2:**206*f*, **2:**207

Digestive system *(Continued)*
  radiography of, **2:**192–270
  radiologic apparatus for, **2:**205, **2:**205*f*
  sample exposure technique chart routine projections for, **2:**188*t*
  summary of pathology of, **2:**190*t*–191*t*
  summary of projections for, **2:**170, **2:**170*t*
Digit(s)
  anatomy of, **1:**143, **1:**143*f*
  second through fifth
    anatomy of, **1:**143, **1:**143*f*
    lateral projection of, **1:**154–155, **1:**155*b*
      central ray for, **1:**155
      collimation for, **1:**155
      position of part for, **1:**154, **1:**154*f*
      position of patient for, **1:**154
      structures shown on, **1:**155, **1:**155*f*
    PA oblique projection in, lateral rotation of, **1:**156
      central ray for, **1:**156
      collimation for, **1:**156
      evaluation criteria for, **1:**156*b*
      medial rotation of second digit in, **1:**157*f*
      position of part for, **1:**156, **1:**156*f*
      position of patient for, **1:**156
      structures shown on, **1:**156, **1:**157*f*
    PA projection of, **1:**152–153
      central ray for, **1:**153
      collimation for, **1:**153
      computed radiography for, **1:**153
      evaluation criteria for, **1:**153*b*
      position of part for, **1:**152, **1:**152*f*
      position of patient for, **1:**152–153
      structures shown in, **1:**153, **1:**153*f*
Digital breast tomosynthesis (DBT), **2:**354–355, **2:**355*f*
Digital radiographic absorptiometry, **2:**488, **2:**488*f*
Digital radiography (DR), **2:**2, **2:**3*f*, **1:**14
  of cervical spine, lateral projection, in right or left dorsal decubitus position, **2:**24
  of femur
    AP projection, **2:**21
    lateral projection, in mediolateral or lateromedial projection, **2:**22
Digital subtraction angiography, **3:**323–324
  acquisition rate in, **3:**323
  biplane imaging system for, **3:**324, **3:**324*f*, **3:**403
  "bolus chase" or "DSA stepping" method for, **3:**323
  of common carotid artery, **3:**324*f*
  historical development of, **3:**313
  magnification in, **3:**325
  misregistration in, **3:**324
  post-processing, **3:**324
  procedure for, **3:**324
  three-dimensional intraarterial, **3:**326, **3:**326*f*
Digitally reconstructed radiograph (DRR), in radiation oncology, **3:**493, **3:**493*f*
Dignity, of parents/children, **3:**73
Diphenhydramine hydrochloride (Benadryl), **2:**316*t*
Diploë, **2:**4*f*–5*f*, **2:**5, **1:**59
Direct coronal image, in CT, **3:**266
Direct metal laser sintering (DMLS), **3:**225–226
Discordance, in DXA, **2:**471, **2:**491
Diskography, provocative, **2:**166, **2:**166*f*
Dislocation, **2:**143*t*, **1:**151*t*, **1:**225*t*, **1:**282*t*, **1:**379*t*
Displaced fracture, **1:**64
Display FOV (DFOV), in CT, **3:**246
Display monitor, for CT, **3:**237–238, **3:**238*f*
Distal, definition of, **1:**65, **1:**65*f*
Distal convoluted tubule, **2:**277, **2:**277*f*
Distal humerus
  AP projection of, **1:**198
    in acute flexion, **1:**200, **1:**200*b*, **1:**200*f*
    in partial flexion, **1:**198, **1:**198*b*, **1:**198*f*
  PA axial projection of, **1:**207, **1:**207*b*, **1:**207*f*
Distal interphalangeal (DIP) joints
  of lower extremity, **1:**278
  of upper extremity, **1:**147, **1:**147*f*–148*f*
Distal tibiofibular joint, **1:**278*t*, **1:**280, **1:**280*f*
Distance measurement, in CT, **3:**230*f*
Diverticulitis, **2:**190*t*–191*t*
Diverticulosis, **2:**190*t*–191*t*
  in older adults, **3:**157
Documentation
  of medication administration, **2:**325
  for trauma radiography, **2:**115
Dolichocephalic skull, **2:**30, **2:**30*f*

I-10

Dopamine hydrochloride, 2:316t
Dopamine transporter study, 3:455
Doppler effect, 3:433
Doppler ultrasound, 3:433
Dorsal, definition of, 1:65
Dorsal decubitus position, 1:76, 1:76f
Dorsal recumbent position, 1:72f
Dorsal surface of foot, 1:270
Dorsiflexion, 1:79, 1:79f
Dorsoplantar projection, 1:70t
Dorsum, definition of, 1:65
Dorsum sellae, 2:4f, 2:10f–11f, 2:11
   AP axial projection of, 2:43f
   PA axial projection of, 2:38f, 2:47f
   sectional anatomy of, 3:174–175, 3:183
Dose, 3:478
Dose inhomogeneity, in radiation oncology, 3:496
Dose-length product (DLP), 3:256, 3:266
DoseRight, 3:257f
Dosimetry, for radiation oncology, 3:495–497, 3:495f–496f, 3:495t, 3:509
Dotter, Charles, 3:312–313
"Dotter method," for percutaneous transluminal angioplasty, 3:356
Double-contrast arthrography
   of knee, 2:147, 2:147f
   of shoulder, 2:144, 2:144f–145f
DR. See Digital radiography
Dressings, surgical, 1:11
Drug-eluting stent (DES), 3:403
DSA. See Digital subtraction angiography
Dual-energy computed tomography (DECT), 3:234
Dual energy vertebral assessment (DVA), 2:483–484
Dual energy x-ray absorptiometry (DXA), 2:456, 2:491
   accuracy and precision of, 2:469–471, 2:469f–470f
   anatomy, positioning, and analysis for, 2:477–483, 2:478f
   array-beam techniques for, 2:458, 2:468–471, 2:468f
   best practices for, 2:490
   computer competency in, 2:474
   conventional radiography and, 2:457
   cross-calibration of, 2:471
   discordance in, 2:471
   of forearm, 2:482–483, 2:482f
   lateral lumbar spine, 2:483
   least significant change in, 2:470
   longitudinal quality control in, 2:475–476, 2:475f–476f
   mean in, 2:469, 2:469f
   of PA lumbar spine, 2:478–480, 2:478f–479f
   patient care and education for, 2:473
   patient history for, 2:473
   pencil-beam techniques for, 2:458, 2:468–471, 2:468f
   peripheral, 2:487
   physical and mathematic principles of, 2:465–467
      energy-switching system, 2:465f–466f, 2:466
         beam hardening, 2:466
      K-edge filtration systems
         crossover in, 2:466
         scintillating detector pileup in, 2:466
         physics problems of, 2:466
      projectional, or areal, technique, 2:467
      rare-earth, filtered x-ray source, 2:465, 2:465f–466f
      soft tissue compensation in, 2:466, 2:467f
      volumetric density in, 2:467, 2:467f
   of proximal femur, 2:480–481, 2:480f–481f
   radiation protection in, 2:472, 2:472t
   reference population in, 2:471
   regions of interest in, 2:457
   reporting, confidentiality, record keeping, and scan storage in, 2:474
   scanning, 2:472–483
   serial scans in, 2:477–478, 2:477f
   standardized hip reference database in, 2:471
   as subtraction technique, 2:457
   T-scores in, 2:471, 2:472t
   Z-scores in, 2:471
Dual photon absorptiometry (DPA), 2:458, 2:491
Dual-source computed tomography (DSCT), 3:233–234, 3:233f
Ductal carcinoma in situ (DCIS), 2:376t–377t
   calcifications in, 2:374f
Ductal ectasia, 2:376t–377t
Ductography, of breast, 2:436–437, 2:436f–437f
Ductus deferens
   anatomy of, 2:332, 2:332f–333f
   sectional anatomy of, 3:206

Duodenal bulb
   anatomy of, 2:178f, 2:180, 2:181f
   sectional anatomy of, 3:211
Duodenojejunal flexure, 2:180, 2:181f
Duodenum
   anatomy of, 2:171f, 2:178f, 2:180, 2:181f, 2:185f
   AP oblique projection of, 2:220–221, 2:220f–221f, 2:221b
   AP projection of, 2:224
      central ray for, 2:224
      collimation for, 2:224
      evaluation criteria for, 2:224b
      position of part for, 2:224, 2:224f
      position of patient for, 2:224, 2:224b, 2:224f
      respiration during, 2:224
      structures shown on, 2:224, 2:225f
   lateral projection of, 2:222–223, 2:222f–223f, 2:223b
   mucosa of, 2:185f
   PA axial projection of, 2:217, 2:217b, 2:217f
   PA oblique projection of, 2:218–224, 2:218f–219f, 2:219b
   PA projection of, 2:215–224
      body habitus and, 2:215, 2:216f
      central ray for, 2:215
      double-contrast, 2:215f
      evaluation criteria for, 2:216b
      position of part for, 2:215, 2:215f
      position of patient for, 2:215–216
      respiration during, 2:215
      single-contrast, 2:215f
      structures shown on, 2:215–216, 2:216f
   sectional anatomy of
      on axial plane, 3:211–212, 3:212f
      on coronal plane, 3:220
   sectional image of, 2:187f
Duplex imaging, 3:433
Duplex sonography, 3:428, 3:428f
Duplicate collecting system, 2:280t
Dura mater
   anatomy of, 2:153
   defined, 2:167
   sectional anatomy of, 3:175, 3:178–179
Dural sac, 2:153, 2:153f
Dural sinuses, sectional anatomy of, 3:175
Dural venous sinuses, 3:176–177
DXA. See Dual energy x-ray absorptiometry
Dynamic imaging, in nuclear medicine, 3:450, 3:451f
Dynamic rectal examination, 2:262, 2:262f
Dynamic renal scan, 3:457
Dynamic scanning, with CT, 3:247, 3:266
Dyspnea, 3:403

E
Ear, 2:16, 2:17f
   auricle of, 3:182f, 3:183
   external, 2:16, 2:17f
   internal, 2:16, 2:17f
   middle, 2:16, 2:17f
Echocardiography, 3:430
   of congenital heart lesions, 3:432
   indications for, 3:430
   pathology in, 3:430–432, 3:432f
   procedure for, 3:430, 3:431f
Echogenic structure/mass, 3:412, 3:412f, 3:433
Effective dose, for CT, 3:257
Efferent arteriole, of kidney, 2:277, 2:277f
Efferent lymph vessels, 3:318, 3:403
Ejaculatory ducts, 2:332, 2:333f
Ejection fraction, 3:403, 3:449, 3:478
Eklund technique, craniocaudal projection, 2:402f–404f
Elbow, 1:193–206
   AP oblique projection of
      with lateral rotation, 1:197, 1:197b, 1:197f
      with medial rotation, 1:196, 1:196b, 1:196f
   AP projection of, 1:193–197, 1:193b, 1:193f
      with distal humerus
         in acute flexion, 1:200, 1:200b, 1:200f
         in partial flexion, 1:198, 1:198b, 1:198f
      with proximal forearm, in partial flexion, 1:199, 1:199b, 1:199f
   articulations of, 1:149, 1:149f
   Coyle method for, axiolateral projection of, radial head and coronoid fossa of, 1:204–206, 1:204b
      central ray for, 1:205
      collimation for, 1:205

Elbow (Continued)
      evaluation criteria for, 1:206b
      position of part for, 1:204, 1:204f–205f
      position of patient for, 1:204
      structures shown on, 1:206f
   fat pads of, 1:149, 1:149f
   lateromedial projection of, 1:194–195
      central ray for, 1:194
      collimation for, 1:194
      evaluation criteria for, 1:195b
      in partial flexion, for soft tissue image, 1:195b, 1:195f
      position of part for, 1:193f–194f, 1:194
      position of patient for, 1:194
   for radial head, 1:202
      central ray for, 1:203
      collimation for, 1:203
      evaluation criteria for, 1:203b
      four-position series for, 1:202
      position of part for, 1:202, 1:202f
      position of patient for, 1:202–203
      structures shown on, 1:203, 1:203f
   structures shown on, 1:194–195, 1:194f
   PA axial projection of
      with distal humerus, 1:207, 1:207b, 1:207f
      with olecranon process, 1:208, 1:208b, 1:208f
   PA projection with, proximal forearm in, acute flexion of, 1:201, 1:201b, 1:201f
Elder abuse, 3:151, 3:151b
Electron capture, 3:478
Electronic portal imaging devices (EPIDs), 3:498
Electrophysiology (EP), 3:396–401, 3:403
   device implants, 3:400, 3:400f
   diagnostic procedures, 3:397–398, 3:397f
   interventional conduction procedures, 3:399–401
   mapping, 3:398, 3:398f
Ellipsoid (condyloid) joint, 1:62, 1:63f
Embolization, 3:403
Embolization, transcatheter. See Transcatheter embolization
Embolus, 3:364, 3:403
Embryo, 2:331
   defined, 3:433
   diagnostic medical sonography of, 3:424, 3:425f–426f
Emergency department (ED), 2:105
Emphysema, 1:93t
   in older adults, 3:158, 3:158f, 3:160t
Enchondroma, 1:151t, 1:282t
Endocarditis, echocardiography of sub-bacterial, 3:430
Endocardium, 3:316, 3:403
Endocavity coil, in MRI, 3:290, 3:290f
Endocrine studies, 3:456, 3:457f
Endocrine system, nuclear medicine imaging, 3:455–456
Endocrine system disorders, in older adults, 3:159
Endografts, abdominal aortic aneurysm, 3:358–360, 3:358f–359f
Endometrium
   anatomy of, 2:330
   defined, 3:433
   endovaginal ultrasonography of, 3:424, 3:425f
Endomyocardial biopsy, 3:385, 3:385f
Endorectal transducer, 3:432–433
Endoscopic retrograde cholangiopancreatography (ERCP), 2:268, 2:268f–269f
Endosteum, 1:56, 1:56f
Endovaginal transducers, 3:413f, 3:424, 3:424f, 3:432–433
Enema
   barium. See Barium enema
   diagnostic, 2:259–260, 2:259f
Energy-switching system, for DXA, 2:465f–466f, 2:466
Enteroclysis procedure, 2:231
   air-contrast, 2:231, 2:231f
   barium in, 2:231, 2:231f
   CT, 2:231, 2:232f
   iodinated contrast medium for, 2:231, 2:232f
Enterovaginal fistula, 2:340
EOS system, 3:142, 3:142f
Epicardium, 3:316, 3:403
Epicondyle, 1:64
Epididymis, 2:332, 2:332f–333f
Epididymitis, 2:335t
Epidural space, 2:153, 2:167
Epigastrium, 1:50f
Epiglottis, 1:87f, 1:89, 1:89f, 1:98f, 2:175f–176f
Epiglottitis, 1:93t, 3:110
Epilation, due to radiation, 3:483
Epinephrine, 2:316t

I-11

Epiphyseal artery, **1:**57, **1:**57*f*
Epiphyseal line, **1:**56*f*–57*f*, **1:**58
Epiphyseal plate, **1:**57*f*–58*f*, **1:**58, **1:**61*f*
Epiphysis, **1:**57*f*–58*f*, **1:**58
 slipped, **1:**379*t*
Epithelial tissues, cancer arising from, **3:**485, **3:**485*t*, **3:**509
Equipment room, for MRI, **3:**273
ERCP. *See* Endoscopic retrograde cholangiopancreatography
Ergometer, **3:**403
Erythema, due to radiation, **3:**483
Esophageal hiatus, **2:**176, **2:**177*f*
Esophageal stricture, **2:**211, **2:**211*f*
Esophageal varices, **2:**190*t*–191*t*
Esophagogastric junction, **2:**176
Esophagus
 abdominal, **2:**176, **2:**177*f*
 anatomy of, **1:**87*f*–88*f*, **1:**90, **1:**90*f*, **1:**110*f*, **2:**171, **2:**171*f*, **2:**175*f*, **2:**176, **2:**177*f*, **2:**184*f*
 AP oblique projection of, **2:**210, **2:**210*f*
 AP projection of, **2:**208*f*, **2:**210–211, **2:**211*f*
 Barrett, **2:**190*t*–191*t*
 cervical, **2:**176, **2:**177*f*
 contrast media studies of, **2:**207–209, **2:**207*f*
  barium administration and respiration for, **2:**211, **2:**211*f*
  barium sulfate mixture for, **2:**207
  double-contrast, **2:**207, **2:**209, **2:**209*f*
  examination procedures for, **2:**208–209, **2:**208*f*–209*f*
  single-contrast, **2:**207, **2:**208*f*–209*f*
 exposure time for, **2:**206
 lateral projection of, **2:**208*f*, **2:**210–211
 oblique projections of, **2:**211
 opaque foreign bodies in, **2:**209, **2:**209*f*
 PA projection of, **2:**208*f*, **2:**210–211, **2:**211*f*
 sectional anatomy of, **3:**205
 thoracic, **2:**176, **2:**177*f*
Estrogen, for osteoporosis, **2:**462*t*
Ethics, **1:**2–3
Ethmoid bone
 anatomy of, **2:**3*f*–5*f*, **2:**8, **2:**8*f*–9*f*
 in orbit, **2:**21, **2:**21*f*
 sectional anatomy of, **3:**174
Ethmoidal air cells, **2:**7*f*, **2:**8, **2:**22*f*
 submentovertical projection of, **2:**49*f*
Ethmoidal notch, **2:**7, **2:**7*f*
Ethmoidal sinuses, **2:**8, **2:**8*f*, **2:**22*f*–23*f*, **2:**23
 CT of, **2:**8*f*
 lateral projection of, **2:**93*f*
 PA axial projection of (Caldwell method), **2:**38*f*, **2:**67*f*, **2:**94–95, **2:**94*f*–95*f*, **2:**95*b*
 parietoacanthial projection of, **2:**97*f*
 sectional anatomy of, **3:**174, **3:**183, **3:**187*f*
 submentovertical projection of, **2:**100–101, **2:**100*f*–101*f*, **2:**101*b*
Etiology, **3:**509
Eustachian tube, **2:**16, **2:**17*f*
Evacuation proctography, **2:**262, **2:**262*f*
Evert/eversion, **1:**78, **1:**78*f*
Ewing sarcoma, **1:**151*t*, **1:**282*t*
 in children, **3:**137, **3:**137*f*
ExacTrac system, **3:**499
Exaggerated craniocaudal projection, **2:**417–418, **2:**417*f*
 labeling codes for, **2:**385*t*–390*t*
Excretory cystography
 AP axial projection for, **2:**309*f*
 AP oblique projection for, **2:**311*f*
Excretory system, **2:**275
Excretory urography (EU), **2:**283, **2:**283*f*
 contrast media for, **2:**286, **2:**287*f*
 equipment for, **2:**290
 radiation protection for, **2:**293
 radiographic procedure for, **2:**294–295, **2:**294*f*–295*f*
 ureteral compression for, **2:**292, **2:**292*f*
Exercise
 for older adults, **3:**153
 weight-bearing, for osteoporosis, **2:**464
Exostosis, **1:**282*t*
Expiration, **1:**14, **1:**501
Explosive trauma, **2:**105
Exposure factors
 or obese patients, **1:**42–44
 for trauma radiography, **2:**109, **2:**109*f*

Exposure techniques
 adaptation to patients, **1:**20
 anatomic programmers in, **1:**20, **1:**22*f*
 charts of, **1:**20, **1:**21*f*
 foundation, **1:**20
Exposure time, **1:**18
 for gastrointestinal radiography, **2:**206
Extension, **1:**78, **1:**78*f*
External, definition of, **1:**65
External acoustic meatus, **2:**4*f*, **2:**17*f*, **2:**19*f*
 axiolateral oblique projection of, **2:**88*f*
 as lateral landmark, **2:**29*f*
 lateral projection of, **2:**35*f*–36*f*, **2:**59*f*
 sectional anatomy of, **3:**189*f*
 sphenoid bone and, **2:**10–11
 temporal bone, **2:**14*f*–15*f*, **2:**17*f*
External auditory canal, **2:**15*f*, **2:**16, **3:**184, **3:**185*f*
External-beam therapy, **3:**487, **3:**509
External iliac arteries, **3:**317
 sectional anatomy of, **3:**206, **3:**215–216, **3:**215*f*–216*f*
External oblique muscle, sectional anatomy of, on axial plane
 at level B, **3:**207, **3:**208*f*
 at level C, **3:**209*f*
 at level D, **3:**210*f*
 at level E, **3:**212
 at level G, **3:**213
 at level I, **3:**215
External occipital protuberance, **2:**4*f*, **2:**12, **2:**12*f*–13*f*
 sectional anatomy of, **3:**174
External radiation detector, **3:**478
Extravasation, **2:**324, **3:**327, **3:**403
 in CT, **3:**266
Extremity
 mobile radiography procedures, in operating room, **3:**61–64, **3:**64*b*
  for ankle fracture, **3:**61*f*
  for ankle with antibiotic beads, **3:**62*f*
  for fifth metatarsal nonhealing fracture, **3:**63*f*
  for forearm fracture, **3:**62*f*
  for hip joint replacement, **3:**61*f*
  for tibial plateau fracture, **3:**62*f*
  for total shoulder arthroplasty, **3:**63*f*
  for wrist, **3:**64*f*
 MRI scanner, **3:**275, **3:**275*f*
Extremity magnets, **3:**278, **3:**278*f*
Eye
 acanthioparietal projection of, **2:**65*f*
 lateral projection of, **2:**55, **2:**55*b*, **2:**55*f*
 localization of foreign bodies within, **2:**54–57, **2:**54*f*
 PA axial projection of, **2:**55*b*–56*b*, **2:**56, **2:**56*f*
 parietoacanthial projection (modified Waters method), **2:**57, **2:**57*b*, **2:**57*f*
 preliminary examination of, **2:**54
 radiography of, **2:**52–53, **2:**53*f*
Eyeball, **2:**52, **2:**53*f*

F

Fabella, of femur, **1:**275
Facet(s), **1:**64, **1:**413
Facial bones, **2:**3, **2:**18–21, **2:**18*f*–19*f*
 acanthioparietal projection of
  alternative, **2:**65, **2:**65*f*
  reverse Waters method, **2:**64, **2:**64*b*, **2:**64*f*–65*f*
 hyoid bone as, **2:**3, **2:**21, **2:**21*f*
 inferior nasal concha as, **2:**18*f*, **2:**19
 lacrimal bones as, **2:**18, **2:**18*f*–19*f*
 lateral projection of, **2:**58–67, **2:**58*f*–59*f*, **2:**59*b*
 mandible as, **2:**18*f*, **2:**20, **2:**20*f*
  axiolateral and axiolateral oblique projection of, **2:**79–82, **2:**79*b*, **2:**79*f*–81*f*, **2:**81*b*
  PA axial projection of body of, **2:**78, **2:**78*b*, **2:**78*f*
  PA axial projection of rami of, **2:**76, **2:**76*b*, **2:**76*f*, **2:**78*f*
  PA projection of body of, **2:**77–78, **2:**77*b*, **2:**77*f*
  PA projection of rami of, **2:**75, **2:**75*b*, **2:**77*f*
  panoramic tomography of, **2:**89, **2:**89*f*
  submentovertical projection of, **2:**101*f*
 maxillary bones as, **2:**18
 modified parietoacanthial projection of (modified Waters method), **2:**62, **2:**62*f*–63*f*
 nasal bones as, **2:**5*f*, **2:**18
  lateral projection of, **2:**68, **2:**68*f*–69*f*, **2:**69*b*
 orbits as, **2:**21, **2:**21*f*
  acanthioparietal projection of, **2:**65*f*

Facial bones *(Continued)*
 lateral projection of, **2:**55, **2:**55*b*, **2:**55*f*
 PA axial projection of, **2:**55*b*–56*b*, **2:**56, **2:**56*f*
 parietoacanthial projection (modified Waters method), **2:**57, **2:**57*b*, **2:**57*f*
 preliminary examination of, **2:**54
 PA axial projection of (Caldwell method), **2:**66, **2:**66*f*–67*f*, **2:**67*b*
 palatine bones as, **2:**5*f*, **2:**19
 parietoacanthial projection of (Waters method), **2:**60, **2:**60*b*, **2:**60*f*–61*f*
 vomer as, **2:**5*f*, **2:**18*f*, **2:**19
 submentovertical projection of, **2:**101*f*
 zygomatic bones as, **2:**19
 modified parietoacanthial projection of, **2:**63*f*
Facial trauma, acanthioparietal projection (reverse Waters method) for, **2:**132, **2:**132*f*
Falciform ligament, anatomy of, **2:**184, **2:**185*f*
Fall(s), osteoporosis and, **2:**463, **2:**463*f*
Fallopian tubes
 anatomy of, **2:**329, **2:**329*f*–330*f*
 hydrosalpinx of, **2:**336*f*
 hysterosalpingography of, **2:**336–337, **2:**336*f*–337*f*, **2:**337*b*
 sectional anatomy of, **3:**206
False ribs, **1:**498
Falx cerebri, **3:**178–179
 anatomy of, **2:**153
 defined, **2:**167
 sectional anatomy of, **3:**175
  on axial plane, **3:**178*f*
  on coronal plane, **3:**189*f*
Familial adenomatous polyposis, colon cancer and, **3:**485
Familial cancer research, **3:**485
Family education, for older adults, **3:**161
Faraday cages, **3:**275
Faraday's law of induction, **3:**271
Fat necrosis, **2:**376*t*–377*t*
Fat pads, of elbow, **1:**149, **1:**149*f*
Fat suppression, **3:**306
Female contraceptive devices, **2:**338, **2:**338*f*–339*f*
Female cystourethrography, **2:**314, **2:**314*f*
Female pelvis
 anatomy of, **1:**376, **1:**376*f*, **1:**376*t*
 AP projection of, **1:**382*f*
 transabdominal ultrasonography of, **3:**423–424, **3:**423*f*
Female reproductive system, **2:**329–333
 anatomy of
  fetal development in, **2:**331, **2:**331*f*
  ovaries in, **2:**329, **2:**329*f*–330*f*
  summary of, **2:**334*b*
  uterine tubes in, **2:**329, **2:**329*f*
  uterus in, **2:**330, **2:**330*f*
  vagina in, **2:**330
 radiography of, **2:**336–345
  for imaging of female contraceptive devices, **2:**338, **2:**338*f*–339*f*
  in nonpregnant patient, **2:**336–341
   appointment date and care of patient for, **2:**336
   contrast media for, **2:**336
   hysterosalpingography for, **2:**336–337, **2:**336*f*–337*f*, **2:**337*b*
   pelvic pneumography for, **2:**336, **2:**340, **2:**340*f*
   preparation of intestinal tract for, **2:**336
   radiation protection for, **2:**336
   vaginography for, **2:**336, **2:**340–341, **2:**340*f*–341*f*, **2:**341*b*
  in pregnant patient, **2:**342
   fetography for, **2:**342, **2:**342*f*
   pelvimetry for, **2:**342
   placentography for, **2:**342
   radiation protection for, **2:**342
 sectional anatomy of, **3:**206
Femoral arteries, sectional anatomy of, **3:**206
Femoral arteriogram, **3:**54*b*, **3:**55–56, **3:**55*f*–56*f*, **3:**56*b*
Femoral head
 accurate localization of, **1:**377
 anatomy of, **1:**372*f*, **1:**373, **1:**382*f*, **1:**385*f*
 sectional anatomy of, **3:**217–218, **3:**217*f*
Femoral neck
 accurate localization of, **1:**377
 anatomy of, **1:**372*f*, **1:**373
 angulation of, **1:**374, **1:**374*f*
 AP oblique projection of, **1:**386–389
  bilateral, **1:**386, **1:**386*f*
  evaluation criteria for, **1:**387*b*

Femoral neck *(Continued)*
  position of part for, **1:**386
  position of patient for, **1:**386
  structures shown on, **1:**387, **1:**387*f*
  unilateral, **1:**386–387, **1:**386*f*
 AP projection of, **1:**381, **1:**381*f*
 axiolateral projection of, **1:**388–389, **1:**388*f*
  evaluation criteria for, **1:**389*b*
  structures shown on, **1:**389, **1:**389*f*
 sample exposure technique chart routine projections for, **1:**379*t*
Femoral vein, sectional anatomy of, **3:**206
Femorotibial joint, **1:**278*t*
Femur, **1:**356–359, **1:**373
 anatomy of, **1:**274–275, **1:**274*f*
 AP projection of, **1:**356–359, **1:**356*f*–357*f*
  evaluation criteria for, **1:**357*b*
  mediolateral projection of, **1:**357*f*–359*f*, **1:**358–359, **1:**359*b*
 mobile radiography of, **2:**20–23
  AP projection, **2:**20–23, **2:**20*f*–21*f*, **2:**21*b*
  lateral projection, in mediolateral or lateromedial projection, **2:**22–23, **2:**22*f*–23*f*, **2:**23*b*
 proximal
  anatomy of, **1:**372*f*, **1:**373–374
  AP oblique projection of, **1:**386–389
  AP projection of, **1:**381–385
  radiography of, **1:**381–385
 sample exposure technique chart routine projections for, **1:**379*t*
 summary of pathology, **1:**379*t*
Femur length, fetal ultrasound for, **3:**426, **3:**426*f*
Femur nail, **3:**48–50, **3:**50*b*
 antegrade, **3:**48
 evaluation criteria for, **3:**50*b*
 method for, **3:**49, **3:**49*f*–50*f*
 position of patient and C-arm, **3:**48–49, **3:**48*f*
 retrograde, **3:**49, **3:**49*f*
 structures shown on, **3:**50, **3:**50*f*
Ferguson method
 for AP axial or PA axial projection
  of lumbosacral junction, **1:**466, **1:**466*b*, **1:**466*f*–468*f*
  of sacroiliac joint, **1:**476–477, **1:**476*f*–477*f*, **1:**477*b*
 for PA projection, of scoliosis, **1:**488–489, **1:**488*f*–489*f*, **1:**489*b*
Ferromagnetic detection system (FMDS), **3:**307
Fetal development, **2:**331, **2:**331*f*
Fetography, **2:**342, **2:**342*f*
Fetus, **2:**331, **2:**331*f*
 defined, **3:**433
 diagnostic medical sonography of, **3:**424, **3:**426*f*–427*f*
Fibrillation, **3:**403
Fibroadenoma, **2:**366*f*, **2:**376*t*–377*t*
 diagnostic medical sonography of, **3:**420*f*
Fibroid, **2:**335*t*, **2:**337*f*
 MRI of, **3:**298*f*
Fibrous capsule, **1:**62
Fibrous joints, **1:**60*t*, **1:**61
Fibrous syndesmosis, **1:**500
Fibula
 anatomy of, **1:**273, **1:**273*f*, **1:**276*f*
 AP projection of, **1:**330–334, **1:**330*b*, **1:**330*f*–331*f*
 joints of, **1:**280*f*
 lateral projection of, **1:**332*f*–333*f*
Fibular collateral ligament, **1:**276*f*
Fibular notch, **1:**272*f*
Fick cardiac output, **3:**403
Field, **3:**509
Field light size, with obese patients, **1:**41, **1:**41*f*
Field of view (FOV), in CT, **3:**234, **3:**266
Fifth metatarsal nonhealing fracture, mobile radiography procedures for, in operating room, **3:**63*f*
Film terminale, **2:**153, **2:**167
Fimbriae
 anatomy of, **2:**329, **2:**329*f*
 sectional anatomy of, **3:**206
Fine-needle aspiration biopsy (FNAB), of breast, **2:**438
Fisk modification, for tangential projection, of intertubercular (bicipital) groove, of proximal humerus, **1:**247–248, **1:**247*f*–248*f*, **1:**248*b*
Fission, **3:**478
Fissure, **1:**64
Fistula, **2:**190*t*–191*t*
 abdominal, **2:**270, **2:**270*f*
 rectovaginal, **2:**335*t*, **2:**340, **2:**340*f*–341*f*
 in urinary system, **2:**280*t*

Flat bones, **1:**59, **1:**59*f*
Flat-panel CT (FP-CT), **3:**233
Flexion, **1:**78, **1:**78*f*
 plantar, **1:**79, **1:**79*f*
Flexor retinaculum, **1:**144–145, **1:**144*f*
Flexor tendons, **1:**144–145
Floating ribs, **1:**498
Flocculation-resistant preparations
 for alimentary canal imaging, **2:**203
 for large intestine contrast media studies, **2:**234
Flow, in MRI, **3:**272, **3:**272*f*
Fluid-attenuated inversion recovery (FLAIR), **3:**288, **3:**289*f*
Fluorine-18 (^{18}F), in nuclear medicine, **3:**442*t*
Fluorine-18 (^{18}F)-2-fluoro-2-deoxy-D-glucose (^{18}F-FDG), **3:**478
Fluoroscopic equipment, for alimentary canal, **2:**205, **2:**205*f*
Fluoroscopic image receptor, **1:**14, **1:**15*f*
Fluoroscopic procedures, for operating room, **3:**39–56
 of cervical spine (anterior cervical diskectomy and fusion), **3:**43, **3:**43*b*, **3:**43*f*
 chest (line placement, bronchoscopy), **3:**42, **3:**42*b*, **3:**42*f*
 femoral/tibial arteriogram as, **3:**54*b*, **3:**55–56, **3:**55*f*–56*f*, **3:**56*b*
 femur nail as, **3:**48–50, **3:**50*b*
  antegrade, **3:**48
  evaluation criteria for, **3:**50*b*
  method for, **3:**49, **3:**49*f*–50*f*
  position of patient and C-arm, **3:**48–49, **3:**48*f*
  retrograde, **3:**49, **3:**49*f*
  structures shown on, **3:**50, **3:**50*f*
 of hip (cannulated hip screws or hip pinning), **3:**46–47, **3:**46*f*–47*f*, **3:**47*b*
 of humerus, **3:**53–54, **3:**53*f*–54*f*, **3:**54*b*
 of lumbar spine, **3:**44–45, **3:**44*f*–45*f*, **3:**45*b*
 operative (immediate) cholangiography as, **3:**39–41, **3:**40*f*, **3:**41*b*
 tibia (nail) as, **3:**51–52, **3:**52*b*
  evaluation criteria for, **3:**52*b*
  position of C-arm for, **3:**51, **3:**51*f*
  position of patient for, **3:**51–52
  structures shown on, **3:**52, **3:**52*f*
Focal spot, in obese patients, **1:**42
Focused assessment with sonography in trauma (FAST), **2:**137, **2:**139*f*–140*f*
Folia
 anatomy of, **2:**152
 sectional anatomy of, **3:**176
Folio method, for PA projection, of first MCP joint of thumb, **1:**164, **1:**164*b*, **1:**164*f*–165*f*
Follicular cysts, diagnostic medical sonography of, **3:**424, **3:**433
Fontanelles, **2:**6, **2:**7*f*
Foot, **1:**292–302
 anatomy of, **1:**270–280, **1:**270*f*
 AP oblique projection of, **1:**298*f*–299*f*
  evaluation criteria for, **1:**297*b*
  in lateral rotation, **1:**297*f*–298*f*, **1:**299*b*
  in medial rotation, **1:**296–297, **1:**296*b*, **1:**296*f*
 AP or AP axial projection, **1:**292, **1:**292–300, **1:**293*f*
  central ray for, **1:**292*f*, **1:**293
  collimation for, **1:**293
  composite, **1:**305–306, **1:**305*f*–306*f*
  evaluation criteria for, **1:**294*b*, **1:**304*b*, **1:**306*b*
  position of part, **1:**293
  position of patient, **1:**292–294
  structures shown on, **1:**293–294, **1:**294*f*–295*f*
  weight-bearing method for, **1:**304
   for both feet, **1:**304*f*
 calcaneus of, **1:**270, **1:**270*f*
  axial projection of
   dorsoplantar, **1:**312–313, **1:**312*f*–313*f*
   plantodorsal, **1:**311, **1:**311*f*
   weight-bearing coalition (Harris-Beath) method for, **1:**313, **1:**313*f*
  lateromedial oblique projection (weight-bearing) of, **1:**315, **1:**315*f*
  mediolateral projections of, **1:**314, **1:**314*b*, **1:**314*f*
 congenital club-
  defined, **1:**282*t*
  Kandel method for, dorsoplantar axial projection, **1:**310, **1:**310*f*
  Kite method for, mediolateral projection of, **1:**308–309, **1:**308*f*–309*f*
 dorsum, **1:**270

Foot *(Continued)*
 fore-, **1:**270
 hind-, **1:**270
 joints of, **1:**280*f*
 lateral projection of, **1:**300, **1:**300*b*, **1:**300*f*–301*f*
 lateromedial weight-bearing projection of, **1:**302*f*–303*f*
 longitudinal arch of
  anatomy of, **1:**270, **1:**270*f*
  weight-bearing method for lateromedial projection, **1:**302*b*, **1:**302*f*–303*f*
 mediolateral projection of, **1:**301*f*
 metatarsals of, **1:**270*f*, **1:**271
 mid-, **1:**270
 phalanges of, **1:**270
 plantar surface of, **1:**270
 sesamoids of, **1:**272, **1:**290–291
  tangential projection of
   Holly method for, **1:**290, **1:**291*f*
   Lewis method for, **1:**290, **1:**290*f*
 subtalar joint of
  anatomy of, **1:**279*f*, **1:**280
  Isherwood method for, AP axial oblique projection of
   evaluation criteria for, **1:**316*b*–318*b*
   with lateral rotation ankle, **1:**318, **1:**318*f*
   with medial rotation ankle, **1:**317, **1:**317*f*
  Isherwood method for, lateromedial oblique projection with medial rotation foot of, **1:**316, **1:**316*f*
 summary of pathology, **1:**282*t*
 tarsals, **1:**270*f*, **1:**271, **1:**271*t*
 transverse arch of, **1:**270
Foramen(mina), **2:**4*f*, **1:**57, **1:**64
Foramen lacerum, **2:**4*f*, **2:**14
Foramen magnum, **2:**4*f*, **2:**12, **2:**12*f*–13*f*
 AP axial projection of, **2:**43*f*
 myelogram of, **2:**163*f*
 PA axial projection of, **2:**47*f*
 sectional anatomy of, **3:**174
Foramen of Luschka, **2:**155
Foramen of Magendie, **2:**155
Foramen of Monro, **2:**154
Foramen ovale, **2:**4*f*, **2:**10*f*, **2:**11
Foramen rotundum, **2:**10*f*, **2:**11
Foramen spinosum, **2:**4*f*, **2:**10*f*, **2:**11
 submentovertical projection of, **2:**49*f*
Forearm, **1:**190–192
 anatomy of, **1:**145, **1:**145*f*
 AP projection of, **1:**190–192
  central ray for, **1:**191
  collimation for, **1:**191
  evaluation criteria for, **1:**191*b*
  position of part for, **1:**189*f*–190*f*, **1:**190
  position of patient for, **1:**190–191
  structures shown on, **1:**191, **1:**191*f*
 DXA of, **2:**482–483, **2:**482*f*
 lateromedial projection of, **1:**192, **1:**192*b*, **1:**192*f*
 proximal
  AP projection in, partial flexion of, **1:**199, **1:**199*b*, **1:**199*f*
  PA projection in, acute flexion of, **1:**201, **1:**201*b*, **1:**201*f*
 trauma radiography of, **2:**133*f*
Forearm fracture, mobile radiography procedures for, in operating room, **3:**62*f*
Forebrain, **2:**152
Forefoot, **1:**270
Foreign bodies, **2:**190*t*–191*t*
 aspiration of, **1:**93*t*
 in children
  airway, **3:**112*f*
  ingested, **3:**112, **3:**113*f*
  inserted, **3:**114, **3:**114*f*
 in orbit
  lateral projection of, **2:**55, **2:**55*b*, **2:**55*f*
  localization of within, **2:**54–57, **2:**54*f*
  PA axial projection of, **2:**55*b*–56*b*, **2:**56, **2:**56*f*
  parietoacanthial projection (modified Waters method), **2:**57, **2:**57*b*, **2:**57*f*
  preliminary examination of, **2:**54
Forward planning, in radiation oncology, **3:**496
Fossa, **2:**13*f*, **1:**64
Four-dimensional imaging, diagnostic medical sonography for, **3:**410
Fourth ventricle
 anatomy of, **2:**154*f*, **2:**155
 sectional anatomy of, **3:**176, **3:**181*f*, **3:**183, **3:**190*f*
Fovea capitis, **1:**372*f*–373*f*, **1:**373

Fowler position, **1:**72, **1:**73*f*
Fractional flow reserve (FFR), **3:**391, **3:**403
Fractionation, **3:**504, **3:**509
Fracture(s), **1:**64
　of bony thorax, **1:**504*t*
　in chest, **3:**101–102
　in children, **3:**101–102
　　due to child abuse, **3:**127–131, **3:**127*f*–130*f*
　　due to osteogenesis imperfecta, **3:**134, **3:**134*f*
　　greenstick, **1:**64, **1:**64*f*, **3:**102
　　growth plate, **3:**103
　　pathologic, **3:**135–137
　　plastic or bow, **3:**102
　　Salter-Harris, **3:**102, **3:**102*f*
　　supracondylar, **3:**103, **3:**103*f*
　　toddler's, **3:**102–103
　　torus, **3:**102
　classification of, **1:**64*f*
　compression, **1:**64*f*
　　in older adults, **3:**156, **3:**156*f*, **3:**160*t*
　of cranium, **2:**26*t*
　defined, **1:**64
　fragility, **2:**461, **2:**491
　　overall risk of, **2:**488, **2:**491
　general terms for, **1:**64
　greenstick, **1:**64*f*
　of lower extremity, **1:**282*t*
　mobile radiography in, **2:**8
　osteoporosis and, **2:**463, **2:**463*f*
　pathologic, **3:**135–137
　of pelvis and hip, **1:**379*t*
　risk models, **2:**489–490
　of shoulder girdle, **1:**225*t*
　of upper extremity, **1:**151*t*
　of vertebral column, **1:**424*t*
Fragility fractures, **2:**461, **2:**491
　overall risk of, **2:**488, **2:**491
Frank et al. method, for PA and lateral projection, of scoliosis, **1:**484–489, **1:**485*f*–487*f*, **1:**486*b*
FRAX tool, **2:**489, **2:**491
French size, **3:**403
Frenulum of tongue, **2:**172, **2:**172*f*
Frequency
　in diagnostic medical sonography, **3:**433
　in MRI, **3:**271, **3:**307
Fringe field, **3:**274, **3:**307
Frontal angle, of parietal bone, **2:**9*f*
Frontal bone
　anatomy of, **2:**7, **2:**7*f*, **2:**53*f*
　location of, **2:**3*f*–5*f*
　in orbit, **2:**21, **2:**21*f*
　PA axial projection of, **2:**38*f*
　sectional anatomy of, **3:**174, **3:**178*f*
Frontal eminence, **2:**7, **2:**7*f*
Frontal lobe, sectional anatomy of
　on axial plane
　　at level C, **3:**179–180, **3:**180*f*
　　at level D, **3:**181*f*
　　at level E, **3:**182*f*
　　at level F, **3:**184*f*
　on midsagittal plane, **3:**187*f*
Frontal sinus, **2:**5*f*, **2:**7, **2:**7*f*, **2:**22*f*–23*f*, **2:**23, **2:**53*f*
　lateral projection of, **2:**59*f*, **2:**93*f*
　PA axial projection of (Caldwell method), **2:**38*f*, **2:**67*f*
　parietoacanthial projection of, **2:**97*f*
　sectional anatomy of, **3:**185–186
　　on axial plane, **3:**184*f*–185*f*
　　on midsagittal plane, **3:**187*f*
Frontal squama, **2:**7, **2:**7*f*
Fuchs method, for AP projection, of dens, **1:**427, **1:**427*b*, **1:**427*f*
Full-field digital mammography (FFDM), **2:**353
　labeling for, **2:**384
　manual technique chart for, **2:**376*t*
Functional age, age-specific competencies by, **1:**8
Functional image, **3:**478
Functional magnetic resonance imaging, **3:**305
Fundus
　of stomach, **2:**177*f*–178*f*, **2:**178
　of uterus, **2:**330, **2:**330*f*
Fungal disease of lung, **1:**93*t*

G

Gadolinium, as contrast agent, **3:**291, **3:**291*f*
Galactocele, **2:**376*t*–377*t*

Gallbladder
　anatomy of, **2:**184*f*–186*f*, **2:**186
　biliary drainage procedure and stone extraction for, **2:**265, **2:**265*f*
　body habitus and, **2:**186, **2:**186*f*
　cholangiography of
　　percutaneous transhepatic, **2:**264–265, **2:**264*f*
　　postoperative (T-tube), **2:**266–267, **2:**266*f*–267*f*
　diagnostic medical sonography of, **3:**411*f*, **3:**415–416, **3:**416*f*
　endoscopic retrograde cholangiopancreatography of, **2:**268, **2:**268*f*–269*f*
　MRI of, **3:**296*f*
　prefixes associated with, **2:**263, **2:**263*t*
　radiographic techniques for, **2:**263
　sectional anatomy of, **3:**209
　　on axial plane, **3:**210*f*–211*f*, **3:**211
　　on coronal plane, **3:**220, **3:**220*f*
Gallium-67 (^{67}Ga), in nuclear medicine, **3:**442*t*
Gallstone(s)
　diagnostic medical sonography of, **3:**416*f*
　extraction of, **2:**265, **2:**265*f*
Gamma camera, **3:**445–447, **3:**445*f*, **3:**478
Gamma Knife, **3:**488–489, **3:**489*f*
Gamma ray(s), **3:**478
Gamma ray source, for radiation oncology, **3:**487, **3:**509
Gantry, for CT, **3:**235*f*, **3:**236, **3:**266
Garth method, for AP axial oblique projection, of glenoid cavity, **1:**246, **1:**246*b*, **1:**246*f*
Gas bubble, **2:**178
Gas-ionization detectors, for CT, **3:**266
Gastric antrum, diagnostic medical sonography of, **3:**415*f*
Gastric artery, sectional anatomy of, **3:**211
Gastritis, **2:**190*t*–191*t*
Gastroesophageal reflux, **2:**190*t*–191*t*
Gastrografin (meglumine diatrizoate), for simulation in radiation oncology, **3:**492
Gastrointestinal (GI) intubation, **2:**233, **2:**233*f*
Gastrointestinal (GI) series, **2:**212, **2:**212*f*
　barium sulfate suspension for, **2:**212
　biphasic, **2:**214
　double-contrast, **2:**214, **2:**214*f*
　preliminary preparation for, **2:**212
　preparation of patient for, **2:**212
　single-contrast, **2:**213, **2:**213*f*
Gastrointestinal (GI) studies, in children, **3:**89–90, **3:**89*t*
Gastrointestinal system, nuclear medicine imaging, **3:**456–457
Gastrointestinal (GI) transit, **2:**202
Gastroschisis, fetal ultrasound of, **3:**427*f*
Gastroview (meglumine diatrizoate), for simulation in radiation oncology, **3:**492
Gated radionuclide angiography (RNA), **3:**449*f*, **3:**454
Gating
　cardiac, for MRI, **3:**292, **3:**292*f*
　for MRI, **3:**307
　respiratory, for radiation oncology, **3:**499
Gauss (G), in MRI, **3:**275, **3:**307
Gaynor-Hart method, for tangential projection, of wrist, **1:**188
　evaluation criteria for, **1:**189*b*
　inferosuperior, **1:**188–189, **1:**188*f*
　superoinferior, **1:**189, **1:**189*f*
Genant grading system, **2:**484
Generator system, **3:**439–440, **3:**478
Genetic mutations, cancer and, **3:**484
Genitourinary nuclear medicine, **3:**457
Genitourinary studies, **3:**457
　in children, **3:**89–90, **3:**89*t*
　indications for, **3:**89*t*
　with vesicoureteral reflux, **3:**90, **3:**90*f*–91*f*
Genitourinary system disorders, in older adults, **3:**159
Geriatric radiography, **3:**147–170
　best practices in, **3:**168
Geriatrics
　age-related competencies in, **3:**162
　attitudes toward older adult, **3:**151–152
　contrast agent administration in, **3:**162
　defined, **3:**148
　demographics and social effects of aging in, **3:**148–168, **3:**148*f*, **3:**150*f*
　and elder abuse, **3:**151, **3:**151*b*
　Joint Commission criteria for, **3:**162
　patient care in, **3:**161–162
　　communication in, **3:**161

Geriatrics *(Continued)*
　　patient and family education in, **3:**161
　　skin care in, **3:**161
　　transportation and lifting in, **3:**161
　physical, cognitive, and psychosocial effects of, **3:**152–154, **3:**153*b*, **3:**153*f*
　physiology of, **3:**154–159
　　endocrine system disorders in, **3:**159
　　gastrointestinal system disorders in, **3:**157, **3:**157*f*
　　genitourinary system disorders in, **3:**159
　　hematologic system disorders in, **3:**159
　　immune system decline in, **3:**158
　　integumentary system disorders in, **3:**154, **3:**155*f*
　　musculoskeletal system disorders in, **3:**156, **3:**156*f*–157*f*
　　nervous system disorders in, **3:**154–155
　　respiratory system disorders in, **3:**158, **3:**158*f*
　　sensory system disorders in, **3:**155
　　summary of, **3:**159
　radiographer's role in, **3:**162–163
　radiographic positioning of, **3:**163–167
　　for chest, **3:**163–164, **3:**164*f*
　　for lower extremity, **3:**167, **3:**167*f*
　　for pelvis and hip, **3:**165, **3:**165*f*
　　for spine, **3:**164–165, **3:**165*f*
　　technical factors in, **3:**167
　　for upper extremity, **3:**166, **3:**166*f*
Gerontology, **3:**148
Gestational age, **3:**424, **3:**426
Gestational sac, diagnostic medical sonography of, **3:**424, **3:**426*f*, **3:**433
Gestational weeks, **3:**424, **3:**433
Giant cell tumor, **1:**282*t*
Gianturco, Cesare, **3:**312–313
Glabella, **2:**7*f*
　in anterior aspect of cranium, **2:**3*f*–4*f*
　as anterior landmark, **2:**29*f*
　as lateral landmark, **2:**29*f*
Glabelloalveolar line, **2:**29*f*
Glasgow Coma Scale (GCS), **2:**114, **2:**137
Glenoid cavity, **1:**229–230
　anatomy of, **1:**220*f*, **1:**221
　AP oblique projection of, **1:**229–230
　Apple method for, AP oblique projection of, **1:**231–232, **1:**231*f*–232*f*, **1:**232*b*
　Garth method for, AP axial oblique projection of, **1:**246, **1:**246*b*, **1:**246*f*
　Grashey method for, AP oblique projection of, **1:**229–230, **1:**229*f*–230*f*, **1:**230*b*
Gliding (plane) joint, **1:**62, **1:**63*f*
Glomerular capsule, **2:**277, **2:**277*f*
Glomerulonephritis, **2:**280*t*
Glomerulus, **2:**277, **2:**277*f*
Glottis, **1:**89, **2:**176
Gloves, **1:**5, **3:**33
Glucagon, **2:**186, **2:**316*t*
Gluteus maximus muscle, **3:**215, **3:**215*f*–218*f*
Gluteus medius muscle, **3:**215*f*–216*f*
Gluteus minimus muscle, **3:**216*f*
Gomphosis, **1:**60*f*, **1:**61
Gonad(s), **2:**332
Gonad shielding, **1:**20
　for children, **3:**80, **3:**80*f*
Gonion, **2:**19*f*–20*f*, **2:**20
　as anterior landmark of skull, **2:**29*f*
　as lateral landmark, **2:**29*f*
　as surface landmark, **1:**51*f*
Gout, **1:**151*t*, **1:**282*t*
Gowns
　for patient, **1:**11, **1:**11*f*
　for personnel, **1:**5
　starched, **1:**11
Graafian follicle, **2:**329, **2:**329*f*
Gradient echo sequence, **3:**288, **3:**307
Grandy method, for lateral projection, of cervical vertebrae, **1:**434, **1:**434*b*–435*b*, **1:**434*f*–435*f*
Granulomatous disease, of lung, **1:**93*t*
Grashey method, for AP oblique projection, of glenoid cavity, **1:**229–230, **1:**229*f*–230*f*, **1:**230*b*
Gray matter, **2:**152
Gray (Gy) units, in radiation oncology, **3:**495, **3:**509
Grayscale image
　in CT, **3:**237, **3:**266
　in diagnostic medical sonography, **3:**410, **3:**433

Great saphenous vein, diagnostic medical sonography of, **3**:429*f*
Great vessels, origins of, anomalous, **3**:343
Greater curvature, of stomach, anatomy of, **2**:178, **2**:178*f*
Greater duodenal papilla, **2**:180
Greater sciatic notch, anatomy of, **1**:371*f*, **1**:372, **1**:374*f*
Greater trochanter
　anatomy of, **1**:274*f*, **1**:372*f*, **1**:373, **1**:374*f*, **1**:377*f*, **1**:382*f*
　with obese patients, **1**:39
　sectional anatomy of, **3**:217–218, **3**:217*f*
　as surface landmark, **1**:51*f*
Greater tubercle
　anatomy of, **1**:146*f*, **1**:147
　defined, **1**:56*f*
Greater wing of sphenoid
　anatomy of, **2**:4*f*, **2**:10*f*–11*f*, **2**:11
　sectional anatomy of, **3**:180–181, **3**:182*f*, **3**:184*f*
Greenstick fracture, **1**:64*f*, **3**:102
Grenz rays, **3**:509
Grids, **1**:17–18, **1**:17*f*
　for mammography, **2**:351
　in mobile radiography, **2**:3–4, **2**:4*f*
　for obese patients, **1**:42, **1**:42*f*
　in trauma radiography, **2**:106
Groove, **1**:64
Ground state, **3**:439, **3**:478
Growth plate fractures, **3**:103
Grüntzig, Andreas, **3**:312
Guidewires
　for angiography, **3**:329, **3**:329*f*, **3**:403
　for cardiac catheterization, **3**:375
"Gull wing" sign, **1**:384
Gynecography, **2**:336, **2**:340, **2**:340*f*
Gynecologic applications, of diagnostic medical sonography, **3**:422–424
　anatomic features and, **3**:422, **3**:422*f*
　endovaginal transducers for, **3**:413*f*, **3**:424, **3**:424*f*, **3**:433
　indications for, **3**:423–424
　of ovaries, **3**:411*f*, **3**:413*f*, **3**:424, **3**:425*f*
　transabdominal, **3**:423, **3**:423*f*
　of uterus, **3**:423*f*–425*f*, **3**:424
Gynecomastia, **2**:407
Gyri, **3**:178–179

H

Haas method, for PA axial projection of skull, **2**:46–47, **2**:46*f*
　central ray, **2**:46
　collimation of, **2**:47
　position of part, **2**:46, **2**:46*f*
　position of patient in, **2**:46
　structures shown in, **2**:47, **2**:47*b*, **2**:47*f*
Half-life (T1/2), **3**:439, **3**:478
Half-value layer, **3**:509
Hamartoma, **2**:367*f*, **2**:376*t*–377*t*
Hamate, **1**:143*f*, **1**:144
Hamulus, **1**:64
Hand
　anatomy of, **1**:143–149, **1**:143*f*–144*f*
　articulations of, **1**:148*f*–149*f*
　fan lateral projection of, **1**:170–171
　　evaluation criteria for, **1**:171*b*
　　position of part for, **1**:170, **1**:170*f*
　　position of patient for, **1**:170, **1**:170*f*
　　structures shown on, **1**:171, **1**:171*f*
　lateromedial projection in flexion of, **1**:172, **1**:172*b*, **1**:172*f*
　mediolateral or lateromedial projection in extension of, **1**:170–171
　　evaluation criteria for, **1**:171*b*
　　position of part for, **1**:170, **1**:170*f*
　　position of patient for, **1**:170, **1**:170*f*
　　structures shown on, **1**:171, **1**:171*f*
　Norgaard method, for AP oblique projection, in medial rotation of, **1**:172–173
　　evaluation criteria for, **1**:173*b*
　　position of part of, **1**:172–173, **1**:173*f*
　　position of patient for, **1**:172
　　structures shown on, **1**:173, **1**:173*f*
　PA oblique projection in, lateral rotation of, **1**:168–169
　　evaluation criteria for, **1**:169*b*
　　position of part for, **1**:168
　　　to show joint spaces, **1**:168, **1**:168*f*
　　　to show metacarpals, **1**:168, **1**:168*f*
　　position of patient for, **1**:168

Hand *(Continued)*
　　structures shown on, **1**:169, **1**:169*f*
　PA projection of, **1**:166–173
　　evaluation criteria for, **1**:166*b*
　　position of part for, **1**:166, **1**:166*f*
　　position of patient for, **1**:166
　　special techniques for, **1**:166*b*
　　structures shown on, **1**:166, **1**:167*f*
　position, effects on proximal humerus, **1**:227*t*
　reverse oblique projection of, **1**:169*b*
　tangential oblique projection of, **1**:169*b*
Handwashing, **1**:5
Hangman's fracture, **1**:424*t*
Hard palate, anatomy of, **2**:172, **2**:172*f*, **2**:174, **2**:175*f*
Harris-Beath method for axial projection of calcaneus, **1**:313, **1**:313*f*
Haustra, **2**:182, **2**:182*f*
Haustral folds, **3**:216
Head
　of bone, **1**:64
　　three-dimensional CT of, **3**:172*f*
　trauma, CT of, **2**:114, **2**:114*f*
Head circumference, fetal ultrasound for, **3**:426, **3**:426*f*
Health Insurance Portability and Accountability Act of 1996 (HIPAA), **2**:491
Hearing impairment, in older adults, **3**:155
Heart, **3**:316
　AP oblique projection of, **1**:112–113
　CT angiography for, **3**:250–252, **3**:251*f*–252*f*
　echocardiography of, **3**:430–432
　　for congenital heart lesions, **3**:432
　　indications for, **3**:430
　　pathology in, **3**:430–432, **3**:432*f*
　　procedure for, **3**:430, **3**:431*f*
　lateral projection with barium of, **1**:107
　PA chest radiographs with barium of, **1**:105
　PA oblique projection with barium of, **1**:111
　in radiography of sternum, **1**:506
　sectional anatomy of, **3**:192, **3**:197–200
Heart shadows, **1**:108*f*
Heat trauma, **2**:105
Heel, bone densitometry of, **2**:489*f*
Helical CT, **3**:266
　multislice, **3**:233, **3**:249–250, **3**:249*f*–250*f*
　single-slice, **3**:233
Helix, **2**:16, **2**:17*f*
Hematologic system disorders, in older adults, **3**:159
Hematoma, **2**:376*t*–377*t*, **3**:403
　during catheterization, **3**:332
Hematopoietic tissue, cancer arising from, **3**:485*t*
Hemodynamics, **3**:403
Hemostasis, **3**:403
Hepatic arteriogram, **3**:337, **3**:337*f*
Hepatic artery
　anatomy of, **2**:184
　diagnostic medical sonography of, **3**:415*f*
Hepatic ducts, anatomy of, **2**:185
Hepatic flexure
　anatomy of, **2**:182*f*, **2**:183
　sectional anatomy of, on coronal plane, **3**:212*f*, **3**:220, **3**:220*f*
Hepatic veins
　anatomy of, **2**:184, **2**:185*f*
　sectional anatomy of, **3**:207, **3**:207*f*
Hepatic venography, **3**:355, **3**:355*f*
Hepatitis B virus (HBV), cancer and, **3**:484
Hepatitis C virus, cancer and, **3**:484
Hepatopancreatic ampulla
　anatomy of, **2**:180, **2**:181*f*, **2**:185, **2**:185*f*
　sphincter of, **2**:185, **2**:185*f*
Hereditary nonpolyposis colorectal cancer syndrome, **3**:485
Hernia, hiatal
　AP projection of, **2**:224, **2**:225*f*
　PA oblique projection of (Wolf method), **2**:226, **2**:226*b*–227*b*, **2**:226*f*–227*f*
　upright lateral projection of, **2**:225*f*
Herniated nucleus pulposus (HNP), **3**:293*f*, **1**:413, **1**:424*t*
Heterogeneous structure/mass, in diagnostic medical sonography, **3**:412, **3**:412*f*, **3**:433
Hiatal hernia, **2**:190*t*–191*t*
　AP projection of, **2**:224, **2**:225*f*
　PA oblique projection of (Wolf method), **2**:226, **2**:226*b*–227*b*, **2**:226*f*–227*f*
　upright lateral projection of, **2**:225*f*

Hickey method, for mediolateral projection, of hip, **1**:392, **1**:392*b*, **1**:392*f*–393*f*
Hickman catheter placement, **3**:42*f*
High-dose-rate (HDR) brachytherapy, **3**:487, **3**:509
Highlighting, in CT, **3**:230*f*
High-osmolality contrast agents (HOCAs), in children, **3**:89
High-resolution scans, in CT, **3**:245–246, **3**:246*f*, **3**:266
Hill-Sachs defect, **1**:225*t*, **1**:235
Hilum, **1**:85–86, **1**:85*f*, **1**:92*f*
Hindbrain, **2**:152, **2**:167
Hindfoot, **1**:270
Hinge (ginglymus) joint, **1**:62, **1**:63*f*
Hip(s), **1**:369–408
　abbreviations in, **1**:378*b*
　alternative positioning landmark for, **1**:378
　anatomy of, **1**:371–378, **1**:378*b*
　AP projection of, **1**:390–397, **1**:390*f*
　　evaluation criteria for, **1**:391*b*
　　structures shown in, **1**:391, **1**:391*f*
　axiolateral projection of
　　Clements-Nakayama modification for, **1**:396–397, **1**:396*f*–397*f*, **1**:397*b*
　　Danelius-Miller method for, **1**:394–395, **1**:394*f*–395*f*, **1**:395*b*
　in children, **3**:98
　　developmental dysplasia of, **3**:126, **3**:126*f*
　　general principles of, **3**:98
　　image evaluation for, **3**:96*t*
　　initial images in, **3**:98
　　positioning and immobilization for, **3**:93*f*, **3**:98
　　preparation and communication for, **3**:98
　congenital dislocation of
　　Andren-von Rosén approach for, **1**:389
　　AP projection of, **1**:383, **1**:383*f*
　developmental dysplasia of, **2**:143*t*
　fluoroscopic procedures for, **3**:46–47, **3**:46*f*–47*f*, **3**:47*b*
　in geriatric patients, **3**:165, **3**:165*f*
　lateral projection of, **1**:384–385, **1**:384*f*–385*f*, **1**:385*b*
　localizing anatomic structures in, **1**:377–378, **1**:377*f*
　mediolateral projection of, Lauenstein and Hickey methods for, **1**:392, **1**:392*b*, **1**:392*f*–393*f*
　MRI of, **3**:299*f*
　radiation protection for, **1**:380
　radiography of, **1**:380–405
　sample exposure technique chart routine projections for, **1**:379*t*
　summary of projections for, **1**:370, **1**:370*t*
　trauma radiography of
　　axiolateral projection (Danelius-Miller method) in, **2**:126–127, **2**:126*f*
　　modified axiolateral projection (Clements-Nakayama modification) in, **2**:127, **2**:127*f*
Hip arthrography, **2**:148, **2**:148*f*–149*f*
　AP, **2**:149*f*
　axiolateral "frog,", **2**:148*f*
　with congenital dislocation, **2**:148*f*
　digital subtraction technique for, **2**:148, **2**:149*f*
Hip bone, anatomy of, **1**:371–378, **1**:371*f*
Hip fractures, in osteoporosis, **2**:463
Hip joint, **1**:375
　replacement, mobile radiography procedures for, in operating room, **3**:61*f*
　sectional anatomy of, **3**:221*f*
Hip pads, **2**:463
Hip pinning, **3**:46–47, **3**:46*f*–47*f*, **3**:47*b*
Hip prosthesis, contrast arthrography of, **2**:149*f*
Hip screws, cannulated, **3**:46–47, **3**:46*f*–47*f*, **3**:47*b*
HIPAA. *See* Health Insurance Portability and Accountability Act of 1996
Hirschsprung disease, **2**:190*t*–191*t*
Histogram, in CT, **3**:230*f*
Histoplasmosis, **1**:93*t*
History, for trauma patient, **2**:111
Holly method, for tangential projection, of sesamoids, **1**:290, **1**:291*f*
Holmblad method, for PA axial projection, of intercondylar fossa, **1**:344–345, **1**:344*f*
　evaluation criteria for, **1**:345*b*
　position of part for, **1**:345, **1**:345*f*
　position of patient for, **1**:344, **1**:344*f*
　structures shown on, **1**:345, **1**:345*f*
Homeostasis, **3**:438, **3**:478
Homogeneous structure/mass, in diagnostic medical sonography, **3**:412, **3**:412*f*, **3**:433

Hook of hamate, **1:**144, **1:**144*f*
Horizontal fissure, of lungs, **1:**85*f*, **1:**86
Horizontal plane, **1:**46, **1:**46*f*
Horizontal plates, of palatine bones, **2:**19
Horizontal ray method for contrast arthrography, of knee, **2:**147, **2:**147*f*
Hormone therapy, for osteoporosis, **2:**462*t*
Horn, **1:**64
Horseshoe kidney, **2:**280*t*
Host computer, for CT, **3:**235, **3:**266
Hot lab, **3:**444, **3:**478
Hot spots, in radiation oncology, **3:**496
Hounsfield units, **3:**234, **3:**234*t*, **3:**266
Hughston method, for tangential projection, of patella and patellofemoral joint, **1:**351, **1:**351*f*
Human papillomavirus (HPV), cancer and, **3:**484
Humeral condyle, **1:**146, **1:**146*f*
Humeroradial joint, **1:**149, **1:**149*f*
Humeroulnar joint, **1:**149, **1:**149*f*
Humerus, **1:**209–214
  anatomy of, **1:**146, **1:**146*f*, **1:**221, **1:**221*f*
  AP projection of
    recumbent, **1:**212, **1:**212*b*, **1:**212*f*
    for trauma, **2:**134*f*
    upright, **1:**209, **1:**209*b*, **1:**209*f*
  distal
    AP projection of
      in acute flexion, **1:**200, **1:**200*b*, **1:**200*f*
      in partial flexion, **1:**198, **1:**198*b*, **1:**198*f*
    PA axial projection of, **1:**207, **1:**207*b*, **1:**207*f*
  fluoroscopic procedures for, **3:**53–54, **3:**53*f*–54*f*, **3:**54*b*
  lateromedial projection of
    recumbent, **1:**213, **1:**213*b*, **1:**213*f*
    recumbent or lateral recumbent, **1:**214, **1:**214*b*, **1:**214*f*
    upright, **1:**210–211, **1:**210*f*–211*f*, **1:**211*b*
  mediolateral projection of, **1:**210–211, **1:**210*f*–211*f*, **1:**211*b*
  proximal
    anatomic neck of, **1:**221, **1:**221*f*
    anatomy of, **1:**221, **1:**221*f*
    body of, **1:**221, **1:**221*f*
    greater tubercle of, **1:**221, **1:**221*f*
    head of, **1:**221, **1:**221*f*
    intertubercular (bicipital) groove of
      anatomy of, **1:**221, **1:**221*f*
      Fisk modification for, tangential projection of, **1:**247–248, **1:**247*f*–248*f*, **1:**248*b*
    lesser tubercle of, **1:**221, **1:**221*f*
    Stryker notch method for, AP axial projection of, **1:**245, **1:**245*b*, **1:**245*f*
    superior aspect of, **1:**221*f*
    surgical neck of, **1:**221, **1:**221*f*
Hutchison-Gilford progeria syndrome, **3:**139
Hyaline membrane disease, **1:**93*t*
Hybrid imaging, in nuclear medicine, **3:**437, **3:**475–476, **3:**476*f*
Hybrid-MRI environments, **3:**280–282, **3:**280*f*–282*f*
Hydrogen, magnetic properties of, **3:**271, **3:**271*f*
Hydronephrosis, **2:**280*t*
  diagnostic medical sonography of, **3:**419*f*
  fetal, **3:**427*f*
Hydrosalpinx, **2:**336*f*
Hydroxyzine hydrochloride (Vistaril), **2:**316*t*
Hyoid bone, **2:**3, **2:**21, **2:**21*f*, **1:**87*f*, **1:**88, **1:**89*f*, **1:**98*f*
  anatomy of, **2:**174, **2:**175*f*–176*f*
  axiolateral oblique projection of, **2:**80*f*
  as surface landmark, **1:**51*f*
Hyperechoic structure/mass, **3:**433
Hyperextension, **1:**78, **1:**78*f*
Hyperflexion, **1:**78, **1:**78*f*
Hyperparathyroidism, **2:**462, **2:**491
Hypersthenic body habitus, **1:**52*f*, **1:**53*b*, **1:**54, **1:**54*f*
  gallbladder and, **2:**186, **2:**186*f*
  skull radiography with, **2:**32*f*–33*f*
  stomach and duodenum and, **2:**179, **2:**179*f*
  thoracic viscera and, **1:**83*f*
Hypertension, renal, **2:**280*t*
Hypochondrium, **1:**50*f*
Hypodermic needles, **2:**318*f*, **2:**319
Hypoechoic structure/mass, **3:**433
Hypofractionation, **3:**509
Hypogastric artery, **3:**317
Hypogastrium, **1:**50*f*
Hypoglossal canals, **2:**4*f*, **2:**13, **2:**13*f*
Hyposmia, **3:**155

Hyposthenic body habitus, **1:**52*f*, **1:**53, **1:**53*b*
  gallbladder and, **2:**186, **2:**186*f*
  skull radiography with, **2:**32*f*–33*f*
  stomach and duodenum and, **2:**179, **2:**179*f*
  thoracic viscera and, **1:**83*f*
Hypothalamus, sectional anatomy of, **3:**181–182
Hysterosalpingography, **2:**336–337, **2:**337*f*
  of bicornuate uterus, **2:**337*f*
  of fibroid, **2:**337*f*
  of hydrosalpinx, **2:**336*f*
  of IUD, **2:**338*f*

I

Iatrogenic, definition of, **3:**403
Identification, of radiographs, **1:**34, **1:**34*f*
Ileocecal studies, **2:**229, **2:**230*f*
Ileocecal valve, anatomy of, **2:**182, **2:**182*f*
Ileum, anatomy of, **2:**180, **2:**181*f*–182*f*
Ileus, **1:**129*t*, **2:**190*t*–191*t*
Iliac arteries, MRA of, **3:**302*f*
Iliac bifurcation, MRA of, **3:**302*f*
Iliac crest
  anatomy of, **1:**371*f*, **1:**372, **1:**374*f*, **1:**382*f*
  sectional anatomy of, **3:**214
  as surface landmark, **1:**51*f*
Iliac fossa, **1:**371*f*, **1:**372
Iliac vessels, as sonographic landmark, **3:**411, **3:**411*f*
Iliac wings, **3:**221
Iliacus muscle, **3:**215, **3:**215*f*
Ilioischial column, **1:**400, **1:**401*b*
  anatomy of, **1:**371, **1:**371*f*
Iliopectineal line, **3:**422, **3:**433
Iliopsoas muscles, **3:**217, **3:**217*f*
Iliopubic column, **1:**371, **1:**371*f*, **1:**400, **1:**400*b*
Ilium, **1:**372
  anatomy of, **1:**371, **1:**371*f*, **1:**375*f*–376*f*
  AP and PA oblique projections of, **1:**405, **1:**405*b*, **1:**405*f*–406*f*
Image coregistration, **3:**438, **3:**478
Image enhancement methods, for mammography, **2:**408
  magnification technique in, **2:**409–411, **2:**409*b*, **2:**409*f*–410*f*
  spot compression technique in, **2:**410–411, **2:**410*f*–411*f*, **2:**411*b*
Image flow, in mobile radiography, **2:**26
Image magnification, in CT, **3:**230*f*
Image manipulation, in CT, **3:**229, **3:**230*f*
Image misregistration, in CT, **3:**247–249, **3:**266
Image receptor, **1:**14
  dimensions of, **1:**14, **1:**14*t*
  holders, for trauma radiography, **2:**106
  orientation of anatomy on, **1:**22, **1:**23*f*
  placement of anatomy on, **1:**22, **1:**23*f*
  size of
    for obese patients, **1:**40–41, **1:**41*f*
    for trauma radiography, **2:**115
Image-guided radiation therapy (IGRT), **3:**498, **3:**509
Immobilization devices, **1:**13, **1:**13*f*
  in mobile radiography, **2:**26
  for simulation, in radiation oncology, **3:**491–492, **3:**492*f*–493*f*
  for trauma radiography, **2:**109, **2:**109*f*
Immobilization techniques
  for abdominal radiography, **1:**131, **1:**132*f*
  for children
    for abdominal radiography, **3:**86, **3:**86*f*
    for chest radiography, **3:**92–97
    for gastrointestinal and genitourinary studies, **3:**89–90, **3:**89*t*
    for limb radiography, **3:**99–103, **3:**99*f*–101*f*
    for pelvis and hip radiography, **3:**98
  for trauma radiography, **2:**113
Immune system decline, in older adults, **3:**158
Immunotherapy, **3:**509
Impacted fracture, **1:**64*f*
Implant displacement, for mammography, **2:**385*t*–390*t*
Implantation, **2:**331
Implanted cardioverter defibrillator (ICD), **3:**401, **3:**401*f*
In vitro, definition of, **3:**478
In vivo, definition of, **3:**453, **3:**478
Incontinence, in older adults, **3:**159
Incus, **2:**16
Independent jaws, of linear accelerators, **3:**490*f*, **3:**491, **3:**509
Indexing, in CT, **3:**236, **3:**266

Indium-111 (^{111}In), in nuclear medicine, **3:**442*t*
Infant, development of, **3:**74
Infection control
  for MRI, **3:**286
  for venipuncture, **2:**318
Infection studies, **3:**458
Inferior articular process, **1:**413, **1:**415
Inferior costal margin, as surface landmark, **1:**51*f*
Inferior horn, **2:**154, **2:**154*f*
Inferior mesenteric arteriogram, **3:**338, **3:**338*f*
Inferior mesenteric artery, **3:**206
Inferior mesenteric vein
  anatomy of, **2:**185*f*
  sectional anatomy of, **3:**206–207
Inferior nasal conchae
  anatomy of, **2:**18*f*, **2:**19
  sectional anatomy of, **3:**185*f*, **3:**186, **3:**187*f*
Inferior orbital fissure, **2:**18*f*, **2:**50*f*, **2:**51
Inferior orbital margin, **2:**38*f*
  modified parietoacanthial projection of, **2:**63*f*
  PA axial projection of, **2:**38*f*
Inferior ramus, **1:**371*f*, **1:**372
Inferior sagittal sinus, **3:**179–180, **3:**189–190
Inferior thoracic aperture, **1:**83, **1:**83*f*
Inferior vena cava (IVC)
  anatomy of, **2:**185*f*, **3:**275*f*
  diagnostic medical sonography of, **3:**414*f*–415*f*
  sectional anatomy, in abdominopelvic region of, **3:**200
    on axial plane
      at level A, **3:**207, **3:**207*f*
      at level B, **3:**207, **3:**208*f*
  sectional image of, **2:**187*f*
Inferior venacavogram, **3:**353, **3:**354*f*
Inferolateral-superomedial oblique view, labeling codes for, **2:**385*t*–390*t*
Inferomedial-superolateral oblique view, labeling codes for, **2:**385*t*–390*t*
Inferosuperior projection, **1:**70*t*
Infiltration, **2:**324
Inflammatory carcinoma, **2:**376*t*–377*t*
Infraglottic cavity, **1:**96*f*, **1:**98*f*
Inframammary crease, **2:**361*f*
Infraorbital foramen, **2:**18, **2:**18*f*
Infraorbital margin, **2:**5*f*, **2:**29*f*
Infraorbitomeatal line (IOML), **2:**130
Infrapatellar bursa, **1:**62*f*
Infundibulum, **2:**329, **2:**329*f*
Ingested foreign body, **3:**112, **3:**113*f*
Inguinal hernia, **2:**190*t*–191*t*
Inguinal ligament, **3:**217
Inguinal region, **1:**50*f*
Inion, **2:**12, **2:**12*f*–13*f*
Inkjet printing, **3:**226
Innominate artery, anatomy of, **3:**343, **3:**403
Innominate bone. *See* Hip bone
In-profile view, **1:**71
Inserted foreign body, **3:**114, **3:**114*f*
Inspiration, **1:**14, **1:**501
Instant vertebral analysis (IVA), **2:**483–484
Instant wave-free ratio (IFR), **3:**391, **3:**403
In-stent restenosis, **3:**403
Insula, **3:**174*f*, **3:**180*f*
Insulin, **2:**186
Integumentary system disorders, in older adults, **3:**154, **3:**155*f*
IntelliBeam adjustable filter, **3:**258*f*
Intensity-modulated proton therapy (IMPT), **3:**502
Intensity-modulated radiation therapy (IMRT), **3:**491, **3:**509
Intensive care units (ICUs), in mobile radiography, **2:**26–27
Intercarpal articulations, **1:**148, **1:**148*f*
Interchondral joints, **1:**500
Intercondylar eminence, **1:**272, **1:**277*f*
Intercondylar fossa, **1:**344–348
  anatomy of, **1:**275, **1:**275*f*
  Béclère method for AP axial projection of, **1:**348, **1:**348*b*, **1:**348*f*
  PA axial (tunnel) projection of
    Camp-Coventry method for, **1:**346, **1:**346*b*, **1:**346*f*–347*f*
    Holmblad method for, **1:**344–345, **1:**344*f*
      evaluation criteria for, **1:**345*b*
      position of part for, **1:**345, **1:**345*f*
      position of patient for, **1:**344, **1:**344*f*
      structures shown on, **1:**345, **1:**345*f*

Intercostal spaces, 1:498
Intercuneiform joint, 1:278t, 1:279f
Interhemispheric fissure, 2:152
Iliac plane, 1:48, 1:48f–49f
Intermembranous ossification, 1:57
Intermetatarsal joints, 1:279f
Internal, definition of, 1:65
Internal acoustic meatus, 2:5f, 2:14, 2:14f, 2:17f
Internal capsule, 3:174f, 3:181, 3:189f
Internal carotid arteries
  MR angiography of, 3:302f
  sectional anatomy of, 3:183, 3:184f–185f, 3:187f
Internal iliac arteries, 3:317
  sectional anatomy of, 3:206
Internal jugular vein, sectional anatomy of, 3:184–185, 3:184f
Internal mammary lymph nodes, 2:360
Internal occipital protuberance
  anatomy of, 2:12, 2:13f
  sectional anatomy of, 3:174, 3:181f
Interpeduncular cistern, 3:175, 3:181–182, 3:181f
Interphalangeal (IP) joints, 1:278, 1:278t
  of upper extremity, 1:147, 1:148f
Interpupillary line, 2:29f
Intersinus septum, 2:22f, 2:23
Interstitial implant technique, for brachytherapy, 3:487
Interstitial pneumonitis, 1:93t
Intertrochanteric crest, 1:372f, 1:373
Intertrochanteric line, 1:372f, 1:373
Intertubercular groove, 1:146f, 1:147
Intervention, 3:403
Interventional pain management, 2:166, 2:166f
Interventional procedures, computed tomography for, 3:240, 3:240f–242f
Interventional radiography, 3:311–406
  best practices in, 3:402
  defined, 3:356
  historical development of, 3:312–313
  nonvascular interventional procedures for, 3:370, 3:370f
  other procedures for, 3:370
  percutaneous transluminal angioplasty, 3:356–371
    balloon angioplasty in, 3:356, 3:356f
    of common iliac artery, 3:357f
    Dotter method for, 3:356
    of renal artery, 3:357f
    for stent placement, 3:358, 3:358f
  present and future, 3:371, 3:371f, 3:401
Interventional radiology, in children, 3:144–145, 3:144f–145f
Interventricular foramen, 2:154, 2:154f
Interventricular septal integrity, 3:404
Interventricular septum, 3:192, 3:200, 3:200f–201f
Intervertebral disk, 1:413
Intervertebral foramina
  anatomy of, 1:413, 1:415f–416f, 1:416
  positioning rotations needed to show, 1:416t
Intervertebral joints, 1:422
  lumbar, PA projection of (weight-bearing method), 1:482, 1:482f, 1:483b
Intestinal intubation, 2:233, 2:233f
Intestinal tract preparation
  for contrast media studies
    of colon, 2:236, 2:236f
    of urinary system, 2:288–289, 2:288f–289f
  for female radiography, 2:336
Intima, 3:404
  diagnostic medical sonography of, 3:419
Intraaortic balloon pump (IABP), 3:392, 3:404
Intracavitary implant technique, for brachytherapy, 3:487
Intracoronary stent, 3:404
Intramammary lymph node, 2:361f
Intrathecal injections, 2:160, 2:167
Intrauterine devices (IUDs)
  diagnostic medical sonography of, 3:425f
  imaging of, 2:338, 2:338f–339f
Intravascular lithotripsy (IVL), 3:388, 3:404
Intravascular ultrasound (IVUS), 3:378t, 3:389–390, 3:390f, 3:404
Intravenous urography (IVU), 2:283
Introducer sheaths, for angiography, 3:331–332, 3:332f, 3:404
Intubation examination procedures, for small intestine, 2:233, 2:233f
Intussusception, 2:190t–191t
  in children, 3:87, 3:87f

Invasive ductal carcinoma, 2:376t–377t
  architectural distortion in, 2:375f
Invasive lobular carcinoma, 2:376t–377t
Inversion recovery, in MRI, 3:288, 3:307
Invert/inversion, 1:78f, 1:79
Involuntary muscles, motion and control of, 1:13
Involution, of breast, 2:360
Iodinated contrast media
  adverse reactions to, for urinary system radiology, 2:288
  for alimentary canal imaging, 2:203, 2:203f–204f
  for angiography, 3:322
  for large intestine studies, 2:235
Iodine-123 (^{123}I), in nuclear medicine, 3:442t
Iodine-123 (^{123}I) thyroid uptake measurement, 3:456, 3:456f
Iodine-131 (^{131}I) scan, 3:456
Ionization, 3:486, 3:509
Ionizing radiation, cancer and, 3:484, 3:509
Ipsilateral, definition of, 1:65
Iris, 2:52f, 2:53
Irregular bones, 1:59, 1:59f
Ischial ramus, 1:371f, 1:372
Ischial spine
  anatomy of, 1:371f, 1:372, 1:374f
  sectional anatomy of, 3:218
Ischial tuberosity, 1:385f
  anatomy of, 1:371f, 1:372, 1:374f
  as bony landmark, 1:377f
Ischium, anatomy of, 1:371–372, 1:371f, 1:374f, 1:376f
Isherwood method
  for AP axial oblique projection of subtalar joint
    evaluation criteria for, 1:316b–318b
    with lateral rotation ankle, 1:318, 1:318f
    with medial rotation ankle, 1:316, 1:316f
  for lateromedial oblique projection, with medial rotation foot, 1:316, 1:316f
Ishimore, Shoji, 3:313
Islet cells, 2:186
Islets of Langerhans, 2:186
Isocentric machine, cobalt-60 unit as, 3:488, 3:509
Isodose line/curve, in radiation oncology, 3:495, 3:509
Isoechoic structure/mass, 3:433
Isolation unit
  in mobile radiography, 2:7
  standard precautions for patient in, 1:5
Isotopes, 3:439, 3:478
  in radiation oncology, 3:488, 3:509
Isotropic emission, 3:469, 3:478
Isotropic spatial resolution, in CT, 3:266
Isthmus
  of thyroid, 1:88, 1:88f
  of uterine tubes, 2:329, 2:329f
  of uterus, 2:330, 2:330f
IUDs. See Intrauterine devices

J

Jefferson fracture, 1:424t
Jejunum, anatomy of, 2:180, 2:181f
Jewelry, of patient, 1:11, 1:12f
Joint(s), 1:60
  cartilaginous, 1:61, 1:61f
  fibrous, 1:60t, 1:61
  functional classification of, 1:61
  in long bone studies, 1:22, 1:23f
  structural classification of, 1:60t, 1:61–62
  synovial, 1:60t, 1:62, 1:62f–63f
Joint capsule tear, 2:143t
Joint effusion, 1:151t
Joint Review Committee on Education in Radiologic Technology (JRCERT), 1:8–9
Jones fracture, 1:282t
Judet method, for AP oblique projection, of acetabulum, 1:400, 1:400b–401b, 1:400f–401f
Judkins, Melvin, 3:312
Jugular foramen, 2:4f, 2:13
Jugular notch, 1:497–498
  in obese patients, 1:39, 1:40f
  sectional anatomy of, 3:195
  as surface landmark, 1:51f
Jugular process, 2:13f

K

Kandel method, for dorsoplantar axial projection, of clubfoot, 1:310, 1:310f
K-edge filtration systems, 2:466

Kidney(s)
  anatomy of, 2:185f, 2:276–277
  CT angiography for, 3:250–252, 3:251f
  CT of, 2:282, 2:282f
  diagnostic medical sonography of, 3:418–419, 3:418f–419f
  functions of, 2:275
  horseshoe, 2:280t
  imaging of, 2:282–289, 2:283f
  location of, 2:275f
  nephrotomography of
    AP projection in, 2:301, 2:301f
    percutaneous renal puncture for, 2:302, 2:302f
  pelvic, 2:280t
  polycystic, 2:280t
  sectional anatomy of, 3:204f, 3:205
    on axial plane, 3:210, 3:212–213, 3:212f–213f
    on coronal plane, 3:221, 3:221f
  sectional image of, 2:187f
  US of, 2:282, 2:283f
Kidney stone, diagnostic medical sonography of, 3:419f
Kilovoltage peak (kVp), 1:18
  for obese patients, 1:42
Kinetics, 3:460, 3:478–479
Kite method
  for AP projection of clubfoot, 1:307, 1:307f
  for mediolateral projection of clubfoot, 1:308–309, 1:308f–309f
Kleinschmidt, Otto, 2:350
Knee
  contrast arthrography of, 2:146
    double-contrast (horizontal ray method), 2:147, 2:147f
    vertical ray method for, 2:146, 2:146f
  MRI of, 3:275f, 3:300f
Knee joint, 1:278t, 1:335–339
  anatomy of, 1:276–277, 1:276f, 1:278t
  AP oblique projection of
    in lateral rotation, 1:342, 1:342b, 1:342f, 1:342t
    in medial rotation, 1:343, 1:343b, 1:343f, 1:343t
  AP projection of, 1:335–339, 1:335f–336f, 1:335t
    evaluation criteria for, 1:335b
    weight-bearing method for, 1:340, 1:340b, 1:340f
  mediolateral projection of, 1:338–339, 1:338f–339f, 1:339b
  PA projection of, 1:337, 1:337f
    evaluation criteria for, 1:337b
  Rosenberg weight-bearing method for, 1:341, 1:341b, 1:341f
Knowledge, for mobile radiography, 2:26
Knuckles, 1:143
KUB projection, of abdomen, 1:132
kVp. See Kilovoltage peak
Kyphoplasty
  balloon, 2:463, 2:463f
  defined, 2:167
Kyphosis, 1:412, 1:412f, 1:424t, 2:491
  in older adults, 3:156f, 3:160t
Kyphotic curve, 1:411f, 1:412

L

L5-S1 lumbosacral junction, lateral projection of, 1:464–466, 1:464f–465f, 1:465b
Labyrinths
  anatomy of, 2:8, 2:8f
  sectional anatomy of, 3:174, 3:174f
Lacrimal bones, 2:18, 2:18f–19f
  in orbit, 2:21, 2:21f
  sectional anatomy of, 3:175
Lacrimal foramen, 2:18
Lacrimal sac, 2:52f
Lactation, breast during, 2:362f–363f
Lactiferous ductules, 2:360, 2:361f
Lambda, 2:4f, 2:6, 2:6f
Lambdoidal suture, 2:4f, 2:21t
Laminae
  of typical cervical vertebra, 1:415
  of vertebral arch, 1:413
Laminated object manufacturing (LOM), 3:226
Landmarks, with obese patients, 1:39–40, 1:40f
Laquerrière-Pierquin method, for tangential projection, of scapular spine, 1:265, 1:265b, 1:265f
Large intestine
  anatomy of, 2:171, 2:171f, 2:182–183, 2:182f–184f
  sectional anatomy of, 3:205
Large-core needle biopsy (LCNB), of breast, 2:438

Larmor frequency, in MRI, **3:**271
Laryngeal cavity, **1:**89, **1:**98*f*, **2:**176
Laryngeal pharynx, **1:**87*f*, **1:**88
 anatomy of, **2:**174, **2:**175*f*
Laryngeal vestibule, **1:**89, **1:**96*f*, **1:**98*f*, **2:**176
Laryngopharynx, **2:**175*f*
Larynx
 anatomy of, **1:**87*f*, **1:**89, **1:**89*f*, **2:**175*f*–176*f*, **2:**176
 AP projection of, **2:**200, **2:**200*f*–201*f*, **2:**201*b*
 lateral projection of, **2:**198*f*–199*f*, **2:**199, **2:**199*b*
Lateral, definition of, **1:**65
Lateral apertures, **2:**155, **2:**155*f*
Lateral collateral ligament, **1:**278*f*
Lateral condyle
 of femur, **1:**274*f*, **1:**275
 of tibia, **1:**272, **1:**272*f*
Lateral decubitus position, **1:**76
Lateral epicondyle
 of femur, **1:**274*f*, **1:**275
 of humerus, **1:**146, **1:**146*f*
Lateral fissure, **3:**180*f*, **3:**189*f*
Lateral intercondylar tubercle, **1:**272, **1:**272*f*
Lateral lumbar spine DXA, **2:**483
Lateral malleolus, **1:**272*f*
Lateral meniscus
 anatomy of, **1:**276*f*–277*f*, **1:**277
 double-contrast arthrography of, **2:**147, **2:**147*f*
Lateral position, **1:**73, **1:**73*f*
Lateral projection, of obese patients, **1:**40
Lateral pterygoid lamina, **2:**11*f*, **2:**12
Lateral recumbent position, **1:**72*f*
Lateral resolution, in diagnostic medical sonography, **3:**433
Lateral rotation, **1:**75, **1:**75*f*
Lateral ventricles
 anatomy of, **2:**152, **2:**154
 anterior horn of, **3:**174*f*, **3:**180*f*, **3:**181
 posterior horn of, **3:**174*f*, **3:**180*f*
 sectional anatomy of
  on coronal plane, **3:**189*f*–190*f*
  on midsagittal plane, **3:**187*f*–188*f*
 temporal horn of, **3:**180*f*–181*f*
Lateral vertebral assessment (LVA), **2:**483–484
Lateromedial lateral view, labeling codes for, **2:**385*t*–390*t*
Lateromedial oblique projection, **2:**432–433, **2:**432*f*
Lateromedial projection, **1:**69, **1:**69*f*, **1:**70*t*
Latissimus dorsi, sectional anatomy of, in abdominopelvic region, **3:**200, **3:**200*f*, **3:**207, **3:**207*f*–208*f*
Lauenstein and Hickey methods, for mediolateral projection, of hip, **1:**392, **1:**392*b*, **1:**392*f*–393*f*
Lauterbur, Paul, **3:**270
Lawrence method, for shoulder girdle
 for inferosuperior axial projection, of shoulder girdle, **1:**235, **1:**235*f*–236*f*, **1:**236*b*
 for transthoracic lateral projection, **1:**233–234, **1:**233*f*–234*f*, **1:**234*b*
Le Fort fracture, of cranium, **2:**26*t*
Lead shields, **1:**17, **1:**17*f*
Least significant change (LSC), **2:**470, **2:**491
Left anterior oblique (LAO) position, **1:**74, **1:**74*f*
Left atrial appendage occlusion device, **3:**395, **3:**395*f*, **3:**404
Left colic flexure, anatomy of, **2:**182*f*, **2:**183
Left common carotid artery, sectional anatomy of, **3:**195
Left lower quadrant (LLQ), **1:**50, **1:**50*f*
Left posterior oblique (LPO) position, **1:**77
Left semiprone oblique position, **1:**72, **1:**73*f*
Left upper quadrant (LUQ), **1:**50, **1:**50*f*
Leg
 anatomy of, **1:**272–273
 AP oblique projection of, medial and lateral rotations of, **1:**334, **1:**334*b*, **1:**334*f*
 AP projection of, **1:**330–334, **1:**330*b*–331*b*
 lateral projection of, **1:**332–333, **1:**333*b*
Legg-Calvé-Perthes disease, **1:**379*t*
Lengthwise position, **1:**22, **1:**23*f*
Lens, sectional anatomy of, **3:**174*f*
Lentiform nucleus, **3:**174*f*, **3:**180*f*, **3:**189*f*
Lenz force, **3:**307
Lesion, **3:**404, **3:**509
Lesser curvature, of stomach, anatomy of, **2:**178, **2:**178*f*
Lesser sciatic notch, **1:**371*f*, **1:**372
Lesser trochanter, **1:**274*f*, **1:**372*f*, **1:**373, **1:**382*f*
Lesser tubercle, anatomy of, **1:**146*f*, **1:**147
Lesser wings of sphenoid
 anatomy of, **2:**4*f*, **2:**10*f*–11*f*, **2:**11
 sectional anatomy of, **3:**174–175

Level 1 MRI personnel, **3:**307
Level 2 MRI personnel, **3:**307
Level I trauma center, **2:**105
Level II trauma center, **2:**105
Level III trauma center, **2:**105
Level IV trauma center, **2:**105
Lewis method, for tangential projection of sesamoids, **1:**290, **1:**290*f*
Life stage, age-specific competencies by, **1:**8
Lifting, of older adults, **3:**161
Ligament of Treitz, **2:**180, **2:**181*f*
Ligament tear, **2:**143*t*
Ligamentum capitis femoris, **1:**373, **1:**373*f*
Light pipe, **3:**446, **3:**479
Lindblom method, for AP axial projection, of pulmonary apices, **1:**116–117
 central ray for, **1:**116, **1:**118
 collimation for, **1:**117–118
 evaluation criteria for, **1:**117*b*–118*b*
 position of part for, **1:**116, **1:**116*f*, **1:**118
 position of patient for, **1:**116, **1:**118
 respiration, **1:**116, **1:**118
 SID for, **1:**116
 structures shown on, **1:**117*f*, **1:**118
Line, **1:**64
Line of response (LOR), **3:**469, **3:**479
Line placement, **3:**42, **3:**42*b*, **3:**42*f*
Linear accelerators (linacs), for radiation oncology, **3:**487, **3:**489–491, **3:**490*f*
Linear energy transfer (LET), **3:**486, **3:**509
Linear fracture, of cranium, **2:**26*t*
Linen, **1:**5
Lingula
 anatomy of, **1:**86
 sectional anatomy of, **3:**192, **3:**200
Lipoma, **2:**367*f*, **2:**376*t*–377*t*
Lithotomy position, **1:**72, **1:**73*f*
Liver
 anatomy of, **2:**171, **2:**184–186, **2:**184*f*–186*f*
 diagnostic medical sonography of, **3:**411*f*–412*f*, **3:**414*f*–416*f*, **3:**415–416
 functions of, **2:**184
 with hemangioma, **3:**295*f*
 lobes of, **2:**184, **2:**185*f*
 MRI of, **3:**296*f*–297*f*
 nuclear medicine imaging of, **3:**456–457
 sectional anatomy of, in abdominopelvic region, **3:**207, **3:**207*f*–208*f*
 sectional image of, **2:**187*f*
Lobar pneumonia, **1:**93*t*
 in children, **3:**137
Lobes, of breast, **2:**360
Lobular carcinoma in situ (LCIS), **2:**376*t*–377*t*
Lobular pneumonia, **1:**93*t*
Lobules, of breast, **2:**360, **2:**361*f*
Long bone(s), **1:**59
 anatomy of, **1:**56
 vessels and nerves of, **1:**57*f*
Long bone(s), supine scanogram procedure, **1:**363–364, **1:**363*f*–364*f*, **1:**364*b*
Long bone measurement, **1:**360
 procedure, **1:**360–364
 techniques, **1:**365–366, **1:**365*f*–366*f*
 upright leg, **1:**361–362, **1:**361*f*–362*f*, **1:**362*b*
Long bone studies
 joints in, **1:**22, **1:**23*f*
 in tall patients, **1:**22
Longitudinal angulation, **1:**68
Longitudinal arch
 anatomy of, **1:**270, **1:**270*f*
 lateromedial projection of, weight-bearing method for, **1:**302*b*, **1:**302*f*–303*f*
Longitudinal cerebral fissure, sectional anatomy of, **3:**178–179
Longitudinal fissure, **3:**175, **3:**179–180
Longitudinal plane, in MRI, **3:**271, **3:**307
Longitudinal quality control, in DXA, **2:**475–476, **2:**475*f*–476*f*, **2:**491
Longitudinal sulcus, **2:**152
Loop of Henle, **2:**277, **2:**277*f*
Loop recorder, **3:**401, **3:**404
Lordosis, **1:**412, **1:**424*t*
Lordotic curve, **1:**411*f*, **1:**412
Lordotic position, **1:**76, **1:**77*f*
Low-dose-rate (LDR) brachytherapy, **3:**487, **3:**509

Lower esophageal sphincter (LES), **2:**177*f*, **2:**179
Lower extremity, **1:**267–368
 abbreviations for, **1:**281*b*
 anatomy of, **1:**270–280, **1:**283*t*
  articulations in, **1:**278–280, **1:**278*f*, **1:**278*t*
  femur, **1:**274–275, **1:**274*f*
  fibula, **1:**273, **1:**273*f*
  knee joint, **1:**276–277, **1:**276*f*, **1:**278*t*
  patella, **1:**275, **1:**275*f*
  summary of, **1:**281*b*
  tibia, **1:**272–273, **1:**272*f*
 ankle. *See* Ankle
 arteriograms of, **3:**340, **3:**340*f*
 calcaneus of
  axial projection of
   dorsoplantar, **1:**312–313, **1:**312*f*–313*f*
   plantodorsal, **1:**311, **1:**311*f*
   weight-bearing coalition (Harris-Beath) method for, **1:**313, **1:**313*f*
  lateromedial oblique projection (weight-bearing) of, **1:**315, **1:**315*f*
  mediolateral projection of, **1:**300, **1:**320, **1:**320*b*, **1:**320*f*–321*f*
 femur, **1:**356–359
  anatomy of, **1:**274–275, **1:**274*f*
  AP projection of, **1:**356–359, **1:**356*f*–357*f*
  evaluation criteria for, **1:**357*b*
  mediolateral projection of, **1:**358–359, **1:**358*f*–359*f*, **1:**359*b*
 fibula
  anatomy of, **1:**273, **1:**273*f*
  AP projection of, **1:**330–334, **1:**330*b*, **1:**330*f*–331*f*
  lateral projection of, **1:**332*f*–333*f*
 of geriatric patients, **3:**167*f*
 intercondylar fossa of, **1:**344–348
  Béclère method for AP axial projection of, **1:**348, **1:**348*f*
  PA axial (tunnel) projection of
   Camp-Coventry method for, **1:**346, **1:**346*f*–347*f*
   Holmblad method for, **1:**344–345, **1:**344*f*
 knee joint, **1:**278*t*, **1:**335–339
  anatomy of, **1:**276–277, **1:**276*f*, **1:**278*t*
  AP oblique projection of
   in lateral rotation, **1:**342, **1:**342*f*, **1:**342*t*
   in medial rotation, **1:**343, **1:**343*f*, **1:**343*t*
  AP projection of, **1:**335–339, **1:**335*f*–336*f*, **1:**335*t*
   evaluation criteria for, **1:**335*b*
   weight-bearing method for, **1:**340, **1:**340*f*
  mediolateral projection of, **1:**338–339, **1:**338*f*–339*f*, **1:**339*b*
  PA projection of, **1:**337, **1:**337*f*
   evaluation criteria for, **1:**337*b*
  Rosenberg weight-bearing method for, **1:**341, **1:**341*f*
 long bone measurement. *See* Long bone measurement
 patella, **1:**349–350
  evaluation criteria for, **1:**349*b*
  mediolateral projection of, **1:**350, **1:**350*b*, **1:**350*f*
  PA projection of, **1:**349–350, **1:**349*f*
  tangential projection of
   Hughston method for, **1:**351, **1:**351*f*
   Merchant method for, **1:**352–353, **1:**352*f*–353*f*
   Settegast method for, **1:**354–355, **1:**354*f*–355*f*, **1:**355*b*
 patellofemoral joint of, **1:**351–355
  anatomy of, **1:**280, **1:**280*f*
  evaluation criteria for, **1:**351*b*
  tangential projection of
   Hughston method for, **1:**351, **1:**351*f*
   Merchant method for, **1:**352–353, **1:**352*f*–353*f*
   Settegast method for, **1:**354–355, **1:**354*f*–355*f*, **1:**355*b*
 radiation protection for, **1:**360, **1:**360*f*
 radiography for, **1:**284–366
 sample exposure technique chart routine projections for, **1:**282*t*
 subtalar joint of
  Isherwood method for, AP axial oblique projection of
   evaluation criteria for, **1:**316*b*, **1:**318*b*
   with lateral rotation ankle, **1:**318, **1:**318*f*
   with medial rotation ankle, **1:**317, **1:**317*f*
  Isherwood method for, AP for lateromedial oblique projection with medial rotation foot of, **1:**316, **1:**316*f*
 summary of projections in, **1:**268, **1:**268*t*–269*t*

Lower extremity *(Continued)*
  tibia
    anatomy of, **1:**272–273, **1:**272*f*
    AP projection of, **1:**330–334, **1:**330*b*, **1:**330*f*–331*f*
    lateral projection of, **1:**332*f*–333*f*
  trauma radiography of
    patient position considerations for, **2:**135, **2:**135*f*–136*f*
    structures shown on, **2:**136, **2:**136*f*–138*f*
    trauma positioning tips for, **2:**135–136, **2:**135*f*
  venograms of, **3:**353, **3:**354*f*
Lower limb arteries, duplex sonography of, **3:**429
Lower limb veins, duplex sonography of, **3:**429, **3:**429*f*
Low-osmolality contrast agents (LOCAs), in children, **3:**89
Lumbar curve, **1:**411*f*
Lumbar fusion, **3:**45
Lumbar puncture, **2:**164, **2:**164*f*
  defined, **2:**167
Lumbar ribs, **1:**498
Lumbar vein, diagnostic medical sonography of, **3:**415*f*
Lumbar vertebrae, **1:**411, **1:**419–420, **1:**420*f*
  anatomy of, **1:**411*f*, **1:**419*f*
    accessory process in, **1:**419
    pars interarticularis, **1:**419, **1:**419*f*
    superior aspect of, **1:**419*f*
    transverse process in, **1:**419, **1:**419*f*
  AP/PA projection of, **1:**458–463, **1:**458*f*–461*f*, **1:**460*b*
  fluoroscopic procedures for, **3:**44–45, **3:**44*f*–45*f*, **3:**45*b*
  intervertebral foramina of
    anatomy of, **1:**419
    positioning rotations needed to show, **1:**416*t*
  lateral projection of, **1:**452–455, **1:**452*f*–455*f*, **1:**454*b*–455*b*, **1:**462–463, **1:**462*b*–463*b*, **1:**462*f*–463*f*
    for trauma, **2:**120, **2:**120*b*, **2:**120*f*
  mobile radiography procedures, in operating room, **3:**59, **3:**59*b*, **3:**59*f*–60*f*
  MRI of, **3:**293*f*
  sectional anatomy of, **3:**204
    on axial plane, **3:**212–214, **3:**218
    on coronal plane, **3:**221
    on sagittal plane, **3:**219*f*
  spinal fusion in
    AP projection of, **1:**490–494, **1:**490*f*–491*f*, **1:**491*b*
    lateral projection of, **1:**492–494, **1:**492*f*–493*f*, **1:**493*b*
  spondylolysis, **1:**420, **1:**424*t*
  trauma radiography of, **2:**120
  zygapophyseal joints of, **1:**419, **1:**420*f*
    angle of, **1:**420*t*
    AP oblique projection of, **1:**468, **1:**468*b*–469*b*, **1:**468*f*–470*f*
    PA oblique projection of, **1:**470, **1:**470*b*, **1:**470*f*–471*f*
    positioning rotations needed to show, **1:**416*t*
Lumbar vertebral body, CT of, for needle biopsy of infectious spondylitis, **3:**240*f*
Lumbosacral angle, **1:**412
Lumbosacral joint, **1:**385*f*
Lumbosacral vertebrae
  AP/PA projection of, **1:**458–463, **1:**458*f*–461*f*, **1:**460*b*
  lateral projection of, **1:**452–455, **1:**452*f*–455*f*, **1:**454*b*–455*b*, **1:**462–463, **1:**462*b*–463*b*, **1:**462*f*–463*f*
  at L5-S1 junction, **1:**464–466, **1:**464*f*–465*f*, **1:**465*b*
Lumbrosacral junction, AP axial or PA axial projection of (Ferguson method), **1:**466, **1:**466*b*, **1:**466*f*–468*f*
Lunate, **1:**143*f*, **1:**144
Lung(s)
  anatomy of, **1:**85–86, **1:**85*f*–86*f*
  AP oblique projection for, **1:**112–113
    central ray for, **1:**113
    collimation for, **1:**113
    evaluation criteria for, **1:**113*b*
    position of part for, **1:**112, **1:**112*f*
    position of patient for, **1:**112
    SID for, **1:**112
    structures shown on, **1:**113, **1:**113*f*
  AP projection of, **1:**114–115
    central ray for, **1:**114
    collimation for, **1:**114
    evaluation criteria for, **1:**115*b*
    with pleura, **1:**120–123, **1:**120*f*–121*f*
    position of part for, **1:**114, **1:**114*f*
    position of patient for, **1:**114
    respiration, **1:**114
    SID for, **1:**114
    structures shown on, **1:**115, **1:**115*f*
  apex of, **1:**85–86, **1:**85*f*
  coal miner (black), **1:**93*t*

Lung(s) *(Continued)*
  lateral projection of, **1:**106–107
    cardiac studies with barium in, **1:**107
    central for, **1:**106
    collimation for, **1:**106
    evaluation criteria for, **1:**107*b*
    foreshortening in, **1:**106, **1:**107*f*
    forward bending in, **1:**106, **1:**107*f*
    with pleura, **1:**122*f*
    position of part for, **1:**106, **1:**106*f*–107*f*
    position of patient for, **1:**106
    SID for, **1:**106
    structures shown on, **1:**106–107, **1:**107*f*–108*f*
  lobes of, **1:**84*f*–85*f*, **1:**86
  PA oblique projection of, **1:**109–111
    barium studies in, **1:**111
    central ray for, **1:**109
    collimation for, **1:**109
    evaluation criteria for, **1:**111*b*
    LAO position for, **1:**109–110, **1:**109*f*–110*f*
    position of part for, **1:**109, **1:**109*f*
    position of patient for, **1:**109
    RAO position for, **1:**109–111, **1:**109*f*, **1:**111*f*
    SID for, **1:**109
    structures shown on, **1:**110–111
  PA projection of, **1:**99–115
    breasts in, **1:**103*f*
    cardiac studies with barium in, **1:**105
    central ray for, **1:**104–105
    collimation for, **1:**104–105
    evaluation criteria for, **1:**105*b*
    with pleura, **1:**120–123, **1:**120*f*, **1:**121*b*
    position of part for, **1:**103, **1:**103*f*–104*f*
    position of patient for, **1:**103–105
    respiration, **1:**99–115, **1:**104*f*
    SID for, **1:**103
    structures shown on, **1:**105, **1:**105*f*
  primary lobules of, **1:**91
  pulmonary apices of, **1:**116–119
    AP axial projection for, **1:**116–119, **1:**118*f*
      in lordotic position (Lindblom method), **1:**116–117, **1:**116*f*–117*f*
    PA axial projection for, **1:**119, **1:**119*b*, **1:**119*f*
Lung cancer
  in older adults, **3:**158
  radiation oncology for, **3:**505, **3:**505*f*
Lung markings, in radiography of sternum, **1:**506
Lymph, **3:**314, **3:**404
Lymph nodes, **3:**318, **3:**319*f*
Lymph vessels, **3:**318, **3:**404
Lymphatic system, **3:**314, **3:**318, **3:**319*f*
Lymphocytes, **3:**318
Lymphography, **3:**318
Lymphoreticular tissue, cancer arising from, **3:**485*t*
Lysis, **3:**404

M
Macroaggregated albumin (MAA), **3:**441–442, **3:**441*f*
Magnet, for MRI, **3:**274
Magnet room, for MRI, **3:**274, **3:**274*f*–275*f*
Magnetic field strength, for MRI, **3:**275
Magnetic resonance (MR), **3:**307
Magnetic resonance angiography (MRA), **3:**302, **3:**302*f*
Magnetic resonance cholangiopancreatography (MRCP), **3:**296*f*
Magnetic resonance imaging (MRI), **3:**269–310, **3:**479
  of abdomen, **3:**295–297, **3:**295*f*–297*f*
  artificial intelligence for, **3:**288, **3:**288*f*
  best practices for, **3:**306
  body planes in, **1:**47, **1:**47*f*
  of breast, **3:**294, **3:**294*f*, **2:**400–401
  cardiac, **3:**294*f*
  of central nervous system, **3:**293
    of brain, **3:**293, **3:**293*f*
    of spine, **3:**293
      lumbar, **3:**293*f*
      thoracic, **3:**293*f*
  of chest, **3:**294, **3:**294*f*
  in children, **3:**142–143, **3:**143*f*
  clinical applications of, **3:**293–302
  coils for, **3:**274, **3:**290, **3:**290*f*, **3:**306
  conditional, **3:**307
  contrast media for, **3:**291–292, **3:**291*f*–292*f*
  conventional radiography vs., **3:**270
  diffusion and perfusion for, **3:**303, **3:**303*f*

Magnetic resonance imaging (MRI) *(Continued)*
  equipment for, **3:**273–282
    console as, **3:**273, **3:**273*f*
    equipment room in, **3:**273
    magnet room as, **3:**274, **3:**274*f*–275*f*
  extremity, **3:**275, **3:**275*f*
  functional, **3:**305
  gating for, **3:**292, **3:**292*f*
  historical development of, **3:**270
  imaging parameters for, **3:**287, **3:**287*f*
  infection control for, **3:**286
  of musculoskeletal system, **3:**299, **3:**299*f*–301*f*
  neurography, **3:**305
  patient monitoring for, **3:**291
  of pelvis, **3:**298, **3:**298*f*
  positioning for, **3:**290
  principles of, **3:**270–308
  pulse sequences for, **3:**272, **3:**288, **3:**289*f*
  safety of, **3:**283–286, **3:**307
    biologic effects, **3:**285, **3:**285*f*
    hazards, **3:**285–286, **3:**286*f*
    labeling, **3:**284, **3:**284*f*
    personnel, **3:**284
    pregnancy, **3:**286
    quench, **3:**286
    zones, **3:**283, **3:**283*f*
  scanners
    closed, **3:**275, **3:**275*f*
    extremity magnets, **3:**278, **3:**278*f*
    hybrid-MRI environments, **3:**280–282, **3:**280*f*–282*f*
    open, **3:**276–277, **3:**276*f*–277*f*
    point-of-care, **3:**278–279, **3:**279*f*
  sectional anatomy, **3:**173
  signal production in, **3:**271, **3:**271*f*
  significance of signal in, **3:**272, **3:**272*f*
  slice thickness in, **3:**287
  spectroscopy for, **3:**304, **3:**304*f*
  three-dimensional, **3:**287, **3:**287*f*
  unsafe, **3:**307
  of vessels, **3:**302, **3:**302*f*
  whole-body, **3:**305, **3:**305*f*
Magnetic resonance spectroscopy (MRS), **3:**304, **3:**304*f*
Magnetohydrodynamic effect, **3:**285, **3:**307
Magnetophosphenes, **3:**285, **3:**307
Magnification
  in angiography, **3:**325
  in mammography, **2:**385*t*–390*t*
Magnification radiography, **1:**22
Magnification technique, for mammography, **2:**409–411, **2:**409*b*, **2:**409*f*–410*f*
Main lobar fissure, as sonographic landmark, **3:**411, **3:**411*f*
Main trunk vessels, **3:**315, **3:**315*f*
Major calyces, **2:**277, **2:**277*f*
Major duodenal papilla, **2:**181*f*, **2:**185, **2:**185*f*
Malabsorption syndrome, **2:**190*t*–191*t*
Male
  breast
    calcifications of, **2:**408
    disease, epidemiology of, **2:**407
    routine projections of, **2:**407–408, **2:**407*f*–408*f*
  mammography in, **2:**407
  osteoporosis in, **2:**461
Male cystourethrography, **2:**313, **2:**313*f*
Male pelvis
  anatomy of, **1:**376, **1:**376*f*, **1:**376*t*
  AP projection of, **1:**382*f*
Male reproductive system
  anatomy of, **2:**332–333
    ductus deferens in, **2:**332, **2:**332*f*–333*f*
    ejaculatory ducts in, **2:**332, **2:**332*f*
    prostate in, **2:**332*f*–333*f*, **2:**333
    seminal vesicles in, **2:**332, **2:**333*f*
    summary of, **2:**334*b*
    testes in, **2:**332, **2:**332*f*
  radiography of, **2:**343–345
    of prostate, **2:**345, **2:**345*f*
    of seminal duct, **2:**343, **2:**343*f*–344*f*
  sectional anatomy of, **3:**206
Malignancy, **3:**484, **3:**509
Malleolus, **1:**64
Malleus, **2:**16
Mammary fat, **2:**361*f*
Mammillary bodies, sectional anatomy of, **3:**181–182
Mammillary process, **1:**419

I-19

Mammography, **2:**347–454
  artifacts on, **2:**378, **2:**378f–379f
  of augmented breast, **2:**402–408, **2:**402f
    complications of, **2:**400–401
    craniocaudal projection
      with full implant, **2:**402–408, **2:**402b, **2:**402f
      with implant displaced, **2:**403–404, **2:**403f–404f, **2:**404b
    mediolateral oblique projection
      with full implant, **2:**405, **2:**405b
      with implant displaced, **2:**406, **2:**406b
    MRI and, **2:**400–401
    ultrasonography and, **2:**400–401
  automatic exposure control in, **2:**391
  best practices in, **2:**393
  breast cancer screening, **2:**357
    diagnostic vs., **2:**358
    risk versus benefit, **2:**357–358
  compression in, **2:**384
  descriptive terminology for lesion location, **2:**394, **2:**394b–395b
  equipment for, **2:**351–352, **2:**351f
  evolution of, system, **2:**351, **2:**351f
  examination procedures for, **2:**382–391
  full-field digital, **2:**353
    labeling for, **2:**384
    manual technique chart, **2:**376t
  grids for, **2:**351
  historical development of, **2:**349–350, **2:**349f
  image enhancement methods for, **2:**408
    magnification technique in, **2:**409–411, **2:**409b, **2:**409f
    spot compression technique in, **2:**410–411, **2:**410f–411f, **2:**411b
  labeling of, **2:**385t–390t
  during lactation, **2:**362f–363f
  male, **2:**407
  method of examination for, **2:**378–394
  "mosaic" imaging or tiling in, **2:**382, **2:**383f
  of oversized breast, **2:**382, **2:**383f
  pathologic and mammographic findings in, **2:**365–375
    architectural distortions as, **2:**375, **2:**375f
    calcifications as, **2:**370–375, **2:**370f–374f
    masses as, **2:**365–368, **2:**365f–369f
      spiculated, **2:**366, **2:**369f
  patient preparation for, **2:**378, **2:**378f–381f
  posterior nipple line in, **2:**391, **2:**392f
  principles of, **2:**349–359
  procedures for, **2:**383f
  respiration during, **2:**391
  risk factors for, **2:**358–359
  routine projections, **2:**394
    craniocaudal, **2:**396–399
      central ray in, **2:**397
      evaluation criteria for, **2:**397, **2:**397b
      position of part for, **2:**396, **2:**396f
      position of patient for, **2:**396–397
      structures shown on, **2:**397
    mediolateral oblique, **2:**398–399
      evaluation criteria for, **2:**399, **2:**399b
      position of part for, **2:**398, **2:**398f
      position of patient for, **2:**398–399
      structures shown on, **2:**399
    summary of, **2:**394
  standards for, **2:**351
  summary of projections in, **2:**348t, **2:**394
  supplemental projections in, **2:**412–435
    applications of, **2:**412t
    axilla projection, for axillary tail, **2:**431
      evaluation criteria for, **2:**431, **2:**431b
      position of part for, **2:**431, **2:**431f
      position of patient for, **2:**431
      structures shown on, **2:**431
    captured lesion or coat-hanger, **2:**425, **2:**425b, **2:**425f–426f
    caudocranial, **2:**427–428
      evaluation criteria for, **2:**428b
      position of part for, **2:**427, **2:**427f
      position of patient for, **2:**427–428
      structures shown on, **2:**428
    craniocaudal projection for cleavage, **2:**419–420
      evaluation criteria for, **2:**420, **2:**420b
      position of part for, **2:**419, **2:**419f
      position of patient for, **2:**419–420
      structures shown on, **2:**420
    craniocaudal projection with roll lateral/roll medial, **2:**421–422, **2:**421f

Mammography (Continued)
      evaluation criteria for, **2:**422b
      position of part for, **2:**419f, **2:**421
      position of patient for, **2:**421–422, **2:**421f
      structures shown on, **2:**422, **2:**422f
    exaggerated craniocaudal, **2:**417–418
      evaluation criteria for, **2:**418, **2:**418b
      position of part for, **2:**417, **2:**417f
      position of patient for, **2:**417–418
      structures shown on, **2:**418
    lateromedial oblique, **2:**432–433
      evaluation criteria for, **2:**433, **2:**433b
      position of part for, **2:**432, **2:**432f
      position of patient for, **2:**432–433
      structures shown on, **2:**433
    mediolateral oblique, for axillary tail, **2:**429–430
      evaluation criteria for, **2:**430, **2:**430b
      position of part for, **2:**429, **2:**429f
      position of patient for, **2:**429–430
      structures shown on, **2:**430
    90-degree lateromedial, **2:**415–416
      evaluation criteria for, **2:**416b
      position of part for, **2:**413f, **2:**415, **2:**415f
      position of patient for, **2:**415–416
      structures shown on, **2:**416, **2:**416f
    90-degree mediolateral, **2:**413–414
      evaluation criteria for, **2:**414, **2:**414b
      position of part for, **2:**413–414, **2:**413f
      position of patient for, **2:**413–414
      structures shown on, **2:**414
    superolateral to inferomedial oblique, **2:**434–435
      evaluation criteria for, **2:**435b
      position of part for, **2:**434, **2:**434f
      position of patient for, **2:**434–435
      structures shown on, **2:**435, **2:**435f
    tangential, **2:**423
      evaluation criteria for, **2:**423b
      position of part for, **2:**423, **2:**423f–424f
      position of patient for, **2:**423
      structures shown on, **2:**423, **2:**424f
  xerography, **2:**350, **2:**350f
Mammography Quality Standards Act (MQSA), **2:**351
MammoSite applicator, **3:**507
Mandible, **2:**18f, **2:**20, **2:**20f, **2:**174f
  alveolar portion of, **2:**20, **2:**20f
  axiolateral and axiolateral oblique projection of, **2:**79–82, **2:**79b
    evaluation criteria for, **2:**81b
    position of part of, **2:**79, **2:**79f–80f
    position of patient in, **2:**79–81
    structures shown in, **2:**79–81, **2:**80f–81f
  body of, **2:**20, **2:**20f
    axiolateral oblique projection of, **2:**80f–81f
    axiolateral projection of, **2:**81f
    PA axial projection of, **2:**78, **2:**78b, **2:**78f
    PA projection of, **2:**75f, **2:**77–78, **2:**77b, **2:**77f
  condyle, **3:**184, **3:**184f
  lateral projection of, **2:**59f
  modified parietoacanthial projection of, **2:**63f
  panoramic tomography of, **2:**89, **2:**89f
  rami of, **2:**20, **2:**20f
    AP axial projection of, **2:**74f, **2:**84f
    axiolateral oblique projection of, **2:**80f
    axiolateral projection of, **2:**81f
    lateral projection of, **2:**36f
    PA axial projection of, **2:**76, **2:**76b, **2:**76f, **2:**78f
    PA projection of, **2:**75, **2:**75b, **2:**75f, **2:**77f
    submentovertical projection of, **2:**82f
  sectional anatomy of, **3:**175
  submentovertical projection of, **2:**49f, **2:**82, **2:**82b, **2:**82f, **2:**101f
  symphysis of, **2:**20, **2:**20f
    axiolateral oblique projection of, **2:**81f
    PA axial projection of, **2:**78f
    PA projection of, **2:**77f
    submentovertical projection of, **2:**82f
Mandibular angle, **2:**19f–20f
  as anterior landmark of skull, **2:**29f
  axiolateral oblique projection of, **2:**80f
  axiolateral projection of, **2:**81f
  as lateral landmark, **2:**29f
  PA projection of, **2:**77f
  parietoacanthial projection of, **2:**61f
Mandibular condyle, **2:**10f, **2:**19f–20f
  submentovertical projection of, **2:**49f

Mandibular fossa, **2:**14, **2:**14f, **2:**20f
  axiolateral oblique projection of, **2:**88f
Mandibular notch, **2:**19f–20f, **2:**20
Mandibular ramus, **2:**173f, **3:**185f
Mandrel, **3:**404
Manifold, for cardiac catheterization, **3:**376, **3:**376f
Manubriosternal joint, **1:**500
Manubrium, **1:**497–498
  sectional anatomy of, **3:**196–197, **3:**196f
Mapping, in maximum intensity projection, **3:**252, **3:**266
Marginal lymph sinus, **3:**318
Markers
  anatomic, **1:**27–28, **1:**27f, **1:**28b
  of bone turnover, **2:**462
  for trauma radiography, **2:**110, **2:**110f
Masks, **3:**33
Mass, Dierk, **3:**312–313
Masseters, **3:**186
Mastoid air cells, **2:**14, **2:**15f, **2:**17f, **3:**183
  PA axial projection of, **2:**47f
  PA projection of, **2:**75f
  parietoacanthial projection of, **2:**97f
Mastoid angle, of parietal bone, **2:**9f
Mastoid antrum, **2:**14, **2:**15f, **2:**16, **2:**17f
Mastoid fontanels, **2:**6, **2:**6f
Mastoid process, **2:**4f, **2:**14f–15f
  submentovertical projection of, **2:**49f
Mastoid tip, as surface landmark, **1:**51f
Mastoiditis, **2:**26t
Matrix, in CT, **3:**228, **3:**266
Maxillary bones, **2:**5f, **2:**18
  inferior portions of, **3:**184
  lateral projection of, **2:**59f
  in orbit, **2:**21, **2:**21f, **2:**53f
  parietoacanthial projection of, **2:**61f
Maxillary sinuses, **2:**18, **2:**22, **2:**22f–23f, **2:**53f
  acanthioparietal projection of, **2:**65f
  lateral projection of, **2:**59f, **2:**93f
  parietoacanthial projection of
    modified, **2:**63f
    open-mouth Waters method, **2:**98–99, **2:**98f–99f, **2:**99b
    Waters method, **2:**61f, **2:**96, **2:**96f, **2:**97b
  sectional anatomy of, **3:**184
  submentovertical projection of, **2:**49f, **2:**101f
Maximum aperture diameter, **1:**36t
Maximum intensity projection (MIP), **3:**222–223, **3:**223f, **3:**252, **3:**266
Mean, **2:**491
Mean glandular dose, **2:**354
Meatus, **1:**64
Mechanical thrombectomy, **3:**369, **3:**369f
Meckel diverticulum, **2:**190t–191t
Medial, definition of, **1:**65
Medial collateral ligament, **1:**278f
Medial condyle
  of femur, **1:**274, **1:**274f
  of tibia, **1:**272, **1:**272f
Medial epicondyle, of humerus, **1:**146, **1:**146f
Medial intercondylar tubercle, **1:**272f, **1:**345f
Medial malleolus, **1:**272f, **1:**273
Medial meniscus
  anatomy of, **1:**276f–277f, **1:**277
  double-contrast arthrography of, **2:**147, **2:**147f
Medial orbital wall, **2:**8f
Medial pterygoid lamina, **2:**11f, **2:**12
Medial rotation, **1:**75, **1:**75f
Medial-lateral oblique view, labeling codes for, **2:**385t–390t
Median aperture, **2:**155
Median nerve, **1:**144–145, **1:**144f
Mediastinal structures, in radiography of sternum, **1:**506
Mediastinum
  anatomy of, **1:**90–92, **1:**90f–91f
  CT of, **1:**92f, **1:**93t
  defined, **1:**83
  sectional anatomy of, **3:**192, **3:**202
Medical dosimetrist, **3:**509
Medical imaging, practice standards for, **1:**2
Medical physicist, **3:**509
Medical terminology, **1:**80, **1:**80t
Mediolateral lateral view, labeling codes for, **2:**385t–390t
Mediolateral oblique projection
  for axillary tail, **2:**429–430, **2:**429f
  with full implant, **2:**405, **2:**405b
  with implant displaced, **2:**406, **2:**406b

Mediolateral projection, 1:69, 1:70t
Medulla oblongata
　anatomy of, 2:152, 2:152f–153f
　sectional anatomy of, 3:184–185, 3:184f–185f, 3:187f
Medullary cavity, 1:56, 1:56f
Meglumine diatrizoate (Gastrografin, Gastroview), for simulation in radiation oncology, 3:492
Membranous labyrinth, 2:16
Membranous urethra, 2:279, 2:279f
Meninges, 3:404
　anatomy of, 2:153
　sectional anatomy of, 3:175
Meniscus, 1:62, 1:62f
Meniscus tear, 2:143t
Menstrual cycle, 2:330
Mental foramen, 2:19f–20f, 2:20
Mental point, 2:29f
Mental protuberance, 2:18f, 2:20, 2:20f
Mentomeatal line, 2:64f
Meperidine hydrochloride (Demerol), 2:316t
Merchant method, for tangential projection of patella and patellofemoral joint, 1:352–353, 1:352f–353f, 1:353b
Mesentery, 1:127, 1:127f
Mesocephalic skull, 2:30, 2:30f
Mesovarium, 2:329
Metabolic neurologic study, 3:474
Metacarpals, 1:143, 1:143f
Metacarpophalangeal (MCP) joints
　anatomy of, 1:147, 1:148f
　folio method, for first, 1:164, 1:164b, 1:164f–165f
Metal objects, 1:11, 1:12f
Metastable technetium-99 (^{99m}Tc), 3:439–440, 3:479
Metastasis
　to abdomen, 1:129t
　to bony thorax, 1:504t
　to cranium, 2:26t
　definition of, 3:509
　to hip, 3:379t
　to lower extremity, 1:282t
　radiation oncology for, 3:483, 3:509
　to shoulder girdle, 1:225t
　to thoracic viscera, 1:93t
　to upper extremity, 1:151t
　to vertebral column, 1:424t
Metatarsals, anatomy of, 1:270f, 1:271
Metatarsophalangeal (MTP) articulations, 1:278t, 1:280
Method, 1:77
Microbial fallout, 3:69
Micropuncture access sets, for angiography, 3:330, 3:330f
Microspheres, 3:362
Micturition, 2:278
Midaxillary plane, 1:46, 1:46f
Midazolam hydrochloride (Versed), 2:316t
Midbrain
　anatomy of, 2:152, 2:152f
　sectional anatomy of, 3:187f
Midcoronal plane, 1:46, 1:46f
Middle cerebral arteries
　CT angiography of, 3:251f
　MRI of, 3:303f
　sectional anatomy of, on axial plane, 3:180–181, 3:181f
Middle cranial fossa, 2:6
Middle hepatic vein, as sonographic landmark, 3:411, 3:411f
Middle nasal conchae
　anatomy of, 2:8, 2:8f
　sectional anatomy of, 3:174
Middle phalanges, 1:278
Midfoot, 1:270
Midsagittal plane, 2:29f, 1:46, 1:46f
Milk ducts, examination of, 2:436–437, 2:436f–437f
Milk of calcium, 2:373, 2:373f
Miller-Abbott tube, 2:233
Milliamperage (mA), 1:18
Minimum intensity projection (MINIP), 3:222–223
Minor calyces, 2:277, 2:277f
Misregistration, in digital subtraction angiography, 3:324, 3:404
Mobile radiography, 2:1–28
　of abdomen, 2:14–17
　　AP or PA projection, in left lateral decubitus position, 2:16–17, 2:16f–17f, 2:17b
　　AP projection, 2:14–17, 2:14b, 2:14f–15f
　of cervical spine, 2:24–27
　　best practices in, 2:26–27

Mobile radiography (Continued)
　　lateral projection, in right or left dorsal decubitus position, 2:24–25, 2:24f–25f, 2:25b
　of chest, 2:10–13
　　AP or PA projection, in right or left lateral decubitus position, 2:12–13, 2:12f–13f, 2:13b
　　AP projection, in upright or supine position, 2:10–13, 2:10f–11f, 2:11b
　digital, 2:2, 2:3f
　　of cervical spine, lateral projection, in right or left dorsal decubitus position, 2:24
　examination in, 2:7–8
　of femur, 2:20–23
　　AP projection, 2:20–23, 2:20f–21f, 2:21b
　　lateral projection, in mediolateral or lateromedial projection, 2:22–23, 2:22f–23f, 2:23b
　initial procedures in, 2:7, 2:7b
　isolation considerations with, 2:7
　machines for, 2:2, 2:3f
　for obese patients, 1:43
　for operating room, 3:57–64
　　of cervical spine, 3:57, 3:57b, 3:57f–58f
　　of extremity, 3:61–64, 3:64b
　　　for ankle fracture, 3:61f
　　　for ankle with antibiotic beads, 3:62f
　　　for fifth metatarsal nonhealing fracture, 3:63f
　　　for forearm fracture, 3:62f
　　　for hip joint replacement, 3:61f
　　　for tibial plateau fracture, 3:62f
　　　for total shoulder arthroplasty, 3:63f
　　　for wrist, 3:64f
　　of thoracic or lumbar spine, 3:59, 3:59b, 3:59f–60f
　patient considerations with, 2:8–9
　　fractures as, 2:8
　　interfering devices as, 2:8, 2:9f
　　patient mobility as, 2:8
　　positioning and asepsis as, 2:9
　of pelvis, 2:18–19
　　AP projection, 2:18–19, 2:18f–19f, 2:19b
　principles of, 2:2–9, 2:2f
　radiation safety with, 2:6–7, 2:6f
　technical considerations for, 2:3–5, 2:3f
　　anode heel effect as, 2:5, 2:5t
　　grid as, 2:3–4, 2:4f
　　radiographic technique charts as, 2:5, 2:5f
　　source-to-image receptor distance as, 2:5
Mobility, in mobile radiography, 2:8
Modified barium swallow study (MBSS), 2:197
　contrast set up for, 2:198f
　team members of, 2:198–201
Modified Seldinger technique, 3:404
Mold technique, for brachytherapy, 3:487
Molecular imaging, 3:435–480
Moore method, for PA oblique projection, of sternum, 1:510, 1:510f–511f, 1:511b
Morphine sulfate, 2:316t
Morphometric x-ray absorptiometry, 2:484f, 2:491
Mortise joint
　AP oblique projection in medial rotation of, 1:324–325, 1:324f–325f
　evaluation criteria for, 1:325b
Motion control, 1:12–13, 1:12f
　in involuntary muscles, 1:13
　in obese patients, 1:42
　in voluntary muscles, 1:13
Mouth
　anatomy of, 2:171–172, 2:172f
　salivary glands of. See Salivary glands
MR-guided radiation therapy, 3:282, 3:282f
MRI. See Magnetic resonance imaging
MRI conditional implants, 3:284
MRI medical director (MRMD), 3:307
MRI safe implants, 3:284
MRI safety expert (MRSE), 3:284, 3:307
MRI safety officer (MRSO), 3:284, 3:307
Mucosa, of vagina, 2:330
Multihead gamma camera systems, 3:446–447
Multi-infarct dementia, 3:155
Multileaf collimation (MLC), 3:491, 3:491f, 3:509
Multiplanar reconstruction, in CT, 3:239, 3:239f, 3:266
Multiplanar reformatting (MPR), 3:222, 3:222f
Multiple exams, in mobile radiography, 2:26
Multiple imaging windows, in CT, 3:230f
Multiple myeloma, 1:379t, 1:424t
　of bony thorax, 1:504t
　of cranium, 2:26t

Multiple scan average dose (MSAD), 3:256, 3:266
Multislice detectors, 3:233
Multislice helical CT, 3:233
Musculoskeletal system
　diagnostic medical sonography of, 3:419, 3:419f
　MRI of, 3:299, 3:299f–301f
Musculoskeletal system disorders, in older adults, 3:156, 3:156f–157f
Mutations, cancer and, 3:484
Mycoplasma pneumonia, 3:138
Myelography, 2:160–164
　cervical, 2:163f
　contrast media for, 2:160–161, 2:160f
　conus projection in, 2:162
　of dentate ligament, 2:163f
　examination procedure for, 2:161–163, 2:161f
　foramen magnum, 2:163f
　lumbar, 2:162f
　preparation of examining room for, 2:161, 2:161f
　subarachnoid space, 2:160, 2:163f
Myeloma, multiple, 1:379t, 1:424t
　of bony thorax, 1:504t
　of cranium, 2:26t
Myocardial infarction, 3:404
　echocardiography after, 3:430, 3:432f
Myocardium, 3:316, 3:404
Myometrium, diagnostic medical sonography of, 3:424

N
Nasal bones, 2:5f, 2:18
　lateral projection of, 2:55f, 2:59f, 2:68, 2:68f–69f, 2:69b
　sectional anatomy of, 3:175, 3:183
Nasal concha, sectional anatomy of, 3:174
Nasal septum, 2:19, 1:87f
　anatomy of, 2:175f
　modified parietoacanthial projection of, 2:63f
Nasal spine, 2:7, 2:7f
Nasion, 2:7, 2:7f, 2:29f
　as lateral landmark, 2:29f
Nasopharynx, 2:17f, 1:87f, 1:88, 3:185f
　anatomy of, 2:174, 2:175f
National Council on Radiation Protection (NCRP), 1:20
Navicular bone, 1:271
Naviculocuneiform articulation, 1:278t, 1:279f
Neck
　AP projection of
　　central ray for, 1:95
　　collimation for, 1:95
　　evaluation criteria for, 1:96b
　　position of part for, 1:95, 1:95f
　　position of patient for, 1:95–96
　　structures shown on, 1:96, 1:96f
　lateral projection of, 1:97–98
　　central ray for, 1:98, 1:98f
　　collimation for, 1:98
　　evaluation criteria for, 1:98b
　　position of part for, 1:97, 1:97f
　　position of patient for, 1:97
　　structures shown on, 1:98
　radiography of
　　AP projection of pharynx and larynx in, 2:200, 2:200f–201f, 2:201b
　　deglutition in, 2:197
　　soft palate, pharynx, and larynx in, 2:197
　　technical considerations in, 2:197, 2:197f
　　soft tissue, in children, 3:110–111, 3:110f–111f
Neck brace, trauma radiography with, 2:109f
Needle(s)
　for angiography, 3:329, 3:329f
　handling of, 1:4, 1:4f
　for venipuncture, 2:318–319
　　anchoring of, 2:323, 2:323f
　　discarding of, 2:324, 2:324f
Needle-wire localization, of breast, 2:438
Neer method, for tangential projection, of supraspinatus "outlet," of shoulder girdle, 1:242–243, 1:242f–243f, 1:242t, 1:243b
Neointimal hyperplasia, 3:404
Neonatal intensive care unit (NICU), mobile considerations for, 3:115–123
　elements of an acceptable image, 3:115
　neonate nuances in, 3:116–117, 3:116f
　neonate soft tissue landmarks, 3:115, 3:115f
　safe environment, practicing, 3:124, 3:124f
　team-based approach in, 3:115

I-21

Neonate
　abdomen
　　portable, **3:**119, **3:**119*b*, **3:**119*f*
　　　for line placement, **3:**122–123, **3:**122*b*, **3:**122*f*–123*f*
　　portable decubitus, **3:**120, **3:**120*b*, **3:**120*f*
　　portable dorsal decubitus, **3:**121, **3:**121*b*, **3:**121*f*
　chest
　　portable, for line placement, **3:**122–123, **3:**122*b*, **3:**122*f*–123*f*
　　portable AP, **3:**117, **3:**117*b*, **3:**117*f*
　　portable decubitus, **3:**118, **3:**118*b*, **3:**118*f*
　　portable dorsal decubitus, **3:**121, **3:**121*b*, **3:**121*f*
　cranium of, **2:**6, **2:**6*f*
　development of, **3:**73
　nuances of, **3:**116–117, **3:**116*f*
　soft tissue landmarks of, **3:**115, **3:**115*f*
Nephrogram phase, of kidney, **2:**294
Nephron, **2:**277, **2:**277*f*
Nephron loop, **2:**277, **2:**277*f*
Nephroptosis, **2:**280*t*
Nephrostogram, **2:**303, **2:**303*f*
Nephrotomography, **2:**301
　AP projection in, **2:**301, **2:**301*f*
　percutaneous renal puncture for, **2:**302, **2:**302*f*
Nephrotoxic, definition of, **3:**404
Nephrourography, infusion, equipment for, **2:**290
Nerve tissue, cancer arising from, **3:**485*t*
Nervous system disorders, in older adults, **3:**154–155
Neuroma, acoustic, **2:**26*t*
NICU. *See* Neonatal intensive care unit
Nipple
　anatomy of, **2:**360, **2:**361*f*
　ductography of, **2:**436–437, **2:**436*f*–437*f*
　in mammography, **2:**384
　in profile spot compression, **2:**385*t*–390*t*
Nitrogen-13 (^{13}N), in nuclear medicine, **3:**442*t*
Noctec (chloral hydrate), **2:**316*t*
Noise
　in CT, **3:**244, **3:**266
　in MRI, **3:**307
Nonaccidental trauma, to children, **3:**127–131, **3:**127*f*–130*f*
　imaging protocol for, **3:**131, **3:**131*b*, **3:**132*f*–133*f*
Nondisplaced fracture, **1:**64
Noninvasive imaging, **3:**404
Noninvasive technique, diagnostic medical sonography as, **3:**408, **3:**433
Non-MRI personnel, **3:**307
Nonocclusive, definition of, **3:**404
Nonsterile team members, **3:**32
Nonvascular interventional procedures, **3:**370, **3:**370*f*
Norgaard method, for AP oblique projection, in medial rotation of hand, **1:**172–173
　evaluation criteria for, **1:**173*b*
　position of part of, **1:**172–173, **1:**173*f*
　position of patient for, **1:**172
　structures shown on, **1:**173, **1:**173*f*
Notch, **1:**64
Notification values, for CT, **3:**256
Nuclear cardiology, in nuclear medicine, **3:**454–455
Nuclear magnetic resonance (NMR) imaging, **3:**270, **3:**307
Nuclear medicine, **3:**435–480
　best practices for, **3:**477
　clinical, **3:**453–459
　　bone scintigraphy, **3:**453–454
　　central nervous system imaging, **3:**455
　　endocrine system imaging, **3:**455–456
　　gastrointestinal system imaging, **3:**456–457
　　genitourinary nuclear medicine, **3:**457
　　imaging for infection, **3:**457–458
　　nuclear cardiology, **3:**454–455
　　respiratory imaging, **3:**458
　　sentinel node imaging, **3:**458
　　special imaging procedures, **3:**459
　　therapeutic nuclear medicine, **3:**459
　　tumor imaging, **3:**459
　defined, **3:**436
　future of, **3:**475–476
　　hybrid imaging, **3:**471*f*, **3:**475–476, **3:**476*f*
　　radioimmunotherapy, **3:**475
　general, **3:**436
　historical development of, **3:**436
　imaging methods, **3:**449–453
　　combined SPECT and CT imaging, **3:**453, **3:**453*f*
　　dynamic imaging, **3:**450, **3:**451*f*
　　SPECT imaging, **3:**451–452, **3:**451*f*–452*f*

Nuclear medicine *(Continued)*
　　static/planar imaging, **3:**449
　　whole-body imaging, **3:**450, **3:**450*f*
　instrumentation in, **3:**445–449
　　modern-day gamma camera, **3:**445–447, **3:**445*f*
　　processing systems, **3:**447–448, **3:**447*f*–448*f*
　　quantitative analysis, **3:**449, **3:**449*f*
　physical principle of, **3:**438*f*, **3:**439–442
　　basic nuclear physics, **3:**439
　　nuclear pharmacy, **3:**440*f*–441*f*, **3:**442*t*
　principles of, **3:**436–480
　radiation safety in, **3:**444, **3:**444*f*
Nuclear particle accelerator, **3:**463, **3:**479
Nuclear pharmacy, **3:**439–442, **3:**440*f*–441*f*, **3:**442*t*
Nuclear physics, **3:**439, **3:**440*f*
Nuclear reactors, **3:**436, **3:**479
　in radiation oncology, **3:**488
Nucleus, atomic, **3:**271, **3:**307
Nucleus pulposus, **3:**293*f*
　anatomy of, **1:**413
　herniated, **1:**413
　sectional anatomy of, **3:**191–192
Nuclide, **3:**439, **3:**479
Nulliparous uterus, **2:**330
Nutrient artery, **1:**57, **1:**57*f*
Nutrient foramen, **1:**57, **1:**57*f*

O

Obese patients, working effectively with, **1:**34–44, **1:**35*f*
　automatic exposure control and anatomically programmed radiography systems in, **1:**42
　Bucky grid in, **1:**42, **1:**42*f*
　communication in, **1:**38
　equipment for, **1:**35–36, **1:**35*f*, **1:**36*t*
　exposure factors in, **1:**42–44
　field light size, **1:**41, **1:**41*f*
　focal spot in, **1:**42
　image receptor sizes and collimation in, **1:**40–41, **1:**41*f*
　imaging challenges in, **1:**38–41, **1:**38*f*–39*f*
　landmarks in, **1:**39–40, **1:**40*f*
　mobile radiography, **1:**43
　oblique and lateral projections in, **1:**40
　radiation dose for, **1:**43–44
　technical considerations for, **1:**43*b*
　transportation in, **1:**36–37, **1:**37*f*
Object-to-image receptor distance (OID), **3:**325
Oblique fissures of lungs
　anatomy of, **1:**85*f*, **1:**86
　sectional anatomy of, **3:**200, **3:**200*f*
Oblique fracture, **1:**64*f*
Oblique plane, **1:**46*f*, **1:**47
　pancreas in, **3:**417, **3:**433
Oblique position, **1:**74–75, **1:**74*f*–75*f*
Oblique projection, **1:**67*t*, **1:**69, **1:**70*f*, **1:**74*f*
　of obese patients, **1:**40
Obstetric ultrasonography, **3:**424–427
　in first trimester, **3:**424, **3:**425*f*–426*f*
　history of, **3:**409
　in second trimester, **3:**426, **3:**426*f*–427*f*
　in third trimester, **3:**426–427
Obturator foramen, anatomy of, **1:**371*f*, **1:**372, **1:**382*f*
Obturator internus muscle, **3:**217, **3:**217*f*
Occipital angle, of parietal bone, **2:**9*f*
Occipital bone, **2:**4*f*–5*f*, **2:**12–13, **2:**12*f*–13*f*, **1:**414*f*
　AP axial projection of, **2:**43*f*
　PA axial projection of, **2:**47*f*
　sectional anatomy of, **3:**174, **3:**180–181
　submentovertical projection of, **2:**49*f*
Occipital condyles, **2:**12*f*, **2:**13, **1:**414
Occipital lobe, **3:**180–181
　sectional anatomy of, on midsagittal plane, **3:**187*f*
Occipitoatlantal joints, **2:**13
Occlusal plane, **1:**48, **1:**48*f*–49*f*
Occlusion, **3:**404
OctreoScan, **3:**459
Odontoid process, **2:**12*f*, **1:**414
　submentovertical projection of, **2:**49*f*
Oil cyst, **2:**367*f*
Older adults. *See also* Aging
　age-related competencies, **3:**162
　attitudes toward, **3:**151–152
　chronic conditions of, **3:**150, **3:**150*b*
　contrast agent administration in, **3:**162
　demographics of, **3:**148–168, **3:**148*f*, **3:**150*f*
　economic status of, **3:**149, **3:**149*f*

Older adults *(Continued)*
　exercise for, **3:**153
　health care budget for, **3:**149
　health complaints of, **3:**153, **3:**153*b*
　patient care for, **3:**161–162
　　communication in, **3:**161
　　patient and family education in, **3:**161
　　skin care in, **3:**161
　　transportation and lifting in, **3:**161
　radiographer's role with, **3:**162–163
　radiographic positioning of, **3:**163–167
　　for chest, **3:**163–164, **3:**164*f*
　　for lower extremity, **3:**167, **3:**167*f*
　　for pelvis and hip, **3:**165, **3:**165*f*
　　for spine, **3:**164–165, **3:**165*f*
　　technical factors in, **3:**167
　　for upper extremity, **3:**166, **3:**166*f*
　summary of pathology in, **3:**160*t*
　tips for working with, **3:**161*b*
Olecranon fossa, anatomy of, **1:**146, **1:**146*f*
Olecranon process
　anatomy of, **1:**145, **1:**145*f*
　PA axial projection of, **1:**208, **1:**208*b*, **1:**208*f*
Omenta, **1:**127, **1:**127*f*
Oncologist, **3:**509
Oncology, radiation. *See* Radiation oncology
Opaque arthrography, **2:**142–143, **2:**142*f*
Open fracture, **1:**64, **1:**64*f*
Open scanners, in MRI, **3:**276–277, **3:**276*f*–277*f*
Open surgical biopsy, of breast, **2:**438
Open-mouth technique, for atlas and axis, **1:**428–429, **1:**428*f*–429*f*, **1:**429*b*
Operating room
　contamination control in, **1:**6, **1:**6*f*–7*f*
　dance of, **3:**34–36, **3:**34*f*
Operating room attire, **3:**32*f*, **3:**33
Operating room suite, **3:**32*f*
Operative (immediate) cholangiography, **3:**39–41, **3:**40*f*, **3:**41*f*
Operator's console
　for CT, **3:**237, **3:**237*f*
　for MRI, **3:**273, **3:**273*f*
Optic canal, **2:**4*f*, **2:**50*f*, **2:**52*f*
　sectional anatomy of, **3:**174–175
　sphenoid canal and, **2:**10*f*–11*f*, **2:**11
Optic chiasm, **3:**184*f*, **3:**189*f*
Optic foramen, **2:**3*f*
　anatomy of, **2:**11, **2:**11*f*, **2:**18*f*, **2:**50, **2:**50*f*, **2:**52*f*
　sectional anatomy of, **3:**184*f*
Optic groove, **2:**4*f*, **2:**10*f*, **2:**11
Optic nerve
　anatomy of, **2:**52*f*–53*f*
　sectional anatomy of, **3:**183, **3:**188*f*
Optic tracts, sectional anatomy of, **3:**181–182
Optical coherence tomography (OCT), **3:**378*t*, **3:**391, **3:**391*f*, **3:**404
Oral cavity. *See* Mouth
Oral vestibule, anatomy of, **2:**172
Orbit(s), **2:**21, **2:**21*f*
　acanthioparietal projection of, **2:**65*f*
　apex of, **2:**50
　blowout fracture of, **2:**51*f*
　lateral projection of, **2:**55, **2:**55*b*, **2:**55*f*
　localization of foreign bodies within, **2:**54–57, **2:**54*f*
　PA axial projection of, **2:**56, **2:**56*b*, **2:**56*f*
　parietoacanthial projection of, **2:**51*f*, **2:**61*f*
　preliminary examination of, **2:**54
　radiography of, **2:**50–51, **2:**50*f*
　roof of, lateral projection of, **2:**36*f*
　root of, **3:**184*f*–185*f*
Orbital fat, **2:**52*f*
Orbital mass, needle biopsy of, CT for, **3:**240*f*
Orbital plate, **2:**4*f*, **2:**7, **2:**7*f*
Orbital wall, medial, **2:**8*f*
Orbitomeatal line (OML), **2:**130
Organified, definition of, **3:**455, **3:**479
Oropharynx, **1:**87*f*, **1:**88
　anatomy of, **2:**172, **2:**174, **2:**174*f*–175*f*
Orthopedic metal artifact reduction (OMAR), **3:**245, **3:**245*f*
Os coxae. *See also* Hip bone
　anatomy of, **1:**371
Osgood-Schlatter disease, **1:**282*t*
Ossification, **1:**57
　endochondral, **1:**57
　intermembranous, **1:**57

Ossification (Continued)
primary, **1**:57, **1**:57f
secondary, **1**:57f, **1**:58
Ossification centers, primary and secondary, **1**:57, **1**:57f
Osteoarthritis, **1**:379t
of lower extremity, **1**:282t
in older adults, **3**:156, **3**:160t
of shoulder girdle, **1**:225t
of upper extremity, **1**:151t
of vertebral column, **1**:424t
Osteoblasts, **2**:459, **2**:459f, **2**:491
Osteochondroma, **1**:282t
in children, **3**:135, **3**:135f
Osteoclastoma, **1**:282t
Osteoclasts, **2**:459, **2**:459f, **2**:491
Osteogenesis imperfecta (OI), **3**:134, **3**:134f
Osteoid osteoma, **1**:282t
in children, **3**:136, **3**:136f
Osteology, **1**:46, **1**:55–59
appendicular skeleton in, **1**:55, **1**:55f, **1**:55t
axial skeleton in, **1**:55, **1**:55f, **1**:55t
bone development in, **1**:57–58
bone vessels and nerves in, **1**:57, **1**:57f
classification of bones in, **1**:59, **1**:59f
fractures of, **1**:64, **1**:64f
general bone features in, **1**:56, **1**:56f
markings and features of, **1**:64
Osteoma, osteoid, **1**:282t
in children, **3**:136, **3**:136f
Osteomalacia, **1**:282t, **2**:462, **2**:491
Osteomyelitis, **2**:26t, **1**:151t, **1**:282t, **1**:504t
Osteopenia, **2**:471, **2**:488, **2**:491
Osteopetrosis
of lower extremity, **1**:282t
of shoulder girdle, **1**:225t
of skull, **2**:26t, **1**:379t
of upper extremity, **1**:151t
of vertebral column, **1**:424t
Osteophytosis, **2**:491
Osteoporosis, **2**:26t, **1**:282t, **2**:461–464, **2**:491
biochemical markers for, **2**:462
bone densitometry for, **2**:456
bone health recommendations for, **2**:464, **2**:464t
of bony thorax, **1**:504t
cause of, **2**:461
in children, **2**:487
definition of, **2**:461
fractures and falls in, **2**:463, **2**:463f
medicines for, **2**:462, **2**:462t
in men, **2**:461
in older adults, **3**:156, **3**:160t
of pelvis and proximal femora, **1**:379t
primary, **2**:462, **2**:492
risk factors for, **2**:461
secondary, **2**:462, **2**:492
of shoulder girdle, **1**:225t
type I, **2**:462, **2**:492
type II, **2**:462, **2**:492
of upper extremity, **1**:151t
of vertebral column, **1**:424t
Osteosarcoma, **1**:151t, **1**:282t
in children, **3**:137
Ottonello method, for AP projection, of cervical vertebrae, **1**:442–443, **1**:442f–443f, **1**:443b
Outer canthus, **2**:29f
Oval window, **2**:16, **2**:17f
Ovarian cyst
CT of, **3**:241f
diagnostic medical sonography of, **3**:413f, **3**:424
Ovarian follicles, **2**:329, **2**:329f
Ovarian ligament, **2**:330f
Ovaries
anatomy of, **2**:329, **2**:329f–330f
diagnostic medical sonography of, **3**:411, **3**:411f, **3**:413f, **3**:424, **3**:425f
sectional anatomy of, **3**:206
Over-the-needle cannula, **2**:318f, **2**:319
Ovulation, **2**:329
Ovum, **2**:329
Oximetry, **3**:404
Oxygen saturation, **3**:404
Oxygen-15 (^{15}O), in nuclear medicine, **3**:442t

P

PA lumbar spine, DXA of, **2**:478–480, **2**:478f–479f
PACS. *See* Picture archiving communication system

Paget disease
of bony thorax, **1**:504t
of breast, **2**:376t–377t
of cranium, **2**:26t
of lower extremity, **1**:282t
of pelvis and hip, **1**:379t
of vertebral column, **1**:424t
Pain management, interventional, **2**:166, **2**:166f
Palatine bones, **2**:5f, **2**:19
in orbit, **2**:21, **2**:21f
sectional anatomy of, **3**:175
Palliation, **3**:509
Palmar, definition of, **1**:65
Palmaz, Julio, **3**:312–313
Pancreas
anatomy of, **2**:171, **2**:171f, **2**:181f, **2**:184f–185f, **2**:186, **2**:187f
diagnostic medical sonography of, **3**:415f, **3**:417, **3**:417f
endocrine, **2**:186
exocrine, **2**:186
sectional anatomy of
on axial plane, **3**:210, **3**:210f–212f
on coronal plane, **3**:221f
sectional image of, **2**:187f
Pancreatic duct, anatomy of, **2**:181f, **2**:185f, **2**:186
Pancreatic juice, **2**:186
Pancreatic pseudocyst, **2**:190t–191t
Pancreatitis, **2**:190t–191t
Pangynecography, **2**:336, **2**:340, **2**:340f
Panoramic tomography of mandible, **2**:89, **2**:89f
Pantomography of mandible, **2**:89
Papilloma, **2**:376t–377t
Paramagnetic contrast agent, **3**:291, **3**:307
Parametric image, **3**:460, **3**:479
Paranasal sinuses, **2**:22–23, **2**:22f
in children, **3**:105f, **3**:108, **3**:109f
development of, **2**:22
ethmoidal, **2**:8f, **2**:22f–23f, **2**:23
CT of, **2**:8f
lateral projection of, **2**:93f
PA axial projection of, **2**:38f, **2**:67f, **2**:94–95, **2**:94f–95f, **2**:95b
parietoacanthial projection of, **2**:97f
submentovertical projection of, **2**:100–101, **2**:100f–101f, **2**:101b
frontal, **2**:5f, **2**:7f, **2**:22f–23f, **2**:23, **2**:53f
lateral projection of, **2**:59f, **2**:93f
PA axial projection of, **2**:38f, **2**:67f, **2**:94–95, **2**:94f–95f, **2**:95b
parietoacanthial projection of, **2**:97f
functions of, **2**:22
lateral projection of, **2**:92, **2**:92b, **2**:92f–93f
maxillary, **2**:22, **2**:22f–23f, **2**:53f
acanthioparietal projection of, **2**:65f
lateral projection of, **2**:59f, **2**:93f
parietoacanthial projection of
modified, **2**:63f
open-mouth Waters method, **2**:98–99, **2**:98f–99f, **2**:99b
Waters method, **2**:61f, **2**:96, **2**:96f, **2**:97b
submentovertical projection of, **2**:49f, **2**:101f
PA axial projection of (Caldwell method), **2**:67f
sphenoidal, **2**:5f, **2**:10–11, **2**:10f, **2**:22f–23f, **2**:23
lateral projection of, **2**:36f, **2**:93f
PA axial projection of, **2**:47f, **2**:95f
parietoacanthial projection of, open-mouth Waters method for, **2**:98–99, **2**:98f–99f, **2**:99b
submentovertical projection of, **2**:49f, **2**:100–101, **2**:100f–101f, **2**:101b
technical considerations for radiography of, **2**:90–91, **2**:90f–91f
Parathyroid glands, **1**:88, **1**:88f
Parathyroid hormone, in osteoporosis, **2**:462t
Parenchyma, **1**:85–86
diagnostic medical sonography of, **3**:414, **3**:433
Parent nuclide, **3**:439, **3**:479
Parents, discussing radiation risks and benefits with, **3**:80–81
Parietal, definition of, **1**:65
Parietal bones
anatomy of, **2**:3f–5f, **2**:9, **2**:9f
AP axial projection of, **2**:43f
PA axial projection of, **2**:38f
sectional anatomy of, **3**:174f, **3**:178f, **3**:179–180
Parietal eminence, **2**:9, **2**:9f

Parietal lobe, sectional anatomy of, **3**:178f, **3**:179–180
on axial plane, **3**:178f
on midsagittal plane, **3**:187f
Parietal peritoneum, **1**:127, **1**:127f
Parietal pleura, **1**:86
Parietoacanthial projection, **1**:70t
of facial bones, **2**:60, **2**:60b, **2**:60f–61f
modified, **2**:62, **2**:62f–63f
of maxillary sinuses
open-mouth Waters method, **2**:98–99, **2**:98f–99f, **2**:99b
Waters method, **2**:96, **2**:96f, **2**:97b
of orbit, **2**:57, **2**:57b, **2**:57f
Parotid duct
anatomy of, **2**:173, **2**:173f
sialography of, **2**:192f
Parotid gland
anatomy of, **2**:171f, **2**:173, **2**:173f–174f
lateral projection of, **2**:195–196, **2**:195f–196f, **2**:196b
sectional anatomy of, **3**:189–190, **3**:189f
sialography of, **2**:192f
tangential projection of, **2**:193–194
central ray for, **2**:194
collimation for, **2**:194
evaluation criteria for, **2**:194b
position of patient for, **2**:193–194
in prone body position, **2**:193, **2**:193f
respiration during, **2**:193
structures shown on, **2**:194, **2**:194f
in supine body position, **2**:193, **2**:193f
Pars interarticularis, **1**:419, **1**:419f
Partial volume averaging, in CT, **3**:266–267
Particle accelerator, **3**:463, **3**:479
Passive shielding, in MRI, **3**:307
Passively scattered particle therapy, **3**:502, **3**:509
Patella, **1**:349–350
anatomy of, **1**:275, **1**:275f
evaluation criteria for, **1**:349b
mediolateral projection of, **1**:350, **1**:350b, **1**:350f
PA projection of, **1**:349–350, **1**:349f
tangential projection of
Hughston method for, **1**:351, **1**:351f
Merchant method for, **1**:352–353, **1**:352f–353f
Settegast method for, **1**:354–355, **1**:354f–355f, **1**:355b
Patellar surface, **1**:274f
anatomy of, **1**:275, **1**:275f
of knee joint, **1**:276f
Patellofemoral joint, **1**:351–355
anatomy of, **1**:278t, **1**:280, **1**:280f
evaluation criteria for, **1**:351b
tangential projection of
Hughston method for, **1**:351, **1**:351f
Merchant method for, **1**:352–353, **1**:352f–353f
Settegast method for, **1**:354–355, **1**:354f–355f, **1**:355b
Patency, definition of, **3**:404
Patent ductus arteriosus, cardiac catheterization for, **3**:396
Patent foramen ovale, **3**:396
Patent foramen ovale closure (PFO), **3**:393, **3**:404
Pathogen contamination, control of, **1**:4
Pathologic fractures, in children, **3**:135–137
Pathologist, **3**:509
Patient(s)
clothing, jewelry, and surgical dressings of, **1**:11, **1**:11f
ill or injured, **1**:7–8, **1**:8f
interacting with, **1**:7–8
preexposure instructions to, **1**:14
Patient care, for trauma patient, **2**:111, **2**:112t
Patient education, for older adults, **3**:161
Patient positioning, for trauma radiography, **2**:110, **2**:110f
pDXA. *See* Peripheral dual energy x-ray absorptiometry
Peak bone mass, **2**:460–461, **2**:491
Pearson method, for bilateral AP projection, of acromioclavicular articulation, **1**:249–250, **1**:249f–250f, **1**:250b
Pectoralis major, anatomy of, **2**:360, **2**:360f
Pectoralis minor, anatomy of, **2**:360f
Pediatric imaging, **3**:71–146
Pediatric sonography, **3**:421, **3**:421f
Pedicles
of typical cervical vertebra, **1**:415
of vertebral arch, **1**:413
Pelvic cavity, **1**:49, **1**:49f, **1**:127, **1**:376, **1**:376f
Pelvic curve, **1**:411f
Pelvic girdle, **1**:371
Pelvic kidney, **2**:280t
Pelvic pneumography, **2**:336, **2**:340, **2**:340f

I-23

Pelvic sacral foramina, **1:**421
Pelvicaliceal system, **2:**275
  retrograde urography of, **2:**304–305, **2:**304*f*–305*f*
Pelvimetry, **2:**342
Pelvis, **1:**369–408
  abbreviations in, **1:**378*b*
  alternative positioning landmark for, **1:**378
  anatomy of, **1:**371–378
    female, **1:**376, **1:**376*f*, **1:**376*t*, **1:**382*f*
    male, **1:**376, **1:**376*f*, **1:**376*t*, **1:**382*f*
  anterior bones of
    AP axial outlet projection of, Taylor method for, **1:**402–403, **1:**402*f*–403*f*, **1:**403*b*
    superoinferior axial inlet projection of, Bridgman method for, **1:**404, **1:**404*b*, **1:**404*f*
  AP projection of, **1:**381–385, **1:**382*f*
    for congenital dislocation of hip, **1:**383, **1:**383*f*
    evaluation criteria for, **1:**383*b*
    for trauma, **2:**125, **2:**125*f*
  articulations of, **1:**375
  brim of, **1:**376, **1:**376*f*
  in children, **3:**98
    general principles of, **3:**98
    image evaluation for, **3:**96*t*
    initial images in, **3:**98
    positioning and immobilization for, **3:**93*f*, **3:**98
    preparation and communication for, **3:**98
  false or greater, **1:**376, **1:**376*f*, **3:**422, **3:**433
  in geriatric patients, **3:**165, **3:**165*f*
  inferior aperture or outlet, **1:**376, **1:**376*f*
  joints of, **1:**375*f*, **1:**375*t*
  lateral projection of, **1:**384–385, **1:**384*f*–385*f*, **1:**385*b*
  localization planes of, **1:**390*f*
  localizing anatomic structures in, **1:**377–378, **1:**377*f*
  mobile radiography of, **2:**18–19, **2:**18*f*–19*f*
  MRI of, **3:**298, **3:**298*f*
  radiation protection for, **1:**380
  radiography of, **1:**380–405
  sample exposure technique chart routine projections for, **1:**379*t*
  summary of pathology of, **1:**379*t*
  summary of projections for, **1:**370, **1:**370*t*
  trauma radiography of, **2:**125, **2:**125*f*
  true or lesser, **1:**376, **1:**376*f*, **3:**422, **3:**434
Pencil beam scanning (PBS), **3:**502, **3:**503*f*, **3:**509
Pencil-beam techniques, for DXA, **2:**458, **2:**468–471, **2:**468*f*, **2:**491
Penetrating trauma, **2:**105
Penis, **2:**332, **2:**333*f*
Percent coefficient of variation, **2:**492
Percutaneous, definition of, **3:**404
Percutaneous antegrade pyelography, **2:**303
Percutaneous antegrade urography, **2:**283
Percutaneous coronary intervention (PCI), **3:**386–387, **3:**386*f*–387*f*
Percutaneous left ventricular support device, **3:**392, **3:**392*f*, **3:**404
Percutaneous mitral valve repair, **3:**393, **3:**404
Percutaneous renal puncture, **2:**302, **2:**302*f*
Percutaneous transhepatic cholangiography (PTC), **2:**264–265, **2:**264*f*
Percutaneous transluminal angioplasty, **3:**356–371, **3:**404
  balloon angioplasty in, **3:**356, **3:**356*f*
  of common iliac artery, **3:**357*f*
  Dotter method for, **3:**356
  historical development of, **3:**312
  of renal artery, **3:**357*f*
  for stent placement, **3:**358, **3:**358*f*
Percutaneous transluminal coronary angioplasty (PTCA), **3:**358, **3:**404
Percutaneous transluminal coronary rotational atherectomy (PTCRA), **3:**404
Percutaneous vertebroplasty, **2:**164, **2:**164*f*–165*f*
Perfusion study
  for computed tomography angiography, of brain, **3:**250–252, **3:**252*f*
  in MRI, **3:**303, **3:**307
Pericardial cavity, **1:**49*f*, **1:**83, **3:**316
Pericardial sac, **3:**316
Pericardium
  anatomy of, **3:**316, **3:**404
  sectional anatomy of, **3:**192
Periosteal arteries, **1:**57*f*
Periosteum, **1:**56, **1:**56*f*
Peripheral, definition of, **1:**65

Peripheral angiography, **3:**340–341
  lower limb arteriograms, **3:**340, **3:**340*f*
  lower limb venograms, **3:**353, **3:**354*f*
  upper limb arteriograms, **3:**341, **3:**341*f*
  upper limb venograms, **3:**353, **3:**353*f*
Peripheral dual energy x-ray absorptiometry (pDXA), **2:**487, **2:**492
Peripheral lymph sinus, **3:**318
Peripheral nerve stimulation (PNS), **3:**285, **3:**307
Peripheral quantitative computed tomography (pQCT), **2:**487, **2:**492
Peripheral skeletal measurements, **2:**488, **2:**488*f*–489*f*
Peripherally inserted central catheters (PICCs), **3:**144, **3:**144*f*
Peristalsis, **1:**13, **2:**202
Peritoneal cavity, **1:**127, **1:**127*f*
Peritoneum, **1:**127, **1:**127*f*
  sectional anatomy of, **3:**205
Permanent magnets, for MRI, **3:**274, **3:**307
Permanent pacemaker (PPM), **3:**400, **3:**404
Perpendicular plate
  anatomy of, **2:**8, **2:**8*f*
  sectional anatomy of, **3:**174, **3:**174*f*
Personal hygiene, in surgical radiography, **3:**33
Personal protective equipment (PPE), **1:**4
Personal space and body awareness, in children, **3:**78
PET/CT scanners, **3:**253–255, **3:**255*f*
PET-MRI, **3:**281, **3:**281*f*
Petrosa, submentovertical projection of, **2:**49*f*, **2:**101*f*
Petrous apex, **2:**14, **2:**15*f*
Petrous portion, **2:**4*f*, **2:**15*f*
Petrous pyramid, **2:**14
Petrous ridge, **2:**14, **2:**15*f*
  acanthioparietal projection of, **2:**65*f*
  AP axial projection of, **2:**43*f*
  modified parietoacanthial projection of, **2:**63*f*
  PA axial projection of, **2:**5*f*, **2:**38*f*, **2:**47*f*
  parietoacanthial projection of, **2:**61*f*, **2:**97*f*
  sectional anatomy of, **3:**183
  submentovertical projection of, **2:**82*f*
Phalanges
  of foot, **1:**270, **1:**270*f*
  of hand, **1:**143, **1:**143*f*
Pharmaceuticals, **3:**440, **3:**479
Pharmacologic thrombolysis, **3:**369
Pharyngeal tonsil, **1:**87*f*, **1:**88
  anatomy of, **2:**174, **2:**175*f*
Pharyngoesophageal constriction, **2:**176
Pharynx, **1:**88
  anatomy of, **2:**171, **2:**171*f*, **2:**174, **2:**175*f*, **2:**177*f*, **2:**184
  AP projection of, **2:**200, **2:**200*f*–201*f*, **2:**201*b*
  lateral projection of, **2:**198*f*–199*f*, **2:**199, **2:**199*b*
  sectional anatomy of, **3:**187*f*
  submentovertical projection of, **2:**101*f*
Phase-contrast (PC) imaging, **3:**302
Phasic flow, **3:**433
Phenergan (promethazine hydrochloride), **2:**316*t*
Philips Medical's iDose4, **3:**245, **3:**245*f*
Phleboliths, **2:**280*t*
Photomultiplier tube (PMT), **3:**436, **3:**479
Photopenia, **3:**441–442, **3:**479
Photostimulable storage phosphor image plate (PSP IP), **1:**3
Physician assistant, **3:**31
Physiology, defined, **1:**46
Pia mater
  anatomy of, **2:**153
  sectional anatomy of, **3:**175
Pica, **3:**112, **3:**113*f*
Picture archiving communication system (PACS)
  in bone densitometry, **2:**492
  for digital subtraction angiography, **3:**324
Picture element (pixels), **3:**234, **3:**234*f*
Piezoelectric effect, **3:**410, **3:**433
Pigg-O-Stat, for chest imaging, **3:**92, **3:**92*f*
Pilot image, in radiation oncology, **3:**492–493
Pineal gland, **3:**187*f*
Piriform recess, **1:**87*f*, **1:**89, **2:**175*f*, **2:**176
Pisiform, **1:**143*f*–144*f*, **1:**144
Pituitary adenoma, **2:**26*t*
Pituitary gland
  anatomy of, **2:**10–11, **2:**152
  sectional anatomy of, **3:**183, **3:**187*f*, **3:**189*f*
Pituitary stalk, **3:**181–182, **3:**181*f*
Pivot joint, **1:**62, **1:**63*f*
Pixel (picture element), **3:**234, **3:**234*f*, **3:**267, **3:**472, **3:**479

Placenta
  anatomy of, **2:**331, **2:**331*f*
  diagnostic medical sonography of, **3:**425*f*
  previa, **2:**331, **2:**331*f*
Placentography, **2:**342
Planimetry, **3:**379–381, **3:**404
Plantar, definition of, **1:**65
Plantar flexion, **1:**79, **1:**79*f*
Plantar surface, **1:**270
Plantodorsal projection, **1:**70*t*
Plastic fractures, **3:**102
Pledget, **3:**404
Pleura
  anatomy of, **1:**84*f*, **1:**86
  AP or PA projection of, **1:**120–123, **1:**120*f*–121*f*
  lateral projection of, **1:**122*f*
Pleural cavities, **1:**49*f*, **1:**83, **1:**86
Pleural effusion, **1:**93*t*
  mobile radiograph in, **2:**13*f*
Pleural space, **1:**84*f*
Plural word endings, in medical terminology, **1:**80, **1:**80*t*
Plural word forms, frequently misused, **1:**80, **1:**80*t*
Pneumoarthrography, **2:**142–143
Pneumococcal (lobar) pneumonia, **3:**138
Pneumoconiosis, **1:**93*t*
Pneumonia, **1:**93*t*
  in children, **3:**137–138, **3:**138*f*
  in older adults, **3:**158, **3:**158*f*
Pneumonitis, **1:**93*t*
Pneumoperitoneum, **1:**129*t*
  in children, **3:**88, **3:**88*f*
Pneumothorax, **1:**93*t*, **1:**101
Point-of-care MRI scanners, **3:**278–279, **3:**279*f*
Polonium, **3:**436
Polycystic kidney, **2:**280*t*
Polyembolokoilamania, **3:**114, **3:**114*f*
Polyjet printing, **3:**226
Polyp, **2:**190*t*–191*t*
  cranial, **2:**26*t*
  endometrial, **2:**335*t*
Pons, **2:**5*f*, **3:**181*f*–182*f*, **3:**183, **3:**184*f*
  anatomy of, **2:**152, **2:**152*f*–153*f*
  defined, **2:**167
  sectional anatomy of, on midsagittal plane, **3:**187*f*
Pontine cistern, **3:**175, **3:**183
Popliteal artery, diagnostic medical sonography of, **3:**429*f*
Popliteal surface, of femur, **1:**274*f*
Popliteal vein, diagnostic medical sonography of, **3:**429*f*
Port(s), in children, **3:**145
Porta hepatis
  anatomy of, **2:**184
  diagnostic medical sonography of, **3:**414*f*, **3:**434
Portable placement, in mobile radiography, **2:**26
Portal hypertension, **3:**368
Portal system, **2:**184, **2:**185*f*, **3:**315, **3:**315*f*, **3:**404
Portal vein
  anatomy of, **2:**184, **2:**185*f*
  sectional anatomy of
    on axial plane, **3:**209, **3:**209*f*
    on coronal plane, **3:**220–221, **3:**220*f*
Portal venous system, sectional anatomy of, **3:**206–207
Portsman, Werner, **3:**312
Positioning, **1:**71*b*
  general body, **1:**72
  lateral, **1:**73, **1:**73*f*
  left semiprone oblique, **1:**72, **1:**73*f*
  lithotomy, **1:**72, **1:**73*f*
  lordotic, **1:**76, **1:**77*f*
  for mobile radiography, **2:**26
  note to educators, student, and clinicians, **1:**77
  oblique, **1:**74–75, **1:**74*f*–75*f*
  prone, **1:**72, **1:**72*f*, **1:**74
  recumbent, **1:**72
  seated, **1:**72
  supine, **1:**72, **1:**72*f*
  for trauma radiography, **2:**113
  upright, **1:**66*f*, **1:**72
Positive beam limitation (PBL), **1:**25
Positron(s), **3:**460–462, **3:**460*t*, **3:**461*f*, **3:**462*t*, **3:**479
Positron emission tomography (PET), **3:**476, **3:**479
  clinical, **3:**472–475, **3:**472*f*–473*f*
    cardiology imaging, **3:**474–475
    ^{18}F-FDG oncologic study, **3:**473–474
    neurologic imaging, **3:**474
    oncology imaging, **3:**473, **3:**473*f*

Positron emission tomography (PET) *(Continued)*
  comparison with other modalities, **3**:437–438, **3**:437*t*, **3**:438*f*–439*f*
  detectors for, **3**:436
  future of, hybrid imaging as, **3**:437
  historical development of, **3**:436
  imaging, **3**:470, **3**:470*f*
  principles and facilities in, **3**:460–472, **3**:460*f*
    data and image acquisition, **3**:469–470, **3**:470*f*
    image reconstruction and image processing, **3**:471–472, **3**:471*f*
    positrons, **3**:460–462, **3**:460*t*, **3**:461*f*, **3**:462*t*
    radionuclide production, **3**:462*t*, **3**:463–464, **3**:463*f*–464*f*
    radiopharmaceutical production, **3**:465–468, **3**:465*f*
  radionuclides in, **3**:444
  sensitivity of, **3**:468
  septa, **3**:437, **3**:468
  2-dimensional, **3**:468, **3**:468*f*
Posterior, definition of, **1**:65
Posterior acoustic enhancement, **3**:434
Posterior acoustic shadowing, **3**:413*f*, **3**:434
Posterior arches, anatomy of, **2**:172, **2**:172*f*
Posterior cerebral artery, CT angiography of, **3**:251*f*
Posterior circulation, cerebral angiography of, **3**:351–352
  axial projection, **3**:352, **3**:352*f*
  lateral projection, **3**:351–352, **3**:351*f*
Posterior clinoid process, **2**:4*f*, **2**:10*f*–11*f*
  AP axial projection of, **2**:43*f*
  PA axial projection of, **2**:47*f*
  sectional anatomy of, **3**:174–175
Posterior communicating artery
  arteriography of, **3**:346*f*
  CT angiography of, **3**:251*f*
Posterior cranial fossa, **2**:6
Posterior cruciate ligament, **1**:276*f*, **1**:278*f*
Posterior fat pad, of elbow, **1**:149, **1**:149*f*
Posterior fontanel, **2**:6, **2**:6*f*
Posterior horn, **2**:154, **2**:154*f*
Posterior inferior iliac spine, **1**:371*f*
Posterior nipple line (PNL), in mammography, **2**:391, **2**:392*f*
Posterior superior iliac spine, **1**:371*f*
Posteroanterior (PA) axial oblique projection, **1**:67*t*
Posteroanterior (PA) axial projection, **1**:67*t*, **1**:69
Posteroanterior (PA) oblique projection, **1**:67*t*
Postoperative cholangiography, **2**:266–267, **2**:266*f*–267*f*
Post-processing
  in digital subtraction angiography, **3**:324, **3**:404
  in three-dimensional imaging, **3**:252, **3**:267
Pott fracture, **1**:282*t*
Pouch of Douglas, **3**:422, **3**:422*f*
Power injector, for intravenous contrast media, **3**:243, **3**:243*f*
Precession, **3**:271, **3**:271*f*, **3**:307
Preexposure instructions, **1**:14
Pregnancy
  breast during, **2**:363*f*
  female radiography during, **2**:342
    fetography for, **2**:342, **2**:342*f*
    pelvimetry for, **2**:342
    placentography for, **2**:342
    radiation protection for, **2**:342
Premature infants, development of, **3**:73
Presbycusis, **3**:155
Presbyopia, **3**:155
Preschoolers, development of, **3**:74–76, **3**:74*f*–75*f*
Pressure injector, for cardiac catheterization, **3**:376, **3**:376*f*
Pressure sores, in older adults, **3**:161
Pressure transducer, **3**:404
Pressure wire, for cardiac catheterization, **3**:378*t*
Primary bronchi, sectional anatomy of, **3**:197–199
Primary curves, **1**:412
Primary data, in CT, **3**:228, **3**:267
Primary ossification, **1**:57, **1**:57*f*
Primary osteoporosis, **2**:462, **2**:492
Procedure book, **1**:16
Processes, **1**:64
Processing systems, in gamma camera systems, **3**:447–448, **3**:447*f*–448*f*
Proctography, evacuation, **2**:262, **2**:262*f*
Professionalism
  in mobile radiography, **2**:27
  for trauma radiography, **2**:113
Profile spot compression, nipple in, **2**:385*t*–390*t*

Progeria, **3**:139, **3**:139*f*
Projection(s), **1**:66–71, **1**:67*t*, **1**:70*t*, **1**:71*b*
  anteroposterior (AP), **1**:66, **1**:66*f*, **1**:67*t*
  axial, **1**:67*t*, **1**:68, **1**:68*f*
  axiolateral, **1**:69, **1**:70*t*
  axiolateral oblique, **1**:70*t*
  of bone, **1**:64
  complex, **1**:69
  craniocaudal, **1**:70*t*
  defined, **1**:66
  entrance and exit points of, **1**:66
  in-profile, **1**:71
  lateral, of obese patients, **1**:40
  lateromedial and mediolateral, **1**:69, **1**:70*t*
  note to educators, student, and clinicians, **1**:77
  oblique, of obese patients, **1**:40
  tangential, **1**:68, **1**:68*f*, **1**:70*t*
  transthoracic, **1**:69, **1**:70*t*
  true, **1**:71
  view vs., **1**:77
Projectional (or areal) technique, **2**:492
Promethazine hydrochloride (Phenergan), **2**:316*t*
Promontory, **2**:15*t*
Pronate/pronation, **1**:79, **1**:79*f*
Prophylactic surgery, for breast cancer, **3**:484, **3**:509
Prophylaxis, **1**:5
Prostate, **2**:333
  anatomy of, **2**:279, **2**:279*f*
  MRI of, **3**:298
  radiologic examination of, **2**:306
  sectional anatomy of, **3**:206
Prostate cancer, **2**:335*t*
  in older adults, **3**:159
  radiation oncology for, **3**:498, **3**:505
Prostatic hyperplasia, benign, **2**:280*t*
  in older adults, **3**:159, **3**:160*t*
Prostatic urethra, **2**:279, **2**:279*f*
Prostatography, **2**:306, **2**:345, **2**:345*f*
Protective eyewear, **3**:33
Protocol
  in CT, **3**:267
  in mobile radiography, **2**:27
Protocol book, **1**:16
Proton(s), magnetic properties of, **3**:271, **3**:271*f*
Proton beam therapy, **3**:502–503, **3**:502*f*–503*f*
Proton density, in MRI, **3**:272, **3**:307
Protuberance, **1**:64
Provocative diskography, **2**:166, **2**:166*f*
Proximal, definition of, **1**:65, **1**:65*f*
Proximal convoluted tubule, **2**:277, **2**:277*f*
Proximal femur
  anatomy of, **1**:372*f*, **1**:373–374
  AP oblique projection of, **1**:386–389
    bilateral, **1**:386, **1**:386*f*
    evaluation criteria for, **1**:387*b*
    position of part for, **1**:386
    position of patient for, **1**:386
    structures shown on, **1**:387, **1**:387*f*
    unilateral, **1**:386–387, **1**:386*f*
  AP projection of, **1**:381–385, **1**:383*b*
  DXA of, **2**:480–481, **2**:480*f*–481*f*
  radiography of, **1**:381–385
  sample exposure technique chart routine projections for, **1**:379*t*
  summary of pathology, **1**:379*t*
Proximal humerus, **1**:247–248
  anatomic neck of, **1**:221, **1**:221*f*
  anatomy of, **1**:221, **1**:221*f*
  body of, **1**:221, **1**:221*f*
  greater tubercle of, **1**:221, **1**:221*f*
  head of, **1**:221, **1**:221*f*
  intertubercular (bicipital) groove of, **1**:247–248
    anatomy of, **1**:221, **1**:221*f*
    Fisk modification for, tangential projection of, **1**:247–248, **1**:247*f*–248*f*, **1**:248*b*
    tangential projection of, **1**:247–248
  lesser tubercle of, **1**:221, **1**:221*f*
  Stryker notch method for, AP axial projection of, **1**:245, **1**:245*b*, **1**:245*f*
  superior aspect of, **1**:221*f*
  surgical neck of, **1**:221, **1**:221*f*
Proximal interphalangeal (PIP) joints
  of lower extremity, **1**:278
  of upper extremity, **1**:147, **1**:148*f*
Proximal phalanges, **1**:270

Proximal tibiofibular joint, **1**:278*t*, **1**:280, **1**:280*f*
Psoas muscle, sectional anatomy of, **3**:213, **3**:213*f*
PTA. *See* Percutaneous transluminal angioplasty
PTC. *See* Percutaneous transhepatic cholangiography
PTCA. *See* Percutaneous transluminal coronary angioplasty
Pterion, **2**:4*f*
Pterygoid hamulus, **2**:5*f*, **2**:11*f*, **2**:12
Pterygoid process
  anatomy of, **2**:11*f*, **2**:12
  sectional anatomy of, **3**:174–175
Pubic symphysis, **1**:54*f*
  anatomy of, **1**:375, **1**:375*f*–377*f*, **1**:382*f*
  in obese patients, **1**:39, **1**:40*f*
  superior margin of, **1**:377*f*, **1**:390*f*
  as surface landmark, **1**:51*f*
Pubis, anatomy of, **1**:371*f*, **1**:372, **1**:374*f*
Pulmonary apices, **1**:116–119
  AP axial projection for, **1**:116–119, **1**:118*f*
    in lordotic position (Lindblom method), **1**:116–117, **1**:116*f*–117*f*
  PA axial projection for, **1**:119, **1**:119*b*, **1**:119*f*
Pulmonary arteries, **1**:92*f*
  sectional anatomy of, **3**:193, **3**:197–199
Pulmonary arteriography, **3**:339, **3**:339*f*
Pulmonary circulation, **3**:315, **3**:315*f*, **3**:404
Pulmonary edema, **1**:93*t*
Pulmonary trunk, sectional anatomy of, **3**:197–199
Pulmonary valve, **3**:317
Pulmonary vein, sectional anatomy of, **3**:193, **3**:200, **3**:200*f*
Pulse, **3**:307, **3**:318, **3**:404
Pulse height analyzer, **3**:446, **3**:479
Pulse oximetry, **3**:404
Pulse sequence, in MRI, **3**:272, **3**:288, **3**:307
Pulse wave transducers, for diagnostic medical sonography, **3**:410
Pulse wave ultrasound, for diagnostic medical sonography, **3**:434
Pupil, **2**:52*f*
Purcell, Edward, **3**:270
Pushed-up CC, labeling codes for, **2**:385*t*–390*t*
Pyelography, **2**:283
Pyelonephritis, **2**:280*t*
Pyloric antrum, anatomy of, **2**:178, **2**:178*f*
Pyloric canal, anatomy of, **2**:178, **2**:178*f*
Pyloric orifice, **2**:178*f*, **2**:179
Pyloric portion, of stomach, **2**:178, **2**:181*f*
Pyloric sphincter, anatomy of, **2**:178*f*, **2**:179
Pyloric stenosis, **2**:190*t*–191*t*
Pyrogen-free radiopharmaceuticals, **3**:441, **3**:479

Q

Quadrants of abdomen, **1**:50, **1**:50*f*
Quadratus lumborum muscles, **3**:213, **3**:213*f*
Quadrigeminal cistern, **3**:175
Quality, for trauma radiography, **2**:113
Quantitative analysis, **3**:449, **3**:449*f*, **3**:479
Quantitative computed tomography (QCT), for bone densitometry, **2**:458, **2**:483, **2**:492
Quantitative ultrasound (QUS), **2**:488, **2**:489*f*, **2**:492
Quantum noise, in CT, **3**:244, **3**:267
Quench, during MRI, **3**:286, **3**:307

R

Radial force, **3**:404
Radial fossa, **1**:146, **1**:146*f*
Radial head
  Coyle method for, axiolateral projection of, **1**:204–206, **1**:204*b*
    central ray for, **1**:205
    collimation for, **1**:205
    evaluation criteria for, **1**:206*b*
    position of part for, **1**:204, **1**:204*f*–205*f*
    position of patient for, **1**:204
    structures shown on, **1**:206, **1**:206*f*
  lateromedial projection of, **1**:202–203
    central ray for, **1**:203
    collimation for, **1**:203
    evaluation criteria for, **1**:203*b*
    four-position series for, **1**:202
    position of part for, **1**:202, **1**:202*f*
    position of patient for, **1**:202–203
    structures shown on, **1**:203, **1**:203*f*
Radial notch, **1**:145, **1**:145*f*
Radial scar, **2**:376*t*–377*t*
Radial styloid process, **1**:145, **1**:145*f*

Radial tuberosity, **1:**145, **1:**145*f*
Radiation, **3:**439, **3:**479
 direct effects of, **3:**509
 indirect effects of, **3:**486, **3:**509
 tolerance doses to, **3:**495, **3:**495*t*
Radiation badge, **3:**33
Radiation exposure considerations, for surgical radiography, **3:**39, **3:**39*f*
Radiation fields, **3:**488–489
 collimation of, **1:**25–26, **1:**25*f*–26*f*
Radiation oncologist, **3:**509
Radiation oncology, **3:**481–512
 best practices for, **3:**504
 cancer and, **3:**483–485
  common types of, **3:**483–484, **3:**484*t*
  risk factors for, **3:**484–485, **3:**484*t*
  tissue origins of, **3:**485, **3:**485*t*
 clinical applications of, **3:**505–507
  for breast cancer, **3:**506–507, **3:**506*f*
  for cervical cancer, **3:**505, **3:**505*f*
  for head and neck cancers, **3:**505
  for Hodgkin lymphoma, **3:**506
  for laryngeal cancer, **3:**507
  for lung cancer, **3:**505, **3:**505*f*
  for medulloblastoma, **3:**507, **3:**507*f*
  for prostate cancer, **3:**498, **3:**505
  for skin cancer, **3:**507
 for cure, **3:**482
 defined, **3:**482
 dose depositions in, **3:**487, **3:**487*f*
 equipment for, **3:**487–491
  cobalt-60 units as, **3:**488–489, **3:**489*f*
  linear accelerators (linacs) as, **3:**487, **3:**489–491, **3:**490*f*
  multileaf collimation system as, **3:**491, **3:**491*f*
 external-beam therapy and brachytherapy in, **3:**487
 fractionation in, **3:**482, **3:**509
 future trends for, **3:**508, **3:**508*f*
 historical development of, **3:**483, **3:**483*t*
 for palliation, **3:**482
 principles of, **3:**482–510
 skin-sparing effect of, **3:**488, **3:**488*f*
 steps in, **3:**491–501
  contrast administration, **3:**492, **3:**493*f*
  creation of treatment fields as, **3:**493, **3:**494*f*
  CyberKnife as, **3:**501, **3:**501*f*
  dosimetry as, **3:**482, **3:**495–497, **3:**495*f*–496*f*, **3:**495*t*
  immobilization devices as, **3:**491–492, **3:**492*f*
  reference isocenter as, **3:**492–493
  simulation as, **3:**491–493, **3:**492*f*
  TomoTherapy, **3:**500, **3:**500*f*
  treatment as, **3:**497–501, **3:**498*f*–499*f*
 theory of, **3:**486, **3:**486*t*
Radiation protection
 for children, **3:**80–83, **3:**80*f*, **3:**81*t*
  dose and diagnostic information, **3:**80–83
  for gastrointestinal and genitourinary studies, **3:**89–90, **3:**89*t*
  holding as, **3:**82
  for limb radiography, **3:**101, **3:**101*f*
 for cranium, **2:**33
 with DXA, **2:**472, **2:**472*t*
 for female radiography, **2:**336
  during pregnancy, **2:**342
 for gastrointestinal radiography, **2:**206*f*, **2:**207
 for hip, **1:**380
 for pelvis, **1:**380
 for thoracic viscera, **1:**102, **1:**103*f*
 for trauma radiography, **2:**111
 for urinary system, **2:**293
Radiation safety
 with C-arm, **3:**39, **3:**39*f*
 with mobile radiography, **2:**6–7, **2:**6*f*
 in nuclear medicine, **3:**444, **3:**444*f*
Radiation therapist, **3:**482, **3:**510
Radiation therapy
 defined, **3:**482, **3:**510
 image-guided, **3:**498
 intensity-modulated, **3:**491, **3:**509
 practice standards for, **1:**2
 stereotactic, **3:**500, **3:**510
 treatment planning, CT for, **3:**253, **3:**254*f*
Radio frequency (RF), in MRI, **3:**271, **3:**307
Radioactive, definition of, **3:**436, **3:**479, **3:**510
Radioactive source, in radiation oncology, **3:**487

Radioactivity, **3:**436, **3:**479
Radiocarpal articulation, **1:**148, **1:**148*f*
Radiocurable, definition of, **3:**510
Radioembolization, **3:**362
Radiofrequency (RF) ablation, **3:**399, **3:**404
Radiofrequency (RF) antennas, for MRI, **3:**274
Radiogrammetry, **2:**457, **2:**492
Radiograph(s), **1:**28, **1:**29*f*
 anatomic position, **1:**30–34, **1:**30*f*–31*f*
 display of, **1:**30–34
 identification of, **1:**34, **1:**34*f*
 lateral, **1:**33, **1:**33*f*
 oblique, **1:**33, **1:**33*f*
 posteroanterior and anteroposterior, **1:**31–32, **1:**31*f*–32*f*
Radiographer, **1:**2–44, **3:**79
Radiographic absorptiometry, **2:**457, **2:**488, **2:**492
Radiographic positioning terminology, **1:**45–80
 for method, **1:**77
 for position, **1:**71–77, **1:**71*b*
  decubitus, **1:**76, **1:**77*f*
  Fowler, **1:**72
  general body, **1:**72
  lateral, **1:**73, **1:**73*f*
  left semiprone oblique, **1:**72, **1:**73*f*
  lithotomy, **1:**72, **1:**73*f*
  note to educators, students, and clinicians on, **1:**77
  oblique, **1:**74–75, **1:**74*f*–75*f*
  prone, **1:**72, **1:**72*f*
  recumbent, **1:**72, **1:**72*f*
  supine, **1:**72, **1:**72*f*
  Trendelenburg, **1:**72, **1:**72*f*
  upright, **1:**66*f*, **1:**72
 for projection, **1:**66–71, **1:**67*t*, **1:**70*t*, **1:**71*b*
  AP, **1:**66, **1:**66*f*, **1:**67*t*
  axial, **1:**67*t*, **1:**68, **1:**68*f*
  complex, **1:**69
  in-profile, **1:**71
  lateral, **1:**69, **1:**69*f*
  note to educators, students, and clinicians on, **1:**77
  oblique, **1:**64*f*
  PA, **1:**66, **1:**66*f*, **1:**67*t*
  tangential, **1:**68, **1:**68*f*, **1:**70*t*
  true, **1:**71
 for view, **1:**77
Radiographic procedure, **1:**16
 accessory equipment in, **1:**17–18, **1:**17*f*
 common steps for, **1:**16–17, **1:**16*t*
 initial or routine, **1:**16
Radiographic room
 care in, **1:**3
 gowns and disposable gloves in, **1:**5
 preparation of, **1:**3, **1:**3*f*
Radiographic technique charts, in mobile radiography, **2:**5, **2:**5*f*
Radiography
 in children, **3:**142, **3:**142*f*–143*f*
 conventional, DXA and, **2:**457
 defined, **1:**65
 for lower extremity, **1:**284–366
 mobile, **2:**1–28
  of abdomen, **2:**14–17
  of cervical spine, **2:**24–27
  of chest, **2:**10–13
  digital, **2:**2, **2:**3*f*
  examination in, **2:**7–8
  of femur, **2:**20–23
  initial procedures in, **2:**7, **2:**7*b*
  isolation considerations with, **2:**7
  machines for, **2:**2, **2:**3*f*
  patient considerations with, **2:**8–9
  of pelvis, **2:**18–19
  principles of, **2:**2–9, **2:**2*f*
  radiation safety with, **2:**6–7, **2:**6*f*
  technical considerations for, **2:**3–5, **2:**3*f*
 preliminary steps in, **1:**1–44
Radioimmunotherapy, **3:**475
Radioindicator, **3:**436
Radioisotope, **3:**479
Radiologic technology, defined, **1:**2
Radiologic vertebral assessment (RVA), **2:**483–484
Radiologist assistant (RA), **1:**3
Radiology department, minor surgical procedures in, **1:**5
Radiology practitioner assistant (RPA), **1:**3
Radionuclide, **3:**439–441, **3:**441*f*, **3:**479
 production, **3:**463–464

Radionuclide angiography, **3:**454
Radiopaque markers, for trauma radiography, **2:**110, **2:**110*f*
Radiopaque object, **1:**11, **1:**12*f*
Radiopharmaceuticals, **3:**436, **3:**441*f*, **3:**474, **3:**479
 dose of, **3:**443, **3:**443*f*
 production, **3:**465–468, **3:**465*f*
Radiosensitivity, **3:**486, **3:**510
Radiotracer, **3:**436, **3:**479
Radioulnar joint, **1:**148*f*
Radium (Ra), **3:**436, **3:**510
Radius, of arm, **1:**143*f*, **1:**145, **1:**145*f*
Radon, **3:**436
Rafert-Long method, for PA and PA axial projections, of scaphoid, **1:**184, **1:**184*b*, **1:**184*f*–185*f*
Random coincidence event, **3:**469*f*, **3:**479
Range modulator wheel, **3:**502
RANK ligand (RANKL), in osteoporosis, **2:**462*t*
Rapid film changers, **3:**313
Rapid serial radiographic imaging, **3:**323
Rare-earth filtered system, in DXA, **2:**465, **2:**466*f*
Raw data, in MRI, **3:**273, **3:**308
Ray, **3:**479
Reactor, **3:**510
Real time, **3:**253, **3:**267
Real-time imaging, **3:**434
Receiving coil, in MRI, **3:**271
Recombinant tissue plasminogen activators, **3:**312–313
Reconstruction
 for CT, **3:**235, **3:**267
  multiplanar, **3:**239, **3:**239*f*
 for PET, **3:**436, **3:**479
Rectal ampulla, **2:**183, **2:**183*f*
Rectal examination, dynamic, **2:**262, **2:**262*f*
Rectouterine pouch, diagnostic medical sonography of, **3:**422, **3:**422*f*, **3:**434
Rectouterine recess, diagnostic medical sonography of, **3:**424*f*
Rectovaginal fistula, **2:**341*f*
Rectum
 anatomy of, **2:**171*f*, **2:**182*f*–183*f*, **2:**183
 defecography of, **2:**262, **2:**262*f*
 diagnostic medical sonography of, **3:**422
 sectional anatomy of
  on axial plane, **3:**216–218, **3:**216*f*–218*f*
  on midsagittal plane, **3:**219*f*
Rectus abdominis muscle, sectional anatomy of, **3:**207
 on axial plane
  at level B, **3:**208*f*
  at level C, **3:**209*f*
  at level D, **3:**210*f*
  at level E, **3:**212
  at level G, **3:**213
  at level I, **3:**215
  at level J, **3:**216, **3:**216*f*
 on midsagittal plane, **3:**219*f*
Recumbent position, **1:**72, **1:**72*f*
Red marrow, **1:**56
Reference isocenter, in simulation in radiation oncology, **3:**492–493
Reference population, in DXA, **2:**471, **2:**492
Reflection, in diagnostic medical sonography, **3:**410*f*, **3:**434
Refraction, in diagnostic medical sonography, **3:**410*f*, **3:**434
Region of interest (ROI)
 in CT, **3:**267
 in DXA, **2:**457, **2:**492
 in PET, **3:**479
Regional enteritis, **2:**190*t*–191*t*
Registered diagnostic cardiac sonographers (RDCSs), **3:**408
Registered diagnostic medical sonographers (RDMSs), **3:**408, **3:**408*f*
Registered vascular technologists (RVTs), **3:**408
Regurgitation, cardiac valvular, **3:**408, **3:**430
Relative biologic effectiveness (RBE), **3:**486, **3:**510
Relaxation times, in MRI, **3:**270, **3:**308
Renal arteries
 diagnostic medical sonography of, **3:**415*f*
 MRA of, **3:**302*f*
 sectional anatomy of, **3:**206
Renal arteriogram, **3:**339, **3:**339*f*
Renal calculus, **2:**280*t*, **2:**282*f*
Renal calyces, anatomy of, **2:**277, **2:**277*f*
Renal capsule, **2:**276, **2:**277*f*
Renal cell carcinoma, **2:**280*t*

Renal columns, 2:277, 2:277f
Renal corpuscle, 2:277
Renal cortex, 2:277, 2:277f
Renal cyst, 2:302f
Renal failure, in older adults, 3:160t
Renal fascia, anatomy of, 2:276
Renal hilum, 2:276, 2:277f
Renal hypertension, 2:280t
Renal medulla, 2:277, 2:277f
Renal obstruction, 2:280t
Renal papilla, 2:277, 2:277f
Renal parenchyma, nephrotomography of, 2:301
    AP projection in, 2:301, 2:301f
    percutaneous renal puncture for, 2:302, 2:302f
Renal pelvis, 2:275, 2:277, 2:277f
Renal puncture, percutaneous, 2:302, 2:302f
Renal pyramids, 2:277, 2:277f
Renal sinus, 2:276, 2:277f
Renal transplant, diagnostic medical sonography of, 3:419
Renal tubule, 2:277
Renal vein, sectional anatomy of, 3:206
Renal venography, 3:355, 3:355f
Rendering, in three-dimensional imaging, 3:252, 3:267
Reperfusion, 3:404
Reproductive system, 2:327–346
    abbreviations for, 2:335b
    female. See Female reproductive system
    male. See Male reproductive system
    summary of pathology of, 2:335t
    summary of projections for, 2:328t
Resistive magnets, for MRI, 3:274, 3:308
Resolution
    of collimator, 3:446
    definition of, 3:479
    in diagnostic medical sonography, 3:410, 3:434
Resonance, in MRI, 3:271, 3:308
Resorption, of bone, 2:459, 2:459f
Respect, for parents and children, 3:73
Respiration, 1:517
Respiratory distress syndrome, 1:93t
Respiratory gating, for radiation oncology, 3:499
Respiratory movement, 1:501, 1:501f
    diaphragm in, 1:502, 1:502f
Respiratory studies, 3:458
Respiratory syncytial virus (RSV), 3:137
Respiratory system
    anatomy of, 1:83–86
        alveoli of, 1:84f, 1:85
        bronchial tree of, 1:84, 1:84b, 1:84f
        lungs of, 1:85–86, 1:85f–86f
        trachea of, 1:84, 1:84b, 1:84f
    nuclear medicine imaging in, 3:458
    pleura in
        AP or PA projection of, 1:120–123, 1:120f–121f
        lateral projection of, 1:122f
Respiratory system disorders, in older adults, 3:158, 3:158f
Restenosis, 3:404
Restricted area, 3:69
Retina, 2:52f, 2:53
Retrieval, in three-dimensional imaging, 3:267
Retroareolar cyst, 2:366f
Retrograde cystography, 2:306
    AP axial or PA axial projection for, 2:308–312, 2:308b–309b, 2:308f–309f
    AP oblique projection for, 2:310–311, 2:310f–311f, 2:311b
    contrast injection technique for, 2:306, 2:307f
    indications and contraindications for, 2:306
    injection equipment for, 2:306
    lateral projection for, 2:312, 2:312b, 2:312f
    preliminary preparations for, 2:306
Retrograde femoral nailing, 3:49, 3:49f
Retrograde urography, 2:285
    AP projection for, 2:304–305, 2:304f–305f
    contrast media for, 2:286, 2:287f
    defined, 2:285
    preparation of patient for, 2:289
Retromammary fat, 2:361f
Retroperitoneal cavity, diagnostic medical sonography of, 3:417–418
Retroperitoneum, 1:127, 1:128f
    diagnostic medical sonography of, 3:414–419, 3:414f–415f
    sectional anatomy of, 3:205

Reverse Waters method, for facial bones, 2:64, 2:64b, 2:64f–65f, 2:132, 2:132f
Rheolytic thrombectomy, 3:378t
Rheumatoid arthritis, 1:151t, 1:225t
Rhomboid major muscle, 3:193
Rhomboid minor muscle, 3:193
Ribs, 1:498
    anatomy of, 1:498, 1:498f–499f, 1:517
    anterior, 1:517–519
        PA projection of, 1:518–519, 1:518f–519f, 1:519b
    articulations, 1:500f
    axillary, 1:522–525
        AP oblique projection of, 1:522–525, 1:522f–523f, 1:523b
        PA oblique projection of, 1:524–525, 1:524f–525f, 1:525b
    cervical, 1:498
    false, 1:498
    floating, 1:498
    fractures of, 1:517
    lumbar, 1:498
    posterior, 1:517, 1:520–521
        AP projection of, 1:520–521, 1:520f–521f, 1:521b
        in radiography of sternum, 1:506
    sectional anatomy of, in abdominopelvic region, 3:220
    true, 1:498
Rickets, 1:282t
Right anterior oblique (RAO) position, 1:74, 1:74f
Right colic flexure, 2:182f, 2:183
Right common carotid artery, sectional anatomy of, 3:195
Right jugular trunk, 3:318
Right lower quadrant (RLQ), 1:50, 1:50f
Right lymphatic duct, 3:318
Right posterior oblique (RPO) position, 1:69
Right subclavian artery, sectional anatomy of, 3:195
Right upper quadrant (RUQ), 1:50, 1:50f
Rima glottidis, 1:87f, 1:89f, 1:96f, 2:175f–176f, 2:176
Robert method, for AP projection, of CMC joints, 1:160–161
    central ray for, 1:161, 1:161f
    collimation for, 1:161
    evaluation criteria for, 1:161b
    Lewis modification of, 1:161, 1:161f
    Long and Rafert modification of, 1:161, 1:161f
    position of part for, 1:160, 1:160f
    position of patient for, 1:160, 1:160f
    structures shown on, 1:161, 1:161f
Rods, 2:53
Rolled lateral view, labeling codes for, 2:385t–390t
Rolled medial view, labeling codes for, 2:385t–390t
Rosenberg method for weight-bearing PA projection of knee, 1:341, 1:341f
Rotablator, 3:378t
Rotate/rotation, 1:79, 1:79f
Rotational atherectomy, 3:388–389, 3:388f–389f
Rotational burr atherectomy, 3:404
Rotational force (torque), in MRI, 3:285, 3:308
Rotational tomography of mandible, 2:89
Rotator cuff, sectional anatomy of, 3:193
Rotator cuff tear, 2:143t
    contrast arthrography of, 2:144f
Round ligament
    anatomy of, 2:329f–330f
    diagnostic medical sonography of, 3:415f
Round window, 2:16, 2:17f
Rubidium-82 (^{82}Rb), in nuclear medicine, 3:442t
Rugae
    of stomach, 2:178, 2:178f
    of urinary bladder, 2:278

S
Sacral canal, 1:421
Sacral cornua, 1:421
Sacral foramina, 1:421
Sacral promontory, 1:376f, 1:421
Sacral teratoma, fetal ultrasound of, 3:427f
Sacral vertebrae, 1:411
Sacroiliac (SI) joints
    anatomy of, 1:375, 1:375f, 1:382f
    AP axial or PA axial projection of (Ferguson method), 1:476–477, 1:476f–477f, 1:477b
    AP oblique projection of, 1:472–477, 1:472f–473f, 1:473b
    PA oblique projection of, 1:474–475, 1:474f–475f, 1:475b

Sacrum, 1:371, 1:382f, 1:385f, 1:411
    anatomy of, 2:183f, 1:374f–376f, 1:411f, 1:421f
    AP axial and PA axial projections of, 1:478–481, 1:478f–479f, 1:479b
    lateral projection of, 1:480–481, 1:480f–481f, 1:481b
    sectional anatomy of
        on axial plane, 3:216, 3:216f, 3:218
        on midsagittal plane, 3:219f
Saddle (sellar) joint, 1:62, 1:63f
Sagittal plane, 1:46, 1:46f
    kidneys in, 3:418, 3:434
    in sectional anatomy, 3:200–201
Sagittal sutures, 2:5, 2:21t
Salivary duct obstruction, 2:190t–191t
Salivary glands
    anatomy of, 2:171, 2:173–174, 2:173f–174f
    sialography of, 2:192, 2:192f
Salomon, Albert, 2:350
Salter-Harris fractures, 3:102, 3:102f
Sarcoidosis, 1:93t
Sarcoma
    of breast, 2:376t–377t
    Ewing, 1:151t
        in children, 3:137, 3:137f
Scan
    in CT, 3:267
    in PET, 3:474
Scan diameter, in CT, 3:246, 3:267
Scan duration
    in CT, 3:267
    for CT angiography, 3:250
Scan field of view (SFOV), in CT, 3:246
Scan times, in CT, 3:246, 3:267
Scaphoid, 1:182
    anatomy of, 1:143f, 1:144
    Rafert-Long method for, scaphoid series (PA and PA axial projections with ulnar deviation), 1:184, 1:184b, 1:184f–185f
    Stecher method for, PA axial projection of, 1:182–183, 1:182b, 1:182f–183f
Scapula, 1:257–263
    acromion of, 1:220, 1:220f
    AP oblique projection of, 1:261, 1:261b, 1:261f–262f
    AP projection of, 1:257–261, 1:257b–258b, 1:257f
    coracoid process of, 1:263
        anatomy of, 1:220, 1:220f
        AP axial projection of, 1:263b, 1:263f–264f
    costal (anterior) surface of, 1:220, 1:220f
    crest of spine of, 1:220, 1:220f
    dorsal (posterior) surface of, 1:220, 1:220f
    glenoid cavity of, 1:220–221, 1:220f
    inferior angle of, 1:51f, 1:220–221, 1:220f
    infraspinous fossa of, 1:220, 1:220f
    lateral angle of, 1:221
    lateral border of, 1:220, 1:220f
    lateral projection of, 1:258, 1:258b, 1:258f–260f
    medial border of, 1:220, 1:220f
    neck of, 1:220f, 1:221
    subscapular fossa of, 1:220, 1:220f
    superior angle of, 1:220–221, 1:220f
    superior border of, 1:220, 1:220f
    supraspinous fossa of, 1:220, 1:220f
Scapular notch, 1:220, 1:220f
Scapular spine, Laquerrière-Pierquin method for, tangential projection of, 1:265, 1:265b, 1:265f
Scapular Y, of shoulder girdle, PA oblique projection, 1:240–241
    central ray for, 1:240, 1:242t
    collimation for, 1:240
    evaluation criteria for, 1:241b
    position of part for, 1:240, 1:240f
    position of patient for, 1:240
    respiration for, 1:240
    structures shown on, 1:241, 1:241f
Scapulohumeral articulation, 1:222–224, 1:222f–223f
Scattered coincidence event, 3:469f, 3:479
Scattered radiation, in CT, 3:244
Scattering, in diagnostic medical sonography, 3:434
Scheuermann disease, 1:424t
School-age children, development of, 3:76
Schüller method, for submentovertical projection of cranial base, 2:48–49, 2:48b–49b
    central ray of, 2:49
    position of part in, 2:48–49, 2:48f
    position of patient in, 2:48
    structures shown in, 2:49, 2:49b, 2:49f

Sciatic nerve, **3:**216, **3:**216*f*
Scintillate, definition of, **3:**445
Scintillating detector pileup, in K-edge filtration systems, **2:**466
Scintillation camera, **3:**436, **3:**479
Scintillation counter, **2:**458, **2:**492
Scintillation crystals, **3:**446
Scintillation detectors, **3:**267, **3:**445, **3:**479
Scintillator, **3:**436, **3:**479
Sclera, **2:**53
Scoliosis, **3:**139–141, **1:**412*f*, **1:**424*t*
  Cobb angle in, **3:**141, **3:**141*f*
  congenital, **3:**140
  estimation of rotation in, **3:**141
  idiopathic, **3:**140
  imaging of, **3:**140, **3:**140*f*
  lateral bends with, **3:**141
  neuromuscular, **3:**140
  PA and lateral projection of, **1:**484–489, **1:**485*f*–487*f*, **1:**486*b*
  PA projection of (Ferguson method), **1:**488–489, **1:**488*f*–489*f*, **1:**489*b*
  patterns of, **3:**141
  skeletal maturity with, **3:**141
  symptoms of, **3:**139*f*
  treatment options for, **3:**141
Scottie dog
  in AP oblique projection, **1:**468, **1:**468*f*
  in PA oblique projection, **1:**470*f*
Scout image
  of abdomen, **1:**132
  in radiation oncology, **3:**492–493
Screening mammography, **2:**358
Scrotum, **2:**332
Scrub nurse, **3:**31
Seated position, **1:**72
Secondary curves, **1:**412
Secondary ossification center, **1:**57*f*
Secondary osteoporosis, **2:**462, **2:**492
Sectional anatomy, **3:**171–226
  of abdominopelvic region, **3:**204–221, **3:**204*f*, **3:**206*f*
    on axial plane
      at level A, **3:**207*f*
      at level B, **3:**208*f*
      at level C, **3:**209*f*
      at level D, **3:**210*f*
      at level E, **3:**211*f*
      at level F, **3:**212*f*
      at level G, **3:**213*f*
      at level H, **3:**214*f*
      at level I, **3:**215*f*
      at level J, **3:**216*f*
      at level K, **3:**217*f*–218*f*
    on cadaveric image, **3:**204*f*
    on coronal plane, **3:**220*f*–221*f*
    on midsagittal plane, **3:**219*f*
  advanced visualization for, **3:**222–223, **3:**222*f*–224*f*
  axial planes in, **3:**172
  of cadaveric sections, **3:**173, **3:**174*f*
  coronal planes in, **3:**172
  of cranial region, **3:**174–190
  of CT, **3:**173
  of MRI, **3:**173
  oblique planes in, **3:**172
  overview of, **3:**172–226
  sagittal planes in, **3:**172
  of thoracic region, **3:**191–203
    on cadaveric image, **3:**191, **3:**191*f*
    on coronal plane, **3:**202–203, **3:**203*f*
      level A, **3:**203*f*
      level B, **3:**203*f*
      level C, **3:**203*f*
    on posterior plane, **3:**203
    on sagittal plane, **3:**200–201, **3:**201*f*
      level A, **3:**202*f*
      level B, **3:**202*f*
      level C, **3:**202*f*
      median, **3:**200–201
  3D printing for, **3:**224–226, **3:**224*f*–225*f*
Segmentation
  shaded surface display in, **3:**252
  in 3D printing, **3:**224
  in three-dimensional imaging, **3:**252, **3:**267
Seldinger technique, **3:**312
Selective coronary angiography, **3:**381, **3:**382*f*–383*f*, **3:**384*t*

Selective laser sintering (SLS), **3:**225
Self-efficacy, **3:**152
Sella turcica, **2:**4*f*, **2:**10–11, **2:**10*f*–11*f*
  lateral projection of, **2:**35*f*–36*f*, **2:**59*f*, **2:**93*f*
  sectional anatomy of, **3:**174–175, **3:**182*f*, **3:**183
Semicircular canals, **2:**15*f*, **2:**16, **2:**17*f*
Seminal ducts, radiography of, **2:**343, **2:**343*f*–344*f*
Seminal vesicle(s)
  anatomy of, **2:**332, **2:**333*f*
  sectional anatomy of, **3:**206
Seminal vesicle duct, **2:**333*f*
Seminoma, **2:**335*t*
Semirestricted area, **3:**69
Sensitivity, **3:**479
  of collimator, **3:**446
Sensory system disorders, in older adults, **3:**155
Sentinel node imaging, **3:**458
Septa, **3:**479
Septum pellucidum, sectional anatomy of, **3:**179–180, **3:**188–189, **3:**189*f*
Serial imaging, **3:**313, **3:**404
Serial scans, in DXA, **2:**477–478, **2:**477*f*, **2:**492
Serous membranes, **1:**83
Serratus anterior muscles, **3:**207, **3:**207*f*
  anatomy of, **2:**360
  sectional anatomy of, **3:**193, **3:**200, **3:**200*f*
Sesamoid bones, **1:**59, **1:**59*f*, **1:**270*f*, **1:**272
  of foot, **1:**290–291, **1:**291*f*
    evaluation criteria for, **1:**291*b*
    tangential projection of
      Holly method for, **1:**290, **1:**291*f*
      Lewis method for, **1:**290, **1:**290*f*
  of hand, **1:**143, **1:**143*f*
Settegast method, for tangential projection, of patella and patellofemoral joint, **1:**354–355, **1:**354*f*–355*f*, **1:**355*b*
  evaluation criteria for, **1:**355*b*
  position of part, **1:**354–355
  position of patient, **1:**354, **1:**354*f*
  structures shown on, **1:**355
Shaded surface display (SSD), **3:**223, **3:**223*f*, **3:**252, **3:**267
Shading, in three-dimensional imaging, **3:**252, **3:**267
Sheaths, for cardiac catheterization, **3:**375, **3:**375*f*
Shewhart Control Chart rules, **2:**475, **2:**492
Shielding
  dose reduction and, **3:**80
  gonad, **1:**20
  for children, **3:**80, **3:**80*f*
Shoe covers, **3:**33
Short bones, **1:**59, **1:**59*f*
Short tau inversion recovery (STIR), **3:**288
Shoulder, **1:**226–228
  AP oblique projection for, trauma of, **2:**133, **2:**134*f*
  AP projection of, **1:**226–228, **1:**226*b*
    central ray for, **1:**226
    collimation for, **1:**226
    evaluation criteria for, **1:**228*b*
    external, neutral, internal rotation humerus, **1:**226–228
    with humerus
      in external rotation, **1:**226, **1:**226*f*, **1:**227*t*
      in internal rotation, **1:**226, **1:**226*f*, **1:**227*t*
      in neutral rotation, **1:**226, **1:**227*t*
    position of part, **1:**226, **1:**227*t*
    position of patient, **1:**226
    respiration for, **1:**226
    structures shown on, **1:**228, **1:**228*f*
  Lawrence method for, transthoracic lateral projection of, **1:**233, **1:**233–234, **1:**233*f*–234*f*, **1:**234*b*
  trauma radiography of, **2:**133, **2:**134*f*
Shoulder arthrography
  CT after, **2:**145, **2:**145*f*
  double-contrast, **2:**144, **2:**144*f*–145*f*
  MRI in, **2:**145*f*
  single-contrast, **2:**144, **2:**144*f*–145*f*
Shoulder girdle, **1:**217–266
  abbreviations, **1:**224*b*
  acromioclavicular articulation of, **1:**249–252
    Alexander method for, AP axial projection of, **1:**251–252, **1:**251*f*–252*f*, **1:**252*b*
    anatomy of, **1:**224, **1:**224*b*, **1:**224*f*
    Pearson method for, bilateral AP projection of, **1:**249–250, **1:**249*f*–250*f*, **1:**250*b*
  anatomy of, **1:**219–224, **1:**219*f*, **1:**224*b*
  articulations, **1:**222–224
  clavicle, **1:**253–256
    anatomy of, **1:**219, **1:**219*f*

Shoulder girdle *(Continued)*
    AP axial projection of, **1:**254–255, **1:**254*b*–255*b*, **1:**254*f*–255*f*
    AP projection of, **1:**253–256, **1:**253*b*, **1:**253*f*
    PA axial projection of, **1:**256, **1:**256*f*
    PA projection of, **1:**256, **1:**256*f*
  definition of, **1:**219
  glenoid cavity of, **1:**229–230
    anatomy of, **1:**220*f*, **1:**221
    Apple method for, AP oblique projection of, **1:**231–232, **1:**231*f*–232*f*, **1:**232*b*
    Garth method for, AP axial oblique projection of, **1:**246, **1:**246*b*, **1:**246*f*
    Grashey method for, AP oblique projection of, **1:**229–230, **1:**229*f*–230*f*, **1:**230*b*
  inferosuperior axial projection of, **1:**235–239
    Lawrence method for, **1:**235, **1:**235*f*–236*f*, **1:**236*b*
    Rafert et al. modification in, **1:**235–236
    West Point method for, **1:**237–238, **1:**237*f*–238*f*, **1:**238*b*
  Lawrence method for, transthoracic lateral projection of, **1:**233, **1:**233–234, **1:**233*f*–234*f*, **1:**234*b*
  sample exposure technique chart routine projections for, **1:**225*t*
  scapula, **1:**220–221, **1:**220*f*
    acromion of, **1:**220, **1:**220*f*
    anatomy of, **1:**220
    AP axial projection of coracoid process of, **1:**263*b*, **1:**263*f*–264*f*
    AP axial projection of, **1:**261, **1:**261*b*, **1:**261*f*–262*f*
    AP projection of, **1:**257–261, **1:**257*b*–258*b*, **1:**257*f*
    costal (anterior) surface of, **1:**220, **1:**220*f*
    crest of spine of, **1:**220, **1:**220*f*
    dorsal (posterior) surface of, **1:**220, **1:**220*f*
    glenoid cavity of, **1:**220–221, **1:**220*f*
    inferior angle of, **1:**220–221, **1:**220*f*
    infraspinous fossa of, **1:**220, **1:**220*f*
    Laquerrière-Pierquin method for, tangential projection of, spine of, **1:**265, **1:**265*b*, **1:**265*f*
    lateral angle of, **1:**221
    lateral border of, **1:**220, **1:**220*f*
    lateral projection of, **1:**258, **1:**258*b*, **1:**258*f*–260*f*
    medial border of, **1:**220, **1:**220*f*
    neck of, **1:**220*f*, **1:**221
    scapular notch of, **1:**220, **1:**220*f*
    subscapular fossa of, **1:**220, **1:**220*f*
    superior angle of, **1:**220–221, **1:**220*f*
    superior border of, **1:**220, **1:**220*f*
    supraspinous fossa of, **1:**220, **1:**220*f*
  summary of pathology, **1:**225*t*
  summary of projections, **1:**218, **1:**218*t*
  superoinferior axial projection of, **1:**239, **1:**239*b*, **1:**239*f*
  supraspinatus "outlet" of, **1:**242–244
    AP axial projection of, **1:**244, **1:**244*b*, **1:**244*f*
    Neer method for, tangential projection of, **1:**242–243, **1:**242*f*–243*f*, **1:**242*t*, **1:**243*b*
Shoulder joint
  glenoid cavity of, **1:**246
    Apple method for, AP oblique projection of, **1:**231–232, **1:**231*f*–232*f*, **1:**232*b*
    Garth method for, AP axial oblique projection of, **1:**246, **1:**246*b*, **1:**246*f*
    Grashey method for, AP oblique projection of, **1:**229–230, **1:**229*f*–230*f*, **1:**230*b*
  inferosuperior axial projection of
    Lawrence method, **1:**235, **1:**235*f*–236*f*, **1:**236*b*
    West Point method for, **1:**237–238, **1:**237*f*–238*f*, **1:**238*b*
  proximal humerus of, **1:**245
  scapular Y, PA oblique projection of, **1:**240–241
    central ray for, **1:**240, **1:**242*t*
    collimation for, **1:**240
    evaluation criteria for, **1:**241*b*
    position of part, **1:**240, **1:**240*f*
    position of patient for, **1:**240
    structures shown as, **1:**241, **1:**241*f*
  structural classification, **1:**222*t*
  Stryker notch method for, AP axial projection of, proximal humerus of, **1:**245, **1:**245*b*, **1:**245*f*
  superoinferior axial projection of, **1:**239, **1:**239*b*, **1:**239*f*
  supraspinatus "outlet" of, **1:**242–244
    AP axial projection of, **1:**244, **1:**244*b*, **1:**244*f*
    Neer method for, tangential projection of, **1:**242–243, **1:**242*f*–243*f*, **1:**242*t*, **1:**243*b*
Sialography, **2:**192, **2:**192*f*

SID protocol, **1:**517
Sieverts (Sv), **2:**492
Sigmoid sinuses, **3:**176–177, **3:**184*f*
   sectional anatomy of, **3:**184–185
Signal, in MRI, **3:**308
   production of, **3:**271
   significance of, **3:**272, **3:**272*f*
Silicosis, **1:**93*t*
Simple fracture, **1:**64*f*
Simulation, in radiation oncology, **3:**491–493, **3:**492*f*
   contrast materials for, **3:**492, **3:**493*f*
   creation of treatment fields in, **3:**493, **3:**494*f*
   CT simulator in, **3:**491, **3:**491*f*
   immobilization devices for, **3:**491–492, **3:**492*f*–493*f*
   reference isocenter in, **3:**492–493
Simulator, CT, for radiation oncology, **3:**491–493, **3:**491*f*, **3:**510
Single energy x-ray absorptiometry (SXA), **2:**484, **2:**492
Single photon absorptiometry (SPA), **2:**458, **2:**492
Single photon emission computed tomography (SPECT), **3:**479
   combined with CT, **3:**453, **3:**453*f*
   in nuclear medicine, **3:**451–452, **3:**451*f*–452*f*
   processing systems for, **3:**447–448, **3:**447*f*
Single word forms, frequently misused, **1:**80, **1:**80*t*
Single-slice helical CT (SSHCT), **3:**233
Singular word endings, in medical terminology, **1:**80, **1:**80*t*
Sinuses
   abdominal, **2:**270, **2:**270*f*
   defined, **1:**64
Sinusitis, **2:**26*t*
Skeletal health assessment, in children, **2:**487–488, **2:**487*f*
Skeleton
   appendicular, **1:**55, **1:**55*f*, **1:**55*t*
   axial, **1:**55, **1:**55*f*, **1:**55*t*
Skin care, for older adults, **3:**161
Skin-sparing effect, in radiation oncology, **3:**488, **3:**488*f*, **3:**510
Skull
   anatomy of, **2:**3–23, **2:**3*b*
   AP axial projection of (Towne method), **2:**41, **2:**43*b*
      central ray for, **2:**43
      for pathologic condition or trauma, **2:**44, **2:**44*f*–45*f*
      position of part for, **2:**41, **2:**41*f*–42*f*, **2:**44*f*
      position of patient for, **2:**41
      structures shown in, **2:**43, **2:**43*f*
      variations of, **2:**41*b*
   AP projection of, **2:**40, **2:**40*b*, **2:**40*f*
   articulations of, **2:**21, **2:**21*t*
   brachycephalic, **2:**30, **2:**30*f*
   in children, **3:**101*f*, **3:**104–108, **3:**106*f*–107*f*
      AP axial Towne projection for, **3:**106–108, **3:**106*f*, **3:**108*t*
      AP projection for, **3:**106–108, **3:**106*f*
      with craniosynostosis, **3:**104
      with fractures, **3:**104
      lateral projection for, **3:**106–108, **3:**109*f*
      summary of projections of, **3:**108*t*
   cranial bones of. *See* Cranial bones
   CT localizer, **3:**188*f*
   CT of, **2:**114, **2:**114*f*
   dolichocephalic, **2:**30, **2:**30*f*
   ear in, **2:**16, **2:**17*f*
   eye in, **2:**52–53, **2:**53*f*–54*f*
      acanthioparietal projection of, **2:**65*f*
      lateral projection of, **2:**55, **2:**55*b*, **2:**55*f*
      localization of foreign bodies within, **2:**54–57, **2:**54*f*
      PA axial projection of, **2:**56, **2:**56*f*
      parietoacanthial projection (modified Waters method), **2:**57, **2:**57*b*, **2:**57*f*
      preliminary examination of, **2:**54
   facial bones of. *See* Facial bones
   floor of, **2:**3
   lateral decubitus position of
      for pathologic conditions, trauma or deformity, **2:**44
      for stretcher and bedside examinations, **2:**39, **2:**39*f*
   lateral projection of, in right or left position, **2:**34–37, **2:**34*b*, **2:**34*f*–36*f*
   mesocephalic, **2:**30, **2:**30*f*
   morphology of, **2:**30, **2:**30*f*
   PA axial projection of
      Caldwell method for, **2:**37–39, **2:**37*f*–38*f*
      evaluation criteria for, **2:**39*b*
      position of patient for, **2:**37–39
      structures shown in, **2:**38*f*, **2:**39

Skull *(Continued)*
   Haas method, **2:**46–47, **2:**46*f*
      central ray, **2:**46
      collimation of, **2:**47
      position of part, **2:**46, **2:**46*f*
      position of patient in, **2:**46
      structures shown in, **2:**47, **2:**47*b*, **2:**47*f*
   position of part for, **2:**37–39
   sagittal images of, **3:**186*f*
   sinuses of. *See* Paranasal sinuses
   summary of pathology of, **2:**26*t*
   topography of, **2:**29–33
   trauma radiography of, **2:**128–131
      AP axial projection (reverse Caldwell method and Towne method) in, **2:**130–131, **2:**130*f*–131*f*
      lateral projection in, **2:**128–131, **2:**128*f*–129*f*
Slice
   in CT, **3:**228, **3:**267
   in MRI, **3:**308
Slice thickness, in CT, **3:**257
Slip ring, in CT, **3:**267
Slipped disk, **1:**413
Slipped epiphysis, **1:**379*t*
Small bowel series, **2:**228
Small intestine
   anatomy of, **2:**171, **2:**171*f*, **2:**180, **2:**181*f*, **2:**184*f*
   complete reflux examination of, **2:**231, **2:**231*f*
   enteroclysis procedure for, **2:**231
      air-contrast, **2:**231, **2:**231*f*
      barium in, **2:**231, **2:**231*f*
      CT, **2:**231, **2:**232*f*
      iodinated contrast medium for, **2:**231, **2:**232*f*
   exposure time for, **2:**206
   intubation examination procedures for, **2:**233, **2:**233*f*
   PA or AP projection of, **2:**229
      central ray for, **2:**229
      collimation for, **2:**229
      evaluation criteria for, **2:**229*b*
      ileocecal studies in, **2:**229, **2:**230*f*
      position of part for, **2:**229, **2:**229*f*
      position of patient for, **2:**229
      respiration during, **2:**229
      structures shown on, **2:**229, **2:**229*f*–230*f*
   radiologic examination of, **2:**228–233
      oral method for, **2:**228
      preparation for, **2:**228–233
   sectional anatomy of, **3:**205
      on axial plane
         at level E, **3:**211, **3:**211*f*
         at level F, **3:**212, **3:**212*f*
         at level G, **3:**213, **3:**213*f*
         at level H, **3:**214, **3:**214*f*
         at level I, **3:**215, **3:**215*f*
         at level J, **3:**216, **3:**216*f*
      on coronal plane, **3:**218, **3:**220*f*
SmartShape wedges, for CT, **3:**255–256, **3:**255*f*
Smith fracture, **1:**151*t*
Smooth muscular tissue, **1:**13
Soft palate, **1:**87*f*, **1:**88
   anatomy of, **2:**172, **2:**172*f*, **2:**174, **2:**175*f*
Soft tissue(s)
   compensation, in DXA, **2:**467*f*
   diagnostic medical sonography of, **3:**420
Soft tissue neck (STN), in children, **3:**110–111, **3:**110*f*–111*f*
Solid-state digital detector, **1:**14
Sonar, **3:**409
Sonogram, **3:**479
Sound, velocity of, **3:**410
Sound waves
   defined, **3:**410, **3:**434
   properties of, **3:**410, **3:**410*f*
Source-to-image receptor distance (SID), **1:**24–25, **1:**24*f*, **3:**325
   in mobile radiography, **2:**5, **2:**5*f*
Source-to-object distance (SOD), **3:**325
Source-to-skin distance, **1:**25
Spatial resolution, for CT, **3:**244, **3:**267
Special needs, children with, **3:**77–79
Special planes, **1:**48
SPECT. *See* Single photon emission computed tomography
Spectroscopy, magnetic resonance, **3:**304, **3:**304*f*, **3:**308
Speed
   for mobile radiography, **2:**26
   for trauma radiography, **2:**113
Speed of sound (SOS), **2:**488

Spermatic cord, **3:**206
Sphenoid angle, of parietal bone, **2:**9*f*
Sphenoid bones
   anatomy of, **2:**3*f*–4*f*, **2:**10–12, **2:**10*f*–11*f*
   greater wing of, **2:**4*f*, **2:**10*f*–11*f*, **2:**11
   lesser wing of, **2:**4*f*, **2:**10*f*–11*f*, **2:**11
   in orbit, **2:**21, **2:**21*f*
   sectional anatomy of, **3:**174–175
Sphenoid strut, **2:**11
Sphenoidal fontanel, **2:**6, **2:**6*f*
Sphenoidal sinuses, **2:**5*f*, **2:**10–11, **2:**10*f*, **2:**22*f*–23*f*, **2:**23
   lateral projection of, **2:**36*f*, **2:**93*f*
   PA axial projection of, **2:**47*f*, **2:**95*f*
   parietoacanthial projection of, open-mouth Waters method, **2:**98–99, **2:**98*f*–99*f*, **2:**99*b*
   sectional anatomy of, **3:**183, **3:**185*f*, **3:**199*f*
      on coronal plane, **3:**189*f*
      on midsagittal plane, **3:**187*f*
   submentovertical projection of, **2:**49*f*, **2:**100–101, **2:**100*f*–101*f*, **2:**101*b*
Sphincter of Oddi, **2:**185
Spin echo pulse sequence, **3:**288, **3:**308
Spina bifida, **1:**413, **1:**424*t*
Spinal cord, **2:**5*f*
   anatomy of, **2:**153, **2:**153*f*, **2:**173*f*
   defined, **2:**167
   interventional pain management, **2:**166, **2:**166*f*
   myelography of
      cervical, **2:**163*f*
      contrast media for, **2:**160–161, **2:**160*f*
      foramen magnum, **2:**163*f*
   provocative diskography of, **2:**166, **2:**166*f*
   vertebral augmentation of, **2:**164–165, **2:**164*f*–165*f*
Spinal fusion
   AP projection of, **1:**490–494, **1:**490*f*–491*f*, **1:**491*b*
   lateral projection of, **1:**492–494, **1:**492*f*–493*f*, **1:**493*b*
Spinal nerves, **2:**156, **2:**156*f*–158*f*
Spine, of bone, **1:**64
Spine DXA scans, lateral lumbar, **2:**483
Spine examinations, for geriatric patients, **3:**164–165
Spin-lattice relaxation, **3:**272, **3:**308
Spinous process, **1:**413
Spin-spin relaxation, **3:**272, **3:**308
Spiral fracture, **1:**64*f*
Spleen
   anatomy of, **2:**171, **2:**171*f*, **2:**181*f*, **2:**184*f*–185*f*, **2:**186, **2:**187*f*
   diagnostic medical sonography of, **3:**414*f*, **3:**418, **3:**418*f*
   sectional anatomy of, **3:**205
      abdominopelvic region
         on coronal plane, **3:**220–221, **3:**221*f*
         at level B, **3:**207*f*–208*f*
         at level C, **3:**209, **3:**209*f*
         at level D, **3:**210, **3:**210*f*
         at level E, **3:**211, **3:**211*f*
         at level F, **3:**212, **3:**212*f*
   sectional image of, **2:**187*f*
Splenic arteriogram, **3:**337, **3:**337*f*
Splenic artery
   diagnostic medical sonography of, **3:**414*f*
   sectional anatomy of
      on axial plane, **3:**210*f*–211*f*, **3:**211
      on coronal plane, **3:**220*f*
Splenic flexure, anatomy of, **2:**182*f*, **2:**183
Splenic vein
   anatomy of, **2:**185*f*
   diagnostic medical sonography of, **3:**417, **3:**417*f*
Splenomegaly, diagnostic medical sonography of, **3:**418*f*
Spondylitis, infectious, needle biopsy of, CT for, **3:**240*f*
Spondylolisthesis, **1:**420, **1:**420*f*, **1:**424*t*
Spondylolysis, **1:**420, **1:**424*t*
Spongy bone, **1:**56, **1:**56*f*
Spongy urethra, **2:**279, **2:**279*f*
Spot compression technique, for mammography, **2:**410–411, **2:**410*f*–411*f*, **2:**411*b*
Squama, of occipital bone, **2:**12, **2:**12*f*–13*f*
Squamous cell carcinoma, **3:**485
Squamous sutures
   anatomy of, **2:**4*f*, **2:**5, **2:**21*t*
   sectional anatomy of, **3:**175
Standard deviation, **2:**492
Standard precautions, **1:**4*b*, **1:**4*f*, **1:**5
   in mobile radiography, **2:**26
   in trauma radiography, **2:**113
Standardized hip reference database, in DXA, **2:**471

Stapes, **2:**16, **2:**17*f*
Starburst artifacts, in CT, **3:**245, **3:**245*f*
Static/planar imaging, in nuclear medicine, **3:**449
Statscan, **2:**106, **2:**107*f*–108*f*
Stecher method, for PA axial projection, of scaphoid, **1:**182–183, **1:**182*b*, **1:**182*f*–183*f*
Stenosis, **2:**190*t*–191*t*, **3:**320, **3:**404
  in urinary system, **2:**280*t*
Stents, for cardiac catheterization, **3:**376, **3:**404
Stereolithography (SLA), **3:**225, **3:**225*f*
Stereotactic imaging, biopsy procedures and, **2:**442–448, **2:**448*f*
  equipment for, **2:**443, **2:**443*f*–444*f*
  images, **2:**442, **2:**443*f*, **2:**445*f*
  three-dimensional localization, **2:**442, **2:**442*f*
  X, Y, and Z coordinates, **2:**442, **2:**442*f*–443*f*
Stereotactic radiosurgery (SRS), **3:**488–489, **3:**510
Sterile, definition of, **3:**69
Sterile arthrogram tray, **2:**143, **2:**143*f*
Sterile field, in surgical radiography
  enemies of, **3:**36
  image receptor handling in, **3:**35–36, **3:**35*f*–36*f*
Sterile team members, **3:**30–32, **3:**31*f*
Sternal angle, **1:**51*f*, **1:**498
Sternal extremity, of clavicle, **1:**219, **1:**219*f*
Sternoclavicular (SC) articulation, **1:**224, **1:**224*f*
  anatomy of, **1:**514–516
  PA oblique projection of
    body rotation method, **1:**515, **1:**515*b*, **1:**515*f*
    CR angulation method, **1:**516, **1:**516*b*, **1:**516*f*
  PA projection of, **1:**514–516, **1:**514*b*, **1:**514*f*
  sectional anatomy of, **3:**192
Sternoclavicular joints, **1:**499
Sternocleidomastoid muscles, **3:**194
Sternocostal joints, **1:**500
Sternum, **1:**107*f*
  breasts and, **1:**506
  heart and, **1:**506
  lateral projection of, **1:**512, **1:**512*b*, **1:**512*f*–513*f*
  PA oblique projection of, **1:**508–512
    Moore method for, **1:**510, **1:**510*f*–511*f*, **1:**511*b*
    in RAO position, **1:**508–509, **1:**508*b*–509*b*, **1:**508*f*–509*f*
  posterior ribs and lung markings and, **1:**506
  radiography of, **1:**506–512, **1:**506*f*–507*f*, **1:**506*t*
  sectional anatomy of, **3:**191–192
  thoracic vertebrae and, **1:**506
Steroids, for osteoporosis, **2:**462*t*
Sthenic body habitus, **1:**52*f*, **1:**53, **1:**54*f*
  gallbladder and, **2:**186, **2:**186*f*
  stomach and duodenum and, **2:**179, **2:**179*f*
  thoracic viscera and, **1:**83*f*
Stomach
  anatomy of, **2:**171, **2:**171*f*, **2:**177*f*–179*f*, **2:**178–179, **2:**181*f*
  AP oblique projection of, **2:**220–221, **2:**220*f*–221*f*, **2:**221*b*
  AP projection of, **2:**224
    central ray for, **2:**224
    collimation for, **2:**224
    evaluation criteria for, **2:**224*b*
    position of part for, **2:**224, **2:**224*f*
    position of patient for, **2:**224, **2:**224*b*, **2:**224*f*
    respiration during, **2:**224
    structures shown on, **2:**224, **2:**225*f*
  body habitus and, **2:**179, **2:**179*f*
  body of, **2:**178, **2:**178*f*
  contrast studies of, **2:**213–214
    barium sulfate suspension for, **2:**203, **2:**203*f*–204*f*
    biphasic, **2:**214
    double-contrast, **2:**214, **2:**214*f*
    single-contrast, **2:**213, **2:**213*f*
    water-soluble, iodinated solution for, **2:**203, **2:**203*f*–204*f*
  diagnostic medical sonography of, **3:**414*f*
  exposure time for, **2:**206
  gastrointestinal series for, **2:**212, **2:**212*f*
  lateral projection of, **2:**222–223, **2:**222*f*–223*f*, **2:**223*b*
  PA axial projection of, **2:**217, **2:**217*b*, **2:**217*f*
  PA oblique projection of, **2:**218–224, **2:**218*f*–219*f*, **2:**219*b*
    Wolf method for, **2:**226, **2:**226*b*–227*b*, **2:**226*f*–227*f*
  PA projection of, **2:**215–224
    body habitus and, **2:**215, **2:**216*f*
    central ray for, **2:**215

Stomach (*Continued*)
    double-contrast, **2:**215*f*
    evaluation criteria for, **2:**216*b*
    position of part for, **2:**215, **2:**215*f*
    position of patient for, **2:**215–216
    respiration during, **2:**215
    single-contrast, **2:**215*f*
    structures shown on, **2:**215–216, **2:**216*f*
  radiographic imaging procedure, **2:**214
  sectional anatomy of, **3:**205
    on axial plane
      at level A, **3:**207
      at level B, **3:**207, **3:**208*f*
      at level C, **3:**209, **3:**209*f*
      at level D, **3:**210*f*
      at level E, **3:**211, **3:**211*f*
    on coronal plane, **3:**220, **3:**220*f*
    sectional image of, **2:**187*f*
Stopcocks, **3:**376
Straight sinus, **3:**176–177, **3:**177*f*, **3:**182*f*, **3:**186–187
Streak artifacts, in CT, **3:**245, **3:**245*f*, **3:**267
Striated muscular tissue, motion control of, **1:**13
Stryker notch method, for AP axial projection, of proximal humerus, **1:**245, **1:**245*b*, **1:**245*f*
Styloid process
  anatomy of, **2:**4*f*, **2:**14, **2:**14*f*–15*f*, **1:**64
  sectional anatomy of, **3:**174–175
Subacromial bursa, **1:**222
Subarachnoid cisterns, **2:**153
Subarachnoid space, **3:**175
  anatomy of, **2:**153
  myelogram of, **2:**163*f*
Sub-bacterial endocarditis, echocardiography for, **3:**430
Subclavian trunk, **3:**318
Subclavian vein, sectional anatomy of, **3:**195, **3:**195*f*
Subdural space, **2:**153
Sublingual ducts, anatomy of, **2:**173*f*, **2:**174
Sublingual fold, anatomy of, **2:**172, **2:**172*f*
Sublingual gland, anatomy of, **2:**171*f*, **2:**173–174, **2:**173*f*–174*f*, **2:**184*f*
Sublingual space, anatomy of, **2:**172, **2:**172*f*
Subluxation, **1:**424*t*
Submandibular duct
  anatomy of, **2:**172*f*–173*f*, **2:**174
  sialography of, **2:**192*f*
Submandibular gland
  anatomy of, **2:**171*f*, **2:**173–174, **2:**173*f*–174*f*, **2:**184*f*
  lateral projection of, **2:**195–196, **2:**195*f*–196*f*, **2:**196*b*
  sialography of, **2:**192*f*
Submentovertical projection, **1:**70*t*
Submentovertical (SMV) projection
  of cranial base, **2:**48–49
    central ray of, **2:**49
    position of part in, **2:**48–49, **2:**48*f*
    position of patient in, **2:**48
    structures shown in, **2:**49, **2:**49*b*, **2:**49*f*
  of ethmoidal and sphenoidal sinus, **2:**100–101, **2:**100*f*–101*f*, **2:**101*b*
  of mandible, **2:**82, **2:**82*b*, **2:**82*f*
  of zygomatic arch, **2:**70–74, **2:**70*f*–71*f*, **2:**71*b*
Subscapularis muscle, sectional anatomy of, **3:**193
Subtalar joint, **1:**278*t*, **1:**316–318
  anatomy of, **1:**279*f*, **1:**280
  evaluation criteria of, **1:**316*b*
  Isherwood method for
    AP axial oblique projection of
      evaluation criteria for, **1:**316*b*–318*b*
      with lateral rotation ankle, **1:**318, **1:**318*f*
      with medial rotation ankle, **1:**317, **1:**317*f*
    lateromedial oblique projection with medial rotation foot of, **1:**316, **1:**316*f*
Subtraction technique, DXA as, **2:**457, **2:**492
Sulcus
  defined, **1:**64
  sectional anatomy of, **3:**175–176, **3:**178*f*
Superciliary arch, **2:**7, **2:**7*f*
Superconductive magnet, **3:**274, **3:**308
Superficial, definition of, **1:**65
Superficial structures, diagnostic medical sonography of, **3:**420, **3:**420*f*
Superimposition, of coordinates, in CT, **3:**230*f*
Superinferior projection, **1:**70*t*
Superior, definition of, **1:**65
Superior articular process, **1:**413, **1:**415, **1:**421

Superior cistern, **3:**181, **3:**190*f*
Superior lobes, sectional anatomy of, **3:**200, **3:**200*f*
Superior mesenteric arteriogram, **3:**338, **3:**338*f*
Superior mesenteric artery (SMA)
  diagnostic medical sonography of, **3:**414*f*, **3:**417, **3:**417*f*
  sectional anatomy of, **3:**206
Superior mesenteric vein
  anatomy of, **2:**185*f*
  diagnostic medical sonography of, **3:**415*f*
  sectional anatomy of, **3:**206–207
Superior nasal conchae, **2:**8, **2:**8*f*
Superior orbital fissure, **2:**11, **2:**11*f*, **2:**18*f*, **2:**50*f*, **2:**51
  location of, **2:**3*f*
  PA axial projection of, **2:**38*f*
Superior orbital margin
  lateral projection of, **2:**55*f*
  PA axial projection of, **2:**38*f*
Superior ramus, **1:**371*f*, **1:**372
Superior sagittal sinus, sectional anatomy of, **3:**177*f*–178*f*, **3:**178–179
  on coronal plane, **3:**189–190, **3:**189*f*
  on midsagittal plane, **3:**187*f*
Superior thoracic aperture, **1:**83, **1:**83*f*
Superior vena cava, sectional anatomy of, **3:**195, **3:**197, **3:**197*f*
Superior venacavogram, **3:**353, **3:**354*f*
Superolateral-inferomedial oblique view, labeling codes for, **2:**385*t*–390*t*
Supinate/supination, **1:**79, **1:**79*f*
Supinator fat pad, of elbow, **1:**149, **1:**149*f*
Supine position, **1:**72, **1:**72*f*
Supracondylar fracture, **3:**103, **3:**103*f*
Supraorbital foramen, **2:**3*f*, **2:**7, **2:**7*f*
Supraorbital margins, **2:**7, **2:**7*f*
  lateral projection of, **2:**35*f*
  PA axial projection of, **2:**38*f*
Suprapatellar bursa, **1:**62*f*
Suprarenal glands
  anatomy of, **2:**275, **2:**275*f*
  diagnostic medical sonography of, **3:**414*f*
Surgeon, **3:**31
Surgical assistant, **3:**31
Surgical attire, **3:**32–69
Surgical bed, **3:**482, **3:**510
Surgical dressings, **1:**11
Surgical neck, of humerus, **1:**146–147, **1:**146*f*
Surgical radiography, **3:**29–70
  aseptic techniques in, **3:**36*b*
  attire for, **3:**32–69
  equipment for, **3:**37, **3:**37*f*–38*f*
  cleaning of, **3:**38
  fluoroscopic procedures in, **3:**39–56
    of cervical spine (anterior cervical diskectomy and fusion), **3:**43, **3:**43*b*, **3:**43*f*
    chest (line placement, bronchoscopy), **3:**42, **3:**42*b*, **3:**42*f*
    femoral/tibial arteriogram as, **3:**54*b*, **3:**55–56, **3:**55*f*–56*f*, **3:**56*b*
    femur nail as, **3:**48–50, **3:**50*b*
      antegrade, **3:**48
      evaluation criteria for, **3:**50*b*
      method for, **3:**49, **3:**49*f*–50*f*
      position of patient and C-arm, **3:**48–49, **3:**48*f*
      retrograde, **3:**49, **3:**49*f*
      structures shown on, **3:**50, **3:**50*f*
    of hip (cannulated hip screws or hip pinning), **3:**46–47, **3:**46*f*–47*f*, **3:**47*b*
    of humerus, **3:**53–54, **3:**53*f*–54*f*, **3:**54*b*
    of lumbar spine, **3:**44–45, **3:**44*f*–45*f*, **3:**45*b*
    operative (immediate) cholangiography as, **3:**39–41, **3:**40*f*, **3:**41*b*
    tibia (nail) as, **3:**51–52, **3:**52*b*
      evaluation criteria for, **3:**52*b*
      position of C-arm for, **3:**51, **3:**51*f*
      position of patient for, **3:**51–52
      structures shown on, **3:**52, **3:**52*f*
  mobile radiography procedures in, **3:**57–64
    of cervical spine, **3:**57, **3:**57*b*, **3:**57*f*–58*f*
    of extremity, **3:**61–64, **3:**64*b*
      for ankle fracture, **3:**61*f*
      for ankle with antibiotic beads, **3:**62*f*
      for fifth metatarsal nonhealing fracture, **3:**63*f*
      for forearm fracture, **3:**62*f*
      for hip joint replacement, **3:**61*f*
      for tibial plateau fracture, **3:**62*f*

Surgical radiography *(Continued)*
  for total shoulder arthroplasty, **3:**63f
  for wrist, **3:**64f
  of thoracic or lumbar spine, **3:**59, **3:**59b, **3:**59f–60f
 O-arm equipment, **3:**65, **3:**66f–68f
 in operating room, **3:**34–36, **3:**34f
 operating room attire for, **3:**33, **3:**33f
 personal hygiene in, **3:**33
 practices in, **3:**69
 radiation exposure considerations for, **3:**39, **3:**39f
 scope of, **3:**30, **3:**30b
 sterile field in
  enemies in, **3:**36
  image receptor handling in, **3:**35–36, **3:**35f–36f
Surgical team
 nonsterile team members of, **3:**32
 sterile team members of, **3:**30–32, **3:**31f
Survey image, of abdomen, **1:**132
Suspensory muscle, of duodenum, **2:**180, **2:**181f
Sustentaculum tali, **1:**271, **1:**271f
Sutures, **2:**5, **1:**60f, **1:**61
Swimmer's technique, for lateral projection, of cervicothoracic region, **1:**448–449, **1:**448b–449b, **1:**448f–449f
Symphysis, **1:**61, **1:**61f
Synarthroses, **1:**61
Synchondrosis, **1:**61, **1:**61f
Syndesmosis, **1:**60f, **1:**61
Synostosis, **3:**104
Synovial ball-and-socket joint, **1:**375
Synovial double-gliding joint, **1:**224
Synovial ellipsoidal joints, **1:**422
Synovial fluid, **1:**62, **1:**62f
Synovial gliding joints, **1:**224, **1:**422, **1:**499–500
Synovial irregular gliding joints, **1:**375
Synovial joints, **1:**60t, **1:**62, **1:**62f–63f
Synovial membrane, **1:**62, **1:**62f
Synovial pivot articulation, **1:**422
Syringes, for venipuncture, **2:**318–319, **2:**318f
 recapping of, **2:**319, **2:**319f
System noise, in CT, **3:**267
Systemic arteries, **3:**315
Systemic circulation, **3:**315, **3:**315f, **3:**404
Systemic disease, **3:**482
Systemic veins, **3:**316
Systole, **3:**405

T

Table, for CT, **3:**235f, **3:**236
Table increments, in CT, **3:**267
Table pad, **1:**13
Table speed, for CT angiography, **3:**250, **3:**267
Tachyarrhythmia, **3:**405
Tachycardia, **3:**405
Taeniae coli, **2:**182, **2:**182f
Tall patients, long bone studies in, **1:**22
Talocalcaneal articulation, **1:**278f, **1:**278t
Talocalcaneonavicular articulation, **1:**278f, **1:**278t
Talofibular joint, **1:**278t, **1:**280
Talus, **1:**270f
Tangential projection, **1:**68, **1:**68f, **1:**70t, **2:**423, **2:**423f–424f
 labeling codes for, **2:**385t–390t
Target, **3:**479
Targeted lesion, **3:**405
Tarsals, anatomy of, **1:**270f, **1:**271, **1:**271t
Tarsometatarsal (TMT) articulations, **1:**278t, **1:**280
Taylor method, for AP axial outlet projection, of anterior pelvic bones, **1:**402–403, **1:**402f–403f, **1:**403b
Teamwork, **3:**69
Technetium-99m (⁹⁹ᵐTc), in nuclear medicine, **3:**442t
Technetium-99m (⁹⁹ᵐTc) microaggregated albumin (MAA) lung perfusion scan, **3:**458
Technetium-99m (⁹⁹ᵐTc) sestamibi myocardial perfusion imaging (MPI), **3:**454
Technetium-99m (⁹⁹ᵐTc) tetrofosmin myocardial perfusion imaging (MPI), **3:**454
Technical factors, **1:**18, **1:**19f
Teeth, anatomy of, **2:**172
Teletherapy, **3:**510
Temporal bones, **2:**4f, **2:**14, **2:**14f–15f
 CT scan through, **2:**15f
 location of, **2:**3f
 mastoid portion of, sectional anatomy of, **3:**175, **3:**181f–182f

Temporal bones *(Continued)*
 petromastoid portion of, **2:**14, **2:**17f
 petrous portion of, **2:**5f, **2:**14f–15f
  lateral projection of, **2:**35f–36f
  sectional anatomy of, **3:**175, **3:**189–190
 sectional anatomy of, **3:**175
 squamous portion of, **2:**5f, **2:**14, **2:**14f–15f
  sectional anatomy of, **3:**175, **3:**180–181
 tympanic portion of, **2:**14, **2:**14f
  sectional anatomy of, **3:**175
 zygomatic arch of, **2:**19
  acanthioparietal projection of, **2:**65f
  AP axial projection of (modified Towne method), **2:**74, **2:**74b, **2:**74f
  parietoacanthial projection of, **2:**61f
  submentovertical projection of, **2:**70–74, **2:**70f–71f, **2:**71b
  tangential projection of, **2:**72–73, **2:**72f–73f, **2:**73b
 zygomatic process of, sectional anatomy of, **3:**175
Temporal lobe, sectional anatomy of, **3:**174–175, **3:**174f
 on axial plane
  at level C, **3:**180f
  at level F, **3:**184f
  at level G, **3:**185f
Temporal process, **2:**19, **2:**19f
Temporal resolution, for CT, **3:**244, **3:**267
Temporalis muscle, sectional anatomy of, **3:**174f, **3:**180–181, **3:**180f–181f
Temporary transvenous pacemaker (TTVP), **3:**392, **3:**392f, **3:**405
Temporomandibular joint, **2:**14, **2:**20, **2:**21f, **3:**175
 AP axial projection of, **2:**83–88, **2:**83f–84f, **2:**84b
 axiolateral oblique projection of, **2:**87–88, **2:**87f–88f, **2:**88b
 axiolateral projections of, **2:**81f, **2:**85–86, **2:**85f–86f, **2:**86b
 lateral projection of, **2:**35f–36f
 panoramic tomography of, **2:**89, **2:**89f
Temporomandibular joint (TMJ) syndrome, **2:**26t
Tendinitis, **1:**225t
Tentorium cerebelli
 anatomy of, **2:**153, **2:**167
 sectional anatomy of, **3:**175, **3:**181–182, **3:**190f
Teres minor muscle, sectional anatomy of, **3:**195
Tesla (T), **3:**271, **3:**308
Testicular torsion, **2:**335t
Testis
 anatomy of, **2:**332, **2:**332f
 diagnostic medical sonography of, **3:**420, **3:**420f
Teufel method, for PA axial oblique projection, of acetabulum, **1:**398–399, **1:**398f–399f, **1:**399b
Thalamus, sectional anatomy of, **3:**181, **3:**187f, **3:**189f
Thallium-201 (²⁰¹Tl), in nuclear medicine, **3:**442t
Thallium-201 (²⁰¹Tl) myocardial perfusion imaging, **3:**454–455, **3:**454b
Therapeutic nuclear medicine, **3:**459
Thermodilution cardiac output, **3:**405
Thermography, of breast, **2:**451
Thermoluminescent dosimeters, for CT, **3:**256
Thin-film transistor (TFT) array, **1:**14
Third ventricle
 anatomy of, **2:**152, **2:**154, **2:**154f
 sectional anatomy of, **3:**180f, **3:**181
 on coronal plane, **3:**189f
Thoracic aortography, **3:**334, **3:**334f
Thoracic cavity, **1:**49, **1:**49f, **1:**83, **1:**83f
Thoracic curve, **1:**411f
Thoracic duct, **3:**318, **3:**319f
Thoracic inlet, **3:**191
Thoracic region, sectional anatomy of, **3:**191–203, **3:**193f
 on cadaveric image, **3:**191, **3:**191f
 on coronal plane, **3:**202–203, **3:**203f
  level A, **3:**203f
  level B, **3:**203f
  level C, **3:**203f
 posterior plane, **3:**203
 on sagittal plane, **3:**200–201, **3:**201f
  level A, **3:**202f
  level B, **3:**202f
  level C, **3:**202f
 median, **3:**200–201
Thoracic vertebrae, **1:**411, **1:**418f
 anatomy of, **1:**411f, **1:**417–418
  costal facets and demifacets in, **1:**417, **1:**418t
  posterior oblique aspect in, **1:**417f

Thoracic vertebrae *(Continued)*
 superior and lateral aspects of, **1:**417, **1:**417f
 AP projection of, **1:**450–455, **1:**450f–451f, **1:**451b
 computed tomography of, **1:**451f
 intervertebral foramina of
  anatomy of, **1:**417f, **1:**418
  positioning rotations needed to show, **1:**416t
 lateral projection of, **1:**452–455, **1:**452f–455f, **1:**454b–455b
 for trauma, **2:**120, **2:**120b, **2:**120f
 mobile radiography procedures, in operating room, **3:**59, **3:**59b, **3:**59f–60f
 MRI of, **3:**293f
 in radiography of sternum, **1:**506
 sectional anatomy of, **3:**191–192
 transverse process of, **1:**418
 trauma radiography of, **2:**120
 upper
  lateral projection of, swimmer's technique for, **1:**448–449, **1:**448b–449b, **1:**448f–449f
  vertebral arch (pillars), **1:**446f, **1:**447b
   AP axial oblique projection of, **1:**446–447, **1:**446f–447f
   AP axial projection of, **1:**444–445, **1:**444b–445b, **1:**444f–445f
 zygapophyseal joints of
  anatomy of, **1:**417f–418f, **1:**418
  AP or PA oblique projection of, **1:**456–457, **1:**456f–457f, **1:**457b
  positioning rotations needed to show, **1:**416t
Thoracic viscera, **1:**81–124
 anatomy of, **1:**83–92
  body habitus and, **1:**83–92, **1:**83f
  mediastinum in, **1:**90–92, **1:**90f–91f
  neck in, **1:**87–89, **1:**87f
  respiratory system in, **1:**83–86
   alveoli of, **1:**84f, **1:**85
   bronchial tree of, **1:**84, **1:**84b, **1:**84f
   lungs of, **1:**85–86, **1:**85f–86f
   trachea of, **1:**84, **1:**84b, **1:**84f
  summary of, **1:**91b
  thoracic cavity in, **1:**83, **1:**83f
 breathing instructions for, **1:**100f, **1:**101
 CT of, **1:**92f, **1:**93t
 general positioning considerations for, **1:**99
  for lateral criteria, **1:**99, **1:**99f
  for oblique criteria, **1:**99
  for PA criteria, **1:**99, **1:**100f
  prone, **1:**99f
  upright, **1:**99f
 grid technique for, **1:**101, **1:**102f
 heart as
  lateral projection with barium of, **1:**107
  PA chest radiographs with barium of, **1:**105
  PA oblique projection with barium of, **1:**111
 pleura as
  AP or PA projection of, **1:**120–123, **1:**120f–121f
  lateral projection of, **1:**122f
 sample exposure technique chart routine projections for, **1:**94t
 SID for, **1:**101, **1:**101f
 summary of pathology of, **1:**93t
 summary of projections for, **1:**82, **1:**82t
 technical procedure for, **1:**101, **1:**101f–102f
Thoracolumbar spine, scoliosis of
 PA and lateral projection of (Frank et al. method), **1:**484–489, **1:**485f–487f, **1:**486b
 PA projection of (Ferguson method), **1:**488–489, **1:**488f–489f, **1:**489b
3D printing, for sectional anatomy, **3:**224–226, **3:**224f–225f
Three-dimensional imaging
 CT for, **3:**252–253
 diagnostic medical sonography for, **3:**410
 for intraarterial angiography, **3:**326, **3:**326f
Three-dimensional imaging, for MRI, **3:**287, **3:**287f
Threshold values, in shaded surface display, **3:**252, **3:**267
Thrombectomy, mechanical, **3:**369, **3:**369f
Thrombogenesis, **3:**405
Thrombolysis, pharmacologic, **3:**369
Thrombolytic, **3:**405
Thrombosis, **3:**405
Thrombus, definition of, **3:**405
Thumb, **1:**158–164
 anatomy of, **1:**143f, **1:**154
 AP projection of, **1:**158

Thumb *(Continued)*
　　evaluation criteria for, **1:**159*b*
　　position of part for, **1:**158, **1:**158*f*
　　position of patient for, **1:**158
　　structures shown on, **1:**159, **1:**159*f*
　first carpometacarpal joint of, **1:**160
　　Burman method for, AP projection of, **1:**162–163, **1:**162*f*–163*f*, **1:**163*b*
　　Robert method for, AP projection of, **1:**160–161
　　　central ray for, **1:**161, **1:**161*f*
　　　collimation for, **1:**161
　　　evaluation criteria for, **1:**161*b*
　　　Lewis modification of, **1:**161, **1:**161*f*
　　　Long and Rafert modification of, **1:**161, **1:**161*f*
　　　position of part for, **1:**160, **1:**160*f*
　　　position of patient for, **1:**160, **1:**160*f*
　　　structures shown on, **1:**161, **1:**161*f*
　folio method for, PA projection of, first metacarpophalangeal joint of, **1:**164, **1:**164*b*, **1:**164*f*–165*f*
　lateral projection of, **1:**158
　　evaluation criteria for, **1:**159*b*
　　position of part for, **1:**158, **1:**158*f*
　　position of patient for, **1:**158
　　structures shown on, **1:**159, **1:**159*f*
　PA oblique projection of, **1:**159
　　central ray for, **1:**159
　　collimation for, **1:**159
　　evaluation criteria for, **1:**159*b*
　　position of part for, **1:**159, **1:**159*f*
　　position of patient for, **1:**159
　　structures shown on, **1:**159, **1:**159*f*
　PA projection of, **1:**158
　　evaluation criteria for, **1:**159*b*
　　position of part for, **1:**158, **1:**158*f*
　　position of patient for, **1:**158
　　structures shown on, **1:**159, **1:**159*f*
Thymus gland, **1:**83, **1:**91
Thyroid cartilage, **1:**87*f*–89*f*, **1:**89, **1:**98*f*
　anatomy of, **2:**175*f*–176*f*
　as surface landmark, **1:**51*f*
Thyroid gland
　anatomy of, **1:**88, **1:**88*f*
　diagnostic medical sonography of, **3:**413*f*, **3:**420*f*
Thyroid scan, **3:**455–456, **3:**456*b*
Tibia
　anatomy of, **1:**272–273, **1:**272*f*
　AP projection of, **1:**330–334, **1:**330*b*, **1:**330*f*–331*f*
　joints of, **1:**280*f*
　lateral projection of, **1:**332*f*–333*f*
　nail, **3:**51–52, **3:**52*b*
　　evaluation criteria for, **3:**52*b*
　　position of C-arm for, **3:**51, **3:**51*f*
　　position of patient for, **3:**51–52
　　structures shown on, **3:**52, **3:**52*f*
Tibial arteriogram, **3:**54*b*, **3:**55–56, **3:**55*f*–56*f*, **3:**56*b*
Tibial collateral ligament, **1:**276*f*
Tibial plafond, **1:**273*f*
Tibial plateau, **1:**272, **1:**272*f*, **1:**277*f*
Tibial plateau fracture, mobile radiography procedures for, in operating room, **3:**62*f*
Tibial tuberosity, **1:**272, **1:**272*f*, **1:**277*f*
Tibiofibular joint, **1:**278*t*
Tibiotalar joint, **1:**278*t*
Tilt, **1:**79, **1:**79*f*
Time-of-flight (TOF) imaging, **3:**302
TNM classification, **3:**485, **3:**485*t*
Toddlers, development of, **3:**74
Toddler's fracture, **3:**102–103
Toes
　anatomy of, **1:**270
　AP axial projections of, **1:**284, **1:**284*b*, **1:**285*f*
　AP oblique projection of, **1:**287, **1:**287*b*, **1:**287*f*
　evaluation criteria for, **1:**284*b*
　lateral projections of, **1:**288–289, **1:**288*b*
　　central ray, **1:**289
　　collimation, **1:**289
　　evaluation criteria for, **1:**289*b*
　　for fifth toe, **1:**288, **1:**288*f*–289*f*
　　for fourth toe, **1:**288, **1:**288*f*–289*f*
　　for great toe, **1:**288, **1:**288*f*
　　position of part for, **1:**288
　　position of patient for, **1:**288
　　for second toe, **1:**288, **1:**288*f*
　　structures shown on, **1:**289, **1:**289*f*

Toes *(Continued)*
　　for third toe, **1:**288, **1:**288*f*–289*f*
　PA projection of, **1:**286
　　evaluation criteria for, **1:**286*b*, **1:**286*f*
　radiography, **1:**284–289
Tolerance doses, to radiation, **3:**495, **3:**495*t*
TomoTherapy, **3:**500, **3:**500*f*
Tongue, anatomy of, **2:**171*f*–173*f*, **2:**172, **2:**184*f*
Tonsil
　anatomy of, **2:**172, **2:**172*f*
　palatine, **2:**172
　pharyngeal, **1:**87*f*, **1:**88
Top of ear attachment (TEA), **2:**14, **2:**17*f*
　as lateral landmark, **2:**29*f*
　as surface landmark, **1:**51*f*
Torus fracture, **3:**102, **1:**151*t*
Total body less head (TBLH), **2:**492
Total joint replacement, in older adults, **3:**156, **3:**157*f*
Total shoulder arthroplasty, mobile radiography procedures for, in operating room, **3:**63*f*
Total-body iodine-123 (^{123}I) (TBI) scan, **3:**456
Tourniquet, for venipuncture
　application of, **2:**322*f*, **2:**323
　release of, **2:**323, **2:**323*f*
Towne method, for AP axial projection
　of skull, **2:**41, **2:**43*b*, **2:**130–131, **2:**130*f*–131*f*
　　central ray for, **2:**43
　　in children, **3:**106–108, **3:**106*f*, **3:**108*t*
　　position of part for, **2:**41, **2:**41*f*–42*f*
　　position of patient for, **2:**41
　　structures shown in, **2:**43, **2:**43*f*
　　variations of, **2:**41*b*
　of zygomatic arches, **2:**74, **2:**74*b*, **2:**74*f*
Trabeculae, **1:**56, **1:**56*f*
Trabecular bone, **2:**492
　bone densitometry and, **2:**459, **2:**459*t*
Trabecular bone score (TBS), **2:**489–490, **2:**492
Tracer, **3:**436, **3:**479–480
Trachea
　anatomy of, **1:**84, **1:**84*b*, **1:**84*f*, **2:**175*f*–177*f*
　inferior portion of, **1:**83, **1:**83*f*
　magnified, **1:**113*f*
　sectional anatomy of, **3:**195
Tragus, **2:**16, **2:**17*f*
Transabdominal ultrasonography, of female pelvis, **3:**423, **3:**423*f*
Transcatheter aortic valve replacement (TAVR), **3:**393, **3:**394*f*, **3:**405
Transcatheter embolization, **3:**360–362, **3:**362*f*–363*f*
　in cerebral vasculature, **3:**362, **3:**362*f*
　embolic agents in, **3:**360*b*, **3:**360*t*
　in hypervascular uterine fibroid, **3:**362, **3:**363*f*
　lesions amenable to, **3:**360*b*
　stainless steel coils for, **3:**361–362, **3:**361*f*
Transducer, **3:**405
　for diagnostic medical sonography, **3:**410, **3:**410*f*, **3:**434
Transesophageal echocardiogram (TEE), **3:**405
Transesophageal transducer, **3:**432–433
Transjugular intrahepatic portosystemic shunt (TIPS), **3:**368, **3:**368*f*
Translational force (missile effect), **3:**285, **3:**308
Transmission scan, **3:**438, **3:**480
Transportation
　of obese patients, **1:**36–37, **1:**37*f*
　of older adults, **3:**161
Transposition of great arteries, **3:**405
Transthoracic projection, **1:**69, **1:**70*t*
Transverse abdominal muscle, **3:**212
Transverse arch, of foot, **1:**270
Transverse atlantal ligament, **1:**414
Transverse fracture, **1:**64*f*
Transverse plane, **1:**46, **1:**46*f*
　in MRI, **3:**271, **3:**308
　pancreas in, **3:**417, **3:**434
　in sectional anatomy, **3:**172
Transverse processes, **1:**413
Transverse sinuses, **3:**183, **3:**190*f*
Trapezium
　anatomy of, **1:**143*f*–144*f*, **1:**144
　Clements-Nakayama method for, PA axial oblique projection of, **1:**186, **1:**186*b*, **1:**186*f*
Trapezoid, **1:**143*f*–144*f*, **1:**144
Trauma
　blunt, **2:**105
　defined, **2:**105

Trauma *(Continued)*
　explosive, **2:**105
　heat, **2:**105
　imaging procedures in, **2:**137–139
　　CT as, **2:**106, **2:**137–139
　　diagnostic medical sonography as, **2:**139
　penetrating, **2:**105
　statistics, **2:**105
Trauma center, **2:**105
Trauma patients, handling of, **1:**7
Trauma radiography, **2:**103–140
　abbreviations for, **2:**115*b*
　of abdomen
　　AP projection in, **2:**122–124, **2:**122*f*
　　　in left lateral decubitus position, **2:**123, **2:**123*f*
　　lateral projection in, **2:**124, **2:**124*f*
　best practices in, **2:**113
　breathing instructions for, **2:**115
　　with immobilization devices, **2:**115
　central ray, part, and image receptor alignment in, **2:**115
　of cervical spine, **2:**116
　　AP axial oblique projection in, **2:**119, **2:**119*b*, **2:**119*f*
　　AP axial projection in, **2:**118–119, **2:**118*b*, **2:**118*f*
　　lateral projection in, **2:**116, **2:**116*b*, **2:**116*f*
　of cervicothoracic region, lateral projection in, dorsal decubitus position in, **2:**117, **2:**117*b*, **2:**117*f*
　of chest, AP projection in, **2:**121, **2:**121*f*
　collimated field for, **2:**115
　diagnostic imaging procedures of, **2:**111
　documentation of, **2:**115
　exposure factors for, **2:**109, **2:**109*f*
　of facial bones, acanthioparietal projection (reverse Waters method) in, **2:**132, **2:**132*f*
　grids and IR holders for, **2:**106
　of hip
　　axiolateral projection (Danelius-Miller method) in, **2:**126–127, **2:**126*f*
　　modified axiolateral projection (Clements-Nakayama modification) in, **2:**127, **2:**127*f*
　image evaluation in, **2:**115
　with immobilization devices, **2:**109, **2:**109*f*
　of lower extremity
　　patient position considerations for, **2:**135, **2:**135*f*–136*f*
　　structures shown on, **2:**136, **2:**136*f*–138*f*
　　trauma positioning tips for, **2:**135–136, **2:**135*f*
　patient care in, **2:**111, **2:**112*t*
　patient preparation for, **2:**114
　of pelvis, AP projection in, **2:**125, **2:**125*f*
　positioning aids for, **2:**106
　positioning of patient for, **2:**110, **2:**110*f*
　procedures in, **2:**114–115, **2:**114*f*
　radiation protection for, **2:**111
　of skull, **2:**128–131
　　AP axial projection (reverse Caldwell method and Towne method) in, **2:**130–131, **2:**130*f*–131*f*
　　lateral projection in, **2:**128–131, **2:**128*f*–129*f*
　specialized equipment for, **2:**106
　　dedicated C-arm-type trauma radiographic room as, **2:**106*f*
　　mobile fluoroscopic C-arm a, **2:**106, **2:**107*f*
　　Statscan as, **2:**106, **2:**107*f*–108*f*
　standard precautions in, **2:**113
　summary of projections for, **2:**104–115, **2:**104*t*
　of thoracic and lumbar spine, **2:**120
　　lateral projections in, **2:**120, **2:**120*b*, **2:**120*f*
　of upper extremity, **2:**133–134
　　patient position considerations for, **2:**133
　　for forearm, **2:**133*f*
　　for humerus, **2:**134*f*
　　for shoulder, **2:**133, **2:**134*f*
　　structures shown on, **2:**135–136
　　trauma positioning tips for, **2:**133–134, **2:**133*f*
Trauma team, radiographer's role as part of, **2:**111
Treatment fields, in radiation oncology, **3:**493, **3:**494*f*, **3:**510
Trendelenburg position, **1:**72, **1:**72*f*
Trigone, **2:**278, **2:**278*f*
Tripod fracture, of cranium, **2:**26*t*
Triquetrum, **1:**143*f*–144*f*, **1:**144
Trochanter, defined, **1:**64
Trochlea, **1:**271, **1:**271*f*
Trochlear groove, of femur, **1:**275, **1:**275*f*
Trochlear notch, **1:**145, **1:**145*f*
Trochlear surface, of foot, **1:**271
Trochoid joint, **1:**62, **1:**63*f*

True coincidence event, **3:**469, **3:**469f, **3:**480
"True pelvis,", **1:**127
True projections, **1:**71
True ribs, **1:**498
T-score, in DXA, **2:**471, **2:**472t, **2:**492
T-tube cholangiography, **2:**266–267, **2:**266f–267f
Tube angles, in mobile radiography, **2:**26
Tubercles, **1:**56, **1:**64
Tuberculosis, **1:**93t
Tuberculum sellae
   anatomy of, **2:**4f, **2:**10f, **2:**11
   sectional anatomy of, **3:**174–175
Tuberosities, **1:**56, **1:**64
Tumor, **1:**93t, **2:**190t–191t, **2:**335t, **3:**482
   of abdomen, **1:**129t
   of bone, **1:**282t
   of bony thorax, **1:**504t
   of cranium, **2:**26t
   of shoulder girdle, **1:**225t
Tumor imaging, in nuclear medicine, **3:**459
Tumor studies, **3:**459
Tumor/target volume, **3:**495, **3:**510
Tunneled catheters, in children, **3:**145, **3:**145f
T1 weighted image, **3:**272, **3:**288, **3:**289f, **3:**308
T2 weighted image, **3:**272, **3:**288, **3:**289f, **3:**308
Twining method, in mobile radiography, of cervical spine, **2:**25b
Tympanic cavity, **2:**16, **2:**17f
Tympanic membrane, **2:**16, **2:**17f

U

Ulcer, **2:**190t–191t
   decubitus, in older adults, **3:**161
Ulcerative colitis, **2:**190t–191t
Ulna, **1:**143f, **1:**145, **1:**145f
Ulnar styloid process, **1:**145, **1:**145f
Ultrasonography. *See also* Diagnostic medical sonography
   of breast, **2:**400–401
   of children, **3:**143
   defined, **3:**434
   quantitative, **2:**488, **2:**489f, **2:**492
Umbilical region, **1:**50f
Undifferentiation, **3:**486, **3:**510
Unrestricted area, **3:**69
Upper esophageal sphincter (UES), **2:**176, **2:**177f
Upper extremity, **1:**141–216
   abbreviations for, **1:**151b
   anatomy of, **1:**143–149, **1:**150b
   arm, anatomy of, **1:**146–147, **1:**146f
   arteriograms of, **3:**341, **3:**341f
   articulations, **1:**147–149, **1:**147t, **1:**148f–149f
   elbow
      articulations of, **1:**149, **1:**149f
      fat pads of, **1:**149, **1:**149f
      radiography of, **1:**193b, **1:**193f–197f, **1:**196b–197b
   first carpometacarpal joint, radiography of, **1:**160, **1:**160f–163f, **1:**161b, **1:**163b
   first digit (thumb)
      anatomy of, **1:**143, **1:**143f
      radiography of, **1:**158–164, **1:**158f–159f
   first metacarpophalangeal joint, radiography of, **1:**164, **1:**164b, **1:**164f–165f
   forearm
      anatomy of, **1:**145, **1:**145f
      radiography of, **1:**199, **1:**199b, **1:**199f, **1:**201, **1:**201b, **1:**201f
   general procedures for, **1:**152, **1:**152f
   of geriatric patients, **3:**166f
   hand
      anatomy of, **1:**143–149, **1:**143f–144f
      articulations of, **1:**148f–149f, **1:**150b
      radiography of, **1:**166–173, **1:**166f–173f, **1:**172b
   humerus
      anatomy of, **1:**146, **1:**147f
      distal
         anatomy of, **1:**146
         radiography of, **1:**198, **1:**198b, **1:**198f, **1:**200, **1:**200b, **1:**200f, **1:**207, **1:**207b, **1:**207f
      radiography of, **1:**209–214, **1:**209b, **1:**209f–214f, **1:**211b–212b, **1:**214b
   olecranon process
      anatomy of, **1:**145, **1:**145f
      radiography of, **1:**208, **1:**208b, **1:**208f
   radial head, radiography of, **1:**202, **1:**202f–203f, **1:**203b
   sample exposure technique chart routine projection for, **1:**150t

Upper extremity *(Continued)*
   scaphoid series, radiography of, **1:**184, **1:**184b, **1:**184f–185f
   second through fifth digits
      anatomy of, **1:**143, **1:**143f
      radiography of, **1:**152–214, **1:**152f–157f, **1:**153b, **1:**156b
   summary of pathology of, **1:**151t
   summary of projections for, **1:**142, **1:**142t
   trapezium, radiography of, **1:**186, **1:**186b, **1:**186f
   trauma radiography of, **2:**133–134, **2:**133f
      patient position considerations for, **2:**133
         for forearm, **2:**133f
         for humerus, **2:**134f
         for shoulder, **2:**133, **2:**134f
      structures shown on, **2:**135–136
      trauma positioning tips for, **2:**133–134, **2:**133f
   wrist
      anatomy of, **1:**144, **1:**144f
      articulations of, **1:**148f
      radiography of, **1:**174–187, **1:**174f–181f, **1:**177b–180b
Upper limb arteries, duplex sonography of, **3:**429
Upper limb veins, duplex sonography of, **3:**429
Upright positions, **1:**66f, **1:**72
Ureteral compression, for excretory urography, **2:**292, **2:**292f
Ureterocele, **2:**280t
Ureteropelvic junction (UPJ), **2:**277
Ureterovesical junction (UVJ), **2:**278
Ureters
   anatomy of, **2:**275f, **2:**278, **2:**278f
   radiologic examination of, **2:**306
   retrograde urography of, **2:**304–305, **2:**304f–305f
Urethra
   anatomy of, **2:**278f–279f, **2:**279
   radiologic examination of, **2:**306
Urethral orifice, **2:**330, **2:**330f
Urinary bladder
   anatomy of, **2:**275f, **2:**278, **2:**278f
   cystourethrography of, **2:**285, **2:**285f
      female, **2:**314, **2:**314f
      male, **2:**313, **2:**313f
      voiding, **2:**307f, **2:**314f
   diagnostic medical sonography of, **3:**418–419, **3:**422f
   location of, **2:**275f
   MRI of, **3:**298
   radiologic examination of, **2:**306
   retrograde cystography
      AP axial or PA axial projection for, **2:**308–312, **2:**308b–309b, **2:**308f–309f
      AP oblique projection for, **2:**310–311, **2:**310f–311f, **2:**311b
      lateral projection for, **2:**312, **2:**312b, **2:**312f
   sectional anatomy of, **3:**206
   on coronal plane, **3:**220
Urinary incontinence, in older adults, **3:**160t
Urinary system, **2:**273–326
   abbreviations for, **2:**281b
   anatomy of, **2:**275–279, **2:**275f
      kidneys in, **2:**275f–276f, **2:**276–277
      prostate in, **2:**279, **2:**279f
      summary of, **2:**279b
      suprarenal glands in, **2:**275, **2:**275f
      ureters in, **2:**275f, **2:**278
      urethra in, **2:**279
      urinary bladder in, **2:**275f, **2:**278, **2:**278f
   AP oblique projection of, **2:**298, **2:**298b, **2:**298f
   AP projection of, **2:**296–300, **2:**296b
      central ray for, **2:**296
      collimation for, **2:**296
      evaluation criteria for, **2:**297b
      position of part for, **2:**296
      position of patient for, **2:**292f, **2:**296–297, **2:**296f
      respiration for, **2:**296
      structures shown on, **2:**296–297, **2:**297f
   cystography of. *See* Cystography
   excretory. *See* Excretory urography
   lateral projection of, **2:**299
      in dorsal decubitus position, **2:**300, **2:**300b, **2:**300f
      in right or left position, **2:**299, **2:**299b, **2:**299f
   nephrotomography of, **2:**301
      AP projection in, **2:**301, **2:**301f
      percutaneous renal puncture for, **2:**302, **2:**302f
   pelvicaliceal system in, retrograde urography of, **2:**304–305, **2:**304f–305f

Urinary system *(Continued)*
   preliminary examination of, **2:**291f, **2:**293
   radiation protection for, **2:**293
   radiography, **2:**282–314
      adverse reactions to iodinated media for, **2:**288
      antegrade filling for, **2:**283, **2:**283f
      contrast media for, **2:**286, **2:**287f
      CT in, **2:**282, **2:**282f
      equipment for, **2:**290, **2:**290f–291f
      image quality and exposure technique for, **2:**291, **2:**291f
      motion control for, **2:**291
      overview of, **2:**282–295, **2:**282f
      preparation of intestinal tract for, **2:**288–289, **2:**288f–289f
      preparation of patient for, **2:**289
      procedure for, **2:**291–292
      respiration for, **2:**292
      retrograde filling for, **2:**284f, **2:**285
      ureteral compression for, **2:**292, **2:**292f
      US in, **2:**282, **2:**283f
   sample exposure technique chart routine projections for, **2:**281t
   sectional anatomy of, **3:**205
   summary of pathology of, **2:**280t
   summary of projections for, **2:**274, **2:**274t
   urography. *See* Urography
Urography, **2:**282
   percutaneous antegrade, **2:**283
   retrograde, **2:**285
      AP projection for, **2:**304–305, **2:**304f–305f
      contrast media for, **2:**286, **2:**287f
      defined, **2:**285
      preparation of patient for, **2:**289
Uterine fibroid, **3:**298f, **2:**335t, **2:**337f
Uterine ostium, **2:**330, **2:**330f
Uterine tubes
   anatomy of, **2:**329, **2:**329f–330f
   hydrosalpinx of, **2:**336f
   hysterosalpingography of, **2:**336–337, **2:**336f–337f, **2:**337b
   obstruction of, **2:**335t
   sectional anatomy of, **3:**206
Uterus
   anatomy of, **2:**330, **2:**330f
   bicornuate, **2:**337f
   diagnostic medical sonography of, **3:**422f, **3:**424, **3:**425f
   hysterosalpingography of, **2:**336–337, **2:**336f–337f, **2:**337b
   sectional anatomy of, **3:**206
Uvula, **1:**87f, **1:**88
   anatomy of, **2:**172, **2:**172f, **2:**174, **2:**175f

V

Vacuum-assisted biopsies, **2:**446
Vacuum bag immobilization device, for radiation oncology, **3:**493f
Vagina
   anatomy of, **2:**330
   diagnostic medical sonography of, **3:**422f
   sectional anatomy of, **3:**206
Vaginal orifice, **2:**330, **2:**330f
Vaginal vestibule, **2:**330
Vaginography, **2:**336, **2:**340–341, **2:**340f–341f, **2:**341b
Valium (diazepam), **2:**316t
Valsalva maneuver, **1:**88, **2:**174
Valvular competence, **3:**405
Varices, **3:**405
   esophageal, **2:**190t–191t
   venous, **3:**368
Vascular access devices, in children, **3:**144
Vascular access needles, for angiography, **3:**329, **3:**329f
Vasoconstricting drugs, for transcatheter embolization, **3:**361
Vasoconstriction, **3:**405
Veins, **3:**405
   coronary, **3:**317f
   systemic, **3:**316
Velocity of sound, **3:**410, **3:**434
Vena cava filter placement, **3:**364–367, **3:**364f–367f
Venipuncture, **2:**315–325
   discarding needles after, **2:**324, **2:**324f
   documentation of, **2:**325
   infection control during, **2:**318
   medication preparation for, **2:**319–320, **2:**319f

Venipuncture *(Continued)*
 from bottle or vial, **2:**319, **2:**319*f*
 identification and expiration date in, **2:**320, **2:**320*f*
 nonvented tubing in, **2:**320, **2:**320*f*
 recapping of syringe in, **2:**319, **2:**319*f*
 tube clamp in, **2:**320, **2:**320*f*
 vented tubing in, **2:**320, **2:**320*f*
 medications administered via, **2:**316*t*, **2:**324, **2:**324*f*
 needles and syringes for, **2:**318–319, **2:**318*f*
 patient assessment for, **2:**318
 patient education on, **2:**315
 procedure for, **2:**320–324
 professional and legal considerations for, **2:**315–325
 reactions to and complications of, **2:**325
 removing IV access after, **2:**324, **2:**324*f*
 site preparation for, **2:**322, **2:**322*f*
 site selection for, **2:**320–321, **2:**321*f*
 technique for, **2:**322
  anchoring needle in, **2:**323, **2:**323*f*
  applying tourniquet in, **2:**322*f*, **2:**323
  direct (one-step), **2:**322
  gloves and cleaning of area in, **2:**322*f*, **2:**323
  indirect (two-step), **2:**322
  local anesthetic in, **2:**323
  releasing tourniquet in, **2:**323, **2:**323*f*
  stabilizing skin and entering vein in, **2:**323, **2:**323*f*
  verifying venous access in, **2:**323
Venography, **3:**353–355, **3:**405
 inferior venacavogram in, **3:**353, **3:**354*f*
 peripheral, **3:**320
  of lower limb, **3:**353, **3:**354*f*
  of upper limb, **3:**353, **3:**353*f*
 superior venacavogram in, **3:**353, **3:**354*f*
 visceral, **3:**355, **3:**355*f*
  hepatic, **3:**355, **3:**355*f*
  renal, **3:**355, **3:**355*f*
Venotomy, **3:**405
Venous insufficiency, diagnostic medical sonography of, **3:**429
Venous varices, **3:**368
Ventral, definition of, **1:**65
Ventral decubitus position, **1:**76
Ventral recumbent position, **1:**72*f*
Ventricles, **3:**405
 cardiac, **3:**316
  sectional anatomy of, **3:**192, **3:**200, **3:**200*f*
 cerebral, sectional anatomy of, **3:**176
Ventricular function, echocardiography of, **3:**430
Ventricular system, **2:**154–155, **2:**154*f*
Ventriculomegaly, diagnostic medical sonography of, **3:**421*f*
Venules, **3:**315, **3:**405
Vermiform appendix, anatomy of, **2:**171*f*, **2:**182, **2:**182*f*
Vermis
 anatomy of, **2:**152
 defined, **2:**167
 sectional anatomy of, **3:**176
Versed (midazolam hydrochloride), **2:**316*t*
Vertebra prominens, as surface landmark, **1:**51*f*
Vertebrae
 defined, **1:**411
 false, **1:**411
 true, **1:**411
 typical, **1:**413
Vertebral arch
 anatomy of, **1:**413
 AP axial oblique projection of, **1:**446–447, **1:**446*f*–447*f*, **1:**447*b*
 AP axial projection of, **1:**444–445, **1:**444*b*–445*b*, **1:**444*f*–445*f*
Vertebral arteries
 anatomy of, **3:**342, **3:**342*f*
 junction of, **3:**184*f*
 sectional anatomy of, **3:**184–185, **3:**185*f*
Vertebral articulations, **1:**422, **1:**422*f*
Vertebral augmentation, **2:**164–165, **2:**164*f*–165*f*
Vertebral body, **1:**110*f*
Vertebral canal, **1:**413
Vertebral column, **1:**113*f*, **1:**409–494
 abbreviations for, **1:**423*b*
 anatomy of, **1:**411–422
  cervical vertebrae in, **1:**414–416
  coccyx in, **1:**421*f*, **1:**422
  curvature of, **1:**411*f*–412*f*, **1:**412
  lumbar vertebrae, **1:**419–420

Vertebral column *(Continued)*
 sacrum in, **1:**421, **1:**421*f*
 summary of, **1:**423*b*
 thoracic vertebrae in, **1:**417–418, **1:**418*f*
 typical vertebra in, **1:**413, **1:**413*f*
 vertebral articulations, **1:**422, **1:**422*f*
 defined, **1:**411
 function of, **1:**411
 joints of, **1:**423*t*
 sample exposure technique chart routine projections for, **1:**425*t*
 summary of pathology of, **1:**424*t*
 summary of projections for, **1:**410, **1:**410*t*
 oblique, **1:**426*t*
Vertebral compression fractures (VCFs), **2:**164
Vertebral foramen, **1:**413
Vertebral fracture assessment (VFA), **2:**483–484, **2:**485*f*, **2:**492
Vertebral fractures, in osteoporosis, **2:**463
Vertebral notches, **1:**413
Vertebroplasty
 defined, **2:**167
 for vertebral fractures, **2:**463
Vertical plates, of palatine bones, **2:**19
Vertical ray method for contrast arthrography, of knee, **2:**146, **2:**146*f*
Vesicoureteral reflux, **2:**280*t*
 in children, **3:**90, **3:**90*f*–91*f*
Vesicovaginal fistula, **2:**340
Vessel, MRI of, **3:**302, **3:**302*f*
Vestibular folds, **1:**89, **1:**89*f*, **2:**176, **2:**176*f*
Vestibule, **2:**16
Videofluoroscopic swallow study (VFSS), **2:**197
View, **1:**77
Villi, **2:**180, **2:**181*f*
Viral pneumonitis, **1:**93*t*
Virtual bronchoscopy, **3:**261*f*
Virtual colonoscopy, **3:**223, **2:**234, **2:**235*f*, **3:**259, **3:**260*f*
Virtual CT bronchoscopy, **3:**261*f*
Virtual simulations, in radiation oncology, **3:**491–492, **3:**491*f*
Visceral, definition of, **1:**65
Visceral arteriography
 celiac, **3:**336, **3:**336*f*
 hepatic, **3:**337, **3:**337*f*
 inferior mesenteric, **3:**338, **3:**338*f*
 other, **3:**339
 renal, **3:**339, **3:**339*f*
 splenic, **3:**337, **3:**337*f*
 superior mesenteric, **3:**338, **3:**338*f*
Visceral pericardium, **3:**316
Visceral peritoneum, **1:**127, **1:**127*f*
Visceral pleura, **1:**86
Visceral venography, **3:**355, **3:**355*f*
 hepatic, **3:**355, **3:**355*f*
 renal, **3:**355, **3:**355*f*
Vision, in older adults, **3:**155
Vistaril (hydroxyzine hydrochloride), **2:**316*t*
Vitamin D, adequate intake of, for osteoporosis, **2:**464
Vocal cords, **1:**87*f*, **2:**175*f*
 false, **1:**89, **1:**89*f*
 true, **1:**89, **1:**89*f*
Vocal folds, **1:**87*f*, **1:**89, **1:**89*f*, **2:**176, **2:**176*f*
Voiding cystourethrogram (VCUG), **2:**307*f*, **2:**314*f*
 in children, **3:**90, **3:**90*f*–91*f*
Volume CT (VCT), **3:**233
 multislice spiral CT for, **3:**249–250
 single slice spiral CT for, **3:**247, **3:**248*f*
Volume element (voxels), **3:**234, **3:**234*f*
Volume rendering (VR), **3:**223, **3:**224*f*, **3:**252–253, **3:**253*f*
Volume scanning, **3:**410
Volumetric density, in DXA, **2:**467, **2:**467*f*, **2:**492
Volumetric modulated arc therapy (VMAT), **3:**497
Voluntary muscles, motion and control of, **1:**13, **1:**13*f*
Volvulus, **2:**190*t*–191*t*
Vomer
 anatomy of, **2:**5*f*, **2:**18*f*, **2:**19
 sectional anatomy of, **3:**175, **3:**184
 submentovertical projection of, **2:**101*f*
Voxels (volume element), **3:**234, **3:**234*f*, **3:**267

W

Waiting room, for children, **3:**72, **3:**72*f*
Wallsten, Hans, **3:**312–313

Ward triangle, **2:**492
Warren, Stafford, **2:**350
Washout, **3:**458, **3:**480
Waters method
 for facial bones, **2:**60, **2:**60*b*, **2:**60*f*–61*f*
 for maxillary sinuses, in children, **3:**108, **3:**109*f*
 modified
  for facial bone, **2:**62, **2:**62*f*–63*f*
  for orbits, **2:**57, **2:**57*b*, **2:**57*f*
 open-mouth, for parietoacanthial projection of maxillary sinuses, **2:**98–99, **2:**98*f*–99*f*, **2:**99*b*
 for parietoacanthial projection of maxillary sinuses, **2:**96, **2:**96*f*, **2:**97*b*
 reverse
  for cranial trauma, **2:**132, **2:**132*f*
  for facial bones, **2:**64, **2:**64*b*, **2:**65*f*
Water-soluble iodinated contrast media
 for alimentary canal imaging, **2:**203, **2:**203*f*–204*f*
 for large intestine studies, **2:**235
Wedge filter, for radiation oncology, **3:**496, **3:**496*f*, **3:**510
Weight-bearing exercise, for osteoporosis, **2:**464
Weight-bearing method, for PA projection, of lumbar intervertebral joints, **1:**482, **1:**482*f*, **1:**483*b*
West Point method, for inferosuperior axial projection, of shoulder girdle, **1:**237–238, **1:**237*f*–238*f*, **1:**238*b*
White matter
 anatomy of, **2:**152
 sectional anatomy of, **3:**178–179
Whole-body imaging, in nuclear imaging, **3:**450, **3:**450*f*
Whole-body MRI, **3:**305, **3:**305*f*
Wilms tumor, **2:**280*t*
Window level, **3:**238, **3:**238*t*, **3:**267
Window width, in CT, **3:**238, **3:**238*t*, **3:**267
Wolf method, for PA oblique projection, of superior stomach and distal esophagus, **2:**226, **2:**226*b*–227*b*, **2:**226*f*–227*f*
Wrist, **1:**174–187
 anatomy of, **1:**144, **1:**144*f*
 AP oblique projection in, medial rotation of, **1:**178*f*–179*f*, **1:**179, **1:**179*b*
 AP projection of, **1:**175, **1:**175*b*, **1:**175*f*
 articulations of, **1:**144, **1:**148*f*
 axiolateral projection, **1:**177*b*, **1:**177*f*
 lateromedial projection of, **1:**176
  with carpal boss, **1:**176*b*, **1:**176*f*
  central ray for, **1:**176
  collimation for, **1:**176
  evaluation criteria for, **1:**176*b*
  position of part for, **1:**176, **1:**176*f*
  position of patient for, **1:**176
  structures shown on, **1:**176, **1:**176*f*
 PA oblique projection in, lateral rotation of, **1:**178, **1:**178*f*
 PA projection of, **1:**174–181, **1:**174*b*, **1:**174*f*
  with radial deviation, **1:**181, **1:**181*b*, **1:**181*f*
  with ulnar deviation, **1:**180, **1:**180*b*, **1:**180*f*
 scaphoid of, **1:**182
  anatomy of, **1:**143*f*, **1:**144
  Rafert-Long method, for scaphoid series (PA and PA axial projections with ulnar deviation), **1:**184, **1:**184*b*, **1:**184*f*–185*f*
  Stecher method for, PA axial projection of, **1:**182–183, **1:**182*b*, **1:**182*f*–183*f*
 surgical radiography of, **3:**64*f*
 tangential projection of
  carpal bridge, **1:**187, **1:**187*b*, **1:**187*f*
  Gaynor-Hart method for, **1:**188
   evaluation criteria for, **1:**189*b*
   inferosuperior, **1:**188–189, **1:**188*f*
   superoinferior, **1:**189, **1:**189*f*
Wrist arthrogram, **2:**150*f*, **2:**150

X

Xenon-133 (^{133}Xe), in nuclear medicine, **3:**442*t*
Xenon-133 (^{133}Xe) lung ventilation scan, **3:**458
Xerography, **2:**350, **2:**350*f*
Xeromammogram, **2:**350, **2:**350*f*
Xiphisternal joints, **1:**500
Xiphoid process
 anatomy of, **1:**497*f*, **1:**498
 as surface landmark, **1:**51*f*
X-ray modified barium swallow, **2:**197

Y

Yellow marrow, **1:**56
Yolk sac, diagnostic medical sonography of, **3:**424, **3:**425f–426f

Z

Zenker diverticulum, **2:**190t–191t
Zone I, in MRI, **3:**283, **3:**308
Zone II, in MRI, **3:**283, **3:**308
Zone III, in MRI, **3:**283, **3:**308
Zone IV, in MRI, **3:**283, **3:**308
Z-score, in DXA, **2:**471, **2:**492
Zygapophyseal joints, **1:**413, **1:**422
  cervical
    anatomy of, **1:**416, **1:**416f
    positioning rotations needed to show, **1:**416t
  lumbar
    anatomy of, **1:**419, **1:**419f–420f, **1:**420t
    AP oblique projection of, **1:**468, **1:**468b–469b, **1:**468f–470f
    PA oblique projection of, **1:**470, **1:**470b, **1:**470f, **1:**472f
    positioning rotations needed to show, **1:**416t, **1:**419f
  sectional anatomy of, **3:**191f, **3:**200–201, **3:**201f
  thoracic
    anatomy of, **1:**417–418, **1:**418f
    AP or PA oblique projection of, **1:**456–457, **1:**456f–457f, **1:**457b
    positioning rotations needed to show, **1:**416t
Zygomatic arch, **2:**19
  anatomy of, **2:**18f, **2:**19, **2:**21, **2:**21f, **2:**52f
  AP axial projection of (modified Towne method), **2:**74, **2:**74b, **2:**74f
  modified parietoacanthial projection of, **2:**63f
  parietoacanthial projection of, **2:**61f
  sectional anatomy of, **3:**185f
  submentovertical projection of, **2:**70–74, **2:**70f–71f, **2:**71b
  tangential projection of, **2:**72–73, **2:**72f–73f, **2:**73b
Zygomatic bones
  acanthioparietal projection of, **2:**65f
  sectional anatomy of, **3:**175, **3:**184
Zygomatic process
  anatomy of, **2:**14, **2:**14f
  sectional anatomy of, **3:**174–175
Zygote, **2:**331

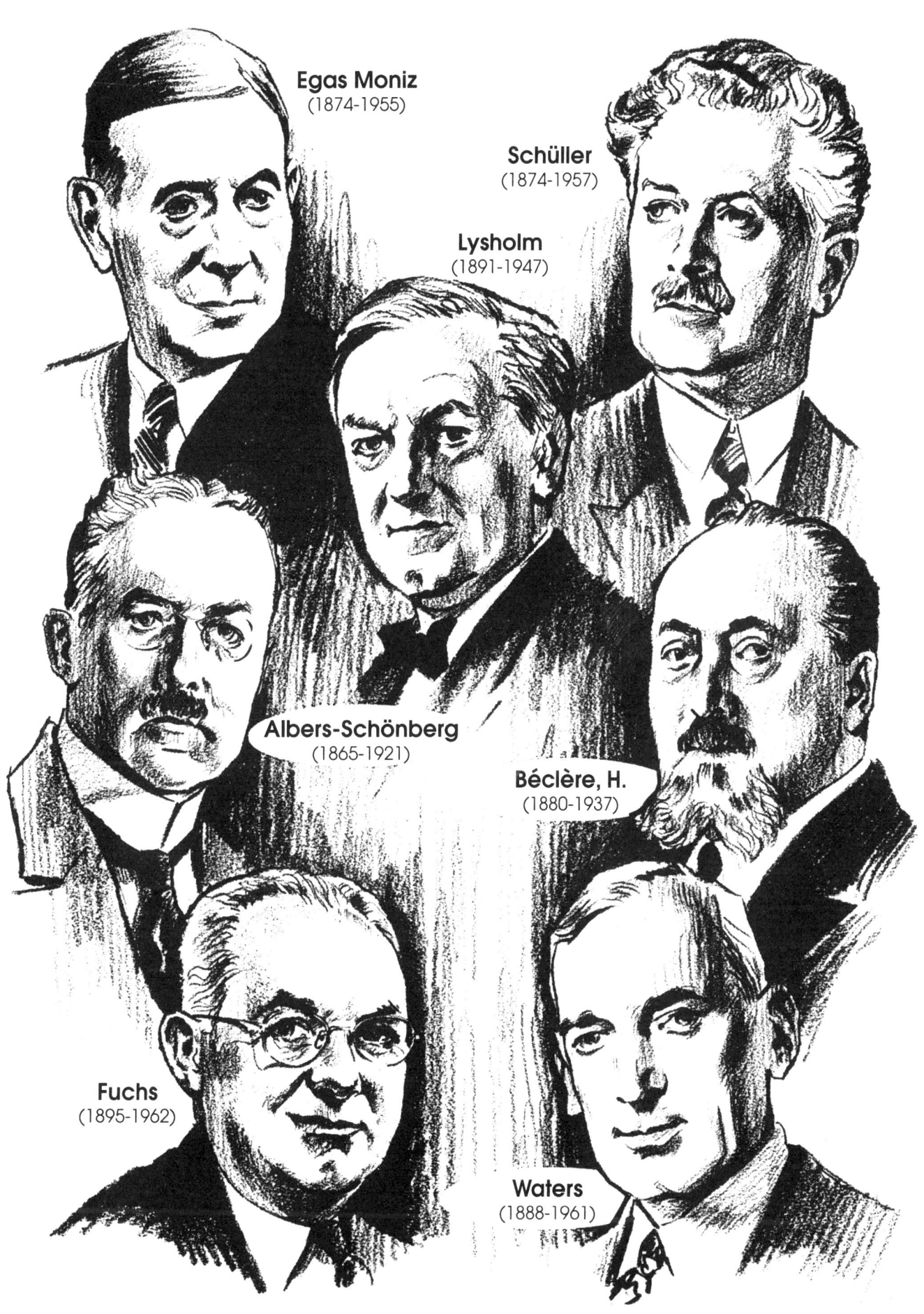